Practical Soft Tissue Pathology

A Diagnostic Approach

A Volume in the Pattern Recognition Series

Pattern Recognition Series
Series editors:
Kevin O. Leslie and Mark R. Wick

Practical Breast Pathology
Kristen A. Atkins and Christina S. Kong

Practical Cytopathology
Andrew S. Field and Matthew A. Zarka

Practical Hepatic Pathology, 2nd Edition
Romil Saxena

Practical Orthopedic Pathology
Andrea T. Deyrup and Gene P. Siegal

Practical Pulmonary Pathology, 2nd Edition
Kevin O. Leslie and Mark R. Wick

Practical Renal Pathology
Donna J. Lager and Neil A. Abrahams

Practical Skin Pathology
James W. Patterson

Practical Soft Tissue Pathology
Jason L. Hornick

Practical Surgical Neuropathology
Arie Perry and Daniel J. Brat

Practical Soft Tissue Pathology

A Diagnostic Approach

A Volume in the Pattern Recognition Series

Edition 2

Jason L. Hornick, MD, PhD
Director of Surgical Pathology and Immunohistochemistry
Department of Pathology
Brigham and Women's Hospital
Professor of Pathology
Harvard Medical School
Boston, Massachusetts

ELSEVIER

1600 John F. Kennedy Blvd.
Ste 1800
Philadelphia, PA 19103-2899

PRACTICAL SOFT TISSUE PATHOLOGY:
A DIAGNOSTIC APPROACH, SECOND EDITION

ISBN: 978-0-323-49714-5

Library of Congress Cataloging-in-Publication Data

Names: Hornick, Jason L., editor.
Title: Practical soft tissue pathology : a diagnostic approach / [edited by]
Jason L. Hornick.
Other titles: Pattern recognition series.
Description: Second edition. | Philadelphia, PA : Elsevier, [2019] |
Series:
Pattern recognition series | Includes bibliographical references and index.
Identifiers: LCCN 2017034576 | ISBN 9780323497145 (hardcover : alk. paper)
Subjects: | MESH: Neoplasms, Connective and Soft Tissue–pathology |
Neoplasms, Connective and Soft Tissue–diagnosis | Neoplasm Grading
Classification: LCC RC280.S66 | NLM QZ 340 | DDC 616.99/474–dc23 LC record
available at https://lccn.loc.gov/2017034576

Content Strategist: Michael Houston
Senior Content Development Specialist: Dee Simpson
Publishing Services Manager: Catherine Jackson
Senior Project Manager: Rachel E. McMullen
Design Direction: Bridget Hoette

Printed in China

Last digit is the print number: 9 8 7 6 5 4 3 2

This book is dedicated to Beryle-Gay Hornick and Jordana Hornick

Contributors

Rita Alaggio, MD
Professor
University of Padua
Institute of Pathologic Anatomy
University of Padua
Padua, Italy

Michele Biscuola, PhD
Institute of Biomedicine of Sevilla (IBiS)
Virgen del Rocio University Hospital/CSIC/University of Sevilla/
CIBERONC
Seville, Spain

Thomas Brenn, MD, PhD, FRCPath
Department of Pathology
Western General Hospital and The University of Edinburgh
Edinburgh, Scotland

Jodi M. Carter, MD, PhD
Assistant Professor
Laboratory Medicine and Pathology
Mayo Clinic
Rochester, Minnesota

Cheryl M. Coffin, MD
Professor Emerita
Pathology, Microbiology, and Immunology
Vanderbilt University Medical Center
Nashville, Tennessee

Enrique de Alava, MD, PhD
Institute of Biomedicine of Sevilla (IBiS)
Virgen del Rocio University Hospital/CSIC/University of Sevilla/
CIBERONC
Seville, Spain

Angelo Paolo Dei Tos, MD
Professor of Pathology
Department of Medicine
University of Padua School of Medicine
Padua, Italy;
Director, Department of Pathology
Azienda ULSS 2 Marca Trevigiana
Treviso, Italy

Leona A. Doyle, MD
Assistant Professor of Pathology
Department of Pathology
Brigham and Women's Hospital and Harvard Medical School
Boston, Massachusetts

Briana C. Gleason, MD
Staff Pathologist
Covenant Surgical Partners
South San Francisco, California

J. Frans Graadt van Roggen, MB ChB, BSc Hons, PhD
Department of Pathology
Alrijne Zorggroep
Leiden, The Netherlands

Pancras C.W. Hogendoorn, MD, PhD
Professor of Pathology
Leiden University Medical Center
Leiden, The Netherlands;
Visiting Professor in Sarcoma Pathology
University of Oxford
Oxford, United Kingdom

Jason L. Hornick, MD, PhD
Director of Surgical Pathology and Immunohistochemistry
Department of Pathology
Brigham and Women's Hospital
Professor of Pathology
Harvard Medical School
Boston, Massachusetts

Vickie Y. Jo, MD
Assistant Professor of Pathology
Department of Pathology
Brigham and Women's Hospital and Harvard Medical School
Boston, Massachusetts

Alexander J. Lazar, MD, PhD
Professor
Departments of Pathology, Genomic Medicine, and Translational Molecular Pathology
The University of Texas M. D. Anderson Cancer Center
Houston, Texas

Bernadette Liegl-Atzwanger, MD
Head of Soft Tissue Pathology Service,
Associate Professor of Pathology
Institute of Pathology Medical University Graz
Graz, Austria

David Marcilla, MD
Institute of Biomedicine of Sevilla (IBiS)
Virgen del Rocio University Hospital/CSIC/University of Sevilla/CIBERONC
Seville, Spain

Adrián Mariño-Enríquez, MD, PhD
Instructor
Department of Pathology
Brigham and Women's Hospital and Harvard Medical School
Boston, Massachusetts

Marisa R. Nucci, MD
Associate Pathologist
Department of Pathology
Brigham and Women's Hospital,
Professor of Pathology
Harvard Medical School
Boston, Massachusetts

André M. Oliveira, MD, PhD
Professor of Laboratory Medicine and Pathology
Department of Laboratory Medicine and Pathology
Mayo Clinic
Rochester, Minnesota

Brian P. Rubin, MD, PhD
Professor and Vice Chair of Research,
Director, Soft Tissue Pathology,
Director, Bone and Soft Tissue Fellowship Program
Robert J. Tomsich Pathology and Laboratory Medicine Institute
Cleveland Clinic
Cleveland, Ohio

Marta Sbaraglia, MD
Department of Pathology
Azienda ULSS 2 Marca Trevigiana
Treviso, Italy

Wei-Lien Wang, MD
Associate Professor
Departments of Pathology and Translational Molecular Pathology
The University of Texas MD Anderson Cancer Center
Houston, Texas

Series Preface

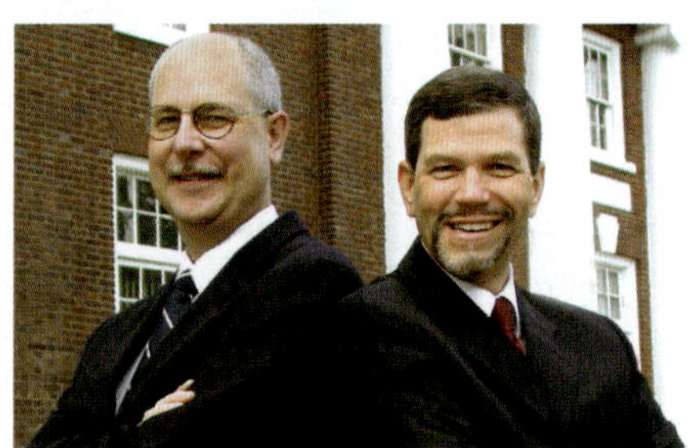

It is often stated that anatomic pathologists come in two forms: "Gestalt"-based individuals, who recognize visual scenes as a whole, matching them unconsciously with memorialized archives; and criterion-oriented people, who work through images systematically in segments, tabulating the results—internally, mentally, and quickly—as they go along in examining a visual target. These approaches can be equally effective, and they are probably not as dissimilar as their descriptions would suggest. In reality, even "Gestaltists" subliminally examine details of an image, and, if asked specifically about particular features of it, they are able to say whether one characteristic or another is important diagnostically.

In accordance with these concepts, in 2004 we published a textbook entitled *Practical Pulmonary Pathology: A Diagnostic Approach* (PPPDA). That monograph was designed around a *pattern-based* method, wherein diseases of the lung were divided into six categories on the basis of their general image profiles. Using that technique, one can successfully segregate pathologic conditions into diagnostically and clinically useful groupings.

The merits of such a procedure have been validated empirically by the enthusiastic feedback we have received from users of our book. In addition, following the old adage that "imitation is the sincerest form of flattery," since our book came out, other publications and presentations have appeared in our specialty with the same approach.

After publication of the PPPDA text, representatives at Elsevier, most notably William Schmitt, were enthusiastic about building a *series* of texts around pattern-based diagnosis in pathology. To this end we have recruited a distinguished group of authors and editors to accomplish that task. Because a panoply of patterns is difficult to approach mentally from a practical perspective, we have asked our contributors to be complete and yet to discuss only principal interpretative images. Our goal is eventually to provide a series of monographs that, in combination with one another, will allow trainees and practitioners in pathology to use salient morphological patterns to reach with confidence final diagnoses in all organ systems.

As stated in the introduction to the PPPDA text, the evaluation of dominant patterns is aided secondarily by the analysis of cellular composition and other distinctive findings. Therefore within the context of each pattern, editors have been asked to use such data to refer the reader to appropriate specific chapters in their respective texts.

We have also stated previously that some overlap is expected between pathologic patterns in any given anatomic site; in addition, specific disease states may potentially manifest themselves with more than one pattern. At first, those facts may seem to militate against the value of pattern-based interpretation. However, pragmatically, they do not. One often can narrow diagnostic possibilities to a very few entities using the pattern method, and sometimes a single interpretation will be obvious. Both of those outcomes are useful to clinical physicians caring for a given patient.

It is hoped that the expertise of our authors and editors, together with the high quality of morphologic images they present in this Elsevier series, will be beneficial to our reader-colleagues.

Kevin O. Leslie, MD
Mark R. Wick, MD

Preface to the First Edition

With its diversity of histologic appearances and the rarity of many types of mesenchymal tumors, soft tissue tumor pathology can be intimidating for pathologists in training and practicing pathologists alike. The current classification system informs the organization of the majority of soft tissue tumor textbooks, emphasizing the line of differentiation exhibited by the tumor cells. Pathologists can relatively easily recognize some mesenchymal tumors as fibroblastic/myofibroblastic, "fibrohistiocytic," smooth muscle, skeletal muscle, vascular, or adipocytic, but for many other soft tissue tumors, the lineage is not intuitively obvious. Immunohistochemistry therefore plays a major role in demonstrating such lineages. However, for some mesenchymal neoplasms, there is no apparent normal cellular counterpart; such tumors (which are both histologically and clinically diverse) are often found in textbooks lumped together in a separate chapter with tumors of uncertain lineage. Despite teaching junior residents to describe tumors based on cytologic findings and histologic patterns, our specialty features surprisingly few pathology textbooks wherein soft tissue tumors are presented in the same manner in which pathologists approach them in daily practice—with tumor cell appearance, architectural arrangements, and stromal characteristics as organizing principles.

This textbook addresses this gap in our literature by taking a pattern-based approach to soft tissue tumor pathology, with chapters devoted to the dominant cytology of the tumor cells (spindle cell tumors, epithelioid tumors, round cell tumors, pleomorphic sarcomas, biphasic tumors, and tumors with mixed patterns), the quality of the extracellular matrix (tumors with myxoid stroma), and other distinguishing features (giant cell–rich tumors, soft tissue tumors with prominent inflammatory cells). Because recognition of many adipocytic, vascular, cartilaginous, and osseous neoplasms is relatively straightforward on histologic grounds alone, separate chapters are devoted to these groups of lesions. Cutaneous, gastrointestinal, and lower genital mesenchymal tumors are also presented in separate chapters, because many distinctive tumor types arise exclusively or predominantly in those anatomic compartments. Because many soft tissue tumors have more than one distinguishing feature (e.g., epithelioid cytology and myxoid stroma, spindle cell morphology and prominent inflammatory cells), quite a few tumors are discussed in multiple chapters to emphasize approaches to differential diagnosis. Although molecular findings are included throughout the textbook when relevant, the final chapter is devoted to molecular testing in soft tissue tumor pathology, both to provide an overview of the methods used (and relative merits of the various techniques) and to give examples of how the application of molecular testing can aid in differential diagnosis.

The main patterns are included in table form in the front of the textbook. This section also includes additional distinguishing findings that can narrow down the differential diagnosis, specific diagnostic considerations within each category, and a reference to the chapter and page number where the particular tumor type can be found. The reader may choose either to use these tables to identify specific tumors in the book based on the dominant pattern and other particular features or to go directly to the chapter or chapters containing tumors with the histologic features recognized. Although these tables are relatively comprehensive, they do not include most vascular, adipocytic, cartilaginous, and osseous tumors, which can be studied in the chapters devoted to those groups of neoplasms.

Jason L. Hornick, MD, PhD

Preface

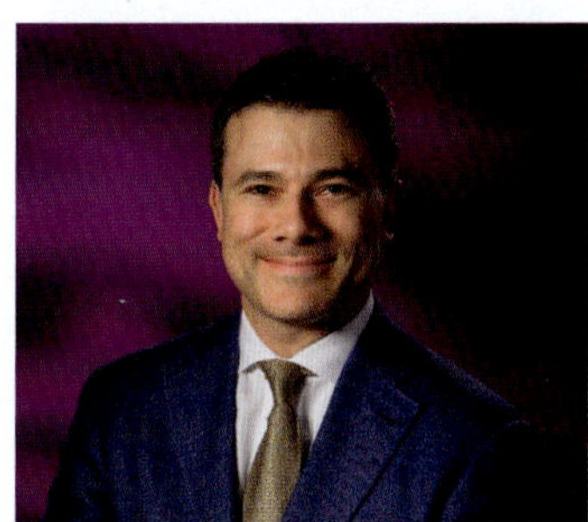

In the 5 years since the publication of the first edition of *Practical Soft Tissue Pathology* and the most recent World Health Organization classification, we have seen remarkable advances in diagnostic soft tissue tumor pathology; the second edition of this book incorporates these changes. New defining molecular genetic alterations continue to be discovered at an astonishing rate. In turn, these findings lead (also with increasing speed) to new diagnostic tests, not only molecular assays but also using immunohistochemistry. In many cases, single-antibody immunohistochemical tests serve as excellent surrogate markers for particular molecular genetic alterations. These novel diagnostic markers have proven to be extremely valuable tools for differential diagnosis, especially in limited biopsy material, such as core needle biopsies and fine needle aspirations, which we encounter every day in clinical practice. In the past, it could be challenging, if not impossible, to render a specific diagnosis in such limited samples; now accurate diagnosis is often possible with the aid of these powerful new markers. These markers have changed our diagnostic approach to both relatively common and rare tumor types, including major histologic categories of soft tissue tumors, such as spindle cell tumors, epithelioid tumors, and round cell sarcomas.

In sarcoma classification, among the most significant recent advances is the emergence of discrete tumor types within the previous category of "undifferentiated round cell sarcomas" based on molecular genetics. After Ewing sarcoma and other well-defined round cell sarcomas were excluded by immunohistochemistry and fluorescence in situ hybridization (FISH), we had no real options beyond this wastebasket category. Now, round cell sarcomas with *CIC* gene rearrangements (most with *CIC-DUX4*) and *BCOR* genetic alterations (most often *BCOR-CCNB3*) are recognized diagnostic categories, with important prognostic implications and, we hope in the near term, distinct systemic therapies. In rapid succession, pathologists have introduced immunohistochemical markers that correlate with these rearrangements, some based on the gene fusions per se (e.g., *CCNB3* and *BCOR*) and others reflecting downstream consequences of these fusions, often discovered by gene expression profiling (such as *ETV4*).

These genetic alterations and emerging diagnostic markers, which have been integrated into the second edition, should improve the accuracy and reproducibility of mesenchymal tumor diagnosis. I hope you find this book useful in your daily clinical practice.

Jason L. Hornick, MD, PhD

Acknowledgment

Many individuals have had a significant impact on my development as a diagnostic pathologist and on the creation of this textbook. I would first like to acknowledge my colleague and friend Christopher Fletcher, without whom I would not have become a surgical pathologist. Without his mentorship and support, this textbook would not exist. Chris generously allowed me to photograph his consult cases, which have greatly enhanced many of the chapters throughout the book. I would like to thank my colleagues and friends who devoted considerable time and effort working on the excellent chapters that they contributed to this project. Their research, writing, and teaching in this field will continue to advance our understanding (and improve the diagnosis) of mesenchymal tumors for a new generation of pathologists and our clinical collaborators.

The residents, fellows, and my colleagues in the pathology department at Brigham and Women's Hospital are an exceptional team of trainees and friends, and I am fortunate to share my passion for surgical pathology with them. My first introduction to monoclonal antibodies was during my doctoral work; I am grateful to Alan Epstein and Clive Taylor for this and for encouraging me to consider a pathology residency. Finally, my wife, Harmony Wu, has provided support and insights during the long journey toward the completion of this textbook, and our children, Hazel and Oscar, have been a source of inspiration and humility and have been (relatively) patient with me along the way.

Jason L. Hornick, MD, PhD

Contents

Pattern-Based Approach to Diagnosis

Pattern	Selected Diseases to Be Considered
Spindle cell	Nodular fasciitis Myofibroma/myopericytoma Cellular benign fibrous histiocytoma Dermatofibrosarcoma protuberans Superficial or desmoid fibromatosis Neurofibroma Schwannoma Leiomyoma Leiomyosarcoma Gastrointestinal stromal tumor Solitary fibrous tumor Spindle cell lipoma Atypical spindle cell lipomatous tumor Soft tissue perineurioma Low-grade fibromyxoid sarcoma Monophasic synovial sarcoma Malignant peripheral nerve sheath tumor Biphenotypic sinonasal sarcoma Dedifferentiated liposarcoma Clear cell sarcoma Nodular Kaposi sarcoma Pseudomyogenic hemangioendothelioma
Epithelioid	Epithelioid hemangioma Epithelioid hemangioendothelioma Epithelioid angiosarcoma Glomus tumor Granular cell tumor Cellular neurothekeoma Myoepithelioma/myoepithelial carcinoma Epithelioid schwannoma Epithelioid malignant peripheral nerve sheath tumor Gastrointestinal stromal tumor Perivascular epithelioid cell tumor (PEComa) Epithelioid sarcoma SMARCA4-deficient thoracic sarcoma Malignant rhabdoid tumor Alveolar soft part sarcoma Clear cell sarcoma Sclerosing epithelioid fibrosarcoma
Pleomorphic	Atypical fibrous histiocytoma Atypical fibroxanthoma "Ancient" schwannoma Dedifferentiated liposarcoma

Pattern	Selected Diseases to Be Considered
Pleomorphic—*cont'd*	Pleomorphic liposarcoma Pleomorphic leiomyosarcoma Pleomorphic rhabdomyosarcoma Myxofibrosarcoma Myxoinflammatory fibroblastic sarcoma Extraskeletal osteosarcoma Undifferentiated pleomorphic sarcoma
Round cell	Ewing sarcoma Embryonal rhabdomyosarcoma Alveolar rhabdomyosarcoma Round cell (high-grade myxoid) liposarcoma Poorly differentiated synovial sarcoma Desmoplastic small round cell tumor Mesenchymal chondrosarcoma *CIC*-rearranged sarcomas *BCOR*-rearranged sarcomas
Biphasic or mixed	Biphasic synovial sarcoma Mixed tumor Glandular malignant peripheral nerve sheath tumor Myoepithelioma/myoepithelial carcinoma Gastrointestinal stromal tumor Ectopic hamartomatous thymoma Dedifferentiated liposarcoma
Myxoid	Intramuscular/cellular myxoma Dermal nerve sheath myxoma Superficial acral fibromyxoma Superficial angiomyxoma Deep angiomyxoma Ossifying fibromyxoid tumor Myoepithelioma/myoepithelial carcinoma Myxofibrosarcoma Pleomorphic liposarcoma Myxoid liposarcoma Extraskeletal myxoid chondrosarcoma Low-grade fibromyxoid sarcoma Myxoinflammatory fibroblastic sarcoma Neurofibroma Soft tissue or reticular perineurioma Malignant peripheral nerve sheath tumor Spindle cell lipoma

Pattern 1 Spindle Cell

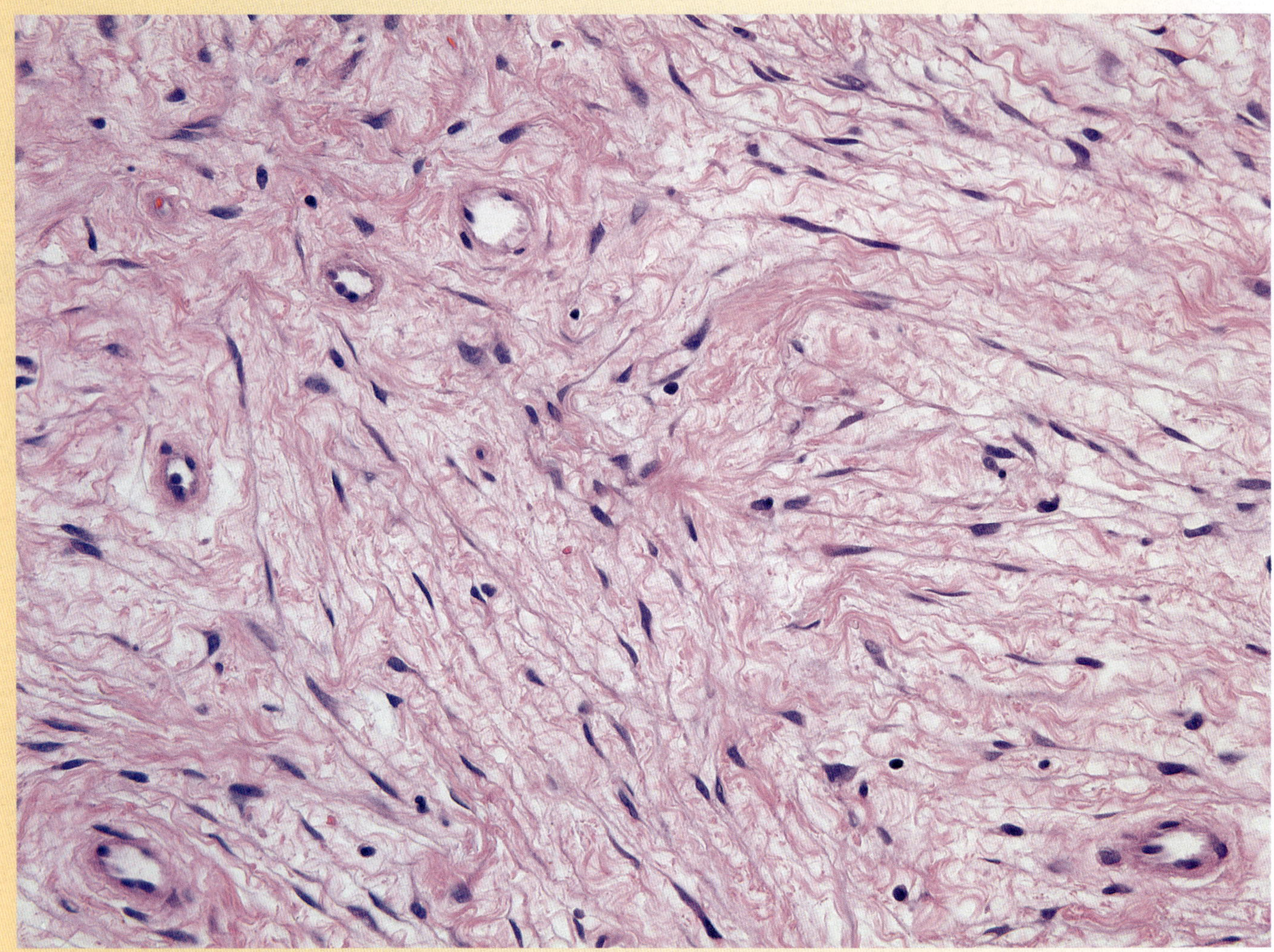

Elements of the pattern: The tumor cells contain pointed or tapering ends.

Pattern 1 Spindle Cell

Additional Findings	Diagnostic Considerations	Chapter:Page
Fascicular architecture	Nodular fasciitis	Ch. 3:20; Ch. 4:102; Ch. 5:158
	Pseudosarcomatous myofibroblastic proliferation	Ch. 3:25
	Myofibroma/myofibromatosis/myopericytoma	Ch. 3:27; Ch. 4:107
	Fibrous hamartoma of infancy	Ch. 4:114
	Calcifying aponeurotic fibroma	Ch. 4:114
	Lipofibromatosis	Ch. 4:115; Ch. 12:313
	Mammary-type myofibroblastoma	Ch. 3:31; Ch. 17:506
	Intranodal palisaded myofibroblastoma	Ch. 3:32
	Cellular benign fibrous histiocytoma	Ch. 15:410
	Dermatomyofibroma	Ch. 15:412
	Superficial fibromatosis	Ch. 3:46
	Desmoid fibromatosis	Ch. 3:47; Ch. 4:109; Ch. 16:481
	Schwannoma	Ch. 3:51; Ch. 16:475
	Cellular schwannoma	Ch. 3:53
	Solitary circumscribed neuroma	Ch. 15:415
	Leiomyoma	Ch. 3:64; Ch. 15:412; Ch. 16:471; Ch. 17:509
	Angioleiomyoma	Ch. 3:66
	Leiomyosarcoma	Ch. 3:66; Ch. 16:474
	Epstein-Barr virus–associated smooth muscle neoplasm	Ch. 3:68
	Lymphangiomyoma	Ch. 3:68
	Inflammatory myofibroblastic tumor	Ch. 4:118; Ch. 10:269; Ch. 16:479
	Gastrointestinal stromal tumor	Ch. 16:460
	Monophasic synovial sarcoma	Ch. 3:72
	Malignant peripheral nerve sheath tumor	Ch. 3:76
	Biphenotypic sinonasal sarcoma	Ch. 3:79
	Atypical fibroxanthoma, spindle cell variant	Ch. 15:449
	Fibrosarcomatous dermatofibrosarcoma protuberans	Ch. 15:418
	Infantile fibrosarcoma	Ch. 4:121
	Infantile rhabdomyofibrosarcoma	Ch. 4:126
	Adult-type fibrosarcoma	Ch. 3:81
	Low-grade myofibroblastic sarcoma	Ch. 3:84; Ch. 4:124
	Cellular fetal rhabdomyoma	Ch. 4:126
	Spindle cell rhabdomyosarcoma	Ch. 3:86; Ch. 4:127
	Clear cell sarcoma	Ch. 3:87
	Nodular Kaposi sarcoma	Ch. 13:382
	Kaposiform hemangioendothelioma	Ch. 13:380
	Spindle cell angiosarcoma	Ch. 13:384
	Pseudomyogenic hemangioendothelioma	Ch. 3:89; Ch. 15:425
Storiform/whorled architecture	Cutaneous benign fibrous histiocytoma	Ch. 15:410
	Deep fibrous histiocytoma	Ch. 3:39
	Dermatofibrosarcoma protuberans	Ch. 15:417
	Storiform collagenoma	Ch. 15:415
	Soft tissue perineurioma	Ch. 3:61; Ch. 15:422
	Hybrid schwannoma/perineurioma	Ch. 15:423
	Low-grade fibromyxoid sarcoma	Ch. 3:81; Ch. 4:124; Ch. 5:153
	Follicular dendritic cell sarcoma	Ch. 10:274
	Dedifferentiated liposarcoma (subset)	Ch. 7:225; Ch. 12:328
Lobulated architecture	Dermal nerve sheath myxoma	Ch. 5:139; Ch. 15:431
	Superficial angiomyxoma	Ch. 5:141; Ch. 15:428
	Myxofibrosarcoma	Ch. 5:148; Ch. 7:218
	Extraskeletal myxoid chondrosarcoma	Ch. 5:151
Plexiform architecture	Plexiform schwannoma	Ch. 3:54
	Plexiform neurofibroma	Ch. 3:59
	Dendritic cell neurofibroma	Ch. 15:424
	Plexiform fibrohistiocytic tumor	Ch. 11:303
	Plexiform fibromyxoma	Ch. 16:484

Pattern 1 Spindle Cell—*cont'd*

Additional Findings	Diagnostic Considerations	Chapter:Page
Nuclear palisading	Intranodal palisaded myofibroblastoma	Ch. 3:32
	Schwannoma	Ch. 3:51
	Monophasic synovial sarcoma (small subset)	Ch. 3:72
	Leiomyoma (subset)	Ch. 3:64
	Gastrointestinal stromal tumor (subset)	Ch. 16:460
Nuclear pleomorphism	"Ancient" schwannoma	Ch. 3:51
	Atypical neurofibroma	Ch. 3:57
	Malignant peripheral nerve sheath tumor	Ch. 3:76
	Pleomorphic lipoma	Ch. 12:316
	Dedifferentiated liposarcoma	Ch. 7:225; Ch. 12:328
	Myxofibrosarcoma	Ch. 5:148; Ch. 7:218
	Myxoinflammatory fibroblastic sarcoma	Ch. 5:155; Ch. 7:217; Ch. 10:286
	Pleomorphic fibroma	Ch. 15:452
	Atypical fibrous histiocytoma	Ch. 15:411
	Atypical fibroxanthoma	Ch. 15:449
Myxoid stroma	Nodular fasciitis (subset)	Ch. 3:20; Ch. 4:102; Ch. 5:158
	Soft tissue perineurioma (subset)	Ch. 5:157
	Reticular perineurioma	Ch. 5:157
	Microcystic/reticular schwannoma	Ch. 5:158
	Solitary fibrous tumor (small subset)	Ch. 5:158
	Monophasic synovial sarcoma (small subset)	Ch. 5:158
	Malignant peripheral nerve sheath tumor (subset)	Ch. 3:76; Ch. 5:158
	Low-grade fibromyxoid sarcoma	Ch. 3:81; Ch. 4:124; Ch. 5:153
	Primitive myxoid mesenchymal tumor of infancy	Ch. 4:123
	Fetal rhabdomyoma	Ch. 4:126
	Embryonal rhabdomyosarcoma (subset)	Ch. 8:242
	Dermal nerve sheath myxoma	Ch. 5:139; Ch. 15:431
	Dermatofibrosarcoma protuberans (small subset)	Ch. 5:158
	Superficial acral fibromyxoma	Ch. 5:140; Ch. 15:427
	Superficial angiomyxoma	Ch. 5:141; Ch. 15:428
	Deep angiomyxoma	Ch. 5:141; Ch. 17:499
	Lipoblastoma	Ch. 12:319
	Spindle cell lipoma (subset)	Ch. 3:50; Ch. 15:405
	Desmoid fibromatosis (subset)	Ch. 3:47; Ch. 4:109; Ch. 16:481
	Plexiform fibromyxoma	Ch. 16:484
	Myxoinflammatory fibroblastic sarcoma	Ch. 5:155; Ch. 7:217; Ch. 10:286
	Myxofibrosarcoma	Ch. 5:148; Ch. 7:218
	Myxoid liposarcoma	Ch. 5:150; Ch. 12:332
	Extraskeletal myxoid chondrosarcoma	Ch. 5:151

Pattern 1 Spindle Cell—*cont'd*

Additional Findings	Diagnostic Considerations	Chapter:Page
Collagenous stroma	Fibroma of tendon sheath	Ch. 3:33
	Desmoplastic fibroblastoma	Ch. 3:34
	Nuchal-type fibroma	Ch. 3:35
	Gardner fibroma	Ch. 4:104
	Fibromatosis colli	Ch. 4:112
	Infantile digital fibroma	Ch. 4:112
	Elastofibroma	Ch. 3:36
	Calcifying fibrous tumor	Ch. 3:37
	Solitary fibrous tumor	Ch. 3:40
	Mammary-type myofibroblastoma	Ch. 3:31; Ch. 17:506
	Hyaline fibromatosis	Ch. 4:118
	Storiform collagenoma	Ch. 15:415
	Superficial fibromatosis	Ch. 3:46
	Desmoid fibromatosis	Ch. 3:47; Ch. 4:109; Ch. 16:481
	Neurofibroma (subset)	Ch. 3:57
	Ganglioneuroma	Ch. 3:63
	Sclerosing perineurioma	Ch. 3:63; Ch. 15:442
	Monophasic synovial sarcoma (subset)	Ch. 3:72
	Low-grade fibromyxoid sarcoma	Ch. 3:81; Ch. 4:124; Ch. 5:153
	Low-grade myofibroblastic sarcoma	Ch. 3:84; Ch. 4:125
Collagen bundles	Intranodal palisaded myofibroblastoma	Ch. 3:32
	Spindle cell lipoma	Ch. 3:50; Ch. 15:453
	Neurofibroma (subset)	Ch. 3:57
	Gastrointestinal stromal tumor (subset)	Ch. 16:460
Prominent inflammatory cells	Calcifying fibrous tumor (lymphocytes)	Ch. 3:37
	Inflammatory myofibroblastic tumor (plasma cells, lymphocytes)	Ch. 4:118; Ch. 10:269; Ch. 16:479
	Leiomyosarcoma (lymphocytes, histiocytes; small subset)	Ch. 10:273
	Epstein-Barr virus–associated smooth muscle neoplasm (lymphocytes)	Ch. 3:68
	Myxoinflammatory fibroblastic sarcoma (neutrophils, lymphocytes)	Ch. 5:155; Ch. 7:217; Ch. 10:286
	Follicular dendritic cell sarcoma (lymphocytes)	Ch. 10:274
	Interdigitating dendritic cell sarcoma (lymphocytes)	Ch. 10:277
	Fibroblastic reticular cell sarcoma (lymphocytes)	Ch. 10:277
	Angiomatoid fibrous histiocytoma (lymphocytes, including germinal centers)	Ch. 3:68; Ch. 10:285
	Gastrointestinal schwannoma (lymphocytes, including germinal centers)	Ch. 16:477
	Inflammatory fibroid polyp (eosinophils)	Ch. 16:482
Prominent or distinctive giant cells	Nodular fasciitis (osteoclast-like; subset)	Ch. 3:20; Ch. 4:102; Ch. 5:158
	Phosphaturic mesenchymal tumor (osteoclast-like)	Ch. 3:30
	Solitary fibrous tumor (floret-type; small subset)	Ch. 3:44
	Pleomorphic lipoma (wreath-like)	Ch. 12:316
	Leiomyosarcoma (osteoclast-like; small subset)	Ch. 11:309
	Clear cell sarcoma (wreath-like)	Ch. 3:87
	Plexiform fibrohistiocytic tumor (osteoclast-like)	Ch. 11:303
	Giant cell fibroblastoma (floret-type)	Ch. 15:421
	Benign fibrous histiocytoma (Touton)	Ch. 15:405
	Soft tissue aneurysmal bone cyst (osteoclast-like)	Ch. 14:397

Pattern 1 Spindle Cell—*cont'd*

Additional Findings	Diagnostic Considerations	Chapter:Page
Adipocytic component	Spindle cell lipoma	Ch. 3:50; Ch. 12:316
	Atypical spindle cell lipomatous tumor	Ch. 3:50; Ch. 12:324
	Lipofibromatosis	Ch. 4:115; Ch. 12:313
	Lipoblastoma	Ch. 12:319
	Myxoid liposarcoma	Ch. 5:150; Ch. 12:332
	Myolipoma	Ch. 3:64; Ch. 12:321
	Mammary-type myofibroblastoma (subset)	Ch. 3:31; Ch. 17:506
	Hemosiderotic fibrolipomatous tumor	Ch. 12:319
	Solitary fibrous tumor (subset)	Ch. 3:44
Calcifications, cartilage, and/or bone/osteoid	Phosphaturic mesenchymal tumor (calcifications, osteoid)	Ch. 3:30
	Calcifying fibrous tumor (calcifications)	Ch. 3:37
	Melanotic schwannoma (calcifications; subset)	Ch. 3:55
	Calcifying aponeurotic fibroma (calcifications)	Ch. 4:114
	Myositis ossificans (bone/osteoid)	Ch. 14:391
	Fasciitis ossificans (bone/osteoid)	Ch. 3:23
	Fibro-osseous pseudotumor (bone/osteoid)	Ch. 14:392
	Soft tissue aneurysmal bone cyst (bone/osteoid; subset)	Ch. 14:397
	Malignant peripheral nerve sheath tumor (cartilage and/or bone; subset)	Ch. 3:76
	Dedifferentiated liposarcoma (cartilage and/or bone; subset)	Ch. 7:225; Ch. 12:328
	Extraskeletal osteosarcoma (bone/osteoid)	Ch. 14:400
Prominent or distinctive blood vessels	Nodular fasciitis (plexiform)	Ch. 3:20; Ch. 4:102; Ch. 5:158
	Myofibroma/myofibromatosis/myopericytoma (dilated, branching)	Ch. 3:27; Ch. 4:107
	Fibroma of tendon sheath (slit-like)	Ch. 3:33
	Nasopharyngeal angiofibroma (dilated, irregular, thin-walled)	Ch. 4:117
	Angiofibroma of soft tissue (small, branching)	Ch. 3:37
	Spindle cell hemangioma (dilated)	Ch. 13:379
	Solitary fibrous tumor (rounded, hyalinized; dilated, branching)	Ch. 3:40
	Monophasic synovial sarcoma (dilated, branching; subset)	Ch. 3:72
	Schwannoma (rounded, hyalinized)	Ch. 3:51
	Angioleiomyoma (thick-walled)	Ch. 3:66
	Lymphangiomyoma (dilated lymphatics)	Ch. 3:68
	Superficial angiomyxoma (elongated)	Ch. 5:141; Ch. 15:428
	Deep angiomyxoma (rounded, medium-sized)	Ch. 5:141; Ch. 17:499
	Cellular angiofibroma (thick-walled, hyalinized, medium-sized)	Ch. 17:504
	Low-grade fibromyxoid sarcoma (elongated)	Ch. 3:81; Ch. 4:124; Ch. 5:153
	Myxoid liposarcoma (plexiform)	Ch. 5:148; Ch. 12:332
	Myxofibrosarcoma (curvilinear)	Ch. 5:148; Ch. 7:218
	Inflammatory fibroid polyp (rounded, small)	Ch. 16:482
	Plexiform fibromyxoma (branching, small)	Ch. 16:484

Pattern 2 Epithelioid

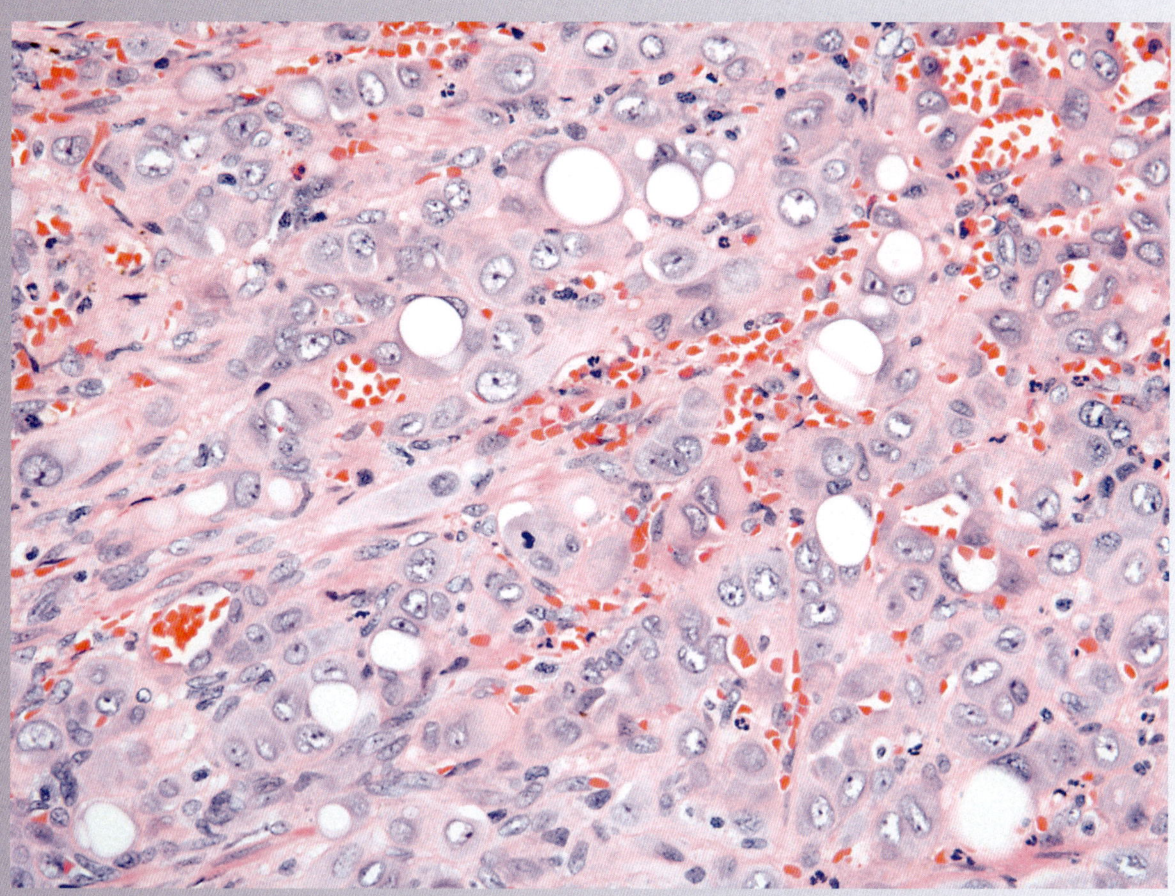

Elements of the pattern: The tumor cells resemble epithelial cells with a rounded or polygonal appearance and at least moderate amounts of cytoplasm.

Pattern 2 Epithelioid

Additional Findings	Diagnostic Considerations	Chapter:Page
Lobulated architecture	Epithelioid hemangioma	Ch. 6:168; Ch. 13:372
	Giant cell tumor of soft tissue	Ch. 11:306
	Myoepithelioma/myoepithelial carcinoma	Ch. 5:145; Ch. 6:173
	Epithelioid schwannoma	Ch. 15:441
	Epithelioid malignant peripheral nerve sheath tumor	Ch. 6:201
	Ossifying fibromyxoid tumor	Ch. 5:143; Ch. 6:185
	Gastrointestinal stromal tumor (subset)	Ch. 16:460
	Ependymoma of soft tissue	Ch. 6:185
	Epithelioid myxofibrosarcoma	Ch. 6:202
Nested architecture	Perivascular epithelioid cell tumor (PEComa)	Ch. 6:177; Ch. 15:439; Ch. 16:485
	Cellular neurothekeoma	Ch. 15:437
	Extracranial meningioma	Ch. 6:184; Ch. 15:443
	Alveolar soft part sarcoma	Ch. 6:186
	Clear cell sarcoma	Ch. 3:87
Trabecular or cord-like architecture	Myoepithelioma/myoepithelial carcinoma (subset)	Ch. 5:145; Ch. 6:173
	Sclerosing PEComa	Ch. 6:178
	Sclerosing perineurioma	Ch. 3:63; Ch. 15:442
	Epithelioid schwannoma (subset)	Ch. 15:441
	Ossifying fibromyxoid tumor	Ch. 5:143; Ch. 6:185
	Extraskeletal myxoid chondrosarcoma	Ch. 5:151
	Epithelioid hemangioendothelioma	Ch. 6:188; Ch. 13:374
	Sclerosing epithelioid fibrosarcoma	Ch. 6:197
Sheet-like architecture	Epithelioid angiomatous nodule	Ch. 13:374
	Epithelioid fibrous histiocytoma	Ch. 15:434
	Cutaneous myoepithelioma	Ch. 15:435
	Reticulohistiocytoma	Ch. 15:446
	Juvenile xanthogranuloma	Ch. 15:444
	Extranodal Rosai-Dorfman disease	Ch. 10:283; Ch. 15:448
	Tenosynovial giant cell tumors	Ch. 11:298
	Glomus tumor	Ch. 6:171; Ch. 16:488
	Adult-type rhabdomyoma	Ch. 6:181
	Granular cell tumor	Ch. 6:182; Ch. 15:432; Ch. 16:490
	Epithelioid sarcoma	Ch. 6:192
	Malignant rhabdoid tumor	Ch. 6:195
	Epithelioid angiosarcoma	Ch. 6:199; Ch. 13:378
	Gastrointestinal stromal tumor	Ch. 16:460
	Gastrointestinal clear cell sarcoma–like tumor (gastrointestinal neuroectodermal tumor)	Ch. 16:477
	Epithelioid inflammatory myofibroblastic sarcoma	Ch. 10:270; Ch. 16:480
	Epithelioid myxofibrosarcoma	Ch. 6:202
	Pleomorphic liposarcoma, epithelioid variant	Ch. 6:202; Ch. 12:334
	Dedifferentiated liposarcoma	Ch. 6:204
Clear cell morphology	Myoepithelioma/myoepithelial carcinoma (subset)	Ch. 5:145; Ch. 6:173
	PEComa	Ch. 6:175; Ch. 15:439; Ch. 16:485
	Distinctive dermal clear cell tumor	Ch. 15:441
	Gastrointestinal stromal tumor (subset)	Ch. 16:460
	Clear cell sarcoma (subset)	Ch. 6:204
	Alveolar rhabdomyosarcoma (rare)	Ch. 8:239
Nuclear pleomorphism	PEComa (subset)	Ch. 6:175; Ch. 16:485
	Epithelioid myxofibrosarcoma	Ch. 6:202
	Pleomorphic liposarcoma, epithelioid variant	Ch. 6:202; Ch. 12:334
Myxoid stroma	Myoepithelioma/myoepithelial carcinoma	Ch. 5:145; Ch. 6:173
	Extraskeletal myxoid chondrosarcoma	Ch. 5:151
	Epithelioid schwannoma (subset)	Ch. 15:441
	Ependymoma of soft tissue	Ch. 6:185
	Ossifying fibromyxoid tumor	Ch. 5:143; Ch. 6:185
	Epithelioid inflammatory myofibroblastic sarcoma	Ch. 10:270; Ch. 16:480
	Epithelioid myxofibrosarcoma	Ch. 6:202

Pattern 2 Epithelioid—*cont'd*

Additional Findings	Diagnostic Considerations	Chapter:Page
Collagenous stroma	Myoepithelioma/myoepithelial carcinoma (subset)	Ch. 6:173
	Granular cell tumor	Ch. 6:182; Ch. 15:432; Ch. 16:490
	Cellular neurothekeoma	Ch. 15:437
	Sclerosing perineurioma	Ch. 3:63; Ch. 15:442
	Sclerosing PEComa	Ch. 6:178
	Sclerosing epithelioid fibrosarcoma	Ch. 6:197
Prominent inflammatory cells	Epithelioid hemangioma (lymphocytes, eosinophils; subset)	Ch. 6:168; Ch. 13:372
	Langerhans cell histiocytosis (eosinophils)	Ch. 10:280
	Indeterminate cell histiocytosis (lymphocytes)	Ch. 10:282
	Extranodal Rosai-Dorfman disease (various)	Ch. 10:283; Ch. 15:448
	Histiocytic sarcoma (lymphocytes, neutrophils)	Ch. 10:283
	Epithelioid inflammatory myofibroblastic sarcoma (neutrophils)	Ch. 10:270; Ch. 16:480
Prominent or distinctive giant cells	Clear cell sarcoma (wreath-like)	Ch. 3:87
	Tenosynovial giant cell tumors (osteoclast-like)	Ch. 11:298
	Giant cell tumor of soft tissue (osteoclast-like)	Ch. 11:306
	Juvenile xanthogranuloma (Touton)	Ch. 15:444
	Reticulohistiocytoma (glassy cytoplasm)	Ch. 15:446
	Gastrointestinal clear cell sarcoma–like tumor (gastrointestinal neuroectodermal tumor) (osteoclast-like; subset)	Ch. 16:477
Prominent or distinctive blood vessels	Epithelioid hemangioma (small- to medium-sized)	Ch. 6:168; Ch. 13:372
	Glomus tumor (capillary-sized; dilated, branching)	Ch. 6:171; Ch. 16:488
	Angiomyofibroblastoma (delicate, thin-walled)	Ch. 17:502
	Epithelioid myxofibrosarcoma (curvilinear)	Ch. 6:202

Pattern 3 Pleomorphic

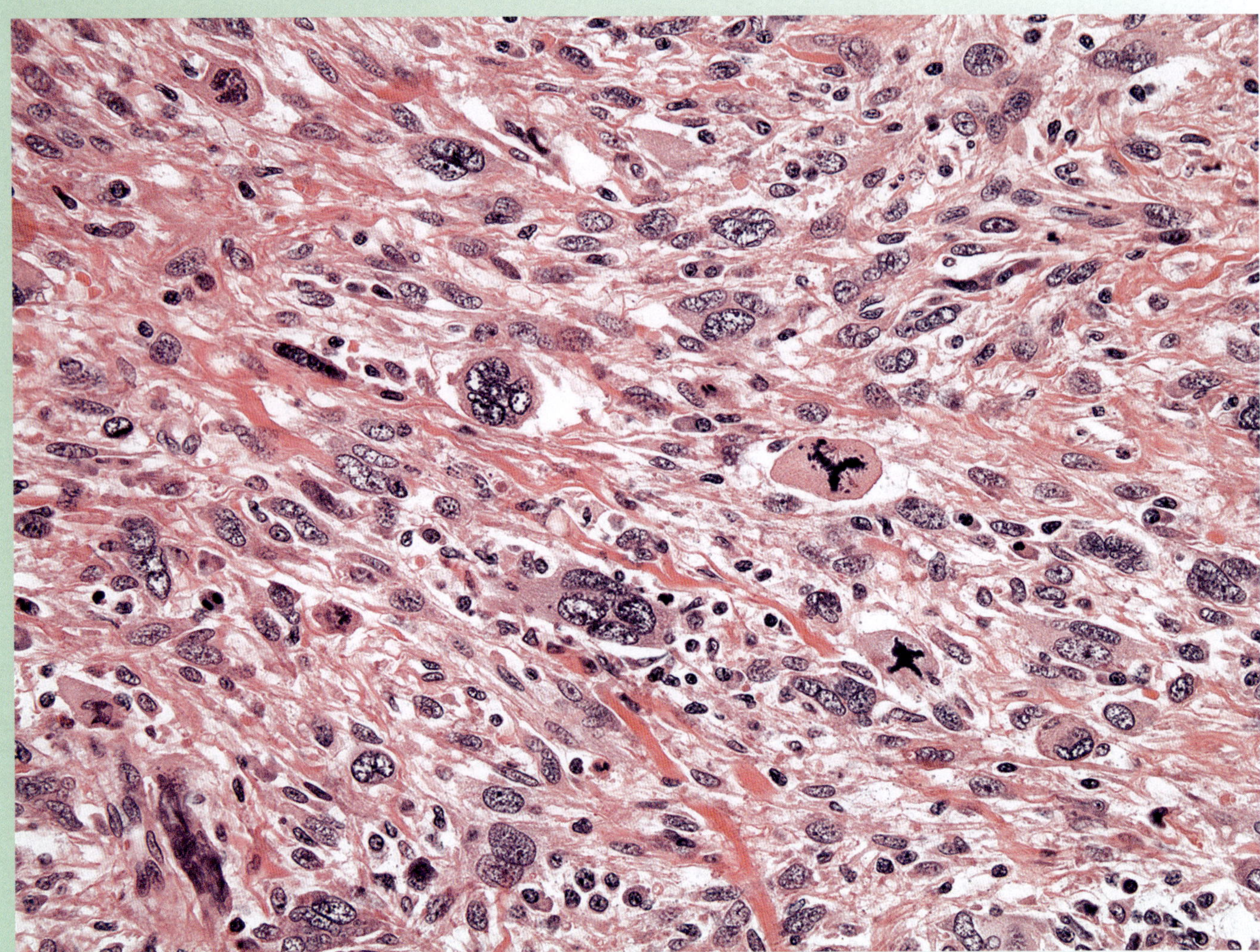

Elements of the pattern: The tumor cells show marked variation in size and shape, often including very large and bizarre forms.

Pattern 3 Pleomorphic

Additional Findings	Diagnostic Considerations	Chapter:Page
Abundant eosinophilic cytoplasm	Pleomorphic leiomyosarcoma Pleomorphic rhabdomyosarcoma Undifferentiated pleomorphic sarcoma (subset)	Ch. 7:221 Ch. 7:221 Ch. 7:212
Cutaneous	Pleomorphic fibroma Atypical fibrous histiocytoma Atypical fibroxanthoma Pleomorphic dermal sarcoma	Ch. 15:452 Ch. 15:411 Ch. 7:210; Ch. 15:449 Ch. 15:451
Myxoid stroma	Myxofibrosarcoma Pleomorphic liposarcoma (subset) Dedifferentiated liposarcoma (subset) Myxoinflammatory fibroblastic sarcoma	Ch. 5:148; Ch. 7:218 Ch. 7:223; Ch. 12:334 Ch. 7:225; Ch. 12:328 Ch. 5:155; Ch. 7:217; Ch. 10:286
Prominent or distinctive giant cells	Pleomorphic leiomyosarcoma (osteoclast-like; subset) Giant cell–rich extraskeletal osteosarcoma (osteoclast-like; subset) Undifferentiated pleomorphic sarcoma (osteoclast-like; subset)	Ch. 11:309 Ch. 11:308 Ch. 11:307
Prominent or distinctive blood vessels	Pleomorphic hyalinizing angiectatic tumor (hyalinized, dilated, thin-walled) "Ancient" schwannoma (hyalinized) Myxofibrosarcoma (curvilinear)	Ch. 7:216 Ch. 3:52 Ch. 5:148; Ch. 7:218
Prominent inflammation	Dedifferentiated liposarcoma (neutrophils, histiocytes; subset) Undifferentiated pleomorphic sarcoma (various; subset) Myxoinflammatory fibroblastic sarcoma (neutrophils, lymphocytes)	Ch. 7:225; Ch. 10:288 Ch. 7:212 Ch. 5:155; Ch. 7:217; Ch. 10:286
Adipocytic component or lipoblasts	Pleomorphic lipoma Pleomorphic liposarcoma Dedifferentiated liposarcoma	Ch. 12:316 Ch. 7:223; Ch. 12:334 Ch. 7:225; Ch. 12:328
Osteoid/bone	Extraskeletal osteosarcoma Dedifferentiated liposarcoma (subset)	Ch. 7:226; Ch. 14:400 Ch. 7:225; Ch. 12:328

Pattern 4 Round Cell

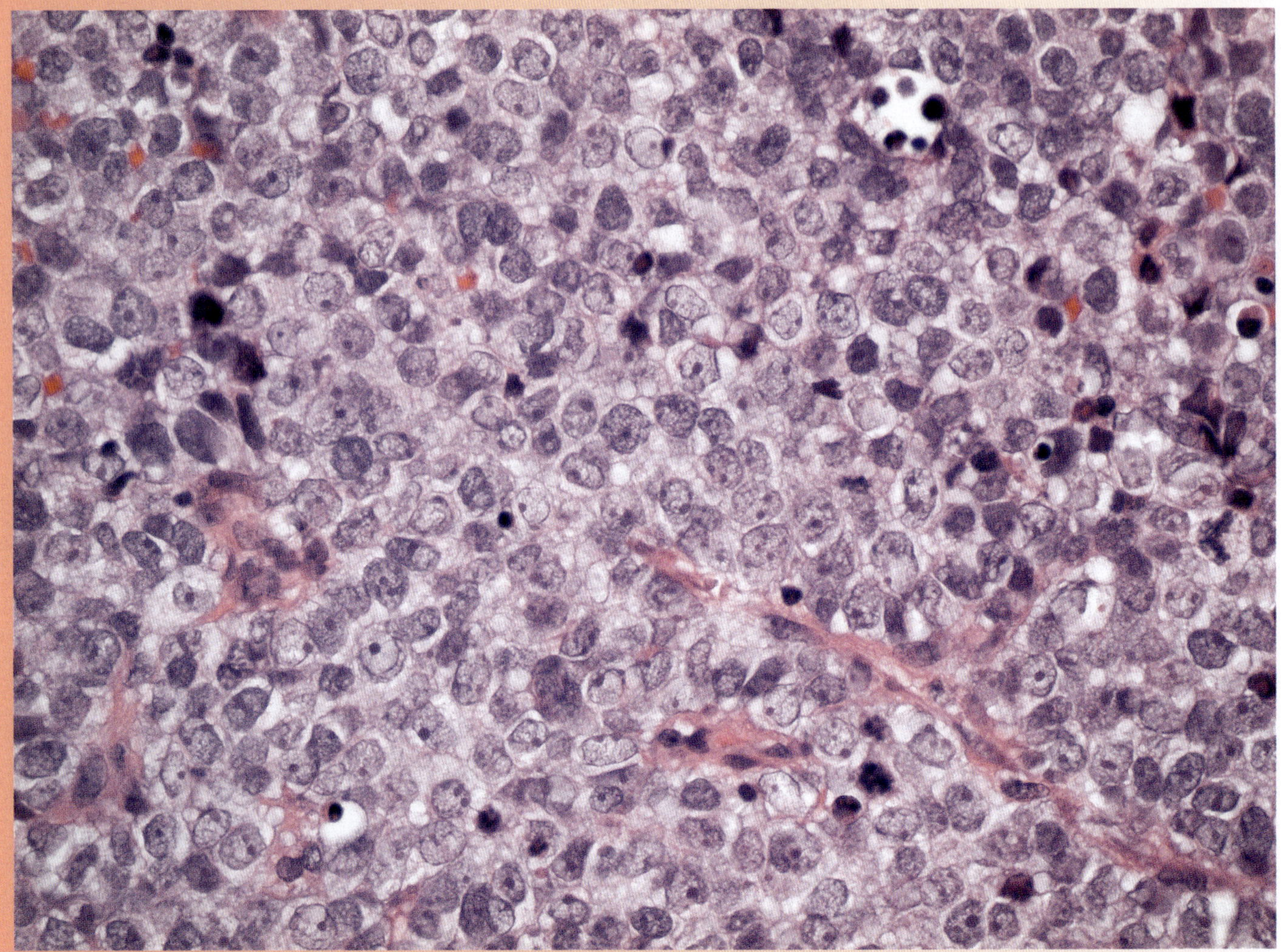

Elements of the pattern: The tumor cells contain round, often uniform nuclei and minimal cytoplasm.

Pattern 4 Round Cell

Additional Findings	Diagnostic Considerations	Chapter:Page
Nested architecture	Alveolar rhabdomyosarcoma (subset)	Ch. 8:239
	Desmoplastic small round cell tumor	Ch. 8:243
Sheet-like architecture	Ewing sarcoma	Ch. 8:235
	Alveolar rhabdomyosarcoma (subset)	Ch. 8:239
	Embryonal rhabdomyosarcoma	Ch. 8:242
	Round cell (high-grade myxoid) liposarcoma (subset)	Ch. 8:243; Ch. 12:332
	Poorly differentiated synovial sarcoma	Ch. 8:244
	Mesenchymal chondrosarcoma	Ch. 14:398
	Gastrointestinal clear cell sarcoma–like tumor (gastrointestinal neuroectodermal tumor)	Ch. 16:477
	CIC-rearranged sarcomas	Ch. 8:245
	BCOR-rearranged sarcomas	Ch. 8:246
Myxoid stroma	Embryonal rhabdomyosarcoma (subset)	Ch. 8:242
	Round cell (high-grade myxoid) liposarcoma (subset)	Ch. 8:243; Ch. 12:332
Collagenous stroma	Desmoplastic small round cell tumor	Ch. 8:243
	Poorly differentiated synovial sarcoma (focal; subset)	Ch. 8:244
Prominent or distinctive blood vessels	Round cell (high-grade myxoid) liposarcoma (plexiform)	Ch. 8:243; Ch. 12:332
	Poorly differentiated synovial sarcoma (dilated, branching; subset)	Ch. 8:244
Prominent or distinctive giant cells	Alveolar rhabdomyosarcoma (wreath-like)	Ch. 8:239
Cartilage	Mesenchymal chondrosarcoma	Ch. 14:398

Pattern 5 Biphasic or Mixed

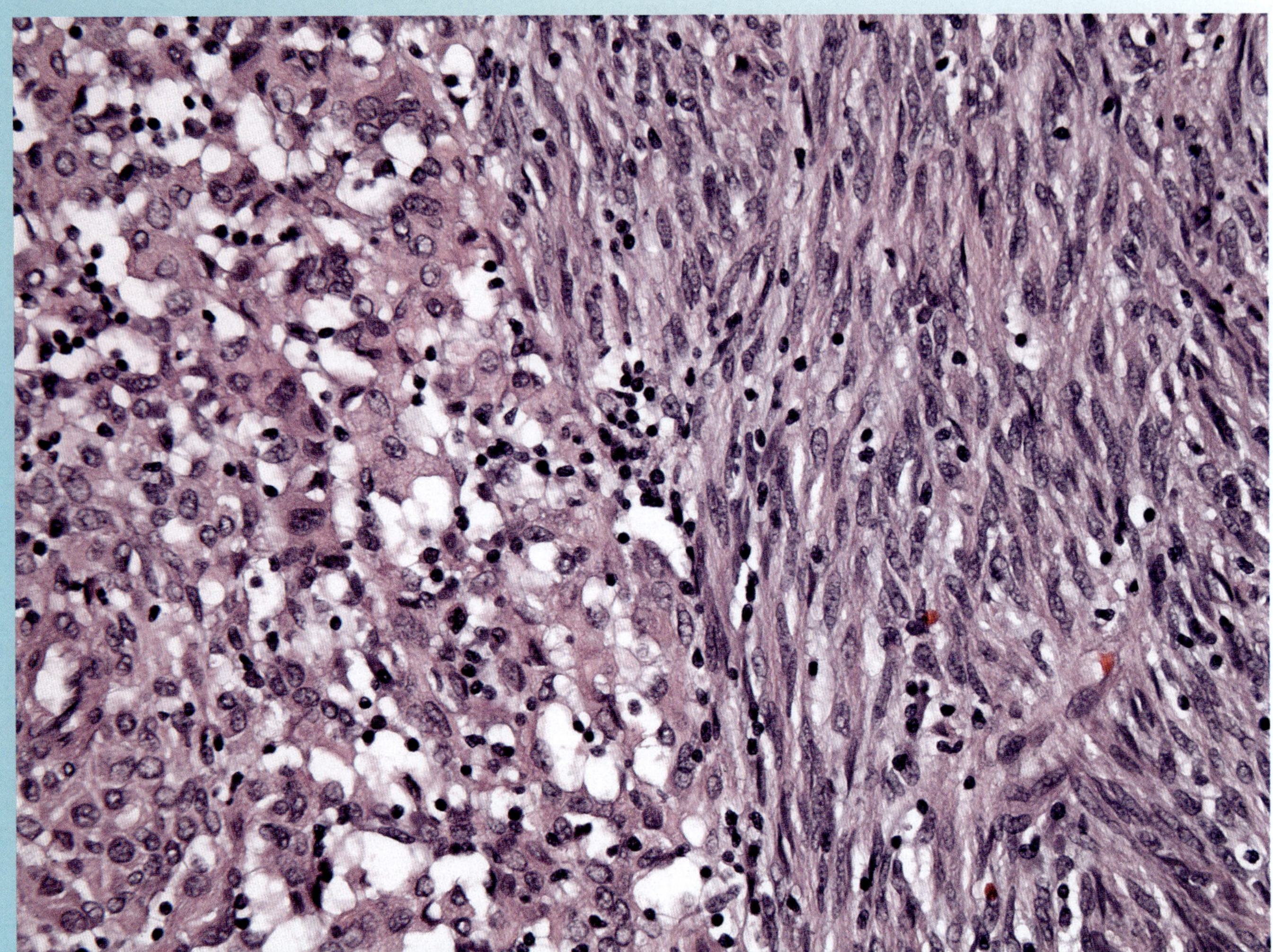

Elements of the pattern: The tumor contains two or more types of cells with distinct morphology, such as spindle cells and epithelioid cells. Some tumors show variation in architecture and stromal composition.

Pattern 5 Biphasic or Mixed

Additional Findings	Diagnostic Considerations	Chapter:Page
Glands or ducts	Biphasic synovial sarcoma	Ch. 9:249
	Mixed tumor	Ch. 9:252
	Glandular malignant peripheral nerve sheath tumor	Ch. 9:254
	Ectopic hamartomatous thymoma	Ch. 9:256
Mixed cytomorphology	Myoepithelioma/myoepithelial carcinoma	Ch. 5:145; Ch. 6:173
	Ectopic hamartomatous thymoma	Ch. 9:256
	Gastrointestinal stromal tumor (subset)	Ch. 9:258; Ch. 16:460
	Dedifferentiated liposarcoma	Ch. 7:225; Ch. 9:259; Ch. 12:328
	Melanotic neuroectodermal tumor of infancy	Ch. 9:262
Myxoid stroma	Myoepithelioma/mixed tumor/myoepithelial carcinoma	Ch. 5:145; Ch. 6:173
Adipocytic component or lipoblasts	Ectopic hamartomatous thymoma (subset)	Ch. 9:256
	Dedifferentiated liposarcoma (subset)	Ch. 7:225; Ch. 9:259; Ch. 12:328
Cartilage and/or bone	Mixed tumor (subset)	Ch. 9:252
	Malignant peripheral nerve sheath tumor (subset)	Ch. 9:254
	Dedifferentiated liposarcoma (subset)	Ch. 7:225; Ch. 9:259; Ch. 12:328

Pattern 6 Myxoid

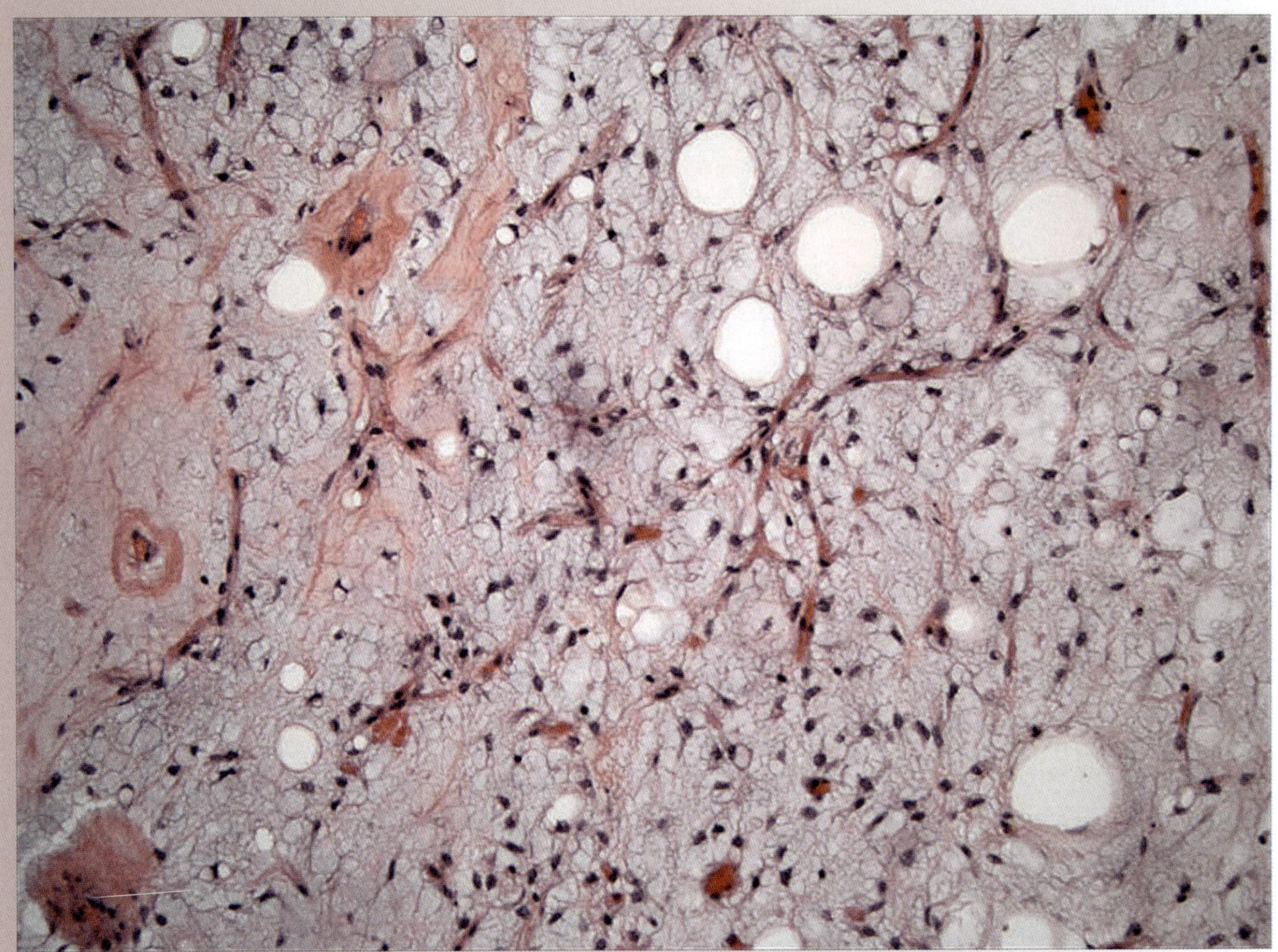

Elements of the pattern: The tumor contains abundant loose extracellular matrix material, often rich in glycosaminoglycans.

Pattern 6 Myxoid

Additional Findings	Diagnostic Considerations	Chapter:Page
Spindle cell cytomorphology	Intramuscular/cellular myxoma	Ch. 5:137
	Juxta-articular myxoma	Ch. 5:138
	Dermal nerve sheath myxoma	Ch. 5:139; Ch. 15:431
	Superficial acral fibromyxoma	Ch. 5:140; Ch. 15:427
	Superficial angiomyxoma	Ch. 5:141; Ch. 15:428
	Deep angiomyxoma	Ch. 5:141; Ch. 17:499
	Plexiform fibromyxoma	Ch. 16:484
	Ossifying fibromyxoid tumor (subset)	Ch. 5:143
	Myxofibrosarcoma	Ch. 5:148; Ch. 7:218
	Myxoid liposarcoma	Ch. 5:150; Ch. 12:332
	Extraskeletal myxoid chondrosarcoma	Ch. 5:151
	Low-grade fibromyxoid sarcoma	Ch. 3:81; Ch. 4:124; Ch. 5:153
	Primitive myxoid mesenchymal tumor of infancy	Ch. 4:123
	Fetal rhabdomyoma	Ch. 4:126
	Embryonal rhabdomyosarcoma	Ch. 8:242
	Neurofibroma	Ch. 5:157
	Soft tissue perineurioma	Ch. 5:157
	Reticular perineurioma	Ch. 5:157
	Microcystic/reticular schwannoma	Ch. 5:158
	Malignant peripheral nerve sheath tumor	Ch. 5:158
	Spindle cell lipoma	Ch. 3:50; Ch. 15:453
	Nodular fasciitis	Ch. 3:20; Ch. 4:102; Ch. 5:158
	Dermatofibrosarcoma protuberans	Ch. 5:158
	Solitary fibrous tumor	Ch. 5:158
	Monophasic synovial sarcoma	Ch. 5:158
Epithelioid cytomorphology	Cellular neurothekeoma	Ch. 15:437
	Ossifying fibromyxoid tumor (subset)	Ch. 5:143; Ch. 6:185
	Myoepithelioma/myoepithelial carcinoma	Ch. 5:145; Ch. 6:173
	Myxofibrosarcoma (subset)	Ch. 6:202
	Extraskeletal myxoid chondrosarcoma (subset)	Ch. 5:151
Pleomorphic cytomorphology	Myxofibrosarcoma	Ch. 5:148; Ch. 7:218
	Pleomorphic liposarcoma	Ch. 7:223; Ch. 12:334
	Myxoinflammatory fibroblastic sarcoma	Ch. 5:155; Ch. 7:217; Ch. 10:286
Lobulated architecture	Dermal nerve sheath myxoma	Ch. 5:139; Ch. 15:431
	Superficial angiomyxoma	Ch. 5:141; Ch. 15:428
	Plexiform fibromyxoma	Ch. 16:484
	Ossifying fibromyxoid tumor	Ch. 5:143; Ch. 6:185
	Myoepithelioma/myoepithelial carcinoma	Ch. 5:145; Ch. 6:173
	Myxofibrosarcoma	Ch. 5:148; Ch. 7:218
	Extraskeletal myxoid chondrosarcoma	Ch. 5:151
Reticular architecture	Reticular perineurioma	Ch. 5:157
	Microcystic/reticular schwannoma	Ch. 5:158
	Extraskeletal myxoid chondrosarcoma	Ch. 5:151
Prominent or distinctive blood vessels	Superficial angiomyxoma (elongated)	Ch. 5:141; Ch. 15:428
	Deep angiomyxoma (rounded, medium-sized)	Ch. 5:141; Ch. 17:499
	Plexiform fibromyxoma (branching, small)	Ch. 16:484
	Myxofibrosarcoma (curvilinear)	Ch. 5:148; Ch. 7:218
	Myxoid liposarcoma (plexiform)	Ch. 5:150; Ch. 12:332

1

Introduction: Tumor Classification and Immunohistochemistry

Jason L. Hornick, MD, PhD

Tumor Classification

Soft tissue tumors have traditionally been classified according to line of differentiation—that is, which normal cell type the neoplastic cells most closely resemble. Such a "lineage" can often be assigned based on a combination of histologic appearances, patterns of protein expression (assessed by immunohistochemistry), and ultrastructural findings (identified by electron microscopy).[1,2] Although electron microscopy once played an important role in the evolution of soft tissue tumor classification, it is now rarely used in clinical practice and has largely been supplanted by immunohistochemistry and molecular genetics. The majority of soft tissue tumors shows mesenchymal or neuroectodermal differentiation. However, a small subset of soft tissue tumors shows unusual lines of differentiation generally reserved for cell types that are usually not found in soft tissues (e.g., epithelial, myoepithelial, or melanocytic). For still other soft tissue tumors, it is not possible to assign a specific line of differentiation even after extensive immunohistochemical (and ultrastructural) evaluation ("undifferentiated" sarcomas). Finally, there exist distinct subtypes of soft tissue sarcomas (most often associated with chromosomal translocations) whose line of differentiation is uncertain.

Assigning a line of differentiation (when appropriate) can be very helpful for the classification of soft tissue tumors. However, tumors within such groups may show highly varied clinical presentations, histologic appearances, and behavior. One such example of this diversity is the group of tumors classified as "rhabdomyosarcomas." The pediatric rhabdomyosarcomas (namely, embryonal and alveolar rhabdomyosarcomas; see Chapter 8) share little, if anything, in common with pleomorphic rhabdomyosarcoma of adults (see Chapter 7). Another such example is the group of tumors designated "liposarcomas." Although well-differentiated/dedifferentiated liposarcoma, myxoid liposarcoma, and pleomorphic liposarcoma are often considered to be "subtypes" of liposarcoma, their clinical presentations, histologic appearances, genetic features, and behavior are entirely different (see Chapter 12). Furthermore, the differential diagnosis of any particular type of soft tissue tumor often does not include other tumors with a shared lineage but instead tumors with similar histologic appearances. As such, although it is conceptually useful to consider groups of tumors with similar lines of differentiation together as a general classification system (as is the case for the World Health Organization classification[3]), for the practicing pathologist, a pattern-based approach to soft tissue tumors is very helpful for arriving at a specific diagnosis. This is the organizational scheme for this textbook.

Some of the chapters approach tumors based on the shape of the tumor cells (spindle cell, epithelioid, round cell, pleomorphic, biphasic or mixed) or the presence of other distinguishing features (myxoid stroma, inflammatory cells, giant cells), whereas separate chapters are dedicated to vascular, adipocytic, and cartilaginous and osseous tumors because the lineage is usually clear for these latter tumor types. Many soft tissue tumors exhibit several such distinguishing features (e.g., spindle cells and inflammatory cells, or epithelioid cells and myxoid stroma); thus some soft tissue tumors are covered in more than one chapter to emphasize approaches to differential diagnosis. Cutaneous, gastrointestinal, and lower genital tract tumors are considered separately, because many distinctive soft tissue tumors are exclusive (or nearly exclusive) to such sites. Although each chapter in the book includes molecular genetic findings of diagnostic relevance to individual tumor types, the final chapter, which is devoted to molecular testing, provides a discussion of methodology and specific examples for which molecular testing is particularly useful in differential diagnosis and serves as a quick reference for the distinguishing genetic features of many tumor types.

Immunohistochemistry

Immunohistochemistry plays a central role in the diagnosis of soft tissue tumors. Although many mesenchymal tumors are characterized by particular patterns of protein expression, for some tumors, the histologic features are sufficiently distinctive such that immunohistochemistry is unnecessary to make a confident diagnosis. In contrast, other types

Box 1.1 Uses of Immunohistochemistry for the Diagnosis of Soft Tissue Tumors

Distinguish among histologically similar tumors
Confirm histologic impression
Support the diagnosis of a rare tumor type
Support the diagnosis when a tumor arises at an unusual anatomic location
Support the diagnosis when a tumor affects a patient of an uncharacteristic age

of soft tissue tumors show considerable morphologic overlap, and immunohistochemistry is an invaluable aid in distinguishing among them. In this latter category, there are often (sometimes subtle) histologic clues that might allow for a specific diagnosis; however, application of a narrow panel of markers can provide reassurance for a more confident diagnosis. For rare tumor types as well as examples arising either at unusual anatomic locations or in patients of uncharacteristic ages—even when the histologic diagnosis is relatively straightforward—immunohistochemical support for the diagnosis can be very helpful (Box 1.1). As mentioned previously, traditional immunohistochemical markers are used to identify specific proteins within tumor cells that indicate a line of differentiation.[2,4] Unfortunately, with rare exceptions, these markers are not particularly lineage specific: there is considerable overlap in the patterns of protein expression shared by various cell types and soft tissue tumors. Over the past decade, markers directed against protein correlates of more specific molecular genetic signatures have become available.[5] Most recently, gene expression profiling has led to the identification of novel, highly specific markers that are proving to be powerful means of confirming the diagnosis of soft tissue tumors, particularly in cases for which specific markers were previously lacking. Although the immunohistochemical markers helpful for diagnosing specific tumor types are covered in the appropriate sections of the other chapters in this book, this chapter discusses these various categories of diagnostic markers in some detail. This is intended to be an introduction to the application of the most commonly used markers, rather than a comprehensive discussion of sensitivity and specificity.

Intermediate Filament Proteins

Antibodies directed against intermediate filament proteins are commonly used in soft tissue tumor diagnosis (Table 1.1).[2] Some of these proteins show relatively limited expression in mesenchymal tumors and are therefore highly valuable, whereas other intermediate filaments are ubiquitously expressed and therefore of dubious utility. Specifically, in this latter category, vimentin is often used as a marker of mesenchymal tumors. However, vimentin expression is not specific for mesenchymal lesions: this protein may also be expressed in a subset of melanomas, lymphomas, and carcinomas. Moreover, vimentin cannot discriminate among various types of soft tissue tumors. As such, vimentin has no real diagnostic value in soft tissue tumor pathology (except perhaps to prove that the tissue has been fixed and processed appropriately to preserve "antigenicity," although many more diagnostically valuable markers can be used for this purpose), and its use in this setting should be discouraged.

PRACTICE POINTS: Vimentin

- Ubiquitously expressed in mesenchymal tumors
- Not specific for mesenchymal tumors; expressed in a subset of carcinomas and melanomas
- No real diagnostic value in soft tissue tumor pathology; its use in this context should be discouraged

Keratins are intermediate filaments widely expressed in epithelial cells. As such, keratins are highly sensitive and specific markers for carcinomas. In contrast, keratins show limited expression in normal mesenchymal cells (other than endothelial cells). Several distinctive types of soft tissue tumors (e.g., epithelioid sarcoma, synovial sarcoma, and myoepithelial tumors) characteristically express keratins, which is a helpful diagnostic feature. However, many other diverse soft tissue tumor types can also express keratins, some relatively commonly and others more rarely. It is important for the surgical pathologist to be aware of the range of keratin-positive soft tissue tumors to avoid potential diagnostic pitfalls (Table 1.2).

Desmin is an intermediate filament of muscle cells. Desmin is expressed in benign and malignant tumors of smooth muscle and skeletal muscle lineages. In addition, desmin may also be expressed in some

Table 1.1 Intermediate Filament Proteins: Utility and Selected Applications in the Diagnosis of Soft Tissue Tumors

Marker	Utility	Applications
Vimentin	None	None
Keratins	Extensive	Differential diagnosis of metastatic carcinoma versus sarcoma; support diagnosis of selected soft tissue tumor types (e.g., epithelioid sarcoma, synovial sarcoma, desmoplastic small round cell tumor)
Desmin	Extensive	Supports diagnosis of leiomyosarcoma, rhabdomyosarcoma, desmoplastic small round cell tumor, and other selected soft tissue tumor types
Glial fibrillary acidic protein	Limited	Supports diagnosis of soft tissue myoepithelioma/myoepithelial carcinoma and malignant peripheral nerve sheath tumor
Neurofilament protein	Limited	Highlights axons in benign peripheral nerve sheath tumors

Table 1.2 Keratin-Positive Soft Tissue Tumors

Tumor Type	Frequency of Staining for Keratin	Extent of Staining for Keratin
Epithelioid sarcoma	Nearly 100%	Usually diffuse
Epithelioid hemangioendothelioma	Up to 50%	Usually focal; occasionally diffuse
Epithelioid angiosarcoma	Up to 50%	Usually diffuse
Extrarenal malignant rhabdoid tumor	Nearly 100%	Usually diffuse
Synovial sarcoma	90%	Limited in monophasic and poorly differentiated (scattered cells); diffuse in glands of biphasic
Leiomyosarcoma	Up to 40%	Usually focal; occasionally diffuse
Schwannoma (retroperitoneal)	70%	Often diffuse
Inflammatory myofibroblastic tumor	30%	Usually patchy
Pseudomyogenic hemangioendothelioma	100%	Usually diffuse
Desmoplastic small round cell tumor	90%	Usually diffuse
Alveolar rhabdomyosarcoma	Up to 50%	Usually patchy
Ewing sarcoma	30%	Usually patchy

Box 1.2 Desmin-Positive Soft Tissue Tumors

Leiomyoma/leiomyosarcoma
Rhabdomyoma/rhabdomyosarcoma
Low-grade myofibroblastic sarcoma
Inflammatory myofibroblastic tumor (subset)
Deep ("aggressive") angiomyxoma
Angiomyofibroblastoma
Mammary-type myofibroblastoma
Desmoplastic small round cell tumor
Angiomatoid fibrous histiocytoma (subset)
Ossifying fibromyxoid tumor (subset)
Tenosynovial giant cell tumors (subset)

myofibroblastic tumors. Desmin expression is also a helpful diagnostic feature of other rare tumor types not generally considered to be myogenic (e.g., desmoplastic small round cell tumor and angiomatoid fibrous histiocytoma) (Box 1.2).

Glial fibrillary acidic protein (GFAP) is a major structural component of astrocytes and is widely used in neuropathology. GFAP may also be expressed in Schwann cells of peripheral nerves and myoepithelial cells. GFAP has a limited role in the diagnosis of soft tissue tumors (peripheral nerve sheath tumors and myoepithelial tumors). Neurofilament protein is expressed in neurons. This marker also has limited diagnostic applications in soft tissue tumor pathology and is most often used for highlighting axons in benign peripheral nerve sheath tumors.

Other Myogenic Markers

Actins are a group of filamentous cytoplasmic proteins that are components of the cytoskeleton and serve multiple cellular functions, including motility and muscle contraction. In soft tissue tumor pathology, α-smooth muscle actin (SMA) is among the most widely used diagnostic markers. In addition to labeling smooth muscle tumors, SMA is also widely expressed in myofibroblastic, myoepithelial, and pericytic/glomus tumors. However, SMA expression is not limited to mesenchymal neoplasms. In fact, almost any tumor showing spindle cell morphology may express SMA to a variable extent, including sarcomatoid carcinomas and spindle cell melanomas. Muscle-specific actin (also known as pan-muscle actin; widely used clone HHF35) shows somewhat overlapping patterns of expression as SMA but in contrast is generally strongly positive in rhabdomyosarcomas, whereas SMA is usually negative or at most shows limited staining in skeletal muscle tumors.

High-molecular-weight or "heavy" caldesmon, or h-caldesmon, is a relatively specific marker for smooth muscle differentiation, which is usually negative in skeletal muscle and myofibroblastic tumors. Few other tumor types consistently express h-caldesmon, including gastrointestinal stromal tumors (GISTs) and glomus tumors.[6] Finally, several skeletal muscle–specific transcription factors are available: myogenin (MYF4) and MYOD1 (MYF3).[7] Both of these markers are extremely useful to confirm the diagnosis of rhabdomyosarcoma as well as the presence of heterologous rhabdomyoblastic differentiation in other tumor types (e.g., dedifferentiated liposarcoma and malignant peripheral nerve sheath tumor [MPNST]). Of note, older antibodies directed against MYOD1 often show nonspecific cytoplasmic background staining, which should be ignored; more recently developed clones show more reliable nuclear staining without such background staining. The lineage-restricted transcription factors that are useful for the diagnosis of soft tissue tumors are listed in Table 1.3.

Endothelial Markers

CD34 and CD31 are the most widely used markers of endothelial differentiation, although neither is entirely specific. In addition to vascular

Table 1.3 Lineage-Restricted Transcription Factors

Markers	Line of Differentiation	Examples of Tumor Types
Myogenin MYOD1	Skeletal muscle	Rhabdomyosarcomas
FLI1 ERG	Endothelium	Angiosarcomas
SOX10	Neuroectoderm	Malignant peripheral nerve sheath tumor
Brachyury	Notochord	Chordoma
SATB2	Osteoblast	Osteosarcoma

Box 1.3 CD34-Positive Soft Tissue Tumors

Solitary fibrous tumor
Dermatofibrosarcoma protuberans
Spindle cell/pleomorphic lipoma
Mammary-type myofibroblastoma
Gastrointestinal stromal tumor
Kaposi sarcoma
Angiosarcoma
Epithelioid hemangioendothelioma
Soft tissue perineurioma
Neurofibroma (subset of cells)
Epithelioid sarcoma (50%)

tumors, CD34 is consistently expressed in solitary fibrous tumor, dermatofibrosarcoma protuberans, and spindle cell lipoma as well as a proportion of GISTs, epithelioid sarcomas, and MPNSTs, to name a few notable tumor types (Box 1.3). CD31 is more sensitive and specific than CD34, although CD31 is also expressed in macrophages[8] and the very rare histiocytic sarcoma. CD31 staining in prominent intratumoral macrophages represents a significant potential diagnostic pitfall. Factor VIII–related antigen is another conventional marker of vascular tumors, but this marker may show considerable background staining, is less sensitive than other endothelial markers, and has therefore largely been abandoned in favor of more reproducible diagnostic markers.

Podoplanin (recognized by the D2-40 monoclonal antibody) is relatively specific for lymphatic differentiation among vascular lesions.[9] Podoplanin is also consistently expressed in Kaposi sarcoma as well as a subset of angiosarcomas and epithelioid hemangioendotheliomas. However, podoplanin is not specific for endothelial differentiation as it is also strongly expressed in several other unrelated tumor types (e.g., mesothelioma, seminoma, and follicular dendritic cell sarcoma).[10,11] In recent years, two ETS family transcription factors have been introduced as markers of vascular differentiation. FLI1 (the most common fusion partner in Ewing sarcoma) shows strong nuclear staining in normal endothelial cells and in nearly all vascular tumors.[12,13] However, FLI1 shows limited specificity; this marker is also positive in lymphocytes, lymphoblastic lymphomas, and a subset of a diverse range of other mesenchymal and nonmesenchymal tumor types.[14,15] Most recently, ERG has emerged as a powerful and highly specific endothelial marker.[16] Similar to FLI1, nearly all vascular lesions show nuclear reactivity for ERG, but the latter marker is much more specific.[15,16] Of note, few other tumor types are also positive for ERG, including 40% to 50% of prostatic adenocarcinomas (i.e., those with *TMPRSS2-ERG* fusion),[17] a subset of Ewing sarcomas (most strongly in those with *EWSR1-ERG* fusion),[18] and some acute myeloid leukemias. These exceptions notwithstanding, ERG is the most sensitive and specific endothelial marker available.

Box 1.4 S-100 Protein-Positive Soft Tissue Tumors

Schwannoma
Neurofibroma
Ganglioneuroma
Granular cell tumor
Dermal nerve sheath myxoma
Malignant peripheral nerve sheath tumor
Clear cell sarcoma
Langerhans cell histiocytosis
Rosai-Dorfman disease
Interdigitating dendritic cell sarcoma
Histiocytic sarcoma (subset)
Myoepithelioma/myoepithelial carcinoma
Ossifying fibromyxoid tumor
Synovial sarcoma (subset)
Extraskeletal myxoid chondrosarcoma (subset)

Box 1.5 Epithelial Membrane Antigen–Positive Soft Tissue Tumors

Epithelioid sarcoma
Synovial sarcoma
Soft tissue perineurioma
Myoepithelioma/myoepithelial carcinoma
Low-grade fibromyxoid sarcoma
Sclerosing epithelioid fibrosarcoma (subset)
Angiomatoid fibrous histiocytoma (subset)
Follicular dendritic cell sarcoma (subset)
Solitary fibrous tumor (subset)

These markers and other endothelial markers are also discussed in Chapter 13.

Schwannian Markers

S-100 protein (S-100B) is the most widely used marker for peripheral nerve sheath tumors. Although S-100 protein is positive in all benign Schwann cell tumors, this marker shows relatively low sensitivity for MPNST (at most, around 50%). Because S-100 protein is also expressed in a variety of other cell types, a range of other tumors are also consistently positive; still other tumor types show variable expression of this marker (Box 1.4). GFAP was discussed previously; this marker is less sensitive than S-100 protein as a Schwann cell marker, although it may be helpful in occasional cases to support a diagnosis of MPNST. SOX10 is a neuroectodermal transcription factor widely used in the diagnosis of melanoma. Similar to S-100 protein, SOX10 is positive in all benign Schwann cell tumors, but the sensitivity of this marker for MPNST is low (around 40%); SOX10 is also expressed in myoepithelial neoplasms of soft tissue.[19,20] CD56 (NCAM1) and CD57 (B3GAT1) are other markers that are sometimes used in soft tissue pathology. However, neither of these antigens is specific for nerve sheath tumors; expression can also be observed in leiomyosarcoma, synovial sarcoma, and some carcinomas, among other tumor types. The editor of this book does not use these markers in the differential diagnosis of soft tissue tumors.

Other Diagnostic Markers

Epithelial membrane antigen (EMA, MUC1) is a transmembrane mucin widely expressed on epithelial cells. As such, along with keratins, EMA is a helpful diagnostic marker for carcinoma. There are a relatively limited range of soft tissue tumors that consistently express EMA (Box 1.5). It is important to remember that EMA is also expressed in plasma cell neoplasms and anaplastic large-cell lymphoma, which may sometimes be considered in the differential diagnosis of soft tissue tumors (as well as carcinomas).

Box 1.6 CD99-Positive Soft Tissue Tumors

Ewing sarcoma
CIC-DUX4 sarcoma
Synovial sarcoma
Mesenchymal chondrosarcoma
Solitary fibrous tumor
Angiomatoid fibrous histiocytoma

Table 1.4 Protein Correlates of Genetic Alterations in Soft Tissue Tumors That Can Be Assessed by Immunohistochemistry

Markers	Tumor Types	Pattern
β-catenin	Desmoid fibromatosis	Aberrant nuclear staining
H3K27me3	MPNST	Loss of nuclear staining
INI1 (SMARCB1)	Malignant rhabdoid tumor Epithelioid sarcoma Epithelioid MPNST	Loss of nuclear staining
MDM2 and CDK4	Well-differentiated liposarcoma Dedifferentiated liposarcoma	Nuclear staining
SDHB and SDHA	Succinate dehydrogenase-deficient GIST	Loss of cytoplasmic staining

GIST, Gastrointestinal stromal tumor; *H3K27me3*, histone H3 with trimethylated lysine 27; *MPNST*, malignant peripheral nerve sheath tumor.

CD99 (recognized by monoclonal antibody O13; also known as MIC2) is a cell surface glycoprotein normally expressed on thymic T lymphocytes. Not surprisingly, CD99 is usually positive in lymphoblastic lymphomas. CD99 is a helpful marker for Ewing sarcoma, in which it usually shows a strong membranous staining pattern. However, occasional cases of Ewing sarcoma show more limited or cytoplasmic staining for CD99 (and are rarely completely negative). Importantly, other tumor types, some of which are in the differential diagnosis with Ewing sarcoma (such as *CIC-DUX4* sarcoma), may also be positive for CD99,[21] although many such cases usually show predominantly cytoplasmic (as opposed to membranous) staining (Box 1.6).

Protein Correlates of Genetic Alterations

With the evolving understanding of the molecular pathogenesis of soft tissue tumors, antibodies directed against protein correlates of specific genetic alterations are increasingly being developed (see also Chapter 18).[22-41] Several of these markers have entered routine diagnostic practice (Table 1.4). This section discusses examples of these markers to illustrate diagnostic applications.

Desmoid fibromatosis is characterized by activation of the Wnt signaling pathway, either by somatic mutations in the *CTNNB1* gene (encoding the β-catenin protein) or as a result of germline mutations in *APC* (in familial adenomatous polyposis). As a result of these mutations, β-catenin, which normally resides on the cell membrane, accumulates in the cytoplasm and nucleus. Immunohistochemistry for β-catenin therefore shows aberrant nuclear staining in the majority (70% to 90%) of cases of desmoid fibromatosis (see Chapters 3, 4, and 16).[22-24] This can be helpful to confirm the diagnosis, particularly in small biopsy samples. However, nuclear staining for β-catenin can also be seen in a subset of other fibroblastic/myofibroblastic tumors, including solitary fibrous tumor and low-grade myofibroblastic sarcoma.[24] The results of immunohistochemistry must therefore be interpreted in the context of the clinical and histologic findings. At the same time, because a subset of desmoid tumors lack this pattern of staining, negative results do not preclude the diagnosis.

Well-differentiated liposarcoma (atypical lipomatous tumor) and dedifferentiated liposarcoma are characterized by ring and giant marker chromosomes, derived from amplified material from chromosome 12q13~15. This amplification event results in overexpression of several proteins whose genes reside within this chromosomal region, including MDM2 and CDK4.[25,26] Immunohistochemistry for MDM2 and CDK4 can be helpful to confirm the diagnosis of well-differentiated liposarcoma (with the differential diagnosis of benign adipocytic neoplasms, particularly when atypia is very subtle) and dedifferentiated liposarcoma (with the differential diagnosis of other pleomorphic and spindle cell sarcomas, especially in small biopsy samples and when a well-differentiated component is absent; see also Chapters 7 and 12).[27] However, overexpression of these markers is not entirely specific for dedifferentiated liposarcoma among high-grade sarcomas. For example, around 60% of MPNSTs are also positive for MDM2 (although CDK4 is almost always negative), and a small subset of myxofibrosarcomas and rhabdomyosarcomas may also express MDM2.[27]

INI1 (also known as SNF5 and SMARCB1) is a member of the SWI/SNF multisubunit chromatin remodeling complex.[28] This complex mobilizes nucleosomes and thereby exposes DNA to transcription factors. INI1 is ubiquitously expressed in the nuclei of normal cells. In contrast, biallelic inactivation of *SMARCB1* is a defining feature of malignant rhabdoid tumor of infancy.[29] Immunohistochemistry for INI1 is therefore very helpful to confirm the diagnosis of this tumor type; loss of nuclear staining for INI1 is nearly always observed in malignant rhabdoid tumors (see Chapter 6).[30,31] Epithelioid sarcoma is also characterized by loss of INI1 expression; this finding is helpful in the differential diagnosis with other epithelioid malignant neoplasms, such as carcinoma and epithelioid endothelial neoplasms (especially epithelioid angiosarcoma), because nearly all other tumor types retain nuclear staining for INI1 (see Chapter 6).[32-34]

Finally, the diagnosis of many translocation-associated sarcomas can now be supported by immunohistochemistry using antibodies directed against protein products of the fusion genes (Table 1.5; see also Chapter 18).[42-56] None of these markers is entirely specific. For example, TFE3 is positive not only in alveolar soft-part sarcoma (see Chapter 6) but also in Xp11 translocation renal cell carcinoma and a small subset of perivascular epithelioid cell tumors (PEComas) and epithelioid hemangioendotheliomas.[42-44] As mentioned in the section on endothelial markers, FLI1 and ERG recognize not only Ewing sarcomas harboring translocations involving these genes[13,14,18] but also nearly all vascular tumors,[12,16] and in the case of FLI1, a subset of many other tumor types. ALK is an excellent diagnostic marker for inflammatory myofibroblastic tumor (see Chapters 4, 10, and 16)[45,46] but is also positive in other tumors with *ALK* gene rearrangements (e.g., anaplastic large-cell lymphoma and pulmonary adenocarcinoma) as well as several other tumor types (e.g., neuroblastoma, alveolar rhabdomyosarcoma, and MPNST).[47,48] Of note, the pattern of ALK staining sometimes correlates with a particular fusion partner (e.g., nuclear membrane staining in epithelioid inflammatory myofibroblastic sarcoma with *RANBP2-ALK* fusion).[49]

Table 1.5 Antibodies Directed Against Protein Products of Translocations

Marker	Translocation-Associated Soft Tissue Tumor	Other Tumor Types
ALK	Inflammatory myofibroblastic tumor	Anaplastic large-cell lymphoma Pulmonary adenocarcinoma (subset) Malignant peripheral nerve sheath tumor (subset) Alveolar rhabdomyosarcoma (subset) Neuroblastoma (subset)
BCOR	*BCOR-CCNB3* sarcoma *BCOR-MAML3* sarcoma	Primitive myxoid mesenchymal tumor of infancy Round cell sarcomas with *BCOR* internal tandem duplication Round cell sarcomas with *YWHAE-NUTM2B*
CAMTA1	Epithelioid hemangioendothelioma	
CCNB3	*BCOR-CCNB3* sarcoma	
ERG	Ewing sarcoma (small subset)	Vascular tumors Prostatic adenocarcinoma (subset) Acute myeloid leukemia (subset)
FLI1	Ewing sarcoma	Vascular tumors Diverse mesenchymal tumors (subset)
FOSB	Pseudomyogenic hemangioendothelioma	Epithelioid hemangioma (subset)
ROS1	Inflammatory myofibroblastic tumor (small subset)	Pulmonary adenocarcinoma (small subset)
STAT6	Solitary fibrous tumor	Dedifferentiated liposarcoma (subset)
TFE3	Alveolar soft part sarcoma	Xp11 translocation renal cell carcinoma PEComa (small subset) Epithelioid hemangioendothelioma (small subset)

Table 1.6 Novel Markers for Soft Tissue Tumors Discovered by Gene Expression Profiling

Marker	Tumor Types
DOG1 (ANO1)	Gastrointestinal stromal tumor
ETV4	*CIC-DUX4* sarcoma
MUC4	Low-grade fibromyxoid sarcoma Sclerosing epithelioid fibrosarcoma
NKX2-2	Ewing sarcoma
TLE1	Synovial sarcoma

ANO1, Anoctamin 1; *DOG1*, discovered on GIST-1; *MUC4*, Mucin 4; *TLE1*, transducin-like enhancer of split 1.

Novel Markers Discovered by Gene Expression Profiling

An emerging application of gene expression profiling is the identification of novel diagnostic markers for immunohistochemistry.[57-68] Several such markers are now used in clinical practice (Table 1.6). DOG1 (**d**iscovered **o**n **G**IST-1) is a highly sensitive and specific marker for GIST (see Chapter 16).[57-61] DOG1, also known as ANO1 (anoctamin 1), is a calcium-activated chloride channel expressed in the interstitial cells of Cajal, the pacemaker cells of the gastrointestinal tract. DOG1 is positive in nearly all KIT-positive GISTs as well as a subset of KIT-negative tumors (including many *PDGFRA*-mutant epithelioid GISTs)[60,61]; therefore DOG1 has become the preferred second-line marker to confirm the diagnosis of GIST. Transducin-like enhancer of split 1 (TLE1) is a transcriptional corepressor that inhibits Wnt signaling. Gene expression profiling studies have shown that high levels of TLE1 expression distinguish synovial sarcoma from other sarcoma types.[62] By immunohistochemistry, diffuse nuclear staining for TLE1 is a sensitive and moderately specific marker for synovial sarcoma (see Chapters 3, 8, and 9).[63-65] However, a subset of tumors in the differential diagnosis of synovial sarcoma (such as MPNST) show positive staining for TLE1, usually with only a weak staining pattern but sometimes more strongly.[63] MUC4 is a high-molecular-weight transmembrane glycoprotein expressed on the cell membrane of many epithelial cells. Recently high levels of MUC4 expression were found to discriminate low-grade fibromyxoid sarcoma from histologic mimics.[66] By immunohistochemistry, nearly all cases of low-grade fibromyxoid sarcoma show strong, diffuse staining for MUC4, whereas MUC4 is completely negative in spindle cell tumors that might be mistaken for this tumor type (e.g., soft tissue perineurioma, low-grade MPNST, myxofibrosarcoma, solitary fibrous tumor, and desmoid fibromatosis; see also Chapters 3 through 5).[67] Recent studies have indicated that some cases of sclerosing epithelioid fibrosarcoma are associated with a histologically distinct component of low-grade fibromyxoid sarcoma and show similar genetic findings (see Chapter 18).[67,68] Around 90% of sclerosing epithelioid fibrosarcomas are strongly positive for MUC4.[69] Before this observation, there were no helpful diagnostic markers for this tumor type. NKX2-2 is a transcription factor involved in neuronal development and glial and neuroendocrine differentiation; NKX2-2 is a downstream target of EWSR1-FLI1 oncogenic signaling in Ewing sarcoma.[70] By immunohistochemistry, nuclear staining for NKX2-2 is a highly sensitive and relatively specific marker for Ewing sarcoma (see Chapter 8); mesenchymal chondrosarcomas are also often positive.[71-73] It is likely that the diagnostic approach to soft tissue tumors will continue to evolve as additional useful markers are discovered using gene expression profiling.

References

1. Fisher C: The comparative roles of electron microscopy and immunohistochemistry in the diagnosis of soft tissue tumours, *Histopathology* 48:32–41, 2006.
2. Doyle LA, Hornick JL: Immunohistology of neoplasms of soft tissue and bone. In Dabbs DJ, editor: *Diagnostic immunohistochemistry: theranostic and genomic applications*, ed 4, Philadelphia, 2014, Saunders/Elsevier.
3. Fletcher CDM, Bridge JA, Hogendoorn PCW, et al, editors: *WHO classification of tumours of soft tissue and bone*, Lyon, France, 2013, IARC Press.
4. Miettinen M: Immunohistochemistry of soft tissue tumours—review with emphasis on 10 markers, *Histopathology* 64:101–118, 2014.
5. Hornick JL: Novel uses of immunohistochemistry in the diagnosis and classification of soft tissue tumors, *Mod Pathol* 27(Suppl 1):S47–S63, 2014.
6. Miettinen MM, Sarlomo-Rikala M, Kovatich AJ, et al: Calponin and h-caldesmon in soft tissue tumors: consistent h-caldesmon immunoreactivity in gastrointestinal stromal tumors indicates traits of smooth muscle differentiation, *Mod Pathol* 12:756–762, 1999.
7. Folpe AL: MyoD1 and myogenin expression in human neoplasia: a review and update, *Adv Anat Pathol* 9:198–203, 2002.
8. McKenney JK, Weiss SW, Folpe AL: CD31 expression in intratumoral macrophages: a potential diagnostic pitfall, *Am J Surg Pathol* 25:1167–1173, 2001.
9. Kahn HJ, Bailey D, Marks A: Monoclonal antibody D2-40, a new marker of lymphatic endothelium, reacts with Kaposi's sarcoma and a subset of angiosarcomas, *Mod Pathol* 15:434–440, 2002.
10. Ordonez NG: Podoplanin: a novel diagnostic immunohistochemical marker, *Adv Anat Pathol* 13:83–88, 2006.
11. Yu H, Gibson JA, Pinkus GS, et al: Podoplanin (D2-40) is a novel marker for follicular dendritic cell tumors, *Am J Clin Pathol* 128:776–782, 2007.
12. Folpe AL, Chand EM, Goldblum JR, et al: Expression of Fli-1, a nuclear transcription factor, distinguishes vascular neoplasms from potential mimics, *Am J Surg Pathol* 25:1061–1066, 2001.
13. Folpe AL, Hill CE, Parham DM, et al: Immunohistochemical detection of FLI-1 protein expression: a study of 132 round cell tumors with emphasis on CD99-positive mimics of Ewing's sarcoma/primitive neuroectodermal tumor, *Am J Surg Pathol* 24:1657–1662, 2000.
14. Rossi S, Orvieto E, Furlanetto A, et al: Utility of the immunohistochemical detection of FLI-1 expression in round cell and vascular neoplasm using a monoclonal antibody, *Mod Pathol* 17:547–552, 2004.
15. McKay KM, Doyle LA, Lazar AJ, et al: Expression of ERG, an ETS family transcription factor, distinguishes cutaneous angiosarcoma from histologic mimics, *Histopathology* 61:989–991, 2012.
16. Miettinen M, Wang ZF, Paetau A, et al: ERG transcription factor as an immunohistochemical marker for vascular endothelial tumors and prostatic carcinoma, *Am J Surg Pathol* 35:432–441, 2011.
17. Shah RB, Chinnaiyan AM: The discovery of common recurrent transmembrane protease serine 2 (TMPRSS2)-erythroblastosis virus E26 transforming sequence (ETS) gene fusions in prostate cancer: significance and clinical implications, *Adv Anat Pathol* 16:145–153, 2009.
18. Wang WL, Patel NR, Caragea M, et al: Expression of ERG, an ETS family transcription factor, identifies ERG-rearranged Ewing sarcoma, *Mod Pathol* 25:1378–1383, 2012.
19. Nonaka D, Chiriboga L, Rubin BP: Sox10: a pan-schwannian and melanocytic marker, *Am J Surg Pathol* 32:1291–1298, 2008.
20. Miettinen M, McCue PA, Sarlomo-Rikala M, et al: Sox10–a marker for not only schwannian and melanocytic neoplasms but also myoepithelial cell tumors of soft tissue: a systematic analysis of 5134 tumors, *Am J Surg Pathol* 39:826–835, 2015.
21. Specht K, Sung YS, Zhang L, et al: Distinct transcriptional signature and immunoprofile of CIC-DUX4 fusion-positive round cell tumors compared to EWSR1-rearranged Ewing sarcomas: further evidence toward distinct pathologic entities, *Genes Chromosomes Cancer* 53:622–633, 2014.
22. Montgomery E, Folpe AL: The diagnostic value of beta-catenin immunohistochemistry, *Adv Anat Pathol* 12:350–356, 2005.
23. Bhattacharya B, Dilworth HP, Iacobuzio-Donahue C, et al: Nuclear beta-catenin expression distinguishes deep fibromatosis from other benign and malignant fibroblastic and myofibroblastic lesions, *Am J Surg Pathol* 29:653–659, 2005.
24. Carlson JW, Fletcher CD: Immunohistochemistry for beta-catenin in the differential diagnosis of spindle cell lesions: analysis of a series and review of the literature, *Histopathology* 51:509–514, 2007.
25. Dei Tos AP, Doglioni C, Piccinin S, et al: Coordinated expression and amplification of the MDM2, CDK4, and HMGI-C genes in atypical lipomatous tumours, *J Pathol* 190:531–536, 2000.
26. Coindre JM, Pedeutour F, Aurias A: Well-differentiated and dedifferentiated liposarcomas, *Virchows Arch* 456:167–179, 2010.
27. Binh MB, Sastre-Garau X, Guillou L, et al: MDM2 and CDK4 immunostainings are useful adjuncts in diagnosing well-differentiated and dedifferentiated liposarcoma subtypes: a comparative analysis of 559 soft tissue neoplasms with genetic data, *Am J Surg Pathol* 29:1340–1347, 2005.
28. Wilson BG, Roberts CW: SWI/SNF nucleosome remodellers and cancer, *Nat Rev Cancer* 11:481–492, 2011.
29. Biegel JA, Zhou JY, Rorke LB, et al: Germ-line and acquired mutations of INI1 in atypical teratoid and rhabdoid tumors, *Cancer Res* 59:74–79, 1999.
30. Hoot AC, Russo P, Judkins AR, et al: Immunohistochemical analysis of hSNF5/INI1 distinguishes renal and extra-renal malignant rhabdoid tumors from other pediatric soft tissue tumors, *Am J Surg Pathol* 28:1485–1491, 2004.
31. Judkins AR: Immunohistochemistry of INI1 expression: a new tool for old challenges in CNS and soft tissue pathology, *Adv Anat Pathol* 14:335–339, 2007.
32. Hollmann TJ, Hornick JL: INI1-deficient tumors: diagnostic features and molecular genetics, *Am J Surg Pathol* 35:e47–e63, 2011.
33. Hornick JL, Dal Cin P, Fletcher CD: Loss of INI1 expression is characteristic of both conventional and proximal-type epithelioid sarcoma, *Am J Surg Pathol* 33:542–550, 2009.
34. Agaimy A: The expanding family of SMARCB1(INI1)-deficient neoplasia: implications of phenotypic, biological, and molecular heterogeneity, *Adv Anat Pathol* 21:394–410, 2014.
35. Gill AJ, Chou A, Vilain R, et al: Immunohistochemistry for SDHB divides gastrointestinal stromal tumors (GISTs) into 2 distinct types, *Am J Surg Pathol* 34:636–644, 2010.
36. Doyle LA, Nelson D, Heinrich MC, et al: Loss of succinate dehydrogenase subunit B (SDHB) expression is limited to a distinctive subset of gastric wild-type gastrointestinal stromal tumours: a comprehensive genotype-phenotype correlation study, *Histopathology* 61:801–809, 2012.
37. Miettinen M, Wang ZF, Sarlomo-Rikala M, et al: Succinate dehydrogenase-deficient GISTs: a clinicopathologic, immunohistochemical, and molecular genetic study of 66 gastric GISTs with predilection to young age, *Am J Surg Pathol* 35:1712–1721, 2011.
38. Wagner AJ, Remillard SP, Zhang YX, et al: Loss of expression of SDHA predicts SDHA mutations in gastrointestinal stromal tumors, *Mod Pathol* 26:289–294, 2013.
39. Miettinen M, Killian JK, Wang ZF, et al: Immunohistochemical loss of succinate dehydrogenase subunit A (SDHA) in gastrointestinal stromal tumors (GISTs) signals SDHA germline mutation, *Am J Surg Pathol* 37:234–240, 2013.
40. Schaefer IM, Fletcher CD, Hornick JL: Loss of H3K27 trimethylation distinguishes malignant peripheral nerve sheath tumors from histologic mimics, *Mod Pathol* 29:4–13, 2016.
41. Prieto-Granada CN, Wiesner T, Messina JL, et al: Loss of H3K27me3 expression is a highly sensitive marker for sporadic and radiation-induced MPNST, *Am J Surg Pathol* 40:479–489, 2016.
42. Argani P, Aulmann S, Illei PB, et al: A distinctive subset of PEComas harbors TFE3 gene fusions, *Am J Surg Pathol* 34:1395–1406, 2010.
43. Argani P, Lal P, Hutchinson B, et al: Aberrant nuclear immunoreactivity for TFE3 in neoplasms with TFE3 gene fusions: a sensitive and specific immunohistochemical assay, *Am J Surg Pathol* 27:750–761, 2003.
44. Antonescu CR, Le Loarer F, Mosquera JM, et al: Novel YAP1-TFE3 fusion defines a distinct subset of epithelioid hemangioendothelioma, *Genes Chromosomes Cancer* 52:775–784, 2013.
45. Cook JR, Dehner LP, Collins MH, et al: Anaplastic lymphoma kinase (ALK) expression in the inflammatory myofibroblastic tumor: a comparative immunohistochemical study, *Am J Surg Pathol* 25:1364–1371, 2001.
46. Coffin CM, Patel A, Perkins S, et al: ALK1 and p80 expression and chromosomal rearrangements involving 2p23 in inflammatory myofibroblastic tumor, *Mod Pathol* 14:569–576, 2001.
47. Corao DA, Biegel JA, Coffin CM, et al: ALK expression in rhabdomyosarcomas: correlation with histologic subtype and fusion status, *Pediatr Dev Pathol* 12:275–283, 2009.
48. Cessna MH, Zhou H, Sanger WG, et al: Expression of ALK1 and p80 in inflammatory myofibroblastic tumor and its mesenchymal mimics: a study of 135 cases, *Mod Pathol* 15:931–938, 2002.
49. Mariño-Enríquez A, Wang WL, Roy A, et al: Epithelioid inflammatory myofibroblastic sarcoma: An aggressive intra-abdominal variant of inflammatory myofibroblastic tumor with nuclear membrane or perinuclear ALK, *Am J Surg Pathol* 35:135–144, 2011.

50. Kao YC, Sung YS, Zhang L, et al: BCOR overexpression is a highly sensitive marker in round cell sarcomas with BCOR genetic abnormalities, *Am J Surg Pathol* 40:1670–1678, 2016.
51. Doyle LA, Fletcher CD, Hornick JL: Nuclear expression of CAMTA1 distinguishes epithelioid hemangioendothelioma from histologic mimics, *Am J Surg Pathol* 40:94–102, 2016.
52. Shibuya R, Matsuyama A, Shiba E, et al: CAMTA1 is a useful immunohistochemical marker for diagnosing epithelioid haemangioendothelioma, *Histopathology* 67:827–835, 2015.
53. Pierron G, Tirode F, Lucchesi C, et al: A new subtype of bone sarcoma defined by BCOR-CCNB3 gene fusion, *Nat Genet* 44:461–466, 2012.
54. Hung YP, Fletcher CD, Hornick JL: FOSB is a useful diagnostic marker for pseudomyogenic hemangioendothelioma, *Am J Surg Pathol* 41:596–606, 2017.
55. Hornick JL, Sholl LM, Dal Cin P, et al: Expression of ROS1 predicts ROS1 gene rearrangement in inflammatory myofibroblastic tumors, *Mod Pathol* 28:732–739, 2015.
56. Doyle LA, Vivero M, Fletcher CD, et al: Nuclear expression of STAT6 distinguishes solitary fibrous tumor from histologic mimics, *Mod Pathol* 27:390–395, 2014.
57. Espinosa I, Lee CH, Kim MK, et al: A novel monoclonal antibody against DOG1 is a sensitive and specific marker for gastrointestinal stromal tumors, *Am J Surg Pathol* 32:210–218, 2008.
58. West RB, Corless CL, Chen X, et al: The novel marker, DOG1, is expressed ubiquitously in gastrointestinal stromal tumors irrespective of KIT or PDGFRA mutation status, *Am J Pathol* 165:107–113, 2004.
59. Lee CH, Liang CW, Espinosa I: The utility of discovered on gastrointestinal stromal tumor 1 (DOG1) antibody in surgical pathology-the GIST of it, *Adv Anat Pathol* 17:222–232, 2010.
60. Miettinen M, Wang ZF, Lasota J: DOG1 antibody in the differential diagnosis of gastrointestinal stromal tumors: a study of 1840 cases, *Am J Surg Pathol* 33:1401–1408, 2009.
61. Liegl B, Hornick JL, Corless CL, et al: Monoclonal antibody DOG1.1 shows higher sensitivity than KIT in the diagnosis of gastrointestinal stromal tumors, including unusual subtypes, *Am J Surg Pathol* 33:437–446, 2009.
62. Terry J, Saito T, Subramanian S, et al: TLE1 as a diagnostic immunohistochemical marker for synovial sarcoma emerging from gene expression profiling studies, *Am J Surg Pathol* 31:240–246, 2007.
63. Foo WC, Cruise MW, Wick MR, et al: Immunohistochemical staining for TLE1 distinguishes synovial sarcoma from histologic mimics, *Am J Clin Pathol* 135:839–844, 2011.
64. Jagdis A, Rubin BP, Tubbs RR, et al: Prospective evaluation of TLE1 as a diagnostic immunohistochemical marker in synovial sarcoma, *Am J Surg Pathol* 33:1743–1751, 2009.
65. Knosel T, Heretsch S, Altendorf-Hofmann A, et al: TLE1 is a robust diagnostic biomarker for synovial sarcomas and correlates with t(X;18): analysis of 319 cases, *Eur J Cancer* 46:1170–1176, 2010.
66. Moller E, Hornick JL, Magnusson L, et al: FUS-CREB3L2/L1-positive sarcomas show a specific gene expression profile with upregulation of CD24 and FOXL1, *Clin Cancer Res* 17:2646–2656, 2011.
67. Doyle LA, Moller E, Dal Cin P, et al: MUC4 is a highly sensitive and specific marker for low-grade fibromyxoid sarcoma, *Am J Surg Pathol* 35:733–741, 2011.
68. Guillou L, Benhattar J, Gengler C, et al: Translocation-positive low-grade fibromyxoid sarcoma: clinicopathologic and molecular analysis of a series expanding the morphologic spectrum and suggesting potential relationship to sclerosing epithelioid fibrosarcoma: a study from the French Sarcoma Group, *Am J Surg Pathol* 31:1387–1402, 2007.
69. Doyle LA, Wang WL, Dal Cin P, et al: MUC4 is a sensitive and extremely useful marker for sclerosing epithelioid fibrosarcoma: association with FUS gene rearrangement, *Am J Surg Pathol* 36:1444–1451, 2012.
70. Smith R, Owen LA, Trem DJ, et al: Expression profiling of EWS/FLI identifies NKX2.2 as a critical target gene in Ewing's sarcoma, *Cancer Cell* 9:405–416, 2006.
71. Yoshida A, Sekine S, Tsuta K, et al: NKX2.2 is a useful immunohistochemical marker for Ewing sarcoma, *Am J Surg Pathol* 36:993–999, 2012.
72. Shibuya R, Matsuyama A, Nakamoto M, et al: The combination of CD99 and NKX2.2, a transcriptional target of EWSR1-FLI1, is highly specific for the diagnosis of Ewing sarcoma, *Virchows Arch* 465:599–605, 2014.
73. Hung YP, Fletcher CD, Hornick JL: Evaluation of NKX2-2 expression in round cell sarcomas and other tumors with EWSR1 rearrangement: imperfect specificity for Ewing sarcoma, *Mod Pathol* 29:370–380, 2016.

2

Biologic Potential, Grading, Staging, and Reporting of Sarcomas

Jason L. Hornick, MD, PhD

Biologic Potential

Among the most important reasons for the accurate classification of soft tissue tumors is the communication of clinical behavior (i.e., assignment into a managerial category). The vast majority of soft tissue tumors can be classified as either benign or malignant. Some benign tumors may occasionally recur, but they typically do so in a nondestructive fashion; simple surgical excision with narrow margins is generally adequate therapy for such tumors. By definition, a benign tumor should not metastasize. However, it is now recognized that in exceptional cases some examples of benign tumors may in fact metastasize (e.g., cutaneous benign fibrous histiocytoma),[1] although the incidence of such an event is likely much less than 1 in 10,000. In contrast, malignant mesenchymal neoplasms (i.e., sarcomas) have a significant potential for local recurrence (including destructive growth through normal tissues) as well as distant metastasis. The risk of metastasis varies widely among different types of sarcomas, sometimes determined by histologic grade (see later discussion).

There is a small group of soft tissue tumors that cannot easily be classified as either benign or malignant. Such tumors (with "intermediate" biologic potential) fall into two main categories: (1) those that exhibit locally aggressive behavior (Box 2.1) and (2) those that may rarely metastasize (Box 2.2).[2,3] Rare tumors fulfill both of these criteria. The prototypical example of a locally aggressive mesenchymal neoplasm is desmoid fibromatosis (see Chapters 3, 4, and 16). Although desmoid tumors do not metastasize, when they arise at particular anatomic sites (e.g., mesentery or neck), because of the proximity to vital structures, they may be associated with significant morbidity and may occasionally result in the patient's death. Several locally aggressive tumor types carry the name *sarcoma* despite the lack of significant metastatic potential. For example, in its conventional form, dermatofibrosarcoma protuberans (DFSP) does not metastasize, although local surgical control may occasionally be difficult. In contrast, the fibrosarcomatous variant of DFSP (representing a form of histologic progression) metastasizes in 10% to 15% of cases (see Chapter 15).[4,5] Most of the tumors that fall into the "rarely metastasizing" category are very uncommon. Although drawing the line between this "intermediate" category and bona fide sarcomas may be somewhat arbitrary, a 2% metastatic risk has been used as a cutoff point.[2,3] For the tumors in these unusual categories, good communication between the pathologist and the treating physicians is critical to convey the clinical significance of the diagnosis, particularly for rare tumor types that are unfamiliar to many clinicians. The remainder of this chapter is devoted to sarcomas.

Sarcoma Grading

In combination with histologic diagnosis, grade is currently the best and most widely used predictor of outcome for the majority of soft tissue sarcomas.[6,7] Grading has relatively limited impact on the rates of local recurrence, although the distinction between low-grade and high-grade sarcomas may influence clinical decision making in terms of primary tumor treatment, especially the administration of radiation therapy, which is often reserved for high-grade sarcomas.[8] In contrast, the primary value of sarcoma grading lies in the prediction of distant metastasis, which (particularly for tumors of the extremities and trunk) is the main determinant of mortality.[6] However, there exists a group of soft tissue sarcomas (many of which harbor translocations) for which grading has generally been thought to have limited (or no) value beyond histologic typing (Boxes 2.3 and 2.4).[7] Several of these sarcoma types have a low rate of metastasis in the first 5 years following surgical excision of the primary tumor but increasing rates of metastasis with long-term follow-up (by 10 or 20 years, in many instances attaining metastatic rates similar to those of high-grade sarcomas). For other sarcoma types (such as dedifferentiated liposarcoma), the metastatic potential is relatively low (15% to 20%). Although conventional wisdom has been that histologic features do not affect outcome for dedifferentiated liposarcoma, recent studies suggest that histologic grade and the presence of heterologous rhabdomyoblastic differentiation predict metastasis and overall survival for this sarcoma type.[9-11] Whether histologic grading is of prognostic significance for malignant peripheral nerve sheath tumors has been a matter of some debate; recent data suggest that assigning French Fédération Nationale des Centres de Lutte Contre le Cancer (FNCLCC) grade is of value for predicting metastasis.[12] Yet other sarcoma types are high grade by definition, with a high risk of distant metastasis, often requiring specific chemotherapeutic protocols.

Box 2.1 Soft Tissue Tumors of Intermediate Biologic Potential, Locally Aggressive

Desmoid fibromatosis
Atypical lipomatous tumor/well-differentiated liposarcoma
Dermatofibrosarcoma protuberans
Myxoinflammatory fibroblastic sarcoma
Tenosynovial giant cell tumor, diffuse type
Kaposiform hemangioendothelioma
Retiform hemangioendothelioma
Composite hemangioendothelioma

Box 2.2 Soft Tissue Tumors of Intermediate Biologic Potential, Rarely Metastasizing

Inflammatory myofibroblastic tumor
Infantile fibrosarcoma
Myxoinflammatory fibroblastic sarcoma
Plexiform fibrohistiocytic tumor
Angiomatoid fibrous histiocytoma
Pseudomyogenic hemangioendothelioma

Box 2.3 Soft Tissue Sarcomas for Which Grading Is of No (or Limited) Value

Alveolar soft part sarcoma
Clear cell sarcoma
Epithelioid sarcoma
Extraskeletal myxoid chondrosarcoma
Low-grade fibromyxoid sarcoma
Sclerosing epithelioid fibrosarcoma

Box 2.4 Soft Tissue Sarcomas That Are High Grade by Definition

Alveolar rhabdomyosarcoma
Angiosarcoma
BCOR-CCNB3 sarcoma
CIC-DUX4 sarcoma
Embryonal rhabdomyosarcoma
Ewing sarcoma
Malignant rhabdoid tumor

For many sarcoma types, the most important parameters for the prediction of metastasis are mitotic activity and necrosis. However, before evaluating these features, a histologic diagnosis should be made. Determination of the mitotic rate without regard to diagnosis can sometimes lead to major diagnostic errors. For example, nodular fasciitis (a benign lesion that often regresses spontaneously) may contain numerous mitotic figures that could lead to an erroneous diagnosis of a high-grade sarcoma. Some other benign mesenchymal tumors (e.g., cellular benign fibrous histiocytoma of the skin) may contain focal necrosis, which is of no clinical consequence. From these examples, it is clear that grading should not be performed before attempting to assign a specific histologic diagnosis, or at least a confident diagnosis of sarcoma, even if the precise classification is uncertain.

PRACTICE POINTS: Mitotic Activity

A diagnosis should be made before the mitotic rate is determined
Benign lesions (such as nodular fasciitis) may have an alarmingly high mitotic rate
Accurate mitotic counting requires well-fixed tissue
The most mitotic area should be identified before beginning to count
Mitotic count should be determined in 10 contiguous high-power fields
Areas of necrosis should be avoided
If the mitotic count is close to the cutoffs between mitotic scores (Table 2.1), the mitotic count should be repeated

Table 2.1 French (Fédération Nationale Des Centres De Lutte Contre Le Cancer) Grading System

Tumor Differentiation	
Score 1	Sarcomas that closely resemble normal adult mesenchymal tissues (e.g., well-differentiated leiomyosarcoma)
Score 2	Sarcomas for which histologic typing is certain
Score 3	Embryonal and undifferentiated sarcomas, synovial sarcoma, and sarcomas of uncertain differentiation
Mitotic Count	
Score 1	0–9 mitoses per 10 HPF
Score 2	10–19 mitoses per 10 HPF
Score 3	≥20 mitoses per 10 HPF
Tumor Necrosis	
Score 0	No necrosis
Score 1	<50% tumor necrosis
Score 2	≥50% tumor necrosis
Histologic Grade (Tumor Differentiation + Mitotic Count + Tumor Necrosis)	
Grade 1 (low grade)	Total score: 2 or 3
Grade 2 (intermediate grade)	Total score: 4 or 5
Grade 3 (high grade)	Total score: 6, 7, or 8

HPF, High-power field.
Modified from Trojani M, Contesso G, Coindre JM, et al: Soft-tissue sarcomas of adults: study of pathological prognostic variables and definition of a histopathological grading system. *Int J Cancer* 33:3742, 1984.

Several different grading systems have been developed. The two most widely used are the US National Cancer Institute (NCI) and the FNCLCC systems, both of which assign sarcomas into three tiers and have demonstrated prognostic value.[13-15] However, the FNCLCC system is more precisely defined and more reproducible.[16] Furthermore, in a large comparative follow-up study, the FNCLCC system has been shown to predict outcome better (with fewer tumors relegated to the intermediate category) than the NCI system.[17] Therefore the FNCLCC system has been recommended by the American Joint Committee on Cancer (AJCC) and the College of American Pathologists (CAP).[18,19] Therefore the FNCLCC grading system is described in this section.

The FNCLCC grading system requires the evaluation of three parameters: tumor differentiation, mitotic count, and tumor necrosis (see Table 2.1).[6,14] Tumor differentiation is the most difficult parameter to apply. In fact, this parameter is a combination of "true" differentiation (i.e., the extent to which tumor cells resemble normal mesenchymal cells) and histologic diagnosis or type. Tumor differentiation scores often cannot be assigned without reference to the specific guidelines of the FNCLCC system (i.e., lists of tumors and corresponding differentiation scores). Some of the tumor differentiation scores according to histologic diagnosis are listed in Table 2.2.[17] This table does not include all the histologic types formally included in the FNCLCC system; some of those tumor types that are high grade by definition, as well as the tumor types for which grading is generally not applied, have been omitted from the table. Mitotic activity is determined by counting mitotic figures in 10 contiguous high-power fields in the most mitotic area. Foci of necrosis should be avoided. If the mitotic count is close to the cutoffs between mitotic scores, the counting of mitoses should be repeated; this parameter is particularly susceptible to interobserver variability and not uncommonly results in changes in grading assignment between pathologists. Tumor necrosis is often assessed on gross examination but must be confirmed histologically; a reasonable guideline is to submit one section from an area of necrotic tumor for confirmation. Hyalinization and hemorrhage should not be included in the assessment of tumor necrosis.[6]

As is evident from this discussion, accurate histologic diagnosis is of fundamental importance in predicting outcome for soft tissue sarcomas. Although it is not practical to develop a separate grading system for each sarcoma type, there are several notable sarcoma types for which particular histologic features (beyond those used in the FNCLCC system) are typically applied for grading. For example, myxoid liposarcoma is graded based on the extent of hypercellular areas, often (although not invariably) accompanied by a transition from spindled to round cell cytomorphology (Fig. 2.1) (see Chapters 5 and 12).[20,21] High-grade ("round cell") myxoid liposarcoma sometimes shows a low mitotic rate and may have limited, if any, necrosis. Similarly, myxofibrosarcoma is typically graded by the extent of myxoid stroma and the presence of cellular areas (see Chapters 5 and 7).[22] Low-grade myxofibrosarcoma shows a hypocellular appearance dominated by myxoid stroma, whereas, in contrast, high-grade myxofibrosarcoma contains hypercellular areas devoid of myxoid matrix (Fig. 2.2). Such areas are indistinguishable from undifferentiated pleomorphic sarcomas.

Table 2.2 Differentiation Scores for Selected Sarcoma Types

Tumor Type	Differentiation Score
Well-differentiated leiomyosarcoma	1
Myxoid liposarcoma	2
Conventional leiomyosarcoma	2
Conventional malignant peripheral nerve sheath tumor	2
Myxofibrosarcoma	2
High-grade myxoid ("round cell") liposarcoma	3
Dedifferentiated liposarcoma	3
Pleomorphic liposarcoma	3
Pleomorphic leiomyosarcoma	3
Synovial sarcoma	3
Malignant peripheral nerve sheath tumor with heterologous rhabdomyoblastic differentiation (malignant Triton tumor)	3
Extraskeletal osteosarcoma	3
Mesenchymal chondrosarcoma	3
Undifferentiated pleomorphic (or spindle cell) sarcoma	3

Modified from Fletcher CDM, Bridge JA, Hogendoorn PCW, et al, eds: *WHO classification of tumours of soft tissue and bone*. Lyon, France, 2013, IARC Press.

Although a 5-year interval from diagnosis to metastasis or survival is often used as a point of comparison in oncology, the natural history of some sarcoma types defies this standard approach. Some such tumors have a low rate of metastasis at 5 years, but metastases continue to develop decades following first diagnosis. Several of the translocation-associated sarcomas for which FNCLCC grading is generally not clinically useful belong to this group (see Box 2.3). A notable example is low-grade fibromyxoid sarcoma (see Chapters 3 and 5). This tumor type shows deceptively bland cytomorphology (mimicking a benign neoplasm) and is invariably low grade based on the FNCLCC system. The 5-year metastatic rate is very low, as might be expected for a low-grade sarcoma. However, with long-term follow-up, many patients (up to 40%) eventually develop pulmonary and pleural metastases, often decades following initial diagnosis (Fig. 2.3).[23]

Sarcoma grading systems were developed based on the evaluation of surgically excised tumors. Incisional biopsy specimens are often sufficiently representative of the tumor as a whole to allow for accurate grading. However, increasingly, core needle biopsy (or even fine needle aspiration) is being used to establish a diagnosis.[24-27] As every surgical pathologist is well aware, it is sometimes not possible to make a firm diagnosis of sarcoma on the basis of limited biopsy material, let alone subclassify sarcomas with certainty. Furthermore, such limited sampling, not surprisingly, may significantly underestimate grade, because many (particularly high-grade) sarcomas show some degree of intratumoral heterogeneity, and mitotic activity may appear deceptively low in a small sample from a tumor. In this setting, some investigators have suggested that the Ki-67 proliferation index (by immunohistochemistry) might be used instead of (or in addition to) mitotic rate in limited biopsies; however, this practice has not been widely adopted.[28] The editor of this book does not use Ki-67 immunohistochemistry for the

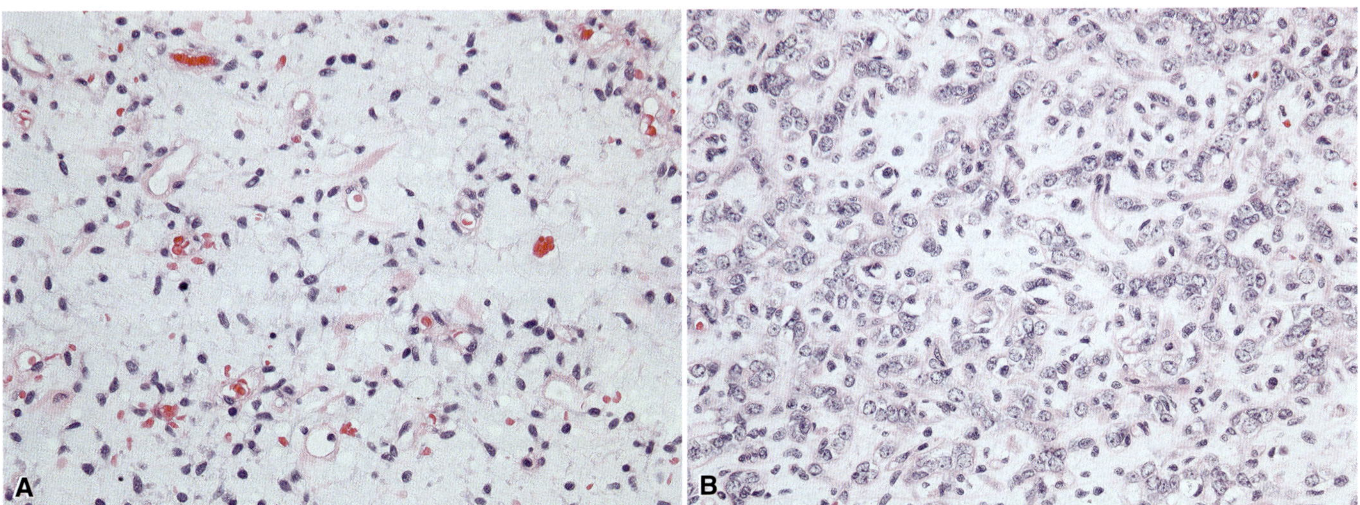

Figure 2.1 Myxoid Liposarcoma. A, Low-grade myxoid liposarcoma composed of bland, uniform short spindle cells in abundant myxoid stroma. **B,** High-grade myxoid liposarcoma usually shows less abundant myxoid stroma and often acquires round cell morphology ("round cell liposarcoma"), sometimes without a high mitotic rate.

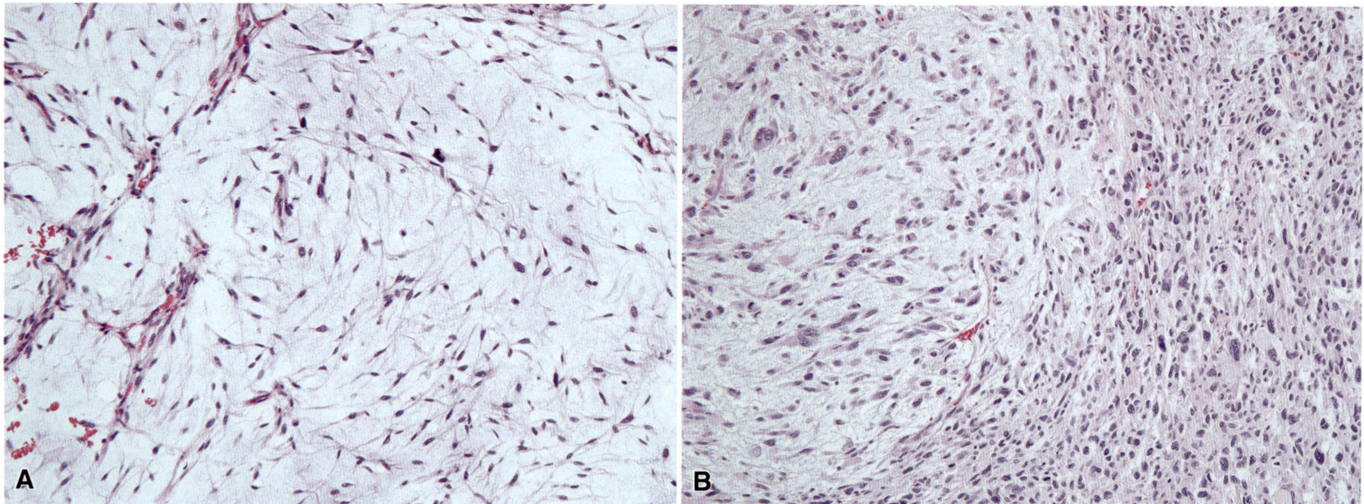

Figure 2.2 Myxofibrosarcoma. **A,** Low-grade myxofibrosarcoma with abundant myxoid stroma and characteristic curvilinear blood vessels. **B,** High-grade myxofibrosarcoma containing highly cellular areas with minimal stroma *(right side)*, indistinguishable from undifferentiated pleomorphic sarcoma.

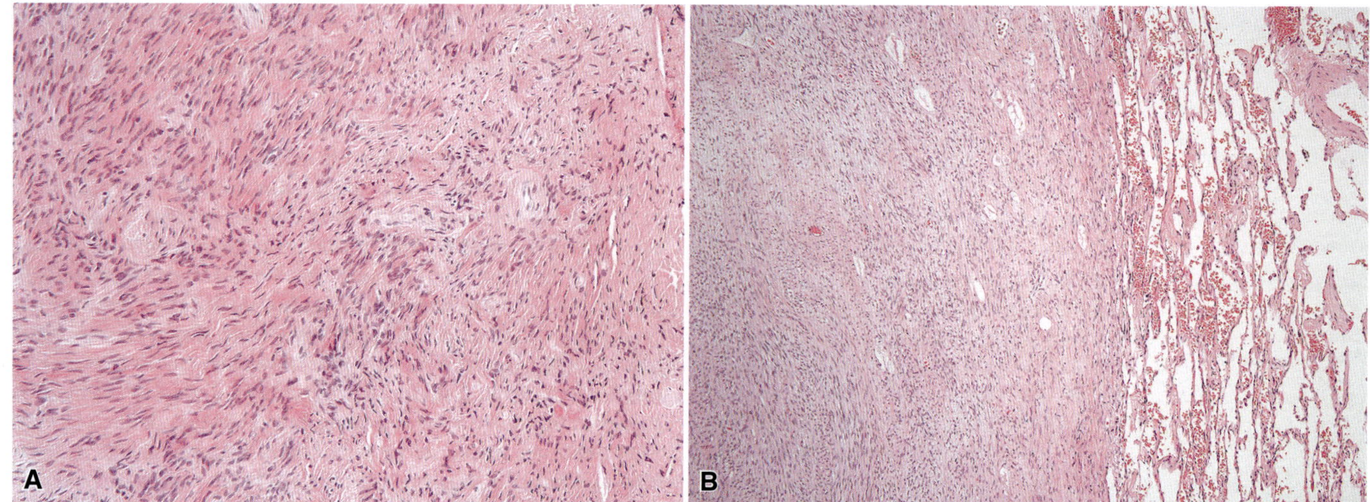

Figure 2.3 Low-Grade Fibromyxoid Sarcoma. **A,** A whorled growth pattern, prominent stromal collagen, and bland spindle cell morphology are characteristic features. This tumor type may easily be mistaken for a benign lesion. **B,** This tumor metastasized to the lung 30 years after initial clinical presentation. Such a natural history is typical of this sarcoma type, despite its low-grade designation.

diagnosis or grading of soft tissue tumors. It is also reasonable to use radiologic imaging to estimate the extent (or at least the presence) of necrosis so as not to give the erroneous impression that a sarcoma is low grade.[6] This is especially important in institutions where preoperative (neoadjuvant) radiation therapy is reserved for high-grade sarcomas. Along these lines, grading of resected sarcomas following neoadjuvant therapy should be discouraged (and is not endorsed by the FNCLCC system), because treatment-related necrosis cannot be distinguished from spontaneous tumor necrosis, and proliferation rate can be affected by prior therapy; however, if the sarcoma is clearly high grade based on a pretreatment biopsy or histologic type, there is no harm in including the high-grade designation in the surgical pathology report of the resected sarcoma.

A molecular grading system has been developed based on gene expression profiling, including a gene set related in large part to genome complexity (Complexity Index in Sarcomas; CINSARC).[29] This gene expression signature has been shown to outperform histologic grade in predicting metastasis for soft tissue sarcomas.[29] The same signature was able to predict outcome for gastrointestinal stromal tumor (GIST), lymphomas, and breast carcinoma. A genomic complexity index based on comparative genomic hybridization has also been demonstrated to predict outcome for patients with GIST better than conventional risk stratification parameters.[30] These techniques are not yet widely used in clinical practice but they illustrate the promise of integrating genomic methodologies into conventional parameters for prognostication.

Sarcoma Staging

As is the case for carcinomas, soft tissue sarcomas may be staged using the tumor-node-metastasis (TNM) system, according to criteria established by the International Union Against Cancer (International Union for Cancer Control; IUCC) and the AJCC (Table 2.3).[18] With several notable exceptions (e.g., alveolar rhabdomyosarcoma, epithelioid sarcoma, and clear cell sarcoma), soft tissue sarcomas only rarely metastasize to lymph nodes, and the N (regional lymph nodes)

Table 2.3 American Joint Committee on Cancer Tumor-Node-Metastasis Classification of Soft Tissue Sarcomas of the Trunk and Extremities and Retroperitoneum

Definition of Primary Tumor (T)	
T Category	**T Criteria**
TX	Primary tumor cannot be assessed
T0	No evidence of primary tumor
T1	Tumor 5 cm or less in greatest dimension
T2	Tumor more than 5 cm and less than or equal to 10 cm in greatest dimension
T3	Tumor more than 10 cm and less than or equal to 15 cm in greatest dimension
T4	Tumor more than 15 cm in greatest dimension
Definition of Regional Lymph Node (N)	
N Category	**N Criteria**
N0	No regional lymph node metastasis or unknown lymph node status
N1	Regional lymph node metastasis
Definition of Distant Metastasis (M)	
M Category	**M Criteria**
M0	No distant metastasis
M1	Distant metastasis
Definition of Grade (G)	
FNCLCC Histologic Grade – see Histologic Grade (G)	
G	**G Definition**
GX	Grade cannot be assessed
G1	Total differentiation, mitotic count and necrosis score of 2 or 3
G2	Total differentiation, mitotic count and necrosis score of 4 or 5
G3	Total differentiation, mitotic count and necrosis score of 6, 7, or 8

From Amin MB, Edge S, Greene F, et al, eds: *AJCC cancer staging manual*, ed 8, New York, 2017, Springer.

Table 2.4 American Joint Committee on Cancer Prognostic Stage Groups for Soft Tissue Sarcomas of the Trunk and Extremities and Retroperitoneum

When T Is...	And N Is...	And M Is...	And Grade Is...	Then the Stage Group Is...
T1	N0	M0	G1, GX	IA
T2, T3, T4	N0	M0	G1, GX	IB
T1	N0	M0	G2, G3	II
T2	N0	M0	G2, G3	IIIA
T3, T4	N0	M0	G2, G3	IIIB
Any T	N1	M0	Any G	IV
Any T	Any N	M1	Any G	IV

From Amin MB, Edge S, Greene F, et al, eds: *AJCC cancer staging manual*, ed 8, New York, 2017, Springer.

designation is therefore rarely relevant. Of note, because the prognostic significance of lymph node and distant metastasis for soft tissue sarcomas is similar, either pathologic N1 or M1 status is categorized as stage IV disease in the eighth edition of the AJCC staging system (Table 2.4).[18] There have been other significant changes from the seventh edition to the eighth edition of the AJCC system. Most notably, the soft tissue sarcoma section has been divided into separate chapters for extremities and trunk, retroperitoneum, head and neck, abdominal and thoracic visceral organs, and "unusual histologies and sites"; in addition, GIST is now included within the soft tissue sarcoma section.[18] The T (primary tumor) categories for extremities and trunk and retroperitoneum are identical (see Table 2.3), whereas the T categories for head and neck, abdominal and thoracic visceral organs, and GIST are distinct. Because sarcomas of the head and neck are usually smaller than those arising at other anatomic sites (with disproportionately high rates of local recurrence), the size cutoffs among T categories for sarcomas at these locations are smaller than for other anatomic sites.[18] Furthermore, depth has been eliminated as a contributor to the T categories in the eighth edition of the AJCC system, following large cohort studies that failed to show a prognostic significance of tumor depth.[18] Finally, a prognostic nomogram (risk-assessment model) has now been included specifically for retroperitoneal sarcomas, based on data sets from several large sarcoma centers and validated by an additional large multiinstitutional study.[31,32] This nomogram includes the following factors: patient age, tumor size, FNCLCC grade, histologic type, multifocality, and extent of resection.[31,32] Unlike AJCC staging for most tumor types, the anatomic staging for soft tissue sarcomas includes not only TNM information but also histologic grade (see Table 2.4).[18] These staging systems have prognostic value for soft tissue sarcomas as a whole, although for some sarcoma types, stage has limited additional predictive value for survival beyond histologic diagnosis.

As discussed in Chapter 16, assessment of risk for progressive disease in GISTs includes mitotic rate, tumor size, and primary anatomic site. This system was established by Miettinen and Lasota.[33] The AJCC has adopted similar categories for a TNM system.[18] Of note, this risk stratification system does not apply to succinate dehydrogenase-deficient GISTs.[34] As mentioned for retroperitoneal sarcomas, nomograms incorporating both pathologic (histologic type, grade, and tumor size) and clinical parameters (age, depth, and anatomic site) have been developed in an attempt to improve prognostication in sarcomas.[35-38] Histologic tumor type–specific nomograms have also been constructed for GISTs, liposarcomas, and synovial sarcoma.[21,39-41] Such systems give varying weights to these various pathologic and clinical parameters and calculate the probability for a given patient dying from sarcoma. These nomograms have been validated using large patient cohorts. However, such nomograms have been generated based on the more common sarcoma types; their utility for rare tumor types is difficult to establish.

Surgical Margins

As discussed earlier in this chapter, the main prognostic value of grading is the prediction of distant metastasis. In contrast, the most important predictor of local recurrence is the status of surgical excision margins.[42,43] Therefore detailed reporting of surgical margins is a critical role of the pathologist. A "marginal" excision is defined as removal of the tumor and its pseudocapsule with minimal (or no) surrounding normal tissue (in such cases, the tumor is often referred to as having been "shelled out"). The margins in such cases often histologically show fibrotic tissue. Marginal excision is assumed to leave microscopic tumor behind and is associated with a significant risk of local recurrence.[43] In contrast, a "wide" excision is defined as removal of the tumor with adjacent normal (healthy) tissue surrounding the tumor. With such "negative" margins, the risk of local recurrence decreases dramatically. "Radical" resection refers to the removal of the tumor and the entire anatomic compartment in which it is located (e.g., the surrounding muscle groups and adjacent fascial planes). As a reasonable guideline, 2 cm is generally considered the optimal distance for negative margins, although anatomic constraints often require narrower margins.[19] The margins should be submitted as perpendicular sections when possible. When the tumor is confined by (and does not invade) a fascial plane, so long as the fascia is resected along with the tumor, such a margin is regarded as oncologically adequate, even when the margins are relatively narrow (in some circumstances, the decision to administer radiation therapy will in part be determined by the presence of intact fascia at close margins). For margins less than 2 cm, the precise distances to the margins should be reported (and whether close margins are bounded by fascia).

PRACTICE POINTS: Surgical Margins

Margins should be taken as perpendicular sections
Precise distances should be reported for margins less than 2 cm
The presence of an intact fascial plane should also be reported for margins less than 2 cm

References

1. Doyle LA, Fletcher CD: Metastasizing "benign" fibrous histiocytoma: a clinicopathologic analysis of 16 cases, *Am J Surg Pathol* 37:484–495, 2013.
2. Fletcher CDM, Bridge JA, Hogendoorn PCW, et al, editors: *WHO classification of tumours of soft tissue and bone*, Lyon, France, 2013, IARC Press.
3. Fletcher CD: The evolving classification of soft tissue tumours: an update based on the new WHO classification, *Histopathology* 48:3–12, 2006.
4. Abbott JJ, Oliveira AM, Nascimento AG: The prognostic significance of fibrosarcomatous transformation in dermatofibrosarcoma protuberans, *Am J Surg Pathol* 30:436–443, 2006.
5. Mentzel T, Beham A, Katenkamp D, et al: Fibrosarcomatous ("high-grade") dermatofibrosarcoma protuberans: clinicopathologic and immunohistochemical study of a series of 41 cases with emphasis on prognostic significance, *Am J Surg Pathol* 22:576–587, 1998.
6. Coindre JM: Grading of soft tissue sarcomas: review and update, *Arch Pathol Lab Med* 130:1448–1453, 2006.
7. Deyrup AT, Weiss SW: Grading of soft tissue sarcomas: the challenge of providing precise information in an imprecise world, *Histopathology* 48:42–50, 2006.
8. Baldini EH, Goldberg J, Jenner C, et al: Long-term outcomes after function-sparing surgery without radiotherapy for soft tissue sarcoma of the extremities and trunk, *J Clin Oncol* 17:3252–3259, 1999.
9. Mussi C, Collini P, Miceli R, et al: The prognostic impact of dedifferentiation in retroperitoneal liposarcoma. A series of surgically treated patients at a single institution, *Cancer* 113:1657–1665, 2008.
10. Keung EZ, Hornick JL, Bertagnolli MM, et al: Predictors of outcomes in patients with primary retroperitoneal dedifferentiated liposarcoma undergoing surgery, *J Am Coll Surg* 218:206–217, 2014.
11. Gronchi A, Collini P, Miceli R, et al: Myogenic differentiation and histologic grading are major prognostic determinants in retroperitoneal liposarcoma, *Am J Surg Pathol* 39:383–393, 2015.
12. Le Guellec S, Decouvelaere AV, Filleron T, et al: Malignant peripheral nerve sheath tumor is a challenging diagnosis: a systematic pathology review, immunohistochemistry, and molecular analysis in 160 patients from the French Sarcoma Group database, *Am J Surg Pathol* 40:896–908, 2016.
13. Costa J, Wesley RA, Glatstein E, et al: The grading of soft tissue sarcomas. Results of a clinicohistopathologic correlation in a series of 163 cases, *Cancer* 53:530–541, 1984.
14. Trojani M, Contesso G, Coindre JM, et al: Soft-tissue sarcomas of adults; study of pathological prognostic variables and definition of a histopathological grading system, *Int J Cancer* 33:37–42, 1984.
15. Coindre JM, Terrier P, Guillou L, et al: Predictive value of grade for metastasis development in the main histologic types of adult soft tissue sarcomas: a study of 1240 patients from the French Federation of Cancer Centers Sarcoma Group, *Cancer* 91:1914–1926, 2001.
16. Coindre JM, Trojani M, Contesso G, et al: Reproducibility of a histopathologic grading system for adult soft tissue sarcoma, *Cancer* 58:306–309, 1986.
17. Guillou L, Coindre JM, Bonichon F, et al: Comparative study of the National Cancer Institute and French Federation of Cancer Centers Sarcoma Group grading systems in a population of 410 adult patients with soft tissue sarcoma, *J Clin Oncol* 15:350–362, 1997.
18. Amin MB, Edge S, Greene F, et al, editors: *AJCC cancer staging manual*, ed 8, New York, 2017, Springer.
19. Rubin BP, Cooper K, Fletcher CD, et al: Protocol for the examination of specimens from patients with tumors of soft tissue, *Arch Pathol Lab Med* 134:e31–e39, 2010.
20. Antonescu CR, Tschernyavsky SJ, Decuseara R, et al: Prognostic impact of p53 status, TLS-CHOP fusion transcript structure, and histological grade in myxoid liposarcoma: a molecular and clinicopathologic study of 82 cases, *Clin Cancer Res* 7:3977–3987, 2001.
21. Dalal KM, Kattan MW, Antonescu CR, et al: Subtype specific prognostic nomogram for patients with primary liposarcoma of the retroperitoneum, extremity, or trunk, *Ann Surg* 244:381–391, 2006.
22. Mentzel T, Calonje E, Wadden C, et al: Myxofibrosarcoma. Clinicopathologic analysis of 75 cases with emphasis on the low-grade variant, *Am J Surg Pathol* 20:391–405, 1996.
23. Evans HL: Low-grade fibromyxoid sarcoma: a clinicopathologic study of 33 cases with long-term follow-up, *Am J Surg Pathol* 35:1450–1462, 2011.
24. Heslin MJ, Lewis JJ, Woodruff JM, et al: Core needle biopsy for diagnosis of extremity soft tissue sarcoma, *Ann Surg Oncol* 4:425–431, 1997.
25. Hoeber I, Spillane AJ, Fisher C, et al: Accuracy of biopsy techniques for limb and limb girdle soft tissue tumors, *Ann Surg Oncol* 8:80–87, 2001.
26. Welker JA, Henshaw RM, Jelinek J, et al: The percutaneous needle biopsy is safe and recommended in the diagnosis of musculoskeletal masses, *Cancer* 89:2677–2686, 2000.
27. Jones C, Liu K, Hirschowitz S, et al: Concordance of histopathologic and cytologic grading in musculoskeletal sarcomas: can grades obtained from analysis of the fine-needle aspirates serve as the basis for therapeutic decisions? *Cancer* 96:83–91, 2002.
28. Hasegawa T, Yamamoto S, Yokoyama R, et al: Prognostic significance of grading and staging systems using MIB-1 score in adult patients with soft tissue sarcoma of the extremities and trunk, *Cancer* 95:843–851, 2002.
29. Chibon F, Lagarde P, Salas S, et al: Validated prediction of clinical outcome in sarcomas and multiple types of cancer on the basis of a gene expression signature related to genome complexity, *Nat Med* 16:781–787, 2010.
30. Lagarde P, Perot G, Kauffmann A, et al: Mitotic checkpoints and chromosome instability are strong predictors of clinical outcome in gastrointestinal stromal tumors, *Clin Cancer Res* 18:826–838, 2012.
31. Gronchi A, Miceli R, Shurell E, et al: Outcome prediction in primary resected retroperitoneal soft tissue sarcoma: histology-specific overall survival and disease-free survival nomograms built on major sarcoma center data sets, *J Clin Oncol* 31:1649–1655, 2013.
32. Raut CP, Miceli R, Strauss DC, et al: External validation of a multi-institutional retroperitoneal sarcoma nomogram, *Cancer* 122:1417–1424, 2016.
33. Miettinen M, Lasota J: Gastrointestinal stromal tumors: pathology and prognosis at different sites, *Semin Diagn Pathol* 23:70–83, 2006.
34. Mason EF, Hornick JL: Conventional risk stratification fails to predict progression of succinate dehydrogenase-deficient gastrointestinal stromal tumors: a clinicopathologic study of 76 cases, *Am J Surg Pathol* 40:1616–1621, 2016.
35. Eilber FC, Brennan MF, Eilber FR, et al: Validation of the postoperative nomogram for 12-year sarcoma-specific mortality, *Cancer* 101:2270–2275, 2004.
36. Kattan MW, Leung DH, Brennan MF: Postoperative nomogram for 12-year sarcoma-specific death, *J Clin Oncol* 20:791–796, 2002.
37. Mariani L, Miceli R, Kattan MW, et al: Validation and adaptation of a nomogram for predicting the survival of patients with extremity soft tissue sarcoma using a three-grade system, *Cancer* 103:402–408, 2005.
38. Ardoino I, Miceli R, Berselli M, et al: Histology-specific nomogram for primary retroperitoneal soft tissue sarcoma, *Cancer* 116:2429–2436, 2010.
39. Gold JS, Gonen M, Gutierrez A, et al: Development and validation of a prognostic nomogram for recurrence-free survival after complete surgical resection of localised primary gastrointestinal stromal tumour: a retrospective analysis, *Lancet Oncol* 10:1045–1052, 2009.
40. Rossi S, Miceli R, Messerini L, et al: Natural history of imatinib-naive GISTs: a retrospective analysis of 929 cases with long-term follow-up and development of a survival nomogram based on mitotic index and size as continuous variables, *Am J Surg Pathol* 35:1646–1656, 2011.
41. Canter RJ, Qin LX, Maki RG, et al: A synovial sarcoma-specific preoperative nomogram supports a survival benefit to ifosfamide-based chemotherapy and improves risk stratification for patients, *Clin Cancer Res* 14:8191–8197, 2008.
42. Collin C, Hajdu SI, Godbold J, et al: Localized operable soft tissue sarcoma of the upper extremity. Presentation, management, and factors affecting local recurrence in 108 patients, *Ann Surg* 205:331–339, 1987.
43. Gronchi A, Lo Vullo S, Colombo C, et al: Extremity soft tissue sarcoma in a series of patients treated at a single institution: local control directly impacts survival, *Ann Surg* 251:506–511, 2010.

3

Spindle Cell Tumors of Adults

Adrián Mariño-Enríquez, MD, PhD, and Jason L. Hornick, MD, PhD

Numerous primary tumors and pseudotumors of soft tissues contain a variable number of spindle cells. In this chapter the authors will discuss only those lesions composed exclusively or predominantly of spindle cells that develop in adult patients and for which the spindle cell component is a key diagnostic feature. Some spindle cell tumors are discussed elsewhere in this book (Table 3.1), if their clinical presentation is restricted to a particular anatomic area with a dedicated chapter (e.g., skin, gastrointestinal tract, or lower genital tract) or if they are better characterized by a prominent histologic feature other than their spindle cell morphology (e.g., myxoid stroma; prominent inflammation; biphasic or mixed appearance; or an adipocytic, vascular, or chondro-osseous line of differentiation). In addition, spindle cell tumors that arise exclusively or substantially more frequently in children are described in Chapter 4.

General Concepts

Approach to the Diagnosis of Spindle Cell Tumors of Soft Tissue

Spindle cell tumors of soft tissue are often a source of diagnostic problems for surgical pathologists. The most common issues include (1) distinguishing a nonmesenchymal malignant spindle cell neoplasm (e.g., spindle

Table 3.1 Spindle Cell Tumors Primarily Covered in Other Chapters

Tumor Type	Chapters Where Discussed
Angiomyofibroblastoma	17
Angiosarcoma, spindle cell type	13
Atypical fibroxanthoma, spindle cell type	15
Benign fibrous histiocytoma and variants	15
Calcifying aponeurotic fibroma	4
Cellular angiofibroma	17
Cranial fasciitis	4
Deep ("aggressive") angiomyxoma	5 and 17
Dendritic cell neurofibroma	15
Dermal nerve sheath myxoma	5 and 15
Dermatofibrosarcoma protuberans	15
Dermatomyofibroma	15
Ectopic hamartomatous thymoma	9
Extraskeletal mesenchymal chondrosarcoma	14
Extraskeletal myxoid chondrosarcoma	5
Extraskeletal osteosarcoma	7 and 14
Fibroblastic reticular cell sarcoma	10
Fibromatosis colli	4
Fibrous hamartoma of infancy	4
Follicular dendritic cell sarcoma	10
Gastrointestinal stromal tumor	16
Gardner fibroma	4
Giant cell fibroblastoma	15
Hemosiderotic fibrolipomatous tumor	12
Hyaline fibromatosis	4
Hybrid schwannoma/perineurioma	15
Infantile digital fibroma	4
Infantile fibrosarcoma	4
Infantile myofibromatosis	4
Infantile rhabdomyofibrosarcoma	4
Interdigitating dendritic cell sarcoma	10
Juvenile nasopharyngeal angiofibroma	4
Kaposi sarcoma	13
Kaposiform hemangioendothelioma	13
Lipofibromatosis	4 and 12
Melanotic neuroectodermal tumor of infancy	9
Myxofibrosarcoma	5 and 7
Myxoid liposarcoma	5 and 12
Ossifying fibromyxoid tumor	5 and 6
Pilar leiomyoma	15
Plexiform fibrohistiocytic tumor	11
Plexiform fibromyxoma	16
Primitive myxoid mesenchymal tumor of infancy	4
Rhabdomyoma, fetal	4
Rhabdomyosarcoma, embryonal	8
Rhabdomyosarcoma, spindle cell (in children)	4
Solitary circumscribed neuroma	15
Spindle cell hemangioma	13
Storiform collagenoma	15
Superficial acral fibromyxoma (digital fibromyxoma)	15
Superficial angiomyxoma	5 and 15

cell carcinoma) from a true sarcoma, (2) discriminating between a benign spindle cell lesion and a malignant one, and (3) classifying (i.e., typing and subtyping) and grading a spindle cell sarcoma. Some particular histologic features (myxoid stroma, prominent inflammatory infiltrate, degenerative changes) may complicate the differential diagnosis. Ancillary techniques, particularly immunohistochemistry and molecular genetics, may be of great help in resolving many diagnostic dilemmas. However, it should be stressed that in many situations the diagnostic approach should be mainly based on knowledge of the relative frequencies of different tumor types and subtypes, an appropriate consideration of the clinical context, and a correct interpretation of morphologic features.

It may not be possible to classify with certainty a subset of spindle cell lesions, both benign and malignant, into established diagnostic categories. In such situations, good communication with the clinical team is mandatory. A descriptive diagnosis that conveys all available information (e.g., status of excision margins, presence of aggressive features, probable line of differentiation, "most likely" diagnosis in that particular clinical context) is usually clinically very helpful and allows for most appropriate patient management.

PRACTICE POINTS: Approach to Spindle Cell Tumors

- Exclude nonmesenchymal spindle cell tumors (especially spindle cell carcinoma and spindle cell melanoma)
- Classify the tumor, if possible
- Determine if the tumor is benign or malignant
- If the tumor is a sarcoma, provide the histologic grade, if appropriate for the tumor type
- Provide clinically relevant information even when the tumor cannot be classified (status of excision margins, probable line of differentiation, presence of aggressive features, most likely diagnosis)

Frequency

Spindle cell tumors account for approximately one-third of all soft tissue tumors that occur in adults. Benign lesions are more common than malignant tumors in this histologic group, among which cutaneous benign fibrous histiocytoma is by far the most frequent example (see Chapter 15).

Clinical Context

Besides the obvious need for clinicopathologic integration for appropriate practice, relatively simple clinical parameters, such as patient age, gender, and anatomic location, can be useful for the diagnosis of some lesions with characteristic clinical or anatomic presentations. Usually, these parameters are helpful in narrowing down a wide differential diagnosis. Occasionally, however, a lesion being considered does not seem to fit the clinical context; such unusual presentations require careful reassessment of the case, integrating all the available information, and, ideally, evaluation by a multidisciplinary team to make sensible decisions for the management of the patient.

Following are some trends in the presentation of soft tissue tumors according to some of these basic clinical parameters:

Patient age. Nodular fasciitis, fibromatoses, synovial sarcoma, and dermatofibrosarcoma protuberans (DFSP) most often arise in young adults, whereas solitary fibrous tumor (SFT), spindle cell lipoma, leiomyosarcoma, angiosarcoma, spindle cell (sarcomatoid) carcinoma, and spindle cell melanoma usually occur in adults 40 years of age or older. Some benign tumors (e.g., benign fibrous histiocytoma, neurofibroma, and schwannoma) may occur at any age.

Previous medical history. For some tumor types, the presence of a particular personal or family medical history, or associated lesions, is significant. A brief summary of some of the associations that may be observed with spindle cell tumors is provided in Box 3.1.

Tumor depth and anatomic location. Tumor depth and location are often important clues to the diagnosis. Although almost every tumor can arise at any location, some tumors have a tendency to occur at specific locations, and others show a relatively restricted anatomic distribution. The preferential locations of some tumor types are shown in Table 3.2.

Box 3.1 Spindle Cell Tumors: Common Clinical Associations

- Trauma: nodular fasciitis and pseudosarcomatous myofibroblastic proliferation (postoperative spindle cell nodule)
- Neurofibromatosis type 1: neurofibroma, GIST, MPNST
- Neurofibromatosis type 2: multiple schwannomas, vestibular schwannoma
- Schwannomatosis: multiple schwannomas
- Carney complex: melanotic schwannoma
- Pregnancy: abdominal fibromatosis
- Familial adenomatous polyposis: desmoid fibromatosis, Gardner fibroma
- Diabetes: palmar fibromatosis, nuchal-type fibroma
- Alport syndrome: esophageal leiomyomatosis
- HIV infection, transplantation, immunodeficiency: Epstein-Barr virus–associated smooth muscle neoplasm, Kaposi sarcoma
- Chronic lymphedema: angiosarcoma
- Radiation therapy: desmoid fibromatosis, angiosarcoma, MPNST, unclassified spindle cell sarcoma

GIST, Gastrointestinal stromal tumor; *HIV*, human immunodeficiency virus; *MPNST*, malignant peripheral nerve sheath tumor.

Table 3.2 Spindle Cell Tumors Occurring at Specific Anatomic Sites

Tumor Type	Location
Pseudosarcomatous myofibroblastic proliferation	Urinary tract
Intranodal palisaded myofibroblastoma	Inguinal lymph nodes
Fibroma of tendon sheath	Hand and foot
Nuchal fibroma	Back of neck
Elastofibroma	Scapular area
Solitary circumscribed neuroma	Face
Spindle cell lipoma	Upper back, shoulder, neck
Superficial fibromatoses	Palmar, plantar, and penile areas
Gastrointestinal stromal tumor	Intraabdominal
Dedifferentiated liposarcoma	Retroperitoneum, paratesticular
Spindle cell angiosarcoma	Head and neck (especially face and scalp)
Spindle cell rhabdomyosarcoma	Paratesticular, head and neck
Biphenotypic sinonasal sarcoma	Nasal cavity and paranasal sinuses

Histologic Parameters

In spindle cell tumors the important morphologic features to evaluate on hematoxylin and eosin–stained sections are similar to those for other mesenchymal neoplasms, including the following:

- Architectural arrangement of the tumor cells (growth pattern): long or short fascicles, whorls, sheets, or haphazard architecture
- Interface between tumor and adjacent tissues: pushing/expansile or infiltrative borders
- Amount and type of extracellular matrix: prominent, scant, or inconspicuous; collagenous, hyalinized, or myxoid

- Intratumoral vascularity: well-developed or inconspicuous; muscular thick-walled or thin-walled vessels, hyalinized vessel walls, branching (hemangiopericytoma [HPC]-like) vessels
- Presence of tumor necrosis
- Cytomorphology: long or short spindle cells, uniformity or pleomorphism, amount and quality of the cytoplasm, nuclear features, degree of atypia
- Mitotic activity

The growth pattern and cytomorphology are key features to help determine the line of differentiation of a spindle cell neoplasm. Infiltrative borders, tumor necrosis, atypical or hyperchromatic nuclei, and mitotic activity may or may not be indicative of malignancy, and they should be interpreted according to the line of differentiation and other features of the lesion. For example, any mitotic activity in a smooth muscle neoplasm of deep soft tissue or in a neurofibroma is usually indicative of a malignant diagnosis, whereas this is not true for myofibroblastic or "fibrohistiocytic" lesions.

Ancillary Techniques

Immunohistochemistry plays a critical role in the diagnosis of spindle cell lesions, both to define lines of differentiation and to identify the expression of proteins that result from molecular genetic alterations specific to particular tumor types. These techniques have essentially replaced ultrastructural studies performed with electron microscopy for the diagnosis of soft tissue tumors, because of widespread availability, ease of application, rapid turnaround time, and cost effectiveness. General aspects of the application of immunohistochemistry for classification of soft tissue tumors are discussed in Chapter 1; the particular immunohistochemical expression patterns are described in the context of each individual tumor type throughout this and the other chapters. Cytogenetic and molecular genetic techniques are also very useful for the diagnosis of soft tissue lesions; they are presented when appropriate for each lesion individually, as well as in some detail in Chapter 18.

Nonmesenchymal Neoplasms With Spindle Cell Cytomorphology

Before considering a final diagnosis of mesenchymal spindle cell tumors, which are relatively infrequent, several nonmesenchymal mimics should be carefully excluded. Among them, spindle cell carcinoma and spindle cell melanoma are the most common, requiring a high degree of suspicion to avoid pitfalls in certain clinical settings. Nonmesenchymal neoplasms that may show spindle cell morphology are listed in Box 3.2. Dendritic cell tumors are discussed in Chapter 10. The most frequently encountered examples are discussed briefly.

Spindle Cell Carcinoma

Spindle cell carcinoma (sarcomatoid carcinoma, including spindle cell squamous cell carcinoma) can occur at virtually any anatomic site. It generally affects middle-aged to elderly adults. Among the most common anatomic sites are sun-exposed skin (face and scalp), lips, upper and lower respiratory tract (mouth, pharynx, larynx, lung), upper and lower digestive tract (esophagus, anal canal), thyroid, breast, urinary tract (urinary bladder, kidney, ureter), and genital tract (endometrium, vulva, penis). Sarcomatoid carcinoma can be encountered in soft tissue in two situations: either as a metastatic deposit (especially from kidney or lung) or as a locoregional extension of a known (or unknown) carcinoma.[1] Thus pertinent previous medical history is crucial. Most sarcomatoid carcinomas are squamous in nature, but adenocarcinomas and other carcinoma types may also occasionally develop a poorly differentiated spindle cell component. The spindle cell growth pattern is usually present de novo but may also appear only at the time of local and/or distant recurrence, sometimes following radiation therapy.

Histologically, most sarcomatoid carcinomas resemble undifferentiated spindle cell/pleomorphic sarcomas (Fig. 3.1), although they may also display storiform, fibrosarcoma-like, leiomyosarcoma-like, nodular fasciitis–like, or HPC-like growth patterns. Foci of heterologous differentiation (such as chondrosarcomatous, osteosarcomatous, rhabdomyosarcomatous, liposarcomatous, or angiosarcomatous elements) may occasionally occur (e.g., in Müllerian carcinosarcoma). Detection of better differentiated, epithelial-like areas and/or an in situ component is crucial to make a proper diagnosis.[2]

By immunohistochemistry, spindled tumor cells in sarcomatoid squamous cell carcinomas often at least focally express broad-spectrum keratins (e.g., MNF116 or AE1/AE3) (see Fig. 3.1C), high-molecular-weight keratins (e.g., clone 34βE12, CK5 or CK5/6), as well as p63 (see Fig. 3.1D). For sarcomatoid carcinomas of visceral sites, it is often necessary to use multiple broad-spectrum keratin antibodies before detecting a positive result. Some sarcomatoid carcinomas can be negative for keratins but may show some reactivity for epithelial membrane antigen (EMA) or p63, which can also be helpful in appropriate clinical settings. Vimentin, which is expressed in both sarcomas and sarcomatoid carcinomas, is not diagnostically useful.

PRACTICE POINTS: Spindle Cell Carcinoma

- Sarcomatoid carcinoma, especially in visceral organs and sun-exposed skin, should be considered before a mesenchymal tumor is diagnosed
- Epithelial-like areas or an in situ component facilitates the diagnosis but may be completely absent
- Even focal expression of keratins, p63, or epithelial membrane antigen can help support the diagnosis
- Multiple broad-spectrum keratin antibodies may be required
- Vimentin is not specific for mesenchymal tumors and is therefore not useful in differential diagnosis

Box 3.2 Nonmesenchymal Spindle Cell Neoplasms

- Spindle cell carcinoma
- Spindle cell/desmoplastic melanoma
- Spindle cell/desmoplastic mesothelioma
- Others
    - Paraganglioma
    - Gliosarcoma (metastasis)
    - Extracranial meningioma
    - Myeloid sarcoma (extramedullary myeloid tumor)
    - Interdigitating dendritic cell sarcoma
    - Mast cell neoplasms (systemic mastocytosis, mastocytoma, mast cell sarcoma)

Spindle Cell Melanoma and Variants

As for spindle cell carcinoma, previous medical history is crucial for the diagnosis of spindle cell melanoma. It usually occurs in soft tissue either as a metastasis or as the extension of locally advanced melanoma. Lymph node metastasis (especially axillary or inguinal) with extracapsular extension into soft tissue is an extremely common presentation. Indeed, an axillary mass showing spindle cell morphology is most likely to be metastatic melanoma (Fig. 3.2). The primary tumor may show either spindle cell or epithelioid cytomorphology. By immunohistochemistry, spindle cell melanomas are generally strongly and diffusely positive for S-100 protein and SOX10 (see Fig. 3.2C), whereas second-line melanocytic markers, such as melan A and HMB-45, are rarely useful, being expressed in less than 10% of cases. Spindle cell melanoma can therefore easily be confused with malignant peripheral nerve sheath tumor (MPNST), as well as with synovial sarcoma, leiomyosarcoma, and undifferentiated spindle cell/pleomorphic sarcoma.[3]

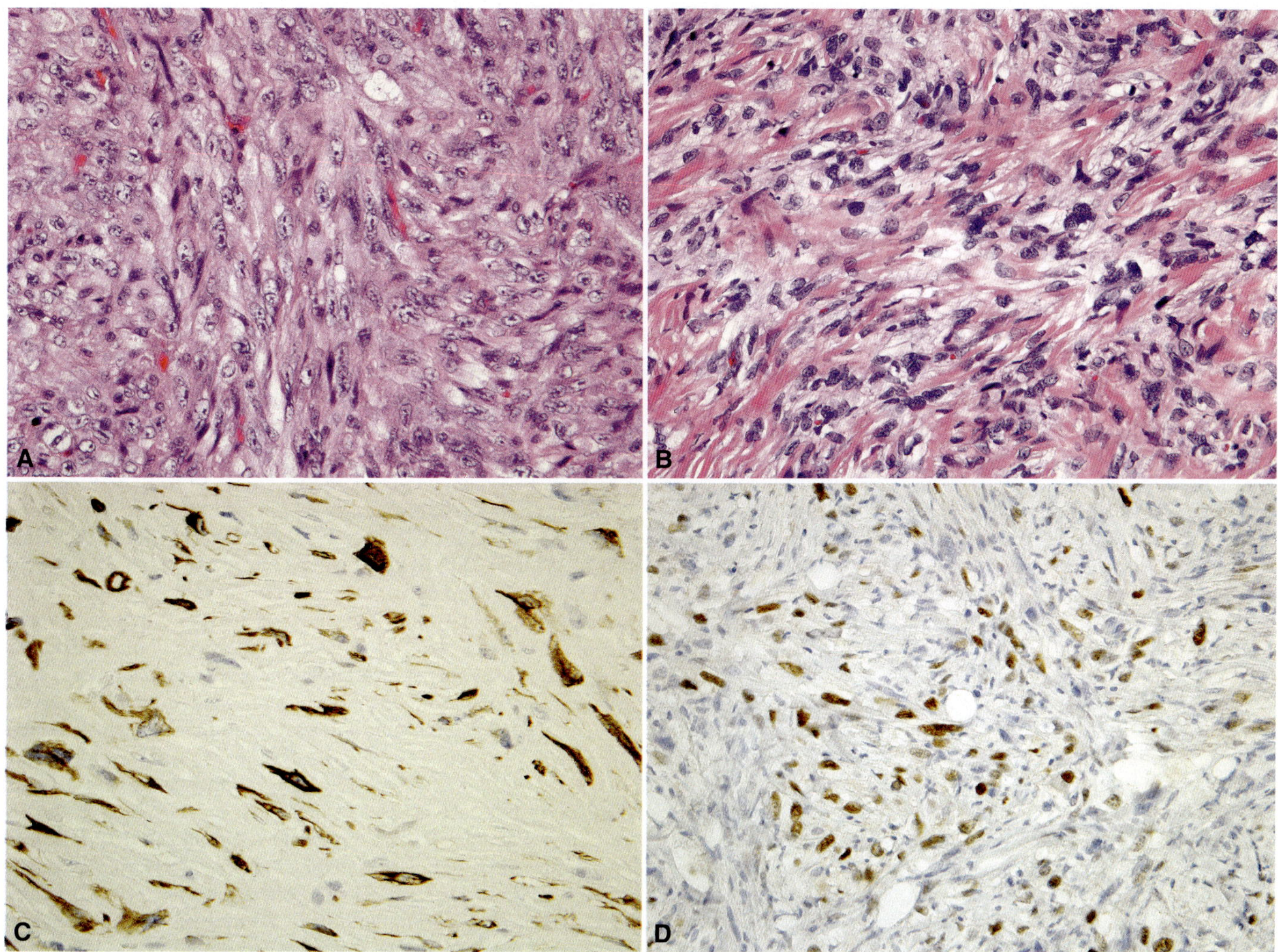

Figure 3.1 Spindle Cell (Sarcomatoid) Carcinoma. (A) Note the polymorphous cytology, including cells with a more polygonal appearance. (B) Sarcomatoid carcinoma of the lung with a haphazard architecture and prominent stromal collagen. (C) Broad-spectrum keratin expression in sarcomatoid carcinoma. (D) Nuclear staining for p63 in sarcomatoid carcinoma.

Desmoplastic melanoma can be considered a distinctive variant of spindle cell melanoma.[4] It tends to occur in older adults (especially men), often in the head and neck area (particularly scalp) and upper back, rarely at mucosal sites (e.g., vulva or gingiva). Spindle cells tend to be arranged in vague fascicles set in an abundant collagenous matrix (see Fig. 3.2D). Melanin production is nearly always absent. Neurotropism (i.e., tumor cells growing within and around nerves at a distance from the main tumor mass), as well as lymphoid aggregates, are frequently observed within and at the periphery of the spindle cell proliferation (see Fig. 3.2D). An atypical or malignant melanocytic proliferation is occasionally seen at the dermal-epidermal junction, a helpful clue to diagnosis. Desmoplastic and spindle cell melanomas share the same immunoprofile, although tumor cells in desmoplastic melanoma are even more frequently negative for HMB-45 and melan A.[5] They can be positive for smooth muscle actin and, very rarely, for keratins.[6,7] Similar to spindle cell melanoma, desmoplastic melanoma may be confused with MPNST (although MPNST is usually only focally positive for S-100 protein and SOX10, in no more than 50% of cases), DFSP, leiomyosarcoma, desmoid fibromatosis, schwannoma, and neurofibroma. Perhaps the most common misdiagnosis for desmoplastic melanoma is hypertrophic scar.

Rare variants of melanoma, such as myxoid melanoma and melanomas with metaplastic changes (including foci of osteosarcomatous, chondrosarcomatous, rhabdomyosarcomatous, or liposarcomatous heterologous differentiation) are difficult to distinguish from some spindle cell sarcomas.[6,7]

PRACTICE POINTS: Spindle Cell and Desmoplastic Melanoma

- Metastatic melanoma, especially in the axilla and groin, should always be considered
- Soft tissue or lymph node metastases may be the initial presentation
- Strong and diffuse expression of S-100 protein and SOX10 is characteristic of melanoma and argues against malignant peripheral nerve sheath tumor
- Second-line melanoma markers (HMB-45, melan A) are usually negative in spindle cell melanoma
- Desmoplastic melanoma may be deceptively bland and is typically paucicellular, mimicking a scar

Malignant Mesothelioma

Localized sarcomatoid mesothelioma can easily be confused with a spindle cell mesenchymal neoplasm (Fig. 3.3), especially MPNST, synovial sarcoma, SFT, spindle cell angiosarcoma, and undifferentiated spindle cell/pleomorphic sarcoma. Hypocellular regions of desmoplastic mesothelioma may resemble a benign fibrosing process or a desmoid tumor,[8] whereas biphasic mesothelioma may mimic biphasic synovial

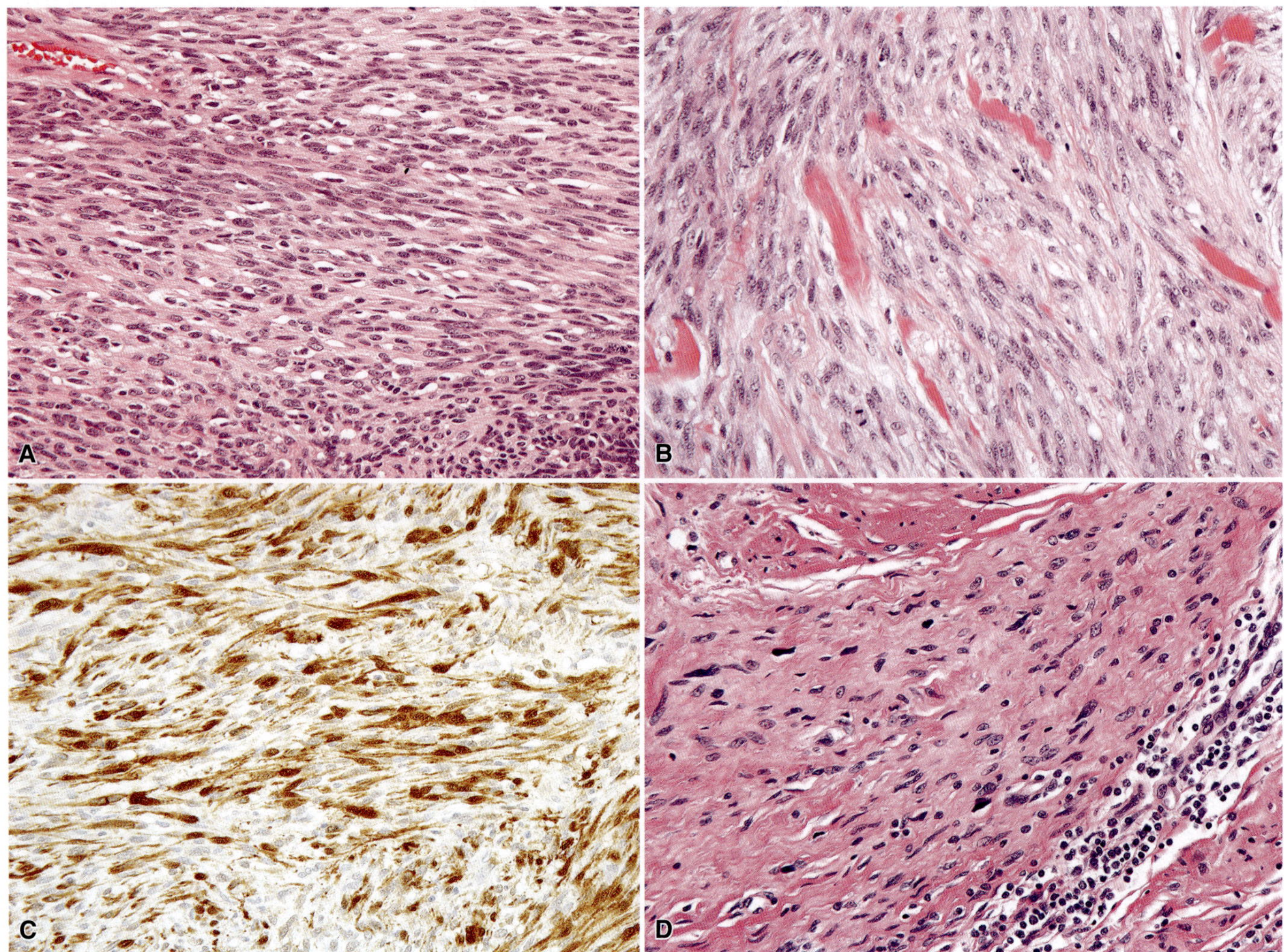

Figure 3.2 Spindle Cell Melanoma. (A) Metastatic melanoma with spindle cell morphology. The patient with this tumor presented with an axillary mass. (B) The tumor cells contain vesicular chromatin and show a high mitotic rate. (C) Strong, diffuse staining for S-100 protein supports the diagnosis of spindle cell melanoma over malignant peripheral nerve sheath tumor. (D) Desmoplastic melanoma composed of vague fascicles of spindle cells with a neural-like appearance in an abundant collagenous stroma. A lymphoid infiltrate is often seen at the periphery of the tumor.

sarcoma. Clues to the diagnosis of mesothelioma are as follows: previous history of asbestos exposure or radiation therapy, recurrent serosal effusions (pleural effusion or ascites), a serosal surface-based mass, and immunoreactivity of tumor cells for keratins (see Fig. 3.3C), EMA, calretinin, WT1 (nuclear pattern), and podoplanin (D2-40), although many sarcomatoid mesotheliomas are negative for mesothelial markers (at least 60% of cases), including calretinin.[8,9] In such cases, WT1 is the most sensitive mesothelial marker (see Fig. 3.3D).

Nodular Fasciitis and Similar Pseudosarcomatous Myofibroblastic Lesions

Nodular Fasciitis

Nodular fasciitis is a self-limited pseudosarcomatous proliferation composed of fibroblasts and myofibroblasts.[10,11] The morphologic spectrum of nodular fasciitis is wide. Several variants have been described under different designations depending on clinical, macroscopic, or particular microscopic features; however, all of these lesions show some overlapping histologic appearances due to their shared myofibroblastic nature. Nodular fasciitis is also discussed in Chapter 4.

Clinical Features

Nodular fasciitis predominates in young to middle-aged adults (20 to 40 years of age) with no gender predilection. It most often occurs as a solitary, small (<2 to 3 cm), sometimes painful subcutaneous nodule that develops rapidly, often in less than 4 to 8 weeks. The anatomic distribution is wide, but the lesion most commonly arises in the upper extremities (40% to 50% of cases), especially the forearm, followed by the head and neck area (where it is most common in children) and the trunk wall. Nodular fasciitis is infrequent in hands and feet, and it is rare in some other sites (e.g., vulva, axilla, lymph node capsule). The depth of nodular fasciitis is variable. Most cases are subcutaneous, but approximately 10% of cases are entirely intramuscular, and a small minority arises in unusual locations such as the skin (intradermal fasciitis), periosteum (parosteal fasciitis and cranial fasciitis), joints (intraarticular fasciitis), or vessels, principally veins (intravascular fasciitis).[12-14] A previous history of trauma is elicited in 10% to 20% of cases.

Pathologic Features

Nodular fasciitis is usually grossly well circumscribed, measuring less than 3 cm in diameter. In the subcutis the nodule tends to develop

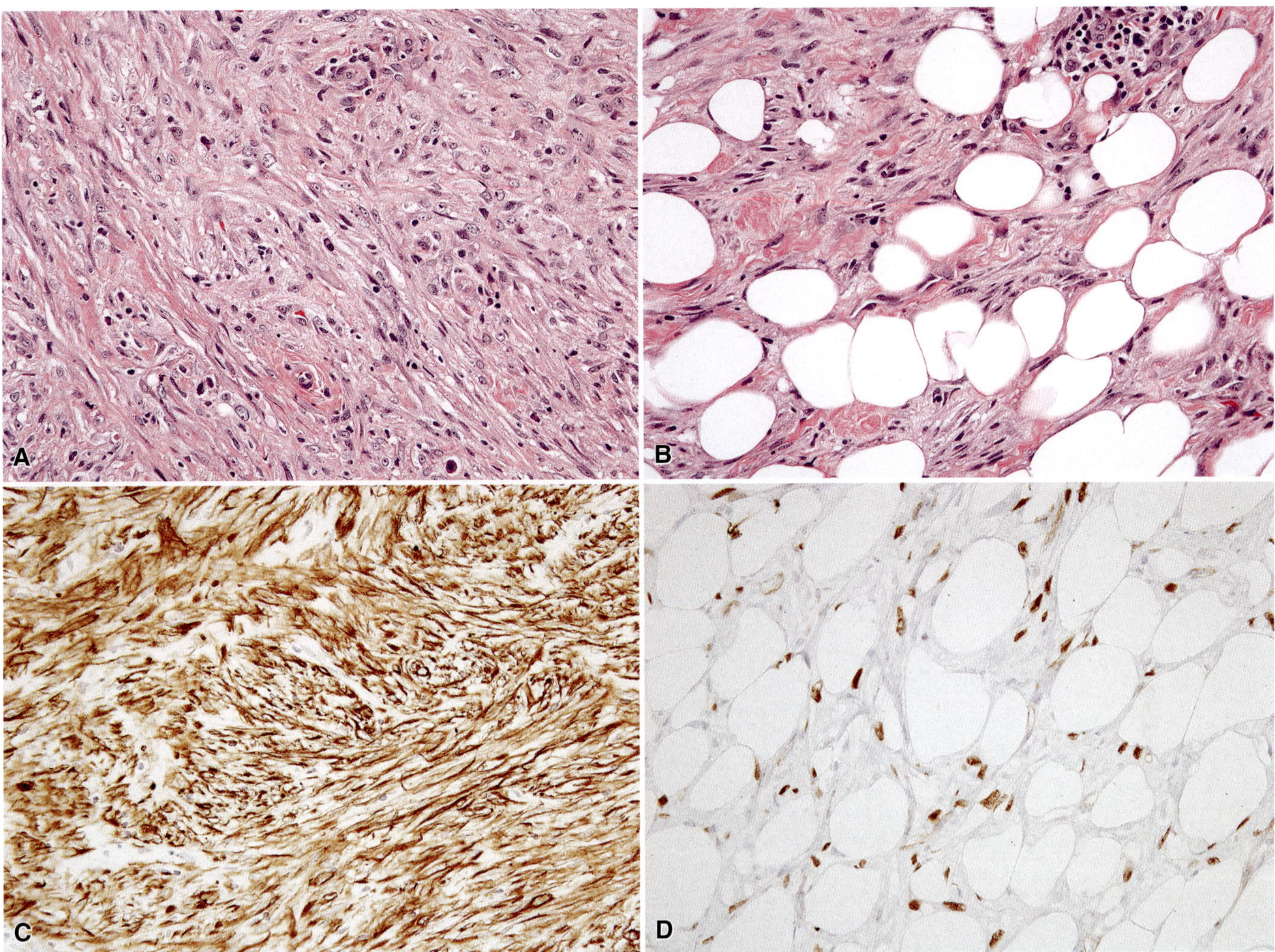

Figure 3.3 Sarcomatoid Mesothelioma. (A) In addition to the clinical presentation, relatively uniform cytology is a clue to the diagnosis of sarcomatoid mesothelioma. (B) Infiltration of adipose tissue of the parietal pleura is a helpful diagnostic feature for mesothelioma. (C) The tumor cells show strong, diffuse staining for broad-spectrum keratins. (D) Nuclear staining for WT1 is a helpful finding.

along fibrous septa, dissecting the adipose tissue. It may also be centered on the superficial aponeurosis (fascial-type nodular fasciitis). In deep soft tissue, especially in skeletal muscle (10% of cases), the lesion tends to be larger than its subcutaneous counterpart. On section, recently developed lesions have a myxoid appearance, whereas older lesions are more fibrous and firmer.

The histologic appearances of nodular fasciitis vary according to the age of the lesion. Early lesions are usually variably cellular, consisting of fibroblasts and myofibroblasts arranged in short irregular fascicles, sometimes with a vaguely storiform pattern, set in a loosely textured myxoid matrix (feathery pattern) or a more collagenous stroma (Fig. 3.4). The cells are plump, with abundant eosinophilic, somewhat fibrillary cytoplasm, resembling cells in tissue culture or granulation tissue. Nuclei are vesicular and contain a single, often prominent nucleolus (see Fig. 3.4C). Mitoses can be numerous and are almost always typical. The lesion tends to extend along the fibrous septa from which it arises and is often surrounded and infiltrated by numerous inflammatory elements (lymphoid aggregates, plasma cells). It may also contain numerous, centripetally oriented capillaries. Mucin pooling, cystic change, interstitial hemorrhage (extravasated erythrocytes), and small collections of intralesional histiocytes are common. Sometimes, the central part of the lesion is markedly hypocellular, contrasting with the hypercellular periphery, resulting in a zonal appearance. Long-standing lesions are less cellular and more fibrotic (see Fig. 3.4D), containing areas of hyalinized fibrosis arranged in dense, refractile, keloid-like collagen bands (see Fig. 3.4E). Approximately 10% of cases of nodular fasciitis contain prominent osteoclast-like multinucleated giant cells (see Chapter 11).

Intramuscular nodular fasciitis is also usually well demarcated. Sometimes, tumor borders are infiltrative, containing some residual entrapped atrophic muscle fibers, akin to desmoid fibromatosis.

Variants of nodular fasciitis and related and similar lesions are as follows:

- Nodular fasciitis with infiltrative borders. Some cases have notably infiltrative borders, more closely mimicking sarcoma.
- Nodular fasciitis with high cellularity. In this form, there is little or no myxoid background and no zonation phenomenon. The lesion is densely cellular, composed of mitotically active spindle cells arranged in short fascicles (see Fig. 3.4F). Such tumors can easily be misdiagnosed as spindle cell sarcomas.
- Cranial fasciitis. This lesion occurs mostly in male infants during the first year of life, frequently following birth trauma (e.g., delivery by forceps) (see Chapter 4). It develops in the soft tissues of the scalp, from the galea aponeurotica, and it may erode and even penetrate the underlying bone with involvement of meninges. It is

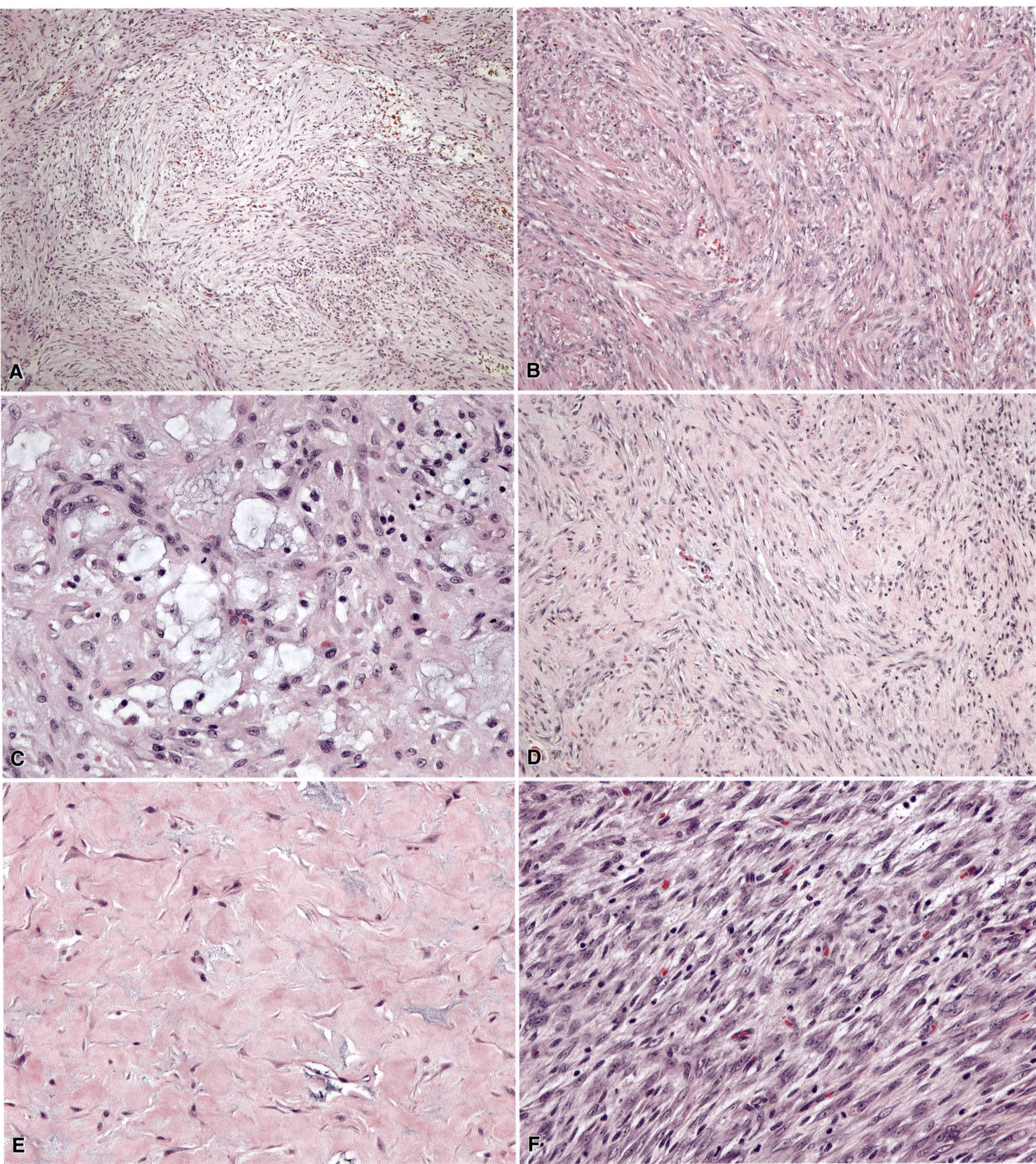

Figure 3.4 **Nodular Fasciitis.** (A) The tumor is composed of loose intersecting fascicles of uniform spindle cells with intervening myxoid stroma producing cleftlike spaces. (B) Nodular fasciitis with collagenous stroma. (C) Plump myofibroblasts with fine chromatin and abundant eosinophilic cytoplasm are characteristic. Note the interspersed small lymphocytes and microcysts. Long-standing lesions often show stromal hyalinization (D), including bundles of keloidal collagen (E). (F) Tumors such as this highly cellular, early lesion without a significant stromal component may be mistaken for spindle cell sarcomas.

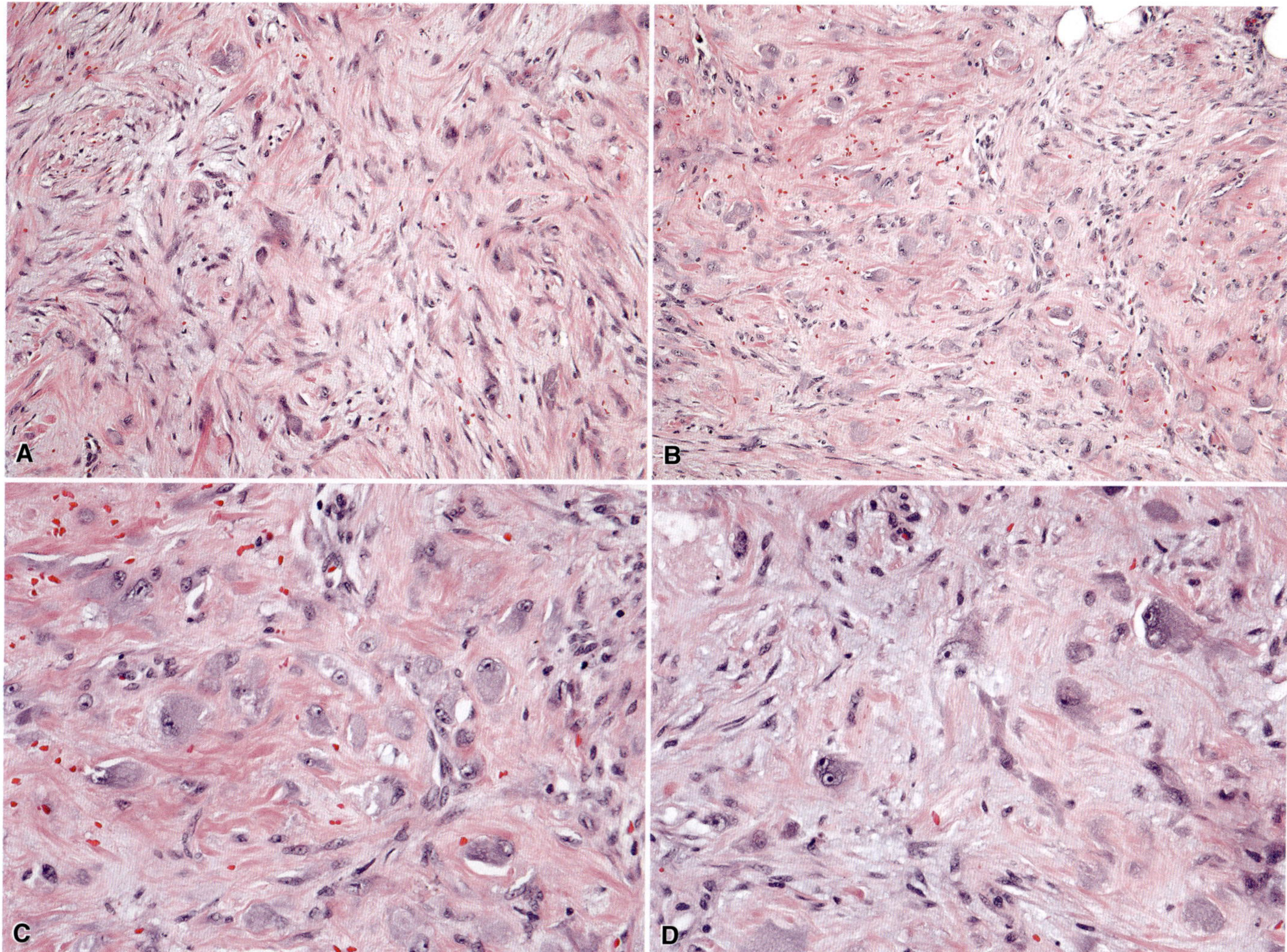

Figure 3.5 Proliferative Fasciitis. The tumor resembles nodular fasciitis (A), except for the presence of ganglion-like cells (B). (C) Large, ganglion-like epithelioid cells with amphophilic cytoplasm and eccentric nuclei are a typical feature. (D) Occasional ganglion-like cells are binucleated. Note the large nucleoli.

often visible on plain radiographs as a lytic lesion of the calvarium. Histologically, it resembles conventional nodular fasciitis but may also contain areas of osseous metaplasia.

- Intravascular fasciitis. This is a rare variant of nodular fasciitis (3% of cases) that grows into and obstructs medium-size veins or, less often, arteries.[14] It may show a multinodular growth pattern inside the same vessel. Intravascular fasciitis tends to be less myxoid and to contain more osteoclast-like giant cells than common nodular fasciitis. It is most often observed in the subcutaneous tissues of the upper limbs or the head and neck.
- Proliferative fasciitis and proliferative myositis, which are morphologically similar lesions.[15,16] Proliferative fasciitis usually occurs in the subcutaneous tissues of the upper limbs (especially forearms) of middle-aged adults (40 to 60 years of age), whereas proliferative myositis mainly affects the flat muscles of the trunk and shoulder girdle. Histologically, in addition to the other findings of nodular fasciitis, the key feature of these two lesions is the presence of unusual large epithelioid cells that resemble ganglion cells or rhabdomyoblasts (Fig. 3.5), containing abundant amphophilic or basophilic cytoplasm and often eccentric, vesicular nuclei with prominent nucleoli (see Fig. 3.5C). Binucleated forms may also be seen (see Fig. 3.5D). The distinctive epithelioid cells tend to form small clusters. In children, proliferative fasciitis may be very cellular and mitotically active, consisting almost exclusively of ganglion-like cells, and thus closely mimic rhabdomyosarcoma. In proliferative myositis, fasciitis-like areas containing ganglion-like cells alternate with foci of atrophic skeletal muscle resulting in a typical "checkerboard" pattern, apparent at low magnification (Fig. 3.6).
- Ischemic fasciitis (also known as "atypical decubital fibroplasia"), which is somewhat similar to proliferative fasciitis because it also contains ganglion-like cells.[17] This lesion usually involves the soft tissues overlying bony prominences, such as the shoulder, the chest wall, and the sacrococcygeal and greater trochanter regions. It occurs over a wide age range, with a peak in elderly adults (70 to 90 years of age); some affected patients are physically debilitated or immobilized.[18] Histologically, ischemic fasciitis characteristically shows a zonal appearance with central areas of fibrinoid necrosis and cystic change, surrounded by granulation tissue and plump amphophilic ganglion-like myofibroblasts (Fig. 3.7).
- Ossifying fasciitis (also known as fasciitis ossificans) is a variant of fasciitis that contains foci of metaplastic bone, but lacking the typical zonation of myositis ossificans (see Chapter 14). When mitotic activity and ossification are prominent, extraskeletal osteosarcoma enters the differential diagnosis.

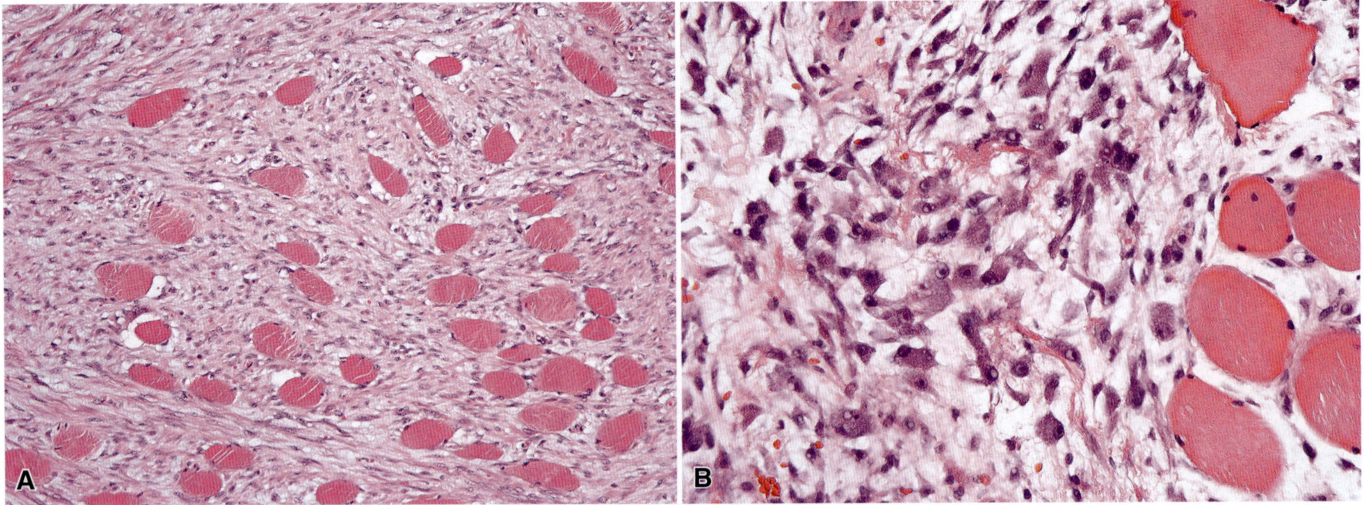

Figure 3.6 Proliferative Myositis. (A) The tumor cells entrap skeletal muscle fibers, imparting a checkerboard-like appearance. (B) Similar to proliferative fasciitis, ganglion-like cells are often present.

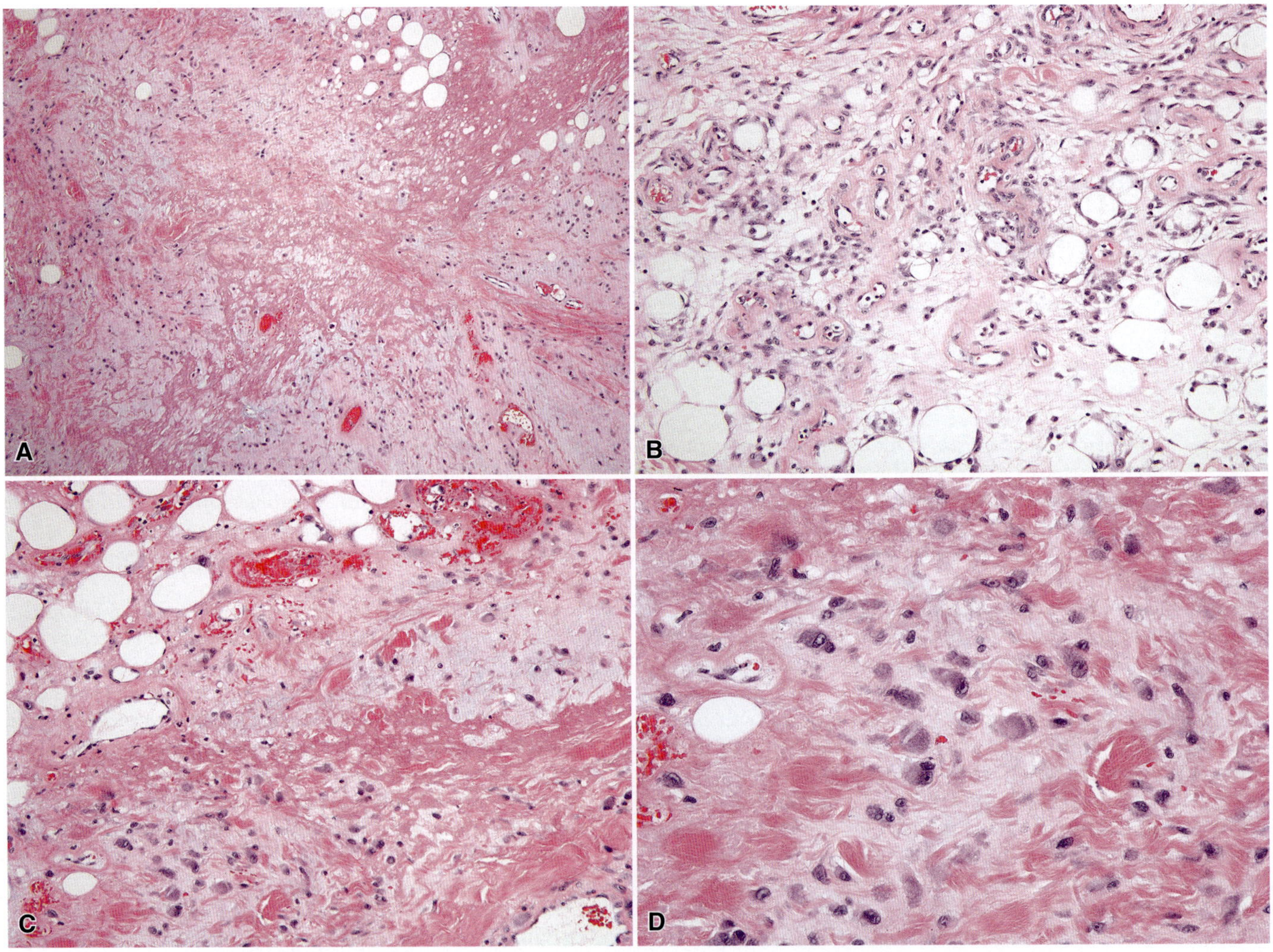

Figure 3.7 Ischemic Fasciitis. The lesion shows a zonal appearance with central areas of fibrinoid necrosis (A) surrounded by granulation tissue (B). (C) A proliferation of plump myofibroblasts is observed adjacent to the area of fibrinoid necrosis. (D) Ganglion-like myofibroblasts are seen, similar to those in proliferative fasciitis.

Fasciitis ossificans, myositis ossificans, panniculitis ossificans, florid reactive periostitis, and fibro-osseous pseudotumor of the digits are related benign ossifying pseudosarcomatous fibroblastic/myofibroblastic proliferations (see Chapter 14). Although zonal maturation is typical of myositis ossificans, other lesions in this family lack such architectural organization.

Immunohistochemistry

Myofibroblasts in nodular fasciitis are usually strongly, diffusely positive for smooth muscle actin, muscle-specific actin (clone HHF35), and calponin. Desmin reactivity is observed in only few scattered cells. Caldesmon, S-100 protein, CD34, and β-catenin are not expressed. Occasional visceral lesions show reactivity for keratins. Intralesional histiocytes and osteoclast-like giant cells express CD68 and other histiocyte markers. Proliferation markers (Ki-67) stain a large number of nuclei, in keeping with high proliferative activity of these lesions. The ganglion-like cells in proliferative fasciitis and proliferative myositis are often negative for muscle markers.

Molecular Genetics

Despite the clinical features that suggest a reactive lesion, nodular fasciitis is a clonal proliferation, as shown by the clonal chromosomal rearrangements detected in lesions analyzed cytogenetically.[19-21] Rearrangements of the *USP6* locus at 17p13 have been detected in greater than 90% of cases of nodular fasciitis. The *MYH9-USP6* gene fusion was detected in 65% of cases, resulting in overexpression of the USP6 oncoprotein by a promoter swap mechanism, similarly to aneurysmal bone cyst (see Chapter 14).[22] An alternative *PPP6R3-USP6* fusion with amplification has been reported in a single unusual aggressive case[23]; other gene fusions remain to be identified.

Differential Diagnosis

Nodular fasciitis is often mistaken for a sarcoma (20% to 30% of cases), mainly because of its high cellularity, poor circumscription, rapid growth, and brisk mitotic activity (Box 3.3). However, in contrast to most sarcomas, nodular fasciitis grows very rapidly (within a few weeks), is generally small and located in subcutis, does not contain enlarged and/or hyperchromatic nuclei, and does not show tumor necrosis or atypical mitotic figures.

Predominantly myxoid examples of nodular fasciitis may be confused with myxofibrosarcoma. As opposed to nodular fasciitis, myxofibrosarcoma occurs in the elderly, tends to be multinodular, often shows alternating cellular and myxoid areas, and, most importantly, contains tumor cells with enlarged hyperchromatic nuclei, which are not a feature of nodular fasciitis. Myxoid forms of nodular fasciitis can also be confused with myxoid DFSP (positive for CD34, negative for smooth muscle actin), myxoid forms of low-grade MPNST (positive for S-100 protein, glial fibrillary acidic protein [GFAP], and/or SOX10 in 40% to 50% of cases), and low-grade fibromyxoid sarcoma (LGFMS) (positive for MUC4 and EMA, negative for smooth muscle actin). Hypercellular forms of nodular fasciitis should be distinguished from leiomyosarcoma (large size, reactivity for desmin and caldesmon, in addition to smooth muscle actin), myofibroblastic sarcoma (expression of smooth muscle actin and desmin, negative for caldesmon), Kaposi sarcoma (expression of CD31, CD34, ERG, and human herpesvirus 8), and spindle cell carcinoma (reactivity for keratins, variable EMA, and p63). Lesions containing a large number of ganglion-like cells or rhabdomyoblast-like cells can mimic embryonal or pleomorphic rhabdomyosarcoma (reactivity for actin, desmin, and myogenin) or other pleomorphic sarcomas, as well as ganglioneuroblastoma. Extraskeletal osteosarcoma is the main differential diagnostic consideration for ossifying fasciitis and related lesions. In contrast to ossifying fasciitis, extraskeletal osteosarcoma usually occurs in patients of advanced age (sometimes following radiation therapy), is composed of atypical tumor cells with hyperchromatic nuclei, may contain areas of tumor necrosis, and tends to show bone maturation in the center of the lesion rather than at its periphery. Osteoid deposition is also usually less organized in osteosarcoma than in ossifying fasciitis. Marked cellular pleomorphism and atypical mitoses are common in osteosarcoma but virtually absent in ossifying fasciitis.

Box 3.3 Differential Diagnosis of Nodular Fasciitis and Similar Lesions

Nodular Fasciitis, Cellular Phase With Myxoid Change
Intramuscular/cellular myxoma
Myxofibrosarcoma
Malignant peripheral nerve sheath tumor
Myxoid dermatofibrosarcoma protuberans
Low-grade fibromyxoid sarcoma

Nodular Fasciitis, Cellular Phase Without Myxoid Change
Benign fibrous histiocytoma
Myofibroma
Cellular schwannoma
Desmoid fibromatosis
Leiomyosarcoma
Kaposi sarcoma
Spindle cell carcinoma
Spindle cell melanoma

Nodular Fasciitis, Fibrotic Phase
Fibroma of tendon sheath
Desmoplastic fibroblastoma
Neurofibroma
Perineurioma

Proliferative Fasciitis
Rhabdomyosarcoma
Pleomorphic sarcomas
Ganglioneuroblastoma

Ossifying Nodular Fasciitis (Fasciitis Ossificans) and Related Ossifying Lesions
Extraskeletal osteosarcoma

Ischemic Fasciitis
Myxofibrosarcoma
Epithelioid sarcoma

Prognosis and Treatment

Nodular fasciitis is a benign, self-limiting process. Simple excision is the treatment of choice. Local recurrences are exceptional (<2% of cases). Spontaneous regression may occur.

PRACTICE POINTS: Nodular Fasciitis

- Presentation is a rapidly growing, usually subcutaneous tumor in young to middle-aged adults
- Forearm and head and neck are the most common sites
- Rarely arises in the skin, joints, or blood vessels
- Initially highly cellular; long-standing lesions become hypocellular and fibrotic
- Myxoid stroma, extravasated erythrocytes, and a tissue culture–like appearance are typical

Pseudosarcomatous Myofibroblastic Proliferation

Lesions somewhat similar to nodular fasciitis have been reported at mucosal sites under various designations: visceral fasciitis, pseudosarcomatous fibromyxoid tumor, pseudomalignant spindle cell proliferation, postoperative spindle cell nodule, and inflammatory pseudotumor. They most often arise in the genitourinary tract. These lesions belong to a clinically and histologically distinct group that is now widely referred to using the descriptive designation *pseudosarcomatous myofibroblastic proliferation* (PMP).[24-29]

Clinical Features

PMP can be observed at any age but predominantly in adults, with no gender predilection. The genitourinary tract is the most common location (urinary bladder, prostate, urethra, vagina, and vulva), but the lesion may occasionally arise at any mucosal site, including the gastrointestinal tract and the head and neck area (larynx, pharynx, nasal cavity, and mouth). In most patients, it arises spontaneously.[25] In a subset of patients the lesion appears following surgery or instrumentation in the same area, in which case the designation *postoperative spindle cell nodule* has been applied.[28] Such cases, which have been described in the vulva, vagina, urinary bladder, and prostatic urethra, typically occur 1 to 3 months after trauma or an invasive procedure (e.g., transurethral resection of the prostate or urinary bladder, or endometrial curettage). Hemorrhage (e.g., gross hematuria for lesions developing in the urinary tract) is the most common presenting symptom.

Pathologic Features

Grossly, PMP (including postoperative lesions) usually presents as exophytic or polypoid, frequently ulcerated masses that have a tendency to bleed easily. They generally measure less than 5 cm in maximal diameter, but lesions up to 7 cm have been reported in the urinary bladder.

Histologically, PMP consists of a spindle cell proliferation in which cellular elements are arranged in loose fascicles (Fig. 3.8), although some examples are densely cellular and fascicular. The spindle cells have abundant, elongated, eosinophilic to amphophilic cytoplasm (see Fig. 3.8B). Strap-shaped cells may be seen in myxoid areas. Tumor cell nuclei are oval- to spindle-shaped with vesicular chromatin and one or two prominent nucleoli. Marked nuclear pleomorphism is absent. Mitotic activity is variable, ranging from low to brisk in some lesions (10 mitoses or more per 10 high-power fields (HPF)). Atypical mitoses and necrosis are usually absent.[25] The spindle cell proliferation may be admixed with a variable number of inflammatory elements, including neutrophils, eosinophils, lymphocytes, and plasma cells. Myxoid and hemorrhagic changes are frequently observed, as well as numerous capillaries, often oriented toward the ulcerated mucosal surface (akin to granulation tissue).

Immunohistochemistry

As in nodular fasciitis, spindle cells in PMP usually express muscle-specific actin (HHF35), smooth muscle actin, and focal desmin. One-third of lesions are at least focally positive for keratins. The lesions are consistently negative for S-100 protein and CD34. Approximately 50% of cases of PMP express anaplastic lymphoma kinase (ALK), thus overlapping with inflammatory myofibroblastic tumor and complicating the differential diagnosis.[30,31]

Molecular Genetics

A large majority of PMPs do not bear specific chromosomal abnormalities, although some inconsistent chromosomal alterations have been reported in several cases. Some authors have reported *ALK* rearrangements in PMP detected by fluorescence in situ hybridization (FISH).[25] In the authors' experience, despite immunohistochemical expression of ALK, PMPs only rarely show *ALK* rearrangements. Most myofibroblastic lesions with *ALK* rearrangements are better classified as inflammatory myofibroblastic tumors (see Chapters 4 and 10).

Differential Diagnosis

The differential diagnosis of PMP is somewhat similar to that of nodular fasciitis (Box 3.4). Highly cellular examples should be differentiated

Box 3.4 Differential Diagnosis of Pseudosarcomatous Myofibroblastic Proliferation

If Predominantly Myxoid
- Myxofibrosarcoma
- Inflammatory myofibroblastic tumor
- Myxoid leiomyosarcoma
- Embryonal rhabdomyosarcoma

If Predominantly Cellular
- Conventional leiomyosarcoma
- Spindle cell rhabdomyosarcoma
- Kaposi sarcoma
- Spindle cell carcinoma
- Spindle cell melanoma

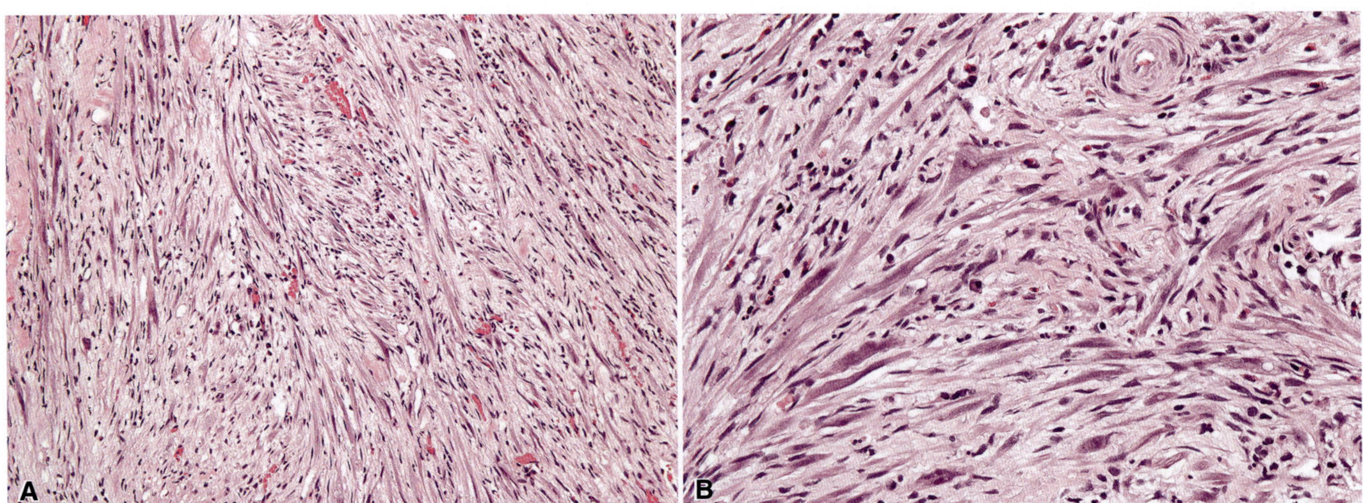

Figure 3.8 Pseudosarcomatous Myofibroblastic Proliferation. (A) This lesion is composed of loose fascicles of plump spindle cells. (B) The tumor cells have elongated cytoplasmic processes with abundant cytoplasm and large nucleoli, which can mimic rhabdomyoblasts.

from leiomyosarcoma, rhabdomyosarcoma, and Kaposi sarcoma. In an appropriate context, spindle cell carcinoma and spindle cell melanoma should also be excluded, especially in patients with a previous history of carcinoma or melanoma.

Making the distinction between PMP and inflammatory myofibroblastic tumor can be difficult, especially for lesions arising in the head and neck region (larynx, mouth) and the genitourinary tract. In the urinary bladder, where PMP predominates, lesions have been reported under various different names (inflammatory pseudotumor, pseudosarcomatous fibromyxoid tumor, inflammatory myofibroblastic tumor, and PMP), illustrating the difficulties encountered in classifying these lesions and, more importantly, in assessing their biologic potential. Some of these tumors bear alterations of the *ALK* gene on 2p23, express ALK by immunohistochemistry, and may recur locally, whereas others do not. In contrast to inflammatory myofibroblastic tumors, PMPs are usually less cellular and less uniformly fascicular, with more prominent myxoid stroma and a sparse inflammatory infiltrate. However, due to the morphologic overlap, a pragmatic approach would be to classify lesions bearing *ALK* gene alterations as inflammatory myofibroblastic tumors and "*ALK*–wild type" lesions as PMPs.[25,30-32] The lack of significant nuclear atypia and hyperchromasia distinguishes PMP from leiomyosarcoma and spindle cell (sarcomatoid) carcinoma. Because the immunophenotypic overlap between PMP and leiomyosarcoma is substantial (including keratin expression), cytologic atypia is the most helpful discriminating feature. If a sarcomatoid carcinoma is considered, expression of p63 or high-molecular-weight keratins would favor a carcinoma, whereas desmin expression would support PMP.

Prognosis and Treatment

PMP usually does not recur after complete excision. However, occasional repeated local recurrences have been reported. Recurring lesions are morphologically similar to nonrecurring cases, and ALK expression does not correlate with recurrence. Worrisome features such as brisk mitotic activity, tumor necrosis, or infiltration of adjacent structures do not correlate with more aggressive behavior either.[25]

Mycobacterial Spindle Cell Pseudotumor

Mycobacterial spindle cell pseudotumors are rare lesions described initially in patients with acquired immunodeficiency syndrome (AIDS), which can also occur in other immunocompromised patients.[33-35] Few cases have been observed in infants after receiving bacille Calmette-Guérin (BCG) vaccination.[36] These pseudotumors mainly occur in lymph nodes and skin but may affect almost any anatomic site (lungs, brain, spleen, nasal cavity). They are composed of a heterogeneous population of fibroblasts, myofibroblasts, and epithelioid to spindled histiocytes, which are laden with numerous acid-fast bacilli (Fig. 3.9). In most instances the organisms represent atypical mycobacteria, especially *Mycobacterium avium-intracellulare*.[33-35] Histoid leprosy, a rare form of lepromatous leprosy, may also display the appearances of a spindle cell tumor, mimicking benign fibrous histiocytoma of the skin.[37]

Myofibroma and Myopericytoma

Myofibroma is a benign neoplasm of superficial soft tissues showing perivascular myoid differentiation. In the context of infantile myofibromatosis (discussed in detail in Chapter 4), solitary or multiple myofibromas present within the first decade of life, usually before 2 years of age.[38] Morphologically identical lesions in adults are more often solitary, although rare examples of multicentric disease have also been described.[39-41] Myofibroma and myofibromatosis lie on a histologic continuum with the other tumor types that show perivascular myoid differentiation, that is, myopericytoma and glomangiopericytoma, the distinction between them sometimes being arbitrary due to considerable morphologic overlap. The designation *perivascular myoma* has been proposed to designate these three lesions collectively.[42,43]

Clinical Features

Adult myofibroma is a solitary painless cutaneous, subcutaneous, or mucosal nodule, most commonly located in the head and neck region or in the lower extremity in adults of any age. Multicentric cases, generally affecting the same anatomic region, are much less frequent in adults than in infants. Cases involving deep-seated locations, including viscera or bone, are extremely rare in adults. Myopericytoma shows a male predominance and also occurs over a wide age range, with a peak in middle-aged adults. Most tumors arise on the extremities, especially the lower limb, and are situated in the subcutaneous tissue or skin.[39-41]

Pathologic Features

Histologically, myofibroma in adults is similar to infantile myofibromatosis. The tumors are well circumscribed but unencapsulated, multinodular, biphasic lesions. They consist of two cellular components (Fig. 3.10): (1) a primitive cellular proliferation of small, ovoid to short spindle cells with scant cytoplasm associated with numerous

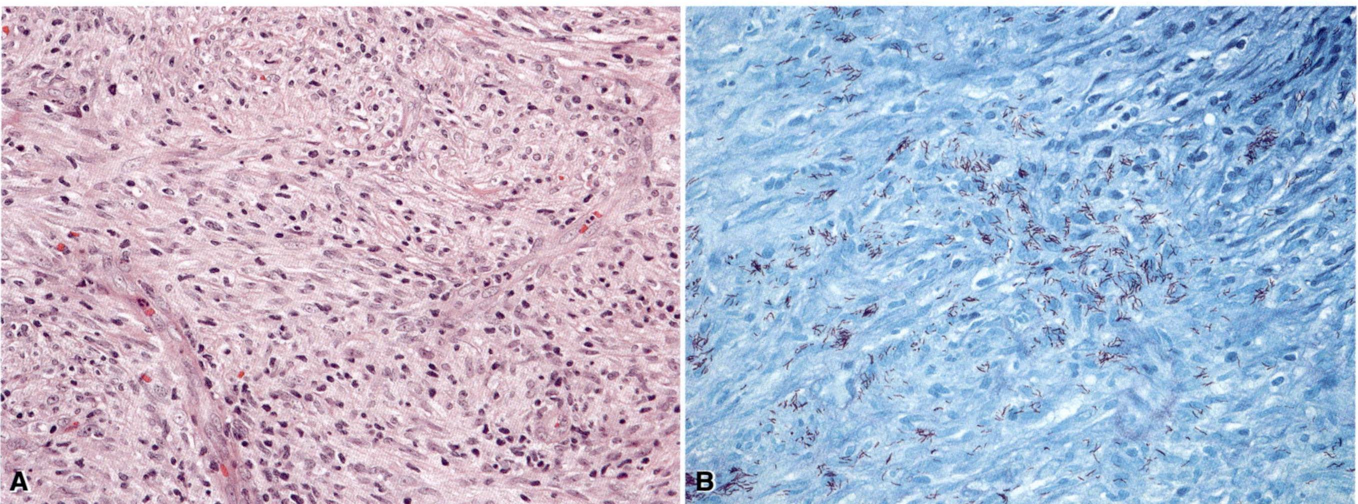

Figure 3.9 Mycobacterial Spindle Cell Pseudotumor. (A) Sheets of spindled to epithelioid histiocytes with pale cytoplasm are typically seen. (B) Numerous mycobacteria can be detected on Ziehl-Neelsen or other acid-fast stains.

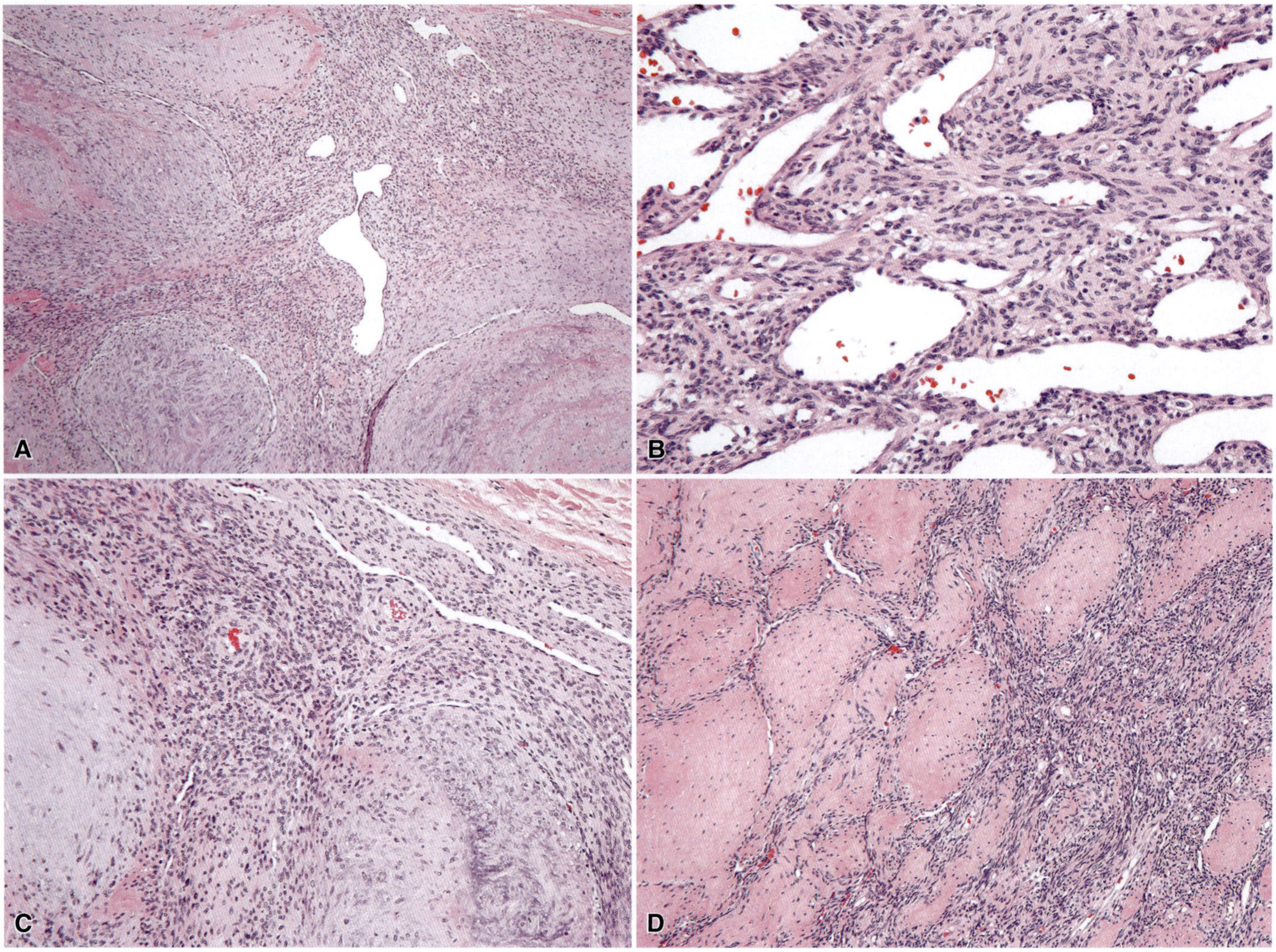

Figure 3.10 Myofibroma. (A) The tumor shows a biphasic appearance: a highly cellular component with prominent thin-walled blood vessels is surrounded by nodular, fascicular areas. (B) The tumor cells in the central area are small and ovoid with a primitive appearance. Note the prominent branching thin-walled blood vessels. (C) A basophilic, pseudochondroid appearance of the myoid nodules is typical. (D) In some myofibromas the myoid nodules show a hyalinized appearance.

thin-walled branching blood vessels (see Fig. 3.10B) and (2) whorled nodules and fascicles of plump spindle cells with tapering nuclei and pale eosinophilic cytoplasm. The two components are present in variable proportions, sometimes haphazardly arranged but more often showing a zonal distribution with the primitive component in the center, surrounded by the myoid whorls. "Reverse zonation" is also possible, with the myoid nodules in the center. The primitive cellular areas are usually less conspicuous than in infantile cases, and some myofibromas are composed nearly exclusively of whorled nodules. The myoid nodules may show a basophilic pseudochondroid appearance (see Fig. 3.10C), as well as prominent stromal hyalinization (see Fig. 3.10D) and calcification, occasionally dominating the lesion and complicating the diagnosis. Similarly, high cellularity and an infiltrative growth pattern are observed in rare cases and should not be overinterpreted as indicators of aggressive behavior.[44] The cytomorphology is consistently bland, and mitotic figures are rare. Tumor nodules typically bulge into thin-walled veins in a subendothelial fashion (Fig. 3.11), often most easily appreciated at the periphery of the lesion; this finding is of no clinical significance.

Myopericytoma is composed of ovoid or plump spindle cells with eosinophilic cytoplasm arranged around numerous thin- and thick-walled blood vessels in a concentric fashion (Fig. 3.12).[45] A typical feature is

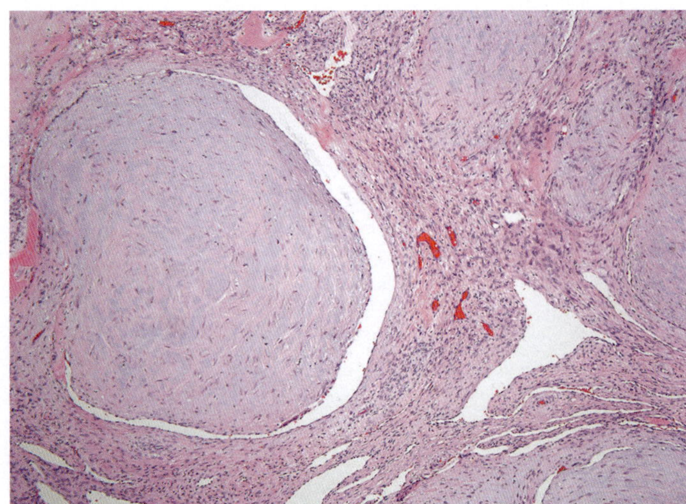

Figure 3.11 Myofibroma. Myoid nodules often protrude into the lumina of thin-walled blood vessels ("telescoping").

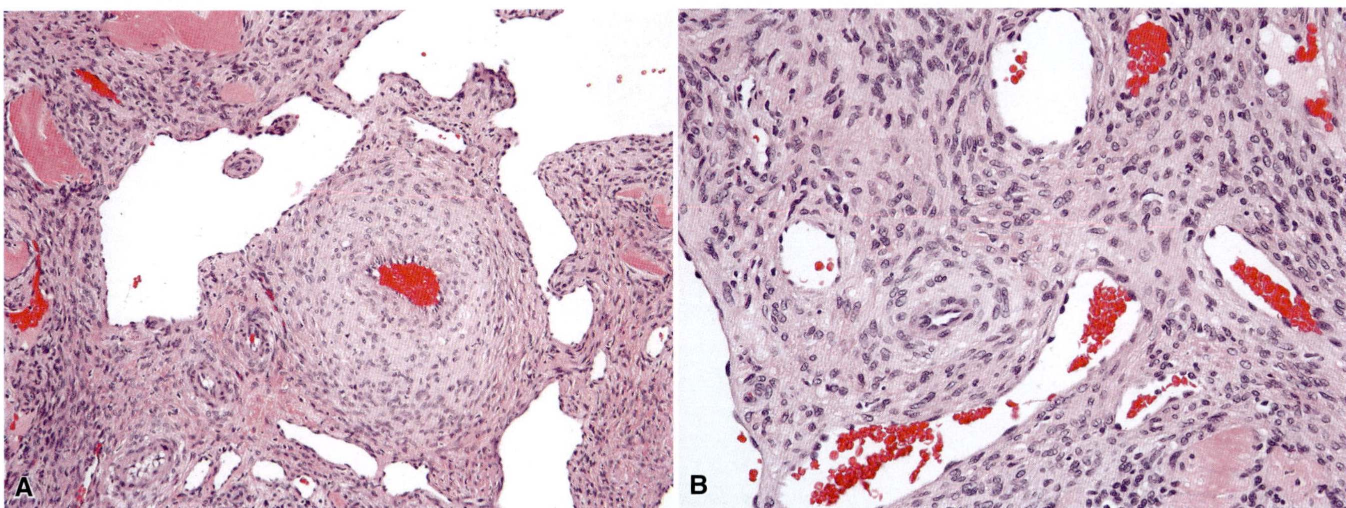

Figure 3.12 Myopericytoma. (A) The tumor is composed of short spindle cells with eosinophilic cytoplasm concentrically arranged around variably thick-walled or dilated, branching blood vessels. (B) The tumor cells contain ovoid to elongated nuclei, pale cytoplasm, and ill-defined cell borders.

the presence of more subtle perivascular cells within the walls of smaller blood vessels beyond the periphery of the main tumor. Occasional examples show areas composed of rounded tumor cells with more sharply defined cell borders (similar to glomus tumor/glomangiopericytoma). Other cases contain perivascular cells that resemble smooth muscle cells (indistinguishable from angioleiomyoma), whereas some tumors contain myoid nodules similar to those of myofibroma. The spectrum of histologic features that may be observed within individual tumors suggests that myofibroma and myopericytoma (and even glomus tumor [see Chapter 6] and angioleiomyoma) lie on a continuum.[41] In terms of nomenclature, tumors that are difficult to separate into one category due to overlapping histology may be designated *myopericytoma/myofibroma*.

Very rarely, myopericytomas show features of malignancy, in the form of marked nuclear atypia and a high mitotic rate. Such tumors may pursue an aggressive clinical course.[46]

Immunohistochemistry

The tumor cells in both myofibroma and myopericytoma are extensively positive for smooth muscle actin and often for h-caldesmon, whereas desmin is focally positive in only a small subset of cases. The primitive, cellular component in myofibroma typically shows less smooth muscle actin expression than the myoid nodules. Tumor cells are negative for S-100 protein, EMA, keratins, and CD34, although CD34 highlights the prominent vascular component.

Molecular Genetics

Myofibromas are characterized by activating *PDGFRB* mutations. Germline heterozygous p.R561C and p.P660T *PDGFRB* mutations were first identified in familial infantile myofibromatosis.[47,48] Subsequently, approximately 70% of sporadic solitary myofibromas were found to harbor gain-of-function mutations in exons 12 and 14 of *PDGFRB*[49]; almost every sporadic case in that study had a combination of two heterozygous *PDGFRB* mutations, an intriguing finding that, if validated, would suggest that transformation in myofibroma requires gain-of-function mutation of both *PDGFRB* alleles or, alternatively, that two mutations *in cis* are required to fully activate *PDGFRB* in this context. Mutations in other genes such as *NOTCH3* have been described, indicating some degree of genetic heterogeneity. A small group of malignant myopericytomas and spindle cell sarcomas with features resembling myofibromatosis show *NTRK1* gene fusions.[50]

Differential Diagnosis

The differential diagnosis of myofibroma includes nodular fasciitis, fibroma of tendon sheath, leiomyoma, dermatomyofibroma, and, as described previously, other perivascular myoid lesions, myopericytoma, and glomangiopericytoma (see Chapter 6). Nodular fasciitis typically contains looser fascicles than myofibroma with variably prominent myxoid stroma and extravasated erythrocytes, and it lacks the biphasic pattern and the prominent thin-walled branching vessels of myofibroma. Fibroma of tendon sheath also lacks the biphasic architecture of myofibroma and usually contains more collagenous stroma with slitlike blood vessels at the tumor periphery. Leiomyoma shows a more homogeneously fascicular growth pattern, with longer spindle cells with brightly eosinophilic cytoplasm. Although both leiomyoma and myofibroma are positive for smooth muscle actin, only leiomyomas show diffuse and strong desmin expression. Dermatomyofibroma (see Chapter 15), which is a plaquelike dermal proliferation of fibroblasts and myofibroblasts arranged parallel to the epidermis, lacks the nodular growth pattern and the biphasic appearance of myofibroma. Other perivascular myoid lesions usually lack the classic biphasic appearance and myoid nodules of myofibroma: in myopericytoma, the short spindle cells are concentrically arranged around vascular lumina in an "onionskin" (multilayered) pattern, whereas glomangiopericytoma tends to have larger, more dilated vessels surrounded by rounded cells with sharp cell borders; however, the morphologic overlap among these lesions is significant and the distinction can sometimes be purely semantic.

Prognosis and Treatment

Adult myofibroma and myopericytoma are benign tumors that rarely recur following marginal or even intralesional excision. Recurrences likely represent continued growth after incomplete excision. Simple surgical excision is adequate treatment. Occasionally, patients develop additional lesions, usually in the same anatomic region. Rare aggressive tumors or extensive lesions not amenable to surgical resection harboring *PDGFRB* mutations or *NTRK1* fusions may benefit from treatment with imatinib, nilotinib, or similar tyrosine kinase inhibitors.[51]

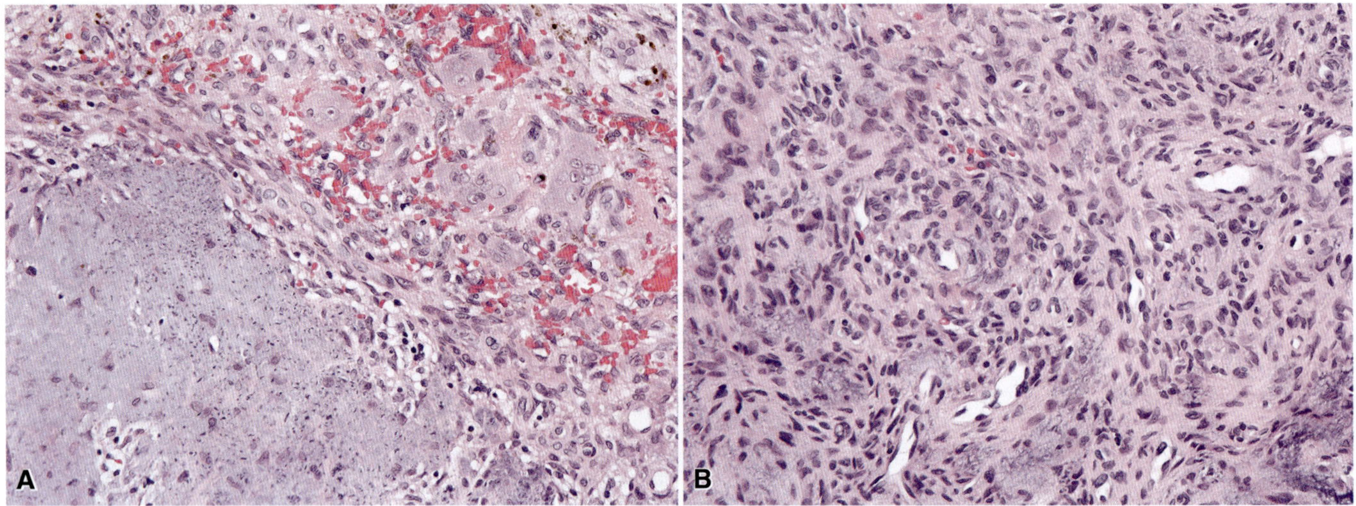

Figure 3.13 **Phosphaturic Mesenchymal Tumor.** (A) The tumor shows a heterogeneous appearance, with spindled-to-stellate cells admixed with osteoclast-like giant cells. The matrix typically contains flocculent ("grungy") calcification. (B) Some phosphaturic mesenchymal tumors contain plumper spindle cells with a myofibroma/myopericytoma-like appearance. Note the arrangement around blood vessels.

PRACTICE POINTS: Myofibroma and Myopericytoma

- Myofibroma and myopericytoma lie on a histologic continuum
- Presentation is a painless subcutaneous nodule, in adults most often solitary but occasionally multiple
- Myofibroma is typically biphasic with small ovoid cells with scant cytoplasm associated with numerous thin-walled blood vessels and whorled nodules of plump myoid spindle cells
- Myoid nodules often show a pseudochondroid appearance
- Myoid nodules typically bulge into the lumina of veins
- Myopericytoma is composed of spindle cells with eosinophilic cytoplasm arranged around thin- and thick-walled blood vessels

Phosphaturic Mesenchymal Tumor

Phosphaturic mesenchymal tumor (PMT), also referred to as "PMT, mixed connective tissue variant," is a rare distinctive mesenchymal neoplasm that may arise in both soft tissue and bone and is characterized by somewhat heterogeneous but recognizable histologic appearances. It frequently elicits a clinical paraneoplastic syndrome consisting of hypophosphatemic (hyperphosphaturic) osteomalacia.[52-54]

Clinical Features

PMT usually affects middle-aged adults with an equal gender distribution. The tumor arises at a wide range of anatomic locations with a predilection for the extremities (especially the thigh and foot). Similar numbers of cases arise primarily in soft tissue (either superficial or deep) and bone. The symptomatology is usually related to long-standing, vitamin D–resistant, severe osteomalacia, leading to stress fractures and pain. Laboratory testing reveals hypophosphatemia and hyperphosphaturia, normocalcemia, and increased serum alkaline phosphatase.[52,53] Rarely, morphologically identical lesions occur without the clinical syndrome or identifiable laboratory abnormalities.[54] Radiologic features are not distinctive.

Pathologic Features

Histologically, PMT has a range of appearances, being composed of variable proportions of bland spindled-to-stellate cells, adipocytes, and osteoclast-type giant cells embedded in an abundant extracellular chondromyxoid to hyalinized matrix with irregular, coarsely granular, or flocculent calcifications (Fig. 3.13). The tumors usually contain a prominent vasculature, consisting of small capillaries and medium-sized blood vessels, some with an ectatic, branching, HPC-like appearance. In some cases the tumor cells focally have a more myoid or glomoid appearance and are situated around blood vessel walls (see Fig. 3.13B). Perivascular hyalinization, osteoid deposition, and microcystic or hemorrhagic changes are common. A rim of ossification may be present at the periphery of the lesion. The tumor cellularity is usually low, and the cytomorphology is bland, with fine chromatin and small nucleoli, and mitotic activity is scant or absent. Very rare cases show increased cellularity, larger nuclear size and pleomorphism, and a mitotic rate greater than 5 per 10 HPF, which may be associated with malignant behavior.

Tumors occurring in bone usually have similar histologic features as the cases affecting soft tissues but may sometimes resemble other bone tumors. These conditions have accordingly been designated *osteoblastoma-like*, *nonossifying fibroma–like*, and *ossifying fibroma–like* variants of PMT.[53]

Immunohistochemistry

Conventional immunohistochemical markers are not useful in the diagnosis of PMT. A minority of tumors shows focal expression of smooth muscle actin. Tumor cells are negative for CD34, desmin, S-100 protein, and keratins. Approximately 80% of PMT express FGFR1, but expression in some morphologic mimics (such as 40% of SFT) reduces the diagnostic value of this marker. Immunohistochemical detection of fibroblast growth factor 23 (FGF23) has been used in research settings; the majority of cases tested have been positive.[54]

Molecular Genetics

Two recurrent gene fusions have been detected in PMT: *FN1-FGFR1* and *FN1-FGF1*, in 40% and 5% of cases, respectively.[55,56] The structure of both fusion proteins suggests an autocrine/paracrine mechanism of activation of the FGFR1 signaling pathway, both by FGF1 and other ligands such as FGF23. Secretion of FGF23 by tumor cells is believed to be responsible for the oncogenic osteomalacia that affects patients with PMT, by inhibiting renal tubular phosphate transport. More than 90% of cases of PMT with oncogenic osteomalacia express FGF23, as well as 75% of histologically identical tumors that present without the clinical paraneoplastic syndrome.[57] Although identifying FGF23 expression by tumor cells may be useful to confirm the diagnosis of PMT and may provide insights into the mechanisms leading to hyperphosphaturia in some cases, its diagnostic value is limited due to the existence of cases of PMT lacking FGF23 expression (likely expressing alternative phosphaturic factors), and, more importantly, the expression of FGF23 by other mesenchymal tumors that do not induce osteomalacia. Detection of a *FGFR1* or *FGF1* rearrangement by FISH will provide strong confirmatory evidence in the appropriate context, albeit with low sensitivity.

Differential Diagnosis

The integration of clinical information and morphologic features allows for the diagnosis of PMT; however, without the suggestive clinical context, the differential diagnosis may be broad given the relative polymorphism of these lesions, including morphologic findings that may be misinterpreted as reactive changes. The vascular pattern in PMT may suggest SFT, which is usually a more cellular lesion that contains more prominent thicker-walled branching blood vessels, lacks the calcified chondromyxoid matrix of PMT, and is usually diffusely positive for CD34 and STAT6. On the other hand, soft tissue chondroma may show a similar calcification pattern and may contain osteoclast-like giant cells; however, it lacks the bland spindled-to-stellate cells and the adipocytic component typical of PMT. Cases with prominent myoid cells may be confused with myofibroma, but the latter tumor type lacks the flocculent calcification and osteoclast-like giant cells of PMT.

Prognosis and Treatment

Most PMT are clinically benign, although occasional cases recur locally.[53,54] Complete resection of the tumor results in recovery of osteomalacia, as well as remission of the clinical symptoms and laboratory abnormalities. Exceptional malignant examples can usually be recognized on morphologic grounds (based on increased cellularity, marked nuclear atypia, and high mitotic activity).[54] Malignant PMT has a significant potential for local recurrence and may also metastasize. The efficacy of FGFR inhibitors to treat PMT and tumor-induced osteomalacia is being tested in clinical trials.

Myofibroblastoma and Variants

Mammary-Type Myofibroblastoma

Primary soft tissue tumors indistinguishable from myofibroblastoma of the breast are designated *mammary-type* or *extramammary myofibroblastoma* (see Chapter 17). Similar to its breast counterparts,[58] mammary-type myofibroblastoma is a benign neoplasm related to spindle cell lipoma, which most frequently affects older male patients and arises in subcutaneous tissue.[59] The anatomic distribution is wide, with approximately 40% of cases located in the groin or inguinal region and 5% to 10% of cases in the trunk or lower extremities; rare cases are deep seated, in intracavitary or visceral locations.[60] The tumor is well circumscribed but unencapsulated and consists of a haphazard arrangement of variably sized fascicles of spindled to ovoid cell, embedded in a collagenous stroma with interspersed thick hyalinized collagen bundles (Fig. 3.14). The cytomorphology is similar to that of spindle cell lipoma, with spindle cells containing short stubby nuclei and ill-defined, scant palely eosinophilic to amphophilic cytoplasm (see Fig. 3.14B). Focal cytologic atypia or occasional multinucleated cells may be seen. An adipocytic component is often present, sometimes predominating, which can show variability in adipocyte size but lacks atypical adipocytes or true lipoblasts. Stromal mast cells can be prominent. Mitoses may be easily identified (sometimes more than 5 per 10 HPF), but atypical mitotic figures are absent. By immunohistochemistry, the lesional cells are usually positive for both desmin and CD34, whereas RB1 expression is lost in approximately 90% of cases.[61] Expression of smooth muscle actin and S-100 is uncommon.[59] The molecular genetic features of mammary-type myofibroblastoma are identical to those of spindle cell lipoma and consist of monoallelic or biallelic deletions of chromosome 13q (in particular 13q14), sometimes in combination with monosomy 16q.[62,63]

The differential diagnosis of mammary-type myofibroblastoma of soft tissue is wide and, depending on the anatomic location, may include benign lesions such as spindle cell lipoma, cellular angiofibroma, angiomyofibroblastoma, soft tissue perineurioma, and SFT, and intermediate and malignant tumors such as DFSP, atypical spindle cell lipomatous tumor, and low-grade MPNST. Spindle cell lipoma shows significant morphologic overlap with mammary-type myofibroblastoma, although subtle differences exist. Mammary-type myofibroblastoma usually contains a less prominent adipocytic component than spindle cell lipoma and shows a more fascicular architecture; the background collagenous stroma is generally more prominent, with thick collagen bundles, sometimes arranged in a zigzag pattern. In contrast to spindle cell lipoma, mammary-type myofibroblastoma is typically positive for desmin in addition to CD34. Cellular angiofibroma contains hyalinized blood

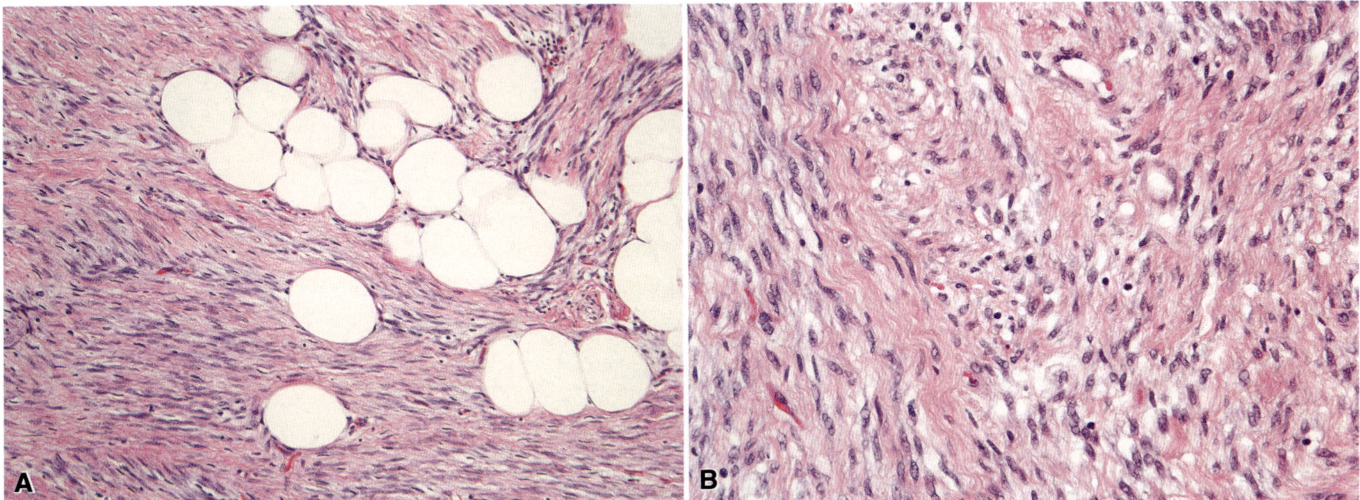

Figure 3.14 Mammary-Type Myofibroblastoma. (A) The lesion is composed of fascicles of spindle cells in a collagenous stroma. Note the adipocytic component. (B) The tumor cells contain short nuclei and scant indistinct cytoplasm, similar to spindle cell lipoma.

vessels, which are not a feature of mammary-type myofibroblastoma. In addition, although CD34 may be positive, desmin and smooth muscle actin are usually negative. Angiomyofibroblastoma mainly affects female patients and is characterized by prominent small vessels and a population of rounded, usually perivascular cells that are typically desmin positive. Particularly in postmenopausal women, angiomyofibroblastoma may have a more hyalinized stroma and a more spindled appearance and thus more closely resemble mammary-type myofibroblastoma. Desmin is often negative in such cases (see Chapter 17). Soft tissue perineurioma is composed of slender spindle cells with long bipolar cytoplasmic processes that are usually arranged in a storiform to whorled (rather than fascicular) pattern and express EMA but are negative for desmin. SFT may also enter the differential diagnosis of mammary-type myofibroblastoma in that it is a well-circumscribed, CD34-positive spindle cell lesion with a ubiquitous anatomic distribution, sometimes containing adipocytes (fat-forming SFT). SFT has a patternless appearance, lacking the fascicular architecture of mammary-type myofibroblastoma, and contains prominent HPC-like branching, dilated vessels. Desmin positivity is rare in SFT and usually very focal when present; STAT6 is specific for SFT in this differential diagnosis.

DFSP potentially may also enter into the differential diagnosis if a small biopsy showing tumor infiltration into fat is examined. DFSP arises in the dermis, rather than deeper soft tissues, is usually markedly hypercellular with a tight storiform architecture, and shows diffuse infiltration of adipose tissue. Although the tumor cells are positive for CD34, they are negative for desmin. Atypical spindle cell lipomatous tumor is generally larger, with more stromal and adipocytic nuclear atypia including scattered hyperchromatic cells and variation in adipocyte size. Lipoblasts can generally be found. The spindle cells of low-grade MPNST typically contain more tapering or buckled nuclei with cytologic atypia and often show perivascular accentuation. Tumor cells are usually negative for desmin, whereas 40% to 50% of MPNSTs are positive for S-100 protein or SOX10 (although the expression is typically only focal in distribution).

Mammary-type myofibroblastoma is a benign lesion, with no potential to recur or metastasize. Simple surgical excision is adequate treatment.[59]

Intranodal Palisaded Myofibroblastoma

So-called *palisaded myofibroblastoma* is a benign intranodal myofibroblastic proliferation with a predilection for the inguinal lymph nodes. It has also been referred to as *intranodal hemorrhagic spindle cell tumor with amianthoid fibers*, reflecting two prominent histologic features: the deposition of abundant extracellular collagen bundles, resulting in stellate crystalline structures, and frequent interstitial hemorrhage. The tumors affect middle-aged adults as a painless mass, males being affected twice as frequently as females. Most cases have been described in the inguinal lymph nodes, some also in a submandibular location.[64,65]

The lesion usually occupies the center of the lymph node, with scattered hemorrhagic areas (Fig. 3.15). Histologically, the most distinctive feature is the presence of abundant deposits of eosinophilic fibrillary material (amianthoid fibers) (Fig. 3.16), composed of collagens type I and III.[66] The fascicles of spindle cells are interspersed within these structures, often with a radial arrangement showing prominent nuclear palisading (see Fig. 3.16). The cells show bland myofibroblastic morphology, with small ovoid nuclei and scant palely eosinophilic cytoplasm. Paranuclear eosinophilic globules may be present. Interstitial hemorrhage with hemosiderin deposition is often prominent.[67] Focal myxoid stroma may be present, resulting in areas reminiscent of nodular fasciitis. Metaplastic bone formation has been described.[68] Hotspot mutations in *CTNNB1* have been identified in intranodal myofibroblastoma, leading to nuclear expression of β-catenin and cyclin D1.[69,70] The tumor cells

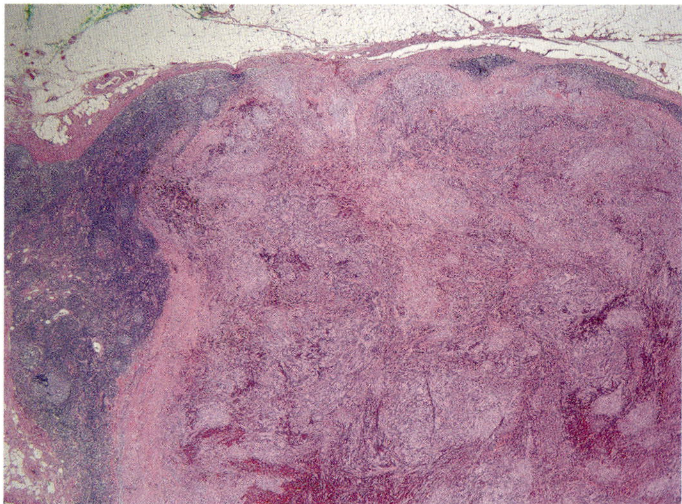

Figure 3.15 Intranodal Palisaded Myofibroblastoma. The tumor is composed of fascicles of myofibroblastic spindle cells. Note the areas of hemorrhage.

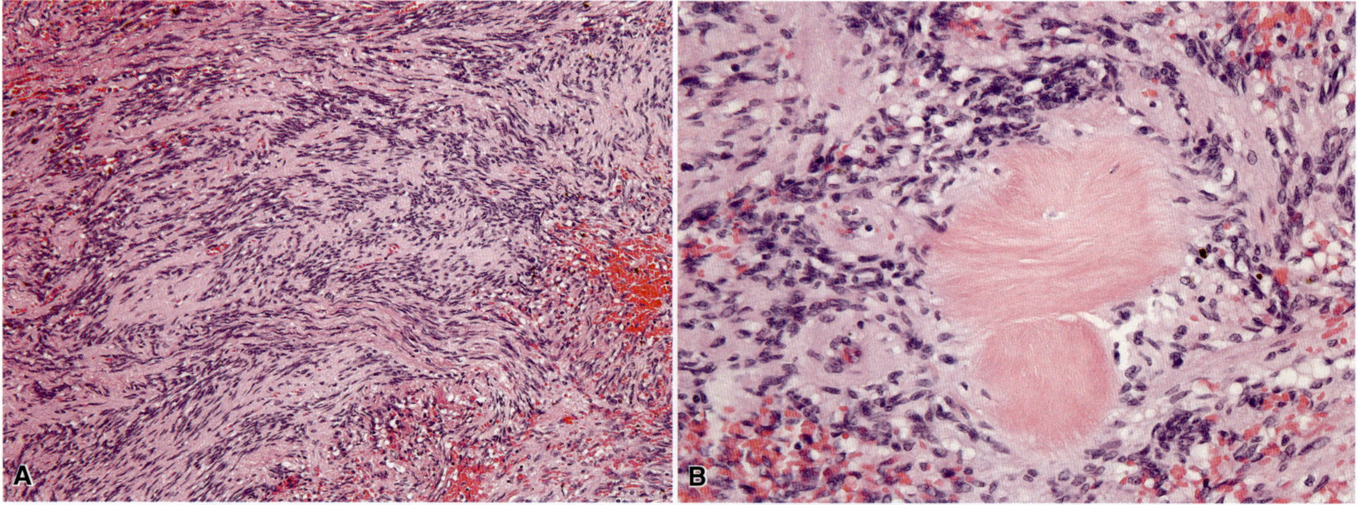

Figure 3.16 Intranodal Palisaded Myofibroblastoma. (A) Nuclear palisading may be striking. (B) Deposits of eosinophilic, fibrillary collagen (amianthoid-like fibers) are a distinctive feature. Note the bland cytology and tapering nuclei.

also express smooth muscle actin but only occasionally desmin, and they are negative for CD34 and S-100.[67]

The diagnosis of intranodal myofibroblastoma is usually straightforward due to the presence of amianthoid fiber–like extracellular material. However, in some cases, schwannoma, dendritic cell sarcomas, and Kaposi sarcoma may conceivably enter the differential diagnosis. Schwannoma typically shows alternating cellular (Antoni A) and hypocellular areas with hyalinization of vessel walls, in addition to diffuse, strong expression of S-100 protein. Dendritic cell sarcomas often show a syncytial growth pattern with prominent intratumoral lymphocytes and at least mild nuclear atypia. Follicular dendritic cell sarcomas are positive for CD21 and CD35, whereas interdigitating dendritic cell sarcomas express S-100 protein. Kaposi sarcoma often shows a fascicular architecture with prominent slitlike spaces and hemorrhage. The clinical context should help in the diagnosis of Kaposi sarcoma (see Chapter 13), in addition to expression of CD34 and human herpesvirus 8, which are absent in intranodal myofibroblastoma.[67,70]

Intranodal myofibroblastoma is a benign lesion, for which simple surgical excision is adequate treatment. Exceptional cases of recurrence and multifocality have been reported.[68,71] The tumor has no potential to metastasize.

Fibroma

The term *fibroma* has been applied to variety of lesions composed of spindle cells set in an abundant collagenous stroma. Many different types of fibroma have been described based on location (e.g., fibroma of tendon sheath, nasopharyngeal fibroma [angiofibroma], nuchal-type fibroma), composition (e.g., sclerotic fibroma [storiform collagenoma] of the skin, desmoplastic fibroblastoma, elastofibroma), or association with specific syndromes (Gardner fibroma). Of note, the nonspecific designation "fibroma" should be avoided because this term does not refer to a specific soft tissue tumor type. The cutaneous lesions (storiform collagenoma/sclerotic fibroma, pleomorphic fibroma) are discussed in Chapter 15. Nasopharyngeal angiofibroma and Gardner fibroma are discussed in Chapter 4.

Fibroma of Tendon Sheath

Clinical Features

Fibroma of tendon sheath is a rare tumor that most often arises in the hands of adults between 20 and 50 years of age, with a 2 : 1 male predominance. It usually occurs as a well-circumscribed, slowly growing, painless nodule attached to tendons. The thumb, index finger, middle finger, and wrist are predominantly affected (80% of cases). Less frequently, it may develop on the sole of the foot or close to the knee. Pain or trigger finger are occasional presenting symptoms.

Despite similarities in clinical presentation and gross appearance, there is no good evidence that fibroma of tendon sheath and localized tenosynovial giant cell tumor (giant cell tumor of tendon sheath) are related.

Pathologic Features

Fibroma of tendon sheath is usually small (0.5 to 2 cm) and firm. Cut section reveals a glistening, gray-white, sometimes multilobulated lesion.

Histologically, fibroma of tendon sheath is a well-delineated hypocellular collagenous lobulated nodule containing spindled to stellate fibroblasts; thin-walled, curvilinear blood vessels; and stromal pseudovascular spaces (Fig. 3.17). Some fibromas of tendon sheath may contain hypercellular areas composed of tightly apposed, bland-appearing fibroblasts, resembling nodular fasciitis (Fig. 3.18). Multinucleated osteoclast-like giant cells are usually absent. Myxoid change, cyst formation, or areas of osseous or cartilaginous metaplasia may occasionally be seen. Rare examples of fibroma of tendon sheath contain few pleomorphic cells (showing degenerative nuclear atypia).

Immunohistochemistry

The tumor cells often express smooth muscle actin but are negative for desmin, CD34, keratins, EMA, and S-100 protein.

Molecular Genetics

A translocation t(2;11)(q31;q12) has been reported in fibroma of tendon sheath.[72] Interestingly, similar chromosomal abnormalities involving the region 11q12 have been observed in desmoplastic fibroblastoma (collagenous fibroma), suggesting a potential relationship between these two entities.[73]

Differential Diagnosis

The differential diagnosis of fibroma of tendon sheath primarily includes nodular fasciitis and superficial fibromatoses, although fibrous histiocytoma, giant cell tumor of tendon sheath, and soft tissue chondroma (if cartilaginous metaplasia is present) may also be considered. Nodular fasciitis rarely arises on the hands and fingers. In contrast to fibroma of tendon sheath, nodular fasciitis is composed of loose fascicles of

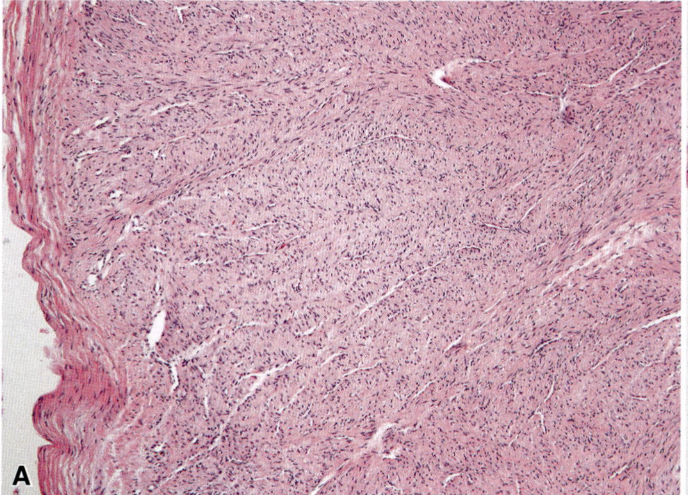

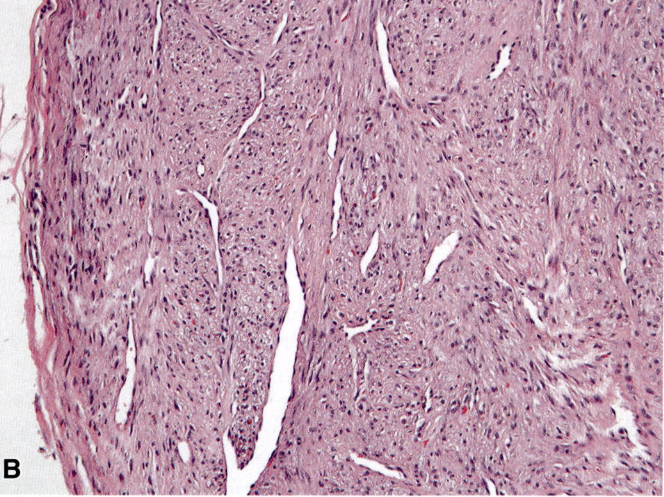

Figure 3.17 Fibroma of Tendon Sheath. (A) The lesion is hypocellular with small spindled fibroblasts and prominent stromal collagen. (B) Slitlike vessels are typically seen at the tumor periphery.

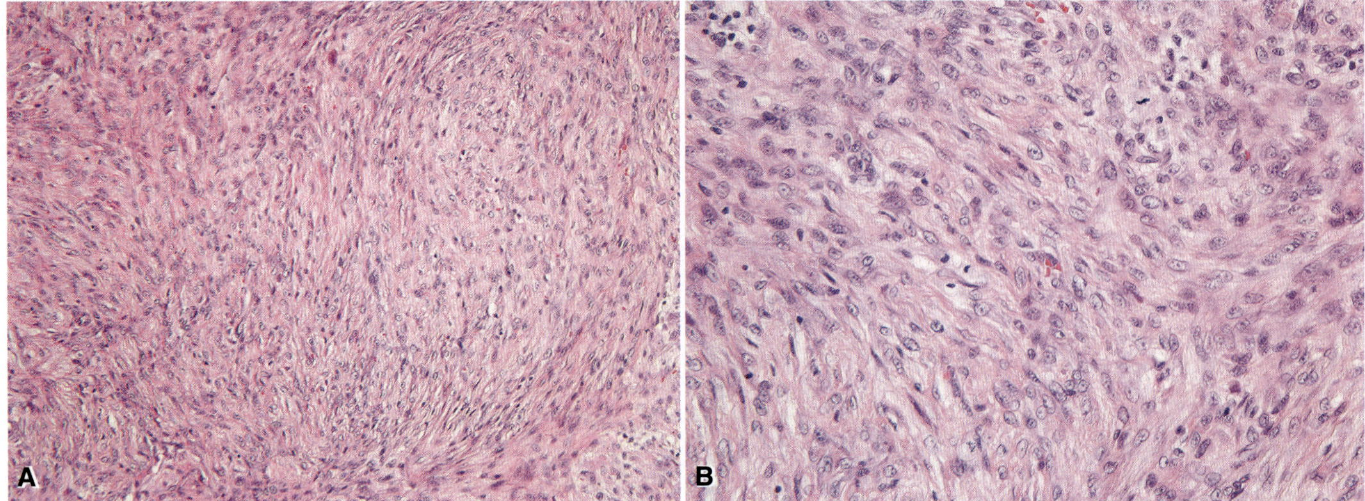

Figure 3.18 **Fibroma of Tendon Sheath.** (A) Some hypercellular examples superficially resemble nodular fasciitis. (B) The tumor is composed of short spindle cells with plump ovoid nuclei and small nucleoli. Note the presence of mitotic activity.

plump spindle cells with a "tissue culture"-like appearance including microcysts and extravasated erythrocytes, and it typically lacks prominent stromal collagen and peripheral slitlike blood vessels. Palmar fibromatosis shows a more nodular, infiltrative growth pattern. Fibrous histiocytoma involves the skin and is composed of a more heterogeneous cellular population with short spindle cells, lymphocytes, and foamy macrophages, and it shows peripheral collagen entrapment. Giant cell tumor of tendon sheath is dominated by small mononuclear histiocytoid cells, instead of spindle cells. Soft tissue chondroma is a uniformly cartilaginous lesion with a multinodular growth pattern.

Prognosis and Treatment

Fibroma of tendon sheath may recur locally after simple excision (up to 20% to 25% of cases) but does not metastasize. Reexcision is usually curative.

Desmoplastic Fibroblastoma (Collagenous Fibroma)

Described by Evans in 1995 desmoplastic fibroblastoma is an uncommon benign soft tissue tumor.[74] The term *collagenous fibroma,* which emphasizes its hypocellular appearance and the presence of marked stromal collagenization, is an alternative designation.[75,76]

Clinical Features

Desmoplastic fibroblastoma usually arises in deep subcutaneous tissue or less often in skeletal muscle (25% of cases) of middle-aged adults, with a male predominance (male-to-female ratio, 3:1). Most patients experience gradual development of a slow growing, painless mass, measuring 3 to 4 cm on average. The lesion can occur at nearly any anatomic site, although the upper extremities (shoulder, upper arm, forearm) are predominantly affected.

Pathologic Features

Grossly, desmoplastic fibroblastoma is a well-delineated, firm, ovoid mass with a gray, sometimes glistening cut surface. Histologically, it is relatively well circumscribed but unencapsulated (Fig. 3.19), with a paucicellular, variably collagenous, sometimes multinodular appearance (Fig. 3.20). Peripheral entrapment of adipose tissue or skeletal muscle is common (see Fig. 3.20A). The key diagnostic feature is the presence of characteristic, widely spaced, spindle-shaped to stellate fibroblasts within edematous to fibromyxoid stroma (see Fig. 3.20B). Tumor cell nuclei are bland with open chromatin and small central nucleoli. Cytologic atypia and tumor necrosis are absent; mitoses are very rare. Intratumoral vessels are scarce.

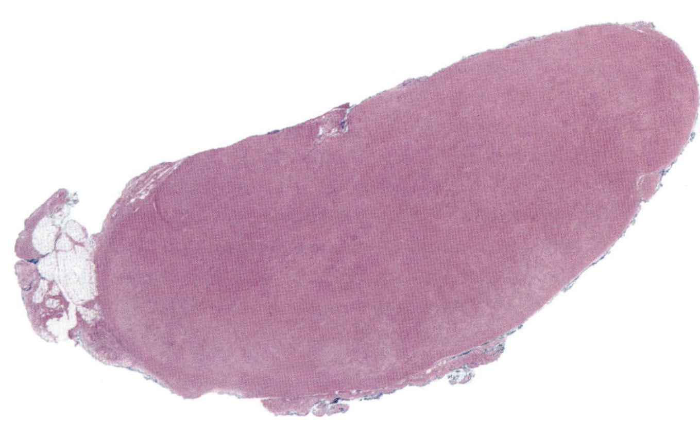

Figure 3.19 **Desmoplastic Fibroblastoma.** The tumor is relatively well circumscribed but may entrap adjacent adipose tissue. Note the ovoid appearance of the tumor nodule.

Immunohistochemistry

The tumor cells may focally express muscle-specific actin (clone HHF35) and smooth muscle actin. They are negative for desmin, CD34, and S-100 protein.[76] Immunohistochemical detection of FOSL1 expression has been used in research settings but has not been yet validated for clinical purposes.[77]

Molecular Genetics

Alterations of the 11q12 region, including translocation t(2;11)(q31;q12) similar to that observed in fibroma of tendon sheath, have been reported in several desmoplastic fibroblastomas.[73,78] *FOSL1*has been proposed as the target gene of the 11q12 rearrangements in desmoplastic fibroblastoma.[79]

Differential Diagnosis

The differential diagnosis of desmoplastic fibroblastoma includes nodular fasciitis, fibroma of tendon sheath (if the lesion is in close proximity to tendons), and desmoid fibromatosis. Nodular fasciitis is generally a

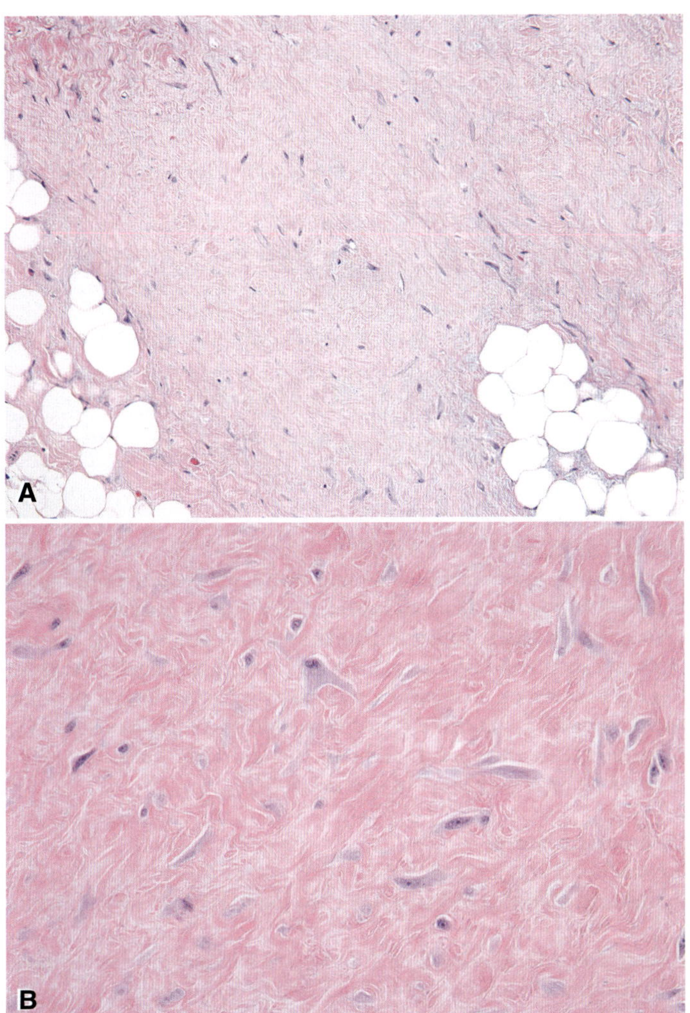

Figure 3.20 Desmoplastic Fibroblastoma. (A) The tumor is hypocellular with a collagenous stroma. Note the entrapped adjacent adipose tissue. (B) The tumor cells show characteristic stellate cytomorphology. Note the fine chromatin and small nucleoli.

more cellular lesion with a more fascicular architecture and microcystic degeneration, and it lacks the typical stellate fibroblasts. Fibroma of tendon sheath is also more cellular and fascicular with prominent stromal collagen and peripheral slitlike blood vessels. Desmoid fibromatosis is composed of long, sweeping fascicles of more elongated spindle cells with medium-sized blood vessels between fascicles. Nuclear staining for β-catenin supports the diagnosis of desmoid fibromatosis.

Prognosis and Treatment

Simple excision is curative. Desmoplastic fibroblastoma shows no tendency for local recurrence.

Nuchal-Type Fibroma

Nuchal-type fibroma is an unusual collagenous lesion that may easily be confused with a nonspecific fibrosing process. This lesion shows histologic overlap with Gardner fibroma (see Chapter 4).

Clinical Features

Nuchal-type fibroma presents as a subcutaneous mass that is localized most frequently, but not exclusively, in the posterior neck region of middle-aged adults (30 to 50 years of age). It has a predilection for men.[80,81] Rare cases have been observed in the face, upper back, or lumbar region. Approximately 40% to 50% of patients with nuchal-type fibroma have diabetes mellitus.[81] Unlike Gardner fibroma, nuchal-type fibroma is not associated with familial adenomatous polyposis or desmoid tumors.

Pathologic Features

Grossly, nuchal-type fibroma generally measures between 2 and 8 cm in maximal diameter (median, 3 to 4 cm) and presents as an ill-defined fibrous mass with a gray to white cut surface.

Histologically, nuchal-type fibroma is paucicellular, composed of an admixture of thick bundles of hyalinized collagen, few bland spindled fibroblasts, and entrapped islands of subcutaneous fatty tissue (Fig. 3.21). A cracking artifact between collagen bundles is common (see Fig. 3.21B). Inflammation is minimal, although stromal mast cells may be observed. The lesion also contains a variable number of elastic fibers (similar to elastofibroma), as well as small blood vessels and small nerves

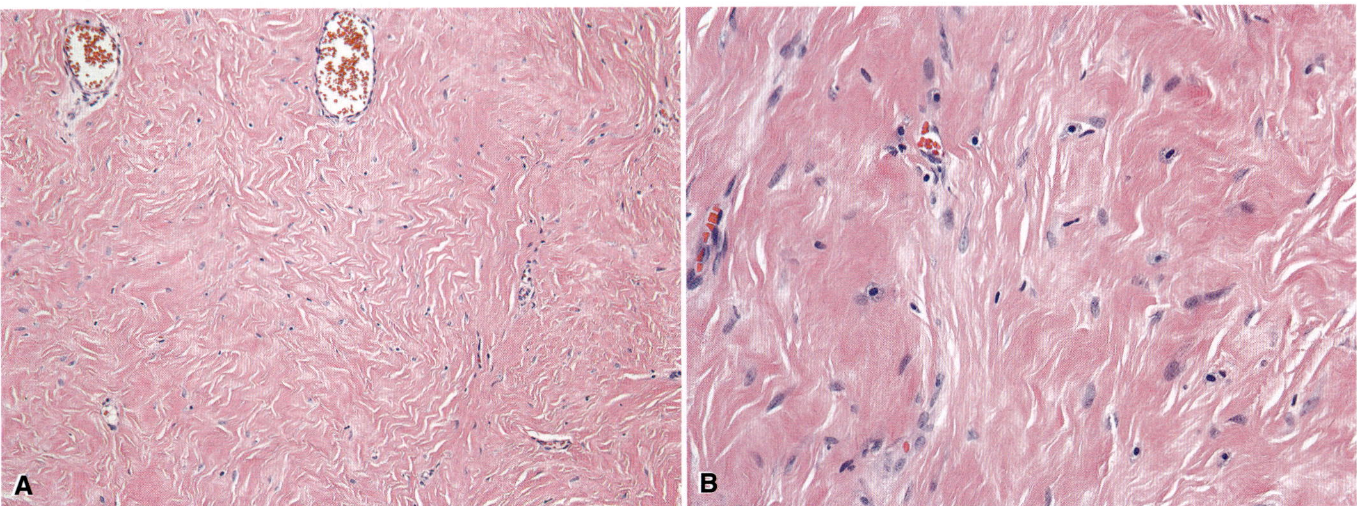

Figure 3.21 Nuchal-Type Fibroma. (A) This lesion is hypocellular with abundant collagenous stroma. (B) A cracking artifact may be seen between collagen bundles. Note the small, nondescript spindled tumor cells and scattered mast cells.

(sometimes resembling traumatic neuroma) (Fig. 3.22). Nuchal-type fibroma may extend into underlying skeletal muscle.

Immunohistochemistry

The lesional fibroblasts usually express CD34 (70% to 80% of cases) and are negative for smooth muscle actin, desmin, S-100 protein, and β-catenin.

Differential Diagnosis

The main differential diagnosis of nuchal-type fibroma is Gardner fibroma (see Chapter 4). The two lesions are nearly indistinguishable morphologically, although the bundles of small nerves typically observed in nuchal-type fibroma are lacking in Gardner fibroma. In contrast to nuchal-type fibroma, Gardner fibroma occurs in infants, children, and adolescents; has no gender predilection; and has no association with diabetes mellitus.[82] Gardner fibroma is highly associated with familial adenomatous polyposis, desmoid fibromatosis, and germline mutations of *APC* (at least 50% to 70% of cases).[82,83] Fibroblasts in both tumor types are positive for CD34, but only Gardner fibroma shows nuclear staining for β-catenin. Any lesion with nuchal-type fibroma morphology that occurs in children should be considered a Gardner fibroma, requiring additional clinical (and familial) investigation.

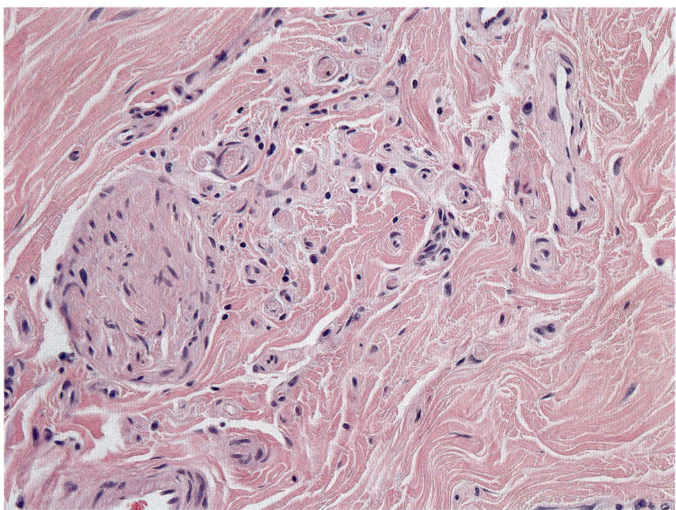

Figure 3.22 Nuchal-Type Fibroma. Clusters of small nerves are often seen within the lesion.

Prognosis and Treatment

Nuchal-type fibroma is benign. Nondestructive local recurrence may occur, but reexcision is usually curative.

PRACTICE POINTS: Nuchal-Type Fibroma

- Typical presentation is on the posterior neck of middle-aged adult men
- Paucicellular lesion with thick hyalinized collagen bundles and few bland spindle cells
- Cracking artifact between collagen bundles is typical
- Entrapped small nerves are often seen
- Essentially indistinguishable from Gardner fibroma

Elastofibroma

Clinical Features

Elastofibroma is an uncommon lesion that develops in the soft tissues between the lower scapula and chest wall of elderly patients (60 to 80 years of age), with a female predominance.[84-86] The lesion can be bilateral (10% of cases) and may occasionally occur in extrascapular locations (e.g., deltoid region, oral cavity). It usually presents as a slow growing, generally painless soft tissue mass. Some patients complain of limitation of motion. Repetitive local trauma is thought to be causative, many patients reporting a history of manual labor.[86]

Pathologic Features

Elastofibroma is as an ill-defined, infiltrative mass measuring 5 to 10 cm in maximal diameter. On sectioning, the lesion is composed of mature adipose tissue intermixed with whitish firm fibrous tissue. Histologically, elastofibroma is composed of a variable admixture of elastic fibers, collagen, mature adipose tissue, and spindled fibroblasts (Fig. 3.23). The hallmark of the lesion is elastic fibers that are characteristically numerous, large, eosinophilic, and fragmented, arranged in cords or globoid structures. They are scattered throughout a hypocellular collagenous stroma. Myxoid and even cystic change can be observed in the collagenous component. The lesion may infiltrate into adjacent tissues (skeletal muscle or periosteum).

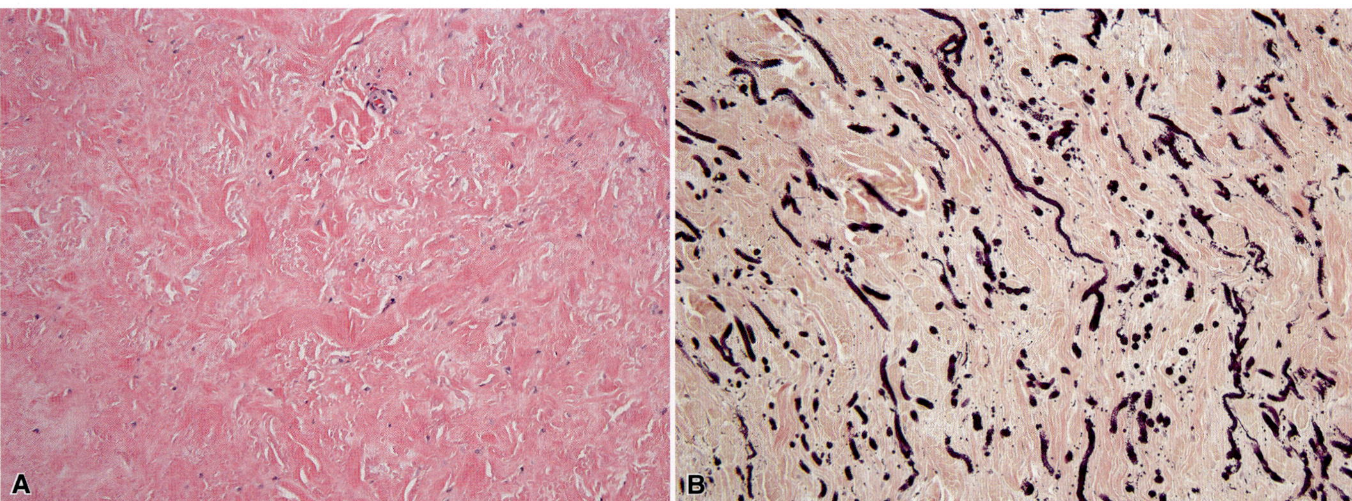

Figure 3.23 Elastofibroma. (A) This hypocellular lesion contains bland spindle cells haphazardly arranged within abundant hyalinized stroma containing collagen and elastic fibers. (B) Numerous large, fragmented elastic fibers are a typical feature that can be highlighted by Verhoeff-van Gieson stain.

Immunohistochemistry

The spindle cells are occasionally positive for smooth muscle actin but negative for desmin, CD34, and S-100 protein. Elastic fibers can be highlighted by special stains (e.g., Verhoeff-van Gieson stain; see Fig. 3.23B).

Differential Diagnosis

The diagnosis of elastofibroma is generally straightforward for a tumor arising on the lower aspect of the scapula, after the characteristic elastic fibers are identified. Desmoplastic fibroblastoma may occasionally be considered, but the typical stellate fibroblasts and lack of fragmented elastic fibers help distinguish this tumor type.

Prognosis and Treatment

Elastofibroma is benign and does not recur. Simple excision is curative.

Calcifying Fibrous Tumor

Calcifying fibrous tumor (previously known as calcifying fibrous pseudotumor) is a paucicellular fibroblastic proliferation that usually affects children and young adults.[87,88] It occurs as a long-standing painless mass in the deep soft tissues or in body cavities, often involving peritoneum or pleura.[89,90] A substantial subset of cases is multifocal at diagnosis.[91] This tumor has previously been interpreted as either reactive in nature or as a late "burned-out" stage of inflammatory myofibroblastic tumor,[92,93] but currently most authors regard it as a distinct fibroblastic neoplasm.[90]

Calcifying fibrous tumor is a firm, well-circumscribed, sometimes lobulated hypocellular lesion composed of dense stromal collagen with psammomatous and dystrophic calcifications and a patchy chronic inflammatory infiltrate (Fig. 3.24). It contains only very few scattered spindled fibroblasts with bland nuclear morphology (see Fig. 3.24B). Most tumors are positive for CD34, occasionally with scattered cells expressing smooth muscle actin and desmin, and ALK and S-100 protein are consistently negative.[90]

Calcifying fibrous tumor is a benign lesion with a low risk of recurrence and no metastatic potential.

Angiofibroma of Soft Tissue

Angiofibroma of soft tissue is a benign soft tissue tumor that is clinically and pathologically distinct from cellular angiofibroma (see Chapter 17) and nasopharyngeal angiofibroma (see Chapter 4).[94]

Clinical Features

Angiofibroma of soft tissue occurs over a wide age range and affects females twice as frequently as males. The tumor most often occurs as a slowly growing painless mass located in the soft tissues of the extremities, mainly the legs, often adjacent to joints or fibrotendinous structures. The tumors may be subcutaneous or deep seated. Unusual anatomic locations include the back, abdominal wall, pelvic cavity, and breast.

Preoperative duration is usually long, up to several years. Most lesions are well circumscribed; however, in some cases, infiltration into adjacent structures (including intraarticular extension) may be detected on imaging. Such findings, combined with the hypervascularity of the lesion, may occasionally raise clinical concerns for malignancy and result in significant overtreatment.

Pathologic Features

Histologically, angiofibroma of soft tissue is composed of relatively uniform bland spindle cells set in a variably myxoid-to-collagenous stroma with a prominent and complex vascular pattern (Fig. 3.25). The tumor is generally well circumscribed but unencapsulated, although focal infiltration of the adjacent soft tissues may be present. The tumors are vaguely lobulated, with alternating myxoid and collagenous areas and regional variation in cellularity. Focal degenerative changes such as ischemic necrosis and edema may be present, perhaps reflecting long preoperative duration. The prominent blood vessels in soft tissue angiofibroma are of variable size and shape. Innumerable small thin-walled branching blood vessels are evenly distributed throughout the lesion, somewhat reminiscent of those seen in myxoid liposarcoma, although larger and even more numerous (see Fig. 3.25B). In addition, less prominent medium-sized or large blood vessels with variably thick walls are noticeable in most tumors; in some instances, these are rounded, occasionally slitlike, but most often with ectatic lumina and staghorn (HPC-like) morphology, resembling the vessels in SFT (see Fig. 3.25C). These larger vessels tend to be located at the periphery of the tumor. Common additional features include collagen deposition around blood vessels and marked hyalinization or fibrinoid necrosis of medium-sized vessel walls.

The cytomorphology of the lesional spindle cells is nondistinctive, with inconspicuous palely eosinophilic cytoplasm and short ovoid or more tapering nuclei, with irregular nuclear contours and fine chromatin with inconspicuous to small nucleoli (see Fig. 3.25D). Cytologic atypia

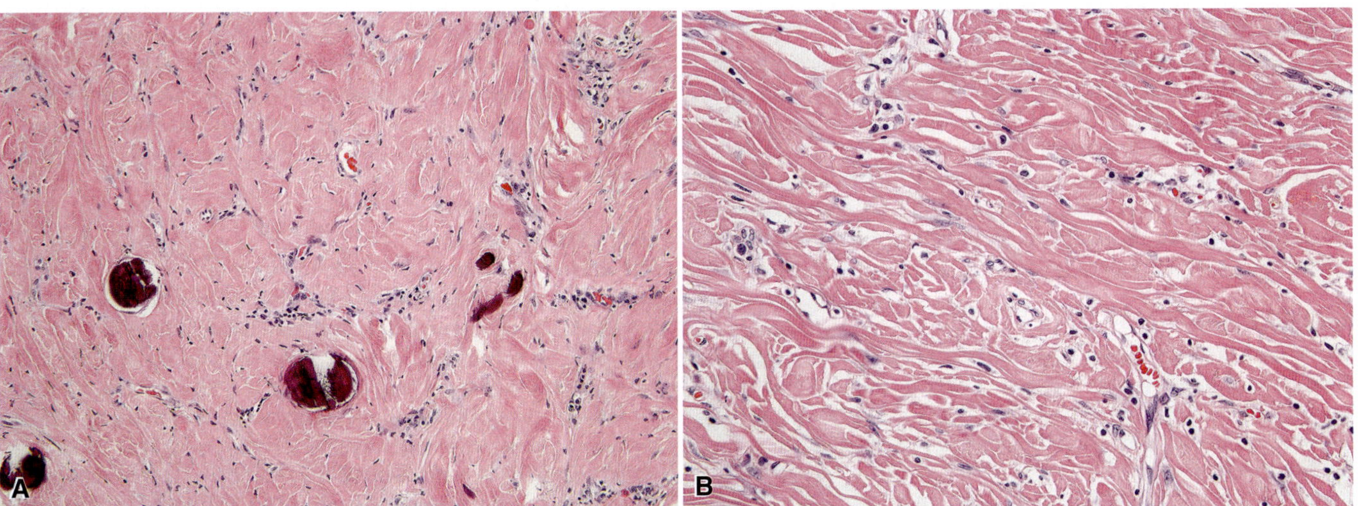

Figure 3.24 Calcifying Fibrous Tumor. (A) The tumor is composed of dense stromal collagen with scattered dystrophic and psammomatous calcifications as well as a sparse chronic inflammatory infiltrate. (B) The small spindled tumor cells are obscured by the dense collagen. Note the scattered lymphocytes and plasma cells.

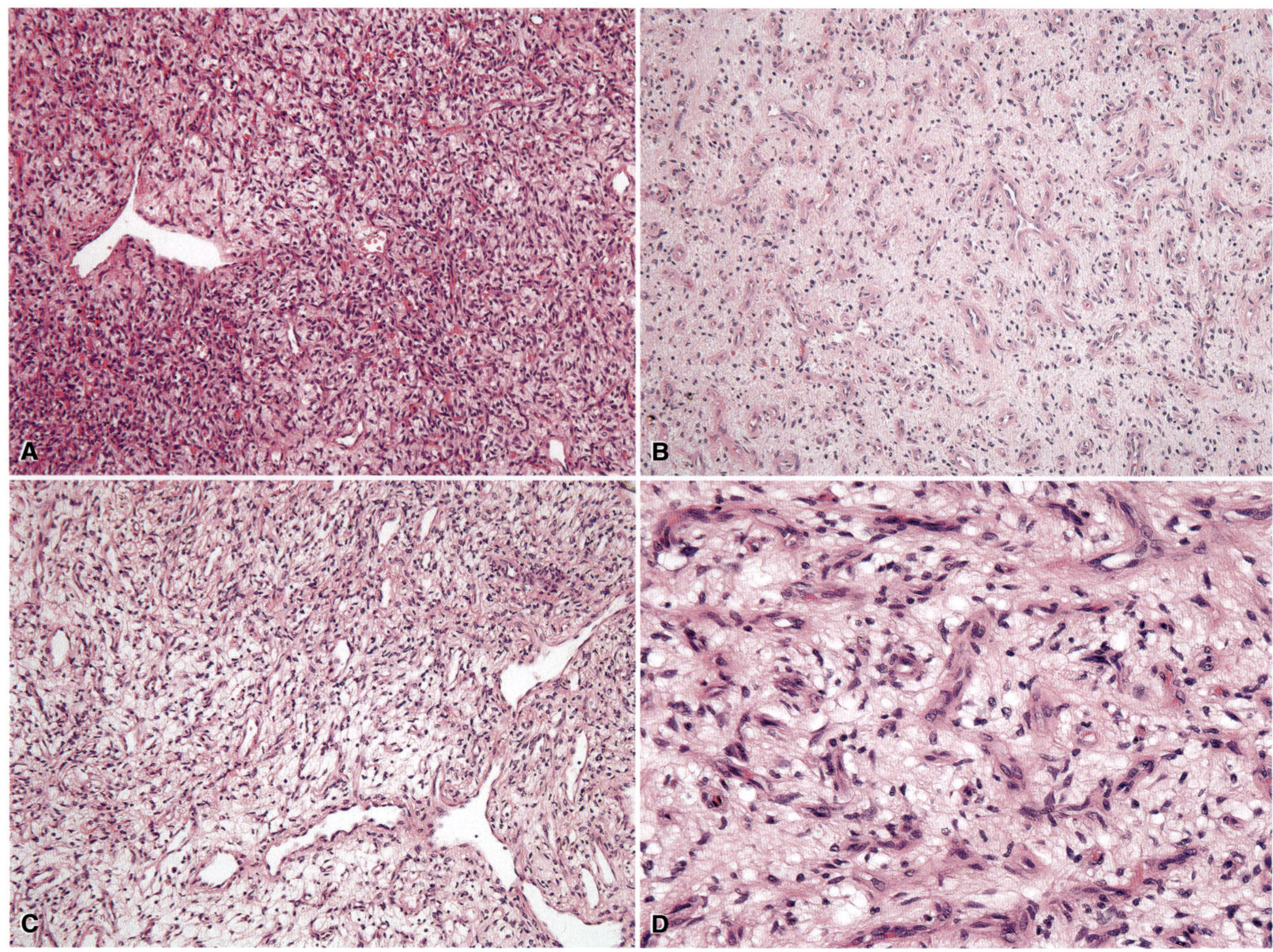

Figure 3.25 Angiofibroma of Soft Tissue. (A) The tumor is composed of uniform spindle cells in a variably collagenous or myxoid stroma with prominent blood vessels. (B) Numerous thin-walled branching blood vessels are typical. (C) Larger blood vessels with a dilated, branching (hemangiopericytoma-like) appearance are often also apparent. (D) The tumor cells are bland and nondescript with short ovoid to tapering hyperchromatic nuclei and indistinct cytoplasm. The numerous branching small blood vessels have thicker walls than those in myxoid liposarcoma.

and nuclear hyperchromasia are absent. Mitotic activity is generally low (<5 per 10 HPF).

There is usually some variation in the tumor stroma, ranging from a loosely myxoid matrix transitioning smoothly into areas of deposition of fine fibrillary or coarsely banded collagen. In some cases, myxoid tumor lobules are sharply demarcated with more abrupt transition to collagenous areas. A variably dense inflammatory infiltrate, comprising mainly small lymphocytes, some mast cells, and occasional neutrophils and plasma cells, is usually noted, sometimes in a perivascular distribution.

Immunohistochemistry

Immunohistochemistry does not play a significant role in the diagnosis of angiofibroma of soft tissue. The tumor cells express EMA in 50% of cases, usually focally but sometimes diffusely. CD34, smooth muscle actin, and desmin may also be focally detected. Tumor cells are negative for S-100 protein.

Molecular Genetics

Soft tissue angiofibroma is characterized by a simple karyotype, usually with a t(5;8)(p15;q12) translocation, resulting in an *AHRR-NCOA2* fusion gene.[94,95] This fusion gene seems to be specific for angiofibroma of soft tissue and may be a useful aid for diagnosis. Alternative gene fusions include *GTF2I-NCOA2*, emphasizing the relevance of NCOA2 in the development of soft tissue angiofibroma.[96] Detection of *NCOA2* rearrangements by FISH may be diagnostically useful,[97] but it should be interpreted with caution, given the involvement of this gene in other spindle cell tumors.

Differential Diagnosis

The differential diagnosis includes a range of benign and low-grade malignant soft tissue tumors, such as cellular angiofibroma, SFT, LGFMS, low-grade myxofibrosarcoma, and myxoid liposarcoma. Other diagnoses that may be considered in more myxoid examples include cellular myxoma and superficial angiomyxoma.

Cellular angiofibroma occurs nearly exclusively in the pelviperineal region and contains more rounded blood vessels. It is usually more uniformly cellular, with short stubby spindle cells resembling those in spindle cell lipoma (see Chapter 17). SFT shows a "patternless" architecture, with pronounced variation in cellularity, prominent thick collagen bundles, and characteristic branching staghorn vessels, which are not accompanied by the abundant smaller vessels typical of angiofibroma of soft tissue. STAT6 expression is specific for SFT in this differential diagnosis.

LGFMS shows alternating collagenous and myxoid areas that may resemble some cases of angiofibroma of soft tissue; however, there is usually a more whorled growth pattern, and the tumors tend to be more uniformly hypocellular. In addition, although LGFMS may contain arcades of thin-walled vessels, vascularity is usually not prominent. Immunohistochemical detection of MUC4 expression or demonstration of *FUS* gene rearrangement can help confirm the diagnosis of LGFMS.

Myxofibrosarcoma shows distinctive histologic features, including a lobulated growth pattern with infiltrative margins and tumor cells with hyperchromatic atypical or pleomorphic nuclei. Obvious cytologic features of malignancy are usually present, and the characteristic curvilinear vessels with perivascular hypercellularity bear no resemblance to the rich vascular network of angiofibroma of soft tissue. Myxoid liposarcoma contains a prominent plexiform network of thin-walled capillaries, but even the smallest vessels in angiofibroma have thicker walls and are more numerous than the delicate capillaries of myxoid liposarcoma. These differences, in addition to the less abundant myxoid stroma and the absence of lipoblasts in angiofibroma of soft tissue, allow distinction between these tumor types.

Prognosis and Treatment

Angiofibroma of soft tissue pursues a benign clinical course, with rare local recurrences and no evident metastatic potential. Simple local excision is adequate treatment.[94]

Fibrous Histiocytoma and Variants

Conventional benign fibrous histiocytoma, as well as cellular, aneurysmal, and atypical variants, most often occur in the skin (see Chapter 15). Deep fibrous histiocytoma, which arises in subcutaneous and deep soft tissue, will be discussed in this section.

Deep Fibrous Histiocytoma

Deep fibrous histiocytoma is an uncommon variant of fibrous histiocytoma. Some examples (especially those expressing CD34) show overlapping features with SFT.

Clinical Features

Deep fibrous histiocytoma is a distinctive form of fibrous histiocytoma that mainly occurs in deep subcutis (90% of cases) and rarely in subfascial soft tissue of adults (median age, 35 to 45 years).[98,99] Men are more often affected than women (male-to-female ratio, 1.5 : 1). The extremities (especially lower limb, one-third of cases) and head and neck region are the most common sites. Rare tumors have also been reported in the retroperitoneum, mediastinum, and pelvis.[99] Most patients present with a slow-growing, painless mass.

Pathologic Features

Deep fibrous histiocytoma is usually well circumscribed but unencapsulated (Fig. 3.26), with an average size of 3 cm.[98,99] Histologically, it is a cellular lesion with a prominent storiform growth pattern (see Fig. 3.26B). Tumor cell nuclei are oval or spindle shaped with fine chromatin and one or two small nucleoli. Extracellular matrix deposition is minimal, with limited areas of stromal hyalinization. Approximately 50% of cases are composed of a relatively uniform population of spindle cells (see Fig. 3.26C), whereas other cases are more heterogeneous in composition, containing variable numbers of osteoclast-like giant cells, foam cells, siderophages, mast cells, and lymphoid aggregates (see Fig. 3.26D). HPC-like blood vessels may be prominent. Mitotic activity is low (<5 per 10 HPF). Focal nuclear pleomorphism may be observed, similar to atypical fibrous histiocytoma of the skin (see Chapter 15). Tumor necrosis is rare. Osseous metaplasia may occasionally be observed.

Box 3.5 Differential Diagnosis of Deep Fibrous Histiocytoma

- Solitary fibrous tumor (cellular variant)
- Mammary-type myofibroblastoma
- Cellular schwannoma
- Soft tissue perineurioma
- Giant cell tumor of tendon sheath
- Dermatofibrosarcoma protuberans
- Unclassified spindle cell/pleomorphic sarcoma

Immunohistochemistry

The immunophenotype of deep fibrous histiocytoma is nonspecific. The tumor cells may show at least focal expression of CD34, smooth muscle actin, and/or CD99, each in approximately 40% to 50% of cases. Desmin is rarely positive.[98,99] Histiocytic markers (i.e., CD68 and CD163) are variably expressed, highlighting admixed histiocytes. The tumor cells are consistently negative for EMA, keratins, and S-100 protein.

Molecular Genetics

Gene fusions involving the protein kinase C genes *PRKCB* and *PRKCD* have been identified in a small percentage of deep fibrous histiocytomas,[100] although these findings have not yet been translated to the clinical management of these tumors.

Differential Diagnosis

The main differential diagnosis for deep fibrous histiocytoma is the cellular variant of SFT (Box 3.5). Both tumor types are well circumscribed, and they have a monomorphous cellular appearance with a prominent HPC-like vascular network, a relative absence of nuclear pleomorphism, and often strong CD34 reactivity. Deep fibrous histiocytoma tends to be smaller than SFT and usually has a more prominent storiform architecture, but in some cases it is almost impossible to distinguish between these two entities on histologic grounds. Expression of STAT6 is helpful to confirm the diagnosis of SFT. Histologic features of malignancy (e.g., a high mitotic rate, atypical mitotic figures, tumor necrosis, cellular pleomorphism, infiltrative borders) are more frequently observed in cellular/malignant SFT than in deep fibrous histiocytoma. In contrast, the presence of multinucleated giant cells, foam cells, and siderophages strongly favors deep fibrous histiocytoma. This distinction has clinical importance, particularly in cases with mitotic activity, because mitotically active cellular (malignant) SFT tends to be more aggressive than deep fibrous histiocytoma in terms of metastatic potential (20% to 30% for malignant SFT vs. 1% to 2% for deep fibrous histiocytoma).

Other tumor types that may be considered in the differential diagnosis with deep fibrous histiocytoma include DFSP (markedly infiltrative borders with honeycomb growth pattern through adipose tissue; more spindled and less pleomorphic tumor cells with scant cytoplasm; lack of multinucleated cells, foam cells, and lymphocytes), cellular schwannoma (strong and diffuse reactivity for S-100 protein), soft tissue perineurioma (whorled growth pattern, slender elongated tumor cells with bipolar cytoplasmic processes, reactivity for EMA), giant cell tumor of tendon sheath (fingers and toes, rounded tumor cells, numerous osteoclast-like giant cells), and unclassified spindle cell/pleomorphic sarcoma (large size, atypical mitotic figures, necrosis, cellular atypia, tumor giant cells, infiltrative borders, usually no expression of CD34).

Prognosis and Treatment

Deep fibrous histiocytoma usually behaves in a benign fashion, with a potential for local recurrence (20%), especially when incompletely

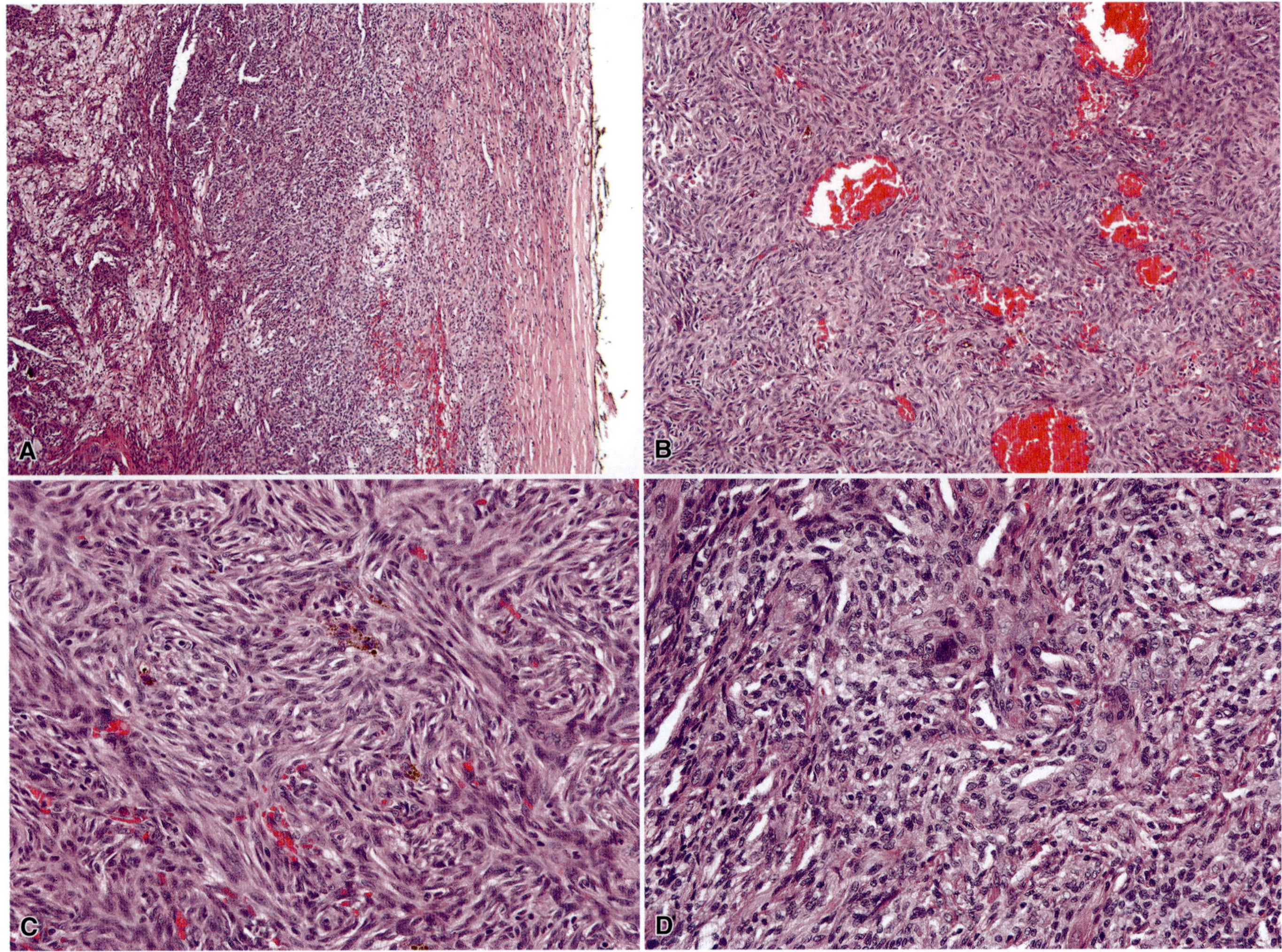

Figure 3.26 **Deep Fibrous Histiocytoma.** (A) In contrast to cutaneous fibrous histiocytoma, deep fibrous histiocytoma is typically well circumscribed. (B) The tumor often shows a storiform architecture with scattered dilated blood vessels. (C) Some tumors are composed of uniform short spindle cells (similar to cutaneous cellular fibrous histiocytoma). (D) Other examples show a more heterogeneous cellular composition, including foam cells and osteoclast-like giant cells.

excised. Rarely, deep fibrous histiocytoma may metastasize. Aggressive treatment of typical cases is not appropriate.[99]

Solitary Fibrous Tumor and Variants

SFT is a fibroblastic neoplasm that most often arises in the pleura but can occur at virtually any anatomic location. In the past, most cases of SFT have been designated *HPC*, a diagnostic category originally established for a neoplasm believed to show perivascular (pericytic) differentiation with a well-developed branching vascular pattern.[101] Although most often seen in SFT, branching ectatic (staghorn) vessels can also be observed in many other unrelated tumor types, such as synovial sarcoma, mesenchymal chondrosarcoma, infantile fibrosarcoma, and PMT, among others, including tumors with true pericytic differentiation (myopericytoma).[102-104] Many examples of these other tumor types were previously buried within the HPC category. Nowadays, the term *HPC* is of limited value, and its use should be discouraged to avoid diagnostic confusion, other than for sinonasal HPC (a distinctive smooth muscle actin–positive sinonasal tumor showing true pericytic differentiation). An HPC-like vascular pattern is just one descriptive feature of SFT and its variants discussed herein.

Solitary Fibrous Tumor

Clinical Features

Originally described in the pleura by Klemperer and Rabin in 1931 (reviewed by Gengler in reference 103), SFT is more frequently encountered at extrapleural sites, including subcutaneous tissue (40% of cases), deep soft tissue, and visceral organs (e.g., thyroid, salivary glands, liver, gastrointestinal tract, urinary bladder, and prostate).[105,106]

SFT has a peak incidence in middle-aged adults, with no gender predilection. It generally presents as a slow-growing mass, which can gradually reach a large size before coming to clinical attention. The retroperitoneum, deep soft tissues of proximal extremities (thigh, axilla), abdominal cavity, trunk, and head and neck (including the orbit and meninges) are the most common extrapleural locations.[107,108]

Approximately 10% of SFTs occur in the head and neck region. Symptoms are mostly related to mass effect, depending on the size and site of the tumor. SFT of the head and neck tends to present relatively early with compression symptoms or local invasion in cases with malignant behavior. Rarely, SFT may cause hypoglycemia due to the production of insulin-like growth factor I or II.[109-111]

Pathologic Features

Grossly, SFT is usually well circumscribed. Tumor size ranges from 1 to 25 cm (median size, 5 to 8 cm).

Histologically, SFT has a wide range of features, ranging from cellular neoplasms to predominantly fibrous lesions, with intermediate forms between the two ends of the spectrum. Fibrous forms of SFT are characterized by alternating hypercellular and hypocellular fibrous areas (Fig. 3.27). The hypercellular areas are composed of rounded-to-spindle cells without a clearly discernible architecture, an appearance often referred to as "patternless."[109,112] Tumor cell nuclei usually have vesicular chromatin, and there may be nuclear pseudoinclusions. Fibrous forms also contain characteristic medium-sized, rounded vessels with thickened and hyalinized walls (see Fig. 3.27B). Amianthoid-like bodies composed of aggregates of extracellular collagen may also be seen.

Cellular forms of SFT resemble what had traditionally been called HPC. In contrast to the more common fibrous form, cellular SFT usually has a monotonous appearance with moderate to high cellularity, little intervening fibrosis, numerous thin-walled "staghorn" branching vessels, and round-to-oval monomorphic tumor cell nuclei (Fig. 3.28). Myxoid or microcystic changes, nuclear palisading, foci of chronic inflammation, and interstitial mast cells are commonly observed in SFT, as well as occasional pseudovascular ("angiectoid") spaces and multinucleated stromal cells, similar to those observed in so-called giant cell angiofibroma (see subsequent discussion). Calcification and ossification are rare. Predominantly myxoid SFT has also been described and is particularly difficult to recognize, leading to problems in differential diagnosis (see Chapter 5).[113]

Mitoses are usually sparse, and necrosis is rare in SFT. Proposed criteria for malignancy (see Prognosis and Treatment) include increased cellularity, mitotic activity (≥4 mitoses per 10 HPF), and necrosis; mitotic activity is the most reliable criterion (Fig. 3.29). Rare SFTs show an alternative type of malignant transformation in the form of dedifferentiation; analogous to other mesenchymal tumors (such as dedifferentiated liposarcoma), there is an abrupt transition to a morphologically non-distinctive anaplastic component, with epithelioid, pleomorphic, round cell, or spindle cell morphology.[114] This phenomenon is usually accompanied by loss of CD34 expression and strong staining for p53 and p16, and is associated with highly aggressive behavior, particularly for large, deep-seated tumors.[114]

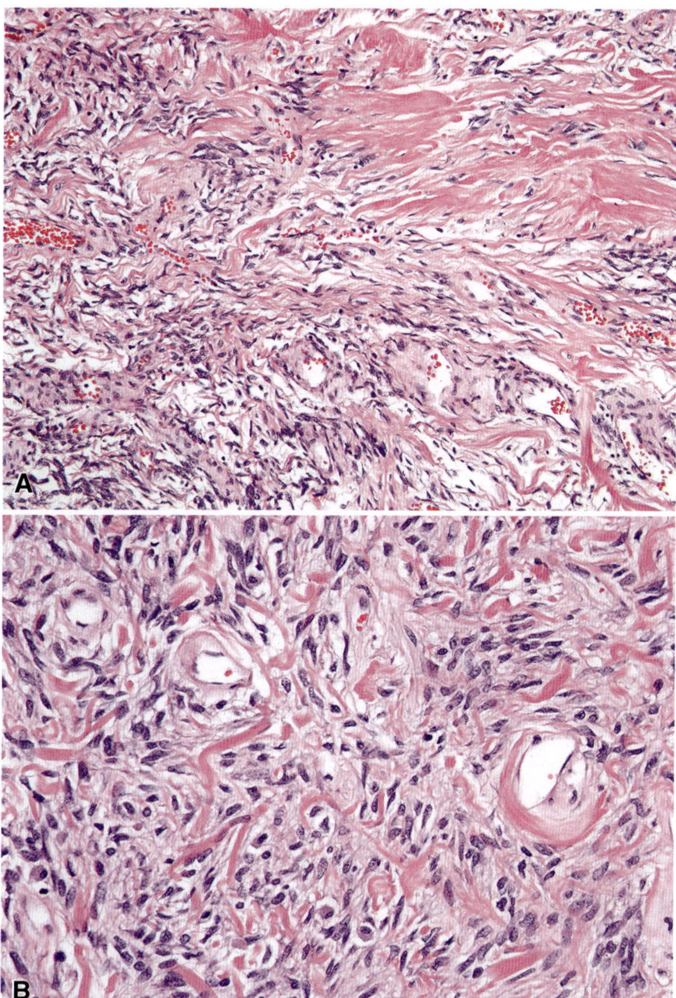

Figure 3.27 Solitary Fibrous Tumor. (A) A typical fibrous example with varying cellularity, collagenous stroma, and a "patternless" architecture. (B) Rounded blood vessels with hyalinized walls are a characteristic feature.

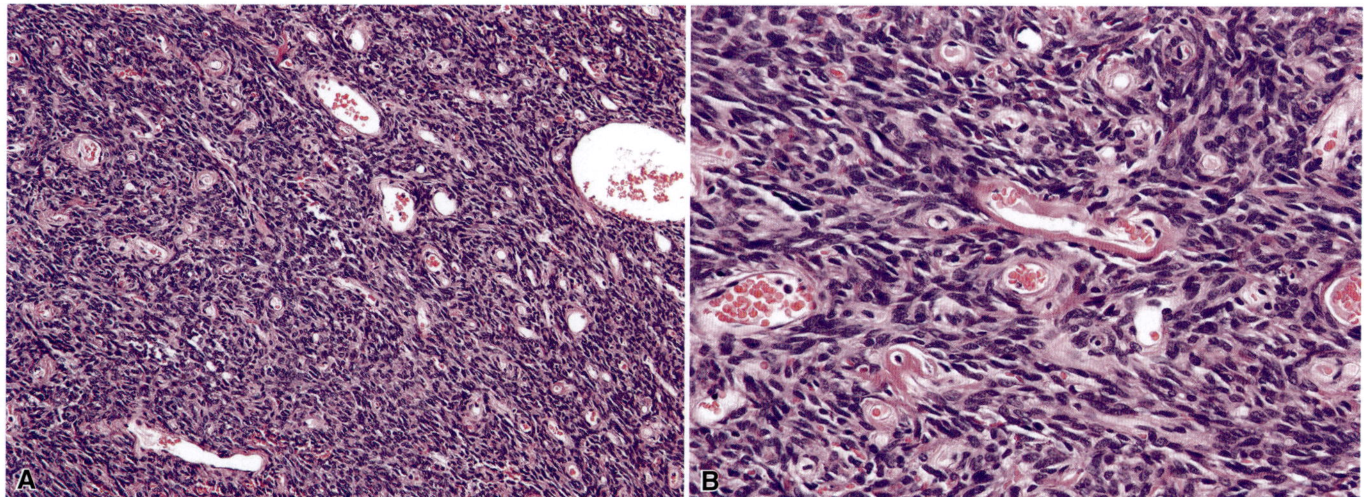

Figure 3.28 Cellular Solitary Fibrous Tumor. (A) The tumor has a monotonous appearance with uniform cellularity, minimal intervening fibrosis, and dilated vessels. (B) The tumor cells are uniform with ovoid nuclei and indistinct cytoplasm. Note the prominent dilated vessels. Such tumors were formerly known as *hemangiopericytoma*.

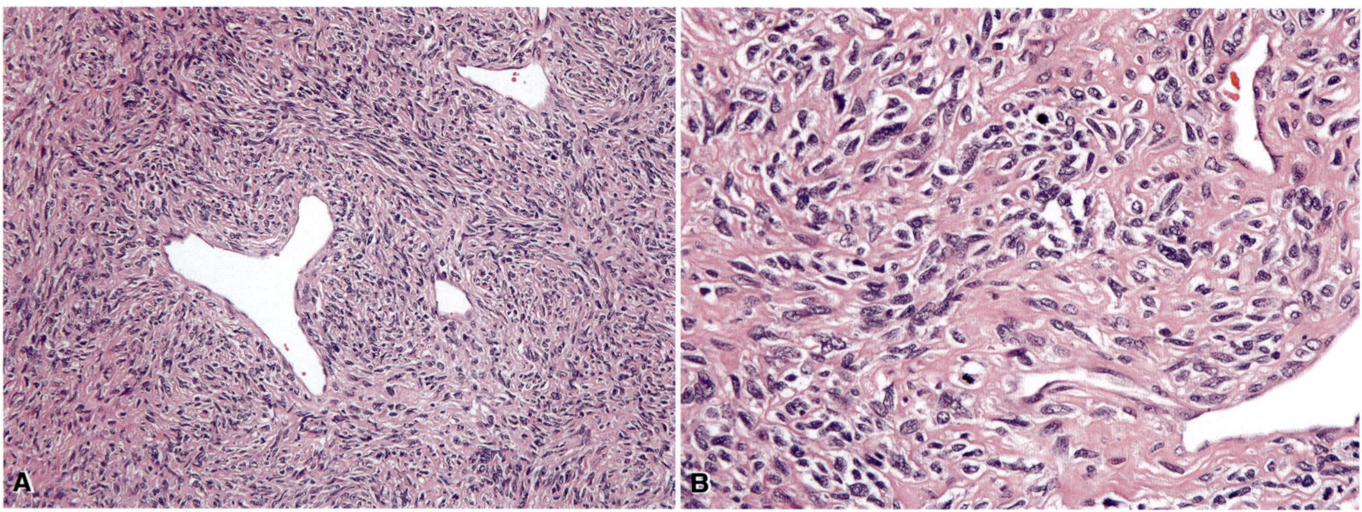

Figure 3.29 Malignant Solitary Fibrous Tumor. (A) On low power the tumor appears similar to cellular solitary fibrous tumor. (B) Nuclear atypia and a high mitotic rate are observed.

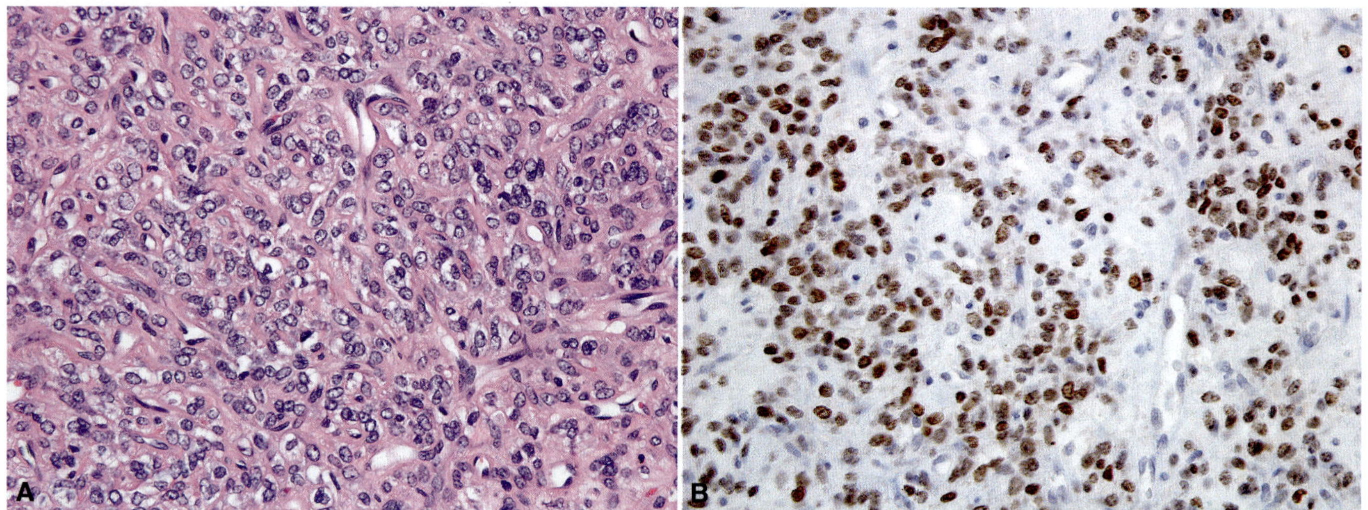

Figure 3.30 Solitary Fibrous Tumor. (A) This example is composed of uniform ovoid to round cells. Note the stromal collagen. (B) Strong and diffuse nuclear staining for STAT6 is a characteristic finding.

Immunohistochemistry

Immunohistochemical detection of STAT6 is the most useful diagnostic marker for SFT.[115] Nuclear expression of STAT6 is seen in more than 95% of SFT and is usually diffuse in distribution and strong in intensity (Fig. 3.30).[115-118] In addition, SFT commonly expresses CD34 (90% to 95% of cases) and CD99 (70%) (Fig. 3.31). A smaller subset of tumors is positive for EMA (20%), smooth muscle actin (20%), and bcl-2 (30%). TLE1 is weakly positive in occasional cases,[119] whereas MUC4 is negative.[120] Only very rare cases show focal staining for S-100 protein or desmin, and tumors are virtually always negative for keratins.[103,121] Cellular and malignant variants of SFT also express STAT6 but are somewhat less often positive for CD34; when positive, the staining is usually weaker and less diffuse than in fibrous SFT.[122,123]

Molecular Genetics

The diagnosis of SFT has been greatly simplified since the discovery of a recurrent *NAB2-STAT6* gene fusion that leads to STAT6 upregulation and overexpression, which can be detected by immunohistochemistry.[124,125] The *NAB2-STAT6* gene fusion is the result of a paracentric inversion affecting the long arm of chromosome 12, within a region in 12q13 too small to be reliably detected for clinical purposes by G-banding or a dual-color FISH assay. There are several variants of the fusion with a range of breakpoints, demonstrating some degree of genotype/phenotype correlation: the predominant fusion variant joins exon 4 of *NAB2* to exons 2 to 4 of *STAT6*, which is most common in "classic" SFT cases, affecting the chest wall of older patients. The second most common variant, joining *NAB2* exon 6 to *STAT6* exon 16/17, is detected in extrathoracic cases affecting younger patients, and collectively pursue a more aggressive clinical course.[126-128] At present, no molecular marker distinguishes benign from malignant lesions, although signs of genetic progression, such as size-related increased copy number changes, *TP53* mutations, and *TERT* promoter mutations, have been described in aggressive cases.[129-131] Among mesenchymal tumors, the highest levels of insulin-like growth factor II expression are detected in SFT both at the protein level and by gene expression profiling, opening the possibility of pharmacologic treatment targeting the insulin-like growth factor II pathway.[132]

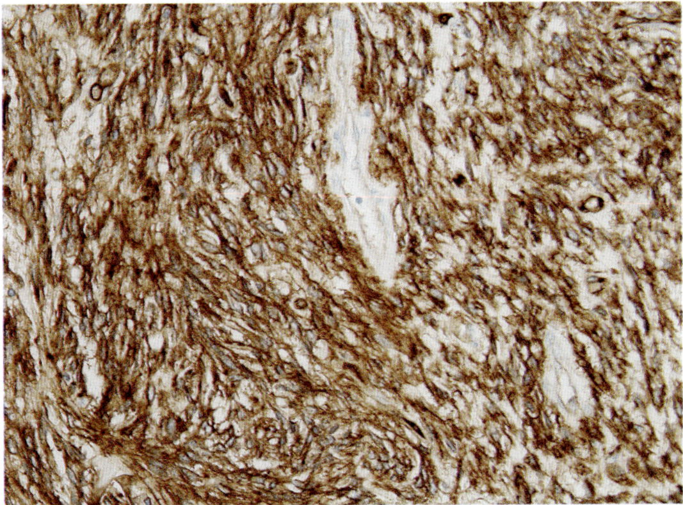

Figure 3.31 **Solitary Fibrous Tumor.** Nearly all cases show diffuse staining for CD34.

Box 3.6 Differential Diagnosis of Solitary Fibrous Tumor

If Predominantly Fibrous

Mammary-type myofibroblastoma
Angiofibroma of soft tissue
Desmoid fibromatosis

If Predominantly Vascular

Hemangioma with prominent stromal hyalinization
Symplastic hemangioma

If Predominantly Cellular (Including Malignant Forms)

Deep fibrous histiocytoma
Spindle cell lipoma
Cellular angiofibroma
Spindle cell thymoma (WHO type A)
Cellular schwannoma
Monophasic synovial sarcoma
Malignant peripheral nerve sheath tumor
Spindle cell/desmoplastic mesothelioma
Spindle cell melanoma
Spindle cell/poorly differentiated carcinoma
Dedifferentiated liposarcoma
Phosphaturic mesenchymal tumor

If Predominantly Myxoid

Low-grade fibromyxoid sarcoma
Low-grade malignant peripheral nerve sheath tumor
Cellular myxoma
Myxoid dermatofibrosarcoma protuberans
Giant cell fibroblastoma
Myxoid liposarcoma
Low-grade myxofibrosarcoma

If Containing Numerous Stromal Giant Cells (Giant Cell Angiofibroma)

Giant cell fibroblastoma

If Containing Mature Fat (Fat-Forming Solitary Fibrous Tumor; Lipomatous Hemangiopericytoma)

Well-differentiated liposarcoma
Dedifferentiated liposarcoma, morphologically low grade
Myolipoma/lipoleiomyoma
Angiomyolipoma
Phosphaturic mesenchymal tumor

If Containing Calcifications

Calcifying synovial sarcoma
Phosphaturic mesenchymal tumor

Differential Diagnosis

The differential diagnosis of SFT can be broad (Box 3.6) but is greatly simplified by the detection of STAT6 expression by immunohistochemistry. At soft tissue sites, SFT should be distinguished from cellular schwannoma, mammary-type myofibroblastoma, deep fibrous histiocytoma, spindle cell lipoma, cellular angiofibroma, angiofibroma of soft tissue, metastasis from spindle cell (sarcomatoid) carcinoma and spindle cell melanoma, LGFMS (especially if myxoid foci are prominent), monophasic synovial sarcoma, MPNST, and dedifferentiated liposarcoma. In occasional cases, sometimes designated *vascular SFT*, thick-walled vessels are so numerous that the lesion may easily be confused with a hemangioma.

In contrast to SFT, cellular schwannoma is strongly and diffusely positive for S-100 protein. The same applies for spindle cell melanoma. In the retroperitoneum and abdominal cavity, SFT may be confused with morphologically low-grade dedifferentiated liposarcoma. However, dedifferentiated liposarcoma is usually less well circumscribed, contains an adjacent well-differentiated adipocytic component in most cases, and is positive for MDM2 and CDK4. Of note, STAT6 is expressed in approximately 15% of well-differentiated/dedifferentiated liposarcomas, which may complicate the evaluation of a spindle cell neoplasm in intraabdominal or retroperitoneal locations.[133] CD34 can also be expressed by both SFT and dedifferentiated liposarcoma, a potentially misleading finding. MPNST is often associated with a large nerve and typically shows a more fascicular architecture than SFT with perivascular hypercellularity, tapering nuclei, and focal expression of S-100 protein, SOX10, or GFAP in 40% to 50% of cases. Although monophasic synovial sarcoma is also commonly positive for CD99 and bcl-2, it usually shows strong nuclear staining for TLE1 and is almost always negative for CD34 (95% of cases); STAT6 is specific for SFT in this differential diagnosis. In difficult cases, FISH for *SS18* rearrangement can be used to confirm the diagnosis. Mammary-type myofibroblastoma is composed of denser fascicles of spindle cells with eosinophilic cytoplasm, separated by thick bundles of hyalinized collagen. They may contain thick-walled vessels and resemble SFT, especially on core biopsy specimen. As opposed to SFT, in addition to CD34, tumor cells in myofibroblastoma are usually diffusely positive for desmin. Spindle cell lipoma typically arises in the upper back, shoulder, or neck of middle-aged men. Similar to SFT, spindle cell lipoma is usually strongly and diffusely positive for CD34. However, spindle cell lipoma typically contains short stubby spindle cells and distinctive ropy collagen bundles, as well as a variable adipocytic component; branching, HPC-like vessels are not a feature of spindle cell lipoma. Cellular examples of spindle cell lipoma lacking fat cells are especially difficult to distinguish from SFT.

Deep fibrous histiocytoma may closely resemble SFT, and sometimes it is nearly impossible to distinguish between these two tumor types; both are well-circumscribed neoplasms that contain HPC-like vessels and may express CD34.[98,99] However, deep fibrous histiocytoma tends to show a predominantly storiform growth pattern rather than the patternless architecture and alternating hypocellular and hypercellular areas typical of SFT. Intratumoral thick-walled hyalinized vessels are also more frequently found in SFT than in deep fibrous histiocytoma. STAT6 is a helpful marker to confirm the diagnosis of SFT in this differential diagnosis.

LGFMS can easily be confused with the myxoid variant of SFT, especially on core biopsies. In contrast to SFT, LGFMS is uniformly positive for MUC4 and almost never expresses CD34.[120] In addition, LGFMS shows *FUS* gene rearrangement, with the specific t(7;16)

translocation in most cases.[134] Other tumors that can occasionally be confused with SFT include hyalinized variants of myoepithelioma and sclerosing epithelioid fibrosarcoma for predominantly hyalinized SFT, myxoid liposarcoma for myxoid forms of SFT, spindle cell thymoma in the mediastinum, and ectopic hamartomatous thymoma.

Prognosis and Treatment

The clinical course of SFT is difficult to predict; although most SFTs pursue a benign clinical course, 5% to 10% recur or metastasize, sometimes years or even decades after excision of the primary tumor. Typical sites of metastasis include the lungs, liver, and bone. The vast majority of SFTs that behave aggressively show histologic features of malignancy, but rarely benign-appearing SFTs give rise to metastases. Published criteria for malignancy in SFT include large tumor size (>5 cm or >15 cm), disseminated disease at presentation, infiltrative margins, high cellularity, nuclear pleomorphism, areas of tumor necrosis, and an increased mitotic rate (≥4 mitoses per 10 HPF).[123,135-138] High mitotic activity is the single most reliable criterion for malignancy. A risk stratification model using age (≥55 years), size (≥15 cm), and mitotic index (≥4 per 10 HPF) defines aggressive tumors with a high risk of metastasis.[138]

Histologically malignant SFT shows a higher metastatic potential than predominantly fibrous SFT (20% to 30% vs. 5%).[114,139] SFTs located in the mediastinum, abdomen, retroperitoneum, and pelvis are generally large, cellular, and mitotic tumors, and therefore tend to be more aggressive than those arising at other sites.[137] Dedifferentiation is associated with a particularly poor prognosis.[114]

Despite these generalizations regarding prognosis, the relationship between morphology and outcome in SFT is notoriously inconsistent; some histologically malignant lesions behave in a benign fashion, whereas rare morphologically innocuous lesions behave aggressively.[109,136,139] Thus, similar to gastrointestinal stromal tumors (GISTs), it is unwise to consider any SFT as certifiably benign, and long-term follow-up is mandatory for all patients.

Optimal treatment of SFT consists of complete excision with tumor-free margins. Adjuvant radiotherapy should be considered to improve local control for large tumors or histologically malignant examples.[114,139,140]

PRACTICE POINTS: Solitary Fibrous Tumor

- Synonymous with the not-recommended term *hemangiopericytoma*
- Mostly affects middle-aged adults with a wide anatomic distribution
- May present with hypoglycemia
- "Patternless" architecture with variable cellularity; prominent stromal collagen; and ectatic, branching ("staghorn") vessels
- Strong and diffuse nuclear STAT6 expression
- Small unpredictable risk of metastasis (for conventional SFT)
- Histologically malignant solitary fibrous tumor: 20% to 30% metastatic rate
- Most reliable criterion for malignancy: increased mitotic activity (≥4 per 10 HPF)

Giant Cell–Rich Solitary Fibrous Tumor (Giant Cell Angiofibroma)

The term *giant cell angiofibroma* was introduced in 1995 to describe a distinctive orbital tumor of middle-aged adults, which contained numerous stromal giant cells, often lining pseudovascular spaces.[141] Following its initial description, similar lesions have been reported in extraorbital locations, and it is now recognized that giant cell angiofibroma is in fact simply a giant cell–rich morphologic variant of SFT.[142]

Giant cell–rich SFT generally occurs as a slow-growing, well-circumscribed but unencapsulated, small mass (median size, 3 cm). It is most often found in the orbital region (sometimes affecting the eyelids) but can also be seen in the scalp, parotid gland, submandibular and parascapular regions, posterior mediastinum, retroperitoneum, and vulva (reviewed by Gengler).[103]

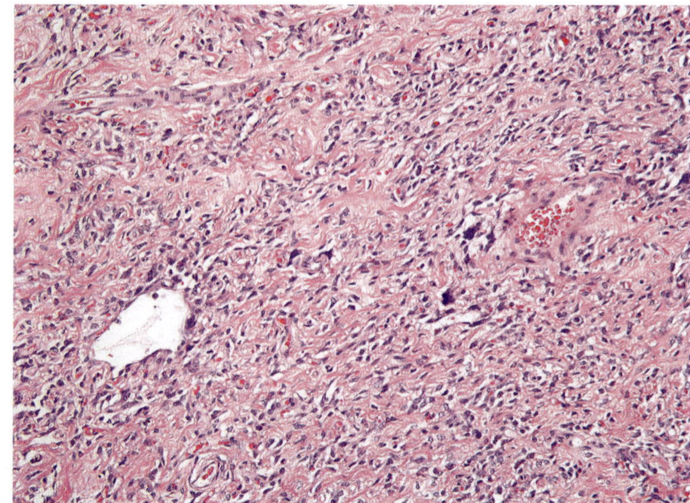

Figure 3.32 Giant Cell–Rich Solitary Fibrous Tumor. In addition to the other typical histologic features of solitary fibrous tumor, the tumor contains multinucleated giant cells, which focally line "angiectoid" spaces. Such tumors were formerly known as *giant cell angiofibroma*.

Histologically, giant cell–rich SFT has similar morphology to conventional SFT, but the giant cell–rich type also contains numerous stromal giant cells, either scattered throughout the lesion or lining pseudovascular ("angiectoid") spaces (Fig. 3.32). These giant cells, which can also be observed in small numbers in conventional SFT, contain multiple nuclei either grouped in the center (leading to nuclear hyperchromasia) or showing a peripheral floretlike arrangement. The immunohistochemical features are similar to conventional SFT (see earlier discussion).

The differential diagnosis of giant cell–rich SFT is approximately the same as conventional SFT. Giant cell fibroblastoma, a recurring but nonmetastasizing neoplasm of childhood related to DFSP, is the greatest histologic mimic. Both lesions are CD34 positive and contain multinucleated stromal giant cells lining pseudovascular spaces. However, giant cell fibroblastoma in its pure form occurs almost exclusively in infants and children, whereas in adults it is usually admixed with foci of conventional DFSP. Giant cell fibroblastoma involves only dermis and subcutaneous tissue; the lesion shows infiltrative margins and does not contain the thick-walled, hyalinized rounded vessels typical of SFT, and it bears specific chromosomal abnormalities, namely the t(17;22) reciprocal translocation or supernumerary ring chromosomes derived from chromosomes 17 and 22, cytogenetic abnormalities that are not found in SFT. Nuclear expression of STAT6 is specific for SFT in this differential diagnosis.

The recurrence rate of giant cell–rich SFT is very low. In the original series, one patient experienced a local recurrence after 5 years.[141] Metastases have not yet been reported.

Fat-Forming Solitary Fibrous Tumor (Lipomatous Hemangiopericytoma)

In 1995 Nielsen and colleagues reported three cases of an unusual tumor composed of mature adipocytes and HPC-like areas, which they considered a distinct morphologic variant of HPC and designated *lipomatous HPC*.[143] Subsequently, additional cases have been reported, and it is now recognized that lipomatous HPC is a variant of SFT showing adipocytic metaplasia.[144,145] Fat-forming SFT occurs as a superficial or deep-seated, well-demarcated mass. They have been reported in the pleura, mediastinum, thyroid,[146] and orbit, but the deep soft tissues of the retroperitoneum and thigh are the most commonly affected sites.

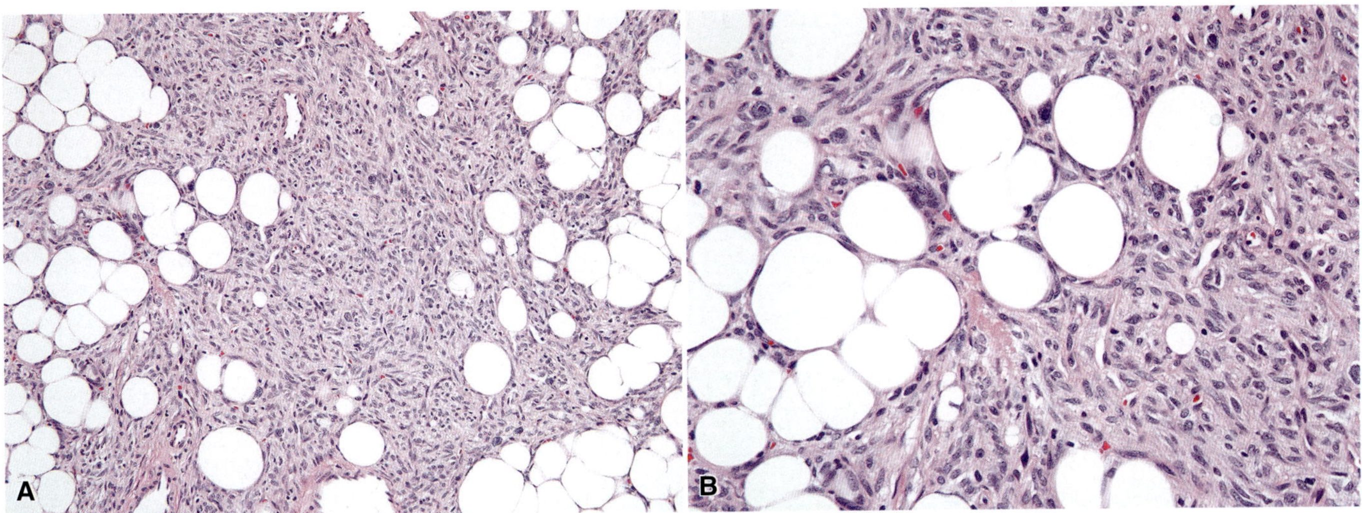

Figure 3.33 Fat-Forming Solitary Fibrous Tumor. (A) Scattered adipocytes are observed in an otherwise typical example of solitary fibrous tumor. Such tumors are also known as *lipomatous hemangiopericytoma*. (B) The tumor cells are uniform and bland.

Similar to conventional SFT, they typically occur in middle-aged adults, with a male predilection.

Histologically, fat-forming SFT resembles the cellular form of SFT, except for the presence of a variable number of mature adipocytes (Fig. 3.33). The immunoprofile is similar to that of conventional SFT, including strong and diffuse expression of STAT6.[147] In addition, the nonadipocytic spindle cell component is positive for CD99, and somewhat less frequently for CD34 (75% of cases). Focal reactivity for smooth muscle actin and EMA has also been reported in a subset of cases, in keeping with the immunophenotypic range of SFT.[145]

The main differential diagnosis of fat-forming SFT includes angiomyolipoma, which in addition to the adipocytic component is characterized by a perivascular arrangement of epithelioid to spindled cells. These cells show variable expression of smooth muscle actin, HMB-45, and melan A and are negative for CD34 and STAT6. Other diagnoses to consider are myolipoma, which typically arises in the pelvis of women and is composed of mature adipocytes admixed with well-differentiated smooth muscle cells that express smooth muscle actin, desmin, and caldesmon[148]; as well as well-differentiated and morphologically low-grade dedifferentiated liposarcomas,[144] which contain enlarged atypical stromal cells with hyperchromatic nuclei and are positive for MDM2 and CDK4. STAT6 is positive in 15% of well-differentiated and dedifferentiated liposarcomas, which is a diagnostic pitfall.

Although fat-forming SFT generally shows benign histology and pursues an indolent clinical course, occasional cases are histologically and clinically malignant. Although experience is limited, it seems that the same criteria for malignancy applied to conventional SFT may be useful in this context. In addition, the presence of lipoblasts and areas resembling atypical lipomatous tumor (ALT)/well-differentiated liposarcoma (WDLPS) is indicative of aggressiveness in this context.[149]

Meningeal Solitary Fibrous Tumor

HPC of cranial and intraspinal meninges has been considered a distinct entity for decades. However, in recent years, analogous to examples at visceral and soft tissue sites, it has been increasingly recognized that meningeal HPC and SFT are in fact histologic variants of the same tumor type; lesions previously designated meningeal HPC are no more than cellular forms of SFT.[150,151] In a comparative study of SFT and conventional HPC of the central nervous system, Tihan and associates observed that two lesions that were initially diagnosed as conventional meningeal HPC recurred as SFT-like neoplasms, a finding in support of a unifying concept.[151] The identification of the *NAB2-STAT6* gene fusion in meningeal HPC confirmed these observations.[118] As in soft tissue, cellular SFT of the central nervous system tends to express CD34 less frequently and to behave more aggressively than fibrous SFT, but both are diffusely positive for STAT6. In fact, meningeal tumors appear to be even more aggressive than their soft tissue counterparts, likely in part because of frequent incomplete surgical excision, showing higher rates of local recurrence (60% to 80%) and metastasis (25% to 65%). The most common metastatic sites include bone, liver, and the gastrointestinal tract.[152,153] Metastases often occur a decade or longer following primary tumor excision. In fact, when a cellular or malignant SFT is encountered in bone or the liver (Fig. 3.34), the possibility of a metastasis from a dural primary tumor should be suggested. Meningeal SFT should primarily be differentiated from fibrous (fibroblastic) meningioma. Although both tumor types may be positive for CD34, fibrous meningiomas usually show uniform diffuse expression of SSTR2

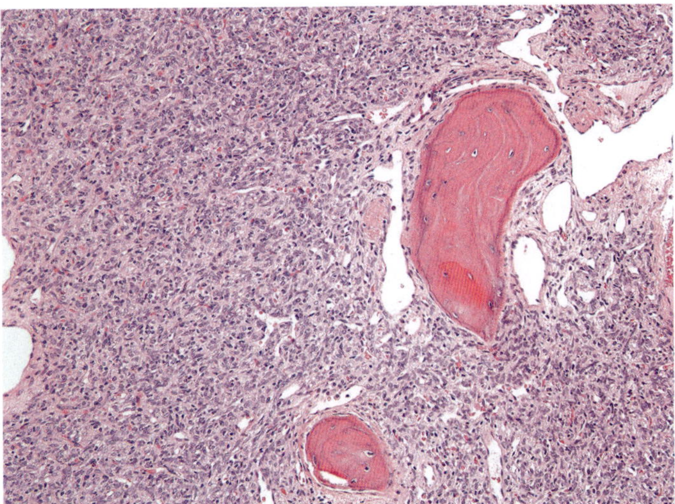

Figure 3.34 Metastatic Cellular Solitary Fibrous Tumor to Bone. This tumor originated in the dura ("meningeal hemangiopericytoma"). Metastases often develop a decade or longer following primary tumor excision at this site. A dural primary should be suspected when a cellular/malignant solitary fibrous tumor is encountered in the bones or liver.

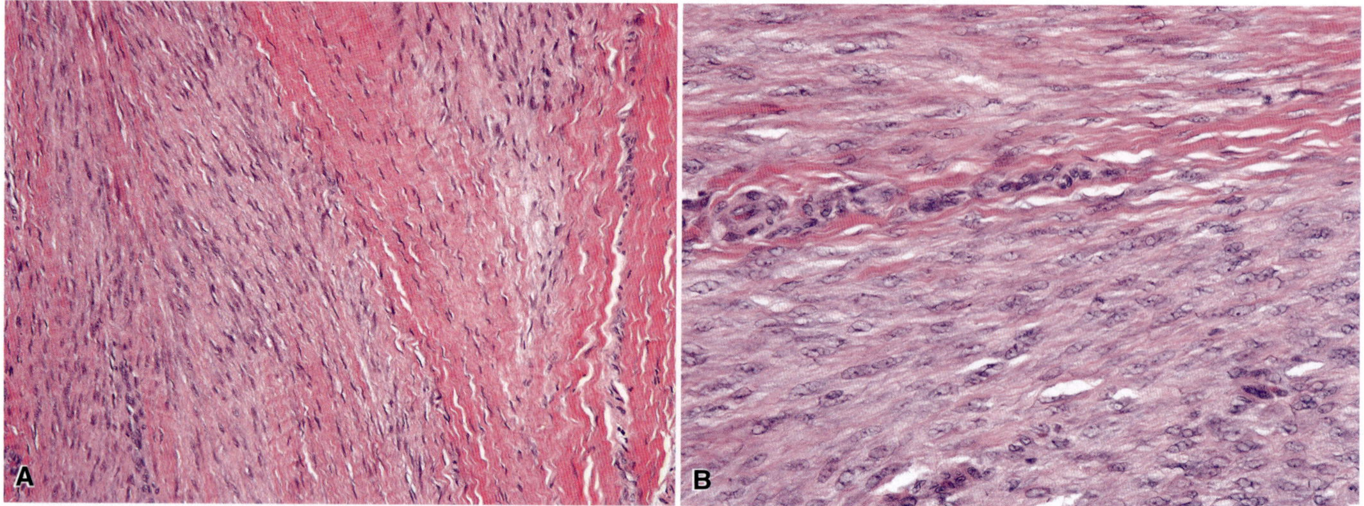

Figure 3.35 Palmar Fibromatosis. (A) Cellular fascicles of bland myofibroblasts infiltrate the palmar fascia. (B) The tumor cells contain vesicular nuclei and palely eosinophilic cytoplasm.

and EMA, in contrast to SFT, which is consistently negative for SSTR2 and is only focally positive for EMA in approximately 20% of cases.[154] STAT6 expression confirms the diagnosis of meningeal SFT. Fibrous meningiomas are also often positive for S-100 protein. In addition, a subset of fibrous meningiomas express the tight junction–associated protein claudin-1, which is consistently negative in SFT.[154]

Fibromatoses

Superficial Fibromatoses

Superficial fibromatoses are benign, recurring but nonmetastasizing, infiltrative fibroblastic lesions arising most commonly within palmar or plantar superficial aponeuroses.[155-157]

Clinical Features

Superficial **palmar fibromatosis** (Dupuytren disease or contracture) is the most common type of fibromatosis.[155,158] This condition mainly affects middle-aged to elderly adults, with a strong predilection for men (male-to-female ratio, 3 to 4:1), and an increasing incidence with advancing age; almost 20% of the general population is affected by 65 years of age.[159] For unknown reasons, palmar fibromatosis occurs most commonly in northern Europeans and is rare in black populations. Patients present with slowly growing small subcutaneous nodules, plaques, or cordlike indurations involving the dermis and underlying fascia of the palm. These nodules may lead to contractures, which usually predominate on the ulnar side of the palm, affecting the fourth and fifth fingers. Dupuytren disease may be bilateral (50% of cases), and the soles of the feet (Ledderhose disease) may be affected simultaneously or metachronously.[156,158,159] There is an association between Dupuytren disease and trauma, alcoholism, diabetes, epilepsy, and chronic lung disease. Coexistence with other superficial fibromatoses (penile fibromatosis, knuckle pads) has also been described but not with deep (desmoid-type) fibromatosis.[156,158]

Plantar fibromatosis (Ledderhose disease) is more common in young adults, children, and adolescents, occurring within the plantar aponeurosis, usually in non–weight-bearing areas.[155,156] The disease usually occurs as solitary or multiple firm nodules that are painful after a long period of standing or walking. Plantar contractures are rare.

Knuckle pads are uncommon, flat or dome-shaped fibrous thickenings of the backs of the proximal interphalangeal or metacarpophalangeal joints.[160] They are frequently associated with palmar and/or plantar fibromatosis.[161] Microscopically, they resemble palmar fibromatosis but do not cause contractures.

Penile fibromatosis (Peyronie disease) is an ill-defined fibrous thickening or mass in the shaft of the penis. Histologically similar to other types of superficial fibromatosis, this lesion will not be discussed further in this chapter.[162]

Pathologic Features

Palmar and plantar fibromatoses consist of single or multiple nodules 0.5 to 2 cm in diameter, attached to a thickened aponeurosis. On cut section, these nodules are firm and grayish in color.

Histologically, the nodules are composed of a monotonous, variably collagenous, fascicular proliferation of bland, uniform fibroblasts (Fig. 3.35). Some mitotic figures may be visible, especially in early (cellular) lesions. The lesion originates from, and blends into, the palmar or plantar aponeurosis and extends into the overlying subcutaneous fat and sometimes dermis. Lesions of long duration are less cellular and more collagenous. Occasional tumors may contain foci of cartilaginous or osseous metaplasia. Plantar fibromatosis is often hypercellular and may be confused with a spindle cell sarcoma (Figs. 3.36 and 3.37) (see later discussion).

Immunohistochemistry

By immunohistochemistry, the spindle cells are variably positive for smooth muscle actin and less frequently for desmin, reflecting myofibroblastic differentiation. Aberrant nuclear staining for β-catenin is commonly observed.[157,163] The cells are negative for CD34, keratins, EMA, and S-100 protein.

Molecular Genetics

Chromosomal abnormalities have been described in palmar fibromatosis, including trisomy 7 and 8 and loss of the Y chromosome.[164] Familial cases have also been reported. Trisomy 8 and 14 have been reported in plantar fibromatosis.[165] Mutations in *APC* and *CTNNB1* are not detected in superficial fibromatoses.[157]

Differential Diagnosis

The diagnosis of palmar and plantar fibromatoses in their conventional forms is usually straightforward. However, some cellular examples, especially in cases of plantar fibromatosis, may be confused with spindle cell sarcomas, including synovial sarcoma and MPNST. In addition to the presence of nuclear atypia, clinical presentation (large tumor size and deep situation for sarcomas), immunohistochemical profile (positivity for epithelial markers and TLE1 in synovial sarcoma, focal reactivity for S-100 protein, GFAP, or SOX10 in MPNST), and the presence of specific gene fusions (e.g., *SS18* rearrangement for synovial sarcoma) are helpful in distinguishing among these possibilities.

Prognosis and Treatment

Superficial fibromatoses have a significant risk of local recurrence. To prevent these recurrences, fasciectomy/aponeurosectomy followed by skin grafting is the recommended treatment whenever possible.

Deep Fibromatosis (Desmoid Fibromatosis)

Desmoid fibromatosis is an infiltrative, fibroblastic/myofibroblastic neoplasm with a significant potential for local recurrence. Dysregulation of the Wnt signaling pathway is characteristic of desmoid fibromatosis, both in the sporadic setting (>90% of cases) and in familial cases.[163,166] Pediatric desmoid fibromatosis is discussed in Chapter 4.

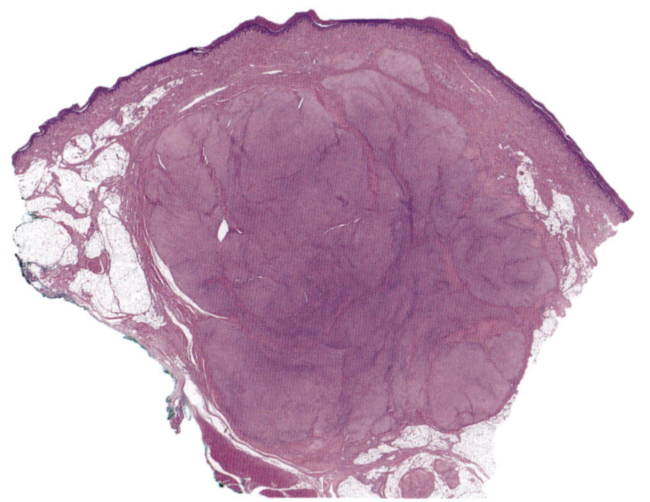

Figure 3.36 Plantar Fibromatosis. This tumor type often has a multinodular appearance.

Clinical Features

The clinical presentation of desmoid fibromatosis varies according to anatomic location. Classically, desmoid fibromatosis is divided into abdominal wall, extraabdominal, and intraabdominal forms.[155,167-170] Abdominal wall desmoid tumors typically involve the rectus abdominis muscles and aponeuroses. They tend to occur in young women during pregnancy or in the first year following childbirth (especially following caesarean section), suggesting possible hormonal and posttraumatic roles in their pathogenesis. Extraabdominal desmoid fibromatosis most often arises in the muscles and aponeuroses of the limb girdles (notably shoulder and pelvic regions), chest wall, back, proximal limbs (especially thigh), and head and neck (20% to 35% of cases) of young to middle-aged adults.

Abdominal wall and extraabdominal desmoid fibromatosis usually occurs as a painless, slowly growing, deep-seated, firm, poorly circumscribed mass. Some tumors come to medical attention because of neurologic compression symptoms or limitation of motion. Desmoid tumors of the head and neck are more frequent in children and tend to be locally aggressive at such sites.[168,171] Desmoid fibromatosis is rarely observed in the hands and feet.[167] In 5% of cases the disease is multicentric, subsequent lesions often developing in the same general anatomic region as the initial tumor (e.g., the same limb). Rarely, extraabdominal and abdominal desmoid tumors may coexist in the same patient. Occasionally, desmoid tumors develop at the site of previous excision of a Gardner fibroma, especially in the paravertebral region (see Chapter 4).

Intraabdominal desmoid fibromatosis develops in the mesentery, pelvis, or retroperitoneum of young to middle-aged adults (peak, 20 to 35 years of age).[168,169] These tumors often remain asymptomatic for a long period of time until they reach a large size (≥10 cm in diameter). Pelvic fibromatosis, which develops mainly in the iliac fossa, is often misdiagnosed as an ovarian neoplasm. These lesions may encroach on the urinary bladder, vagina, or rectum or may compress large vessels, resulting in a wide range of presenting symptoms (e.g., pain, gastrointestinal bleeding, or obstructive symptoms). Retroperitoneal tumors are also often large and asymptomatic unless they compress adjacent structures such as ureters, in which case they may cause hydronephrosis. Trauma is a potential factor in the development of intraabdominal tumors; up to 50% of patients have a history of prior abdominal surgery.[172] Mesenteric fibromatosis (see Chapter 16), the most common form of

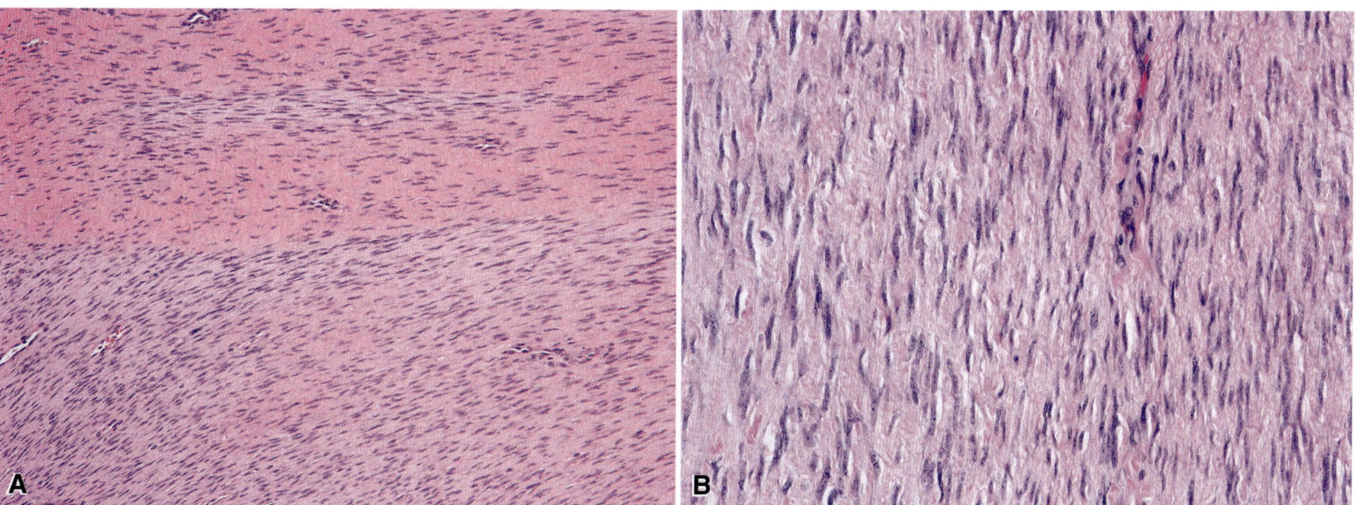

Figure 3.37 Plantar Fibromatosis. (A) The nodules can be hypercellular. (B) The tumor cells contain tapering nuclei and indistinct cytoplasm.

intraabdominal fibromatosis, may be sporadic or associated with Gardner syndrome.[170,173]

Gardner syndrome, a variant of familial adenomatous polyposis, is an autosomal dominant disease. It is more common in women and is usually diagnosed in adults 25 to 35 years of age. The syndrome is defined by the synchronous or metachronous presence of familial adenomatous polyposis, osteomas (especially in the jaw and cranial skeleton), cutaneous epidermoid cysts, and desmoid fibromatosis, among other manifestations.[169,170,173]

Pathologic Features

Most desmoid tumors are solitary, firm, grossly well-circumscribed masses. They typically measure between 5 and 10 cm in greatest dimension. The cut section reveals a whorled, whitish surface resembling a leiomyoma or scar tissue. Myxoid and/or cystic change is occasionally present and may be prominent, especially in intraabdominal tumors. Tumor necrosis is not a feature of desmoid fibromatosis.

Histologically, desmoid tumors are poorly demarcated, uniform tumors composed of spindle-shaped myofibroblasts arranged in long sweeping fascicles (Fig. 3.38). A storiform growth pattern may be present focally. The spindled-to-stellate tumor cells have slightly fibrillary eosinophilic cytoplasm with ill-defined borders and bland nuclei with vesicular chromatin and one to several small nucleoli (see Fig. 3.38B and C). The amount of extracellular matrix observed between the tumor cells is variable, but individual nuclei do not appear to touch each other or overlap. Some lesions can be very cellular, mimicking fibrosarcoma, whereas others are markedly collagenous (see Fig. 3.38D) and sometimes show keloidal hyalinization (see Fig. 3.38E), especially in mesenteric fibromatosis.[174] Well-formed, medium-sized blood vessels with muscular walls are characteristically observed between fascicles in desmoid fibromatosis (see Fig. 3.38F). Mitotic figures are readily identifiable in cellular lesions, but atypical mitoses and cellular pleomorphism are absent. Characteristically, desmoid tumors have infiltrative borders, encroaching on the surrounding skeletal muscle. As a result, atrophic or regenerative skeletal muscle fibers entrapped by the lesion are commonly observed toward the edges of the tumor, along with lymphoid aggregates. Areas of myxoid change resulting in a fasciitis-like morphology are quite common in early lesions, whereas calcifications and metaplastic ossification are occasionally observed in long-standing neoplasms. Small satellite tumor nodules are sometimes observed at the periphery of the main tumor.

Immunohistochemistry

In accordance with myofibroblastic differentiation, desmoid fibromatosis is consistently positive, at least focally, for muscle-specific actin (clone HHF35), smooth muscle actin, and calponin. Focal expression of desmin is also relatively common, often in the form of scattered positive cells. The tumors are usually negative for caldesmon, CD34, keratins, EMA, KIT, and S-100 protein. Approximately 80% of desmoid tumors, whether sporadic or familial, show nuclear and cytoplasmic expression of β-catenin (Fig. 3.39), as a result of a dysregulation of the Wnt signaling pathway.[163,166]

Molecular Genetics

Desmoid fibromatosis presents in two settings: sporadic (90% of cases) and familial. Both forms are characterized by dysregulation of the Wnt signaling pathway. Sporadic cases usually harbor activating mutations in exon 3 of the *CTNNB1* oncogene, coding for β-catenin; sequencing may be used for diagnostic purposes in challenging cases.[175] In contrast, familial cases occurring in the context of Gardner syndrome (familial adenomatous polyposis) show germline inactivating point mutations or allelic deletions of the tumor suppressor *APC* on chromosome 5q.[176] Both mechanisms result in stabilization of β-catenin, as well as its accumulation in the cytoplasm and nucleus of tumor cells, inducing cell proliferation. Tumors without *CTNNB1* or *APC* mutations are very rare and are most likely driven by alternative mechanisms of Wnt/β-catenin activation.[177] Despite initially conflicting observations,[178] sporadic desmoid tumors harboring mutations in codon 45F of exon 3 of *CTNNB1* appear to have an increased tendency for local recurrence[179-181]; *RB1* and *TP53* gene alterations are rarely observed in desmoid tumors. At the cytogenetic level, approximately one-third of desmoid tumors show trisomy of chromosomes 8 and/or 20, together with loss of chromosome Y.[164,182,183]

Differential Diagnosis

Desmoid fibromatosis showing prominent myxoid change may be confused with nodular fasciitis or a reactive myofibroblastic proliferation. This distinction can be made by the large size of the lesion, deep location, and monotonous histologic appearance with a fascicular architecture and low mitotic activity. Highly collagenous lesions should be differentiated from scar tissue. Sometimes this distinction is almost impossible, especially in small biopsy samples and in patients with previous surgery for a desmoid tumor. In such instances, nuclear staining for β-catenin can help confirm the diagnosis, although the clinical relevance of identifying residual tumor cells in reexcisions is unclear (see later discussion). Desmoplastic fibroblastoma and neurofibroma may also be considered in the differential diagnosis. However, desmoplastic fibroblastoma is usually less cellular and less fascicular than desmoid fibromatosis, with stellate fibroblasts, inconspicuous vasculature, and lack of nuclear staining for β-catenin. Neurofibroma shows less uniformly fascicular architecture, and the lesional cells contain wavy, tapering nuclei and show consistent reactivity for S-100 protein.

Cellular variants of desmoid fibromatosis may be confused with sarcomas such as monophasic synovial sarcoma, low-grade myofibroblastic sarcoma, LGFMS, and low-grade MPNST. Desmoid tumors are distinguished from most of these sarcomas by a lack of nuclear atypia. Desmoid fibromatosis is more fascicular than LGFMS and lacks the typical whorled growth pattern and the alternating fibrous and myxoid areas. In addition, the tumor cells in desmoid fibromatosis have plump vesicular nuclei and are consistently and more diffusely positive for smooth muscle actin; they are negative for EMA and MUC4. Nuclear expression of β-catenin is again helpful in this context. Low-grade MPNST often contains cellular and myxoid areas composed of spindle cells with tapering nuclei, which are at least focally positive for S-100 protein or SOX10 in 40% to 50% of cases. In the mesentery and retroperitoneum, desmoid tumors should also be differentiated from idiopathic fibroinflammatory lesions such as sclerosing mesenteritis. The latter is heterogeneous in histologic appearance, showing a variable admixture of cellular fibroblastic and hypocellular fibrotic areas, inflammatory areas containing plasma cells and lymphocytes, and foci of fat necrosis.

Prognosis and Treatment

Desmoid tumors have a strong tendency for local recurrence and may ultimately invade and compromise vital structures, such as large blood vessels and large nerves or viscera, but they do not metastasize. They rarely cause death; the 5-year survival rate is greater than 90%. Complete surgical excision with tumor-free margins is the treatment of choice, but this may result in significant morbidity. Studies suggest that the relationship between margin status and recurrence rate is inconsistent,[184-186] leading to a reevaluation of surgical approaches to desmoid fibromatosis. Less radical surgery with adjuvant systemic therapies may be more beneficial. Antiestrogen agents (tamoxifen) and chemotherapy have been administered with variable success; these approaches may be useful for progressive pediatric cases.[187] Tyrosine kinase inhibitors such as imatinib mesylate have shown some clinical activity, although the biologic basis for this remains unclear and may be limited to aggressive

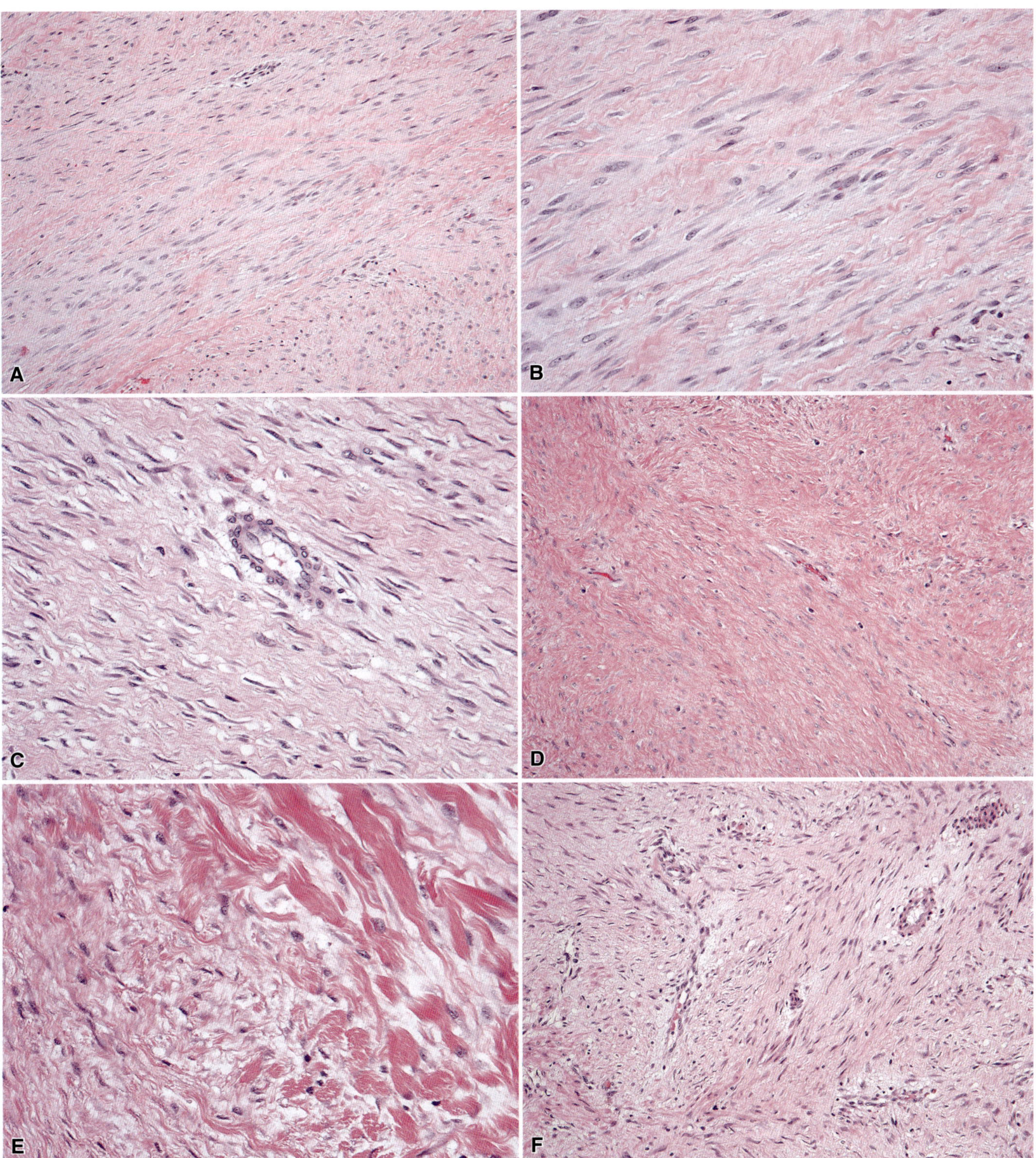

Figure 3.38 Desmoid Fibromatosis. (A) The tumor is composed of long, sweeping fascicles of spindled myofibroblasts. (B) The tumor cells contain eosinophilic, fibrillary cytoplasm and bland nuclei with small nucleoli. Note the collagenous stroma. (C) In some tumors the nuclei have a wavy, neural-like appearance. (D) A hypocellular lesion with stromal hyalinization. (E) Keloidal collagen bundles may be observed. (F) Medium-sized thick-walled blood vessels are typically seen between the tumor fascicles.

cases with *CTNNB1* S45F mutation.[188,189] Radiation therapy is another option for unresectable tumors.[190] The current trend in the treatment of desmoid tumors is to refrain from operating on all but those patients with highly symptomatic tumors. Others receive radiologic follow-up or low doses of methotrexate or doxorubicin (Adriamycin) to stabilize the lesions.[191,192]

PRACTICE POINTS: Desmoid Fibromatosis

- May arise in abdominal wall, extraabdominal, and intraabdominal locations (especially mesentery)
- Mesenteric desmoid fibromatosis in children and young adults may indicate Gardner syndrome (familial adenomatous polyposis)
- Composed of long sweeping fascicles of bland spindle cells arranged in parallel
- Medium-sized blood vessels are typically observed between fascicles
- Stromal collagen is often prominent
- Aberrant nuclear staining for β-catenin is a useful diagnostic feature but is found only in 80% of desmoid tumors and is not entirely specific
- Local recurrences are common, irrespective of margin status

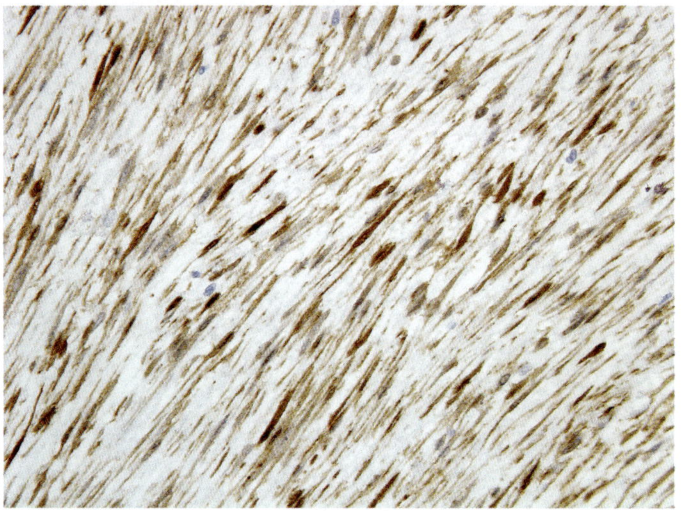

Figure 3.39 **Desmoid Fibromatosis.** Aberrant nuclear staining for β-catenin is a helpful diagnostic feature, although only 80% of cases show such a finding.

Spindle Cell Lipoma

A comprehensive discussion of spindle cell lipoma is provided in Chapter 12. However, some spindle cell lipomas are composed predominantly or exclusively of spindle cells and therefore warrant brief mention in this section. On gross examination, these tumors are usually well circumscribed with a yellowish to whitish cut surface. Histologically, spindle cell lipomas are composed of uniform spindle cells arranged in short bundles (Fig. 3.40). The tumor cells contain short stubby nuclei and scant cytoplasm. Brightly eosinophilic ropy collagen bundles, as well as interstitial mast cells, are commonly seen admixed with the spindle cells (see Fig. 3.40B). The adipocytic component may be minimal or completely absent. Some tumors show prominent myxoid stroma. A cellular variant showing little intervening stroma may expand the differential diagnosis.

By immunohistochemistry, the tumor cells are strongly and diffusely positive for CD34 and negative for smooth muscle actin, desmin, and S-100 protein. Nuclear expression of RB1 is lost,[61] in keeping with the chromosomal abnormalities (mainly deletions) at 13q and 16q consistently present in spindle cell lipoma.

Because of its histologic appearances, spindle cell lipoma can be confused with both benign and malignant neoplasms, including schwannoma, perineurioma, cellular neurofibroma, cellular angiofibroma, nodular fasciitis, desmoid fibromatosis, low-grade MPNST, and spindle cell liposarcoma, although the diagnosis is usually relatively straightforward once the diagnosis is considered.

Atypical Spindle Cell Lipomatous Tumor

Atypical spindle cell lipomatous tumor is a distinctive adipocytic neoplasm that usually affects middle-aged adults and most commonly arises in subcutaneous tissue of the extremities or trunk.[193] Designations such as *spindle cell liposarcoma*,[194,195] *atypical spindle cell lipoma*,[196] and *fibrosarcoma-like lipomatous neoplasm*[197] have been used to describe series of cases of this tumor type, which had been initially classified as a variant of ALT/WDLPS (see Chapter 12); however, due to substantial clinical, histologic, and molecular differences, it is now considered a distinctive low-grade form of liposarcoma.[193,195] Histologically, atypical spindle cell lipomatous tumor is a poorly marginated proliferation of relatively uniform ovoid to elongated spindle cells set in a fibrous or

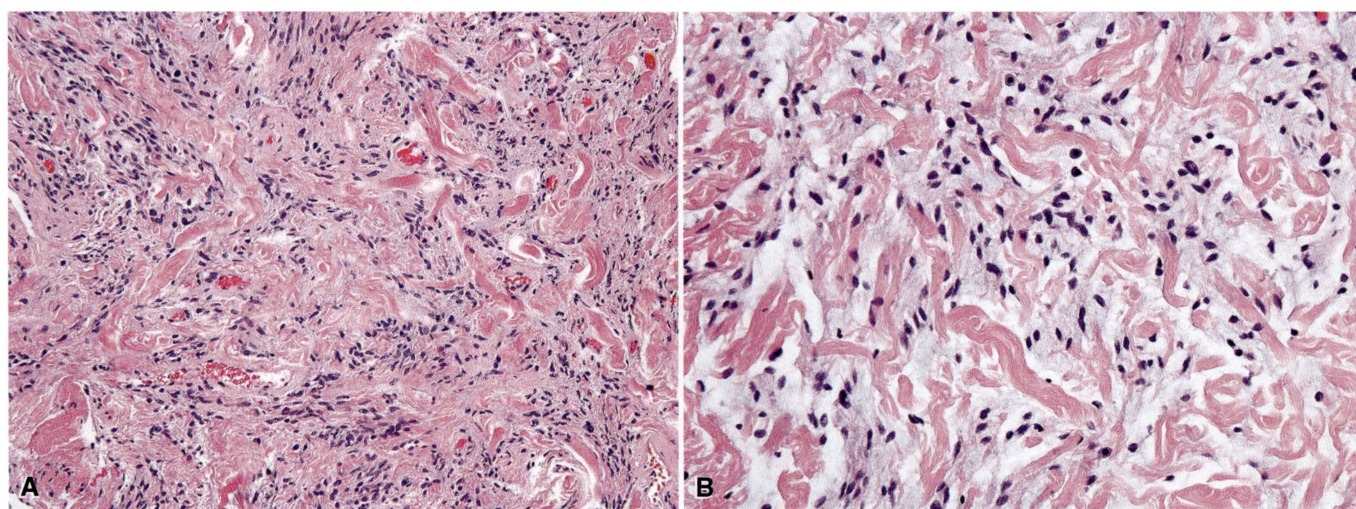

Figure 3.40 **Spindle Cell Lipoma.** (A) The tumor is composed of loose fascicles of bland spindle cells with prominent collagen bundles. This case lacked an adipocytic component. (B) Ropy collagen bundles and prominent mast cells are characteristic features. Note the short spindle cells with hyperchromatic nuclei and myxoid stroma.

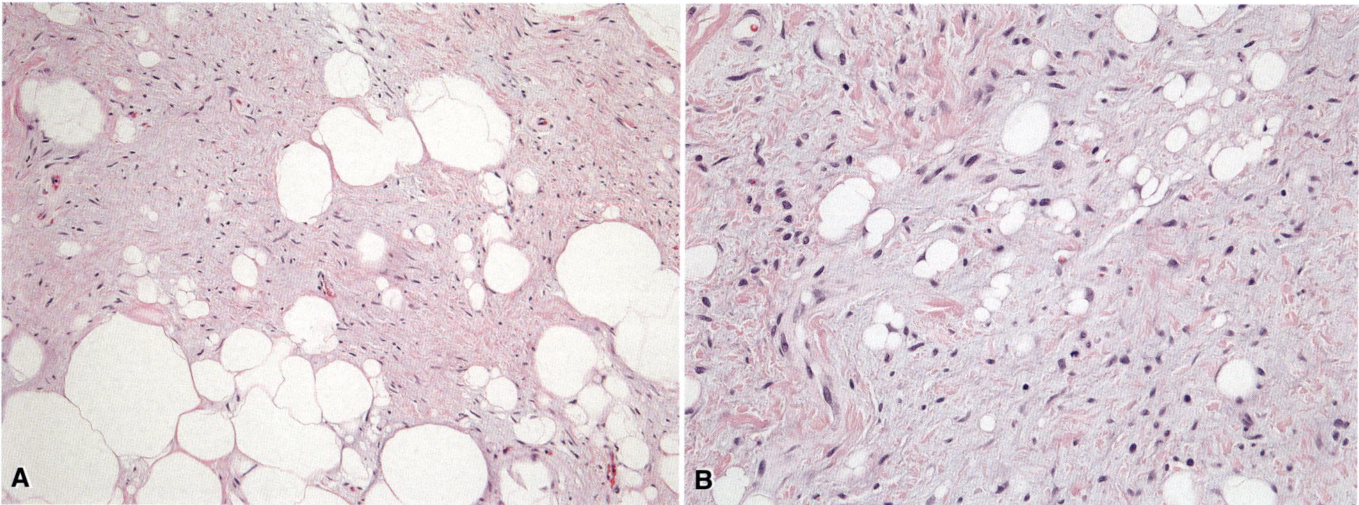

Figure 3.41 **Atypical Spindle Cell Lipomatous Tumor.** (A) Relatively uniform spindle cells are set in a fibrous stroma with scattered adipocytes showing variation in size. (B) Mild nuclear atypia and occasional lipoblasts are observed.

myxoid stroma, with a variable admixed adipocytic component showing variation in adipocyte size, scattered atypical hyperchromatic stromal cells, and occasional univacuolated or multivacuolated lipoblasts (Fig. 3.41). There is usually only mild nuclear hyperchromasia. The variable proportions of spindle cells, adipocytes, and lipoblasts; and cellular elements versus extracellular matrix; as well as the quality of the extracellular matrix (collagenous or myxoid) result in a range of microscopic appearances. As such, the morphology of atypical spindle cell lipomatous tumor is best described as a broad spectrum between the following extremes.(1) Paucicellular tumors, with few cytologically bland spindle cells and minimal nuclear atypia, set in an abundant myxoid matrix with scattered mature adipocytes. These lesions tend to occur in the distal extremities, mainly in the hands and feet, and morphologically may resemble spindle cell lipoma, except for the presence of nuclear atypia and hyperchromasia, the lack of refractile ropy collagen bundles and, in many cases, the anatomic location. (2) Significantly more cellular tumors, composed of numerous spindle cells showing diffuse, mild-to-moderate nuclear atypia, with variable presence of lipoblasts and less extracellular matrix. These lesions could be designated spindle cell ALT/spindle cell liposarcoma, although they behave in a relatively indolent manner.[195]

By immunohistochemistry, the tumor cells are positive for CD34 in approximately 65% of cases; S-100 protein and desmin are also expressed in 20% to 40% of cases. RB1 expression is lost in 60% of cases.[193] In contrast to conventional ALT/WDLPS, MDM2 and CDK4 are negative. These immunohistochemical differences reflect the underlying molecular features of atypical spindle cell lipomatous tumor, which lacks the genomic amplifications of chromosome 12q13–15 characteristic of ALT/WDLPS; atypical spindle cell lipomatous tumor may be biologically closely related to spindle cell lipoma and other tumors showing deletions of chromosome 13q.[193,195]

The differential diagnosis of atypical spindle cell lipomatous tumor includes spindle cell lipoma, neurofibroma, well-differentiated sclerosing liposarcoma, and occasionally low-grade MPNST. Spindle cell lipoma has a limited anatomic distribution (upper back, shoulder, head, and neck) and contains distinctive ropy collagen bundles, which are usually absent in atypical spindle cell lipomatous tumor. In addition, variation in adipocyte size, scattered atypical stromal cells, mild nuclear atypia, and lipoblasts favor atypical spindle cell lipomatous tumor. Similar to atypical spindle cell lipomatous tumor, neurofibroma is characterized by a proliferation of S-100 protein and CD34-positive spindle cells, but the lesional cells typically contain wavy nuclei, adipocytic differentiation is absent, and scattered neurofilament protein–positive axons are usually detected. Well-differentiated sclerosing liposarcoma is composed of bizarre hyperchromatic stromal cells set in a densely collagenous hypocellular stroma, with occasional lipoblasts, and (tumor cells) show nuclear expression of (MDM2 and CDK4). Low-grade MPNST may also express S-100 protein but is usually more cellular than atypical spindle cell lipomatous tumor, and is composed of spindle cells with tapering or wavy nuclei with mild nuclear atypia that characteristically show perivascular accentuation.

Spindle cell liposarcoma recurs locally in 10% to 15% of cases, sometimes repeatedly, if marginally or incompletely excised, but has no potential to metastasize. Dedifferentiation is exceedingly rare.[193]

Schwannoma and Variants

Schwannomas (formerly known as neurilemmomas, a term introduced by Stout in 1935) are common benign peripheral nerve sheath tumors composed of a relatively uniform population of cells showing schwannian differentiation. Many distinct variants have been described, with a wide range of histologic appearances: ancient schwannoma,[198] plexiform schwannoma,[199-201] cellular schwannoma,[202,203] melanotic schwannoma,[204,205] gastric schwannoma,[206,207] microcystic/reticular schwannoma,[208] and epithelioid schwannoma.[209,210] Schwannomas of the gastrointestinal tract are discussed in Chapter 16, and epithelioid schwannoma is discussed in Chapter 6. In addition, rare hybrid nerve sheath tumors showing features of schwannoma combined with another benign nerve sheath tumor have been described, including hybrid schwannoma/neurofibroma and hybrid schwannoma/perineurioma (see Chapter 15). Such tumors may contain histologically discrete areas showing an abrupt transition between different morphologies[211,212] or contain an intimate admixture of the different cell types.[213]

Conventional Schwannoma

Clinical Features

Schwannomas affect patients of all ages but are most common in middle-aged adults, without a clear gender predilection. They frequently arise in the subcutaneous tissues of the distal extremities or the head and neck region, but their anatomic distribution is wide, including retroperitoneal, mediastinal, and visceral locations. Peripheral schwannomas usually

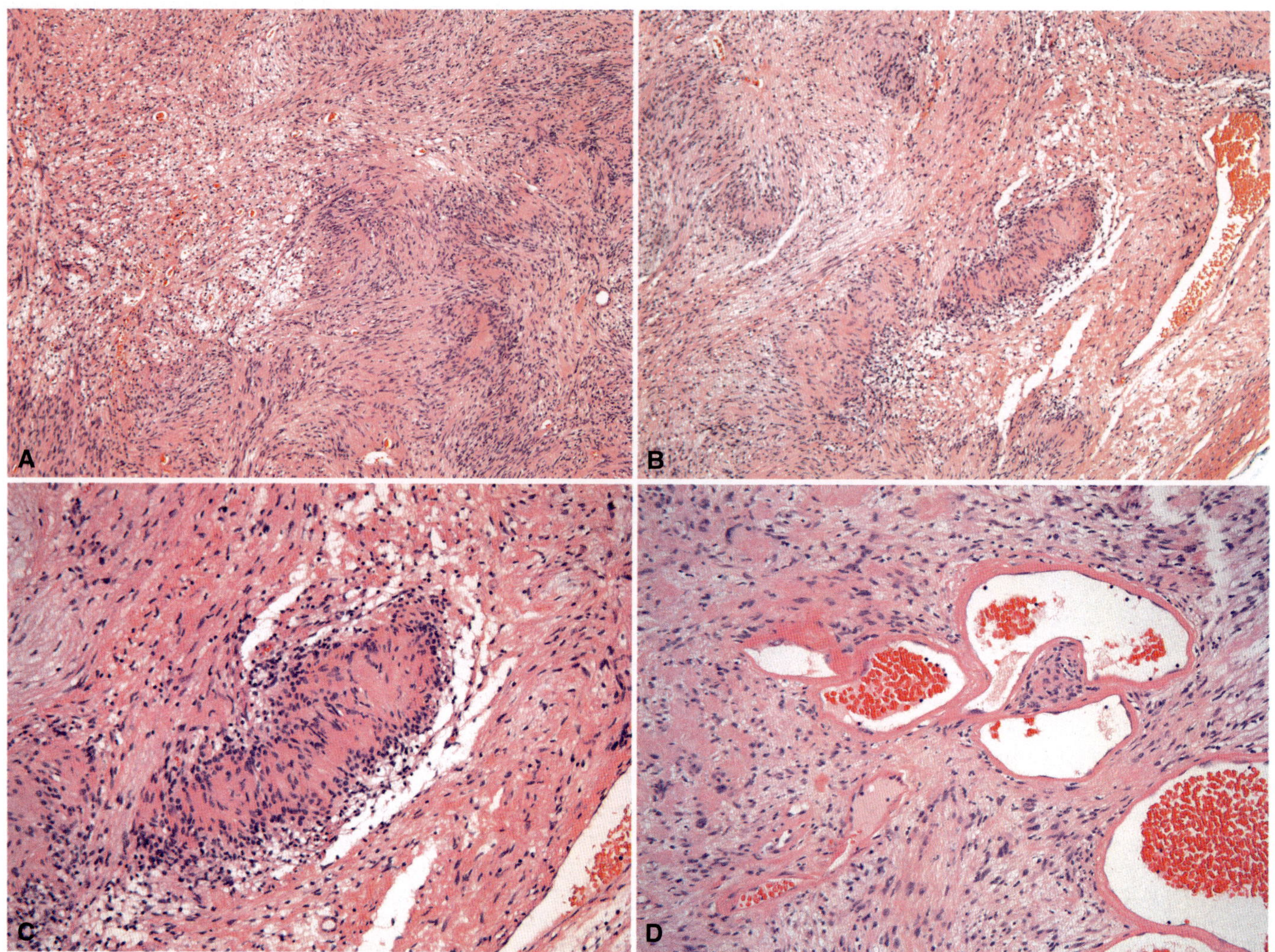

Figure 3.42 **Schwannoma.** A typical example of schwannoma (A) composed of fascicles of plump spindle cells. Many schwannomas show variable cellularity (B), with alternating hypocellular and cellular areas, including foci of nuclear palisading surrounding aggregates of cellular processes (Verocay bodies) (C). Hyalinized, thick-walled blood vessels are characteristic of schwannomas (D) and can be a helpful diagnostic clue in core biopsy specimens.

present as solitary asymptomatic nodules arising eccentrically on sensory nerves. Some schwannomas are associated with the hereditary syndrome neurofibromatosis type 2 (NF2), in such cases frequently arising bilaterally from the intracranial vestibular nerves.

Pathologic Features

Conventional schwannoma grows as a nodular, well-circumscribed, encapsulated mass on the periphery of a nerve. The tumor is usually surrounded by a thick capsule and is composed of fascicles of plump spindle cells with elongated tapering nuclei and moderately abundant, eosinophilic cytoplasm with indistinct cell borders (Fig. 3.42). Focal nuclear atypia and mitotic activity may be present. The cellularity is variable (see Fig. 3.42B) due to a characteristic zonation of alternating hypercellular areas (Antoni A), with distinctive focal nuclear palisading surrounding aggregates of cellular processes (Verocay bodies) (see Fig. 3.42C), and looser hypocellular areas (Antoni B). Thick-walled, hyalinized blood vessels, occasionally with perivascular hemosiderin deposition, are commonly present (see Fig. 3.42D), as well as variable numbers of foamy histiocytes and lymphoid cells. Areas of infarction, stromal hyalinization, cystic degeneration, and edema are frequently found to variable degrees; tumors in which these features are prominent and accompanied by significant degenerative nuclear atypia are often called "ancient" schwannomas (Fig. 3.43). Rare schwannomas, which have been referred to as "neuroblastoma-like," contain abundant small, rounded hyperchromatic Schwann cells forming giant rosettelike structures surrounding collagenous nodules (Fig. 3.44).[214]

Schwannomas occurring in some anatomic locations show distinct morphologic features that may reflect differences in biology. The lack of encapsulation characteristic of schwannomas of the sinonasal and gastrointestinal tract and the prominent lymphoid infiltrate cuffing gastrointestinal (especially gastric) schwannomas (see Chapter 16) are two examples.[206,215,216]

Immunohistochemistry

By immunohistochemistry, tumor cells in schwannomas consistently express S-100 protein, showing strong and diffuse nuclear and cytoplasmic staining (Fig. 3.45), as well as SOX10. The capsule is positive for EMA, which highlights the delicate cytoplasmic processes of perineurial cells.[217] GFAP is often coexpressed by tumor cells, especially in gastrointestinal and retroperitoneal tumors, sometimes diffusely but more commonly focally.[218,219] Keratin staining is commonly detected in deep-seated schwannomas of the retroperitoneum and posterior mediastinum, mainly with AE1/AE3, which has been attributed to cross-reactivity with GFAP.[219,220]

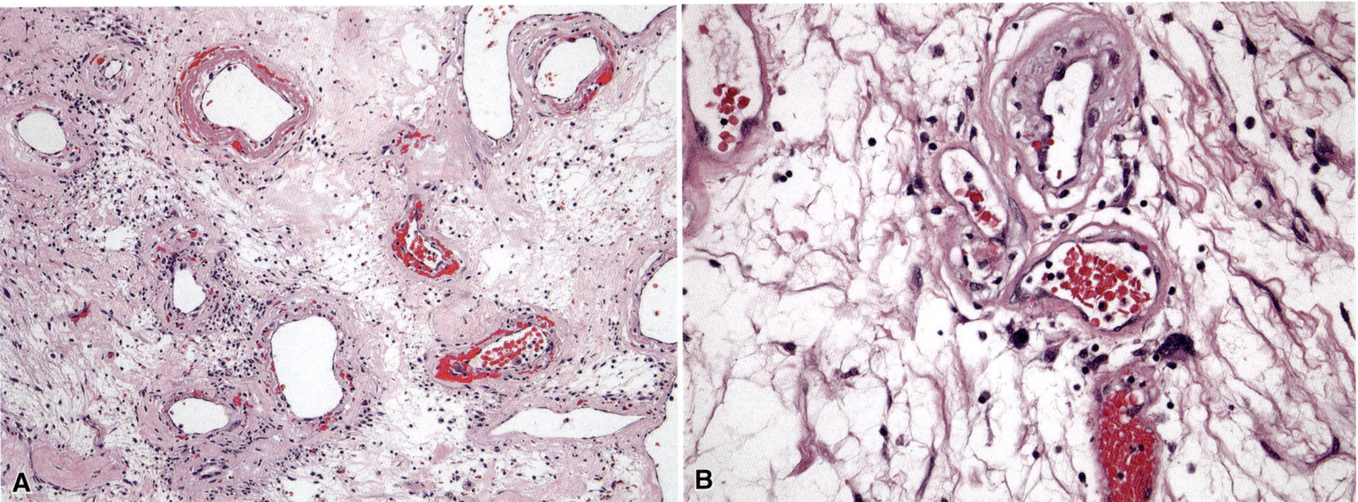

Figure 3.43 **Ancient Schwannoma.** Schwannomas with extensive infarction, stromal hyalinization, and edema (A) often contain pleomorphic tumor cells with degenerative nuclear atypia (B).

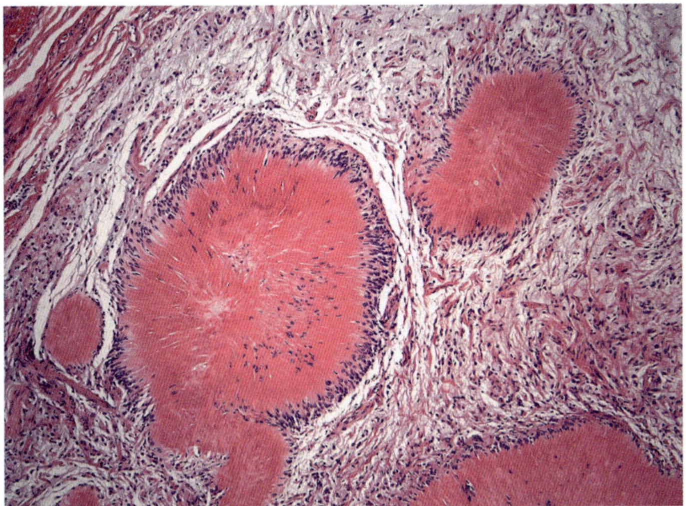

Figure 3.44 **"Neuroblastoma-Like" Schwannoma.** Occasional otherwise typical schwannomas contain giant rosettelike structures, composed of collagenous nodules surrounded by small rounded hyperchromatic cells.

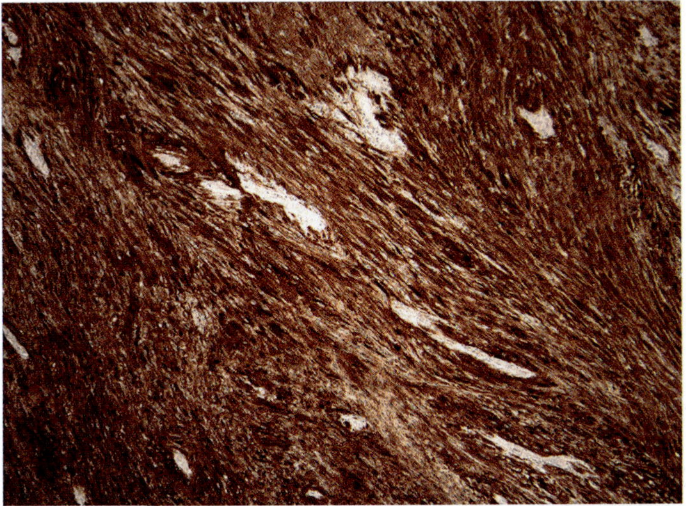

Figure 3.45 **Schwannoma.** The tumor cells show strong, diffuse staining for S-100 protein.

Molecular Genetics

Conventional schwannomas are characterized by loss of expression of the protein merlin, a critical regulator of contact-dependent inhibition of proliferation, cell-to-cell adhesion, transmembrane signaling, and actin cytoskeleton organization. In the context of NF2, the loss of merlin expression is due to loss-of-function mutations of the *NF2* gene, a tumor suppressor gene located at 22q12. Biallelic inactivation of *NF2* is usually due to germline truncating deletions followed by loss of heterozygosity.[221,222] Sporadic conventional schwannomas usually show similar somatic mutations, including common losses of chromosome 22q, but occasionally show other epigenetic or posttranslational events, also resulting in loss of merlin expression.[223,224] Additional recurrent mutations affect *ARID1A*, *ARID1B,* and *DDR.* A recurrent *SH3PXD2A-HTRA1* rearrangement, resulting from a balanced chromosomal inversion on chromosome 10q, is present in approximately 10% of schwannomas and leads to MEK-ERK activation.[225]

Differential Diagnosis

The diagnosis of conventional schwannoma is usually straightforward, in contrast to its morphologic variants that may closely mimic other neoplasms (Box 3.7 and later discussion). Of note, nuclear palisading is a nonspecific finding, occasionally prominent in other tumor types such as synovial sarcoma or GIST. The characteristic strong and diffuse staining for S-100 protein in schwannoma is comparable only to that seen in melanoma, from which schwannoma can usually be differentiated on morphologic grounds, or with the appropriate clinicopathologic correlation. Rarely, schwannomas showing extensive degenerative changes, such as infarction or stromal hyalinization, may be mistakenly classified as reactive or fibrous lesions.

Prognosis and Treatment

Schwannomas only very rarely recur following marginal surgical excision. In the exceedingly rare occasions when malignant transformation occurs, it is most often in the form of sarcomas with epithelioid cytomorphology, either epithelioid angiosarcoma or epithelioid MPNST.[226-228]

Cellular Schwannoma

Most often located in the retroperitoneum or mediastinum, this variant of schwannoma usually occurs as a large, deep-seated mass arising from a large nerve, which may be focally infiltrative and even cause bone erosion, raising the clinical suspicion for malignancy.[229] These tumors

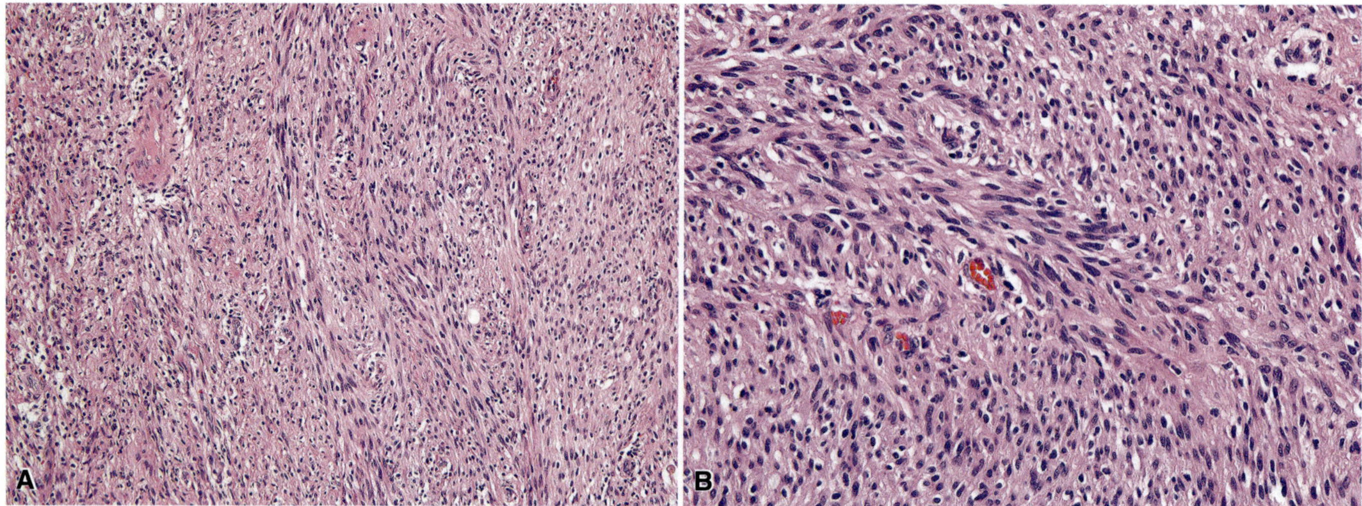

Figure 3.46 **Cellular Schwannoma.** (A) The tumor is composed of dense intersecting fascicles of spindle cells. (B) The tumor cells contain bland tapering nuclei and eosinophilic cytoplasm.

Box 3.7 Differential Diagnosis of Morphologic Variants of Schwannoma

Schwannoma of the Sinonasal Tract
Malignant peripheral nerve sheath tumor
Biphenotypic sinonasal sarcoma
Melanoma

Ancient Schwannoma
Deep fibrous histiocytoma
Symplastic hemangioma

Cellular Schwannoma
Thymoma (spindle cell variant, WHO type A)
Solitary fibrous tumor
Monophasic synovial sarcoma
Malignant peripheral nerve sheath tumor
Dedifferentiated liposarcoma
Spindle cell rhabdomyosarcoma
Sarcomatoid mesothelioma
Spindle cell melanoma
Spindle cell carcinoma

Plexiform Schwannoma
Plexiform neurofibroma

Melanotic Schwannoma
Melanocytoma
Melanoma

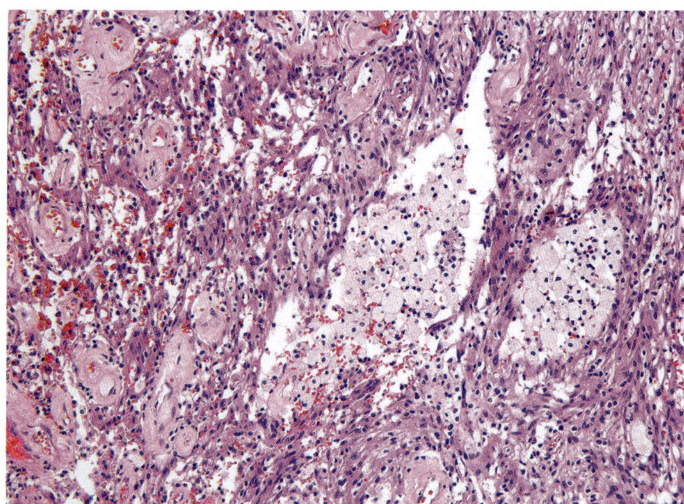

Figure 3.47 **Cellular Schwannoma.** Aggregates of foamy histiocytes are often present. Note the hyalinized vessels.

are slightly more common in women and show an increased rate of local recurrence (up to 25% in some series),[230] mainly attributable to incomplete excision. Histologically, cellular schwannomas are composed of dense fascicles of slender spindle cells with tapering nuclei and eosinophilic cytoplasm (Fig. 3.46). Occasional foci of nuclear palisading may be observed. Mitotic activity may be focally high, and there may be degenerative nuclear atypia. These findings, together with the hypercellularity and the worrisome clinical presentation, may lead to a diagnosis of malignancy. Aggregates of foamy histiocytes and hyalinized vessels are usually at least focally present (Fig. 3.47) and are helpful clues to the correct diagnosis. Combining these morphologic features with diffuse and strong expression of S-100 protein and absence of desmin prevents a misdiagnosis of low-grade MPNST or leiomyosarcoma.[202,203]

Plexiform Schwannoma

This uncommon variant is characterized by its distinctive growth pattern, consisting of multiple discrete encapsulated tumor nodules, with round or elongated shapes (Fig. 3.48) and a similar architecture to the more common plexiform neurofibroma.[231] Unlike the latter, plexiform schwannoma is not associated with neurofibromatosis type 1 (NF1),[199] although rare cases may be associated with NF2.[232] The tumor usually affects children or young adults. Most often located in the trunk, it frequently arises in the dermis and subcutaneous tissue, and rarely in deep soft tissues or visceral locations.[201] Histologically, each tumor nodule is composed mainly of Antoni A–type tissue (see Fig. 3.48), with high cellularity resembling cellular schwannoma, sometimes even raising concerns for malignancy. Similar to conventional schwannoma, the individual tumor nodules are surrounded by an EMA-positive perineurial capsule. In contrast to plexiform neurofibroma (Table 3.3), the intervening

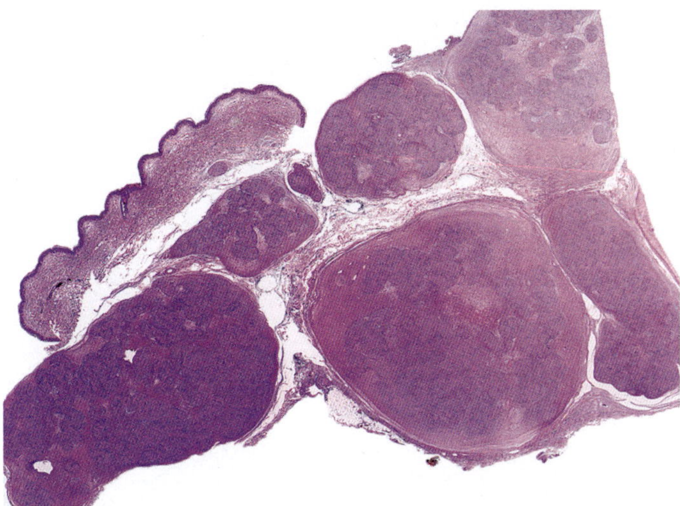

Figure 3.48 Plexiform Schwannoma. The tumor is composed of discontiguous encapsulated nodules. Individual nodules show typical histologic features of schwannoma.

Table 3.3 Comparison Between Plexiform Schwannoma and Plexiform Neurofibroma

Feature	Plexiform Schwannoma	Plexiform Neurofibroma
Age	Wide range	Children
Associated with neurofibromatosis type 1	No	Yes
Depth	Superficial ≫ deep	Superficial ≫ deep
Histology	Sharply circumscribed nodules	Hyperplastic nerves/diffuse neurofibroma-like changes
Extent of S-100 protein	All cells	50%–80% of cells
Epithelial membrane antigen (EMA)	Capsule	Patchy or negative
Neurofilament protein	Negative	Scattered axons
Malignant potential	Essentially none	Yes

tissue between the nodules does not contain a spindle cell proliferation. Plexiform schwannoma shows uniformly benign behavior.[199,233]

The distinctive variant *plexiform cellular schwannoma* usually presents congenitally or in infants as a rapidly growing mass involving the skin and subcutaneous tissues of the extremities, groin, or pelvis.[233] Formerly designated plexiform MPNST,[234] plexiform cellular schwannoma typically has a variably infiltrative or relatively circumscribed growth pattern. It is composed of highly cellular, generally small nodules of cytologically uniform spindle cells with elongated, hyperchromatic nuclei and indistinct cell borders (Fig. 3.49). Mitotic activity may be high (>10 per 10 HPF). This variant has a high rate of local recurrence but does not metastasize.[233,234]

Epithelioid Schwannoma

Epithelioid schwannoma is discussed in Chapter 15.

Melanotic Schwannoma

The rare melanotic schwannoma is a proliferation of Schwann cells with cytoplasmic melanosomes and melanin pigment production.[235,236]

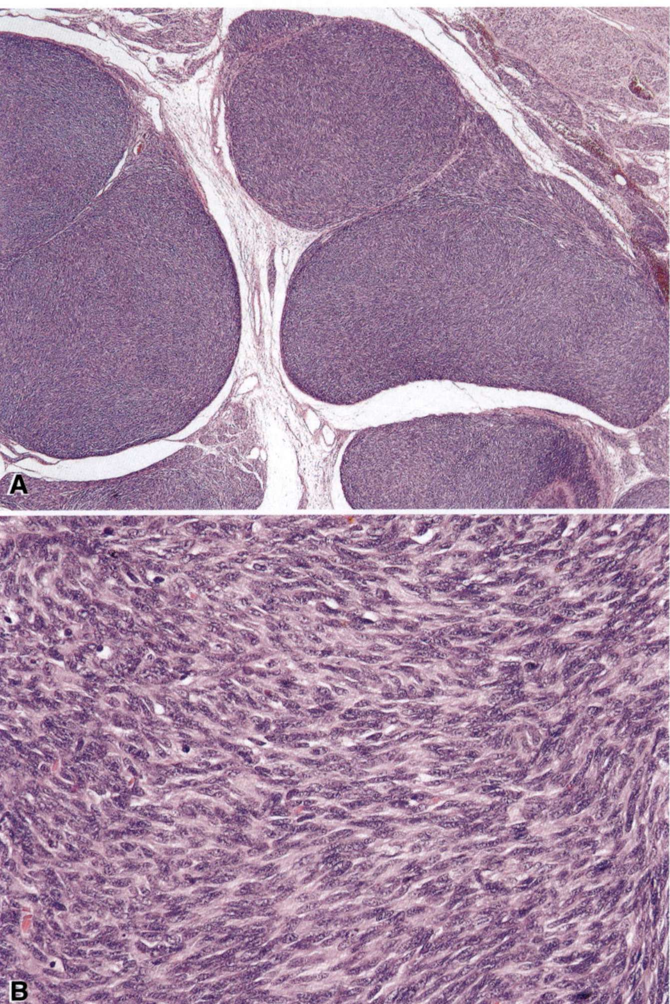

Figure 3.49 Plexiform Cellular Schwannoma. The tumor often shows an infiltrative growth pattern and is composed of highly cellular nodules (A) of uniform hyperchromatic spindle cells with elongated nuclei and indistinct cytoplasm (B).

Clinically, it affects middle-aged adults, arising most commonly from spinal nerve roots, infrequently in the soft tissues of the trunk and extremities, viscera, or bone, with a tendency for local recurrence if incompletely excised.[204,205] The tumors are often, but not always, encapsulated. Histologically, melanotic schwannoma shows a fascicular or vaguely whorled growth pattern, seldom with nuclear palisading. The tumor cells are plump, ranging from short spindle cells to somewhat epithelioid cells, with occasional dendritic processes (Fig. 3.50). Nuclear grooves are a typical finding (see Fig. 3.50B), and nuclear pseudoinclusions may be evident. A considerable number of melanotic schwannomas have spherical multilaminar calcifications and have been designated *psammomatous melanotic schwannoma* (Fig. 3.51); more than half of such tumors are associated with Carney complex (see later discussion).[237] Regardless of its association with Carney complex, most melanotic schwannomas harbor inactivating mutations of *PRKAR1A*.[238] Loss of PRKAR1A protein expression is detectable in a subset of cases.[239] Some melanotic schwannomas have enlarged, atypical nuclei, with prominent nucleoli and a high mitotic rate. These features, together with tumor necrosis, are more often seen in the poorly characterized subset of cases that pursue a malignant clinical course, but the correlation between morphology and clinical behavior is inconsistent. The differential diagnosis with malignant melanoma may be difficult in such cases due

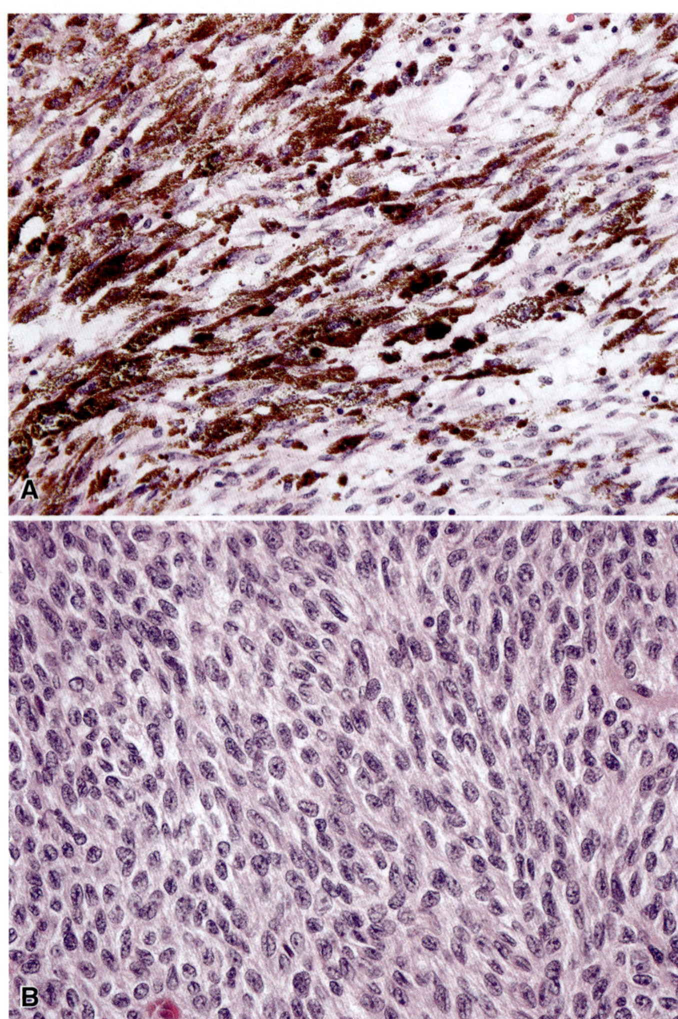

Figure 3.50 Melanotic Schwannoma. (A) The tumor is composed of fascicles and sheets of cells obscured by abundant melanin pigment. (B) In an area devoid of melanin, the ovoid tumor cells with nuclear grooves can be appreciated.

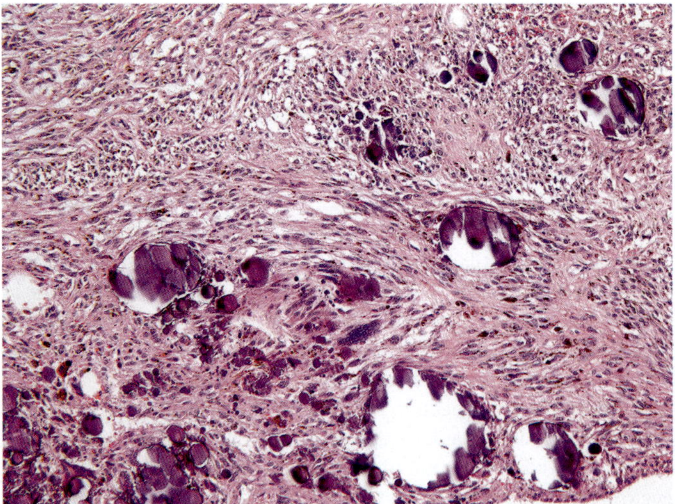

Figure 3.51 Psammomatous Melanotic Schwannoma. Occasionally, melanotic schwannomas contain psammoma bodies. Such tumors are highly associated with Carney complex.

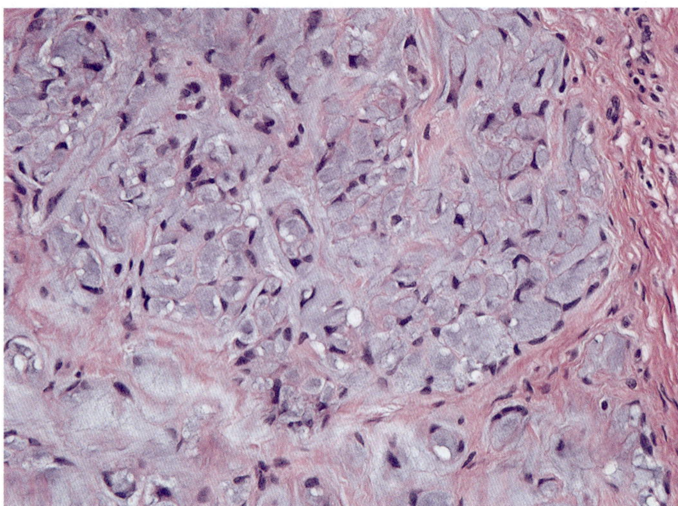

Figure 3.52 Microcystic/Reticular Schwannoma. This variant of schwannoma is composed of anastomosing slender spindle cells with eosinophilic cytoplasm in a myxoid or collagenous stroma.

to clinical and morphologic overlap[240]; loss of *PRKAR1A* expression may be helpful to support melanotic schwannoma.[238]

Microcystic/Reticular Schwannoma

Schwannomas with a striking microcystic and reticular growth pattern arise predominantly at visceral locations (especially gastrointestinal tract).[208] Although clinically comparable to other schwannomas of the gastrointestinal tract (see Chapter 16), the relevance of this morphologic variant lies in the often difficult differential diagnosis that includes much more aggressive entities (see subsequent discussion). Histologically, this variant of schwannoma is composed of anastomosing and intersecting strands of spindle cells with ill-defined eosinophilic cytoplasm in a microcystic and reticular architecture with prominent myxoid or fibrillary collagenous stroma (Fig. 3.52). Similar to other schwannomas of these sites, this tumor can be unencapsulated and even infiltrative when arising in the gastrointestinal or respiratory tracts. The tumor cells show strong nuclear and cytoplasmic positivity for S-100 protein and variably strong GFAP, which in combination with the pertinent negative markers should allow for proper diagnosis.

Microcystic schwannomas in the gastrointestinal tract are usually located in the submucosa but can extend into the mucosa and entrap native crypts. In biopsy specimens, the myxoid matrix in combination with microcystic structures can closely mimic small tubular epithelial structures and signet-ring cells, thereby leading to confusion with adenocarcinoma. The absence of nuclear atypia and immunohistochemical negativity for keratins allows for the distinction between mucinous adenocarcinoma and microcystic schwannoma. Mucosal perineurioma may also be considered in the differential diagnosis, which is easily resolved by the immunohistochemical detection of S-100 protein and GFAP, combined with the lack of EMA expression.

When arising outside the gastrointestinal tract, the differential diagnosis of microcystic schwannoma includes reticular perineurioma, myoepithelial tumors, and extraskeletal myxoid chondrosarcoma. Reticular perineurioma contains slender, elongated spindle cells with bipolar cytoplasmic processes highlighted by EMA staining, and the tumor cells are negative for both S-100 protein and GFAP. Myoepithelial tumors typically show intratumoral architectural and cytologic heterogeneity, including reticular and solid or nested areas, and epithelioid, plasmacytoid, and clear cells. In addition to S-100 protein and GFAP, myoepithelial tumors show immunoreactivity for keratins and EMA.[241] Although the reticular architecture of microcystic/reticular schwannoma is shared with extraskeletal myxoid chondrosarcoma, extraskeletal myxoid chondrosarcoma shows more abundant myxoid stroma, and the tumor cells contain more obvious eosinophilic cytoplasm. In addition, S-100 protein expression is observed in only approximately 20% of extraskeletal myxoid chondrosarcomas and is typically focal, whereas essentially 100% of cells of microcystic/reticular schwannomas show S-100 protein staining.

Schwannomatosis and Genetic Predisposition to Particular Types of Schwannoma

Sporadic schwannomas are much more common than those associated with genetic conditions. However, some schwannomas can present as a manifestation of at least three unrelated clinical conditions characterized by multiple neoplasms due to constitutional loss of tumor suppressor genes: NF2, Carney complex, and schwannomatosis. NF2 is an autosomal dominant disorder characterized by germline loss-of-function mutations in the tumor suppressor gene *NF2*, located at 22q12.[221,222] Schwannomas of the vestibular nerve, diagnostic of NF2 when bilateral, occur in combination with meningiomas and gliomas in relatively young patients. Approximately 15% of patients with the autosomal dominant Carney complex are affected by psammomatous melanotic schwannomas, in association with myxomas, spotty pigmentation, and endocrine overactivity; a subset of affected patients harbors mutations in the tumor suppressor gene *PRKAR1A* at 17q23–24.[242] Schwannomatosis, characterized by multiple peripheral schwannomas, differs from NF2 mainly by the absence of vestibular schwannomas. Approximately 50% of familial and less than 10% of sporadic schwannomatosis patients have germline mutations of *SMARCB1* at 22q11.2, in combination with loss of the contiguous *NF2* gene.[243,244] *LZTR1* is another gene implicated in some cases of schwannomatosis with a similar genetic mechanism as *SMARCB1*,[245] and additional loci are likely yet to be discovered.

Neurofibroma

Neurofibroma is a relatively common benign peripheral nerve sheath tumor composed of a mixed population of Schwann cells, fibroblasts, and perineurial or perineurial-like cells, with scattered intermingled axons.[246-248] It is most often a sporadic tumor, but it can also occur as a manifestation of the genetic syndrome NF1. There are three main morphologic variants of neurofibroma: localized, diffuse, and plexiform.[249,250] The localized variant is the most common, usually presenting as a solitary polypoid or nodular cutaneous lesion on the trunk or neck, only rarely associated with NF1. Diffuse neurofibroma is uncommon and consists of a large ill-defined plaquelike lesion presenting as a subcutaneous thickening, usually in the neck or the trunk; only approximately 10% of cases are associated with NF1. Plexiform neurofibroma, on the other hand, is consistently associated with NF1 and thus considered pathognomonic of the disease; lesions usually present in childhood, often preceding the appearance of other symptoms of the syndrome.

Localized Neurofibroma

Clinical Features

Localized neurofibroma is usually a painless cutaneous nodule or polypoid lesion presenting in adulthood with no clinically distinctive features. Although usually solitary, neurofibromas can occasionally be multiple; this occurrence does not necessarily imply a diagnosis of NF1.[249] The anatomic distribution of localized neurofibroma is wide because it can involve nerves of any size and any location, including deep soft tissues and viscera. Deep-seated tumors are more often associated with NF1 and carry a small risk of malignant transformation that is absent, or negligible, in small superficial lesions.[251]

Pathologic Features

Localized neurofibromas are circumscribed, unencapsulated tumors usually located in the dermis or subcutis. Occasional lesions are completely intraneural, resulting in a fusiform swelling of a peripheral nerve that can be grossly identified on either side of the lesion. Histologically, neurofibroma shows a variety of appearances depending on the relative proportions of its constituent cellular components and variable stroma. The most typical form consists of a haphazard or vaguely whorled proliferation of elongated spindle cells with poorly defined, palely eosinophilic cytoplasmic processes and wavy or buckled hyperchromatic nuclei, admixed with a population of short spindle cells (Fig. 3.53). Scattered throughout are abundant mast cells and occasional nerve fibers. The tumor stroma may be variably myxoid or collagenous, including purely myxoid neurofibromas (sometimes difficult to differentiate

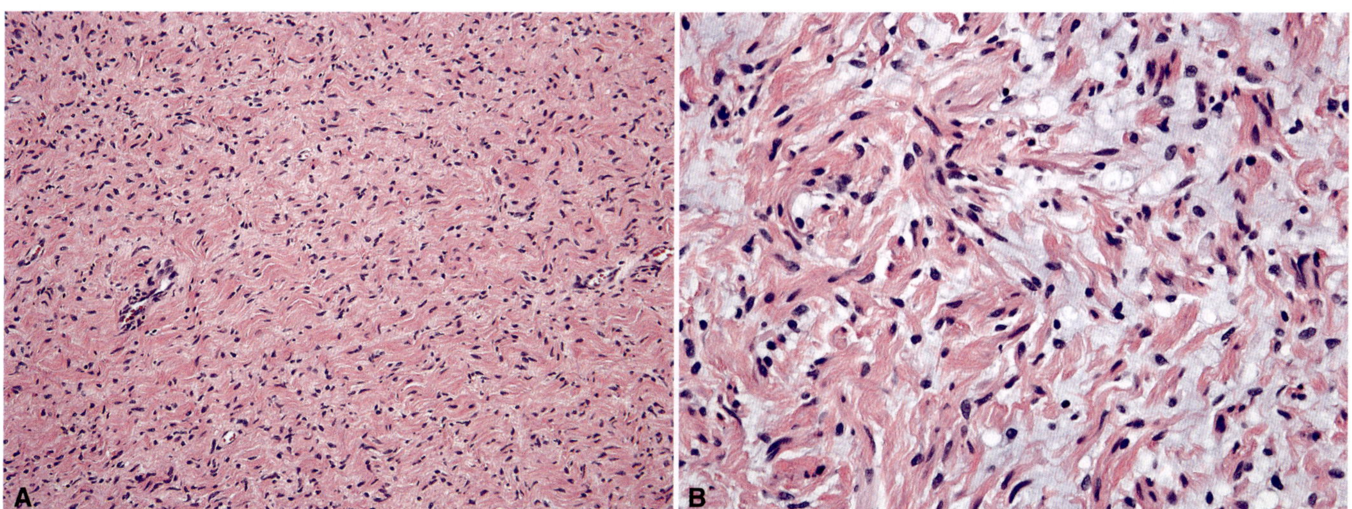

Figure 3.53 Neurofibroma. (A) The tumor is composed of haphazardly arranged spindle cells in a collagenous stroma. (B) The tumor cells contain hyperchromatic nuclei and range from short spindle cells to more elongated cells with buckled nuclei and indistinct cytoplasm. Note the scattered mast cells.

from myxoma) and markedly hyalinized tumors with thick collagen fibers (so-called collagenous neurofibroma), which are often described as having a "shredded carrots" appearance (Fig. 3.54). In any case the cytomorphology is characteristic.

The Schwann cells in neurofibroma may show focal nuclear pleomorphism and degenerative hyperchromasia; cases in which this is a prominent feature have been called "bizarre" or "atypical" neurofibromas, analogous to ancient schwannomas (Fig. 3.55).[252] Cellular atypia alone in an otherwise conventional neurofibroma has no clinical significance. In contrast, the presence of mitotic activity, which usually occurs in combination with nuclear atypia and some increase in cellularity, is very worrisome for malignant transformation.[253]

Rare morphologic variants of localized neurofibroma with no specific clinical connotations have been descriptively termed *epithelioid neurofibroma* and *granular-cell neurofibroma*, in which the Schwann cells show epithelioid morphology with abundant eosinophilic cytoplasm or cytoplasmic periodic acid–Schiff-positive eosinophilic granules, respectively. So-called *dendritic cell neurofibroma* is a rare cutaneous tumor of controversial nosology consisting of nodules or lobules of two main types of S-100 protein–positive cells: large, pale, ganglion-like cells with dendritic processes individually surrounded by more numerous smaller round-to-spindled cells, resulting in rosette-like structures.[254,255] It occurs as a clinically benign solitary papule or nodule affecting adults, with a wide anatomic distribution (see Chapter 15).

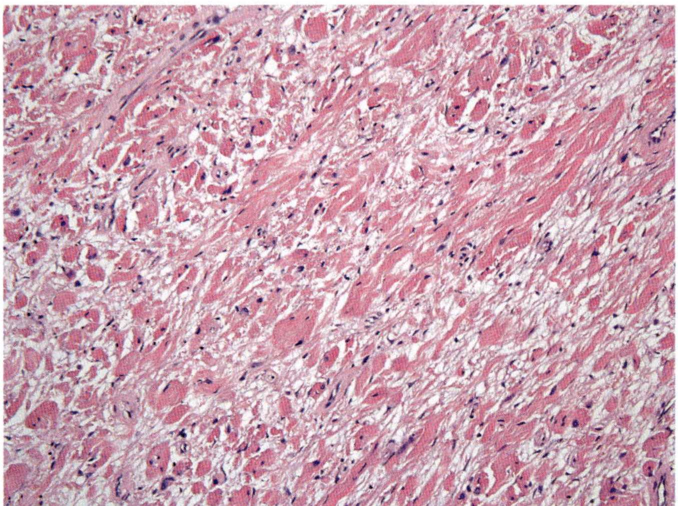

Figure 3.54 Neurofibroma. Some neurofibromas contain numerous thick collagen fibers.

Occasionally, neurofibromas contain discrete nodular foci of schwannomatous differentiation (Fig. 3.56), indistinguishable from schwannoma.[212] Such tumors are designated *hybrid neurofibroma/schwannomas*.

Immunohistochemistry

The heterogeneous cellular composition of neurofibroma is highlighted by immunohistochemistry: S-100 protein stains only a subset of cells, usually 30% to 60% (Fig. 3.57), in contrast to the extensive and intense positivity in schwannomas.[218] CD34-positive admixed fibroblasts are nearly always present (see Fig. 3.57B),[256] although less numerous, and intermingled cells expressing EMA occur in less than 10% of cases.[257] Neurofilament protein usually decorates axons scattered throughout the lesion.[218] The rare hybrid neurofibroma/schwannoma shows strong, diffuse staining for S-100 protein in the schwannomatous foci.

Molecular Genetics

The molecular genetic abnormalities in neurofibroma have been extensively studied in the context of NF1, in which the autosomal dominant germline inactivation of one allele of the *NF1* gene is followed by a second somatic hit in the neurofibromas.[258-261] Anecdotal evidence supports the notion that sporadic neurofibromas have a similar pathogenesis, consisting of biallelic inactivation of *NF1*.[262] *NF1* is a tumor suppressor gene located at 17q11.2 encoding for the ubiquitously expressed protein neurofibromin, a GTPase-activating protein that physiologically downregulates the activity of the RAS signaling pathway. Loss of *NF1* results in cellular effects comparable to those in the presence of an activated RAS oncogene.[263,264] Interestingly, loss of heterozygosity for *NF1* seems to occur in the Schwann cells, which then induce the proliferation of the accompanying cell types by paracrine signals, likely facilitated by the hemizygous dosage of *NF1* in those cells in the hereditary setting.[265-268] Hybrid neurofibroma/schwannoma may show monosomy 22, indicating a biological relationship with schwannoma.[269]

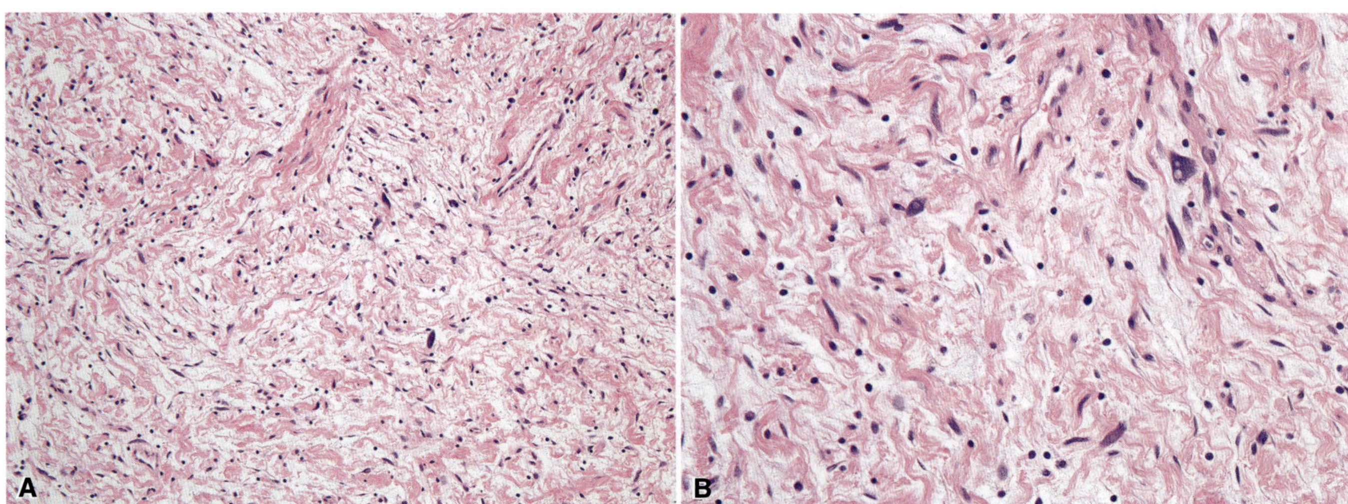

Figure 3.55 Atypical (Bizarre) Neurofibroma. (A) This variant of neurofibroma contains scattered pleomorphic cells showing degenerative nuclear atypia. Such tumors should be carefully examined for mitotic activity. (B) Note the smudgy chromatin and nuclear pseudoinclusions.

Differential Diagnosis

Neurofibroma may be difficult to differentiate from schwannoma in a small biopsy. Schwannoma generally contains less stroma and larger tumor cells; the hyalinized vessels typical of schwannoma are lacking in neurofibroma. The presence of a subset of S-100 protein–negative cells and CD34-positive fibroblasts is usually sufficient to confirm the diagnosis of neurofibroma if the morphology is misleading. The differential diagnosis for neurofibroma variants is discussed later.

Prognosis and Treatment

Sporadic localized neurofibroma has almost no potential for malignant transformation, in contrast to its syndromic counterpart. There is no tendency for local recurrence. Simple surgical excision is adequate treatment.

Diffuse Neurofibroma

Diffuse neurofibroma is a clinically distinctive variant that usually presents in young adults as an ill-defined plaque of subcutaneous and dermal thickening, most commonly in the trunk or head and neck area.

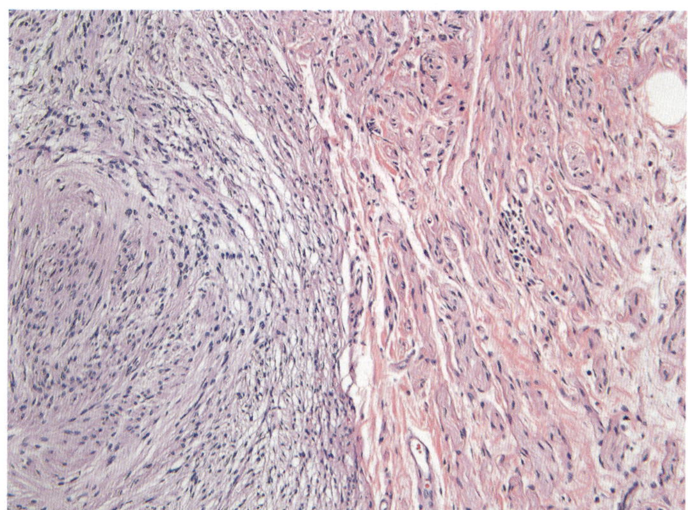

Figure 3.56 Hybrid Neurofibroma/Schwannoma. This tumor shows features of neurofibroma, as well as discrete nodular foci of schwannomatous differentiation *(left side).*

The lesion tends to be large and sometimes disfiguring. The risk of malignant transformation is minimal. The association with NF1 is variable.[250,251] Histologically, diffuse neurofibroma is a markedly infiltrative process, entrapping rather than destroying normal structures. The neurofibromatous tissue expands the dermis and permeates the subcutaneous fat along connective tissue septa and surrounding individual adipocytes, in a manner reminiscent of DFSP (Fig. 3.58). The cytomorphology of diffuse neurofibroma is comparable to that of localized lesions, although some cases tend to be composed of more rounded cells.[250] Foci of pale eosinophilic rounded fibrillary structures similar to Wagner-Meissner tactile corpuscles are a helpful diagnostic clue and may be prominent or very limited in extent (see Fig. 3.58B). The nerves entrapped within the lesion are usually hypertrophic and edematous, and the overlying epidermis may be hyperpigmented. The chief differential diagnostic consideration is DFSP; however, DFSP has a uniformly storiform architecture. Although both tumor types are typically positive for CD34, DFSP lacks Schwann cells that are positive for S-100 protein. Some diffuse neurofibromas contain scattered dendritic cells with melanin pigment that may be focally abundant, in which case the designation *pigmented (melanotic) neurofibroma* may be applied.[270,271] This variant is most often seen in black patients.

Plexiform Neurofibroma

Plexiform neurofibroma is essentially diagnostic of NF1, affecting 20% to 40% of patients with this syndrome.[272,273] It is defined by its growth pattern, consisting of multiple tortuous cords and nodules of variable size that correspond to nerve fascicles replaced and expanded by neurofibromatous tissue. The lesions most often present in children, and they may be deep but are more often superficial. Plexiform neurofibromas commonly arise in the head, skull base, or neck—from cranial nerves or upper cervical nerves. Lesions on the trunk and limbs can be associated with significant hypertrophy of the surrounding soft tissues and bone. Involvement of the skin results in dermal thickening and variable hyperpigmentation.[274] Histologically, multiple juxtaposed hypertrophic nerve fascicles of variable sizes are sectioned at different angles, resulting in a complex picture of rounded to elongated structures composed of usually myxoid neurofibromatous tissue individually surrounded by a fibrous capsule (the EMA-positive perineurial capsule) (Fig. 3.59). Often the tissue between individual abnormal nerves is involved by the neurofibromatous proliferation, similar to diffuse neurofibroma (see Fig. 3.59B). Occasionally, cells with nuclear

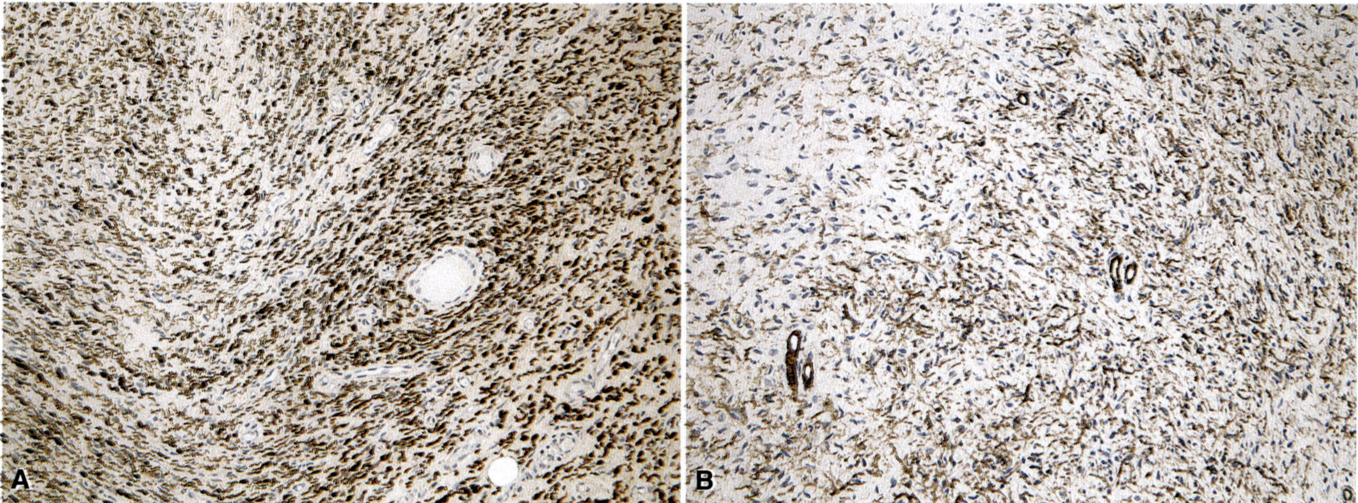

Figure 3.57 Neurofibroma. (A) S-100 protein is usually positive in the majority of cells. (B) CD34 is also usually positive.

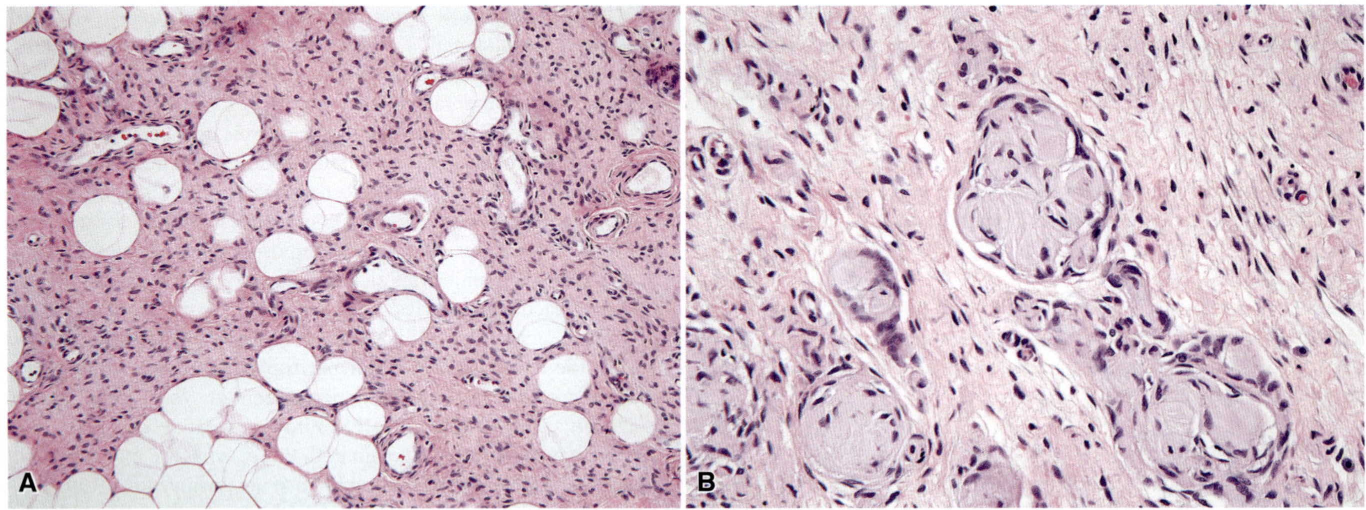

Figure 3.58 Diffuse Neurofibroma. (A) The tumor shows an infiltrative growth pattern through adipose tissue. (B) Wagner-Meissner–like corpuscles are a helpful diagnostic clue.

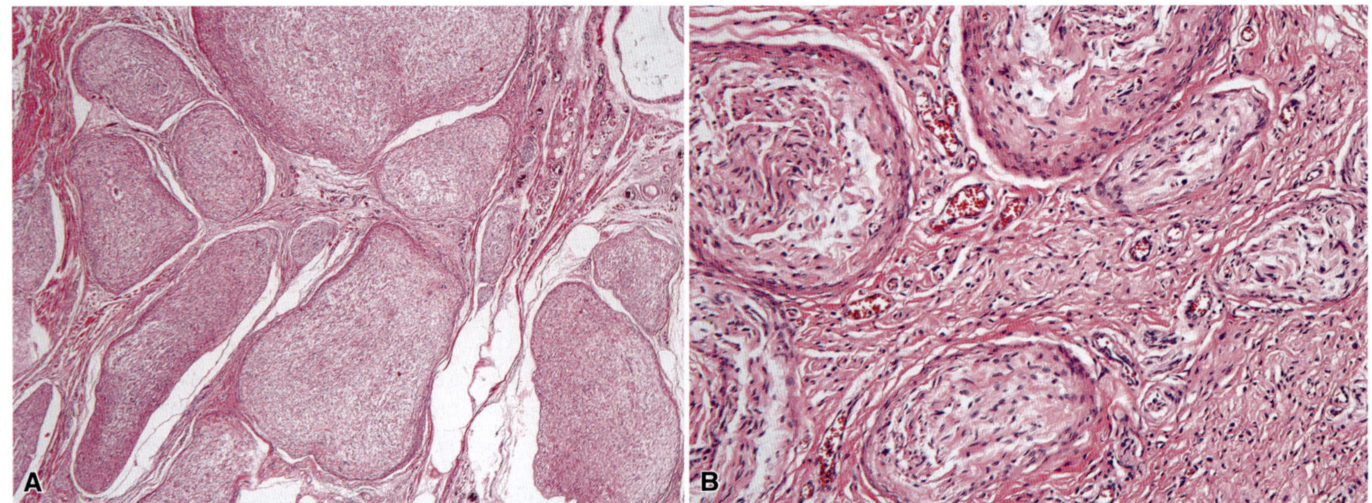

Figure 3.59 Plexiform Neurofibroma. (A) The tumor is composed of multiple, large hypertrophic nerve fascicles, often with somewhat myxoid stroma. (B) A neurofibromatous proliferation is usually seen between the plexiform nodules.

pleomorphism may be present in plexiform neurofibroma ("atypical" or "bizarre" neurofibroma). Mitotic activity, usually in areas of higher cellularity, is indicative of malignant transformation and justifies the diagnosis of MPNST. The pathologic examination of plexiform neurofibroma only rarely leads to difficulties in differential diagnosis; rather, it must be focused on excluding malignant transformation that may be a focal feature in large lesions. The features that distinguish plexiform neurofibroma from plexiform schwannoma are summarized in Table 3.3. Plexiform neurofibroma may pose significant management challenges. The tyrosine kinase inhibitor imatinib may be useful to prevent transformation of plexiform neurofibromas in early stages of the disease progression.[275] Similarly, inhibition of MAPK signaling may be an effective therapeutic strategy for inoperable plexiform neurofibromas in NF1 patients.[276]

Neurofibroma in Neurofibromatosis

Any histologic type of neurofibroma can be found in patients with NF1. Such a neurofibroma should be carefully followed clinically and with imaging techniques to intervene in case of malignant transformation. Numerous cutaneous localized neurofibromas are the hallmark of NF1. However, several localized neurofibromas can occur sporadically and occasionally in some individuals with NF2. Large deep localized neurofibromas may also rarely be sporadic, but these should raise the possibility of NF1 and prompt a detailed clinical evaluation of the patient. With very rare exceptions, plexiform neurofibroma is only seen in patients with NF1.

Malignant Transformation in Neurofibroma

The risk of malignant transformation is variable for different forms of neurofibroma. Localized cutaneous neurofibroma almost never undergoes malignant transformation, and diffuse neurofibroma only rarely does so. When a residual neurofibroma is identified adjacent to MPNST from a patient with NF1, it is usually either a plexiform neurofibroma or a localized intraneural neurofibroma involving a large- or medium-sized nerve or nerve plexus. Malignant transformation of neurofibromas in NF1 is associated with sustained activation of the RAS/MAPK pathway[263] and inactivation of p16 through homozygous deletion of *CDKN2A*.[277,278] At the gene expression level, malignant transformation from neurofibroma to MPNST is associated with loss of expression of a large number of genes and dysregulation of microRNAs involved in the p53 pathway such as miR-34a.[279,280]

The minimal criteria for malignant transformation of a neurofibroma have been somewhat controversial. Some investigators emphasize the significance of mitotic activity, whereas others also require hypercellularity and nuclear atypia (defined as nuclear enlargement and hyperchromasia).[251] As discussed earlier, cellular atypia in isolation has no clinical significance but should prompt a careful search for mitotic figures.[253] In general, these worrisome features usually develop together in malignant lesions; mitotic activity is very unusual in a neurofibroma in the absence of increased cellularity or some degree of nuclear atypia. In individual cases, particularly in patients with NF1, it may be very difficult or even impossible to predict with absolute certainty the clinical behavior of a given lesion; the underlying biology of these proliferations is a continuum that can be captured only partially in morphologic categories. Immunohistochemical markers such as p53, p16, or Ki-67, as well as DNA content or S-phase analysis by flow cytometry, have been explored in small series but are not useful in routine practice at present.[253,277,281,282] Similarly, gene expression profiling of plexiform neurofibromas has revealed a gene expression signature predicting malignant transformation that has yet to be validated for nonresearch purposes.[283]

Perineurioma

Perineuriomas are benign peripheral nerve sheath tumors composed exclusively of perineurial cells, which surround individual nerve fascicles. Much less common than schwannomas and neurofibromas, perineuriomas are not associated with NF and essentially represent the peripheral counterpart of meningiomas, which arise from the arachnoid cap cells.[284-288] There are four main clinicopathologic forms of perineurioma: soft tissue (extraneural) perineurioma, formerly known as storiform perineurial fibroma; intraneural perineurioma, which probably accounts for most cases previously diagnosed as *localized hypertrophic neuropathy* or *hypertrophic interstitial neuritis*; sclerosing perineurioma; and mucosal perineurioma.[289] Mucosal perineuriomas arise almost exclusively in the colon as small sessile polyps and are discussed in Chapter 16.

Benign nerve sheath tumors resembling soft tissue perineurioma but composed of a dual population of perineurial cells and Schwann cells are known as hybrid schwannoma/perineuriomas,[213] which are discussed in Chapter 15. Perineurial or perineurial-like cells are observed in approximately 10% of neurofibromas admixed with the other cellular components, without any clinical significance.[247,257]

Soft Tissue Perineurioma

Clinical Features

Soft tissue perineurioma affects patients over a wide age range, with a peak in middle-aged adults and no gender predilection. It usually occurs as a painless subcutaneous mass in the limbs (although the anatomic distribution is wide).[290] Approximately 25% of cases arise in deep soft tissues, 10% are confined to the skin (see Chapter 15), and tumors rarely arise at central body sites such as the retroperitoneum.

Pathologic Features

Soft tissue perineurioma is grossly well circumscribed but unencapsulated, usually with a tan or white fibrous cut surface. Tumors with abundant myxoid stroma show a more mucoid gross appearance. Histologically, soft tissue perineurioma shows variable cellularity and a whorled, storiform, and lamellar growth pattern (Fig. 3.60). The tumor cells range from the most characteristic slender spindle cells with wavy nuclei and delicate elongated bipolar cytoplasmic processes (see Fig. 3.60C) to slightly plumper cells with more ovoid nuclei (see Fig. 3.60D). The stroma is usually collagenous but may be myxoid in 20% of cases (see Chapter 5). Unusual morphologic features have been described in rare cases, including prominent vacuolization.[291] The presence of mitotic activity, increased cellularity, scattered pleomorphic cells showing degenerative nuclear atypia (analogous to ancient schwannoma and atypical neurofibroma), and focally infiltrative margins has no clinical significance.[290]

Immunohistochemistry

Perineurial cells almost invariably express EMA (Fig. 3.61).[217,292] However, the intensity of EMA staining can be very weak and easily overlooked, due to the extreme thinness of the perineurial bipolar cellular processes, often requiring careful examination at high magnification. In addition to EMA, approximately 65% of perineuriomas are at least focally positive for CD34 (see Fig. 3.61B). Claudin-1 is an extremely specific but relatively insensitive perineurial marker, expressed in approximately 30% of cases.[290,293] GLUT-1 is also expressed in perineuriomas, although it is not specific.[294] S-100 protein is only rarely expressed in soft tissue perineurioma, facilitating the differential diagnosis with schwannoma and hybrid tumors.

Molecular Genetics

Soft tissue perineuriomas show mostly simple diploid or near-diploid karyotypes, characterized by one or few clonal chromosomal abnormalities.[224,295-298] Deletion of material from chromosome 22q is a recurrent but inconsistent finding. Rearrangements and/or deletions of 10q may be a recurrent feature of the sclerosing variant. Loss of material from 22q may be targeting the *NF2* gene locus. Some cases of sclerosing and soft tissue perineurioma have shown missense point mutations in *NF2*, which supports this interpretation.[299]

Differential Diagnosis

The differential diagnosis of soft tissue perineurioma depends on its location and the nature of the tumor stroma (Box 3.8). For superficial tumors, the primary differential diagnosis is DFSP, which can be excluded by the well-circumscribed margins and the expression of EMA in perineurioma. For subcutaneous and deep-seated tumors, the differential diagnosis may be broad and includes other benign nerve sheath tumors (which in contrast to perineurioma show diffuse S-100 protein positivity), SFT, LGFMS, and low-grade MPNST.

SFT is composed of bland ovoid to spindled cells with varying cellularity and a patternless architecture, often with stromal and perivascular hyalinization and HPC-like ectatic, branching blood vessels. SFT lacks the characteristic storiform and whorled architecture and cytomorphology of soft tissue perineurioma and is positive for STAT6. LGFMS may be particularly difficult to differentiate from perineurioma due to significant morphologic and immunophenotypic overlap. LGFMS is usually characterized by sharply demarcated zones of collagenous and myxoid stroma and arcades of small blood vessels. In addition, the cells in LGFMS lack the very long cytoplasmic processes characteristic of perineurioma. Although both tumor types are positive for EMA in most cases, MUC4 is specific for LGFMS in this differential diagnosis.[120]

Box 3.8 Differential Diagnosis of Soft Tissue Perineurioma

- Dermatofibrosarcoma protuberans
- Neurofibroma
- Solitary fibrous tumor
- Low-grade fibromyxoid sarcoma
- Low-grade malignant peripheral nerve sheath tumor
- Cellular myxoma
- Low-grade myxofibrosarcoma

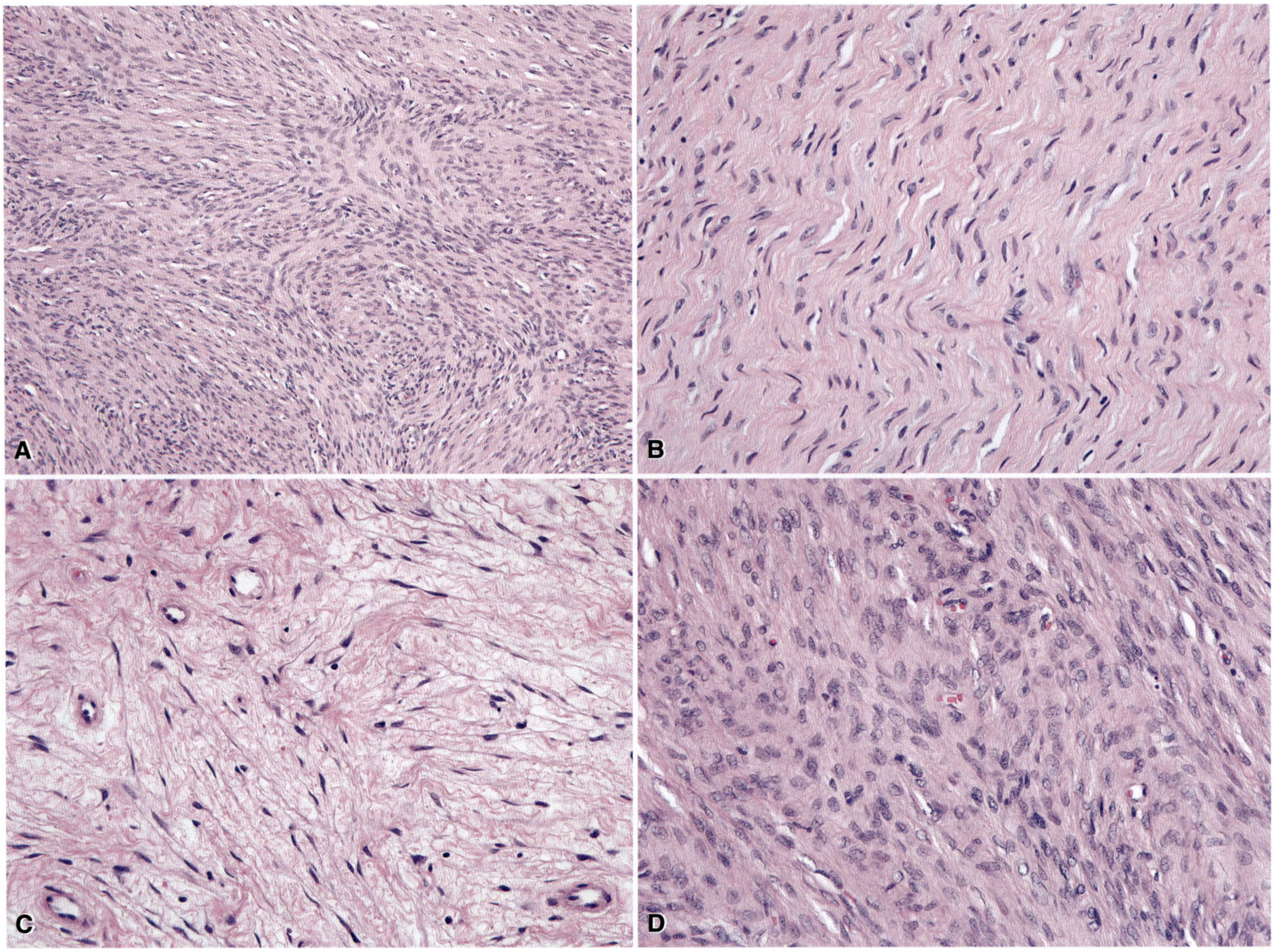

Figure 3.60 **Soft Tissue Perineurioma.** The tumor shows a storiform and whorled (A) or lamellar (B) growth pattern. The tumor is composed of either slender spindle cells with elongated nuclei and delicate bipolar cytoplasmic processes (C) or plumper cells with ovoid nuclei (D).

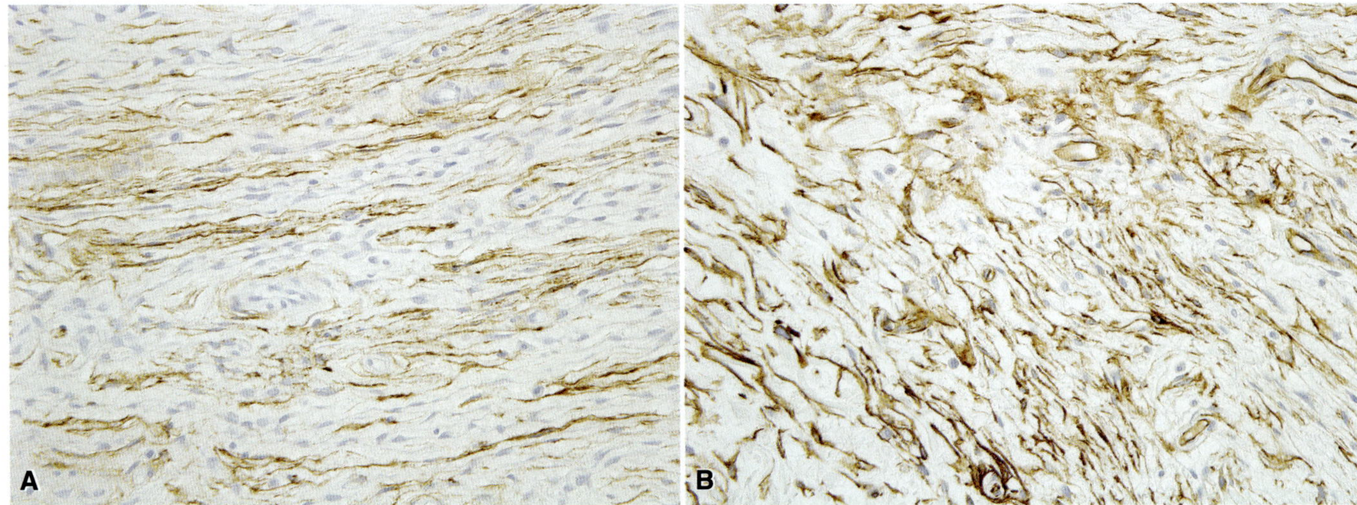

Figure 3.61 **Soft Tissue Perineurioma.** (A) The tumor cells are positive for epithelial membrane antigen, which often highlights the cytoplasmic processes. (B) Approximately two-thirds of perineuriomas are also positive for CD34.

Expression of claudin-1 may be helpful to confirm the diagnosis of perineurioma in some cases.[293] FISH for *FUS* gene rearrangement can also be used to confirm the diagnosis of LGFMS in difficult cases. MPNST may very rarely show perineurial differentiation and demonstrate a storiform and whorled architecture similar to conventional perineurioma, but in contrast it often contains fascicular areas and shows hypercellular perivascular accentuation. Malignancy can be established in such cases based on the presence of significant cytologic atypia and abundant mitoses.[300]

Examples of soft tissue perineurioma with abundant myxoid stroma may be mistaken for cellular myxoma or low-grade myxofibrosarcoma. Cellular myxoma lacks the storiform and whorled architecture and EMA expression of perineurioma. In contrast to soft tissue perineurioma, low-grade myxofibrosarcoma contains elongated, thin-walled, curvilinear blood vessels, occasional vacuolated "pseudolipoblasts," and atypical hyperchromatic pleomorphic cells.

Some cases of soft tissue perineurioma show a prominent reticular growth pattern (see Chapter 5), in which case the differential diagnosis includes myoepithelial tumors, ossifying fibromyxoid tumor, extraskeletal myxoid chondrosarcoma, and myxoid synovial sarcoma.[247,301,302] Myoepithelioma is typically dominated by epithelioid cells, contains solid or nested areas, and is positive for S-100 protein, keratins, and EMA, as well as GFAP (50% of cases). Ossifying fibromyxoid tumor usually shows a lobulated architecture and contains more rounded tumor cells. The majority of cases are positive for S-100 protein, as well as desmin in 50% of tumors. Extraskeletal myxoid chondrosarcoma is usually composed of larger cells with more obvious eosinophilic cytoplasm. In difficult cases, cytogenetic or molecular detection of the t(9;22) translocation or *EWSR1-NR4A3* characteristic of extraskeletal myxoid chondrosarcoma can be used to confirm the diagnosis. Rare examples of myxoid synovial sarcoma may show a reticular growth pattern; however, conventional highly cellular, fascicular spindle cell areas can usually be identified. In addition to EMA, immunohistochemical detection of keratins and TLE1 should facilitate the correct diagnosis.[302]

Prognosis and Treatment

Soft tissue perineuriomas are benign and only rarely recur locally.[290] Conservative simple excision is the appropriate treatment.

Intraneural Perineurioma

Intraneural perineurioma is a very rare tumor that typically affects young adults and is characterized by a symmetric expansion of a major nerve, usually in the extremities, causing clinical symptoms of neurologic deficits.[295,303] Histologically, it consists of a proliferation of bland spindled perineurial cells wrapping around individual axons and residual Schwann cells, resulting in onion bulb–like structures in cross section. There is no cytologic atypia. The clinical course is benign, although nerve compression may have functional consequences.

Sclerosing Perineurioma

Sclerosing perineurioma is an uncommon variant that typically occurs as a painless cutaneous nodule, usually in the fingers or hands of young adults.[294,304] Lesions occurring in extraacral locations are very rare.[305] Histologically, sclerosing perineurioma is a relatively well-circumscribed collagenous nodule containing cords, whorls, and clusters of small rather epithelioid or plump spindled cells with inconspicuous pale eosinophilic cytoplasm and round to ovoid small nuclei (Fig. 3.62). The cellularity is variable within the lesion, but the stroma is homogeneously collagenous throughout. The tumor cells are diffusely positive for EMA, which often highlights cytoplasmic processes. The differential diagnosis of sclerosing perineurioma is discussed in Chapter 15.

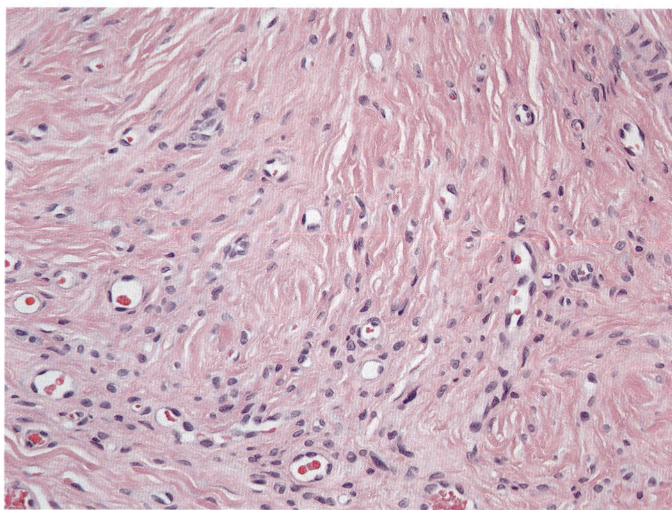

Figure 3.62 Sclerosing Perineurioma. The tumor is composed of cords of small epithelioid to short spindle cells in a dense collagenous stroma.

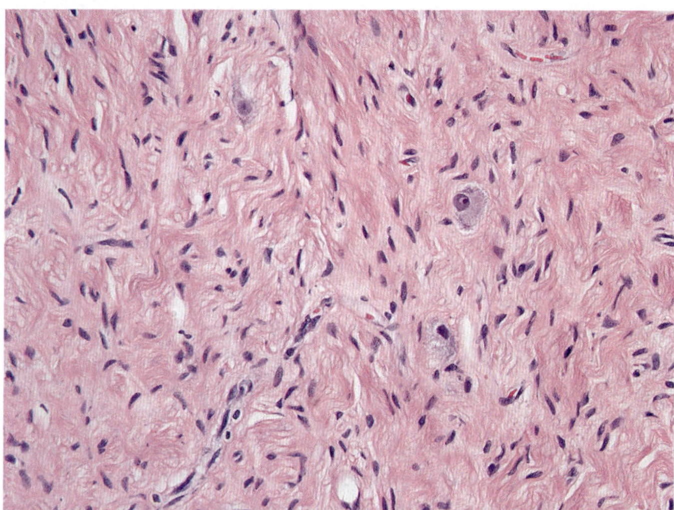

Figure 3.63 Ganglioneuroma. The tumor is composed of haphazardly arranged spindle cells with tapering nuclei and scattered ganglion cells in a collagenous stroma.

Ganglioneuroma

Ganglioneuromas of soft tissue arise most often in the retroperitoneum or posterior mediastinum, although a small proportion of cases occur in the gastrointestinal tract (see Chapter 16). Some ganglioneuromas affect patients with NF1, but most tumors are sporadic. Ganglioneuroma most commonly affects adolescents and young adults between 10 and 40 years of age, with no gender predilection. The tumor presents clinically as a large mass, rarely associated with catecholamine secretion and corresponding systemic symptoms (diarrhea, sweating, or hypertension). On imaging, some ganglioneuromas show extensive calcification, but most are nondescript homogeneous masses.

Grossly, ganglioneuromas are well-circumscribed, encapsulated, rubbery tumors. Histologically, the lesion may have somewhat irregular margins and consists of a proliferation of haphazardly arranged S-100 protein–positive Schwann cells and variably prominent, scattered mature ganglion cells, in a collagenous stroma (Fig. 3.63). Scattered axons can be highlighted by a stain for neurofilament protein.

The chief differential diagnostic considerations are neurofibroma and schwannoma. Neurofibromas rarely arise in the retroperitoneum or posterior mediastinum and lack ganglion cells but are otherwise indistinguishable from ganglioneuroma. For practical purposes, ganglioneuroma should be the favored diagnosis when a core biopsy of a tumor from such anatomic sites shows a neurofibroma-like lesion, even if ganglion cells are not identified. Schwannomas from the retroperitoneum are usually much more cellular, contain larger, plump spindle cells and occasional hyalinized vessels, and show diffuse and strong expression of S-100 protein. Retroperitoneal schwannomas are also commonly positive for keratin.

Ganglioneuromas are benign and do not recur. Rare ganglioneuroblastomas in young children contain a component histologically indistinguishable from ganglioneuroma. Very rarely, ganglioneuromas undergo malignant transformation to MPNST.

Benign Smooth Muscle Tumors

Tumors with smooth muscle differentiation can be categorized for practical purposes according to the anatomic compartment where they occur: skin, subcutis, external genitalia, deep soft tissue (including abdominal cavity, pelvis, and retroperitoneum), and visceral locations (including uterine tumors). The constituent cells have common morphologic and immunohistochemical properties, but many of these tumors form distinct clinicopathologic subsets because clinical behavior and criteria for malignancy relate primarily to location.[306] The very common uterine smooth muscle tumors have been extensively characterized, but they are not discussed in this book; they are usually studied and managed in the context of gynecologic pathology (reviewed by Nucci and Oliva).[307] Cutaneous, gastrointestinal, and external genital smooth muscle tumors are discussed in Chapters 15, 16, and 17, respectively.

Leiomyoma of Deep Soft Tissue and Related Lesions (Myolipoma/Lipoleiomyoma)

Clinical Features

Leiomyomas of deep soft tissue are rare, accounting for no more than 4% of benign soft tissue tumors,[308] and should be diagnosed with caution only after careful exclusion of malignant features. Slow-growing tumors, they form well-circumscribed masses, which can reach a large size. Two distinct subgroups are generally recognized: tumors in deep subcutaneous or subfascial somatic soft tissue and tumors within the abdominal cavity or pelvis. Primary leiomyomas of deep somatic soft tissues are particularly rare. They usually arise in the limbs, with no gender predilection. They are rarely associated with blood vessel walls. In contrast, pelvic and retroperitoneal leiomyomas are more common, and the large majority occur in women. They resemble uterine leiomyomas and, in fact, may be considered part of the same clinical and biologic continuum of hormonally driven tumors characterized by the expression of estrogen and progesterone receptors.[309,310] Like other retroperitoneal tumors, deep leiomyomas of this site are frequently large at presentation.

Pathologic Features

Leiomyomas present as well-circumscribed, white, rubbery nodules that detach easily from surrounding structures. Histologically, deep leiomyomas are composed of intersecting fascicles of elongated spindle cells with abundant brightly eosinophilic cytoplasm and blunt-ended, cigar-shaped nuclei (Fig. 3.64). Nuclear palisading is occasionally prominent. Relatively common stromal features include myxoid change, fibrosis, and occasional osteoclast-like giant cells. Stromal calcification is a typical feature of somatic-type deep leiomyoma, sometimes combined with focal clear cell change. In retroperitoneal or intraabdominal tumors in women, a range of changes similar to those of uterine leiomyoma can be found, including stromal hyalinization, trabecular architecture, focal calcification or ossification, hemorrhage with hemosiderin deposition, and cyst formation (Fig. 3.65). Retroperitoneal leiomyomas are exceptionally rare in men and are more uniformly cellular with a compact appearance.[310] Degenerative nuclear atypia may be seen, in the form of enlarged, irregularly shaped and hyperchromatic nuclei without mitotic activity, and in isolation does not indicate malignancy (see subsequent discussion).[311,312] Tumors with prominent degenerative nuclear atypia have sometimes been referred to as *symplastic leiomyomas*, as in the uterus. Some benign smooth muscle tumors have a component of differentiated adipose tissue without atypia. These can be considered neoplasms with divergent differentiation and are known as *myolipomas*. They occur in the uterus (where they are designated *lipoleiomyomas*), pelvis, retroperitoneum, or groin of middle-aged women.[313] Myolipoma is discussed in Chapter 12.

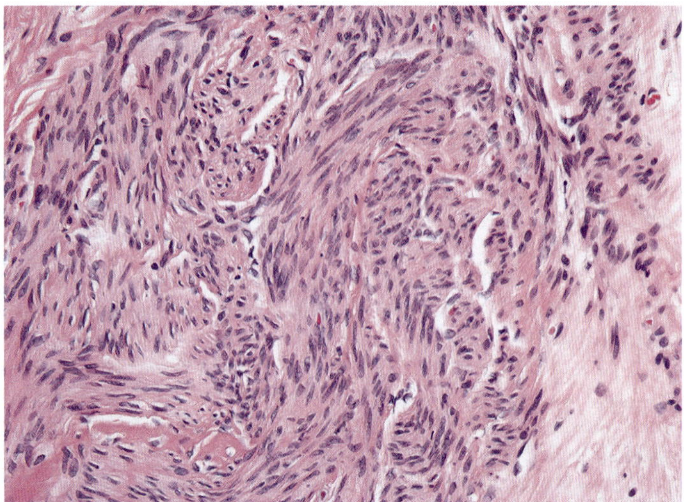

Figure 3.64 Leiomyoma of Deep Soft Tissue. The tumor contains intersecting fascicles of uniform spindle cells with eosinophilic cytoplasm.

Criteria for Malignancy

Surgically excised smooth muscle tumors should be thoroughly sampled. Lesions without any atypia, necrosis, or mitoses can be confidently diagnosed as leiomyoma. In a core or a small biopsy specimen, the diagnosis of a benign deep smooth muscle tumor is especially problematic. In this context the diagnosis of "well-differentiated smooth muscle neoplasm" with no mitotic activity is appropriate, with a comment that distinguishing between leiomyoma and low-grade leiomyosarcoma is difficult in limited biopsy material.

The presence of necrosis in smooth muscle tumors indicates malignancy.[306,308,312,314] In addition, the presence of more than minimal atypia alone or with any mitotic activity can be taken as evidence of leiomyosarcoma.[306,310]

In leiomyoma of deep somatic soft tissue with no nuclear atypia or necrosis, fewer than 1 mitosis per 50 HPF has been considered compatible with the diagnosis of a benign tumor.[309,312] One group reported no malignant behavior in three tumors with up to 4 mitoses per 50 HPF, with a mean follow-up of 58 months.[309] However, recurrences have been reported by others in tumors with 1 mitosis per 50 HPF.[312,315] Well-differentiated smooth muscle tumors of somatic soft tissue with 1 to 5 mitoses per 50 HPF may be regarded as having uncertain malignant potential.[314]

Retroperitoneal, pelvic, and intraabdominal well-differentiated smooth muscle tumors in women with fewer than 5 mitoses per 50 HPF can be diagnosed as leiomyoma. A small number of cases have recurred, but none has metastasized, with median follow-up of 42 and 142 months in two published series.[309,310] Such tumors with 5 to 10 mitoses per 50 HPF in women should probably be considered of uncertain malignant

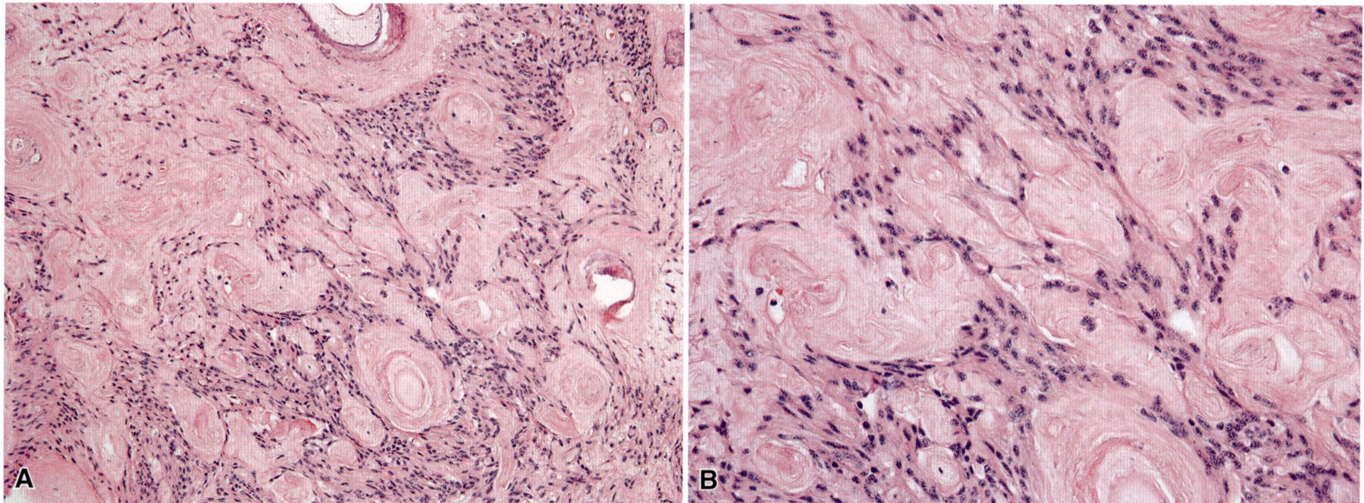

Figure 3.65 Retroperitoneal Leiomyoma. (A) Pelvic and retroperitoneal leiomyomas in women often show similar histologic features as uterine leiomyomas, including stromal hyalinization and a trabecular architecture. (B) Note the uniform nuclei and eosinophilic cytoplasm.

potential. In men, leiomyomas of these sites are so rare that experience is very limited. Any mitotic activity in such a smooth muscle tumor in a man is a worrisome feature; tumors with 1 to 5 mitoses per 50 HPF may be considered of uncertain malignant potential, and any more than 5 should be diagnosed as leiomyosarcoma.

Immunohistochemistry

Leiomyomas are diffusely positive for smooth muscle actin and muscle-specific actin, desmin, and h-caldesmon. Up to 40% of smooth muscle tumors express epithelial markers (keratins and EMA), and occasional cases may express S-100 protein. Some leiomyosarcomas are also positive for CD34 but are consistently negative for KIT.[310] Uterine-type retroperitoneal leiomyomas are occasionally positive for the GIST marker DOG1 (ANO1).[316]

The majority of uterine-type deep leiomyomas show nuclear expression of estrogen and progesterone receptors.[309,310] Deep leiomyomas of somatic soft tissues generally lack these hormone receptors, although limited numbers of cases have been studied; positivity has been reported in a patient with multiple somatic deep leiomyomas associated with uterine fibroids.[317] However, hormone receptors can be expressed in a proportion of uterine leiomyosarcomas and are therefore not a reliable marker of benignity, although they are generally more weakly and focally expressed in retroperitoneal leiomyosarcoma compared with uterine leiomyosarcoma.[318] Moreover, some retroperitoneal leiomyosarcomas that are positive for estrogen and progesterone receptors have a low mitotic rate and can be misinterpreted as benign, especially in a small biopsy sample. Retroperitoneal leiomyomas in males lack estrogen receptors but occasional cases show focal positivity for progesterone receptors.

Molecular Genetics

There is considerable information available about the genetics of uterine leiomyomas, but it is unclear to what extent it applies to soft tissue leiomyomas. Uterine leiomyomas are characterized by hotspot *MED12* mutations,[319] which have been identified at very low frequency in soft tissue leiomyomas.[320-322] The second most common genetic event in uterine leiomyoma is rearrangement of 12q14–q15 affecting *HMGA2*, among other genes.[323,324] Whether such rearrangements are found in the nonhormonally driven soft tissue leiomyomas is unknown. The gene encoding the metabolic enzyme fumarate hydratase is a tumor suppressor, germline mutation of which is responsible for two rare hereditary conditions presenting with multiple cutaneous leiomyomas, namely multiple cutaneous and uterine leiomyomatosis (OMIM 150800) and hereditary leiomyomatosis and renal cell cancer (OMIM 605839),[325] as well as occasional sporadic uterine leiomyomas.[326] Whether fumarate hydratase plays a role in the pathogenesis of soft tissue leiomyomas remains to be demonstrated.

Differential Diagnosis

The histologic criteria that help distinguish deep leiomyoma from low-grade leiomyosarcoma have been discussed previously. Higher-grade examples of leiomyosarcoma show nuclear pleomorphism, mitotic activity often including atypical forms, and necrosis. Epstein-Barr virus (EBV)-associated smooth muscle tumors often arise in a clinical context of severe immunosuppression. They are frequently multiple. Histologically, they may resemble typical smooth muscle tumors but are often composed of less differentiated-appearing ovoid cells with a more prominent lymphoid infiltrate (see later discussion).

Myopericytoma/myofibroma in adults rarely involves the deep soft tissues. Typically, these tumors show a whorled perivascular arrangement of tumor cells with less abundant eosinophilic cytoplasm and areas with dilated blood vessels. Similar to leiomyoma, immunohistochemical staining for smooth muscle actin and h-caldesmon is positive in nearly all cases, but in contrast desmin expression is detected in less than 10% of cases.[45] Cellular schwannoma can closely resemble leiomyoma, especially in a core needle biopsy. However, it is typically encapsulated, diffusely positive for S-100 protein, and generally lacks muscle markers.[203] Low-grade myofibroblastic sarcoma can occur in deep somatic soft tissue of the extremities and trunk, as well as the head and neck and intraabdominal locations. It is composed of fascicles of cells with more tapering nuclei and more palely eosinophilic cytoplasm than smooth muscle tumors. Although low-grade myofibroblastic sarcoma is often positive for both smooth muscle actin and desmin, it is negative for h-caldesmon.[327] Perivascular epithelioid cell tumor (PEComa) can have spindle cell morphology, but it is usually dominated by epithelioid cells and has more granular eosinophilic to clear cytoplasm. Although both leiomyoma and PEComa express smooth muscle actin and desmin, melanocytic markers such as HMB-45 and melan A are positive only in PEComa.[328,329] In the abdomen, GIST can resemble leiomyoma but usually contains more slender nuclei and more palely eosinophilic or basophilic cytoplasm with a fibrillary, syncytial appearance. Similar to leiomyoma, GISTs are often positive for h-caldesmon but rarely express desmin. Most GISTs are positive for KIT and DOG1.

Prognosis and Treatment

By definition, deep leiomyomas do not metastasize, but local recurrences can occasionally occur. In two large series, no deep somatic leiomyomas and only 3 of 64 (2%) retroperitoneal tumors recurred, and none metastasized.[309,310] Long-term follow-up is advisable because tumors may recur after many years.[306]

PRACTICE POINTS: Leiomyoma of Deep Soft Tissue

- Deep leiomyomas are rare
- Complete excision and thorough sampling are indicated to exclude malignancy
- Retroperitoneal and pelvic leiomyomas in women resemble uterine smooth muscle tumors (e.g., stromal hyalinization and trabecular architecture)
- The presence of necrosis and more than minimal nuclear atypia indicate leiomyosarcoma
- In somatic soft tissue, any mitotic activity is a worrisome feature
- In the retroperitoneum, pelvis, and abdomen of women, a low mitotic rate in well-differentiated smooth muscle tumors is compatible with leiomyoma

Angioleiomyoma

Angioleiomyoma is a benign smooth muscle tumor that usually develops in the subcutaneous soft tissues. It affects patients over a wide age range. Clinically, it presents as a solitary, typically painful nodule, usually in the extremities but occasionally in other locations, such as the oral cavity.[330,331] Histologically, angioleiomyomas are composed of fascicles of well-differentiated smooth muscle cells within which abundant vascular channels—either capillary, venous or cavernous—are identified.[330] In focal areas, the tumor cells are concentrically arranged around the larger vessels (Fig. 3.66). Occasional features without clinical relevance are focal nuclear atypia and stromal calcification. Mitotic figures may be detected; recognition of the vascular component is critical for the correct diagnosis because any mitotic activity in a conventional smooth muscle tumor of the soft tissues of the extremities warrants a diagnosis of leiomyosarcoma. Inconsistent structural and chromosomal aberrations of unknown significance have been documented.[332] Angioleiomyomas only rarely recur and do not metastasize; simple surgical excision is hence appropriate treatment.

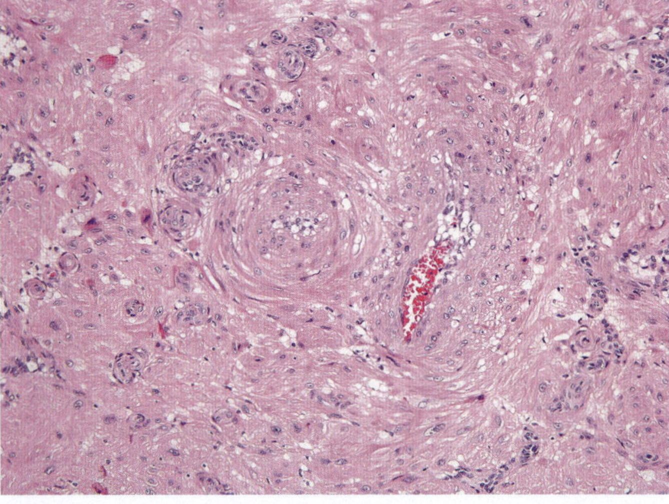

Figure 3.66 Angioleiomyoma. These subcutaneous tumors are composed of fascicles of bland smooth muscle cells, focally arranged around thick-walled blood vessels.

Disseminated Peritoneal Leiomyomatosis, Intravenous Leiomyomatosis, and Benign Metastasizing Leiomyoma

Disseminated peritoneal leiomyomatosis is a rare condition characterized by the development of multiple benign-appearing smooth muscle nodules scattered over the peritoneal surfaces.[333] In contrast, intravenous leiomyomatosis consists of an intravascular growth of benign smooth muscle cells originating in the uterus and extending along the pelvic veins, often reaching in a retrograde fashion into the right atrium.[334] The term *benign metastasizing leiomyoma* is used to describe a rare entity characterized by nodules of benign-appearing smooth muscle in the lung or abdominopelvic lymph nodes.[335] These three entities are hormonally driven benign smooth muscle proliferations often related to uterine leiomyomas, as demonstrated by epidemiologic, clinical, and pathologic overlap,[336] as well as cytogenetic and molecular characteristics.[337-339] They almost exclusively affect women of reproductive age. Despite their frequently alarming clinical presentation, these lesions may be managed conservatively.

Leiomyosarcoma

Leiomyosarcoma accounts for approximately 25% of soft tissue sarcomas; overall, it is the most common sarcoma subtype.[340] As for benign smooth muscle tumors, several clinicopathologic forms of leiomyosarcoma can be categorized according to anatomic location: uterine, retroperitoneal, somatic soft tissue, cutaneous, visceral, gastrointestinal, and major vessel leiomyosarcomas. These forms have been historically treated separately due to significant differences in clinical behavior and biologic potential, but they show considerable overlap morphologically and immunophenotypically. The heterogeneity and molecular pathogenesis of leiomyosarcoma are poorly understood. In general, the diagnosis of leiomyosarcoma is based on the demonstration of malignant histologic features—necrosis, nuclear atypia, and mitotic activity—in a neoplasm showing smooth muscle differentiation.[341]

Clinical Features

Leiomyosarcomas may occur at almost any anatomic location, producing relatively nonspecific symptoms related to local mass effect. Cutaneous leiomyosarcomas occur most frequently in males; when confined to the dermis, such tumors have no metastatic potential and are better termed *atypical intradermal smooth muscle neoplasms* (see Chapter 15).[342] Subcutaneous and intramuscular leiomyosarcomas affect older adults and do not show a gender predilection. Visceral and vascular tumors (excluding uterine leiomyosarcoma) may cause organ-dependent symptoms (e.g., gastrointestinal bleeding in leiomyosarcoma of the colon, vascular thrombosis in inferior vena cava leiomyosarcoma with intraluminal growth). Leiomyosarcoma of the gastrointestinal tract is discussed in Chapter 16. Retroperitoneal tumors are usually large, arising most commonly in middle-aged to elderly adults with a female predominance.

Pathologic Features

Low-grade leiomyosarcomas are tan or white, firm, rubbery masses similar to leiomyomas. Higher-grade, poorly differentiated tumors tend to have a soft, fleshy appearance, with areas of hemorrhage and necrosis. Histologically, leiomyosarcomas are composed of intersecting fascicles of spindle cells (Fig. 3.67). The cells are large and elongated, with abundant brightly eosinophilic cytoplasm, variably blunt-ended (cigar-shaped) nuclei, and well-defined cell borders (see Fig. 3.67B). High-grade tumors may show more variable nuclear features (Fig. 3.68), including some cells with rounded nuclei and an epithelioid appearance. Identification of cells with characteristic nuclear features is critical for proper diagnosis. Variable degrees of nuclei atypia are present, ranging from mild to

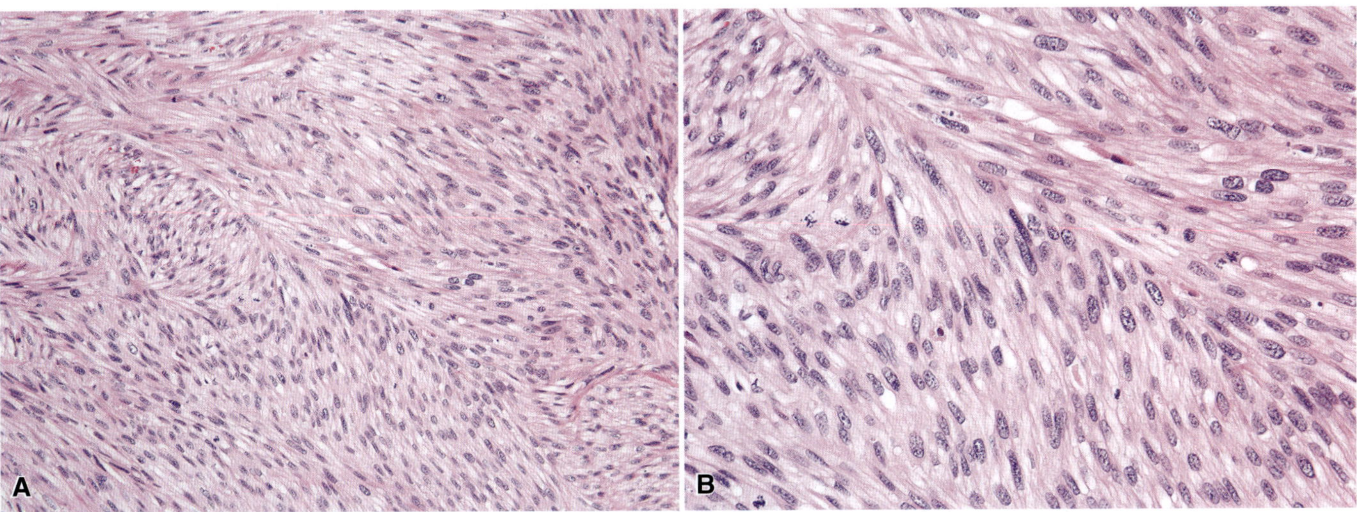

Figure 3.67 Leiomyosarcoma. (A) This well-differentiated leiomyosarcoma is composed of fascicles of eosinophilic spindle cells. (B) The tumor cells contain broad, blunt-ended nuclei and well-defined cell borders. The degree of nuclear atypia and the presence of mitotic activity are diagnostic of leiomyosarcoma.

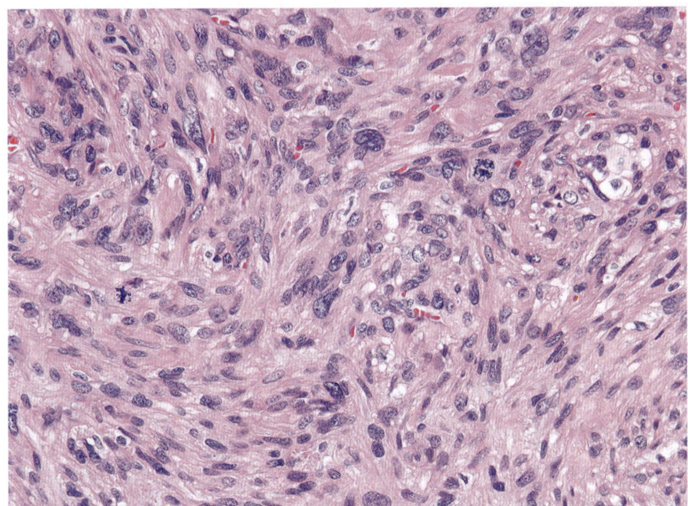

Figure 3.68 Leiomyosarcoma. A less differentiated leiomyosarcoma showing nuclear pleomorphism and a high mitotic rate.

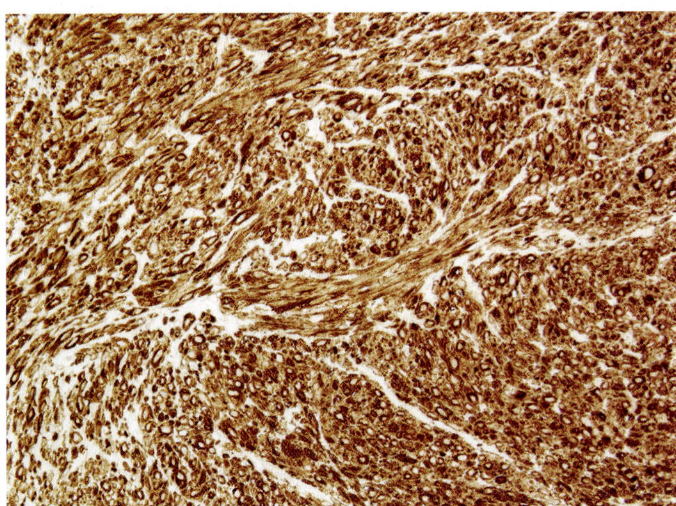

Figure 3.69 Leiomyosarcoma. Most tumors show diffuse expression of desmin.

marked pleomorphism. Cases of leiomyosarcoma dominated by pleomorphic cells are known as *pleomorphic leiomyosarcoma* (see Chapter 7). Mitotic activity is variable and contributes to grading.

Immunohistochemistry

Identification of smooth muscle marker expression is particularly important for the diagnosis of poorly differentiated leiomyosarcoma and examples with overlapping features with other tumor types (see later discussion). Smooth muscle actin and HHF35 are almost invariably positive. Caldesmon is a specific but less sensitive smooth muscle marker. Desmin is usually positive (Fig. 3.69) but may be only focal or even absent in some poorly differentiated tumors. Expression of keratins and EMA is observed in 30% to 40% of leiomyosarcomas.[343,344] The combination of p53, p16, and Ki-67 immunohistochemical staining has been proposed to stratify different risk groups of leiomyosarcomas,[345] but such markers are not widely used in this context.

Molecular Genetics

Leiomyosarcomas are heterogeneous at the genetic level, characterized by complex karyotypes without reproducible characteristic chromosomal aberrations.[346] Preclinical models suggest that the AKT/mammalian target of rapamycin (mTOR) pathway plays a critical role in leiomyosarcoma development.[347,348] Alterations in cell cycle regulators, including the p53 pathway, p16, and Rb, are well-known nonspecific features of leiomyosarcomas.[332] Using an integrative genomic approach combining gene expression profiling and array comparative hybridization, three distinct molecular groups of leiomyosarcomas have been identified, which correlate with immunophenotypic features and prognosis.[349] These findings are not yet routinely applied in clinical practice.

Differential Diagnosis

The characteristic cytomorphology, especially the abundant brightly eosinophilic cytoplasm, usually enables the proper identification of the smooth muscle nature of leiomyosarcomas. The distinction between low-grade leiomyosarcomas and benign smooth muscle tumors is based on the criteria for malignancy previously discussed (see earlier discussion). Other sarcoma types that may enter the differential diagnosis with leiomyosarcoma include low-grade myofibroblastic sarcoma, high-grade myxofibrosarcoma, and dedifferentiated liposarcoma. Low-grade myofibroblastic sarcoma typically shows infiltrative margins and is composed of cells with more tapering nuclei and more palely eosinophilic cytoplasm than leiomyosarcoma. The immunophenotypic features overlap significantly, although myofibroblastic sarcomas are negative for h-caldesmon. The myxoid component of high-grade myxofibrosarcoma may be easily overlooked, and the tumor cells are often arranged in fascicles mimicking high-grade leiomyosarcoma or other high-grade sarcomas. The presence of long, curvilinear blood vessels should raise the possibility of myxofibrosarcoma, which can then be diagnosed through identification of the more typical myxoid areas. Similar to leiomyosarcoma, dedifferentiated liposarcoma typically arises in the retroperitoneum and may show significant histologic and immunophenotypic overlap, including variable expression of smooth muscle actin and desmin, which can lead to misdiagnosis, especially in a core biopsy specimen. However, dedifferentiated liposarcoma typically shows striking morphologic heterogeneity in the dedifferentiated component; identification of a well-differentiated adipocytic component should lead to the correct diagnosis. Immunohistochemical detection of MDM2 and CDK4 or demonstration of *MDM2* gene amplification by FISH is very helpful to support the diagnosis of dedifferentiated liposarcoma.

Prognosis and Treatment

Histologic grade, depth, and anatomic location are strong prognostic factors in leiomyosarcoma. Leiomyosarcomas have a high rate of metastasis, especially to the lung, bone, soft tissues, and liver. This tumor is the most common sarcoma type to metastasize to the skin, especially the scalp.[350] Studies have shown that integrative genomic profiling may be able to predict metastasis and survival in leiomyosarcoma.[349] Likewise, macrophage infiltration and expression of a molecular CSF1-dependent macrophage signature correlate with poor outcome in leiomyosarcoma,[351,352] but these advances have not yet had an impact on clinical practice. Currently, no molecular biomarkers are used in routine prognostication or treatment selection for patients with leiomyosarcoma.

Similarly, no effective targeted therapies directed toward molecular alterations in specific leiomyosarcoma subtypes are available.[349] Clinical management typically consists of surgery with wide margins followed by radiation therapy to decrease the risk of local recurrence. In patients with metastatic disease, doxorubicin-based chemotherapy has shown a marginal association with improved overall survival, sometimes with a modest benefit from the addition of ifosfamide. However, overall response rates are poor in the metastatic setting.[353]

Epstein-Barr Virus–Associated Smooth Muscle Neoplasm

EBV-associated smooth muscle tumors are EBV-driven proliferations that occur in immunocompromised patients of any age, either post-transplantation or in the setting of AIDS.[354-356] The lesions can behave in a benign or malignant fashion, and they often respond to modifications in the patient's immune status. Anatomically, they have been described in soft tissues, gastrointestinal tract, lung, liver, spleen, and adrenal gland, among other sites. They can be multifocal due to clonally distinct tumors.[355,357]

Histologically, EBV-associated smooth muscle neoplasms most often have a spindle cell appearance (Fig. 3.70), but they can also contain more primitive-appearing round cell areas (see Fig. 3.70C). There is often minimal atypia and mitotic activity, as well as a characteristic infiltration by small lymphocytes (see Fig. 3.70B). By immunohistochemistry, the tumor cells are usually positive for smooth muscle actin and less frequently desmin. The presence of EBV can be detected by in situ hybridization for EBV-encoded RNA (EBER) or immunohistochemistry (see Fig. 3.70D). The disease course is variable and seems to be more closely related to the degree of immunosuppression rather than to particular histologic features.[356,357]

Lymphangiomyoma and Lymphangiomyomatosis

Lymphangiomyomatosis (LAM; also known as lymphangioleiomyomatosis) most often involves the lungs but may also affect lymph nodes. The term *lymphangiomyoma* is reserved for a localized mass-forming variant. LAM and lymphangiomyoma are composed of distinctive spindle-shaped perivascular cells and fall on a morphologic and biologic continuum with angiomyolipoma and other soft tissue PEComas (see Chapter 6).[358,359]

LAM is a rare disorder that nearly exclusively affects women of reproductive age. It may be sporadic or arise in the setting of the *tuberous sclerosis complex*, in combination with angiomyolipomas.[360] The localized form (lymphangiomyoma) usually originates in the retroperitoneum, pelvis, or mediastinum. Most patients with an isolated lymphangiomyoma are cured by local excision; however, in some cases, pulmonary LAM is also detected.[361] The pulmonary disease is slowly progressive and eventually fatal. Histologically, lymphangiomyoma is composed of spindle cells arranged in short fascicles adjacent to dilated lymphatics (Fig. 3.71). The cells resemble smooth muscle cells but are plumper in shape and have more granular eosinophilic (or clear) cytoplasm (see Fig. 3.71B). The nuclei are round to oval with fine chromatin and no atypia. The cytomorphology in LAM is identical, although the lesional cells may be subtle, forming small clusters or bundles in the pulmonary interstitium, within the walls of lymphatic channels (Fig. 3.72). Tissue destruction in the lung results in the formation of cysts. Conventional PEComas may occasionally be dominated by spindle cells (Fig. 3.73); such cases can show significant overlap with lymphangiomyoma. Similar to other members of the PEComa family, the cells in LAM variably express both myoid and melanocytic markers, including actin, desmin, and HMB-45 (Fig. 3.74)[359]; smooth muscle markers are more uniformly positive in LAM than in epithelioid PEComas. Mutations in the *TSC2* tumor suppressor gene, resulting in dysregulation of the mTOR pathway, can be demonstrated in both the sporadic and hereditary forms of LAM.[362] Clinical trials have shown that mTOR inhibitors such as sirolimus provide clinical benefit in selected patients.[363]

Angiomatoid Fibrous Histiocytoma

Originally described in 1979 by Enzinger as the angiomatoid variant of malignant fibrous histiocytoma,[364] angiomatoid fibrous histiocytoma (AFH) is a rare neoplasm of uncertain lineage.[365] Large studies have shown that this tumor type may rarely metastasize to regional lymph nodes but has virtually no potential for distant metastasis; as such, AFH is now recognized as a tumor of intermediate biologic potential, and the adjective "malignant" is inappropriate.[366,367] AFH is entirely unrelated to high-grade pleomorphic sarcomas (the lesions previously buried within the "malignant fibrous histiocytoma" category; see Chapter 7). AFH is also unrelated to the aneurysmal variant of fibrous histiocytoma of the skin (see Chapter 15), with which it may be confused owing to the unfortunately similar names. AFH is also discussed in Chapter 10.

Clinical Features

AFH typically occurs in children and young adults, with a mean age of 20 years, but a wide age range has been described.[366,367] The tumor usually presents as a slowly growing mass of the deep dermis and subcutis, most commonly located on the extremities, followed by the trunk and head and neck. Approximately two-thirds of cases occur at sites with abundant lymph nodes, such as the antecubital fossa, popliteal fossa, axilla, and inguinal and supraclavicular areas.[367] The painless mass is often associated with systemic symptoms such as anemia, fever, and weight loss, suggesting cytokine production by the neoplasm. Magnetic resonance imaging is superior to computed tomography in demonstrating

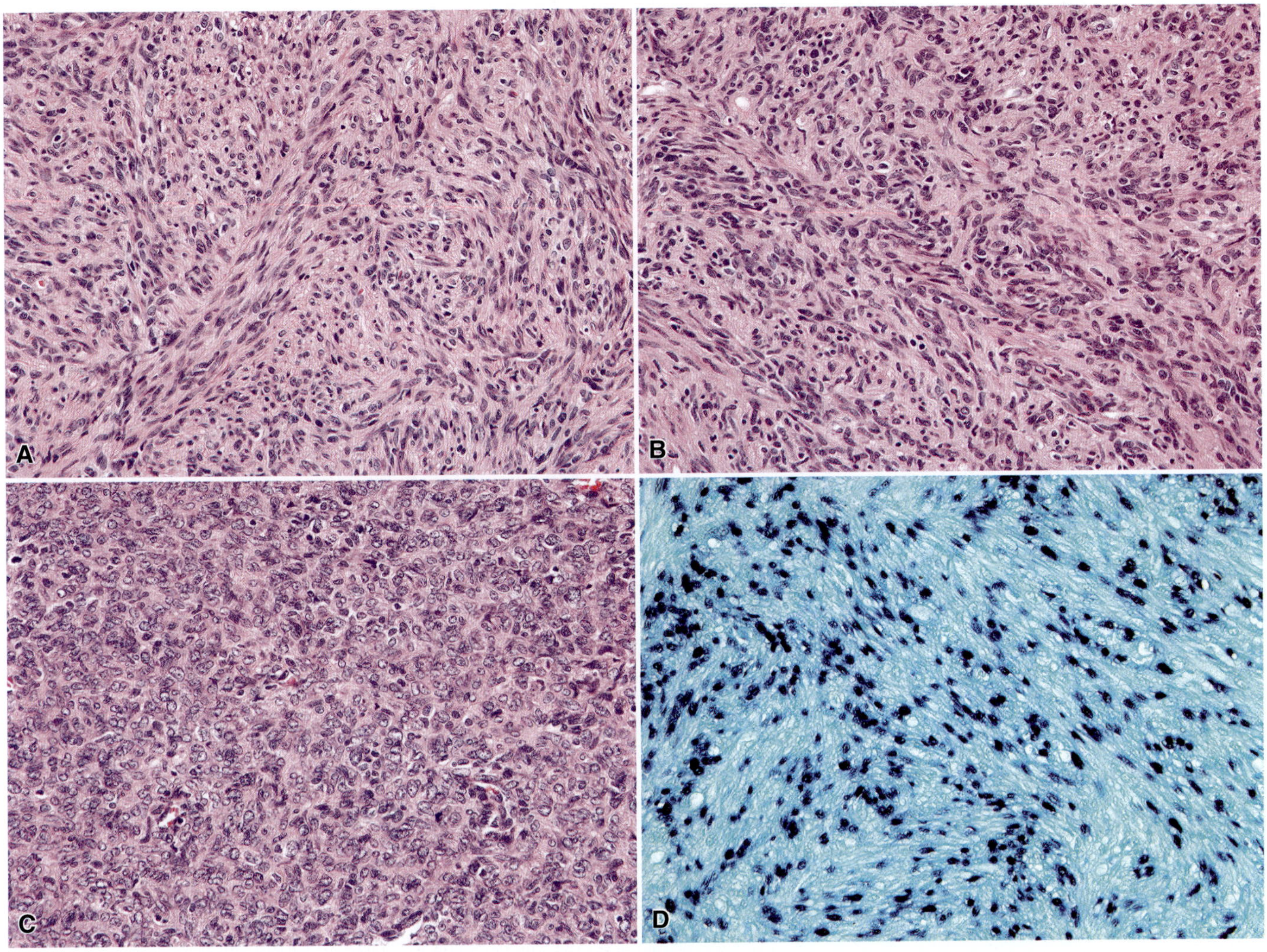

Figure 3.70 **Epstein-Barr Virus-Associated Smooth Muscle Neoplasm.** (A) The tumor is composed of fascicles of spindle cells with eosinophilic cytoplasm and mild nuclear variability. (B) Infiltration by small lymphocytes is typically seen. (C) Some tumors are dominated by primitive-appearing rounded cells. Note the scattered lymphocytes. (D) The presence of Epstein-Barr virus can be detected by in situ hybridization EBV-encoded RNA, which helps confirm the diagnosis.

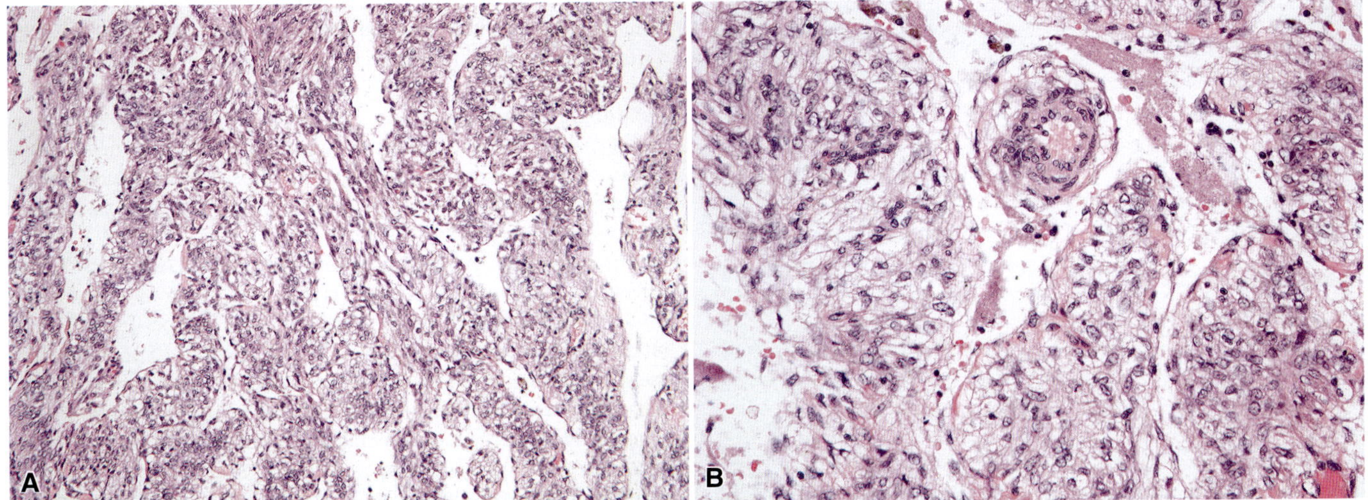

Figure 3.71 **Lymphangiomyoma.** (A) Fascicles of spindle cells abut dilated lymphatic channels. (B) The tumor cells contain granular eosinophilic to clear cytoplasm.

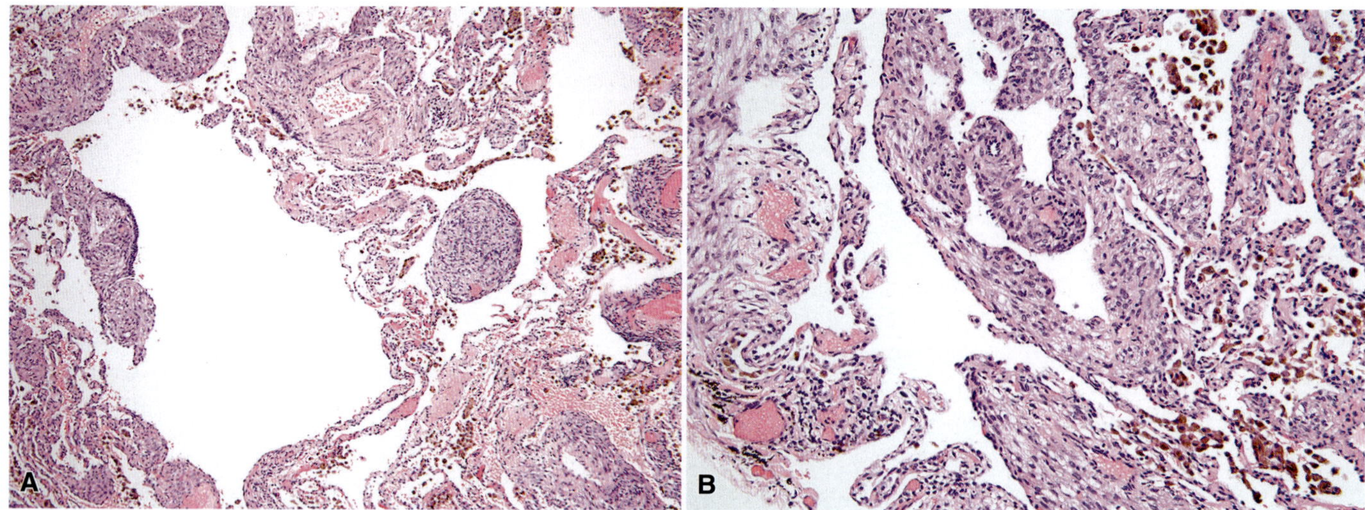

Figure 3.72 Lymphangiomyomatosis. (A) This pulmonary lesion shows a cystic appearance. (B) The interstitium contains clusters of spindled to epithelioid cells with granular eosinophilic to clear cytoplasm.

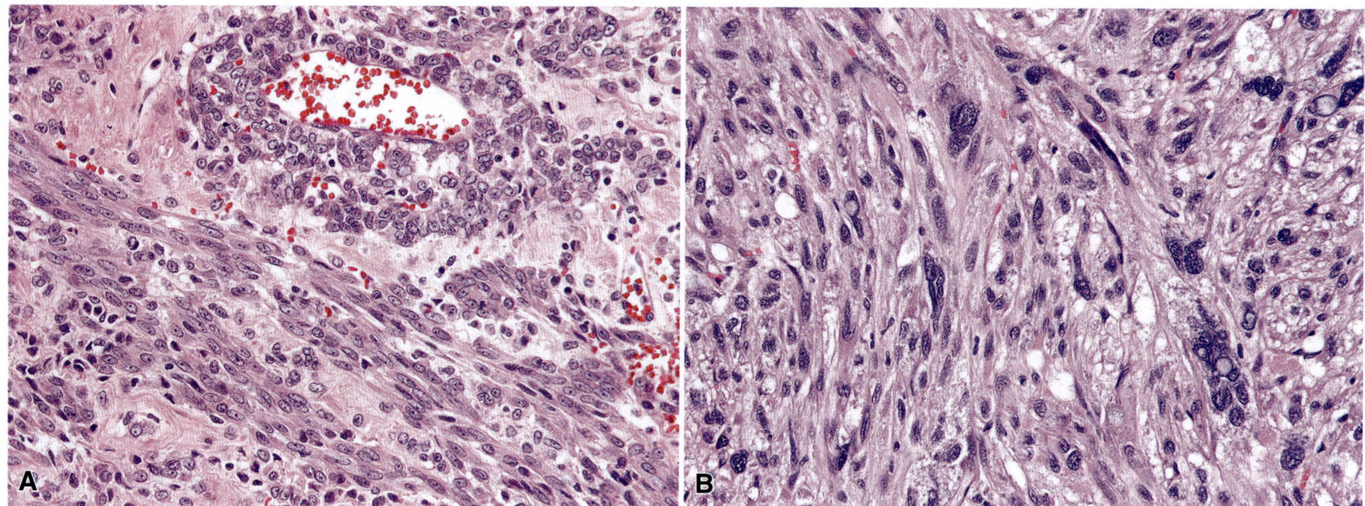

Figure 3.73 Perivascular Epithelioid Cell Tumor. (A) A retroperitoneal perivascular epithelioid cell tumor (PEComa) showing spindle cell morphology. Note the granular eosinophilic cytoplasm and perivascular growth. (B) A malignant PEComa composed of spindle cells with abundant cytoplasm. Note the nuclear pleomorphism.

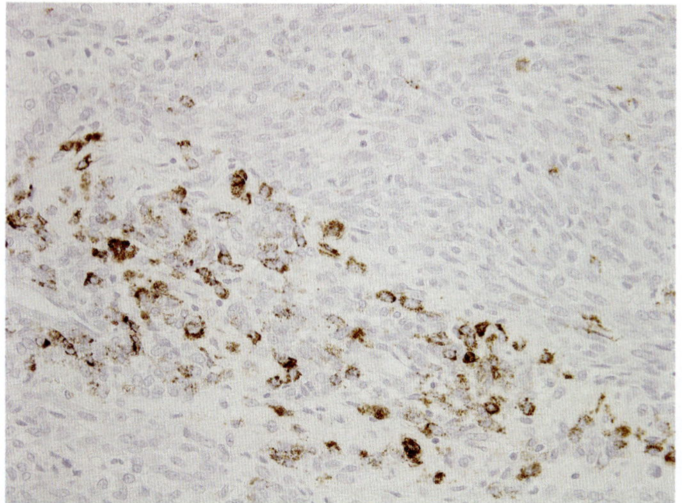

Figure 3.74 Lymphangiomyoma. HMB-45 is typically positive in only few scattered cells.

fluid-fluid levels within the cystic component of the tumor, indicative of intralesional hemorrhage.[368]

Pathologic Features

Grossly, AFH is a firm, well-circumscribed, tan-gray mass, usually measuring 2 to 4 cm in diameter. The cross section usually reveals irregular blood-filled cystic spaces, simulating a hematoma or hemangioma.

Histologically, AFH is typically multinodular, composed of ovoid, histiocyte-like or short spindled myoid cells, often surrounded by a thick fibrous capsule with a variably prominent peripheral chronic inflammatory component (Figs. 3.75 and 3.76).[367] In some examples the surrounding inflammation, composed of lymphocytes and plasma cells with occasional germinal centers (see Fig. 3.76), may mimic a lymph node infiltrated by a metastatic tumor, but subcapsular sinuses and hilar lymphatics, which one would expect to encounter in an actual lymph node, are absent.[364] Foci of intralesional hemorrhage are often seen in the central portion of the tumor, leading to the formation of large blood-filled spaces that may simulate vascular channels. The cystic spaces are lined by flattened tumor cells, not endothelial cells.[366] AFH may occasionally lack cystic spaces (the "solid" variant; see Fig. 3.76B) and peripheral lymphoid tissue, particularly in incisional biopsies.[369]

The cytomorphology is characteristic: AFH is composed of a population of uniform, bland, spindled-to-histiocytoid cells with abundant palely eosinophilic cytoplasm with indistinct cell borders imparting a syncytial appearance (Fig. 3.77). The cytoplasm may contain finely granular hemosiderin pigment, and the nuclei are pale and vesicular. Cellular pleomorphism, mitotic activity, and hyperchromatic giant cells, features not associated with adverse clinical behavior, are occasionally present.[366,369,370] The extracellular matrix is usually scant, but occasional cases show prominent myxoid stromal change.[371]

Immunohistochemistry

Approximately 50% of cases of AFH express desmin and EMA (Fig. 3.78), and they are also often positive for muscle-specific actin (clone HHF35). Occasional staining for other myoid markers has been described

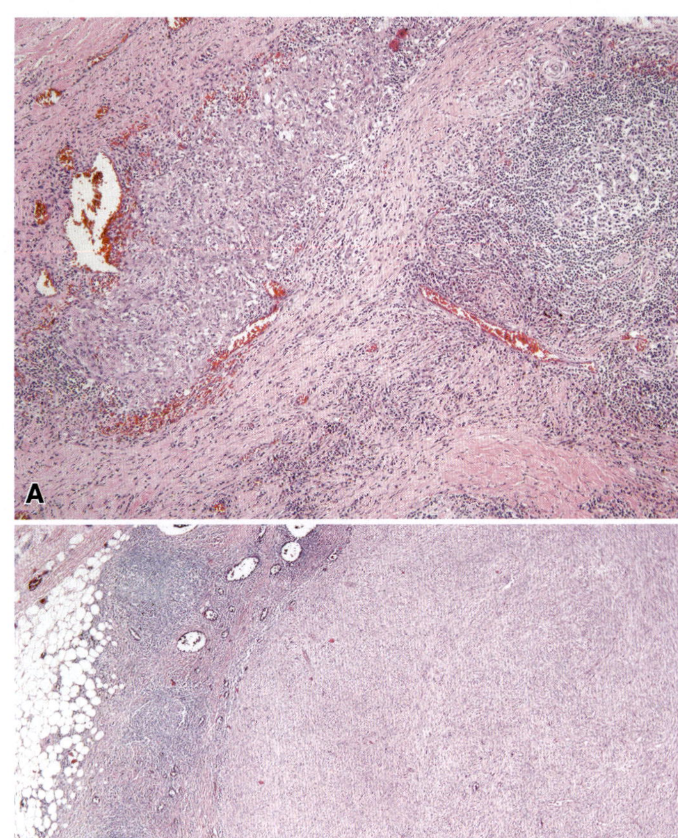

Figure 3.76 Angiomatoid Fibrous Histiocytoma. (A) The periphery of the tumor contains a thick fibrotic pseudocapsule. Note the irregular nodule of tumor cells. (B) "Solid" angiomatoid fibrous histiocytoma lacks cystic spaces. Note the peripheral lymphoid follicles.

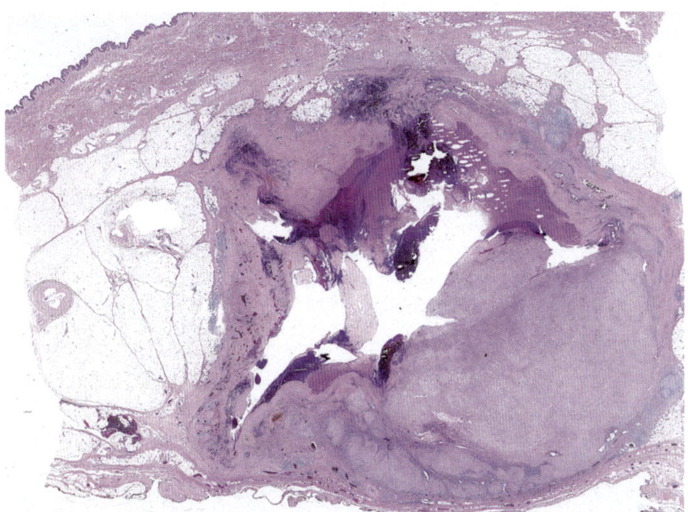

Figure 3.75 Angiomatoid Fibrous Histiocytoma. The tumor shows a multinodular appearance with blood-filled cystic spaces and a peripheral lymphoid infiltrate.

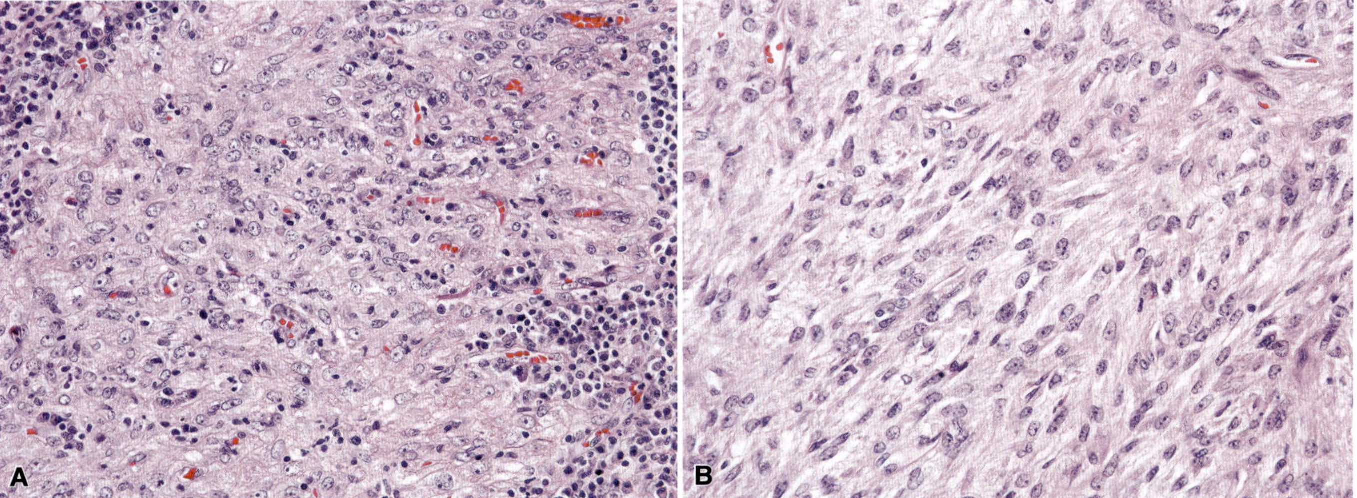

Figure 3.77 Angiomatoid Fibrous Histiocytoma. (A) The tumor nodules are composed of bland histiocytoid cells with abundant palely eosinophilic cytoplasm and ill-defined cell borders. (B) Some tumors show spindle cell morphology. Note the vesicular nuclei, small nucleoli, and pale cytoplasm.

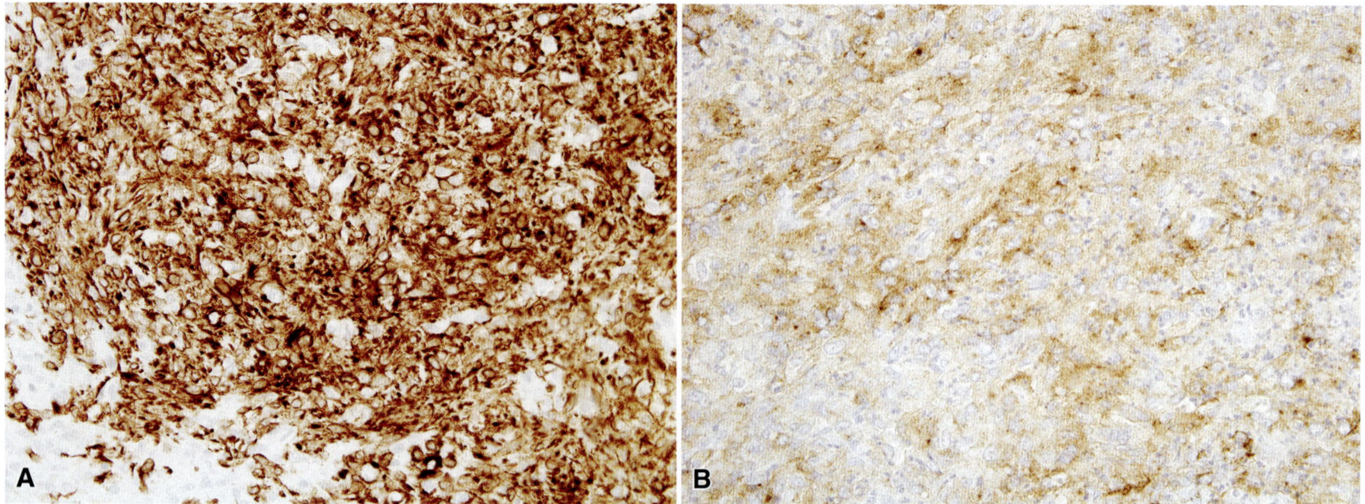

Figure 3.78 Angiomatoid Fibrous Histiocytoma. Expression of both desmin (A) and epithelial membrane antigen (B) is typical of this tumor type, although only approximately 50% of tumors are positive for these markers.

in a small percentage of cases.[365,367,372] Tumor cells are virtually always negative for keratins, S-100 protein, CD34, and follicular dendritic cell markers (CD21, CD35). Immunoreactivity with CD99 is common, often with a strong and diffuse pattern, and it may result in misdiagnosis in cases with predominantly round cell morphology.[373]

Molecular Genetics

The most common translocation in AFH is t(2;22)(q33;q12), which creates an *EWSR1-CREB1* fusion oncogene (see Chapter 18). A subset of cases is characterized by the alternative fusion *EWSR1-ATF1*, resulting from a t(12;22)(q13;q12).[373-375] Interestingly, both of these fusion oncogenes are also detected in clear cell sarcoma (CCS) of soft tissues, a much more aggressive tumor type, and in the CCS-like tumor of the gastrointestinal tract (also known as gastrointestinal neuroectodermal tumor).[375,376] Curiously, the first translocation identified in AFH is the least common one, t(12;16)(q13;p11), leading to an *FUS-ATF1* fusion gene.[374,377]

Differential Diagnosis

AFH is a rare tumor type, which can be difficult to diagnose especially with limited sampling. The immunohistochemical coexpression of desmin and EMA, if present, is very helpful. Aneurysmal benign fibrous histiocytoma may be confused with AFH because of its similar name. A dermal lesion that usually arises in young adults, the aneurysmal variant of fibrous histiocytoma is distinguished by more variable cytomorphology, as well as the characteristic features of conventional dermatofibroma, such as overlying epidermal hyperplasia and peripheral entrapment of collagen bundles.

The dense peripheral lymphoplasmacytic infiltrate occasionally suggests a lymph node metastasis. However, on careful examination, AFH has no true nodal architecture, such as subcapsular or medullary sinuses, and germinal center formation is randomly arranged around the tumor. AFH may occasionally show prominent pleomorphism and a high mitotic rate, in which case it may be confused with a sarcoma, or, when involving the dermis, atypical fibrous histiocytoma.

Prognosis and Treatment

AFH recurs locally in 10% to 15% of patients, whereas lymph node or lung metastases are rare (1%), with exceptional disease-related deaths.[366,367] Local recurrence is more likely in deeply situated tumors and those with infiltrative margins. Wide local surgical excision without adjuvant therapy is the recommended treatment for AFH.[366,378]

PRACTICE POINTS: Angiomatoid Fibrous Histiocytoma

- Typically arises in superficial soft tissues of the extremities of children and young adults
- Characteristic histologic features include multinodularity; blood-filled spaces; a thick fibrous pseudocapsule; and a prominent peripheral lymphoplasmacytic infiltrate, including germinal centers
- Tumor cells are usually uniform and bland with abundant pale, eosinophilic syncytial cytoplasm
- Expression of desmin and epithelial membrane antigen (EMA) is observed in 50% of cases
- *EWSR1* gene rearrangements are identified in the vast majority of cases
- Lymph node metastases are rare

Synovial Sarcoma

Synovial sarcoma is a malignant mesenchymal neoplasm showing epithelial differentiation that includes biphasic, monophasic, and poorly differentiated (round cell) variants.[379] The designation *synovial sarcoma* was originally proposed on the basis of morphologic similarity to the developing synovium; however, synovial sarcoma is entirely unrelated to synovial cells, but its name has been historically retained despite abundant evidence of its inaccuracy.[380] Most often arising in deep soft tissue over a wide anatomic distribution, synovial sarcoma is increasingly recognized in visceral organs (especially lung and pleura) following the development of molecular techniques that can be used to confirm the diagnosis. Biphasic synovial sarcoma is discussed in Chapter 9, whereas poorly differentiated synovial sarcoma is discussed in Chapter 8. This discussion will focus on monophasic spindle cell synovial sarcoma.

Clinical Features

Accounting for 10% to 15% of adult soft tissue sarcomas, synovial sarcomas are most common in adolescents and young adults, although they can also affect older patients and children.[381,382] There is a slight male predominance (male-to-female ratio, 1.2:1). Most synovial sarcomas develop in the deep soft tissues of the proximal or middle part of the extremities or limb girdles, often adjacent to large joints, especially the knee and hip (although very rarely intraarticular). Approximately 25%

of tumors arise in the distal extremities (fingers, hand, or foot). More rarely, synovial sarcomas occur in the head and neck region, abdominal wall, body cavities, or visceral organs.[383] Common presenting symptoms include a long-standing palpable mass, pain or tenderness, paresthesias, and limitation of motion.

A small fraction of cases have been associated with prior radiation therapy.[384,385] A diagnosis of synovial sarcoma may be suspected on imaging studies due to the presence of calcifications in the tumor, and superficial involvement of the underlying bone in the form of a periosteal reaction, erosion, or frank invasion, which is observed in 15% to 20% of cases.[386]

Pathologic Features

Grossly, synovial sarcoma is a well-circumscribed but unencapsulated mass, usually within skeletal muscle or attached to an adjacent tendon sheath or joint capsule. The tumors are typically yellow-tan to gray on cut section and vary from soft to firm. Cystic change may occur. Tumor size varies according to location: synovial sarcoma of the hands and feet are usually small, ranging from 1 to 3 cm, whereas in the proximal extremities, the tumors tend to be larger, measuring up to 15 to 20 cm (median, 7 cm). Large tumors often contain areas of necrosis.

Histologically, synovial sarcoma shows three main patterns: biphasic, monophasic (spindle cell), and poorly differentiated.[383,387] The most common variant is monophasic spindle cell synovial sarcoma. Other less common variants include purely glandular monophasic synovial sarcoma, tumors with prominent bone and calcification (calcifying synovial sarcoma), and myxoid synovial sarcoma.[388-391] Biphasic synovial sarcoma contains distinct but intermingled epithelial and spindle cell components (see Chapter 9). Monophasic synovial sarcoma is composed of highly cellular solid sheets or fascicles of remarkably uniform small spindle cells with a high nuclear-to-cytoplasmic ratio (Fig. 3.79). Some tumors are composed of tight intersecting fascicles with a herringbone (fibrosarcoma-like) appearance (see Fig. 3.79B). The tumor cells contain scant cytoplasm, and the cell margins are usually indistinct, resulting in a syncytial appearance and the impression of overlapping nuclei (see Fig. 3.79C). Synovial sarcoma often contains characteristic hyalinized or wiry collagen bundles (see Fig. 3.79D), which may be variably calcified and sometimes resemble osteoid. Dystrophic calcifications are relatively common (Fig. 3.80A). Mast cells are often prominent (see Fig. 3.80B). Ectatic, branching HPC-like vessels are common (Fig. 3.81). Nuclear palisading, pseudorosette formation, and myxoid stromal change (see Chapter 5) are other potential histologic features. Nuclear pleomorphism

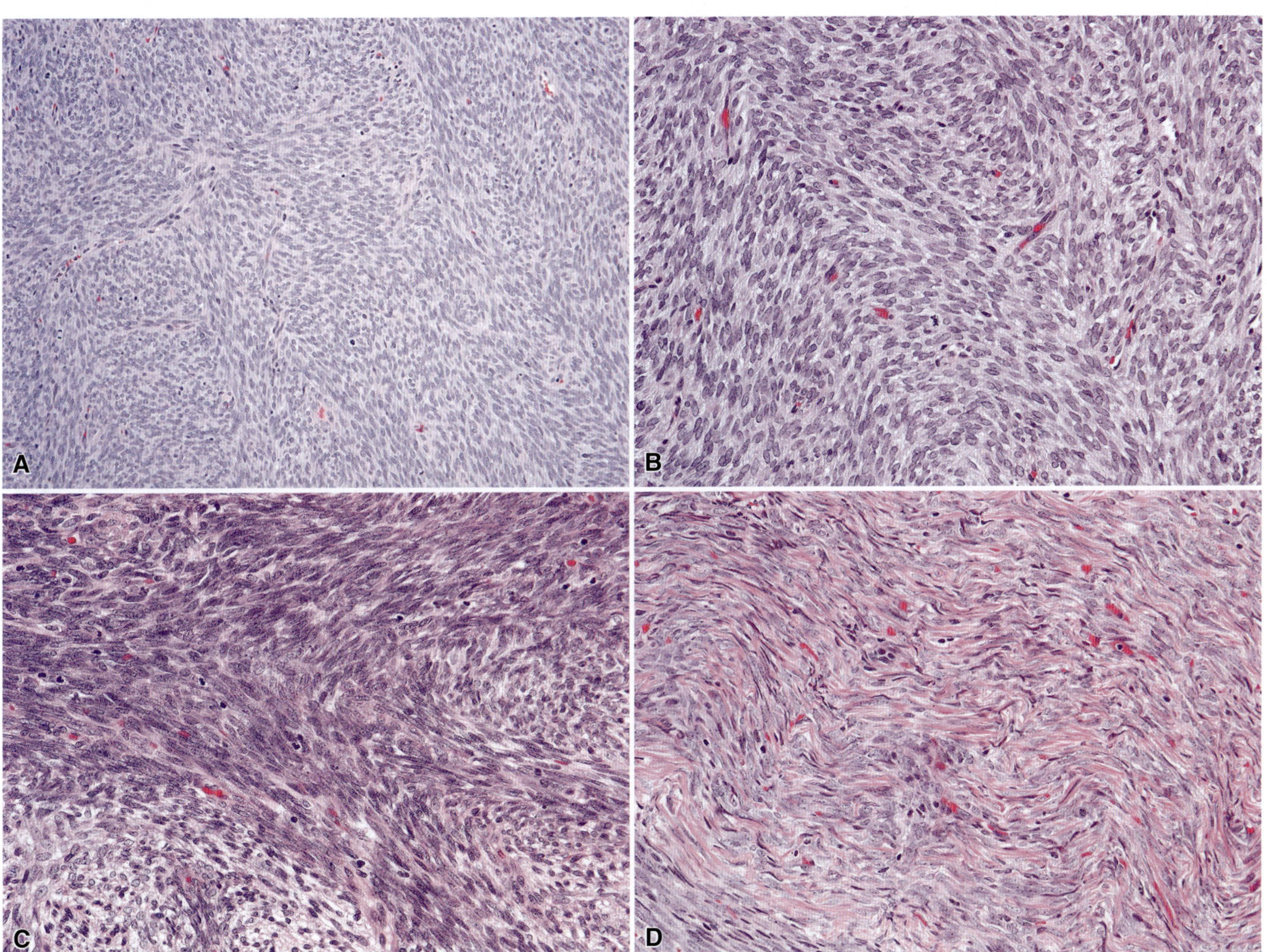

Figure 3.79 Monophasic Synovial Sarcoma. (A) The tumor is composed of highly cellular fascicles of spindle cells. (B) Some tumors have short intersecting fascicles with a herringbone (fibrosarcoma-like) appearance. (C) The tumor cells are remarkably uniform with overlapping nuclei and scant, indistinct cytoplasm. (D) Wiry stromal collagen is a characteristic feature.

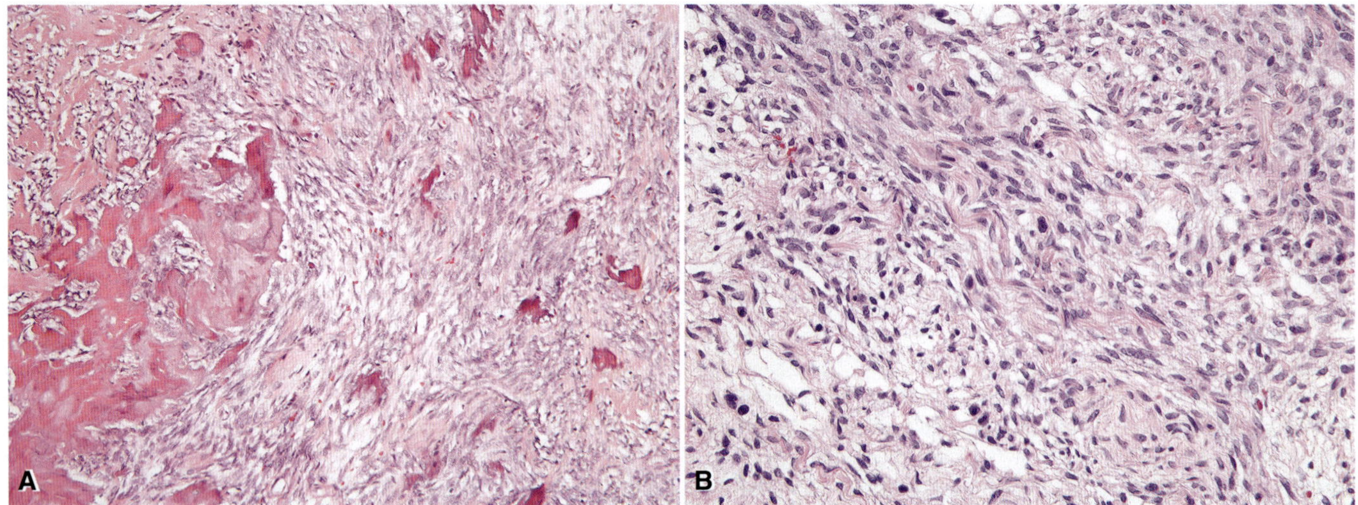

Figure 3.80 **Monophasic Synovial Sarcoma.** (A) Dystrophic calcification may be prominent. (B) A hypocellular example with scattered stromal mast cells.

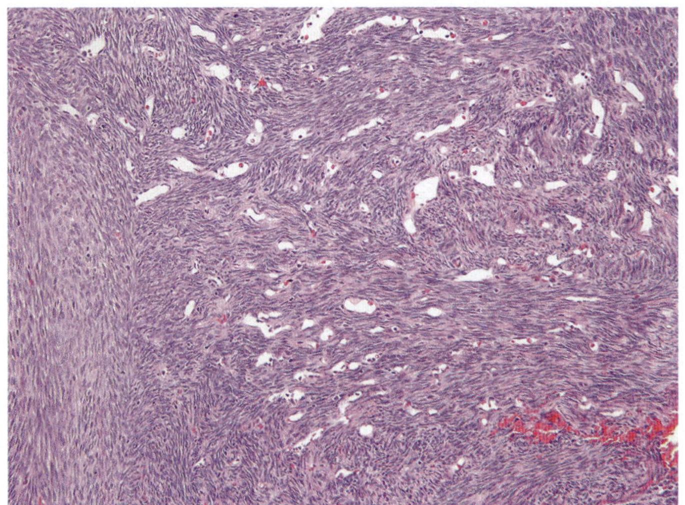

Figure 3.81 **Monophasic Synovial Sarcoma.** This tumor contains dilated, branching, hemangiopericytoma-like vessels.

is highly unusual in synovial sarcoma but may occasionally be seen in tumors excised following preoperative radiation therapy. The mitotic rate is highly variable. Necrosis is common in large and poorly dedifferentiated tumors. Large areas of cystic change are occasionally observed.

Poorly differentiated synovial sarcoma (see Chapter 8) is composed of solid sheets of uniform, closely packed, relatively small round-to-short spindled cells, often with a prominent HPC-like vasculature.[387] Rarely, structures resembling pseudorosettes may be seen, suggesting the possibility of Ewing sarcoma. Mitoses are often numerous, and tumor necrosis is common in this high-grade variant of synovial sarcoma. Poorly differentiated areas may be found focally in up to 20% of otherwise typical monophasic or biphasic synovial sarcomas, but synovial sarcomas may also be entirely poorly differentiated. Rare cases containing numerous rhabdoid cells are best classified as poorly differentiated synovial sarcoma.

Calcifying synovial sarcomas are biphasic or monophasic spindle cell tumors containing large areas of calcification, bone, or, rarely, cartilage.

Immunohistochemistry

Epithelial differentiation in synovial sarcoma is demonstrable by immunohistochemistry and represents an extremely useful diagnostic feature.[379,392] The glandular component of biphasic synovial sarcoma is uniformly and strongly positive for keratins and EMA. In monophasic spindle cell synovial sarcoma, staining for EMA is often patchy or focal (Fig. 3.82A), and keratins are generally expressed in only scattered individual cells. Only 40% to 50% of poorly differentiated synovial sarcomas express keratins, but EMA is positive in most cases.[387,393] In contrast to MPNST and Ewing sarcoma, synovial sarcoma expresses both keratins 7 and 19, which may be useful in differential diagnosis.[394]

CD99 is expressed in 60% to 75% of synovial sarcomas, especially in the poorly differentiated variant, usually in the cytoplasm, but occasionally with a membranous staining pattern.[383,393,395] S-100 protein is detected in approximately 30% of monophasic synovial sarcomas, usually in a focal distribution, and in 10% of poorly differentiated synovial sarcomas.[393] Reactivity for CD57 and CD56 has also been reported, but these markers show limited specificity among sarcomas. Synovial sarcoma is almost always negative for CD34 and desmin.[395,396] Immunostaining for the SYT (SS18) protein has been reported as a marker for synovial sarcoma,[397] but in the experience of the authors and others, this is not specific for synovial sarcoma.

Gene expression profiling studies have identified the transcriptional regulator TLE1 (transducin-like enhancer of split 1) as an excellent discriminator of synovial sarcoma from other sarcoma types. Using specific anti-TLE1 antibodies on paraffin sections, this protein is detected in almost all cases of synovial sarcoma.[119,398] A strong and diffuse nuclear staining pattern for TLE1 is almost always observed in synovial sarcoma (see Fig. 3.82B), whereas only a small subset of tumors in the differential diagnosis, such as MPNST, shows weak or focal expression; however, strong expression may be observed in occasional cases of MPNST.[119,399]

Molecular Genetics

Synovial sarcoma is characterized by a t(X;18) balanced translocation,[400,401] which involves the *SS18 (SYT)* gene on chromosome 18 and either the *SSX1* or the *SSX2* gene on chromosome X[402]; rarely, alternative fusions involving *SSX4* or *SS18L1* may be found (see Chapter 18).[403,404] In any case, the t(X;18) translocation results in the formation of a fusion oncogene that encodes a transcription-activating protein.[402,405]

The t(X;18) translocation and the resulting *SS18-SSX* fusion oncogene are diagnostic markers specific for synovial sarcoma[406] that can be detected by conventional cytogenetics,[401] FISH,[407,408] or reverse transcriptase polymerase chain reaction (RT-PCR).[409-411] FISH or RT-PCR

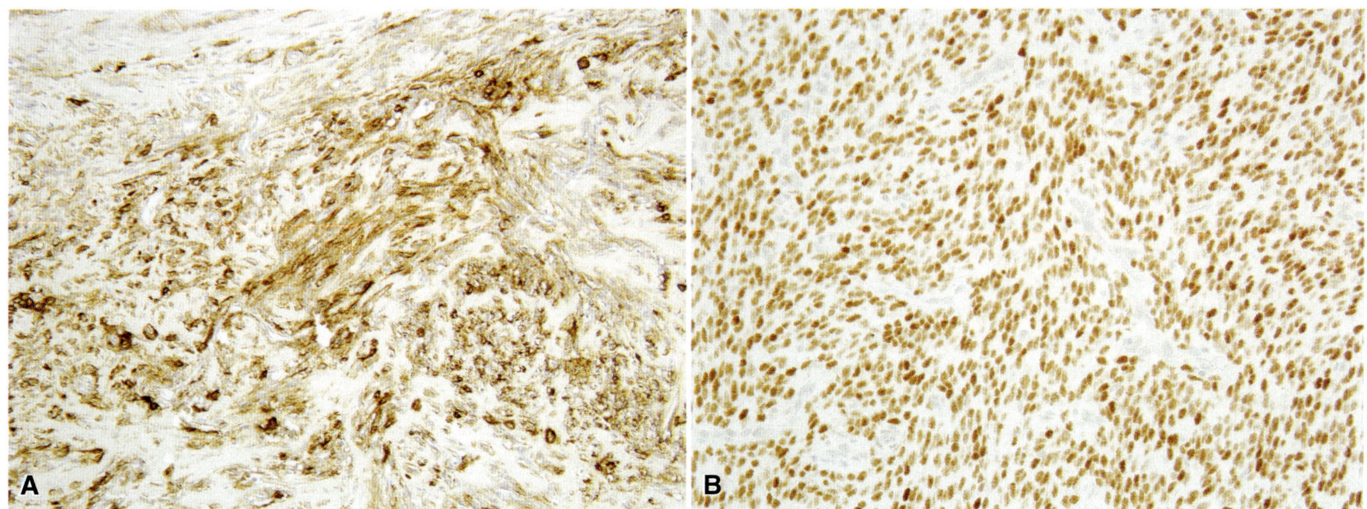

Figure 3.82 Monophasic Synovial Sarcoma. (A) Epithelial membrane antigen is expressed in nearly all cases. (B) Strong nuclear staining for transducin-like enhancer of split 1 (TLE1) is a helpful diagnostic feature.

can be especially helpful when dealing with poorly differentiated synovial sarcoma and tumors occurring at unusual anatomic sites.[395]

There is some correlation between the translocation variant and the morphologic type of synovial sarcoma: biphasic tumors are rarely associated with *SS18-SSX2* fusion transcripts, which are present in monophasic synovial sarcoma.[412,413] The prognostic relevance of the translocation and the clinical impact of the different variants are controversial. Initial studies in small numbers of patients suggested that the fusion variant on its own, or in combination with the complexity of the karyotype, could predict clinical behavior; patients with the *SS18-SSX2* fusion had significantly better metastasis-free survival than patients with *SS18-SSX1*.[412,414,415] However, subsequent larger studies have been unable to confirm these observations. Rather, it seems that the histologic grade and disease stage are the most important prognostic factors,[415,416] with little or no contribution of the translocation variant.

Poorly differentiated synovial sarcoma has a distinctive gene expression profile, when compared with the biphasic and monophasic subtypes.[417]

Differential Diagnosis

Because of its wide anatomic distribution and variable histologic patterns, synovial sarcoma can create substantial diagnostic difficulties. The differential diagnosis of biphasic synovial sarcoma is discussed in Chapter 9, whereas poorly differentiated synovial sarcoma is covered in Chapter 8. Monophasic spindle cell synovial sarcoma should mainly be distinguished from MPNST, SFT, CCS, spindle cell rhabdomyosarcoma, and fibrosarcoma. MPNST can show significant histologic overlap with synovial sarcoma, although MPNST typically features alternating cellularity with areas of myxoid stroma, perivascular accentuation, and buckled or wavy nuclei. Both tumors may be positive for S-100 protein; thus this marker is not particularly useful in differential diagnosis. Loss of H3K27me3 supports MPNST, although this antibody requires careful titration to avoid weak (or absent) staining in cases of synovial sarcoma.[418,419] Epithelial markers are rarely detected in MPNST, and GFAP and SOX10 are consistently negative in synovial sarcoma. Strong nuclear staining for TLE1 is moderately specific for synovial sarcoma in this differential diagnosis; 10% to 20% of MPNST cases are also positive for TLE1. A history of NF1 should suggest MPNST. In occasional cases when immunohistochemical results are equivocal, molecular techniques may be the only reliable means to distinguish between these tumor types.

Synovial sarcomas containing prominent HPC-like vessels and stromal collagen may be confused with SFT. However, SFTs usually lack the fascicular architecture and uniform nuclear morphology of synovial sarcomas. Approximately 20% of SFTs are at least focally positive for EMA, a further potential diagnostic pitfall. Expression of CD34 strongly favors SFT, whereas TLE1 and keratins support synovial sarcoma. STAT6 is specific for SFT in this differential diagnosis. CCS also typically affects young adults and arises at similar anatomic sites as synovial sarcoma. The fascicular architecture and uniform cytology may lead to confusion with synovial sarcoma, although CCS typically shows a more nested architecture, and the tumor cells contain more abundant cytoplasm and more prominent nucleoli. S-100 protein is strongly and diffusely expressed in almost all cases of CCS, and the melanocytic markers HMB-45 and melan A are also usually positive, whereas keratin is negative. Similar to synovial sarcoma, spindle cell rhabdomyosarcoma is composed of uniform spindle cells arranged in fascicles, often with prominent hyalinized stromal collagen. However, occasional cells with brightly eosinophilic cytoplasm (i.e., rhabdomyoblasts) are usually identifiable on careful examination. Diffuse expression of desmin and MYOD1, and more limited staining for myogenin, confirm the diagnosis of spindle cell rhabdomyosarcoma. Fibrosarcoma in adults is exceedingly rare and is a diagnosis of exclusion; most putative examples of "fibrosarcoma" in the older literature can be reclassified as various other tumor types using modern diagnostic criteria and molecular techniques.[420] One of the most common tumor types showing a fibrosarcoma-like pattern is monophasic synovial sarcoma.

Prognosis and Treatment

Synovial sarcoma is an aggressive sarcoma type. Wide excision followed by radiation therapy is standard treatment. Neoadjuvant or adjuvant chemotherapy can also be used in selected patients. Recurrences and metastases usually occur within 2 years after primary excision but may occasionally develop years or even decades later. Local recurrence is mainly related to inadequate local therapy. Metastases occur in approximately 40% of cases, mostly to the lungs, and, less frequently, to bone. Lymph node metastases are rare. Reported 5- and 10-year overall survival rates range from 36% to 76% and from 20% to 63%, respectively.[383,413,415,416,421]

For patients with localized disease at presentation (80% to 90% of synovial sarcomas of the distal extremities), potential prognostic factors include high histologic grade, large tumor size (>5 cm), high mitotic rate (>10 mitoses per 10 HPF), tumor necrosis, poorly differentiated histology, relatively older age at diagnosis (variably reported as older than 20, 25, or 40 years), proximal location, vascular invasion, and invasion of bone and neurovascular structures.[382,421,422] Small tumors on the distal extremities have a favorable prognosis.[416,423,424] There is no consistent prognostic difference between monophasic spindle cell and biphasic synovial sarcoma, whereas poorly differentiated synovial sarcomas are almost always aggressive with a particularly high rate of metastasis. Prominent calcification has been proposed to be a favorable prognostic factor, but this remains to be confirmed in larger studies.

The prognostic relevance of the gene fusion variant in synovial sarcoma is controversial (see earlier discussion) but does not appear to play a significant role. High Ki-67 proliferation index and p53 staining have been reported to correlate with an increased risk of tumor recurrence[425] but are rarely used in clinical practice.

PRACTICE POINTS: Synovial Sarcoma

- Most commonly affects adolescents and young adults
- Calcification on imaging can be a diagnostic clue
- Monophasic synovial sarcoma is composed of fascicles or sheets of remarkably uniform small spindle cells with scant cytoplasm and overlapping nuclei (purple or blue appearance on low magnification)
- Wiry stromal collagen, hemangiopericytoma-like vessels, and prominent mast cells are typical features
- Patchy expression of epithelial membrane antigen and keratins is characteristic
- Strong and diffuse nuclear staining for TLE1 is moderately specific
- t(X;18) translocation is diagnostic

Malignant Peripheral Nerve Sheath Tumor

MPNST is the current designation for a malignant soft tissue tumor showing neuroectodermal differentiation, similar to the cellular constituents of the normal peripheral nerve sheath. Terms such as *neurofibrosarcoma*, *malignant schwannoma*, and *neurogenic sarcoma*, as well as other histogenetic designations, are obsolete; most of these tumors are somewhat heterogeneous in their cellular composition, although Schwannian differentiation usually predominates.[426]

Clinical Features

MPNSTs are generally deep-seated tumors arising most commonly in the proximal lower extremity, followed by the paraspinal region and the proximal upper extremity. The clinical presentation is usually nonspecific, but neurologic symptoms may occur. MPNSTs occur either sporadically or in patients with NF1, in approximately equal numbers. Most sporadic cases affect adults of either gender between 30 and 60 years of age, although the age distribution is wide. In patients with NF1, the lifetime risk of developing MPNST is 2% to 10%; sometimes the tumors develop in childhood, but they are most common during the fourth decade of life, preferentially in males.[427-430] Patients with NF1 should be closely followed; the onset of pain or rapid increase in size in any neurofibroma in this clinical setting should prompt a biopsy or excision, to allow for early detection of malignant transformation. This phenomenon is most common in deep plexiform lesions and only exceptionally occurs in dermal tumors.[251,431] Other neuroectodermal tumors, such as schwannoma or ganglioneuroma, may rarely give rise to secondary MPNST.[226,228,432,433] Approximately 10% of MPNSTs are radiation induced; in the past, this was mainly associated with the use of radiation therapy to treat neurofibromas in patients with NF1, a practice that has been abandoned.[434,435]

Pathologic Features

MPNSTs are usually large lesions that may sometimes cause a fusiform expansion of the nerve from which they arise. In addition, a preexisting neurofibroma may be identified on inspection. Depending on the stroma and cellularity, the tumors can be fibrous, gelatinous, or fleshy in consistency.[436] Histologically, most MPNSTs are composed of highly cellular fascicles of spindle cells, sometimes with a vaguely whorled growth pattern. Although focally epithelioid morphology is not uncommon in high-grade tumors, a distinct subset of MPNSTs is composed predominantly (or entirely) of epithelioid cells (see Chapter 6). Some cases show uniformly high cellularity throughout the tumor, with a fibrosarcoma-like fascicular growth pattern similar to monophasic synovial sarcoma (Fig. 3.83). However, more often, tumors are composed of relatively hypocellular areas alternating with hypercellular areas showing perivascular accentuation, resulting in a marbled appearance at low magnification (see Fig. 3.83B and C). The extracellular matrix in less cellular areas is usually myxoid, which may be abundant in up to 10% of cases (see Chapter 5). There is often a well-developed vascular network, sometimes including HPC-like vessels. Clusters of small rounded blood vessels are commonly seen in high-grade tumors. The spindle cells in MPNST are typically uniform, with palely eosinophilic cytoplasm with indistinct cell borders, and hyperchromatic thin nuclei, with wavy or focally buckled shapes (Fig. 3.84). There is often some degree of nuclear pleomorphism (see Fig. 3.83D). In the more frequent intermediate- and high-grade tumors, mitotic figures are often readily identified (Fig. 3.85A) and geographic necrosis is not uncommon. However, low-grade MPNST may show very scarce mitotic activity. In the context of NF1, the presence of essentially any mitotic activity in a neurofibroma (especially deep-seated tumors with areas of increased cellularity or any nuclear atypia) warrants the diagnosis of MPNST (see "Malignant Transformation in Neurofibroma"). Nuclear palisading is uncommon in MPNST. Approximately 10% to 15% of MPNSTs show heterologous mesenchymal differentiation.[437] The most common divergent elements include chondrosarcomatous, osteosarcomatous, and rhabdomyosarcomatous components; MPNST with heterologous rhabdomyoblastic differentiation is widely known as *malignant Triton tumor*.[437,438] A much smaller percentage of tumors contain angiosarcomatous areas[439] and very rarely epithelial (especially glandular) elements, complicating the differential diagnosis with synovial sarcoma (see Chapter 9); glandular MPNST is highly associated with NF1.[437,440,441]

Immunohistochemistry

Improvements in understanding of MPNST biology (see Molecular Genetics) have led to the identification of H3K27me3 as a diagnostically useful immunohistochemical marker for MPNST, especially high-grade tumors.[442] Loss of H3K27me3 staining is observed in approximately 50% of MPNST overall, including 30% of low-grade tumors and up to 90% of high-grade MPNST (see Fig. 3.85B).[418,443] The specificity of H3K27me3 loss is very high; cases of synovial sarcoma may show loss of H3K27me3 staining under certain technical conditions.[419] In the absence of H3K27me3 loss, it is often difficult to support the diagnosis of MPNST by immunohistochemistry.[444] At most, 40% to 50% of tumors express S-100 protein, typically in only a focal or patchy distribution (Fig. 3.86),[438,445,446] although low-grade MPNST arising in a neurofibroma often shows more consistent staining. GFAP and SOX10 are positive in 30% to 40% of cases. CD34 is often positive, sometimes extensively. EMA may show focal staining, and focal desmin expression is not uncommon. Strong reactivity for desmin (as well as myogenin or MYOD1) may be used to confirm heterologous rhabdomyoblastic differentiation. The synovial sarcoma marker TLE1 shows nuclear staining in a small subset of MPNSTs, occasionally strong and diffuse.

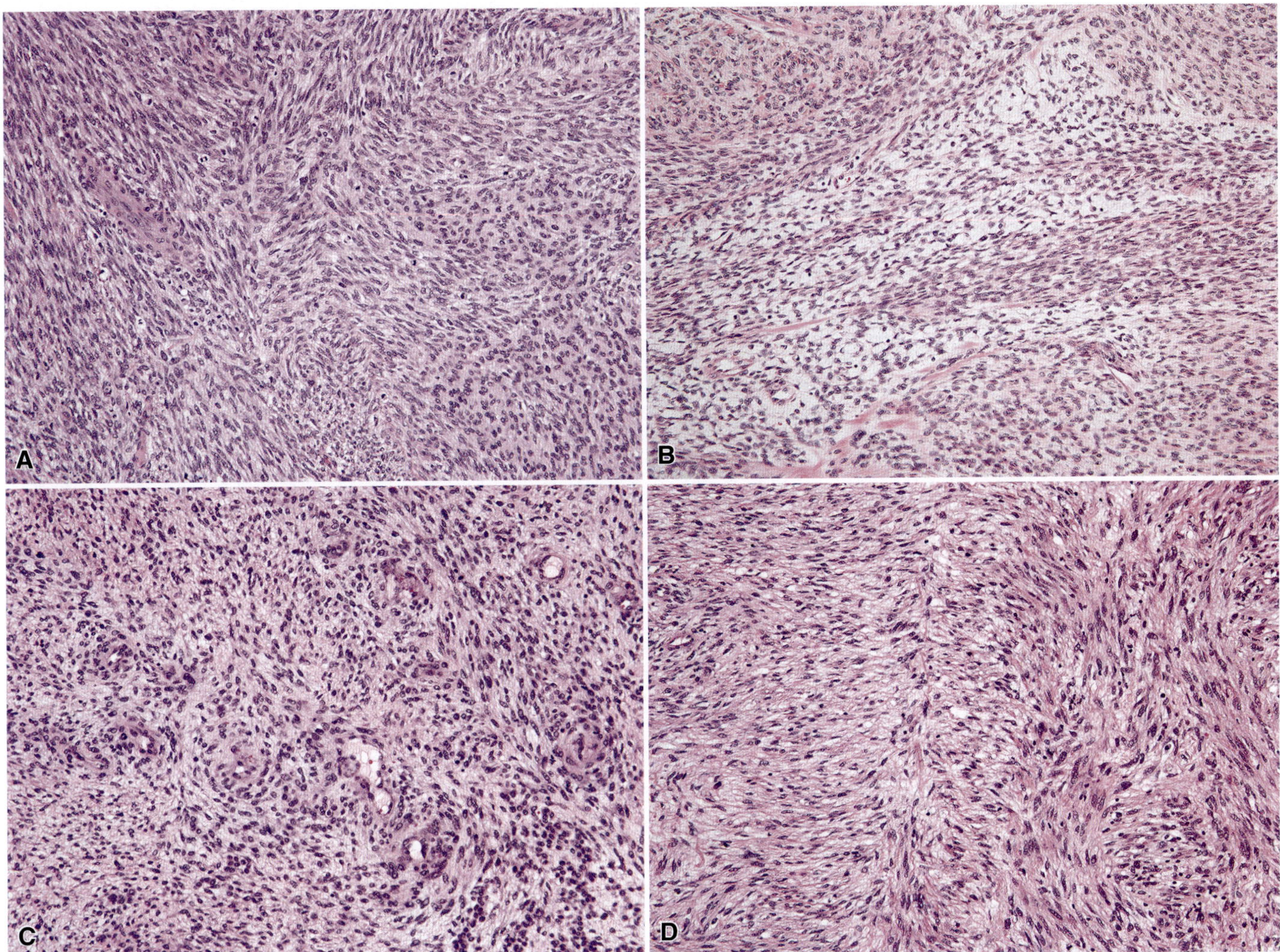

Figure 3.83 **Malignant Peripheral Nerve Sheath Tumor.** (A) The tumor is composed of cellular fascicles of spindle cells. Note the uniform cytomorphology and similarity to synovial sarcoma. (B) Alternating hypercellular and hypocellular, myxoid areas are a typical feature. (C) Perivascular accentuation of cellularity is another helpful diagnostic clue. (D) A tumor with collagenous stroma. Note the variability in nuclear size.

Molecular Genetics

MPNSTs are characterized by clonal chromosomal aberrations resulting in complex karyotypes, with numerous structural and numerical changes.[224] Several seemingly recurrent chromosomal abnormalities have been identified in small number of cases, including monosomy 22 or a focal amplification of distal 17q.

NF1 inactivation and the subsequent upregulation of the RAS family of proteins are likely early events in MPNST development.[447] Inactivation of *TP53* seems to be a key molecular event in MPNST progression and possibly also in its initiation.[448,449] Dysregulation of several other cell cycle–related proteins, including p16 (*CDKN2A*), p19, and p27, has been also implicated in MPNST progression.[277,278] A critical event in MPNST biology is loss of PRC2 function secondary to somatic inactivating mutations of *SUZ12* or *EED*, which encode subunits of the complex. These mutations are present in greater than 90% of sporadic and radiation-associated MPNST, and in approximately 70% of NF1-associated MPNST.[442,450] Loss of function of PRC2 leads to global epigenetic dysregulation that amplifies RAS-driven transcription. The immediate result of PRC2 inactivation is global loss of trimethylation of lysine 27 in histone 3 (H3K27me3), which provides a useful immunohistochemical marker for MPNST.

Differential Diagnosis

High-grade MPNST should be distinguished from monophasic synovial sarcoma, which can show remarkably similar histologic appearances, as well as spindle cell melanoma, dedifferentiated liposarcoma, leiomyosarcoma, and fibrosarcoma. Monophasic synovial sarcoma is more uniform than MPNST, both architecturally and cytologically, composed of cells with characteristic plump overlapping nuclei in contrast to the hyperchromatic, thin, buckled nuclei of MPNST. The presence of wiry stromal collagen and focal calcifications are typical of synovial sarcoma, whereas perivascular accentuation should favor MPNST. Loss of H3K27me3 supports the diagnosis of MPNST. S-100 protein is not helpful in this differential diagnosis, because both tumor types may show variable degrees of positivity. EMA, CD99, and the nuclear protein TLE1 are more commonly expressed in synovial sarcoma.[119,396,445,451] The demonstration of a t(X;18) translocation, or one of the resulting *SS18-SSX* fusion genes by FISH or RT-PCR, is specific for synovial sarcoma.[452,453]

Spindle cell melanoma must be always considered in the differential diagnosis, especially in superficial lesions or in locations such as the axilla or groin, where lymph node metastases from cutaneous melanomas are common.[454] Besides the essential clinicopathologic correlation, in

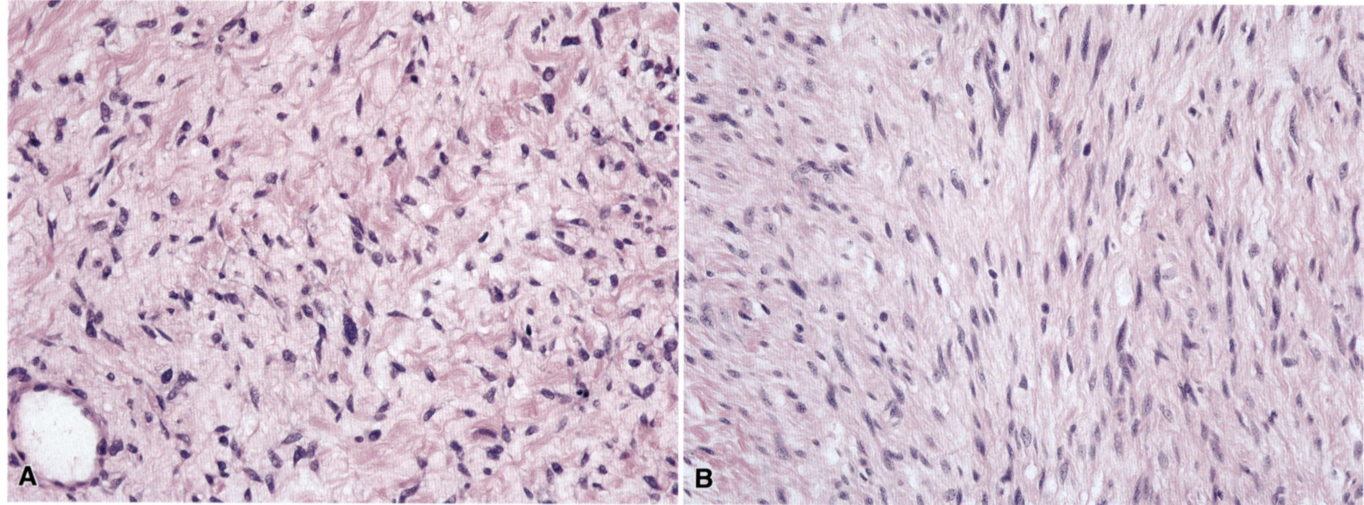

Figure 3.84 Malignant Peripheral Nerve Sheath Tumor. (A) The spindle cells typically contain hyperchromatic, tapering nuclei and indistinct cytoplasm. Note the collagenous stroma. (B) Some tumors contain more elongated nuclei.

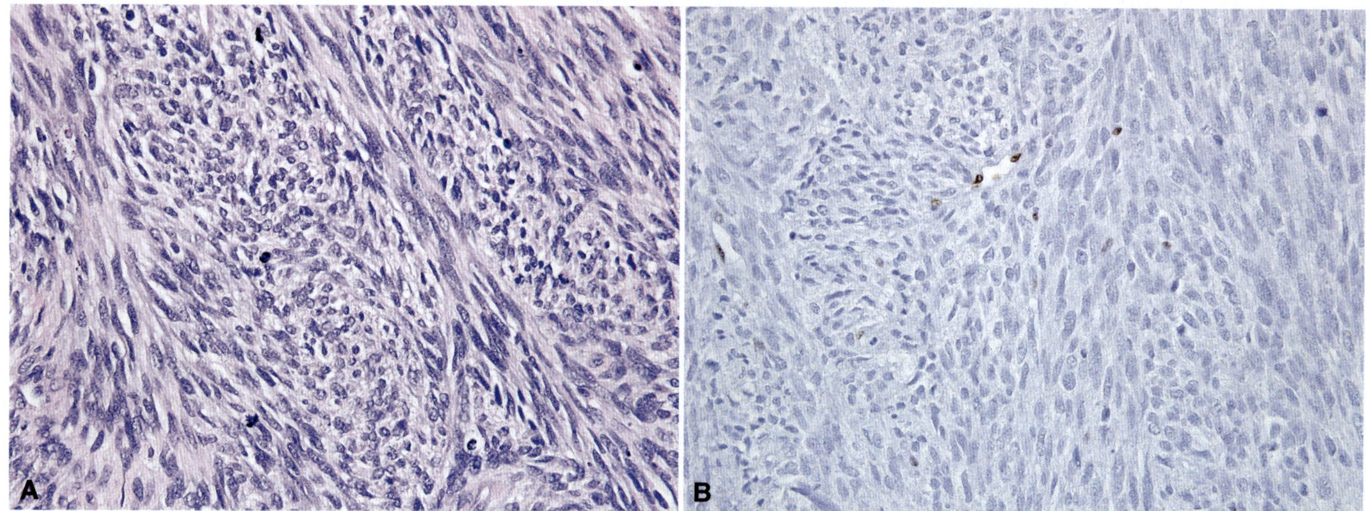

Figure 3.85 Malignant Peripheral Nerve Sheath Tumor. (A) Some examples show a fibrosarcoma-like appearance with intersecting tight fascicles of elongated spindle cells. Note the prominent mitotic activity. (B) Loss of nuclear H3K27me3 is a highly specific finding, seen in 90% of high-grade tumors.

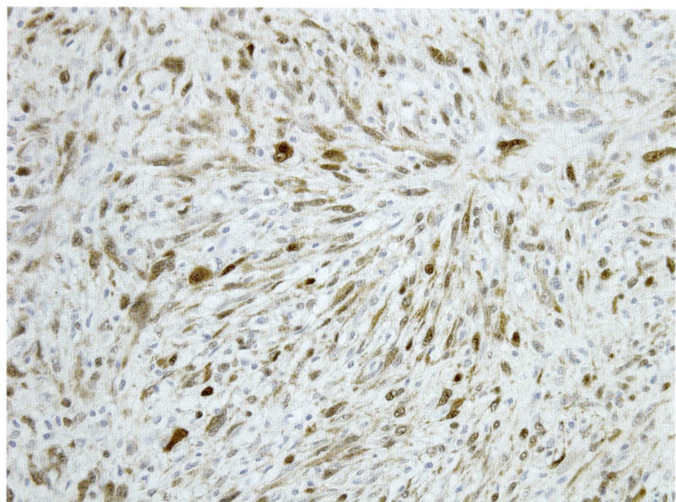

Figure 3.86 Malignant Peripheral Nerve Sheath Tumor. Focal staining for S-100 protein is observed in 40% to 50% of cases.

search of a primary cutaneous melanocytic lesion or past medical history, metastatic melanoma often shows severe nuclear atypia with large nucleoli, an admixture of epithelioid and spindle cells, and a focally nested architecture. In addition, diffuse and intense expression of S-100 protein and SOX10 is rarely seen in MPNST but is a typical feature of melanoma. The expression of second-line melanocytic markers such as HMB-45 or melan A may be helpful in this context, although spindle cell melanomas are usually negative. Loss of H3K27me3 strongly favors MPNST.

Dedifferentiated liposarcoma of the retroperitoneum may be difficult to distinguish from MPNST, particularly in core biopsy samples. Both tumor types may be composed of spindle cells with tapering nuclei and mild nuclear atypia. Heterogeneous architecture and cytology should suggest dedifferentiated liposarcoma over MPNST, and radiologic evidence of an adipocytic component can also be very helpful. MDM2 is overexpressed not only in dedifferentiated liposarcoma but also in approximately 60% of MPNSTs. CDK4 expression is more specific for dedifferentiated liposarcoma in this context. Detection of *MDM2* amplification by FISH is specific for dedifferentiated liposarcoma in this differential diagnosis.

Leiomyosarcoma rarely poses diagnostic difficulties given the presence of spindle cells with brightly eosinophilic cytoplasm and broad, blunt-ended nuclei, although some high-grade tumors can be highly cellular with less abundant cytoplasm and more variable nuclear morphology. In such cases, staining for SMA, desmin, and h-caldesmon supports the diagnosis of leiomyosarcoma.

Fibrosarcoma of adults is an exceedingly rare tumor type that is a diagnosis of exclusion. When MPNSTs lack S-100 protein, SOX10, and GFAP expression, they may be difficult to distinguish from fibrosarcoma. However, the combination of varying cellularity; focally myxoid stroma; perivascular accentuation; and wavy, buckled nuclei should suggest MPNST. Loss of H3K27me3 is more sensitive for MPNST than Schwann cell markers (and highly specific). The fibrosarcoma-like component of fibrosarcomatous DFSP can also mimic MPNST; this distinction should be relatively straightforward with appropriate clinicopathologic correlation (i.e., DFSP is a superficial tumor that invariably contains a cutaneous component) and adequate sampling to identify the conventional storiform DFSP component (see Chapter 15).

Low-grade MPNST may be confused with neurofibroma and LGFMS. The diagnosis of MPNST arising in a neurofibroma relies on the identification of mitotic figures, generally accompanied by increased cellularity and nuclear atypia (see "Neurofibroma"). Histologic clues to LGFMS include sharply demarcated fibrous and myxoid areas, a whorled architecture, and remarkably bland cytomorphology. EMA and MUC4 are typically positive in LGFMS; the latter marker in particular is highly specific for this tumor type.

The distinction between MPNST and cellular schwannoma or cellular SFT may also be occasionally challenging. MPNSTs generally show a higher degree of cellular pleomorphism and nuclear atypia than these other tumor types. Foamy macrophages and hyalinized vessel walls are often seen in cellular schwannoma, which combined with intense S-100 protein expression allow for proper diagnosis. Architectural features of SFT include prominent HPC-like vessels, a "patternless" (not fascicular) growth pattern, and stromal hyalinization. Immunohistochemical detection of CD34 and STAT6 is typical. Loss of H3K27me3 is specific for MPNST in this differential diagnosis.

Prognosis and Treatment

Aggressive surgical resection followed by radiation therapy is often required to achieve local control in patients with MPNST. The prognosis is poor, with overall 5-year survival rates ranging from approximately 50% in sporadic cases to 10% to 15% in NF1-related tumors.[428,436,455] Local recurrence and metastatic rates are high, and common metastatic sites include the lungs, bones, and pleura.[112,436,455] Therapeutic options for metastatic MPNST are limited; chemotherapy has thus far shown little benefit. Large tumor size and a high mitotic rate have been shown to correlate with poor prognosis in some studies.[436] The prognostic significance of grading in MPNST remains controversial, although data suggest grading predicts metastasis (see Chapter 2).[444]

PRACTICE POINTS: Malignant Peripheral Nerve Sheath Tumor

- May be sporadic or affect patients with type 1 neurofibromatosis
- Ten percent of tumors are associated with prior radiation therapy
- Characteristic appearance at low magnification with alternating areas of hypocellularity and hypercellularity, focally myxoid stroma, and perivascular accentuation
- Typically uniform cytology with wavy nuclei and pale cytoplasm
- Heterologous mesenchymal differentiation in 10% to 15% of cases
- Difficult to confirm by immunohistochemistry; 50% of cases overall show loss of the methylation marker H3K27me3 (90% of high-grade tumors); patchy reactivity for S-100 protein, glial fibrillary acidic protein, or SOX10 in less than 50% of cases.

Biphenotypic Sinonasal Sarcoma

Biphenotypic sinonasal sarcoma is a recently recognized locally aggressive sarcoma type with dual neural and myogenic differentiation.[456] Thus far, tumors of this type have only been described in the sinonasal region.

Clinical Features

Biphenotypic sinonasal sarcoma affects adults, with a peak incidence in the fifth decade and a striking female predilection.[456] Most patients present with nasal congestion or pressure; pain is occasionally the presenting symptom. The nasal cavity and ethmoid sinus are the most common sites; involvement of multiple sinuses is frequent.[456] Some tumors extend into the orbit.

Pathologic Features

Biphenotypic sinonasal sarcoma shows infiltrative margins and is composed of long fascicles of uniform spindle cells with bland, elongated nuclei and scant cytoplasm (Fig. 3.87A). Bone invasion is present in approximately 20% of tumors. Entrapment of submucosal glands and invaginated surface epithelium is a typical feature (see Fig. 3.87B). In some cases, strands of collagen may be seen between tumor cells (see Fig. 3.87C). HPC-like vessels are seen in some cases (see Fig. 3.87D). The cellularity of the tumors may be high, but cytologic atypia is mild and mitotic rates are consistently low (see Fig. 3.87C and D).[457] Approximately 5% to 10% of cases contain occasional rhabdomyoblasts with brightly eosinophilic cytoplasm.

Immunohistochemistry

The tumor cells show a characteristic dual neural and myogenic phenotype, expressing S-100 protein (Fig. 3.88A), smooth muscle actin (see Fig. 3.88B), muscle-specific actin (clone HHF35), and calponin. Desmin is less often positive. Expression of myogenin and MYOD1 is limited to few cells in cases with focal rhabdomyoblastic differentiation. Nuclear staining for β-catenin has been described, as well as diffuse expression of TLE1.[457,458] SOX10 is consistently negative.[458]

Molecular Genetics

Biphenotypic sinonasal sarcoma is characterized by consistent *PAX3* gene rearrangements.[457] More than 50% of cases harbor a *PAX3-MAML3* fusion, which upregulates PAX3 and leads to aberrant expression of genes involved in neuroectodermal and myogenic differentiation.[456] Smaller numbers of cases show alternative fusion genes, including *PAX3-NCOA1*[459] and *PAX3-FOXO1*,[460] which is remarkable given the striking pathologic and clinical differences between this tumor type and *PAX3-FOXO1*–positive alveolar rhabdomyosarcoma. Approximately 20% of cases show *PAX3* rearrangements with unknown fusion partners.

Differential Diagnosis

Biphenotypic sinonasal sarcoma should be distinguished chiefly from monophasic synovial sarcoma and MPNST. The histologic appearances of biphenotypic sinonasal sarcoma and monophasic synovial sarcoma in particular can be nearly identical, and there is substantial immunophenotypic overlap between these tumor types as well. Up to 30% of synovial sarcomas express S-100 protein, and biphenotypic sinonasal sarcomas can show diffuse nuclear staining for TLE1. Expression of keratins and EMA is typical of synovial sarcoma but rare in biphenotypic sinonasal sarcoma; expression of desmin and SMA favor biphenotypic sinonasal sarcoma. Molecular analysis (i.e., FISH for *SS18* or *PAX3*) provides a definitive diagnosis. Given the fascicular architecture, elongated nuclei, and consistent expression of S-100 protein, biphenotypic sinonasal sarcoma may easily be mistaken for MPNST. In fact, before the description of this distinctive tumor type, many

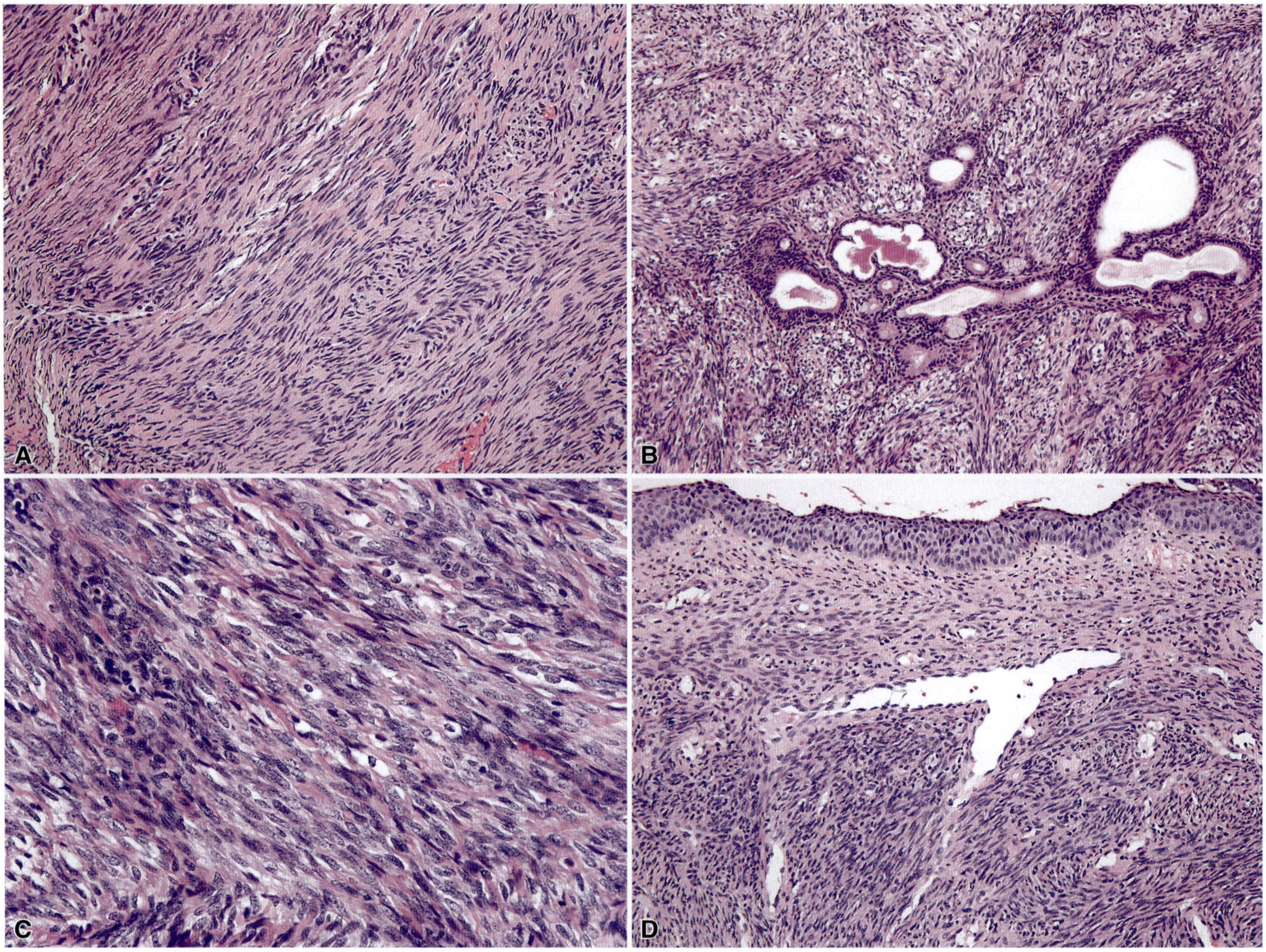

Figure 3.87 Biphenotypic Sinonasal Sarcoma. (A) The tumor is composed of long fascicles of spindle cells. (B) Entrapment of dilated glands is a common finding. (C) The uniform elongated spindle cells show mild nuclear atypia and a low mitotic rate. The occasional presence of intercellular strands of collagen heightens the resemblance to monophasic synovial sarcoma. (D) Some tumors contain dilated, branching (hemangiopericytoma-like) blood vessels.

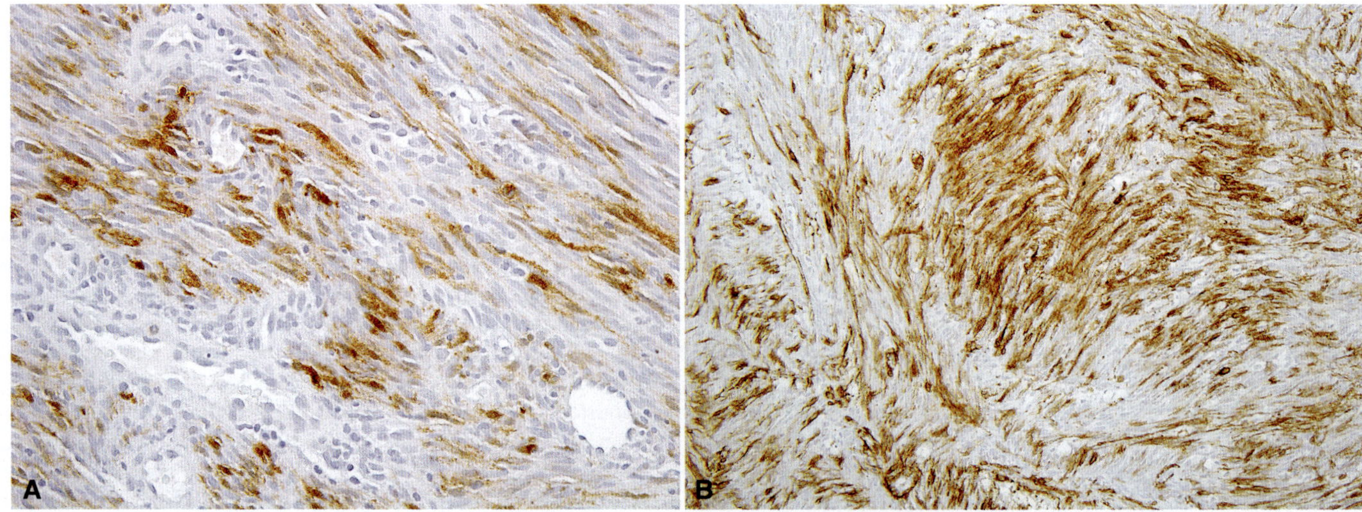

Figure 3.88 Biphenotypic Sinonasal Sarcoma. This distinctive tumor type shows a dual neural and myogenic phenotype. (A) S-100 protein is consistently positive. (B) Most tumors express smooth muscle actin. Desmin is also positive in a subset of tumors (not shown).

examples were diagnosed as low-grade MPNST. The occasional presence of a limited rhabdomyoblastic component heightens the resemblance to MPNST. However, most MPNSTs with heterologous rhabdomyoblastic differentiation ("malignant Triton tumors") are histologically obvious high-grade sarcomas; in contrast, biphenotypic sinonasal sarcomas show only mild nuclear atypia and a low mitotic rate and usually lack necrosis. Demonstration of *PAX3* rearrangement confirms biphenotypic sinonasal sarcoma.

Prognosis and Treatment

Biphenotypic sinonasal sarcoma is an aggressive tumor with a high rate of local recurrence (nearly 50%), but distant metastasis has not yet been reported.

Sarcomas With Fibroblastic Differentiation

Several distinct sarcoma types are composed of cells believed to show fibroblastic differentiation. The designation *fibrosarcoma* theoretically refers to a malignant mesenchymal neoplasm composed solely of fibroblasts. Historically applied to many spindle cell sarcomas with uniform cytomorphology and collagenous stroma (including tumor types now recognized to belong to diverse diagnostic categories with more specific lines of differentiation), this term is currently reserved for four unrelated entities: myxofibrosarcoma, infantile fibrosarcoma (congenital fibrosarcoma), adult-type fibrosarcoma, and sclerosing epithelioid fibrosarcoma.

Myxofibrosarcoma is a relatively common, often superficial sarcoma of older adults, with a predilection for the limbs. It shows a wide range of morphologic appearances, including myxoid stroma–rich low-grade lesions and high-grade tumors with a minor myxoid component (see Chapters 5 and 7).

Infantile fibrosarcoma, in contrast, is a rare mesenchymal neoplasm of infants. It is a highly cellular neoplasm composed of rather primitive spindle cells and is characterized by a t(12;15)(p13;q25) reciprocal translocation and the resulting *ETV6-NTRK3* fusion oncogene (see Chapter 4).

Adult-type fibrosarcoma is vanishingly rare. As the ability to diagnose mesenchymal neoplasms has improved, it has become apparent that most tumors traditionally diagnosed as fibrosarcoma can be reclassified into well-defined diagnostic categories with distinct clinical and pathologic features and behavior. Adult-type fibrosarcoma is now regarded as a diagnosis of exclusion, as discussed subsequently.

Sclerosing epithelioid fibrosarcoma is a rare mesenchymal neoplasm with epithelioid morphology and abundant hyalinized collagenous stroma (see Chapter 6); these tumors are related to LGFMS (see later discussion).

Three additional "fibroblastic" sarcomas deserve mention. Transformation of DFSP to a higher-grade variant is designated *fibrosarcomatous DFSP* (see Chapter 15). Although the diagnosis is generally straightforward when a nondescript fascicular spindle cell sarcoma is seen arising within an otherwise typical DFSP of the skin, fibrosarcomatous DFSP can be diagnostically challenging when only the higher-grade component is biopsied or when a lung metastasis is observed without proper clinical information. *Myxoinflammatory fibroblastic sarcoma* is a distinctive low-grade sarcoma of the distal extremities characterized by a multinodular architecture and small numbers of large, pleomorphic cells with inclusion-like nucleoli within a variably myxoid or fibroinflammatory stromal background (see Chapters 5, 7, and 10). *LGFMS* is a fibroblastic sarcoma with a deceptively bland cytomorphology that usually affects young adults. It is discussed in detail in this section.

Box 3.9 Tumor Types That May Be Misdiagnosed as "Fibrosarcoma"

Monophasic synovial sarcoma
Malignant peripheral nerve sheath tumor
Solitary fibrous tumor
Fibrosarcomatous dermatofibrosarcoma protuberans
Myxofibrosarcoma
Low-grade fibromyxoid sarcoma
Leiomyosarcoma
Low-grade myofibroblastic sarcoma
Undifferentiated pleomorphic sarcoma

Adult-Type Fibrosarcoma

Adult-type fibrosarcoma is exceptionally rare. Conceptually, it represents a malignant tumor composed of fibroblasts showing no other line of differentiation, which translates nowadays into a diagnosis of exclusion. Applying strict morphologic criteria together with modern immunohistochemical stains and molecular techniques, less than 1% of soft tissue sarcomas may represent "true" adult-type fibrosarcomas.[420] Most of the tumors traditionally diagnosed as fibrosarcoma can be correctly reclassified as monophasic synovial sarcoma, SFT, myxofibrosarcoma, MPNST, or undifferentiated pleomorphic sarcoma (Box 3.9). Many postradiation soft tissue sarcomas show no recognizable line of differentiation and might therefore be regarded as fibrosarcoma, although they are histologically heterogeneous and rarely show the classic uniform cytology and tight, intersecting fascicular architecture of fibrosarcoma.

Only one recent study has systematically approached the problem of reclassifying putative cases of fibrosarcoma using strict updated morphologic criteria and a panel of ancillary techniques.[420] After rereview of a large series of cases, the small number of cases of "adult-type fibrosarcoma" remaining affected middle-aged adults, arose in the extremities, trunk, or head and neck region, and were usually deep seated. Histologically, the lesional spindle cells are monomorphic, giving the tumor a uniform appearance, forming homogeneous dense fascicles of hyperchromatic spindle cells, characteristically arranged in a herringbone pattern. Variably prominent parallel collagen fibers may be interspersed between the cells. The tumors may be of low, intermediate, or high grade, with increasing cellularity, nuclear atypia, and mitotic activity, but pleomorphism is not a feature. Immunohistochemical stains do not reveal any specific line of differentiation, by definition.

The differential diagnosis of adult-type fibrosarcoma includes essentially every monotonous, highly cellular spindle cell neoplasm that should be excluded before making the diagnosis (see Box 3.9). These include monophasic synovial sarcoma, SFT, myofibroblastic sarcoma, MPNST, high-grade myxofibrosarcoma, and leiomyosarcoma, among others. Regarding prognosis, fibrosarcoma frequently recurs, in up to 60% of cases, and often metastasizes to the lungs and bones. Disease-specific mortality is approximately 50%.[420] Optimal treatment requires excision with wide margins, followed by adjuvant radiotherapy.

Low-Grade Fibromyxoid Sarcoma and Variants

First described by Evans in 1987,[461] LGFMS is currently considered a specific type of fibrosarcoma with distinctive clinical behavior and genetic features. Because of its deceptively bland cytomorphology, this sarcoma had been previously mistaken for a number of benign and malignant neoplasms, including desmoid fibromatosis and various low-grade sarcomas.[462-465] Since its seminal description, the clinicopathologic and immunohistochemical features of LGFMS have been progressively defined, and significant improvements have been made regarding the molecular characterization of this sarcoma type. In 1997 the morphologic spectrum of LGFMS was expanded to include hyalinizing spindle cell

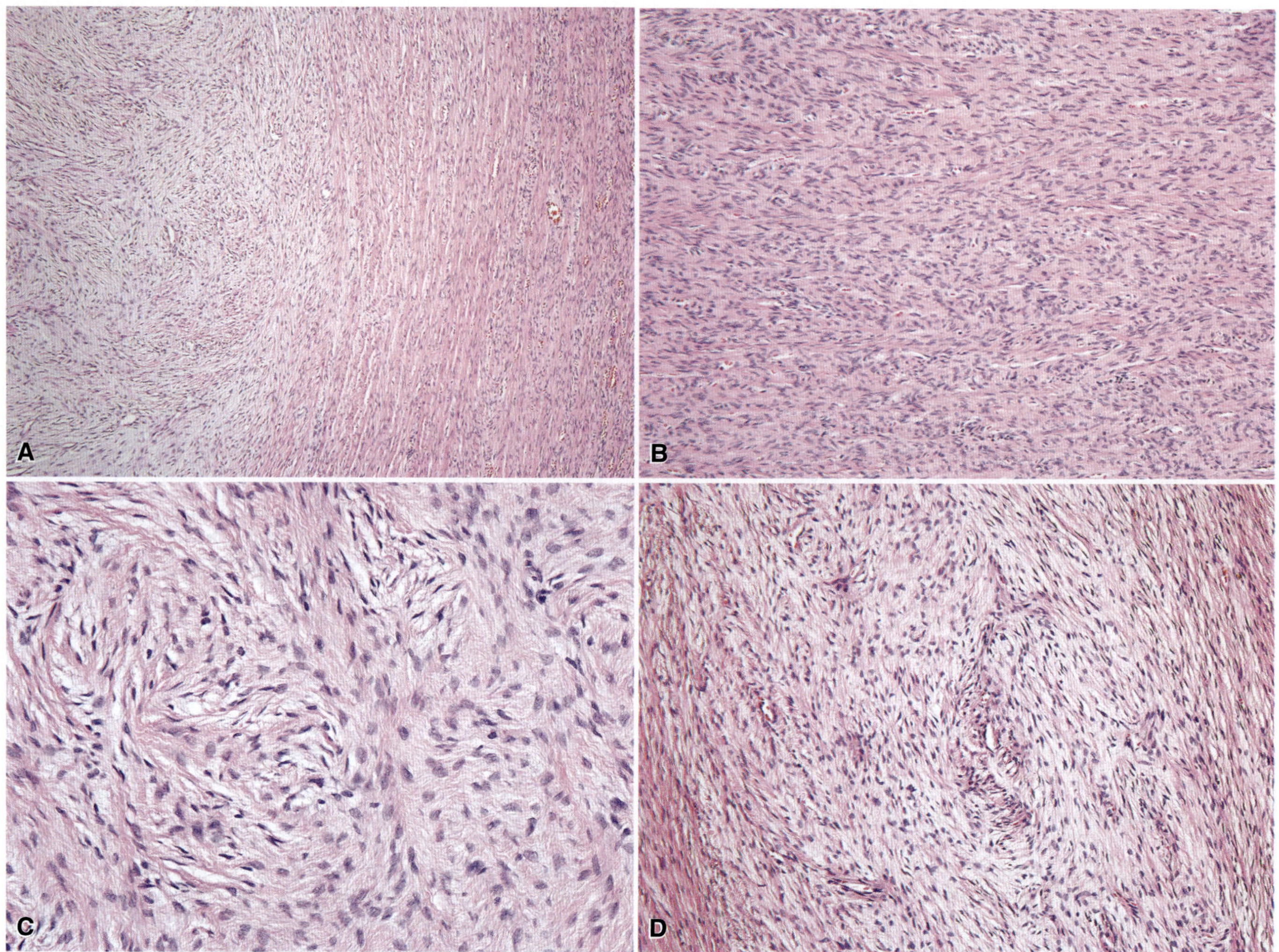

Figure 3.89 Low-Grade Fibromyxoid Sarcoma. (A) The tumor is composed of alternating, sharply demarcated fibrous and myxoid areas. (B) In the fibrous areas the tumor cells often show a storiform growth pattern. (C) The tumor cells are bland and uniform, with ovoid or elongated nuclei with fine chromatin and indistinct cytoplasm. Note the whorled architecture. (D) Elongated blood vessels are typically seen in the more myxoid areas.

tumor with giant rosettes, now recognized to be a histologic variant of LGFMS.[466] LGFMS is also discussed in Chapters 4 and 5.

Clinical Features

LGFMS preferentially affects young adults, with a median age of 35 years. The typical clinical presentation is that of a slowly growing, painless mass in the deep soft tissues with a predilection for the lower extremities, especially the thigh, limb girdle, and trunk. Examples located in superficial soft tissue are more common in childhood.[467]

Pathologic Features

Grossly, LGFMS is usually well circumscribed, with a white, firm appearance on cut section. Histologically, the tumor is characterized by sharply demarcated, alternating fibrous and myxoid areas containing monomorphic spindled to ovoid tumor cells arranged in a fascicular, storiform, or whorled growth pattern (Fig. 3.89). The tumor cells are remarkably bland, with small uniform nuclei, fine chromatin, and ill-defined borders (see Fig. 3.89C). The myxoid areas often contain arcades of small blood vessels (see Fig. 3.89D). Mitotic activity is usually very low, and necrosis is uncommon. Despite the well-circumscribed macroscopic appearance, the tumor often infiltrates into surrounding tissues.

A subset of LGFMS cases contains unusual and often misleading histologic features.[464,466,468] Approximately 10% of tumors contain areas of increased cellularity (Fig. 3.90), giant rosettes (hyalinized collagenous nodular structures surrounded by palisading rounded or ovoid cells) (Fig. 3.91A), or foci of epithelioid cells (see Fig. 3.91B). Rare cases show more notable nuclear atypia or focal pleomorphism (see Fig. 3.91C). In addition, markedly hypocellular (sclerotic) areas with a misleading fibrotic appearance can occasionally be present (see Fig. 3.91D). The latter appearance in particular is a potential diagnostic pitfall, especially when encountered in a core biopsy specimen. Occasional LGFMS cases are associated with a component of sclerosing epithelioid fibrosarcoma.

Immunohistochemistry

LGFMS is characterized by expression of the epithelial mucin MUC4 (Fig. 3.92).[120] Identified through gene expression profiling,[469] MUC4 is a highly sensitive and specific marker that is diffusely and strongly expressed in nearly all cases of LGFMS.[120] EMA is also usually positive in LGFMS (in up to 80% of cases), although expression is often more limited in extent.[120,468,470] LGFMS is often positive for the nonspecific markers CD99 and bcl-2, but these are not helpful in differential diagnosis.[468] Focal expression of SMA, desmin, CD34, or keratin is

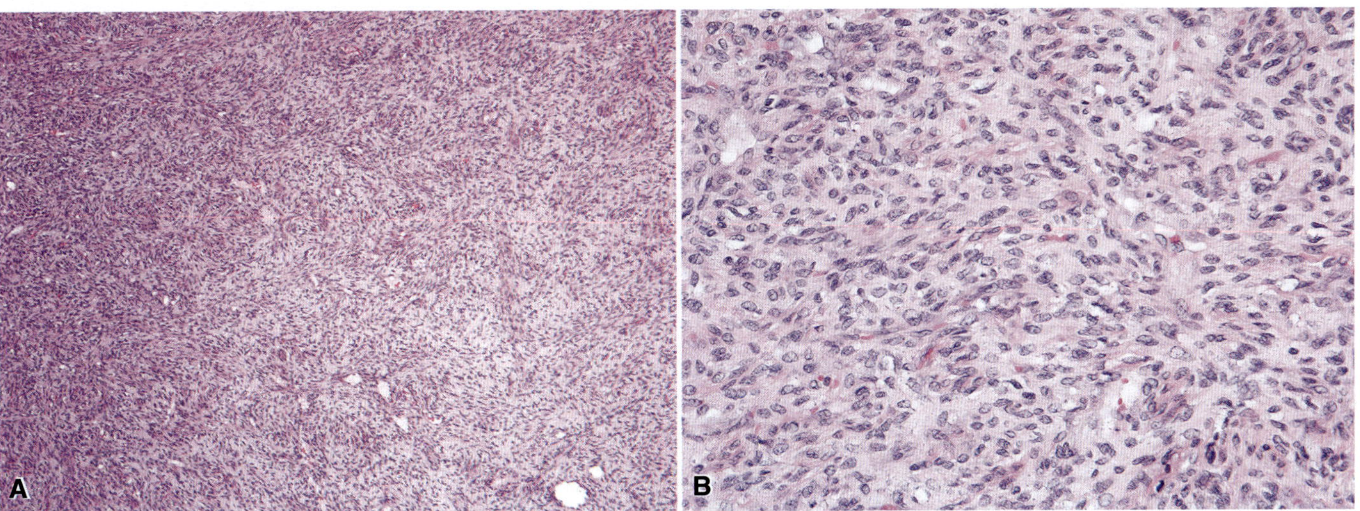

Figure 3.90 Low-Grade Fibromyxoid Sarcoma. (A) Occasional tumors show a more uniformly hypercellular appearance. (B) The ovoid tumor cells are uniform with indistinct cell borders.

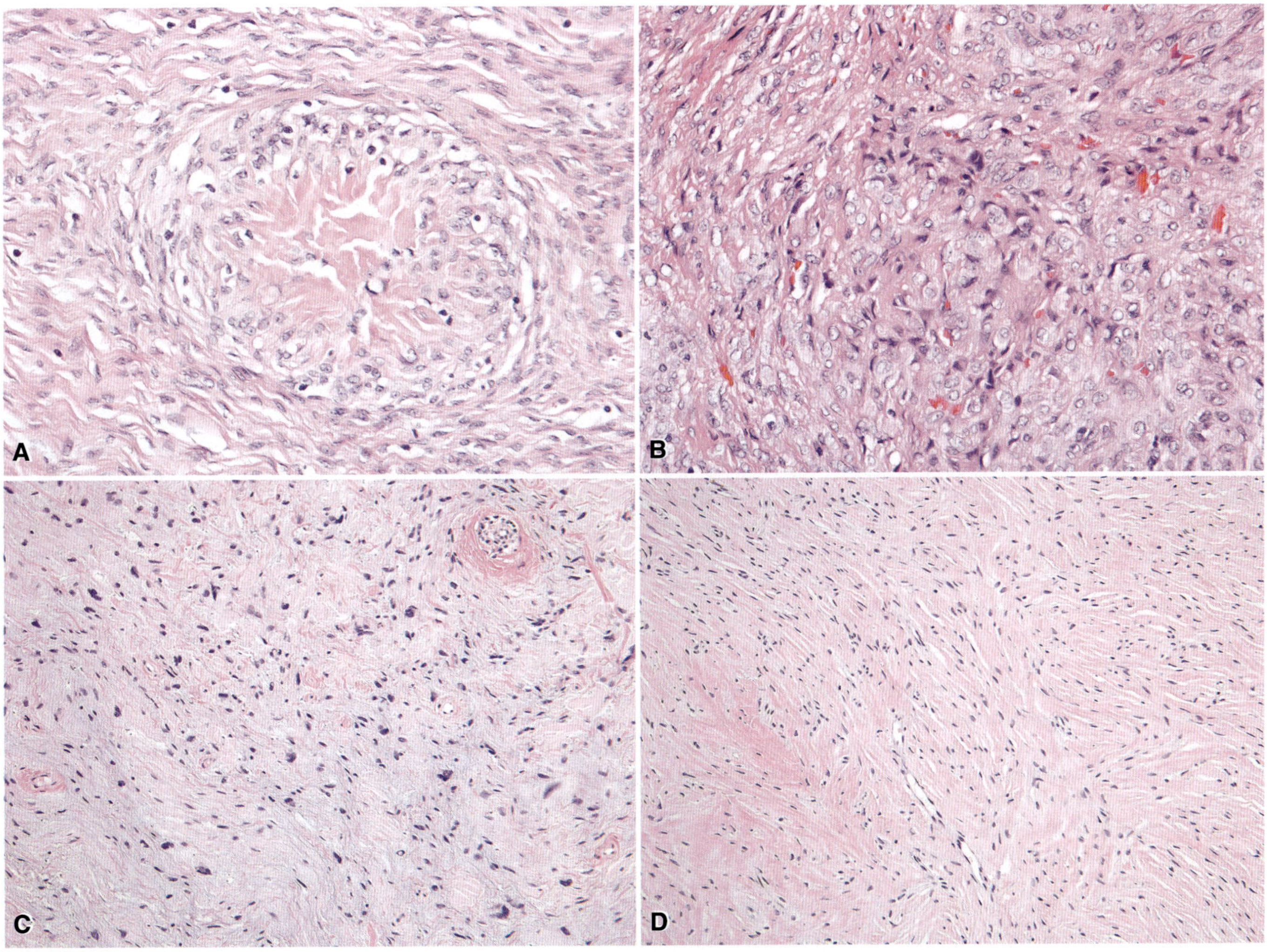

Figure 3.91 Low-Grade Fibromyxoid Sarcoma. (A) Giant collagen rosettes are observed in approximately 10% of cases. (B) Some tumors contain foci of epithelioid cells. (C) Rare tumors show misleading nuclear pleomorphism. (D) Hypocellular examples with dense collagenous stroma are difficult to recognize.

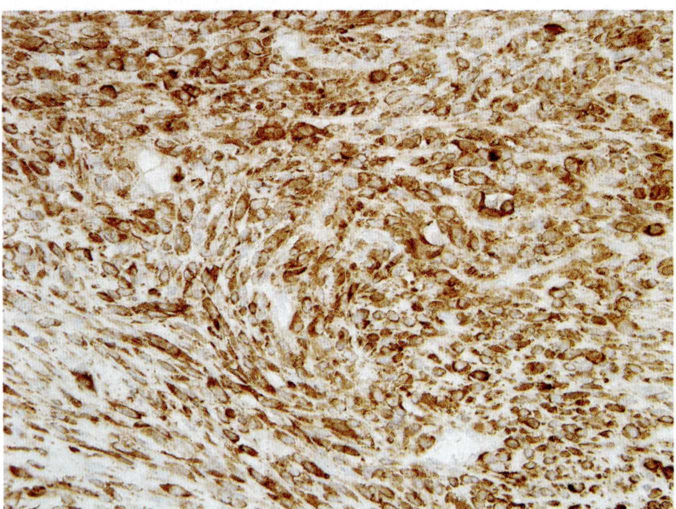

Figure 3.92 Low-Grade Fibromyxoid Sarcoma. Strong cytoplasmic staining for MUC4 is a highly sensitive and specific diagnostic feature.

Box 3.10 Differential Diagnosis of Low-Grade Fibromyxoid Sarcoma

Soft tissue perineurioma
Solitary fibrous tumor
Desmoid fibromatosis
Intramuscular/cellular myxoma
Low-grade myxofibrosarcoma
Low-grade malignant peripheral nerve sheath tumor

rarely seen in LGFMS, whereas the tumor is consistently negative for S-100 protein, GFAP, SOX10, caldesmon, and KIT.[120,134,463,468,470]

Molecular Genetics

LGFMS is characterized by the specific recurrent translocations t(7;16) or t(11;16) (see Chapter 18).[134,470,471] *FUS-CREB3L2* fusion gene transcripts resulting from the t(7;16)(q34;p11) translocation can be detected by RT-PCR in up to 95% of fusion-positive cases.[468,471] Rare LGFMS cases bear the alternative t(11;16)(p11;p11) translocation, which fuses the *FUS* gene at 16p11 to the *CREB3L1* gene at 11p11.[470]

Rearrangements of the *FUS* gene may be detected for diagnosis using FISH or RT-PCR on paraffin-embedded tissue.[472,473] These molecular techniques facilitate the confirmation of unusual histologic variants of LGFMS, such as highly cellular or pleomorphic examples. A subset of sclerosing epithelioid fibrosarcomas (including some tumors showing hybrid features of LGFMS and sclerosing epithelioid fibrosarcoma) has been shown to share the same molecular alterations as LGFMS.[468,474]

Differential Diagnosis

Because of its bland appearances, LFGMS can easily be confused with various benign soft tissue tumors (Box 3.10), including desmoid fibromatosis, soft tissue perineurioma, and cellular myxoma, as well as other low-grade sarcomas, especially low-grade MPNST and low-grade myxofibrosarcoma. A limited panel of markers, including MUC4, EMA, CD34, S-100 protein, SMA, and β-catenin, depending on the specific differential diagnosis, is usually sufficient to reach a specific diagnosis.

Desmoid fibromatosis is composed of uniformly cellular, long sweeping fascicles of spindle cells, in contrast to the alternating myxoid and collagenous areas and whorled growth pattern of LGFMS. Desmoid tumors are usually diffusely positive for SMA, and the majority of cases (approximately 80%) show nuclear staining for β-catenin. They are consistently negative for MUC4 and EMA. Similar to LGFMS, cellular myxoma has a predilection for the deep soft tissues of the thigh and is composed of bland spindle cells in a variably myxoid stroma. However, cellular myxoma is uniformly negative for MUC4. Distinguishing between LGFMS and soft tissue perineurioma used to be particularly challenging because both lesions typically show a whorled growth pattern, some perineuriomas contain variably myxoid stroma, and EMA is usually positive in both tumor types; MUC4 staining can now be used to discriminate easily between these tumor types.

In contrast to LGFMS, low-grade myxofibrosarcoma is usually located in the subcutaneous tissue of older adults, contains more abundant myxoid stroma with distinctive curvilinear blood vessels and pseudolipoblasts, and shows nuclear atypia and pleomorphism. In addition, myxofibrosarcoma is negative for EMA and MUC4. Low-grade MPNST may bear a close resemblance to LGFMS but generally contains tapering, wavy nuclei with more notable nuclear atypia. S-100 protein, GFAP, and SOX10 are each positive in 40% to 50% of cases, and MUC4 is negative.

Prognosis and Treatment

LGFMS has a tendency for late recurrences, occurring in more than 50% of patients with long-term follow-up. Most metastases of LGFMS also develop late in the course of the disease, after a median of 5 years but as late as 45 years after initial diagnosis.[475] The metastatic rate at 10 years is close to 40%; the lungs and pleura are the most common metastatic sites. Up to 40% of patients eventually die of disease after a median of 15 years.[475]

PRACTICE POINTS: Low-Grade Fibromyxoid Sarcoma

- Most common in deep soft tissues of the thigh and trunk of young adults
- Consists of uniform, bland spindle cells in alternating, sharply demarcated fibrous areas with whorled architecture and myxoid areas with arcades of small blood vessels
- Tumor cells typically express epithelial membrane antigen and MUC4
- t(7;16) translocation with *FUS* gene rearrangement is typical
- Follows a protracted clinical course, with late recurrences and metastases to lungs and pleura (10 to 30 years or longer after initial diagnosis)

Low-Grade Myofibroblastic Sarcoma

Low-grade myofibroblastic sarcoma is a rare, recently recognized sarcoma type.[476,477] Myofibroblastic differentiation in a spindle cell sarcoma can be suspected on histologic examination, but immunohistochemistry helps support the diagnosis. Myofibroblasts show characteristic ultrastructural features, but electron microscopy is now rarely used in clinical practice for the diagnosis of soft tissue tumors.[478-480] Intermediate and high-grade spindle cell and pleomorphic sarcomas may show myofibroblastic differentiation; however, such tumors are difficult to diagnose reproducibly and often remain within the small group of unclassified sarcomas. Of note, the dedifferentiated component of dedifferentiated liposarcoma not uncommonly shows myofibroblastic differentiation. Some myofibroblastic sarcomas are related to inflammatory myofibroblastic tumor; these can occur as recurrences of conventional spindle cell inflammatory myofibroblastic tumor (representing a form of tumor progression or transformation) or de novo as the result of the specific *ALK* translocations *RANBP2-ALK* or *RRBP1-ALK* (epithelioid inflammatory myofibroblastic sarcoma) (see Chapters 4, 10, and 16). Only low-grade myofibroblastic sarcoma will be discussed in detail in this section.

Clinical Features

Low-grade myofibroblastic sarcoma has a predilection for the head and neck region (30% of cases), particularly the tongue, face, neck, and

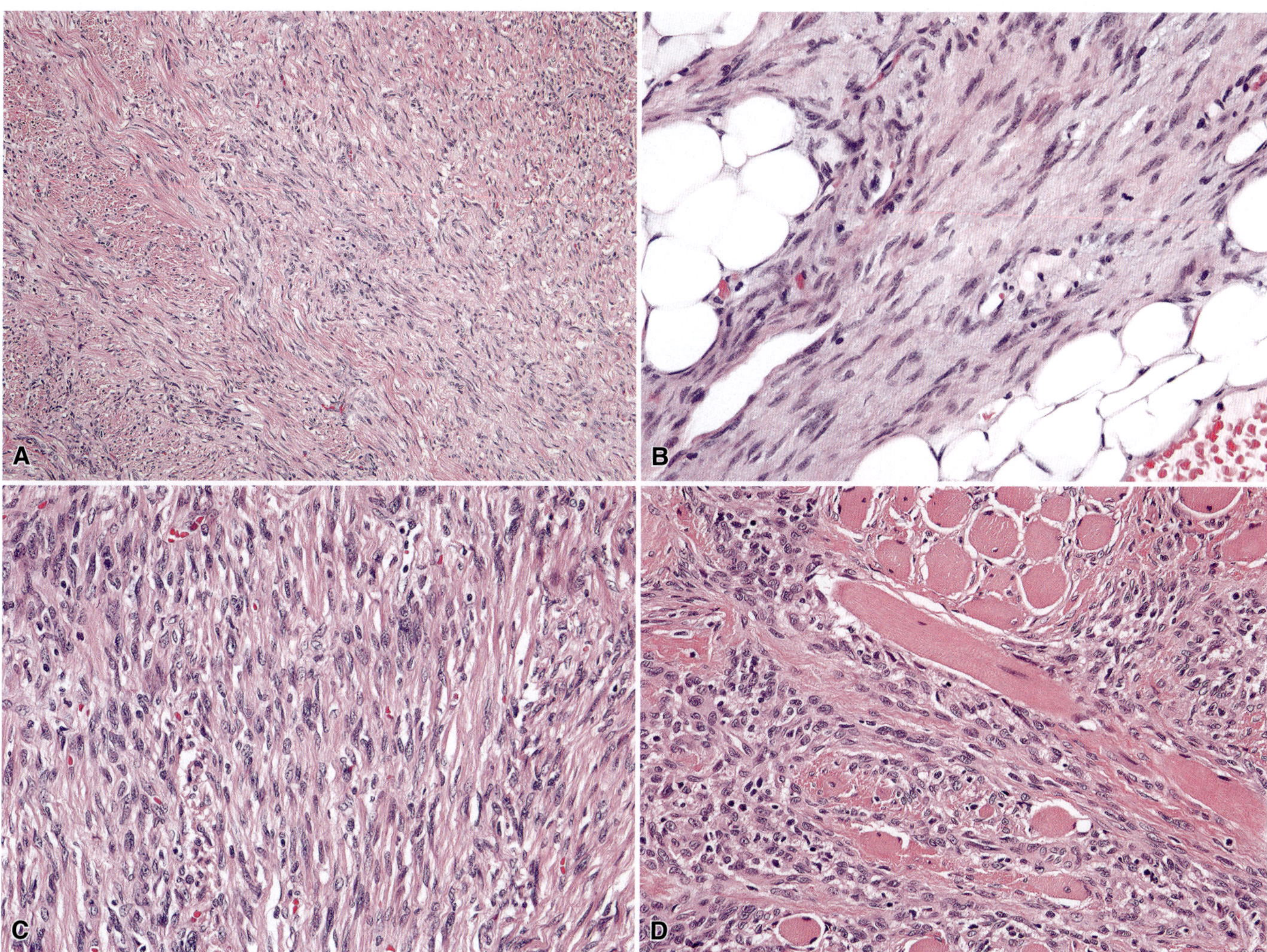

Figure 3.93 Low-Grade Myofibroblastic Sarcoma. (A) The tumor is composed of long fascicles of spindle cells with palely eosinophilic cytoplasm. (B) The tumor cells contain elongated nuclei with tapering ends. Note the mild nuclear atypia. (C) Some tumors show more notable nuclear atypia. (D) The tumor has infiltrative margins into adjacent skeletal muscle.

facial bones, but it shows a wide anatomic distribution. The tumor has a peak incidence in middle-aged adults, with no gender predilection. It often presents as a slowly growing painless mass, which can be superficial or situated in deep soft tissues.[477,480]

Pathologic Features

Grossly, low-grade myofibroblastic sarcoma is generally well circumscribed, with a white firm cut surface.[476,477] Histologically, the tumor is typically composed of long fascicles of relatively uniform spindle cells with abundant, palely eosinophilic, fibrillary cytoplasm and ill-defined cell borders (Fig. 3.93). Stromal collagen is often prominent. The nuclei are slender or wavy with tapering ends and dispersed chromatin, sometimes with a prominent nucleolus (see Fig. 3.93B).[477] The degree of nuclear atypia is usually mild to moderate, but occasional cells with more notable nuclear atypia or pleomorphism may be observed (see Fig. 3.93C). Mitotic activity is typically low (1 to 5 mitoses per 10 HPF) but occasionally higher. Despite its macroscopic appearance, low-grade myofibroblastic sarcoma usually shows ill-defined margins and infiltrates into the surrounding tissues (see Fig. 3.93D).

Immunohistochemistry

Low-grade myofibroblastic sarcoma is usually positive for SMA, desmin, or both. Some tumors show strong and diffuse desmin expression but are negative for SMA. The tumor cells are consistently negative for h-caldesmon, myogenin, CD34, EMA, keratins, and S-100 protein. Tumor cells are also often positive for calponin, and a subset of tumors shows nuclear staining for β-catenin, which can complicate the differential diagnosis with desmoid fibromatosis (see later discussion).

Differential Diagnosis

Low-grade myofibroblastic sarcoma should mainly be distinguished from desmoid fibromatosis, leiomyosarcoma, and spindle cell rhabdomyosarcoma. Similar to low-grade myofibroblastic sarcoma, desmoid fibromatosis is composed of long fascicles of spindle cells with tapering nuclei and prominent stromal collagen. Although both tumor types show irregular margins, low-grade myofibroblastic sarcoma is generally more infiltrative than a desmoid tumor. The most helpful distinguishing feature of low-grade myofibroblastic sarcoma is the presence of nuclear variability and atypia; desmoid fibromatosis is devoid of atypia and does not contain pleomorphic cells. Nuclear staining for β-catenin is not specific for desmoid fibromatosis in this differential diagnosis, but diffuse desmin expression favors low-grade myofibroblastic sarcoma.

Leiomyosarcoma also shows a fascicular architecture, but the fascicles are typically shorter than those in low-grade myofibroblastic sarcoma, and

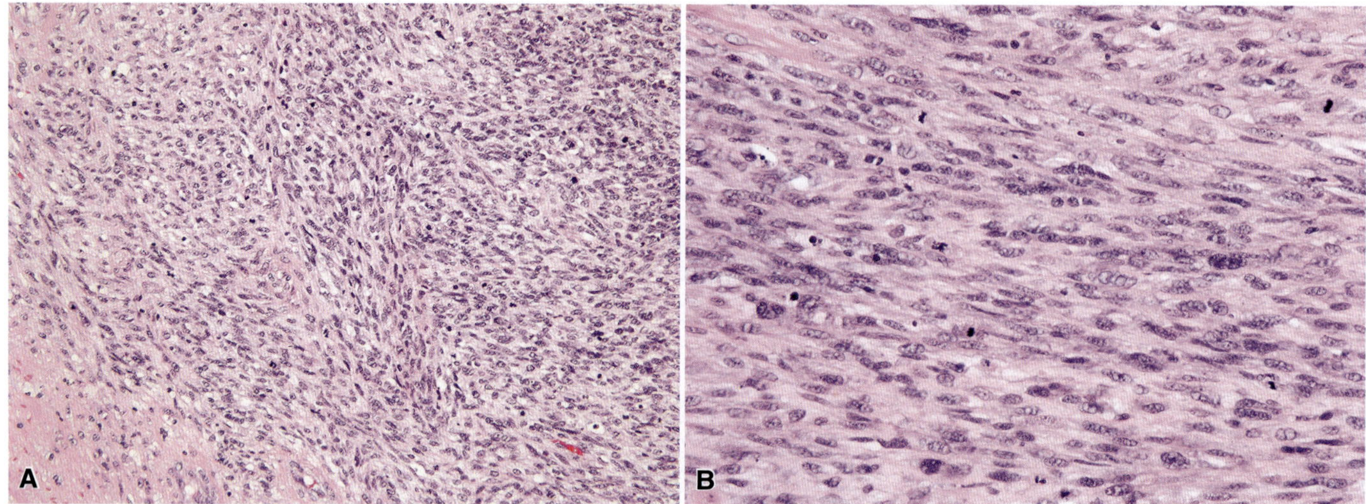

Figure 3.94 Spindle Cell Rhabdomyosarcoma. (A) The tumor is composed of long fascicles of relatively uniform spindle cells. This tumor type may be mistaken for leiomyosarcoma. (B) The tumor cells contain elongated nuclei with vesicular chromatin and pale indistinct cytoplasm. Note the prominent mitotic activity.

the tumor cells contain more brightly eosinophilic cytoplasm; broader, blunt-ended nuclei; and more distinct cell borders. Leiomyosarcoma usually lacks the abundant stromal collagen seen in low-grade myofibroblastic sarcoma. Both tumor types often express SMA and desmin, but h-caldesmon is specific for leiomyosarcoma in this differential diagnosis.

Spindle cell rhabdomyosarcoma also typically arises in the head and neck and shows a fascicular architecture. However, spindle cell rhabdomyosarcoma is usually more hypercellular with less abundant cytoplasm, and occasional rhabdomyoblasts with brightly eosinophilic cytoplasm can be found after careful examination. Diffuse desmin expression is shared by both tumor types, but nuclear staining for the skeletal muscle transcription factors myogenin and MYOD1 is only observed in rhabdomyosarcoma.

Prognosis and Treatment

Low-grade myofibroblastic sarcoma has a relatively favorable prognosis following wide surgical excision. It recurs locally in approximately 30% of cases, usually due to inadequate initial resection. The metastatic rate is low (5% to 10%); the lungs are the most common site of metastases.[476,477]

Spindle Cell Rhabdomyosarcoma

Spindle cell rhabdomyosarcoma is an uncommon, distinct variant of rhabdomyosarcoma. Initially described in children, spindle cell rhabdomyosarcoma was initially considered a histologic subtype of embryonal rhabdomyosarcoma in the pediatric population with a particularly favorable prognosis. At present, it is regarded as a distinct entity that accounts for less than 5% of rhabdomyosarcomas in this age group (see Chapter 4).[481] Examples arising in adulthood behave substantially more aggressively.[482-484] Spindle cell rhabdomyosarcoma is related to, and falls on a morphologic spectrum with, sclerosing rhabdomyosarcoma.[482,483,485]

Clinical Features

In contrast to the striking male predilection of spindle cell rhabdomyosarcoma in children, in adults the gender distribution is more even but still with a 2:1 male predominance. The head and neck region is the most common anatomic site in adults, followed by the extremities and the trunk.[482,484] Paratesticular location can occur but is rare in adults.

Pathologic Features

Grossly, the tumors are nodular or lobulated with a fleshy, sometimes whorled solid cut surface. Histologically, spindle cell rhabdomyosarcoma is composed of long intersecting cellular fascicles of relatively uniform spindle cells with oval to elongated nuclei and mild atypia, vesicular chromatin, small nucleoli, and pale indistinct cytoplasm (Fig. 3.94). Occasionally, the neoplastic cells show more rounded or epithelioid morphology. In addition, scattered throughout the tumor are small numbers of spindled or polygonal-shaped rhabdomyoblasts with hyperchromatic, eccentrically placed nuclei, and abundant brightly eosinophilic cytoplasm. The mitotic rate is highly variable but may be quite low, and atypical mitotic figures may sometimes be identified. Foci of tumor necrosis may occasionally be present. The tumors usually show infiltrative margins. Some tumors contain areas with abundant collagen deposition between tumor cells, imparting a pseudovascular or osteoid-like appearance, identical to the cases described as sclerosing rhabdomyosarcoma (Fig. 3.95).[482,483] In such cases the diagnosis of spindle cell/sclerosing rhabdomyosarcoma is appropriate.

Immunohistochemistry

Similar to other rhabdomyosarcoma subtypes, spindle cell rhabdomyosarcoma is usually diffusely positive for desmin and muscle-specific actin (clone HHF35), whereas nuclear staining for myogenin and MYOD1 ranges from focal to diffuse; MYOD1 is usually more extensively positive than myogenin.[482,486] A small subset of cases is focally positive for broad-spectrum keratins and EMA. CD34 is occasionally expressed, but tumor cells are negative for S-100 protein, GFAP, SOX10, caldesmon, and HMB-45.[482,484]

Molecular Genetics

Spindle cell rhabdomyosarcoma is characterized by a recurrent neomorphic p.L122R mutation in *MYOD1* that occurs in combination with PI3K pathway activation and promotes proliferation through MYC.[487] Identification of similar mutations in sclerosing rhabdomyosarcoma supports the interpretation that these entities are related.[488,489] Several reported cases demonstrated complex karyotypes with inconsistent numerical and structural cytogenetic abnormalities.[490,491] As discussed in Chapter 4, congenital and infantile spindle cell rhabdomyosarcomas are characterized by recurrent gene fusions involving *NCOA2* and

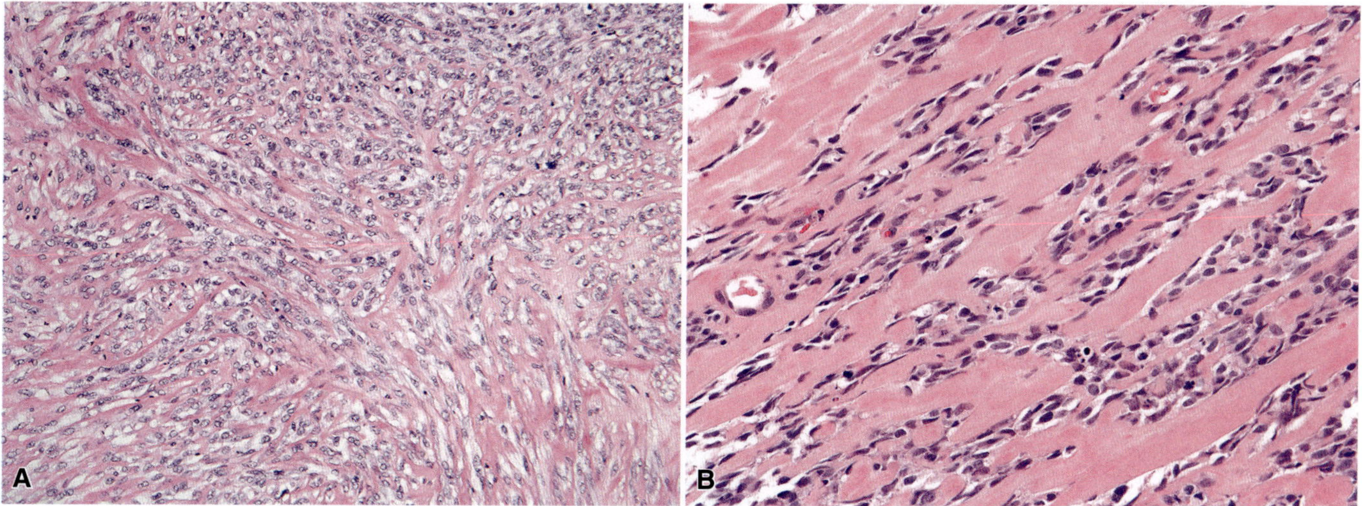

Figure 3.95 Spindle Cell/Sclerosing Rhabdomyosarcoma. (A) Some tumors contain sclerosing areas with abundant hyalinized collagenous stroma. (B) The tumor cells are arranged in nests and small alveolar structures with a pseudovascular appearance. Note the dense sclerotic stroma.

VGLL2.[492,493] Tumors in older children and adults share the abovementioned *MYOD1* and *PIK3CA* mutations.[488]

Differential Diagnosis

The main entities to be considered in the differential diagnosis of spindle cell rhabdomyosarcoma, particularly in the head and neck region, are spindle cell carcinoma, desmoplastic or spindle cell malignant melanoma, leiomyosarcoma, MPNST with heterologous rhabdomyoblastic differentiation, and monophasic synovial sarcoma. Immunohistochemistry is very helpful to exclude most of these diagnostic considerations.

Spindle cell (sarcomatoid) squamous cell carcinoma and spindle cell melanoma are much more common malignant neoplasms affecting the head and neck region of adults. Evidence of conventional squamous cell carcinoma, or an adjacent in situ component, is a helpful diagnostic clue; the diagnosis of carcinoma can be confirmed by the expression of keratins (particularly MNF116 and high-molecular-weight keratins such as CK5) and p63. Spindle cell or desmoplastic melanoma is usually diffusely positive for S-100 protein and SOX10, although second-line melanocytic markers are usually negative.

Spindle cell rhabdomyosarcoma may easily be mistaken for leiomyosarcoma. Both tumor types are composed of long fascicles of spindle cells, although the lesional cells in leiomyosarcoma contain broader, blunt-ended nuclei and abundant eosinophilic cytoplasm. Similar to spindle cell rhabdomyosarcoma, leiomyosarcoma is often diffusely positive for desmin, but SMA and h-caldesmon expression favors leiomyosarcoma, and nuclear staining for myogenin and MYOD1 is specific for rhabdomyosarcoma. MPNST showing heterologous rhabdomyoblastic differentiation may closely resemble spindle cell rhabdomyosarcoma. The clinical context can be very helpful; a history of NF1 or an association with a large nerve suggests MPNST. Most commonly, heterologous differentiation (along with desmin and myogenin expression) is seen only focally within the tumor, and areas of typical MPNST with varying cellularity, focally myxoid stroma, and perivascular accentuation predominate. Monophasic synovial sarcoma is also composed of highly cellular fascicles of spindle cells but shows more monotonous cytomorphology with overlapping nuclei and scant cytoplasm. Expression of TLE1, EMA, and focal keratins supports synovial sarcoma, which is consistently negative for desmin and myogenin.

Prognosis and Treatment

Although spindle cell rhabdomyosarcoma has a favorable prognosis in children, with a 5-year survival of greater than 95%,[486] the prognosis is poor in adults. This is likely due in part to the inability of adults to tolerate high-dose chemotherapy regimens comparable to pediatric protocols and to the difficulty in achieving complete surgical excision in certain anatomic locations.[482,484] However, the prognosis is better than other types of rhabdomyosarcoma, such as the pleomorphic variant, in adults.[484] Surgery is the initial treatment, followed by radiation therapy to prevent local recurrence. Chemotherapy is often of limited benefit, although some patients experience disease palliation.

Clear Cell Sarcoma

CCS is a malignant soft tissue tumor with melanocytic differentiation. First described as *CCS of tendons and aponeuroses*,[494] it had subsequently been widely also referred to as *malignant melanoma of soft parts*.[495,496] Although this designation is convenient to describe the melanocytic nature of CCS,[497,498] it may lead to diagnostic confusion; there are sufficient biologic and clinicopathologic differences to justify a distinct designation. CCS may rarely arise in the gastrointestinal tract, and a distinctive, somewhat similar neuroectodermal tumor lacking melanocytic differentiation also arises at this anatomic site (see Chapter 16).[499,500] Of note, CCS of the kidney is an unrelated pediatric tumor, but CCS of soft tissue type has also been described in this organ.[501]

Clinical Features

CCS mainly affects young adults and adolescents. The peak incidence is between 10 and 40 years, although the age range is wide. CCS usually presents as a slowly growing tender nodule in the distal extremities, with a median size of 2 to 5 cm, most often located around the ankle or foot, followed by the knee, wrist, and hands.[502,503] It is not rare for patients to have painless tumors for years before they seek medical attention. CCS is usually a deep-seated lesion, associated with tendons, tendon sheaths, or aponeuroses, with only occasional involvement of the subcutaneous tissue or dermis.

Pathologic Features

Grossly, CCS shows infiltrative margins, merging with adjacent fibrous tissue of tendons or aponeuroses. Histologically, the tumor is composed

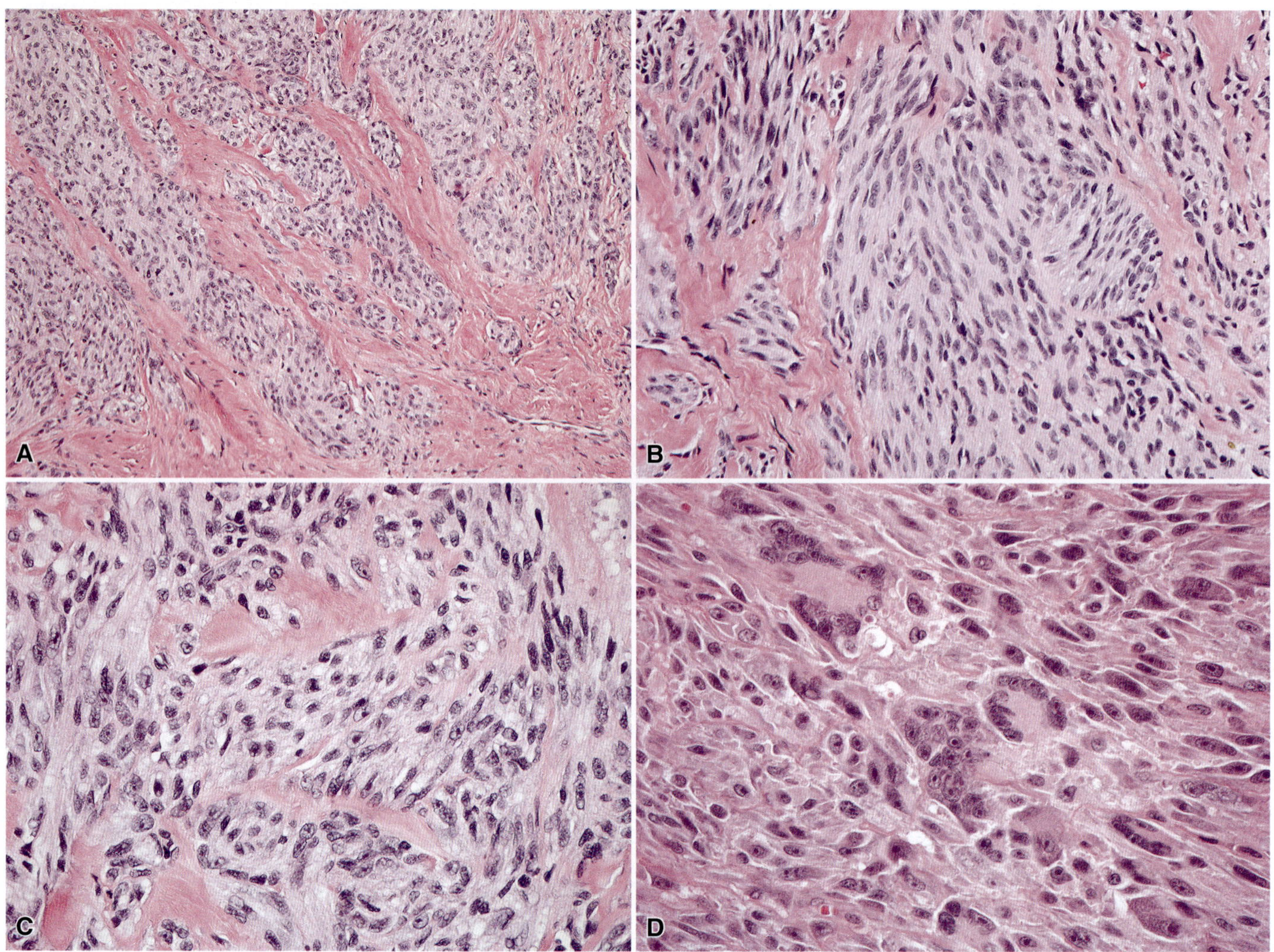

Figure 3.96 **Clear Cell Sarcoma.** (A) The tumor is composed of nests and short fascicles of uniform spindle cells separated by dense fibrous stroma. (B) The tumor cells contain abundant palely eosinophilic cytoplasm. (C) The nuclei are vesicular with large central nucleoli. (D) Wreathlike multinucleated giant cells are a typical feature.

of nests, bundles, and short fascicles of uniform spindled-to-epithelioid cells separated by prominent dense fibrous septa (Fig. 3.96).[494,504] The tumor cells contain abundant cytoplasm that may be clear but is more often palely eosinophilic (see Fig. 3.96B). The nuclei are vesicular, usually with a large central single nucleolus (see Fig. 3.96C). Scattered multinucleated giant cells with peripherally distributed nuclei in a wreath-like pattern are observed in more than half of cases (see Fig. 3.96D). Finely granular melanin pigment can be identified after careful examination in approximately two-thirds of cases of CCS.[495,504] The mitotic rate is usually low, and pleomorphism is absent.

Immunohistochemistry

The tumor cells in CCS express melanocytic markers, including S-100 protein, SOX10, HMB-45, melan A, and microphthalmia transcription factor (MITF).[504-506] In contrast to most cutaneous melanomas, staining for HMB-45 is usually stronger and more diffuse than S-100 protein (Fig. 3.97). Tumor cells may be focally positive for neuron-specific enolase, synaptophysin, and other neuroectodermal markers and are typically negative for EMA, keratins, and desmin.

Molecular Genetics

CCS is characterized by a reciprocal translocation t(12;22)(q13;q12) that results in the *EWSR1-ATF1* fusion oncogene (see Chapter 18).[507-509] *EWSR1-ATF1* functions as a transcriptional regulator that constitutively activates the expression of ATF1 target genes.[510,511] One of these genes is *MITF*, which is overexpressed in CCS cells and is likely responsible, at least in part, for the resulting melanoma-like gene expression profile observed in CCS.[498,512,513] Overexpression of *MITF* is detected at the transcript level[506]; the nuances of the interaction between the melanocytic program in CCS cells and the translocation-related fusion oncoprotein are not understood.

The translocation t(12;22)(q13;q12) and the resulting *EWSR1-ATF1* fusion are also detected in other tumor types, namely, AFH (see "Angiomatoid Fibrous Histiocytoma") and hyalinizing clear cell carcinoma of the salivary gland. Interestingly, the alternative fusion *EWSR1-CREB1* observed in AFH is also found in the CCS-like tumor of the gastrointestinal tract (also known as gastrointestinal neuroectodermal tumor), as well as in a small subset of conventional CCS of somatic soft tissue.[375,504,514] FISH for *EWSR1* or RT-PCR can be used clinically to aid in differential diagnosis with careful attention to the clinical presentation and morphologic features.[506,515]

Differential Diagnosis

Metastatic melanoma can be extremely difficult to distinguish from CCS because the immunophenotypic features are indistinguishable. The clinical context (i.e., a deep-seated infiltrative mass in the distal extremities),

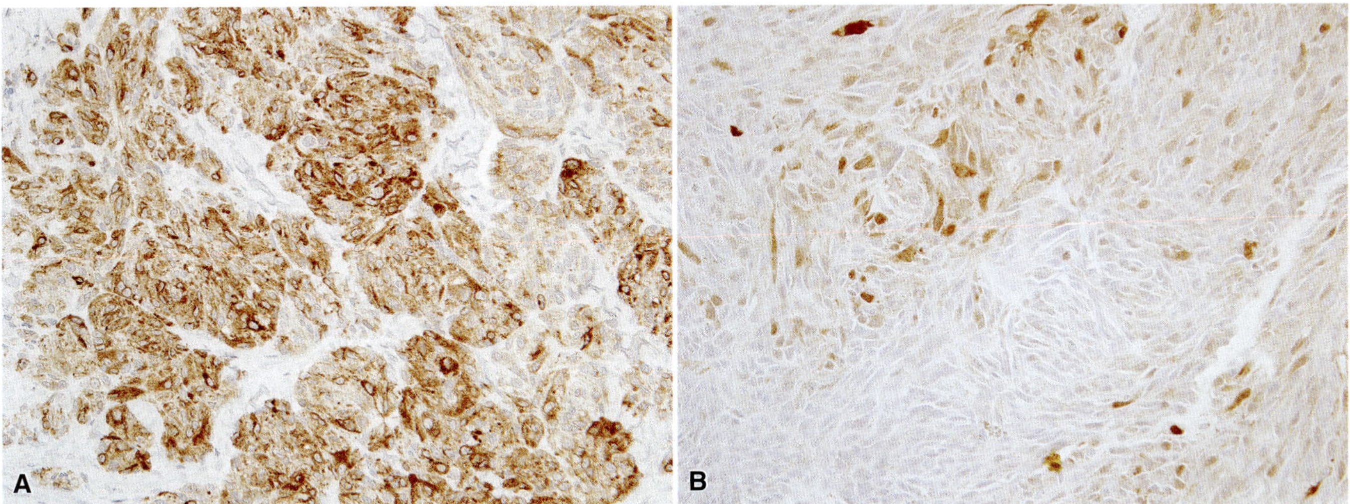

Figure 3.97 Clear Cell Sarcoma. (A) HMB-45 is usually diffusely positive. (B) Expression of S-100 protein is often more limited than other melanocytic markers.

the absence of junctional activity, and the uniform cytomorphology are helpful clues to the diagnosis of CCS, but in some cases detection of the translocation or its gene product is needed.[497,515,516] Distinguishing between CCS and other hypothetical differential diagnostic considerations, such as monophasic synovial sarcoma, MPNST, and leiomyosarcoma, should be relatively straightforward on morphologic and immunohistochemical grounds. Synovial sarcoma lacks the nested architecture, abundant cytoplasm, prominent nucleoli, and melanocytic differentiation of CCS; expression of TLE1, EMA, and keratins supports synovial sarcoma. In contrast to CCS, MPNST is composed of long fascicles of spindle cells with slender, tapering, or wavy nuclei and indistinct cytoplasm; varying cellularity and areas of myxoid stroma are other typical features. Although both tumor types often express S-100 protein, MPNST is negative for HMB-45 and melan A. Leiomyosarcoma shows a fascicular architecture and uniform cellularity without the prominent stroma surrounding individual nests and fascicles typical of CCS, and the tumor cells contain broader nuclei, more brightly eosinophilic cytoplasm, and well-defined cell borders. Expression of SMA, desmin, and h-caldesmon distinguishes leiomyosarcoma from CCS.

PRACTICE POINTS: Clear Cell Sarcoma

- Primary soft tissue sarcoma with melanocytic differentiation
- Most common in deep soft tissues of distal extremities of adolescents and young adults
- Composed of nests and short fascicles of uniform spindled-to-epithelioid cells with pale, eosinophilic cytoplasm and prominent nucleoli, separated by dense fibrous septa
- Occasional multinucleated wreath-like tumor giant cells are typical
- Expression of HMB-45 is usually stronger and more diffuse than S-100 protein
- t(12;22) translocation with *EWSR1-ATF1* fusion is typical
- Prognosis is poor; protracted clinical course with metastases to lymph nodes, lungs, and bone

Prognosis and Treatment

CCS usually follows a protracted clinical course, with frequent local recurrences and late metastases. The long-term prognosis of CCS is poor. Early diagnosis and initial wide excision are essential for local control and a more favorable outcome. Conventional chemotherapy has limited efficacy, as documented by response rates of less than 5% and median progression-free survival of 11 weeks in a retrospective study.[517] Inhibitors of MET and its ligand hepatocyte growth factor (HGF) have shown promising activity in preclinical studies.[513]

CCS metastasizes to regional lymph nodes, lungs, and bone. Five-year survival rates tend to overestimate survival because metastases often develop later. In a large series with long-term follow-up, the survival rates at 5, 10, and 20 years were 67%, 33%, and 10%, respectively.[502] Extended follow-up is therefore mandatory. Unfavorable prognostic factors include large tumor size (>5 cm), the presence of necrosis, early local recurrence, and positive resection margins.[496,503]

Pseudomyogenic Hemangioendothelioma

Pseudomyogenic hemangioendothelioma is a distinctive endothelial neoplasm of intermediate biologic potential, occurring as multiple discrete lesions in different tissue planes of a limb.[518] Originally described as the *fibroma-like variant of epithelioid sarcoma*[519] and later referred to as *epithelioid sarcoma-like hemangioendothelioma*,[520] pseudomyogenic hemangioendothelioma is a vascular neoplasm that histologically closely resembles a myoid tumor. Most patients (75%) present with cutaneous nodules. Pseudomyogenic hemangioendothelioma is also discussed in Chapter 15.

Clinical Features

Pseudomyogenic hemangioendothelioma typically affects young adults; more than 90% of patients are diagnosed between the second and fifth decades of life. There is a striking male predominance (male-to-female ratio, 5:1). The tumors are usually located in the limbs, most commonly in the lower extremities, and occur as a single or multiple nodules, either painless or painful, often affecting multiple tissue planes in the same anatomic region. Patients most often present with superficial nodules involving the skin and subcutaneous tissue. However, on further work-up, intramuscular tumors are detected in approximately 50% of patients, and 20% of patients have multiple lytic bony lesions.[518] Approximately two-thirds of patients have multiple lesions at presentation. Positron emission tomography scan often helps identify deep-seated lesions.

Pathologic Features

Most tumor nodules are 1 to 2 cm in size and are grossly well circumscribed with a tan or white, fibrous to fleshy cut surface. Histologically, pseudomyogenic hemangioendothelioma typically shows irregular, infiltrative margins (Fig. 3.98), sometimes with an almost plexiform appearance. The tumor is composed of loose fascicles and sheets of

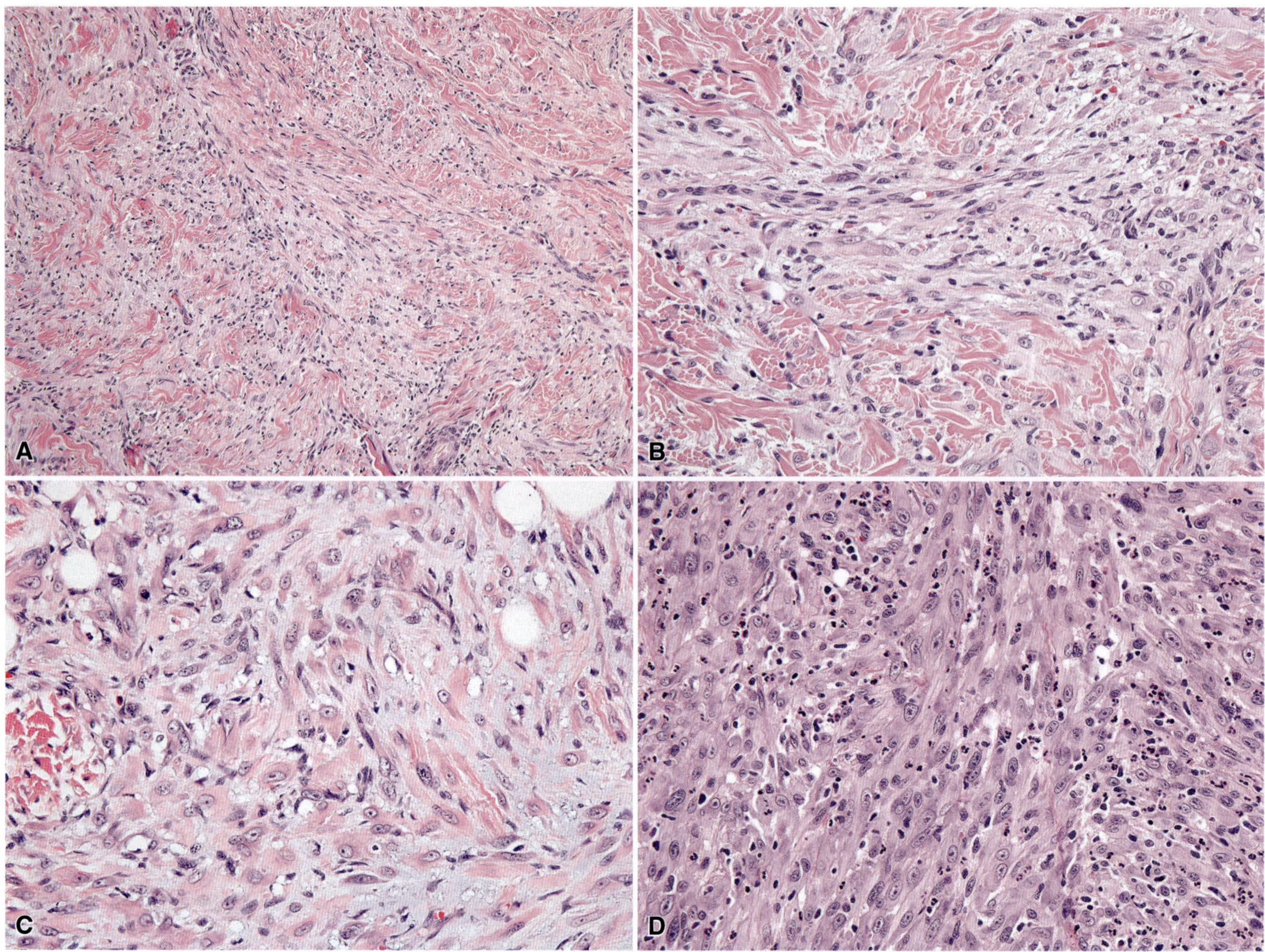

Figure 3.98 Pseudomyogenic Hemangioendothelioma. (A) The tumor typically shows irregular, infiltrative margins. (B) The tumor is composed of loose fascicles and sheets of plump spindle cells with abundant eosinophilic cytoplasm. Note the mild nuclear atypia. (C) Some tumor cells resemble rhabdomyoblasts. Note the scattered cells with a more epithelioid appearance. (D) A prominent neutrophilic inflammatory infiltrate is seen in approximately 50% of cases.

plump spindle cells with vesicular nuclei, variably prominent nucleoli, and abundant eosinophilic cytoplasm (see Fig. 3.98B). In some cases, cells with a strikingly rhabdomyoblast-like appearance are prominent (see Fig. 3.98C). Approximately 50% of tumors contain a prominent neutrophilic inflammatory infiltrate (see Fig. 3.98D). A minority of the tumor cells shows more polygonal or epithelioid cytomorphology. The degree of nuclear atypia is usually mild but may occasionally be moderate or severe. Likewise, cellular pleomorphism is uncommon. Mitotic activity and vascular invasion may be observed with no apparent clinical significance. Some tumors show foci of necrosis.

Immunohistochemistry

The tumor cells are usually diffusely positive for keratin AE1/AE3 and show strong nuclear staining for FLI1 and ERG (Fig. 3.99), supporting endothelial differentiation. However, only 50% of tumors are positive for CD31, and they are consistently negative for CD34. Expression of FOSB, resulting from the gene fusion characteristic of this tumor type, can be detected by immunohistochemistry to further confirm the diagnosis (Fig. 3.100).[521] Tumors are usually negative for EMA and keratin MNF116. Despite the myoid appearance of the tumor cells, they are negative for desmin, although they may be focally positive for smooth muscle actin. They are negative for S-100 protein. Nuclear expression of INI1 is retained in the tumor cells.[518]

Molecular Genetics

Pseudomyogenic hemangioendothelioma is characterized by a balanced t(7;19)(q22;q13) translocation that creates a *SERPINE1-FOSB* fusion gene.[522,523]

Differential Diagnosis

The differential diagnosis of deep-seated pseudomyogenic hemangioendothelioma includes conventional epithelioid sarcoma, epithelioid hemangioendothelioma and epithelioid angiosarcoma, myogenic tumors, and nodular or proliferative fasciitis. Conventional epithelioid sarcoma enters the differential diagnosis due primarily to clinical and immunophenotypic overlap, although the morphology is quite different: epithelioid sarcoma lacks the plump, myoid-appearing spindle cell morphology (instead being dominated by small epithelioid cells), as well as the fascicular and sheetlike growth pattern of pseudomyogenic hemangioendothelioma. The immunophenotypic overlap is limited to the expression of broad-spectrum keratins because epithelioid sarcoma is also positive for EMA and often for CD34,[524] and it almost always shows loss of INI1

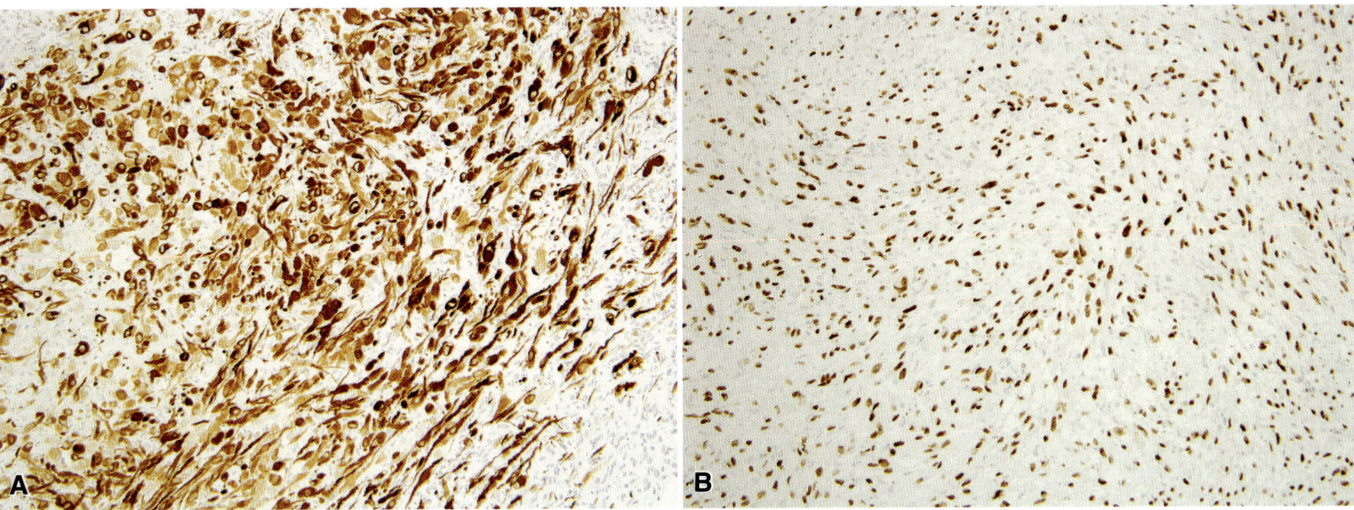

Figure 3.99 Pseudomyogenic Hemangioendothelioma. (A) The tumor cells express keratin AE1/AE3, usually in a strong and diffuse fashion. (B) Nuclear staining for ERG (and FLI1) is consistently observed.

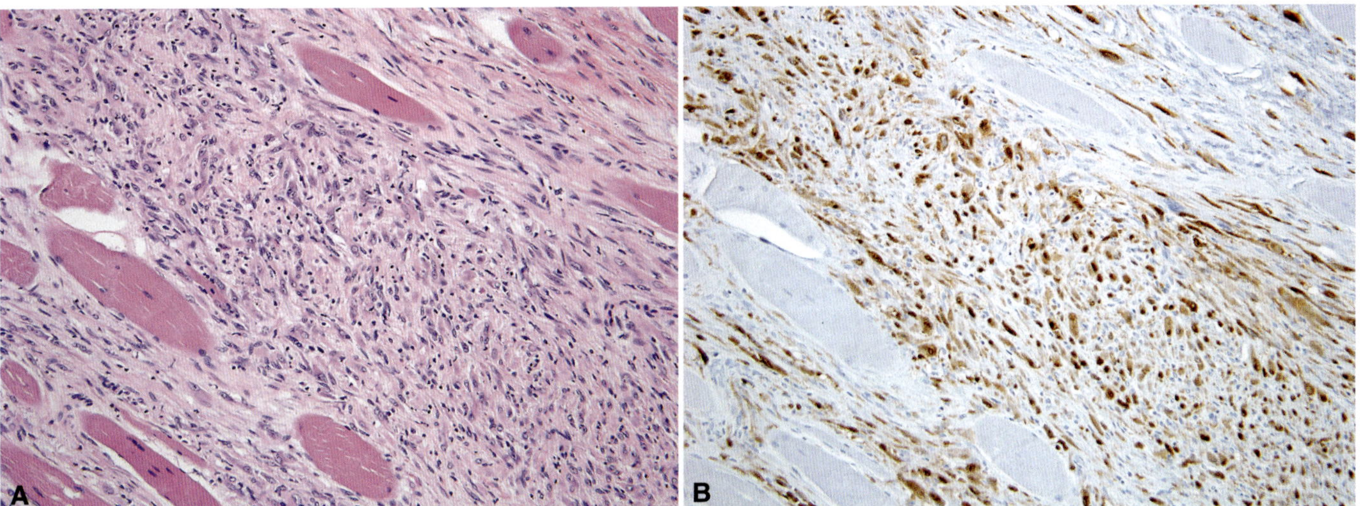

Figure 3.100 Pseudomyogenic Hemangioendothelioma. (A) Plump spindle cells with abundant eosinophilic cytoplasm infiltrate between skeletal muscle fibers. (B) Nuclear staining for FOSB is a characteristic finding, reflecting the underlying *SERPINE1-FOSB* gene fusion.

expression.[525,526] Pseudomyogenic hemangioendothelioma is instead positive for FOSB and ERG and, in 50% of cases CD31, but lacks EMA and CD34 expression and retains INI1.[518] Pseudomyogenic hemangioendothelioma shows some overlapping immunophenotypic features with epithelioid endothelial tumors, although CD34 expression is limited to epithelioid hemangioendothelioma and angiosarcoma, which in turn only occasionally express keratin in such a strong and diffuse fashion. The morphology is completely different: the solid sheets and fascicles of spindle cells in pseudomyogenic hemangioendothelioma contrast with the cords of epithelioid cells with occasional intracytoplasmic vacuoles within a myxohyaline stroma, typical of epithelioid hemangioendothelioma. CAMTA1 expression is specific for epithelioid hemangioendothelioma is this differential diagnosis, whereas FOSB favors pseudomyogenic hemangioendothelioma. Epithelioid angiosarcoma also grows in solid sheets but is often associated with stromal hemorrhage and at least focal evidence of vasoformative architecture. Furthermore, epithelioid angiosarcoma typically consists of larger epithelioid cells with amphophilic cytoplasm and is usually of high nuclear grade, as opposed to the mild atypia and cytoplasmic eosinophilia seen in most examples of pseudomyogenic hemangioendothelioma. Although pseudomyogenic hemangioendothelioma may mimic a myoid tumor histologically (especially a skeletal muscle neoplasm), it lacks expression of desmin and myogenin. The myofibroblastic cells in nodular and proliferative fasciitis generally lack the intense cytoplasmic eosinophilia of pseudomyogenic hemangioendothelioma and show less nuclear atypia. In addition, diffuse keratin expression and reactivity for ERG and CD31 are not seen in nodular or proliferative fasciitis. Of note, a small subset of nodular and proliferative fasciitis cases is also positive for FOSB.[521]

Prognosis and Treatment

Almost 60% of patients develop local recurrences (sometimes multiple) or develop additional tumor nodules in the same general anatomic region, usually within the first few years of follow-up, regardless of the status of the initial resection margins. It appears that conservative surgical treatment is the best therapeutic option, although the multifocality of the disease may raise clinical concerns and prompt aggressive surgical approaches. However, the disease course is usually indolent, with only exceptional distant metastases, which may occur many years after initial presentation.[518]

PRACTICE POINTS: Pseudomyogenic Hemangioendothelioma

- Predominantly affects young adult men
- Often presents as multiple discrete lesions in different tissue planes of a limb (skin, muscle, and bone)
- Positron emission tomography scan helpful to identify clinically inapparent nodules in deep soft tissue
- Composed of loose fascicles and sheets of plump spindle cells with abundant brightly eosinophilic cytoplasm, vesicular nuclei, and usually only mild nuclear atypia
- Tumor cells may mimic rhabdomyoblasts
- Fifty percent of tumors associated with prominent stromal neutrophils
- Tumor cells are diffusely positive for AE1/AE3, FLI1, ERG, and FOSB; 50% express CD31

Unclassified Spindle Cell Sarcomas

Approximately 5% to 10% of spindle cell sarcomas remain unclassifiable even after the application of strict morphologic criteria and ancillary (immunohistochemical and molecular) techniques. This likely heterogeneous group of tumors includes both histologically high-grade and low-grade sarcomas, which may arise in deep or superficial soft tissues. Some such tumors likely represent examples of MPNST, the diagnosis of which is notoriously difficult to confirm in patients without a history of NF1 (because conventional immunohistochemical markers have relatively low sensitivity). Of note, many postradiation sarcomas of deep soft tissue belong to the "unclassified" category (Fig. 3.101). Radiation-associated soft tissue sarcomas pursue a more aggressive clinical course than their sporadic counterparts, independent of histologic type.[527] In addition, the expression of myogenic markers by tumor cells in spindle cell and pleomorphic sarcomas seems to confer a worse prognosis, even in the absence of other features allowing for classification into a specific diagnostic category.[528,529] Finally, use of the term *fibrosarcoma* as a default diagnosis for spindle cell sarcomas that do not fit into other well-defined categories should be discouraged; such a designation seems to imply a cohesive diagnostic group, whereas in actuality unclassified spindle cell sarcomas are both histologically and clinically heterogeneous.

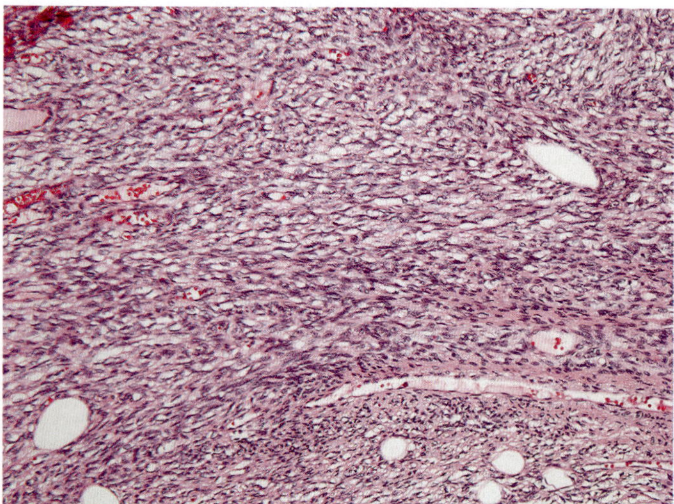

Figure 3.101 Unclassified Spindle Cell Sarcoma. This spindle cell sarcoma arose following radiation therapy. Many postradiation sarcomas cannot be subclassified.

References

1. Guarino M, Tricomi P, Giordano F, et al: Sarcomatoid carcinomas: pathological and histopathogenetic considerations, *Pathology* 28:298–305, 1996.
2. Wick MR, Swanson PE: Carcinosarcomas: current perspectives and an historical review of nosological concepts, *Semin Diagn Pathol* 10:118–127, 1993.
3. Lodding P, Kindblom LG, Angervall L: Metastases of malignant melanoma simulating soft tissue sarcoma. A clinico-pathological, light- and electron microscopic and immunohistochemical study of 21 cases, *Virchows Arch A Pathol Anat Histopathol* 417:377–388, 1990.
4. Wharton JM, Carlson JA, Mihm MC, Jr: Desmoplastic malignant melanoma: diagnosis of early clinical lesions, *Hum Pathol* 30:537–542, 1999.
5. Blessing K, Sanders DS, Grant JJ: Comparison of immunohistochemical staining of the novel antibody melan-A with S-100 protein and HMB-45 in malignant melanoma and melanoma variants, *Histopathology* 32:139–146, 1998.
6. Magro CM, Crowson AN, Mihm MC: Unusual variants of malignant melanoma, *Mod Pathol* 19(Suppl 2):S41–S70, 2006.
7. Banerjee SS, Harris M: Morphological and immunophenotypic variations in malignant melanoma, *Histopathology* 36:387–402, 2000.
8. Travis WD: Sarcomatoid neoplasms of the lung and pleura, *Arch Pathol Lab Med* 134:1645–1658, 2010.
9. Attanoos RL, Dojcinov SD, Webb R, et al: Anti-mesothelial markers in sarcomatoid mesothelioma and other spindle cell neoplasms, *Histopathology* 37:224–231, 2000.
10. Wirman JA: Nodular fasciitis, a lesion of myofibroblasts: an ultrastructural study, *Cancer* 38:2378–2389, 1976.
11. Montgomery EA, Meis JM: Nodular fasciitis. Its morphologic spectrum and immunohistochemical profile, *Am J Surg Pathol* 15:942–948, 1991.
12. Bernstein KE, Lattes R: Nodular (pseudosarcomatous) fasciitis, a nonrecurrent lesion: clinicopathologic study of 134 cases, *Cancer* 49:1668–1678, 1982.
13. Shimizu S, Hashimoto H, Enjoji M: Nodular fasciitis: an analysis of 250 patients, *Pathology* 16:161–166, 1984.
14. Patchefsky AS, Enzinger FM: Intravascular fasciitis: a report of 17 cases, *Am J Surg Pathol* 5:29–36, 1981.
15. Meis JM, Enzinger FM: Proliferative fasciitis and myositis of childhood, *Am J Surg Pathol* 16:364–372, 1992.
16. Chung EB, Enzinger FM: Proliferative fasciitis, *Cancer* 36:1450–1458, 1975.
17. Perosio PM, Weiss SW: Ischemic fasciitis: a juxta-skeletal fibroblastic proliferation with a predilection for elderly patients, *Mod Pathol* 6:69–72, 1993.
18. Liegl B, Fletcher CD: Ischemic fasciitis: analysis of 44 cases indicating an inconsistent association with immobility or debilitation, *Am J Surg Pathol* 32:1546–1552, 2008.
19. Sawyer JR, Sammartino G, Baker GF, et al: Clonal chromosome aberrations in a case of nodular fasciitis, *Cancer Genet Cytogenet* 76:154–156, 1994.
20. Birdsall SH, Shipley JM, Summersgill BM, et al: Cytogenetic findings in a case of nodular fasciitis of the breast, *Cancer Genet Cytogenet* 81:166–168, 1995.
21. Velagaleti GV, Tapper JK, Panova NE, et al: Cytogenetic findings in a case of nodular fasciitis of subclavicular region, *Cancer Genet Cytogenet* 141:160–163, 2003.
22. Erickson-Johnson MR, Chou MM, Evers BR, et al: Nodular fasciitis: a novel model of transient neoplasia induced by MYH9-USP6 gene fusion, *Lab Invest* 91:1427–1433, 2011.
23. Guo R, Wang X, Chou MM, et al: PPP6R3-USP6 amplification: novel oncogenic mechanism in malignant nodular fasciitis, *Genes Chromosomes Cancer* 55:640–649, 2016.
24. Albores-Saavedra J, Manivel JC, Essenfeld H, et al: Pseudosarcomatous myofibroblastic proliferations in the urinary bladder of children, *Cancer* 66:1234–1241, 1990.
25. Harik LR, Merino C, Coindre JM, et al: Pseudosarcomatous myofibroblastic proliferations of the bladder: a clinicopathologic study of 42 cases, *Am J Surg Pathol* 30:787–794, 2006.
26. Jones EC, Clement PB, Young RH: Inflammatory pseudotumor of the urinary bladder. A clinicopathological, immunohistochemical, ultrastructural, and flow cytometric study of 13 cases, *Am J Surg Pathol* 17:264–274, 1993.
27. Lundgren L, Aldenborg F, Angervall L, et al: Pseudomalignant spindle cell proliferations of the urinary bladder, *Hum Pathol* 25:181–191, 1994.
28. Proppe KH, Scully RE, Rosai J: Postoperative spindle cell nodules of genitourinary tract resembling sarcomas. A report of eight cases, *Am J Surg Pathol* 8:101–108, 1984.
29. Ro JY, el Naggar AK, Amin MB, et al: Pseudosarcomatous fibromyxoid tumor of the urinary bladder and prostate: immunohistochemical, ultrastructural, and DNA flow cytometric analyses of nine cases, *Hum Pathol* 24:1203–1210, 1993.
30. Hirsch MS, Dal Cin P, Fletcher CD: ALK expression in pseudosarcomatous myofibroblastic proliferations of the genitourinary tract, *Histopathology* 48:569–578, 2006.
31. Gleason BC, Hornick JL: Inflammatory myofibroblastic tumours: where are we now? *J Clin Pathol* 61:428–437, 2008.
32. Tsuzuki T, Magi-Galluzzi C, Epstein JI: ALK-1 expression in inflammatory myofibroblastic tumor of the urinary bladder, *Am J Surg Pathol* 28:1609–1614, 2004.
33. Wood C, Nickoloff BJ, Todes-Taylor NR: Pseudotumor resulting from atypical mycobacterial infection: a "histoid" variety of *Mycobacterium avium-intracellulare* complex infection, *Am J Clin Pathol* 83:524–527, 1985.
34. Logani S, Lucas DR, Cheng JD, et al: Spindle cell tumors associated with mycobacteria in lymph nodes of HIV-positive patients: 'Kaposi sarcoma with mycobacteria' and 'mycobacterial pseudotumor, *Am J Surg Pathol* 23:656–661, 1999.

35. Umlas J, Federman M, Crawford C, et al: Spindle cell pseudotumor due to *Mycobacterium avium-intracellulare* in patients with acquired immunodeficiency syndrome (AIDS). Positive staining of mycobacteria for cytoskeleton filaments, *Am J Surg Pathol* 15:1181–1187, 1991.
36. Yin HL, Zhou XJ, Wu JP, et al: Mycobacterial spindle cell pseudotumor of lymph nodes after receiving Bacille Calmette-Guerin (BCG) vaccination, *Chin Med J* 117:308–310, 2004.
37. Wade HW: The histoid variety of lepromatous leprosy, *Int J Lepr* 31:129–142, 1963.
38. Chung EB, Enzinger FM: Infantile myofibromatosis, *Cancer* 48:1807–1818, 1981.
39. Daimaru Y, Hashimoto H, Enjoji M: Myofibromatosis in adults (adult counterpart of infantile myofibromatosis), *Am J Surg Pathol* 13:859–865, 1989.
40. Smith KJ, Skelton HG, Barrett TL, et al: Cutaneous myofibroma, *Mod Pathol* 2:603–609, 1989.
41. Beham A, Badve S, Suster S, et al: Solitary myofibroma in adults: clinicopathological analysis of a series, *Histopathology* 22:335–341, 1993.
42. Granter SR, Badizadegan K, Fletcher CD: Myofibromatosis in adults, glomangiopericytoma, and myopericytoma: a spectrum of tumors showing perivascular myoid differentiation, *Am J Surg Pathol* 22:513–525, 1998.
43. Ide F, Mishima K, Yamada H, et al: Perivascular myoid tumors of the oral region: a clinicopathologic re-evaluation of 35 cases, *J Oral Pathol Med* 37:43–49, 2008.
44. Linos K, Carter JM, Gardner JM, et al: Myofibromas with atypical features: expanding the morphologic spectrum of a benign entity, *Am J Surg Pathol* 38:1649–1654, 2014.
45. Mentzel T, Dei Tos AP, Sapi Z, et al: Myopericytoma of skin and soft tissues: clinicopathologic and immunohistochemical study of 54 cases, *Am J Surg Pathol* 30:104–113, 2006.
46. McMenamin ME, Fletcher CD: Malignant myopericytoma: expanding the spectrum of tumours with myopericytic differentiation, *Histopathology* 41:450–460, 2002.
47. Martignetti JA, Tian L, Li D, et al: Mutations in PDGFRB cause autosomal-dominant infantile myofibromatosis, *Am J Hum Genet* 92:1001–1007, 2013.
48. Cheung YH, Gayden T, Campeau PM, et al: A recurrent PDGFRB mutation causes familial infantile myofibromatosis, *Am J Hum Genet* 92:996–1000, 2013.
49. Agaimy A, Bieg M, Michal M, et al: Recurrent somatic PDGFRB mutations in sporadic infantile/solitary adult myofibromas but not in angioleiomyomas and myopericytomas, *Am J Surg Pathol* 41:195–203, 2017.
50. Haller F, Knopf J, Ackermann A, et al: Paediatric and adult soft tissue sarcomas with NTRK1 gene fusions: a subset of spindle cell sarcomas unified by a prominent myopericytic/haemangiopericytic pattern, *J Pathol* 238:700–710, 2016.
51. Arts FA, Chand D, Pecquet C, et al: PDGFRB mutants found in patients with familial infantile myofibromatosis or overgrowth syndrome are oncogenic and sensitive to imatinib, *Oncogene* 35:3239–3248, 2016.
52. Salassa RM, Jowsey J, Arnaud CD: Hypophosphatemic osteomalacia associated with "nonendocrine" tumors, *N Engl J Med* 283:65–70, 1970.
53. Weidner N, Santa Cruz D: Phosphaturic mesenchymal tumors. A polymorphous group causing osteomalacia or rickets, *Cancer* 59:1442–1454, 1987.
54. Folpe AL, Fanburg-Smith JC, Billings SD, et al: Most osteomalacia-associated mesenchymal tumors are a single histopathologic entity: an analysis of 32 cases and a comprehensive review of the literature, *Am J Surg Pathol* 28:1–30, 2004.
55. Lee JC, Jeng YM, Su SY, et al: Identification of a novel FN1-FGFR1 genetic fusion as a frequent event in phosphaturic mesenchymal tumour, *J Pathol* 235:539–545, 2015.
56. Lee JC, Su SY, Changou CA, et al: Characterization of FN1-FGFR1 and novel FN1-FGF1 fusion genes in a large series of phosphaturic mesenchymal tumors, *Mod Pathol* 29:1335–1346, 2016.
57. Bahrami A, Weiss SW, Montgomery E, et al: RT-PCR analysis for FGF23 using paraffin sections in the diagnosis of phosphaturic mesenchymal tumors with and without known tumor induced osteomalacia, *Am J Surg Pathol* 33:1348–1354, 2009.
58. Wargotz ES, Weiss SW, Norris HJ: Myofibroblastoma of the breast. Sixteen cases of a distinctive benign mesenchymal tumor, *Am J Surg Pathol* 11:493–502, 1987.
59. McMenamin ME, Fletcher CD: Mammary-type myofibroblastoma of soft tissue: a tumor closely related to spindle cell lipoma, *Am J Surg Pathol* 25:1022–1029, 2001.
60. Howitt BE, Fletcher CD: Mammary-type myofibroblastoma: clinicopathologic characterization in a series of 143 cases, *Am J Surg Pathol* 40:361–367, 2016.
61. Chen BJ, Marino-Enriquez A, Fletcher CD, et al: Loss of retinoblastoma protein expression in spindle cell/pleomorphic lipomas and cytogenetically related tumors: an immunohistochemical study with diagnostic implications, *Am J Surg Pathol* 36:1119–1128, 2012.
62. Pauwels P, Sciot R, Croiset F, et al: Myofibroblastoma of the breast: genetic link with spindle cell lipoma, *J Pathol* 191:282–285, 2000.
63. Maggiani F, Debiec-Rychter M, Verbeeck G, et al: Extramammary myofibroblastoma is genetically related to spindle cell lipoma, *Virchows Arch* 449:244–247, 2006.
64. Weiss SW, Gnepp DR, Bratthauer GL: Palisaded myofibroblastoma. A benign mesenchymal tumor of lymph node, *Am J Surg Pathol* 13:341–346, 1989.
65. Fletcher CD, Stirling RW: Intranodal myofibroblastoma presenting in the submandibular region: evidence of a broader clinical and histological spectrum, *Histopathology* 16:287–293, 1990.
66. Skalova A, Michal M, Chlumska A, et al: Collagen composition and ultrastructure of the so-called amianthoid fibres in palisaded myofibroblastoma. Ultrastructural and immunohistochemical study, *J Pathol* 167:335–340, 1992.
67. Nguyen T, Eltorky MA: Intranodal palisaded myofibroblastoma, *Arch Pathol Lab Med* 131:306–310, 2007.
68. Creager AJ, Garwacki CP: Recurrent intranodal palisaded myofibroblastoma with metaplastic bone formation, *Arch Pathol Lab Med* 123:433–436, 1999.
69. Laskin WB, Lasota JP, Fetsch JF, et al: Intranodal palisaded myofibroblastoma: another mesenchymal neoplasm with CTNNB1 (beta-catenin gene) mutations: clinicopathologic, immunohistochemical, and molecular genetic study of 18 cases, *Am J Surg Pathol* 39:197–205, 2015.
70. Kleist B, Poetsch M, Schmoll J: Intranodal palisaded myofibroblastoma with overexpression of cyclin D1, *Arch Pathol Lab Med* 127:1040–1043, 2003.
71. Lioe TF, Allen DC, Bell JC: A case of multicentric intranodal palisaded myofibroblastoma, *Histopathology* 24:173–175, 1994.
72. Dal Cin P, Sciot R, De Smet L, et al: Translocation 2;11 in a fibroma of tendon sheath, *Histopathology* 32:433–435, 1998.
73. Sciot R, Samson I, van den Berghe H, et al: Collagenous fibroma (desmoplastic fibroblastoma): genetic link with fibroma of tendon sheath? *Mod Pathol* 12:565–568, 1999.
74. Evans HL: Desmoplastic fibroblastoma. A report of seven cases, *Am J Surg Pathol* 19:1077–1081, 1995.
75. Nielsen GP, O'Connell JX, Dickersin GR, et al: Collagenous fibroma (desmoplastic fibroblastoma): a report of seven cases, *Mod Pathol* 9:781–785, 1996.
76. Miettinen M, Fetsch JF: Collagenous fibroma (desmoplastic fibroblastoma): a clinicopathologic analysis of 63 cases of a distinctive soft tissue lesion with stellate-shaped fibroblasts, *Hum Pathol* 29:676–682, 1998.
77. Kato I, Yoshida A, Ikegami M, et al: FOSL1 immunohistochemistry clarifies the distinction between desmoplastic fibroblastoma and fibroma of tendon sheath, *Histopathology* 69:1012–1020, 2016.
78. Bernal K, Nelson M, Neff JR, et al: Translocation (2;11)(q31;q12) is recurrent in collagenous fibroma (desmoplastic fibroblastoma), *Cancer Genet Cytogenet* 149:161–163, 2004.
79. Macchia G, Trombetta D, Moller E, et al: FOSL1 as a candidate target gene for 11q12 rearrangements in desmoplastic fibroblastoma, *Lab Invest* 92:735–743, 2012.
80. Balachandran K, Allen PW, MacCormac LB: Nuchal fibroma. A clinicopathological study of nine cases, *Am J Surg Pathol* 19:313–317, 1995.
81. Michal M, Fetsch JF, Hes O, et al: Nuchal-type fibroma: a clinicopathologic study of 52 cases, *Cancer* 85:156–163, 1999.
82. Wehrli BM, Weiss SW, Yandow S, et al: Gardner-associated fibromas (GAF) in young patients: a distinct fibrous lesion that identifies unsuspected Gardner syndrome and risk for fibromatosis, *Am J Surg Pathol* 25:645–651, 2001.
83. Coffin CM, Hornick JL, Zhou H, et al: Gardner fibroma: a clinicopathologic and immunohistochemical analysis of 45 patients with 57 fibromas, *Am J Surg Pathol* 31:410–416, 2007.
84. Stemmermann GN, Stout AP: Elastofibroma dorsi, *Am J Clin Pathol* 37:499–506, 1962.
85. Harry RD, Kruger RL, McLaughlin CW: Elastofibroma dorsi. An unusual soft tissue tumor simulating sarcoma, *Am J Surg* 125:713–714, 1973.
86. Nagamine N, Nohara Y, Ito E: Elastofibroma in Okinawa. A clinicopathologic study of 170 cases, *Cancer* 50:1794–1805, 1982.
87. Rosenthal NS, Abdul-Karim FW: Childhood fibrous tumor with psammoma bodies. Clinicopathologic features in two cases, *Arch Pathol Lab Med* 112:798–800, 1988.
88. Fetsch JF, Montgomery EA, Meis JM: Calcifying fibrous pseudotumor, *Am J Surg Pathol* 17:502–508, 1993.
89. Pinkard NB, Wilson RW, Lawless N, et al: Calcifying fibrous pseudotumor of pleura. A report of three cases of a newly described entity involving the pleura, *Am J Clin Pathol* 105:189–194, 1996.
90. Nascimento AF, Ruiz R, Hornick JL, et al: Calcifying fibrous 'pseudotumor': clinicopathologic study of 15 cases and analysis of its relationship to inflammatory myofibroblastic tumor, *Int J Surg Pathol* 10:189–196, 2002.
91. Lee JC, Lien HC, Hsiao CH: Coexisting sclerosing angiomatoid nodular transformation of the spleen with multiple calcifying fibrous pseudotumors in a patient, *J Formos Med Assoc* 106:234–239, 2007.
92. Van Dorpe J, Ectors N, Geboes K, et al: Is calcifying fibrous pseudotumor a late sclerosing stage of inflammatory myofibroblastic tumor? *Am J Surg Pathol* 23:329–335, 1999.
93. Hill KA, Gonzalez-Crussi F, Chou PM: Calcifying fibrous pseudotumor versus inflammatory myofibroblastic tumor: a histological and immunohistochemical comparison, *Mod Pathol* 14:784–790, 2001.
94. Marino-Enriquez A, Fletcher CD: Angiofibroma of soft tissue: clinicopathologic characterization of a distinctive benign fibrovascular neoplasm in a series of 37 cases, *Am J Surg Pathol* 36:500–508, 2012.
95. Jin Y, Möller E, Nord KH, et al: Fusion of the AHRR and NCOA2 genes through a recurrent translocation t(5;8)(p15;q13) in soft tissue angiofibroma results in upregulation of aryl hydrocarbon receptor target genes, *Genes Chromosomes Cancer* 51:510–520, 2012.
96. Arbajian E, Magnusson L, Mertens F, et al: A novel GTF2I/NCOA2 fusion gene emphasizes the role of NCOA2 in soft tissue angiofibroma development, *Genes Chromosomes Cancer* 52:330–331, 2013.
97. Sugita S, Aoyama T, Kondo K, et al: Diagnostic utility of NCOA2 fluorescence in situ hybridization and Stat6 immunohistochemistry staining for soft tissue angiofibroma and morphologically similar fibrovascular tumors, *Hum Pathol* 45:1588–1596, 2014.
98. Fletcher CD: Benign fibrous histiocytoma of subcutaneous and deep soft tissue: a clinicopathologic analysis of 21 cases, *Am J Surg Pathol* 14:801–809, 1990.
99. Gleason BC, Fletcher CD: Deep "benign" fibrous histiocytoma: clinicopathologic analysis of 69 cases of a rare tumor indicating occasional metastatic potential, *Am J Surg Pathol* 32:354–362, 2008.

100. Walther C, Hofvander J, Nilsson J, et al: Gene fusion detection in formalin-fixed paraffin-embedded benign fibrous histiocytomas using fluorescence in situ hybridization and RNA sequencing, *Lab Invest* 95:1071–1076, 2015.
101. Stout AP, Murray MR: Hemangiopericytoma: a vascular tumor featuring Zimmermann's pericytes, *Ann Surg* 116:26–33, 1942.
102. Nappi O, Ritter JH, Pettinato G, et al: Hemangiopericytoma: histopathological pattern or clinicopathologic entity? *Semin Diagn Pathol* 12:221–232, 1995.
103. Gengler C, Guillou L: Solitary fibrous tumour and haemangiopericytoma: evolution of a concept, *Histopathology* 48:63–74, 2006.
104. Verbeke SL, Fletcher CD, Alberghini M, et al: A reappraisal of hemangiopericytoma of bone; analysis of cases reclassified as synovial sarcoma and solitary fibrous tumor of bone, *Am J Surg Pathol* 34:777–783, 2010.
105. Chan JK: Solitary fibrous tumour—everywhere, and a diagnosis in vogue, *Histopathology* 31:568–576, 1997.
106. Goodlad JR, Fletcher CD: Solitary fibrous tumour arising at unusual sites: analysis of a series, *Histopathology* 19:515–522, 1991.
107. Brunnemann RB, Ro JY, Ordonez NG, et al: Extrapleural solitary fibrous tumor: a clinicopathologic study of 24 cases, *Mod Pathol* 12:1034–1042, 1999.
108. Carneiro SS, Scheithauer BW, Nascimento AG, et al: Solitary fibrous tumor of the meninges: a lesion distinct from fibrous meningioma. A clinicopathologic and immunohistochemical study, *Am J Clin Pathol* 106:217–224, 1996.
109. England DM, Hochholzer L, McCarthy MJ: Localized benign and malignant fibrous tumors of the pleura. A clinicopathologic review of 223 cases, *Am J Surg Pathol* 13:640–658, 1989.
110. Strom EH, Skjorten F, Aarseth LB, et al: Solitary fibrous tumor of the pleura. An immunohistochemical, electron microscopic and tissue culture study of a tumor producing insulin-like growth factor I in a patient with hypoglycemia, *Pathol Res Pract* 187:109–113, discussion 114–116, 1991.
111. Fukasawa Y, Takada A, Tateno M, et al: Solitary fibrous tumor of the pleura causing recurrent hypoglycemia by secretion of insulin-like growth factor II, *Pathol Int* 48:47–52, 1998.
112. Fletcher CDM: *Diagnostic histopathology of tumors*, Edinburgh, 2013, Churchill Livingstone Elsevier.
113. de Saint Aubain Somerhausen N, Rubin BP, Fletcher CD: Myxoid solitary fibrous tumor: a study of seven cases with emphasis on differential diagnosis, *Mod Pathol* 12:463–471, 1999.
114. Mosquera JM, Fletcher CD: Expanding the spectrum of malignant progression in solitary fibrous tumors: a study of 8 cases with a discrete anaplastic component—is this dedifferentiated SFT? *Am J Surg Pathol* 33:1314–1321, 2009.
115. Doyle LA, Vivero M, Fletcher CD, et al: Nuclear expression of STAT6 distinguishes solitary fibrous tumor from histologic mimics, *Mod Pathol* 27:390–395, 2014.
116. Cheah AL, Billings SD, Goldblum JR, et al: STAT6 rabbit monoclonal antibody is a robust diagnostic tool for the distinction of solitary fibrous tumour from its mimics, *Pathology* 46:389–395, 2014.
117. Yoshida A, Tsuta K, Ohno M, et al: STAT6 immunohistochemistry is helpful in the diagnosis of solitary fibrous tumors, *Am J Surg Pathol* 38:552–559, 2014.
118. Schweizer L, Koelsche C, Sahm F, et al: Meningeal hemangiopericytoma and solitary fibrous tumors carry the NAB2-STAT6 fusion and can be diagnosed by nuclear expression of STAT6 protein, *Acta Neuropathol* 125:651–658, 2013.
119. Foo WC, Cruise MW, Wick MR, et al: Immunohistochemical staining for TLE1 distinguishes synovial sarcoma from histologic mimics, *Am J Clin Pathol* 135:839–844, 2011.
120. Doyle LA, Möller E, Dal Cin P, et al: MUC4 is a highly sensitive and specific marker for low-grade fibromyxoid sarcoma, *Am J Surg Pathol* 35:733–741, 2011.
121. Westra WH, Gerald WL, Rosai J: Solitary fibrous tumor. Consistent CD34 immunoreactivity and occurrence in the orbit, *Am J Surg Pathol* 18:992–998, 1994.
122. Hanau CA, Miettinen M: Solitary fibrous tumor: histological and immunohistochemical spectrum of benign and malignant variants presenting at different sites, *Hum Pathol* 26:440–449, 1995.
123. Vallat-Decouvelaere AV, Dry SM, Fletcher CD: Atypical and malignant solitary fibrous tumors in extrathoracic locations: evidence of their comparability to intra-thoracic tumors, *Am J Surg Pathol* 22:1501–1511, 1998.
124. Robinson DR, Wu YM, Kalyana-Sundaram S, et al: Identification of recurrent NAB2-STAT6 gene fusions in solitary fibrous tumor by integrative sequencing, *Nat Genet* 45:180–185, 2013.
125. Mohajeri A, Tayebwa J, Collin A, et al: Comprehensive genetic analysis identifies a pathognomonic NAB2/STAT6 fusion gene, nonrandom secondary genomic imbalances, and a characteristic gene expression profile in solitary fibrous tumor, *Genes Chromosomes Cancer* 52:873–886, 2013.
126. Chuang IC, Liao KC, Huang HY, et al: NAB2-STAT6 gene fusion and STAT6 immunoexpression in extrathoracic solitary fibrous tumors: the association between fusion variants and locations, *Pathol Int* 66:288–296, 2016.
127. Tai HC, Chuang IC, Chen TC, et al: NAB2-STAT6 fusion types account for clinicopathological variations in solitary fibrous tumors, *Mod Pathol* 28:1324–1335, 2015.
128. Barthelmess S, Geddert H, Boltze C, et al: Solitary fibrous tumors/hemangiopericytomas with different variants of the NAB2-STAT6 gene fusion are characterized by specific histomorphology and distinct clinicopathological features, *Am J Pathol* 184:1209–1218, 2014.
129. Miettinen MM, el Rifai W, Sarlomo-Rikala M, et al: Tumor size-related DNA copy number changes occur in solitary fibrous tumors but not in hemangiopericytomas, *Mod Pathol* 10:1194–1200, 1997.
130. Akaike K, Kurisaki-Arakawa A, Hara K, et al: Distinct clinicopathological features of NAB2-STAT6 fusion gene variants in solitary fibrous tumor with emphasis on the acquisition of highly malignant potential, *Hum Pathol* 46:347–356, 2015.
131. Bahrami A, Lee S, Schaefer IM, et al: TERT promoter mutations and prognosis in solitary fibrous tumor, *Mod Pathol* 29:1511–1522, 2016.
132. Steigen SE, Schaeffer DF, West RB, et al: Expression of insulin-like growth factor 2 in mesenchymal neoplasms, *Mod Pathol* 22:914–921, 2009.
133. Doyle LA, Tao D, Marino-Enriquez A: STAT6 is amplified in a subset of dedifferentiated liposarcoma, *Mod Pathol* 27:1231–1237, 2014.
134. Reid R, de Silva MV, Paterson L, et al: Low-grade fibromyxoid sarcoma and hyalinizing spindle cell tumor with giant rosettes share a common t(7;16)(q34;p11) translocation, *Am J Surg Pathol* 27:1229–1236, 2003.
135. Hasegawa T, Matsuno Y, Shimoda T, et al: Extrathoracic solitary fibrous tumors: their histological variability and potentially aggressive behavior, *Hum Pathol* 30:1464–1473, 1999.
136. Enzinger FM, Smith BH: Hemangiopericytoma. An analysis of 106 cases, *Hum Pathol* 7:61–82, 1976.
137. Gold JS, Antonescu CR, Hajdu C, et al: Clinicopathologic correlates of solitary fibrous tumors, *Cancer* 94:1057–1068, 2002.
138. Demicco EG, Park MS, Araujo DM, et al: Solitary fibrous tumor: a clinicopathological study of 110 cases and proposed risk assessment model, *Mod Pathol* 25:1298–1306, 2012.
139. Espat NJ, Lewis JJ, Leung D, et al: Conventional hemangiopericytoma: modern analysis of outcome, *Cancer* 95:1746–1751, 2002.
140. Bishop AJ, Zagars GK, Demicco EG, et al: Soft tissue solitary fibrous tumor: combined surgery and radiation therapy results in excellent local control, *Am J Clin Oncol* 2015. [Epub ahead of print].
141. Dei Tos AP, Seregard S, Calonje E, et al: Giant cell angiofibroma. A distinctive orbital tumor in adults, *Am J Surg Pathol* 19:1286–1293, 1995.
142. Guillou L, Gebhard S, Coindre JM: Orbital and extraorbital giant cell angiofibroma: a giant cell-rich variant of solitary fibrous tumor? Clinicopathologic and immunohistochemical analysis of a series in favor of a unifying concept, *Am J Surg Pathol* 24:971–979, 2000.
143. Nielsen GP, Dickersin GR, Provenzal JM, et al: Lipomatous hemangiopericytoma. A histologic, ultrastructural and immunohistochemical study of a unique variant of hemangiopericytoma, *Am J Surg Pathol* 19:748–756, 1995.
144. Folpe AL, Devaney K, Weiss SW: Lipomatous hemangiopericytoma: a rare variant of hemangiopericytoma that may be confused with liposarcoma, *Am J Surg Pathol* 23:1201–1207, 1999.
145. Guillou L, Gebhard S, Coindre JM: Lipomatous hemangiopericytoma: a fat-containing variant of solitary fibrous tumor? Clinicopathologic, immunohistochemical, and ultrastructural analysis of a series in favor of a unifying concept, *Hum Pathol* 31:1108–1115, 2000.
146. Cameselle-Teijeiro J, Manuel Lopes J, Villanueva JP, et al: Lipomatous haemangiopericytoma (adipocytic variant of solitary fibrous tumour) of the thyroid, *Histopathology* 43:406–408, 2003.
147. Creytens D, Ferdinande L: Diagnostic utility of STAT6 immunohistochemistry in the diagnosis of fat-forming solitary fibrous tumors, *Appl Immunohistochem Mol Morphol* 24:e12–e13, 2016.
148. Fukushima M, Schaefer IM, Fletcher CD: Myolipoma of soft tissue: clinicopathologic analysis of 34 cases, *Am J Surg Pathol* 41:153–160, 2017.
149. Lee JC, Fletcher CD: Malignant fat-forming solitary fibrous tumor (so-called "lipomatous hemangiopericytoma"): clinicopathologic analysis of 14 cases, *Am J Surg Pathol* 35:1177–1185, 2011.
150. Perry A, Scheithauer BW, Nascimento AG: The immunophenotypic spectrum of meningeal hemangiopericytoma: a comparison with fibrous meningioma and solitary fibrous tumor of meninges, *Am J Surg Pathol* 21:1354–1360, 1997.
151. Tihan T, Viglione M, Rosenblum MK, et al: Solitary fibrous tumors in the central nervous system. A clinicopathologic review of 18 cases and comparison to meningeal hemangiopericytomas, *Arch Pathol Lab Med* 127:432–439, 2003.
152. Pakasa NM, Pasquier B, Chambonniere ML, et al: Atypical presentations of solitary fibrous tumors of the central nervous system: an analysis of unusual clinicopathological and outcome patterns in three new cases with a review of the literature, *Virchows Arch* 447:81–86, 2005.
153. Mena H, Ribas JL, Pezeshkpour GH, et al: Hemangiopericytoma of the central nervous system: a review of 94 cases, *Hum Pathol* 22:84–91, 1991.
154. Hahn HP, Bundock EA, Hornick JL: Immunohistochemical staining for claudin-1 can help distinguish meningiomas from histologic mimics, *Am J Clin Pathol* 125:203–208, 2006.
155. Allen PW: The fibromatoses: a clinicopathologic classification based on 140 cases, *Am J Surg Pathol* 1:255–270, 1977.
156. Fetsch JF, Laskin WB, Miettinen M: Palmar-plantar fibromatosis in children and preadolescents: a clinicopathologic study of 56 cases with newly recognized demographics and extended follow-up information, *Am J Surg Pathol* 29:1095–1105, 2005.
157. Montgomery E, Lee JH, Abraham SC, et al: Superficial fibromatoses are genetically distinct from deep fibromatoses, *Mod Pathol* 14:695–701, 2001.
158. Ushijima M, Tsuneyoshi M, Enjoji M: Dupuytren type fibromatoses. A clinicopathologic study of 62 cases, *Acta Pathol Jpn* 34:991–1001, 1984.
159. Ross DC: Epidemiology of Dupuytren's disease, *Hand Clin* 15:53–62, vi, 1999.
160. Hueston JT: Some observations on knuckle pads, *J Hand Surg [Br]* 9:75–78, 1984.
161. Caroli A, Zanasi S, Marcuzzi A, et al: Epidemiological and structural findings supporting the fibromatous origin of dorsal knuckle pads, *J Hand Surg [Br]* 16:258–262, 1991.

162. Smith BH: Peyronie's disease, *Am J Clin Pathol* 45:670–678, 1966.
163. Carlson JW, Fletcher CD: Immunohistochemistry for beta-catenin in the differential diagnosis of spindle cell lesions: analysis of a series and review of the literature, *Histopathology* 51:509–514, 2007.
164. De Wever I, Dal Cin P, Fletcher CD, et al: Cytogenetic, clinical, and morphologic correlations in 78 cases of fibromatosis: a report from the CHAMP Study Group. CHromosomes And Morphology, *Mod Pathol* 13:1080–1085, 2000.
165. Breiner JA, Nelson M, Bredthauer BD, et al: Trisomy 8 and trisomy 14 in plantar fibromatosis, *Cancer Genet Cytogenet* 108:176–177, 1999.
166. Bhattacharya B, Dilworth HP, Iacobuzio-Donahue C, et al: Nuclear beta-catenin expression distinguishes deep fibromatosis from other benign and malignant fibroblastic and myofibroblastic lesions, *Am J Surg Pathol* 29:653–659, 2005.
167. Mehrotra AK, Sheikh S, Aaron AD, et al: Fibromatoses of the extremities: clinicopathologic study of 36 cases, *J Surg Oncol* 74:291–296, 2000.
168. Fallen T, Wilson M, Morlan B, et al: Desmoid tumors—a characterization of patients seen at Mayo Clinic 1976–1999, *Fam Cancer* 5:191–194, 2006.
169. Reitamo JJ, Hayry P, Nykyri E, et al: The desmoid tumor. I. Incidence, sex-, age- and anatomical distribution in the Finnish population, *Am J Clin Pathol* 77:665–673, 1982.
170. Burke AP, Sobin LH, Shekitka KM, et al: Intra-abdominal fibromatosis. A pathologic analysis of 130 tumors with comparison of clinical subgroups, *Am J Surg Pathol* 14:335–341, 1990.
171. Hoos A, Lewis JJ, Urist MJ, et al: Desmoid tumors of the head and neck—a clinical study of a rare entity, *Head Neck* 22:814–821, 2000.
172. Hayry P, Reitamo JJ, Totterman S, et al: The desmoid tumor. II. Analysis of factors possibly contributing to the etiology and growth behavior, *Am J Clin Pathol* 77:674–680, 1982.
173. Heiskanen I, Jarvinen HJ: Occurrence of desmoid tumours in familial adenomatous polyposis and results of treatment, *Int J Colorectal Dis* 11:157–162, 1996.
174. Zreik RT, Fritchie KJ: Morphologic spectrum of desmoid-type fibromatosis, *Am J Clin Pathol* 145:332–340, 2016.
175. Le Guellec S, Soubeyran I, Rochaix P, et al: CTNNB1 mutation analysis is a useful tool for the diagnosis of desmoid tumors: a study of 260 desmoid tumors and 191 potential morphologic mimics, *Mod Pathol* 25:1551–1558, 2012.
176. Lips DJ, Barker N, Clevers H, et al: The role of APC and beta-catenin in the aetiology of aggressive fibromatosis (desmoid tumors), *Eur J Surg Oncol* 35:3–10, 2009.
177. Crago AM, Chmielecki J, Rosenberg M, et al: Near universal detection of alterations in CTNNB1 and Wnt pathway regulators in desmoid-type fibromatosis by whole-exome sequencing and genomic analysis, *Genes Chromosomes Cancer* 54:606–615, 2015.
178. Domont J, Salas S, Lacroix L, et al: High frequency of beta-catenin heterozygous mutations in extra-abdominal fibromatosis: a potential molecular tool for disease management, *Br J Cancer* 102:1032–1036, 2010.
179. Lazar AJ, Tuvin D, Hajibashi S, et al: Specific mutations in the beta-catenin gene (CTNNB1) correlate with local recurrence in sporadic desmoid tumors, *Am J Pathol* 173:1518–1527, 2008.
180. Colombo C, Miceli R, Lazar AJ, et al: CTNNB1 45F mutation is a molecular prognosticator of increased postoperative primary desmoid tumor recurrence: an independent, multicenter validation study, *Cancer* 119:3696–3702, 2013.
181. van Broekhoven DL, Verhoef C, Grunhagen DJ, et al: Prognostic value of CTNNB1 gene mutation in primary sporadic aggressive fibromatosis, *Ann Surg Oncol* 22:1464–1470, 2015.
182. Fletcher JA, Naeem R, Xiao S, et al: Chromosome aberrations in desmoid tumors. Trisomy 8 may be a predictor of recurrence, *Cancer Genet Cytogenet* 79:139–143, 1995.
183. Mertens F, Willen H, Rydholm A, et al: Trisomy 20 is a primary chromosome aberration in desmoid tumors, *Int J Cancer* 63:527–529, 1995.
184. Merchant NB, Lewis JJ, Woodruff JM, et al: Extremity and trunk desmoid tumors: a multifactorial analysis of outcome, *Cancer* 86:2045–2052, 1999.
185. Smith AJ, Lewis JJ, Merchant NB, et al: Surgical management of intra-abdominal desmoid tumours, *Br J Surg* 87:608–613, 2000.
186. Gronchi A, Casali PG, Mariani L, et al: Quality of surgery and outcome in extra-abdominal aggressive fibromatosis: a series of patients surgically treated at a single institution, *J Clin Oncol* 21:1390–1397, 2003.
187. Ananth P, Werger A, Voss S, et al: Liposomal doxorubicin: effective treatment for pediatric desmoid fibromatosis, *Pediatr Blood Cancer* 64(7), 2017.
188. Heinrich MC, McArthur GA, Demetri GD, et al: Clinical and molecular studies of the effect of imatinib on advanced aggressive fibromatosis (desmoid tumor), *J Clin Oncol* 24:1195–1203, 2006.
189. Kasper B, Gruenwald V, Reichardt P, et al: Correlation of CTNNB1 mutation status with progression arrest rate in RECIST progressive desmoid-type fibromatosis treated with imatinib: translational research results from a phase 2 study of the German Interdisciplinary Sarcoma Group (GISG-01), *Ann Surg Oncol* 23:1924–1927, 2016.
190. Ballo MT, Zagars GK, Pollack A, et al: Desmoid tumor: prognostic factors and outcome after surgery, radiation therapy, or combined surgery and radiation therapy, *J Clin Oncol* 17:158–167, 1999.
191. Sturt NJ, Clark SK: Current ideas in desmoid tumours, *Fam Cancer* 5:275–285, discussion 287–288, 2006.
192. Hosalkar HS, Fox EJ, Delaney T, et al: Desmoid tumors and current status of management, *Orthop Clin North Am* 37:53–63, 2006.
193. Marino-Enriquez A, Nascimento AF, Ligon AH, et al: Atypical spindle cell lipomatous tumor: clinicopathologic characterization of 232 cases demonstrating a morphologic spectrum, *Am J Surg Pathol* 41:234–244, 2017.
194. Dei Tos AP, Mentzel T, Newman PL, et al: Spindle cell liposarcoma, a hitherto unrecognized variant of liposarcoma. Analysis of six cases, *Am J Surg Pathol* 18:913–921, 1994.
195. Mentzel T, Palmedo G, Kuhnen C: Well-differentiated spindle cell liposarcoma ('atypical spindle cell lipomatous tumor') does not belong to the spectrum of atypical lipomatous tumor but has a close relationship to spindle cell lipoma: clinicopathologic, immunohistochemical, and molecular analysis of six cases, *Mod Pathol* 23:729–736, 2010.
196. Creytens D, van Gorp J, Savola S, et al: Atypical spindle cell lipoma: a clinicopathologic, immunohistochemical, and molecular study emphasizing its relationship to classical spindle cell lipoma, *Virchows Arch* 465:97–108, 2014.
197. Deyrup AT, Chibon F, Guillou L, et al: Fibrosarcoma-like lipomatous neoplasm: a reappraisal of so-called spindle cell liposarcoma defining a unique lipomatous tumor unrelated to other liposarcomas, *Am J Surg Pathol* 37:1373–1378, 2013.
198. Dahl I: Ancient neurilemmoma (schwannoma), *Acta Pathol Microbiol Scand [A]* 85:812–818, 1977.
199. Fletcher CD, Davies SE: Benign plexiform (multinodular) schwannoma: a rare tumour unassociated with neurofibromatosis, *Histopathology* 10:971–980, 1986.
200. Kao GF, Laskin WB, Olsen TG: Solitary cutaneous plexiform neurilemmoma (schwannoma): a clinicopathologic, immunohistochemical, and ultrastructural study of 11 cases, *Mod Pathol* 2:20–26, 1989.
201. Agaram NP, Prakash S, Antonescu CR: Deep-seated plexiform schwannoma: a pathologic study of 16 cases and comparative analysis with the superficial variety, *Am J Surg Pathol* 29:1042–1048, 2005.
202. Fletcher CD, Davies SE, McKee PH: Cellular schwannoma: a distinct pseudosarcomatous entity, *Histopathology* 11:21–35, 1987.
203. White W, Shiu MH, Rosenblum MK, et al: Cellular schwannoma. A clinicopathologic study of 57 patients and 58 tumors, *Cancer* 66:1266–1275, 1990.
204. Font RL, Truong LD: Melanotic schwannoma of soft tissues. Electron-microscopic observations and review of literature, *Am J Surg Pathol* 8:129–138, 1984.
205. Killeen RM, Davy CL, Bauserman SC: Melanocytic schwannoma, *Cancer* 62:174–183, 1988.
206. Daimaru Y, Kido H, Hashimoto H, et al: Benign schwannoma of the gastrointestinal tract: a clinicopathologic and immunohistochemical study, *Hum Pathol* 19:257–264, 1988.
207. Hou YY, Tan YS, Xu JF, et al: Schwannoma of the gastrointestinal tract: a clinicopathological, immunohistochemical and ultrastructural study of 33 cases, *Histopathology* 48:536–545, 2006.
208. Liegl B, Bennett MW, Fletcher CD: Microcystic/reticular schwannoma: a distinct variant with predilection for visceral locations, *Am J Surg Pathol* 32:1080–1087, 2008.
209. Kindblom LG, Meis-Kindblom JM, Havel G, et al: Benign epithelioid schwannoma, *Am J Surg Pathol* 22:762–770, 1998.
210. Laskin WB, Fetsch JF, Lasota J, et al: Benign epithelioid peripheral nerve sheath tumors of the soft tissues: clinicopathologic spectrum of 33 cases, *Am J Surg Pathol* 29:39–51, 2005.
211. Michal M, Kazakov DV, Belousova I, et al: A benign neoplasm with histopathological features of both schwannoma and retiform perineurioma (benign schwannoma-perineurioma): a report of six cases of a distinctive soft tissue tumor with a predilection for the fingers, *Virchows Arch* 445:347–353, 2004.
212. Feany MB, Anthony DC, Fletcher CD: Nerve sheath tumours with hybrid features of neurofibroma and schwannoma: a conceptual challenge, *Histopathology* 32:405–410, 1998.
213. Hornick JL, Bundock EA, Fletcher CD: Hybrid schwannoma/perineurioma: clinicopathologic analysis of 42 distinctive benign nerve sheath tumors, *Am J Surg Pathol* 33:1554–1561, 2009.
214. Goldblum JR, Beals TF, Weiss SW: Neuroblastoma-like neurilemoma, *Am J Surg Pathol* 18:266–273, 1994.
215. Hasegawa SL, Mentzel T, Fletcher CD: Schwannomas of the sinonasal tract and nasopharynx, *Mod Pathol* 10:777–784, 1997.
216. Voltaggio L, Murray R, Lasota J, et al: Gastric schwannoma: a clinicopathologic study of 51 cases and critical review of the literature, *Hum Pathol* 43:650–659, 2012.
217. Ariza A, Bilbao JM, Rosai J: Immunohistochemical detection of epithelial membrane antigen in normal perineurial cells and perineurioma, *Am J Surg Pathol* 12:678–683, 1988.
218. Kawahara E, Oda Y, Ooi A, et al: Expression of glial fibrillary acidic protein (GFAP) in peripheral nerve sheath tumors. A comparative study of immunoreactivity of GFAP, vimentin, S-100 protein, and neurofilament in 38 schwannomas and 18 neurofibromas, *Am J Surg Pathol* 12:115–120, 1988.
219. Gray MH, Rosenberg AE, Dickersin GR, et al: Glial fibrillary acidic protein and keratin expression by benign and malignant nerve sheath tumors, *Hum Pathol* 20:1089–1096, 1989.
220. Fanburg-Smith JC, Majidi M, Miettinen M: Keratin expression in schwannoma; a study of 115 retroperitoneal and 22 peripheral schwannomas, *Mod Pathol* 19:115–121, 2006.
221. Trofatter JA, MacCollin MM, Rutter JL, et al: A novel moesin-, ezrin-, radixin-like gene is a candidate for the neurofibromatosis 2 tumor suppressor, *Cell* 72:791–800, 1993.
222. Rouleau GA, Merel P, Lutchman M, et al: Alteration in a new gene encoding a putative membrane-organizing protein causes neuro-fibromatosis type 2, *Nature* 363:515–521, 1993.
223. Stemmer-Rachamimov AO, Xu L, Gonzalez-Agosti C, et al: Universal absence of merlin, but not other ERM family members, in schwannomas, *Am J Pathol* 151:1649–1654, 1997.
224. Mertens F, Dal Cin P, De Wever I, et al: Cytogenetic characterization of peripheral nerve sheath tumours: a report of the CHAMP study group, *J Pathol* 190:31–38, 2000.
225. Agnihotri S, Jalali S, Wilson MR, et al: The genomic landscape of schwannoma, *Nat Genet* 48:1339–1348, 2016.
226. Woodruff JM, Selig AM, Crowley K, et al: Schwannoma (neurilemoma) with malignant transformation. A rare, distinctive peripheral nerve tumor, *Am J Surg Pathol* 18:882–895, 1994.

227. Mentzel T, Katenkamp D: Intraneural angiosarcoma and angiosarcoma arising in benign and malignant peripheral nerve sheath tumours: clinicopathological and immunohistochemical analysis of four cases, *Histopathology* 35:114–120, 1999.
228. McMenamin ME, Fletcher CD: Expanding the spectrum of malignant change in schwannomas: epithelioid malignant change, epithelioid malignant peripheral nerve sheath tumor, and epithelioid angiosarcoma: a study of 17 cases, *Am J Surg Pathol* 25:13–25, 2001.
229. Woodruff JM, Godwin TA, Erlandson RA, et al: Cellular schwannoma: a variety of schwannoma sometimes mistaken for a malignant tumor, *Am J Surg Pathol* 5:733–744, 1981.
230. Casadei GP, Scheithauer BW, Hirose T, et al: Cellular schwannoma. A clinicopathologic, DNA flow cytometric, and proliferation marker study of 70 patients, *Cancer* 75:1109–1119, 1995.
231. Woodruff JM, Marshall ML, Godwin TA, et al: Plexiform (multinodular) schwannoma. A tumor simulating the plexiform neurofibroma, *Am J Surg Pathol* 7:691–697, 1983.
232. Ishida T, Kuroda M, Motoi T, et al: Phenotypic diversity of neurofibromatosis 2: association with plexiform schwannoma, *Histopathology* 32:264–270, 1998.
233. Woodruff JM, Scheithauer BW, Kurtkaya-Yapicier O, et al: Congenital and childhood plexiform (multinodular) cellular schwannoma: a troublesome mimic of malignant peripheral nerve sheath tumor, *Am J Surg Pathol* 27:1321–1329, 2003.
234. Meis-Kindblom JM, Enzinger FM: Plexiform malignant peripheral nerve sheath tumor of infancy and childhood, *Am J Surg Pathol* 18:479–485, 1994.
235. Mennemeyer RP, Hallman KO, Hammar SP, et al: Melanotic schwannoma. Clinical and ultrastructural studies of three cases with evidence of intracellular melanin synthesis, *Am J Surg Pathol* 3:3–10, 1979.
236. Lowman RM, Livolsi VA: Pigmented (melanotic) schwannomas of the spinal canal, *Cancer* 46:391–397, 1980.
237. Carney JA: Psammomatous melanotic schwannoma. A distinctive, heritable tumor with special associations, including cardiac myxoma and the Cushing syndrome, *Am J Surg Pathol* 14:206–222, 1990.
238. Torres-Mora J, Dry S, Li X, et al: Malignant melanotic schwannian tumor: a clinicopathologic, immunohistochemical, and gene expression profiling study of 40 cases, with a proposal for the reclassification of "melanotic schwannoma, *Am J Surg Pathol* 38:94–105, 2014.
239. Wang L, Zehir A, Sadowska J, et al: Consistent copy number changes and recurrent PRKAR1A mutations distinguish melanotic schwannomas from melanomas: SNP-array and next generation sequencing analysis, *Genes Chromosomes Cancer* 2015. [Epub ahead of print].
240. Krausz T, Azzopardi JG, Pearse E: Malignant melanoma of the sympathetic chain: with a consideration of pigmented nerve sheath tumours, *Histopathology* 8:881–894, 1984.
241. Hornick JL, Fletcher CD: Myoepithelial tumors of soft tissue: a clinicopathologic and immunohistochemical study of 101 cases with evaluation of prognostic parameters, *Am J Surg Pathol* 27:1183–1196, 2003.
242. Kirschner LS, Carney JA, Pack SD, et al: Mutations of the gene encoding the protein kinase A type I-alpha regulatory subunit in patients with the Carney complex, *Nat Genet* 26:89–92, 2000.
243. Jacoby LB, Jones D, Davis K, et al: Molecular analysis of the NF2 tumor-suppressor gene in schwannomatosis, *Am J Hum Genet* 61:1293–1302, 1997.
244. Hulsebos TJ, Plomp AS, Wolterman RA, et al: Germline mutation of INI1/SMARCB1 in familial schwannomatosis, *Am J Hum Genet* 80:805–810, 2007.
245. Piotrowski A, Xie J, Liu YF, et al: Germline loss-of-function mutations in LZTR1 predispose to an inherited disorder of multiple schwannomas, *Nat Genet* 46:182–187, 2014.
246. Lassmann H, Jurecka W, Lassmann G, et al: Different types of benign nerve sheath tumors. Light microscopy, electron microscopy and autoradiography, *Virchows Arch A Pathol Anat Histol* 375:197–210, 1977.
247. Ushigome S, Takakuwa T, Hyuga M, et al: Perineurial cell tumor and the significance of the perineurial cells in neurofibroma, *Acta Pathol Jpn* 36:973–987, 1986.
248. Louis DN, Ohgaki H, Wiestler OD, et al: *Classification of tumours of the central nervous system*, Lyon, France, 2007, IARC Press.
249. Fletcher CD: Peripheral nerve sheath tumors. A clinicopathologic update, *Pathol Annu* 25(Pt 1):53–74, 1990.
250. Megahed M: Histopathological variants of neurofibroma. A study of 114 lesions, *Am J Dermatopathol* 16:486–495, 1994.
251. Woodruff JM: Pathology of tumors of the peripheral nerve sheath in type 1 neurofibromatosis, *Am J Med Genet* 89:23–30, 1999.
252. Jokinen CH, Argenyi ZB: Atypical neurofibroma of the skin and subcutaneous tissue: clinicopathologic analysis of 11 cases, *J Cutan Pathol* 37:35–42, 2010.
253. Lin BT, Weiss LM, Medeiros LJ: Neurofibroma and cellular neurofibroma with atypia: a report of 14 tumors, *Am J Surg Pathol* 21:1443–1449, 1997.
254. Michal M, Fanburg-Smith JC, Mentzel T, et al: Dendritic cell neurofibroma with pseudorosettes: a report of 18 cases of a distinct and hitherto unrecognized neurofibroma variant, *Am J Surg Pathol* 25:587–594, 2001.
255. Woodruff JM, Busam KJ: Histologically benign cutaneous dendritic cell tumor with pseudorosettes, *Am J Surg Pathol* 26:1644–1645, author reply 1645–1648, 2002.
256. Weiss SW, Nickoloff BJ: CD-34 is expressed by a distinctive cell population in peripheral nerve, nerve sheath tumors, and related lesions, *Am J Surg Pathol* 17:1039–1045, 1993.
257. Zamecnik M, Michal M: Perineurial cell differentiation in neurofibromas. Report of eight cases including a case with composite perineurioma-neurofibroma features, *Pathol Res Pract* 197:537–544, 2001.
258. Wallace MR, Marchuk DA, Andersen LB, et al: Type 1 neurofibromatosis gene: identification of a large transcript disrupted in three NF1 patients, *Science* 249:181–186, 1990.
259. Colman SD, Williams CA, Wallace MR: Benign neurofibromas in type 1 neurofibromatosis (NF1) show somatic deletions of the NF1 gene, *Nat Genet* 11:90–92, 1995.
260. Serra E, Puig S, Otero D, et al: Confirmation of a double-hit model for the NF1 gene in benign neurofibromas, *Am J Hum Genet* 61:512–519, 1997.
261. Pemov A, Li H, Patidar R, et al: The primacy of NF1 loss as the driver of tumorigenesis in neurofibromatosis type 1-associated plexiform neurofibromas, *Oncogene* 36:3168–3177, 2017.
262. Storlazzi CT, Von Steyern FV, Domanski HA, et al: Biallelic somatic inactivation of the NF1 gene through chromosomal translocations in a sporadic neurofibroma, *Int J Cancer* 117:1055–1057, 2005.
263. Basu TN, Gutmann DH, Fletcher JA, et al: Aberrant regulation of ras proteins in malignant tumour cells from type 1 neurofibromatosis patients, *Nature* 356:713–715, 1992.
264. Shen MH, Harper PS, Upadhyaya M: Molecular genetics of neurofibromatosis type 1 (NF1), *J Med Genet* 33:2–17, 1996.
265. Kluwe L, Friedrich R, Mautner VF: Loss of NF1 allele in Schwann cells but not in fibroblasts derived from an NF1-associated neurofibroma, *Genes Chromosomes Cancer* 24:283–285, 1999.
266. Serra E, Rosenbaum T, Winner U, et al: Schwann cells harbor the somatic NF1 mutation in neurofibromas: evidence of two different Schwann cell subpopulations, *Hum Mol Genet* 9:3055–3064, 2000.
267. Zhu Y, Ghosh P, Charnay P, et al: Neurofibromas in NF1: Schwann cell origin and role of tumor environment, *Science* 296:920–922, 2002.
268. Yang FC, Ingram DA, Chen S, et al: Nf1-dependent tumors require a microenvironment containing Nf1+/– and c-kit-dependent bone marrow, *Cell* 135:437–448, 2008.
269. Stahn V, Nagel I, Fischer-Huchzermeyer S, et al: Molecular analysis of hybrid neurofibroma/schwannoma identifies common monosomy 22 and alpha-T-catenin/CTNNA3 as a novel candidate tumor suppressor, *Am J Pathol* 186:3285–3296, 2016.
270. Bird CC, Willis RA: The histogenesis of pigmented neurofibromas, *J Pathol* 97:631–637, 1969.
271. Fetsch JF, Michal M, Miettinen M: Pigmented (melanotic) neurofibroma: a clinicopathologic and immunohistochemical analysis of 19 lesions from 17 patients, *Am J Surg Pathol* 24:331–343, 2000.
272. Huson SM, Harper PS, Compston DA: Von Recklinghausen neurofibromatosis. A clinical and population study in south-east Wales, *Brain* 111(Pt 6):1355–1381, 1988.
273. Tonsgard JH, Kwak SM, Short MP, et al: CT imaging in adults with neurofibromatosis-1: frequent asymptomatic plexiform lesions, *Neurology* 50:1755–1760, 1998.
274. Korf BR: Plexiform neurofibromas, *Am J Med Genet* 89:31–37, 1999.
275. Robertson KA, Nalepa G, Yang FC, et al: Imatinib mesylate for plexiform neurofibromas in patients with neurofibromatosis type 1: a phase 2 trial, *Lancet Oncol* 13:1218–1224, 2012.
276. Dombi E, Baldwin A, Marcus LJ, et al: Activity of selumetinib in neurofibromatosis type 1-related plexiform neurofibromas, *N Engl J Med* 375:2550–2560, 2016.
277. Nielsen GP, Stemmer-Rachamimov AO, Ino Y, et al: Malignant transformation of neurofibromas in neurofibromatosis 1 is associated with CDKN2A/p16 inactivation, *Am J Pathol* 155:1879–1884, 1999.
278. Kourea HP, Orlow I, Scheithauer BW, et al: Deletions of the INK4A gene occur in malignant peripheral nerve sheath tumors but not in neurofibromas, *Am J Pathol* 155:1855–1860, 1999.
279. Subramanian S, Thayanithy V, West RB, et al: Genome-wide transcriptome analyses reveal p53 inactivation mediated loss of miR-34a expression in malignant peripheral nerve sheath tumours, *J Pathol* 220:58–70, 2010.
280. Beert E, Brems H, Daniels B, et al: Atypical neurofibromas in neurofibromatosis type 1 are premalignant tumors, *Genes Chromosomes Cancer* 50:1021–1032, 2011.
281. Liapis H, Marley EF, Lin Y, et al: p53 and Ki-67 proliferating cell nuclear antigen in benign and malignant peripheral nerve sheath tumors in children, *Pediatr Dev Pathol* 2:377–384, 1999.
282. McCarron KF, Goldblum JR: Plexiform neurofibroma with and without associated malignant peripheral nerve sheath tumor: a clinicopathologic and immunohistochemical analysis of 54 cases, *Mod Pathol* 11:612–617, 1998.
283. Levy P, Bieche I, Leroy K, et al: Molecular profiles of neurofibromatosis type 1-associated plexiform neurofibromas: identification of a gene expression signature of poor prognosis, *Clin Cancer Res* 10:3763–3771, 2004.
284. Lazarus SS, Trombetta LD: Ultrastructural identification of a benign perineurial cell tumor, *Cancer* 41:1823–1829, 1978.
285. Bilbao JM, Khoury NJ, Hudson AR, et al: Perineurioma (localized hypertrophic neuropathy), *Arch Pathol Lab Med* 108:557–560, 1984.
286. Weidenheim KM, Campbell WG, Jr: Perineural cell tumor. Immunocytochemical and ultrastructural characterization. Relationship to other peripheral nerve tumors with a review of the literature, *Virchows Arch A Pathol Anat Histopathol* 408:375–383, 1986.
287. Tsang WY, Chan JK, Chow LT, et al: Perineurioma: an uncommon soft tissue neoplasm distinct from localized hypertrophic neuropathy and neurofibroma, *Am J Surg Pathol* 16:756–763, 1992.
288. Mentzel T, Dei Tos AP, Fletcher CD: Perineurioma (storiform perineurial fibroma): clinicopathological analysis of four cases, *Histopathology* 25:261–267, 1994.
289. Hornick JL, Fletcher CD: Intestinal perineuriomas: clinicopathologic definition of a new anatomic subset in a series of 10 cases, *Am J Surg Pathol* 29:859–865, 2005.
290. Hornick JL, Fletcher CD: Soft tissue perineurioma: clinicopathologic analysis of 81 cases including those with atypical histologic features, *Am J Surg Pathol* 29:845–858, 2005.
291. Torres-Mora J, Ud Din N, Ahrens WA, et al: Pseudolipoblastic perineurioma: an unusual morphological variant of perineurioma that may simulate liposarcoma, *Hum Pathol* 57:22–27, 2016.

292. Theaker JM, Fletcher CD: Epithelial membrane antigen expression by the perineurial cell: further studies of peripheral nerve lesions, *Histopathology* 14:581–592, 1989.
293. Folpe AL, Billings SD, McKenney JK, et al: Expression of claudin-1, a recently described tight junction-associated protein, distinguishes soft tissue perineurioma from potential mimics, *Am J Surg Pathol* 26:1620–1626, 2002.
294. Yamaguchi U, Hasegawa T, Hirose T, et al: Sclerosing perineurioma: a clinicopathological study of five cases and diagnostic utility of immunohistochemical staining for GLUT1, *Virchows Arch* 443:159–163, 2003.
295. Emory TS, Scheithauer BW, Hirose T, et al: Intraneural perineurioma. A clonal neoplasm associated with abnormalities of chromosome 22, *Am J Clin Pathol* 103:696–704, 1995.
296. Giannini C, Scheithauer BW, Jenkins RB, et al: Soft-tissue perineurioma. Evidence for an abnormality of chromosome 22, criteria for diagnosis, and review of the literature, *Am J Surg Pathol* 21:164–173, 1997.
297. Sciot R, Dal Cin P, Hagemeijer A, et al: Cutaneous sclerosing perineurioma with cryptic NF2 gene deletion, *Am J Surg Pathol* 23:849–853, 1999.
298. Brock JE, Perez-Atayde AR, Kozakewich HP, et al: Cytogenetic aberrations in perineurioma: variation with subtype, *Am J Surg Pathol* 29:1164–1169, 2005.
299. Lasota J, Fetsch JF, Wozniak A, et al: The neurofibromatosis type 2 gene is mutated in perineurial cell tumors: a molecular genetic study of eight cases, *Am J Pathol* 158:1223–1229, 2001.
300. Hirose T, Scheithauer BW, Sano T: Perineurial malignant peripheral nerve sheath tumor (MPNST): a clinicopathologic, immunohistochemical, and ultrastructural study of seven cases, *Am J Surg Pathol* 22:1368–1378, 1998.
301. Michal M: Extraneural retiform perineuriomas. A report of four cases, *Pathol Res Pract* 195:759–763, 1999.
302. Graadt van Roggen JF, McMenamin ME, Belchis DA, et al: Reticular perineurioma: a distinctive variant of soft tissue perineurioma, *Am J Surg Pathol* 25:485–493, 2001.
303. Boyanton BL, Jr, Jones JK, Shenaq SM, et al: Intraneural perineurioma: a systematic review with illustrative cases, *Arch Pathol Lab Med* 131:1382–1392, 2007.
304. Fetsch JF, Miettinen M: Sclerosing perineurioma: a clinicopathologic study of 19 cases of a distinctive soft tissue lesion with a predilection for the fingers and palms of young adults, *Am J Surg Pathol* 21:1433–1442, 1997.
305. Fox MD, Gleason BC, Thomas AB, et al: Extra-acral cutaneous/soft tissue sclerosing perineurioma: an under-recognized entity in the differential of CD34-positive cutaneous neoplasms, *J Cutan Pathol* 37:1053–1056, 2010.
306. Hornick JL, Fletcher CD: Criteria for malignancy in nonvisceral smooth muscle tumors, *Ann Diagn Pathol* 7:60–66, 2003.
307. Nucci MR, Oliva E: *Gynecologic pathology: a volume in the series foundations in diagnostic pathology*, Edinburgh, 2009, Churchill Livingstone/Elsevier.
308. Miettinen M, Fetsch JF: Evaluation of biological potential of smooth muscle tumours, *Histopathology* 48:97–105, 2006.
309. Billings SD, Folpe AL, Weiss SW: Do leiomyomas of deep soft tissue exist? An analysis of highly differentiated smooth muscle tumors of deep soft tissue supporting two distinct subtypes, *Am J Surg Pathol* 25:1134–1142, 2001.
310. Paal E, Miettinen M: Retroperitoneal leiomyomas: a clinicopathologic and immunohistochemical study of 56 cases with a comparison to retroperitoneal leiomyosarcomas, *Am J Surg Pathol* 25:1355–1363, 2001.
311. Kilpatrick SE, Mentzel T, Fletcher CD: Leiomyoma of deep soft tissue. Clinicopathologic analysis of a series, *Am J Surg Pathol* 18:576–582, 1994.
312. Fletcher CD, Kilpatrick SE, Mentzel T: The difficulty in predicting behavior of smooth-muscle tumors in deep soft tissue, *Am J Surg Pathol* 19:116–117, 1995.
313. Meis JM, Enzinger FM: Myolipoma of soft tissue, *Am J Surg Pathol* 15:121–125, 1991.
314. Weiss SW: Smooth muscle tumors of soft tissue, *Adv Anat Pathol* 9:351–359, 2002.
315. Shmookler BM, Lauer DH: Retroperitoneal leiomyosarcoma. A clinicopathologic analysis of 36 cases, *Am J Surg Pathol* 7:269–280, 1983.
316. Miettinen M, Wang ZF, Lasota J: DOG1 antibody in the differential diagnosis of gastrointestinal stromal tumors: a study of 1840 cases, *Am J Surg Pathol* 33:1401–1408, 2009.
317. Horiuchi K, Yabe H, Mukai M, et al: Multiple smooth muscle tumors arising in deep soft tissue of lower limbs with uterine leiomyomas, *Am J Surg Pathol* 22:897–901, 1998.
318. Rao UN, Finkelstein SD, Jones MW: Comparative immunohistochemical and molecular analysis of uterine and extrauterine leiomyosarcomas, *Mod Pathol* 12:1001–1009, 1999.
319. Makinen N, Mehine M, Tolvanen J, et al: MED12, the mediator complex subunit 12 gene, is mutated at high frequency in uterine leiomyomas, *Science* 334:252–255, 2011.
320. Matsubara A, Sekine S, Yoshida M, et al: Prevalence of MED12 mutations in uterine and extrauterine smooth muscle tumours, *Histopathology* 62:657–661, 2013.
321. Ravegnini G, Marino-Enriquez A, Slater J, et al: MED12 mutations in leiomyosarcoma and extrauterine leiomyoma, *Mod Pathol* 26:743–749, 2013.
322. de Graaff MA, Cleton-Jansen AM, Szuhai K, et al: Mediator complex subunit 12 exon 2 mutation analysis in different subtypes of smooth muscle tumors confirms genetic heterogeneity, *Hum Pathol* 44:1597–1604, 2013.
323. Hodge JC, Morton CC: Genetic heterogeneity among uterine leiomyomata: insights into malignant progression, *Hum Mol Genet* 16(Spec1):R7–R13, 2007.
324. Mehine M, Kaasinen E, Heinonen HR, et al: Integrated data analysis reveals uterine leiomyoma subtypes with distinct driver pathways and biomarkers, *Proc Natl Acad Sci USA* 113:1315–1320, 2016.
325. Tomlinson IP, Alam NA, Rowan AJ, et al: Germline mutations in FH predispose to dominantly inherited uterine fibroids, skin leiomyomata and papillary renal cell cancer, *Nat Genet* 30:406–410, 2002.
326. Lehtonen R, Kiuru M, Vanharanta S, et al: Biallelic inactivation of fumarate hydratase (FH) occurs in nonsyndromic uterine leiomyomas but is rare in other tumors, *Am J Pathol* 164:17–22, 2004.
327. Fisher C: Low-grade sarcomas with CD34-positive fibroblasts and low-grade myofibroblastic sarcomas, *Ultrastruct Pathol* 28:291–305, 2004.
328. Folpe AL, Mentzel T, Lehr HA, et al: Perivascular epithelioid cell neoplasms of soft tissue and gynecologic origin: a clinicopathologic study of 26 cases and review of the literature, *Am J Surg Pathol* 29:1558–1575, 2005.
329. Vang R, Kempson RL: Perivascular epithelioid cell tumor ('PEComa') of the uterus: a subset of HMB-45-positive epithelioid mesenchymal neoplasms with an uncertain relationship to pure smooth muscle tumors, *Am J Surg Pathol* 26:1–13, 2002.
330. Hachisuga T, Hashimoto H, Enjoji M: Angioleiomyoma. A clinicopathologic reappraisal of 562 cases, *Cancer* 54:126–130, 1984.
331. Brooks JK, Nikitakis NG, Goodman NJ, et al: Clinicopathologic characterization of oral angioleiomyomas, *Oral Surg Oral Med Oral Pathol Oral Radiol Endod* 94:221–227, 2002.
332. Sandberg AA: Updates on the cytogenetics and molecular genetics of bone and soft tissue tumors: leiomyosarcoma, *Cancer Genet Cytogenet* 161:1–19, 2005.
333. Tavassoli FA, Norris HJ: Peritoneal leiomyomatosis (leiomyomatosis peritonealis disseminata): a clinicopathologic study of 20 cases with ultrastructural observations, *Int J Gynecol Pathol* 1:59–74, 1982.
334. Clement PB, Young RH, Scully RE: Intravenous leiomyomatosis of the uterus. A clinicopathological analysis of 16 cases with unusual histologic features, *Am J Surg Pathol* 12:932–945, 1988.
335. Abell MR, Littler ER: Benign metastasizing uterine leiomyoma. Multiple lymph nodal metastases, *Cancer* 36:2206–2213, 1975.
336. Canzonieri V, D'Amore ES, Bartoloni G, et al: Leiomyomatosis with vascular invasion. A unified pathogenesis regarding leiomyoma with vascular microinvasion, benign metastasizing leiomyoma and intravenous leiomyomatosis, *Virchows Arch* 425:541–545, 1994.
337. Quade BJ, McLachlin CM, Soto-Wright V, et al: Disseminated peritoneal leiomyomatosis. Clonality analysis by X chromosome inactivation and cytogenetics of a clinically benign smooth muscle proliferation, *Am J Pathol* 150:2153–2166, 1997.
338. Ordulu Z, Dal Cin P, Chong WW, et al: Disseminated peritoneal leiomyomatosis after laparoscopic supracervical hysterectomy with characteristic molecular cytogenetic findings of uterine leiomyoma, *Genes Chromosomes Cancer* 49:1152–1160, 2010.
339. Nucci MR, Drapkin R, Dal Cin P, et al: Distinctive cytogenetic profile in benign metastasizing leiomyoma: pathogenetic implications, *Am J Surg Pathol* 31:737–743, 2007.
340. Toro JR, Travis LB, Wu HJ, et al: Incidence patterns of soft tissue sarcomas, regardless of primary site, in the surveillance, epidemiology and end results program, 1978–2001: an analysis of 26,758 cases, *Int J Cancer* 119:2922–2930, 2006.
341. Fletcher CDM, Bridge JA, Hogendoorn PCW, et al, editors: *WHO classification of tumors of soft tissue and bone*, Lyon, France, 2013, IARC Press.
342. Kraft S, Fletcher CD: Atypical intradermal smooth muscle neoplasms: clinicopathologic analysis of 84 cases and a reappraisal of cutaneous "leiomyosarcoma.", *Am J Surg Pathol* 35:599–607, 2011.
343. Miettinen M: Immunoreactivity for cytokeratin and epithelial membrane antigen in leiomyosarcoma, *Arch Pathol Lab Med* 112:637–640, 1988.
344. Iwata J, Fletcher CD: Immunohistochemical detection of cytokeratin and epithelial membrane antigen in leiomyosarcoma: a systematic study of 100 cases, *Pathol Int* 50:7–14, 2000.
345. Lee CH, Turbin DA, Sung YC, et al: A panel of antibodies to determine site of origin and malignancy in smooth muscle tumors, *Mod Pathol* 22:1519–1531, 2009.
346. Mandahl N, Fletcher CD, Dal Cin P, et al: Comparative cytogenetic study of spindle cell and pleomorphic leiomyosarcomas of soft tissues: a report from the CHAMP Study Group, *Cancer Genet Cytogenet* 116:66–73, 2000.
347. Hernando E, Charytonowicz E, Dudas ME, et al: The AKT-mTOR pathway plays a critical role in the development of leiomyosarcomas, *Nat Med* 13:748–753, 2007.
348. Babichev Y, Kabaroff L, Datti A, et al: PI3K/AKT/mTOR inhibition in combination with doxorubicin is an effective therapy for leiomyosarcoma, *J Transl Med* 14:67, 2016.
349. Beck AH, Lee CH, Witten DM, et al: Discovery of molecular subtypes in leiomyosarcoma through integrative molecular profiling, *Oncogene* 29:845–854, 2010.
350. Wang W-L, Bones-Valentin RA, Prieto VG, et al: Sarcoma metastases to the skin: a clinicopathologic study of 65 patients, *Cancer* 118:2900–2904, 2012.
351. Lee CH, Espinosa I, Vrijaldenhoven S, et al: Prognostic significance of macrophage infiltration in leiomyosarcomas, *Clin Cancer Res* 14:1423–1430, 2008.
352. Espinosa I, Beck AH, Lee CH, et al: Coordinate expression of colony-stimulating factor-1 and colony-stimulating factor-1-related proteins is associated with poor prognosis in gynecological and nongynecological leiomyosarcoma, *Am J Pathol* 174:2347–2356, 2009.
353. Collins IM, Thomas DM: Novel approaches to treatment of leiomyosarcomas, *Curr Oncol Rep* 13:316–322, 2011.
354. Chadwick EG, Connor EJ, Hanson IC, et al: Tumors of smooth-muscle origin in HIV-infected children, *JAMA* 263:3182–3184, 1990.
355. van Hoeven KH, Factor SM, Kress Y, et al: Visceral myogenic tumors. A manifestation of HIV infection in children, *Am J Surg Pathol* 17:1176–1181, 1993.
356. McClain KL, Leach CT, Jenson HB, et al: Association of Epstein-Barr virus with leiomyosarcomas in children with AIDS, *N Engl J Med* 332:12–18, 1995.

357. Deyrup AT, Lee VK, Hill CE, et al: Epstein-Barr virus-associated smooth muscle tumors are distinctive mesenchymal tumors reflecting multiple infection events: a clinicopathologic and molecular analysis of 29 tumors from 19 patients, *Am J Surg Pathol* 30:75–82, 2006.
358. Cornog JL, Jr, Enterline HT: Lymphangiomyoma, a benign lesion of chyliferous lymphatics synonymous with lymphangiopericytoma, *Cancer* 19:1909–1930, 1966.
359. Chan JK, Tsang WY, Pau MY, et al: Lymphangiomyomatosis and angiomyolipoma: closely related entities characterized by hamartomatous proliferation of HMB-45-positive smooth muscle, *Histopathology* 22:445–455, 1993.
360. Costello LC, Hartman TE, Ryu JH: High frequency of pulmonary lymphangioleiomyomatosis in women with tuberous sclerosis complex, *Mayo Clin Proc* 75:591–594, 2000.
361. Matsui K, Tatsuguchi A, Valencia J, et al: Extrapulmonary lymphangioleiomyomatosis (LAM): clinicopathologic features in 22 cases, *Hum Pathol* 31:1242–1248, 2000.
362. Carsillo T, Astrinidis A, Henske EP: Mutations in the tuberous sclerosis complex gene TSC2 are a cause of sporadic pulmonary lymphangioleiomyomatosis, *Proc Natl Acad Sci USA* 97:6085–6090, 2000.
363. McCormack FX, Inoue Y, Moss J, et al: Efficacy and safety of sirolimus in lymphangioleiomyomatosis, *N Engl J Med* 364:1595–1606, 2011.
364. Enzinger FM: Angiomatoid malignant fibrous histiocytoma: a distinct fibrohistiocytic tumor of children and young adults simulating a vascular neoplasm, *Cancer* 44:2147–2157, 1979.
365. Fletcher CD: Angiomatoid "malignant fibrous histiocytoma": an immunohistochemical study indicative of myoid differentiation, *Hum Pathol* 22:563–568, 1991.
366. Costa MJ, Weiss SW: Angiomatoid malignant fibrous histiocytoma. A follow-up study of 108 cases with evaluation of possible histologic predictors of outcome, *Am J Surg Pathol* 14:1126–1132, 1990.
367. Fanburg-Smith JC, Miettinen M: Angiomatoid "malignant" fibrous histiocytoma: a clinicopathologic study of 158 cases and further exploration of the myoid phenotype, *Hum Pathol* 30:1336–1343, 1999.
368. Li CS, Chan WP, Chen WT, et al: MRI of angiomatoid fibrous histiocytoma, *Skeletal Radiol* 33:604–608, 2004.
369. Weinreb I, Rubin BP, Goldblum JR: Pleomorphic angiomatoid fibrous histiocytoma: a case confirmed by fluorescence in situ hybridization analysis for EWSR1 rearrangement, *J Cutan Pathol* 35:855–860, 2008.
370. Billings SD, Folpe AL: Cutaneous and subcutaneous fibrohistiocytic tumors of intermediate malignancy: an update, *Am J Dermatopathol* 26:141–155, 2004.
371. Schaefer IM, Fletcher CD: Myxoid variant of so-called angiomatoid "malignant fibrous histiocytoma": clinicopathologic characterization in a series of 21 cases, *Am J Surg Pathol* 38:816–823, 2014.
372. Pettinato G, Manivel JC, De Rosa G, et al: Angiomatoid malignant fibrous histiocytoma: cytologic, immunohistochemical, ultrastructural, and flow cytometric study of 20 cases, *Mod Pathol* 3:479–487, 1990.
373. Rossi S, Szuhai K, Ijszenga M, et al: EWSR1-CREB1 and EWSR1-ATF1 fusion genes in angiomatoid fibrous histiocytoma, *Clin Cancer Res* 13:7322–7328, 2007.
374. Hallor KH, Mertens F, Jin Y, et al: Fusion of the EWSR1 and ATF1 genes without expression of the MITF-M transcript in angiomatoid fibrous histiocytoma, *Genes Chromosomes Cancer* 44:97–102, 2005.
375. Antonescu CR, Dal Cin P, Nafa K, et al: EWSR1-CREB1 is the predominant gene fusion in angiomatoid fibrous histiocytoma, *Genes Chromosomes Cancer* 46:1051–1060, 2007.
376. Antonescu CR, Nafa K, Segal NH, et al: EWS-CREB1: a recurrent variant fusion in clear cell sarcoma—association with gastrointestinal location and absence of melanocytic differentiation, *Clin Cancer Res* 12:5356–5362, 2006.
377. Hallor KH, Micci F, Meis-Kindblom JM, et al: Fusion genes in angiomatoid fibrous histiocytoma, *Cancer Lett* 251:158–163, 2007.
378. Grossman LD, White IVRR, Arber DA: Angiomatoid fibrous histiocytoma, *Ann Plast Surg* 36:649–651, 1996.
379. Fisher C: Synovial sarcoma: ultrastructural and immunohistochemical features of epithelial differentiation in monophasic and biphasic tumors, *Hum Pathol* 17:996–1008, 1986.
380. Miettinen M, Virtanen I: Synovial sarcoma—a misnomer, *Am J Pathol* 117:18–25, 1984.
381. Schmidt D, Thum P, Harms D, et al: Synovial sarcoma in children and adolescents. A report from the Kiel Pediatric Tumor Registry, *Cancer* 67:1667–1672, 1991.
382. Chan JA, McMenamin ME, Fletcher CD: Synovial sarcoma in older patients: clinicopathological analysis of 32 cases with emphasis on unusual histological features, *Histopathology* 43:72–83, 2003.
383. Fisher C: Synovial sarcoma, *Ann Diagn Pathol* 2:401–421, 1998.
384. van de Rijn M, Barr FG, Xiong QB, et al: Radiation-associated synovial sarcoma, *Hum Pathol* 28:1325–1328, 1997.
385. Egger JF, Coindre JM, Benhattar J, et al: Radiation-associated synovial sarcoma: clinicopathologic and molecular analysis of two cases, *Mod Pathol* 15:998–1004, 2002.
386. Jong B, Shahabpour M, Spruyt D, et al: Imaging and differential diagnosis of synovial sarcoma, *J Belge Radiol* 75:335–339, 1992.
387. van de Rijn M, Barr FG, Xiong QB, et al: Poorly differentiated synovial sarcoma: an analysis of clinical, pathologic, and molecular genetic features, *Am J Surg Pathol* 23:106–112, 1999.
388. Farris KB, Reed RJ: Monophasic, glandular, synovial sarcomas and carcinomas of the soft tissues, *Arch Pathol Lab Med* 106:129–132, 1982.
389. Majeste RM, Beckman EN: Synovial sarcoma with an overwhelming epithelial component, *Cancer* 61:2527–2531, 1988.
390. Krane JF, Bertoni F, Fletcher CD: Myxoid synovial sarcoma: an underappreciated morphologic subset, *Mod Pathol* 12:456–462, 1999.
391. Winnepenninckx V, De Vos R, Debiec-Rychter M, et al: Calcifying/ossifying synovial sarcoma shows t(X;18) with SSX2 involvement and mitochondrial calcifications, *Histopathology* 38:141–145, 2001.
392. Miettinen M: Keratin subsets in spindle cell sarcomas. Keratins are widespread but synovial sarcoma contains a distinctive keratin polypeptide pattern and desmoplakins, *Am J Pathol* 138:505–513, 1991.
393. Folpe AL, Schmidt RA, Chapman D, et al: Poorly differentiated synovial sarcoma: immunohistochemical distinction from primitive neuroectodermal tumors and high-grade malignant peripheral nerve sheath tumors, *Am J Surg Pathol* 22:673–682, 1998.
394. Smith TA, Machen SK, Fisher C, et al: Usefulness of cytokeratin subsets for distinguishing monophasic synovial sarcoma from malignant peripheral nerve sheath tumor, *Am J Clin Pathol* 112:641–648, 1999.
395. Coindre JM, Pelmus M, Hostein I, et al: Should molecular testing be required for diagnosing synovial sarcoma? A prospective study of 204 cases, *Cancer* 98:2700–2707, 2003.
396. Pelmus M, Guillou L, Hostein I, et al: Monophasic fibrous and poorly differentiated synovial sarcoma: immunohistochemical reassessment of 60 t(X;18)(SYT-SSX)-positive cases, *Am J Surg Pathol* 26:1434–1440, 2002.
397. He R, Patel RM, Alkan S, et al: Immunostaining for SYT protein discriminates synovial sarcoma from other soft tissue tumors: analysis of 146 cases, *Mod Pathol* 20:522–528, 2007.
398. Terry J, Saito T, Subramanian S, et al: TLE1 as a diagnostic immunohistochemical marker for synovial sarcoma emerging from gene expression profiling studies, *Am J Surg Pathol* 31:240–246, 2007.
399. Kosemehmetoglu K, Vrana JA, Folpe AL: TLE1 expression is not specific for synovial sarcoma: a whole section study of 163 soft tissue and bone neoplasms, *Mod Pathol* 22:872–878, 2009.
400. Reeves BR, Smith S, Fisher C, et al: Characterization of the translocation between chromosomes X and 18 in human synovial sarcomas, *Oncogene* 4:373–378, 1989.
401. Knight J, Reeves B, Smith S, et al: Cytogenetic and molecular analysis of synovial sarcoma, *Int J Oncol* 1:747–752, 1992.
402. Clark J, Rocques PJ, Crew AJ, et al: Identification of novel genes, SYT and SSX, involved in the t(X;18)(p11.2;q11.2) translocation found in human synovial sarcoma, *Nat Genet* 7:502–508, 1994.
403. Skytting B, Nilsson G, Brodin B, et al: A novel fusion gene, SYT-SSX4, in synovial sarcoma, *J Natl Cancer Inst* 91:974–975, 1999.
404. Storlazzi CT, Mertens F, Mandahl N, et al: A novel fusion gene, SS18L1/SSX1, in synovial sarcoma, *Genes Chromosomes Cancer* 37:195–200, 2003.
405. Crew AJ, Clark J, Fisher C, et al: Fusion of SYT to two genes, SSX1 and SSX2, encoding proteins with homology to the Kruppel-associated box in human synovial sarcoma, *EMBO J* 14:2333–2340, 1995.
406. van de Rijn M, Barr FG, Collins MH, et al: Absence of SYT-SSX fusion products in soft tissue tumors other than synovial sarcoma, *Am J Clin Pathol* 112:43–49, 1999.
407. Poteat HT, Corson JM, Fletcher JA: Detection of chromosome 18 rearrangement in synovial sarcoma by fluorescence in situ hybridization, *Cancer Genet Cytogenet* 84:76–81, 1995.
408. Terry J, Barry TS, Horsman DE, et al: Fluorescence in situ hybridization for the detection of t(X;18)(p11.2;q11.2) in a synovial sarcoma tissue microarray using a breakapart-style probe, *Diagn Mol Pathol* 14:77–82, 2005.
409. Tsuji S, Hisaoka M, Morimitsu Y, et al: Detection of SYT-SSX fusion transcripts in synovial sarcoma by reverse transcription-polymerase chain reaction using archival paraffin-embedded tissues, *Am J Pathol* 153:1807–1812, 1998.
410. Lasota J, Jasinski M, Debiec-Rychter M, et al: Detection of the SYT-SSX fusion transcripts in formaldehyde-fixed, paraffin-embedded tissue: a reverse transcription polymerase chain reaction amplification assay useful in the diagnosis of synovial sarcoma, *Mod Pathol* 11:626–633, 1998.
411. Guillou L, Coindre J, Gallagher G, et al: Detection of the synovial sarcoma translocation t(X;18) (SYT;SSX) in paraffin-embedded tissues using reverse transcriptase-polymerase chain reaction: a reliable and powerful diagnostic tool for pathologists. A molecular analysis of 221 mesenchymal tumors fixed in different fixatives, *Hum Pathol* 32:105–112, 2001.
412. Kawai A, Woodruff J, Healey JH, et al: SYT-SSX gene fusion as a determinant of morphology and prognosis in synovial sarcoma, *N Engl J Med* 338:153–160, 1998.
413. Antonescu CR, Kawai A, Leung DH, et al: Strong association of SYT-SSX fusion type and morphologic epithelial differentiation in synovial sarcoma, *Diagn Mol Pathol* 9:1–8, 2000.
414. Panagopoulos I, Mertens F, Isaksson M, et al: Clinical impact of molecular and cytogenetic findings in synovial sarcoma, *Genes Chromosomes Cancer* 31:362–372, 2001.
415. Ladanyi M, Antonescu CR, Leung DH, et al: Impact of SYT-SSX fusion type on the clinical behavior of synovial sarcoma: a multi-institutional retrospective study of 243 patients, *Cancer Res* 62:135–140, 2002.
416. Guillou L, Benhattar J, Bonichon F, et al: Histologic grade, but not SYT-SSX fusion type, is an important prognostic factor in patients with synovial sarcoma: a multicenter, retrospective analysis, *J Clin Oncol* 22:4040–4050, 2004.
417. Nakayama R, Mitani S, Nakagawa T, et al: Gene expression profiling of synovial sarcoma: distinct signature of poorly differentiated type, *Am J Surg Pathol* 34:1599–1607, 2010.
418. Schaefer IM, Fletcher CD, Hornick JL: Loss of H3K27 trimethylation distinguishes malignant peripheral nerve sheath tumors from histologic mimics, *Mod Pathol* 29:4–13, 2016.

419. Cleven AH, Sannaa GA, Briaire-de Bruijn I, et al: Loss of H3K27 tri-methylation is a diagnostic marker for malignant peripheral nerve sheath tumors and an indicator for an inferior survival, *Mod Pathol* 29:582–590, 2016.
420. Bahrami A, Folpe AL: Adult-type fibrosarcoma: a reevaluation of 163 putative cases diagnosed at a single institution over a 48-year period, *Am J Surg Pathol* 34:1504–1513, 2010.
421. Lewis JJ, Antonescu CR, Leung DH, et al: Synovial sarcoma: a multivariate analysis of prognostic factors in 112 patients with primary localized tumors of the extremity, *J Clin Oncol* 18:2087–2094, 2000.
422. Machen SK, Easley KA, Goldblum JR: Synovial sarcoma of the extremities: a clinicopathologic study of 34 cases, including semi-quantitative analysis of spindled, epithelial, and poorly differentiated areas, *Am J Surg Pathol* 23:268–275, 1999.
423. Trassard M, Le Doussal V, Hacene K, et al: Prognostic factors in localized primary synovial sarcoma: a multicenter study of 128 adult patients, *J Clin Oncol* 19:525–534, 2001.
424. Michal M, Fanburg-Smith JC, Lasota J, et al: Minute synovial sarcomas of the hands and feet: a clinicopathologic study of 21 tumors less than 1 cm, *Am J Surg Pathol* 30:721–726, 2006.
425. Antonescu CR, Leung DH, Dudas M, et al: Alterations of cell cycle regulators in localized synovial sarcoma: a multifactorial study with prognostic implications, *Am J Pathol* 156:977–983, 2000.
426. Erlandson RA, Woodruff JM: Peripheral nerve sheath tumors: an electron microscopic study of 43 cases, *Cancer* 49:273–287, 1982.
427. Ducatman BS, Scheithauer BW, Piepgras DG, et al: Malignant peripheral nerve sheath tumors in childhood, *J Neurooncol* 2:241–248, 1984.
428. King AA, Debaun MR, Riccardi VM, et al: Malignant peripheral nerve sheath tumors in neurofibromatosis 1, *Am J Med Genet* 93:388–392, 2000.
429. Evans DG, Baser ME, McGaughran J, et al: Malignant peripheral nerve sheath tumours in neurofibromatosis 1, *J Med Genet* 39:311–314, 2002.
430. McCaughan JA, Holloway SM, Davidson R, et al: Further evidence of the increased risk for malignant peripheral nerve sheath tumour from a Scottish cohort of patients with neurofibromatosis type 1, *J Med Genet* 44:463–466, 2007.
431. Allison KH, Patel RM, Goldblum JR, et al: Superficial malignant peripheral nerve sheath tumor: a rare and challenging diagnosis, *Am J Clin Pathol* 124:685–692, 2005.
432. Fletcher CD, Fernando IN, Braimbridge MV, et al: Malignant nerve sheath tumour arising in a ganglioneuroma, *Histopathology* 12:445–448, 1988.
433. Ghali VS, Gold JE, Vincent RA, et al: Malignant peripheral nerve sheath tumor arising spontaneously from retroperitoneal ganglioneuroma: a case report, review of the literature, and immunohistochemical study, *Hum Pathol* 23:72–75, 1992.
434. Foley KM, Woodruff JM, Ellis FT, et al: Radiation-induced malignant and atypical peripheral nerve sheath tumors, *Ann Neurol* 7:311–318, 1980.
435. Ducatman BS, Scheithauer BW: Postirradiation neurofibrosarcoma, *Cancer* 51:1028–1033, 1983.
436. Hruban RH, Shiu MH, Senie RT, et al: Malignant peripheral nerve sheath tumors of the buttock and lower extremity. A study of 43 cases, *Cancer* 66:1253–1265, 1990.
437. Ducatman BS, Scheithauer BW: Malignant peripheral nerve sheath tumors with divergent differentiation, *Cancer* 54:1049–1057, 1984.
438. Daimaru Y, Hashimoto H, Enjoji M: Malignant "triton" tumors: a clinicopathologic and immunohistochemical study of nine cases, *Hum Pathol* 15:768–778, 1984.
439. Morphopoulos GD, Banerjee SS, Ali HH, et al: Malignant peripheral nerve sheath tumour with vascular differentiation: a report of four cases, *Histopathology* 28:401–410, 1996.
440. Christensen WN, Strong EW, Bains MS, et al: Neuroendocrine differentiation in the glandular peripheral nerve sheath tumor. Pathologic distinction from the biphasic synovial sarcoma with glands, *Am J Surg Pathol* 12:417–426, 1988.
441. Woodruff JM, Christensen WN: Glandular peripheral nerve sheath tumors, *Cancer* 72:3618–3628, 1993.
442. Lee W, Teckie S, Wiesner T, et al: PRC2 is recurrently inactivated through EED or SUZ12 loss in malignant peripheral nerve sheath tumors, *Nat Genet* 46:1227–1232, 2014.
443. Prieto-Granada CN, Wiesner T, Messina JL, et al: Loss of H3K27me3 expression is a highly sensitive marker for sporadic and radiation-induced MPNST, *Am J Surg Pathol* 40:479–489, 2016.
444. Le Guellec S, Decouvelaere AV, Filleron T, et al: Malignant peripheral nerve sheath tumor is a challenging diagnosis: a systematic pathology review, immunohistochemistry, and molecular analysis in 160 patients from the French sarcoma group database, *Am J Surg Pathol* 40:896–908, 2016.
445. Fisher C, Carter RL, Ramachandra S, et al: Peripheral nerve sheath differentiation in malignant soft tissue tumours: an ultrastructural and immunohistochemical study, *Histopathology* 20:115–125, 1992.
446. Hirose T, Hasegawa T, Kudo E, et al: Malignant peripheral nerve sheath tumors: an immunohistochemical study in relation to ultrastructural features, *Hum Pathol* 23:865–870, 1992.
447. Basu TN, Gutmann DH, Fletcher JA, et al: Aberrant regulation of ras proteins in malignant tumour cells from type 1 neurofibromatosis patients, *Nature* 356:713–715, 1992.
448. Zhou H, Coffin CM, Perkins SL, et al: Malignant peripheral nerve sheath tumor: a comparison of grade, immunophenotype, and cell cycle/growth activation marker expression in sporadic and neurofibromatosis 1-related lesions, *Am J Surg Pathol* 27:1337–1345, 2003.
449. Berghmans S, Murphey RD, Wienholds E, et al: Tp53 mutant zebrafish develop malignant peripheral nerve sheath tumors, *Proc Natl Acad Sci USA* 102:407–412, 2005.
450. De Raedt T, Beert E, Pasmant E, et al: PRC2 loss amplifies Ras-driven transcription and confers sensitivity to BRD4-based therapies, *Nature* 514:247–251, 2014.
451. Smith TA, Machen SK, Fisher C, et al: Usefulness of cytokeratin subsets for distinguishing monophasic synovial sarcoma from malignant peripheral nerve sheath tumor, *Am J Clin Pathol* 112:641–648, 1999.
452. Ladanyi M, Woodruff JM, Scheithauer BW, et al: Re: O'Sullivan MJ, Kyriakos M, Zhu X, Wick MR, Swanson PE, Dehner LP, Humphrey PA, Pfeifer JD: Malignant peripheral nerve sheath tumors with t(X;18). A pathologic and molecular genetic study, *Mod Pathol* 13:1336–1346, 2000, *Mod Pathol* 14:733–737, 2001.
453. Coindre JM, Hostein I, Benhattar J, et al: Malignant peripheral nerve sheath tumors are t(X;18)-negative sarcomas. Molecular analysis of 25 cases occurring in neurofibromatosis type 1 patients, using two different RT-PCR-based methods of detection, *Mod Pathol* 15:589–592, 2002.
454. King R, Busam K, Rosai J: Metastatic malignant melanoma resembling malignant peripheral nerve sheath tumor: report of 16 cases, *Am J Surg Pathol* 23:1499–1505, 1999.
455. Ducatman BS, Scheithauer BW, Piepgras DG, et al: Malignant peripheral nerve sheath tumors. A clinicopathologic study of 120 cases, *Cancer* 57:2006–2021, 1986.
456. Wang X, Bledsoe KL, Graham RP, et al: Recurrent PAX3-MAML3 fusion in biphenotypic sinonasal sarcoma, *Nat Genet* 46:666–668, 2014.
457. Fritchie KJ, Jin L, Wang X, et al: Fusion gene profile of biphenotypic sinonasal sarcoma: an analysis of 44 cases, *Histopathology* 69:930–936, 2016.
458. Rooper LM, Huang SC, Antonescu CR, et al: Biphenotypic sinonasal sarcoma: an expanded immunoprofile including consistent nuclear beta-catenin positivity and absence of SOX10 expression, *Hum Pathol* 55:44–50, 2016.
459. Huang SC, Ghossein RA, Bishop JA, et al: Novel PAX3-NCOA1 fusions in biphenotypic sinonasal sarcoma with focal rhabdomyoblastic differentiation, *Am J Surg Pathol* 40:51–59, 2016.
460. Wong WJ, Lauria A, Hornick JL, et al: Alternate PAX3-FOXO1 oncogenic fusion in biphenotypic sinonasal sarcoma, *Genes Chromosomes Cancer* 55:25–29, 2016.
461. Evans HL: Low-grade fibromyxoid sarcoma. A report of two metastasizing neoplasms having a deceptively benign appearance, *Am J Clin Pathol* 88:615–619, 1987.
462. Evans HL: Low-grade fibromyxoid sarcoma. A report of 12 cases, *Am J Surg Pathol* 17:595–600, 1993.
463. Goodlad JR, Mentzel T, Fletcher CD: Low grade fibromyxoid sarcoma: clinicopathological analysis of eleven new cases in support of a distinct entity, *Histopathology* 26:229–237, 1995.
464. Folpe AL, Lane KL, Paull G, et al: Low-grade fibromyxoid sarcoma and hyalinizing spindle cell tumor with giant rosettes: a clinicopathologic study of 73 cases supporting their identity and assessing the impact of high-grade areas, *Am J Surg Pathol* 24:1353–1360, 2000.
465. Zamecnik M, Michal M: Low-grade fibromyxoid sarcoma: a report of eight cases with histologic, immunohistochemical, and ultrastructural study, *Ann Diagn Pathol* 4:207–217, 2000.
466. Lane KL, Shannon RJ, Weiss SW: Hyalinizing spindle cell tumor with giant rosettes: a distinctive tumor closely resembling low-grade fibromyxoid sarcoma, *Am J Surg Pathol* 21:1481–1488, 1997.
467. Billings SD, Giblen G, Fanburg-Smith JC: Superficial low-grade fibromyxoid sarcoma (Evans tumor): a clinicopathologic analysis of 19 cases with a unique observation in the pediatric population, *Am J Surg Pathol* 29:204–210, 2005.
468. Guillou L, Benhattar J, Gengler C, et al: Translocation-positive low-grade fibromyxoid sarcoma: clinicopathologic and molecular analysis of a series expanding the morphologic spectrum and suggesting potential relationship to sclerosing epithelioid fibrosarcoma: a study from the French Sarcoma Group, *Am J Surg Pathol* 31:1387–1402, 2007.
469. Moller E, Hornick JL, Magnusson L, et al: FUS-CREB3L2/L1-positive sarcomas show a specific gene expression profile with upregulation of CD24 and FOXL1, *Clin Cancer Res* 17:2646–2656, 2011.
470. Mertens F, Fletcher CD, Antonescu CR, et al: Clinicopathologic and molecular genetic characterization of low-grade fibromyxoid sarcoma, and cloning of a novel FUS/CREB3L1 fusion gene, *Lab Invest* 85:408–415, 2005.
471. Panagopoulos I, Storlazzi CT, Fletcher CD, et al: The chimeric FUS/CREB3l2 gene is specific for low-grade fibromyxoid sarcoma, *Genes Chromosomes Cancer* 40:218–228, 2004.
472. Matsuyama A, Hisaoka M, Shimajiri S, et al: Molecular detection of FUS-CREB3L2 fusion transcripts in low-grade fibromyxoid sarcoma using formalin-fixed, paraffin-embedded tissue specimens, *Am J Surg Pathol* 30:1077–1084, 2006.
473. Patel RM, Downs-Kelly E, Dandekar MN, et al: FUS (16p11) gene rearrangement as detected by fluorescence in-situ hybridization in cutaneous low-grade fibromyxoid sarcoma: a potential diagnostic tool, *Am J Dermatopathol* 33:140–143, 2011.
474. Doyle LA, Wang W, Dal Cin P, et al: MUC4 is a sensitive and extremely useful marker for sclerosing epithelioid fibrosarcoma: association with FUS gene rearrangement, *Am J Surg Pathol* 36:1444–1451, 2012.
475. Evans HL: Low-grade fibromyxoid sarcoma: a clinicopathologic study of 33 cases with long-term follow-up, *Am J Surg Pathol* 35:1450–1462, 2011.
476. Mentzel T, Dry S, Katenkamp D, et al: Low-grade myofibroblastic sarcoma: analysis of 18 cases in the spectrum of myofibroblastic tumors, *Am J Surg Pathol* 22:1228–1238, 1998.
477. Montgomery E, Goldblum JR, Fisher C: Myofibrosarcoma: a clinicopathologic study, *Am J Surg Pathol* 25:219–228, 2001.
478. Fisher C: Myofibroblastic malignancies, *Adv Anat Pathol* 11:190–201, 2004.
479. Eyden B: Electron microscopy in the study of myofibroblastic lesions, *Semin Diagn Pathol* 20:13–24, 2003.
480. Fisher C: Myofibrosarcoma, *Virchows Arch* 445:215–223, 2004.
481. Cavazzana AO, Schmidt D, Ninfo V, et al: Spindle cell rhabdomyosarcoma. A prognostically favorable variant of rhabdomyosarcoma, *Am J Surg Pathol* 16:229–235, 1992.

482. Nascimento AF, Fletcher CD: Spindle cell rhabdomyosarcoma in adults, *Am J Surg Pathol* 29:1106–1113, 2005.
483. Mentzel T, Katenkamp D: Sclerosing, pseudovascular rhabdomyosarcoma in adults. Clinicopathological and immunohistochemical analysis of three cases, *Virchows Arch* 436:305–311, 2000.
484. Stock N, Chibon F, Binh MB, et al: Adult-type rhabdomyosarcoma: analysis of 57 cases with clinicopathologic description, identification of 3 morphologic patterns and prognosis, *Am J Surg Pathol* 33:1850–1859, 2009.
485. Folpe AL, McKenney JK, Bridge JA, et al: Sclerosing rhabdomyosarcoma in adults: report of four cases of a hyalinizing, matrix-rich variant of rhabdomyosarcoma that may be confused with osteosarcoma, chondrosarcoma, or angiosarcoma, *Am J Surg Pathol* 26:1175–1183, 2002.
486. Leuschner I, Newton WA, Jr, Schmidt D, et al: Spindle cell variants of embryonal rhabdomyosarcoma in the paratesticular region. A report of the Intergroup Rhabdomyosarcoma Study, *Am J Surg Pathol* 17:221–230, 1993.
487. Kohsaka S, Shukla N, Ameur N, et al: A recurrent neomorphic mutation in MYOD1 defines a clinically aggressive subset of embryonal rhabdomyosarcoma associated with PI3K-AKT pathway mutations, *Nat Genet* 46:595–600, 2014.
488. Agaram NP, Chen CL, Zhang L, et al: Recurrent MYOD1 mutations in pediatric and adult sclerosing and spindle cell rhabdomyosarcomas: evidence for a common pathogenesis, *Genes Chromosomes Cancer* 53:779–787, 2014.
489. Rekhi B, Upadhyay P, Ramteke MP, et al: MYOD1 (L122R) mutations are associated with spindle cell and sclerosing rhabdomyosarcomas with aggressive clinical outcomes, *Mod Pathol* 29:1532–1540, 2016.
490. Gil-Benso R, Carda-Batalla C, Navarro-Fos S, et al: Cytogenetic study of a spindle-cell rhabdomyosarcoma of the parotid gland, *Cancer Genet Cytogenet* 109:150–153, 1999.
491. Debiec-Rychter M, Hagemeijer A, Sciot R: Spindle-cell rhabdomyosarcoma with 2q36 approximately q37 involvement, *Cancer Genet Cytogenet* 140:62–65, 2003.
492. Mosquera JM, Sboner A, Zhang L, et al: Recurrent NCOA2 gene rearrangements in congenital/infantile spindle cell rhabdomyosarcoma, *Genes Chromosomes Cancer* 52:538–550, 2013.
493. Alaggio R, Zhang L, Sung YS, et al: A molecular study of pediatric spindle and sclerosing rhabdomyosarcoma: identification of novel and recurrent VGLL2-related fusions in infantile cases, *Am J Surg Pathol* 40:224–235, 2016.
494. Enzinger FM: Clear-cell sarcoma of tendons and aponeuroses. An analysis of 21 cases, *Cancer* 18:1163–1174, 1965.
495. Chung EB, Enzinger FM: Malignant melanoma of soft parts. A reassessment of clear cell sarcoma, *Am J Surg Pathol* 7:405–413, 1983.
496. Sara AS, Evans HL, Benjamin RS: Malignant melanoma of soft parts (clear cell sarcoma). A study of 17 cases, with emphasis on prognostic factors, *Cancer* 65:367–374, 1990.
497. Graadt van Roggen JF, Mooi WJ, Hogendoorn PC: Clear cell sarcoma of tendons and aponeuroses (malignant melanoma of soft parts) and cutaneous melanoma: exploring the histogenetic relationship between these two clinicopathological entities, *J Pathol* 186:3–7, 1998.
498. Segal NH, Pavlidis P, Noble WS, et al: Classification of clear-cell sarcoma as a subtype of melanoma by genomic profiling, *J Clin Oncol* 21:1775–1781, 2003.
499. Zambrano E, Reyes-Mugica M, Franchi A, et al: An osteoclast-rich tumor of the gastrointestinal tract with features resembling clear cell sarcoma of soft parts: reports of 6 cases of a GIST simulator, *Int J Surg Pathol* 11:75–81, 2003.
500. Kosemehmetoglu K, Folpe AL: Clear cell sarcoma of tendons and aponeuroses, and osteoclast-rich tumour of the gastrointestinal tract with features resembling clear cell sarcoma of soft parts: a review and update, *J Clin Pathol* 63:416–423, 2010.
501. Rubin BP, Fletcher JA, Renshaw AA: Clear cell sarcoma of soft parts: report of a case primary in the kidney with cytogenetic confirmation, *Am J Surg Pathol* 23:589–594, 1999.
502. Lucas DR, Nascimento AG, Sim FH: Clear cell sarcoma of soft tissues. Mayo Clinic experience with 35 cases, *Am J Surg Pathol* 16:1197–1204, 1992.
503. Kawai A, Hosono A, Nakayama R, et al: Clear cell sarcoma of tendons and aponeuroses: a study of 75 patients, *Cancer* 109:109–116, 2007.
504. Hisaoka M, Ishida T, Kuo TT, et al: Clear cell sarcoma of soft tissue: a clinicopathologic, immunohistochemical, and molecular analysis of 33 cases, *Am J Surg Pathol* 32:452–460, 2008.
505. Kindblom LG, Lodding P, Angervall L: Clear-cell sarcoma of tendons and aponeuroses. An immunohistochemical and electron microscopic analysis indicating neural crest origin, *Virchows Arch A Pathol Anat Histopathol* 401:109–128, 1983.
506. Antonescu CR, Tschernyavsky SJ, Woodruff JM, et al: Molecular diagnosis of clear cell sarcoma: detection of EWS-ATF1 and MITF-M transcripts and histopathological and ultrastructural analysis of 12 cases, *J Mol Diagn* 4:44–52, 2002.
507. Stenman G, Kindblom LG, Angervall L: Reciprocal translocation t(12;22)(q13;q13) in clear-cell sarcoma of tendons and aponeuroses, *Genes Chromosomes Cancer* 4:122–127, 1992.
508. Reeves BR, Fletcher CD, Gusterson BA: Translocation t(12;22)(q13;q13) is a nonrandom rearrangement in clear cell sarcoma, *Cancer Genet Cytogenet* 64:101–103, 1992.
509. Zucman J, Delattre O, Desmaze C, et al: EWS and ATF-1 gene fusion induced by t(12;22) translocation in malignant melanoma of soft parts, *Nat Genet* 4:341–345, 1993.
510. Fujimura Y, Ohno T, Siddique H, et al: The EWS-ATF-1 gene involved in malignant melanoma of soft parts with t(12;22) chromosome translocation, encodes a constitutive transcriptional activator, *Oncogene* 12:159–167, 1996.
511. Jishage M, Fujino T, Yamazaki Y, et al: Identification of target genes for EWS/ATF-1 chimeric transcription factor, *Oncogene* 22:41–49, 2003.
512. Schaefer KL, Brachwitz K, Wai DH, et al: Expression profiling of t(12;22) positive clear cell sarcoma of soft tissue cell lines reveals characteristic up-regulation of potential new marker genes including ERBB3, *Cancer Res* 64:3395–3405, 2004.
513. Davis IJ, McFadden AW, Zhang Y, et al: Identification of the receptor tyrosine kinase c-Met and its ligand, hepatocyte growth factor, as therapeutic targets in clear cell sarcoma, *Cancer Res* 70:639–645, 2010.
514. Wang WL, Mayordomo E, Zhang W, et al: Detection and characterization of EWSR1/ATF1 and EWSR1/CREB1 chimeric transcripts in clear cell sarcoma (melanoma of soft parts), *Mod Pathol* 22:1201–1209, 2009.
515. Coindre JM, Hostein I, Terrier P, et al: Diagnosis of clear cell sarcoma by real-time reverse transcriptase-polymerase chain reaction analysis of paraffin embedded tissues: clinicopathologic and molecular analysis of 44 patients from the French sarcoma group, *Cancer* 107:1055–1064, 2006.
516. Langezaal SM, Graadt van Roggen JF, Cleton-Jansen AM, et al: Malignant melanoma is genetically distinct from clear cell sarcoma of tendons and aponeurosis (malignant melanoma of soft parts), *Br J Cancer* 84:535–538, 2001.
517. Jones RL, Constantinidou A, Thway K, et al: Chemotherapy in clear cell sarcoma, *Med Oncol* 28:859–863, 2011.
518. Hornick JL, Fletcher CD: Pseudomyogenic hemangioendothelioma: a distinctive, often multicentric tumor with indolent behavior, *Am J Surg Pathol* 35:190–201, 2011.
519. Mirra JM, Kessler S, Bhuta S, et al: The fibroma-like variant of epithelioid sarcoma. A fibrohistiocytic/myoid cell lesion often confused with benign and malignant spindle cell tumors, *Cancer* 69:1382–1395, 1992.
520. Billings SD, Folpe AL, Weiss SW: Epithelioid sarcoma-like hemangioendothelioma, *Am J Surg Pathol* 27:48–57, 2003.
521. Hung YP, Fletcher CD, Hornick JL: FOSB is a useful diagnostic marker for pseudomyogenic hemangioendothelioma, *Am J Surg Pathol* 41:596–606, 2017.
522. Trombetta D, Magnusson L, von Steyern FV, et al: Translocation t(7;19)(q22;q13)—a recurrent chromosome aberration in pseudomyogenic hemangioendothelioma? *Cancer Genet* 204:211–215, 2011.
523. Walther C, Tayebwa J, Lilljebjorn H, et al: A novel SERPINE1-FOSB fusion gene results in transcriptional up-regulation of FOSB in pseudomyogenic haemangioendothelioma, *J Pathol* 232:534–540, 2014.
524. Miettinen M, Fanburg-Smith JC, Virolainen M, et al: Epithelioid sarcoma: an immunohistochemical analysis of 112 classical and variant cases and a discussion of the differential diagnosis, *Hum Pathol* 30:934–942, 1999.
525. Chbani L, Guillou L, Terrier P, et al: Epithelioid sarcoma: a clinicopathologic and immunohistochemical analysis of 106 cases from the French sarcoma group, *Am J Clin Pathol* 131:222–227, 2009.
526. Hornick JL, Dal Cin P, Fletcher CD: Loss of INI1 expression is characteristic of both conventional and proximal-type epithelioid sarcoma, *Am J Surg Pathol* 33:542–550, 2009.
527. Gladdy RA, Qin LX, Moraco N, et al: Do radiation-associated soft tissue sarcomas have the same prognosis as sporadic soft tissue sarcomas?, *J Clin Oncol* 28:2064–2069, 2010.
528. Fletcher CD, Gustafson P, Rydholm A, et al: Clinicopathologic re-evaluation of 100 malignant fibrous histiocytomas: prognostic relevance of subclassification, *J Clin Oncol* 19:3045–3050, 2001.
529. Deyrup AT, Haydon RC, Huo D, et al: Myoid differentiation and prognosis in adult pleomorphic sarcomas of the extremity: an analysis of 92 cases, *Cancer* 98:805–813, 2003.

4

Pediatric Spindle Cell Tumors

Cheryl M. Coffin, MD, and Rita Alaggio, MD

Spindle cell tumors in children and adolescents encompass a wide range of benign, intermediate, and malignant neoplasms, with the predominant phenotypic category being fibroblastic-myofibroblastic tumors. The most frequent spindle cell sarcomas of childhood include spindle cell and embryonal rhabdomyosarcoma (RMS), malignant peripheral nerve sheath tumor, synovial sarcoma, leiomyosarcoma, and various fibroblastic-myofibroblastic sarcomas.[1,2] The majority of the nonrhabdomyosarcomatous spindle cell sarcomas occur more frequently in adults. In this chapter, the focus is on the fibroblastic-myofibroblastic tumors that occur predominantly in children and adolescents, and on several other spindle cell neoplasms that occur principally in younger patients. Round cell tumors are discussed in Chapter 8.

When confronted with a spindle cell tumor in a child or adolescent, the considerations for the pathologist include the following[3]:

1. Appropriate handling and triage of the fresh specimen to optimize diagnosis. For example, acquisition of fresh tissue for cytogenetic analysis, frozen tissue for molecular diagnostic tests, and a sample preserved for ultrastructural analysis may be useful. This is in addition to conventional light microscopy and immunohistochemistry on formalin-fixed, paraffin-embedded tissue.
2. Careful consideration of differential diagnosis. The range of spindle cell tumors includes reactive or pseudosarcomatous proliferations, as well as benign, intermediate, and malignant neoplasms. The pathologic diagnosis is critical for clinical management of these lesions, and morphologic overlap can present a challenge in classification.
3. Ancillary diagnostic techniques. Immunohistochemistry is an important diagnostic adjunct, especially for phenotypic classification, but does not generally allow a distinction between benign and malignant neoplasms within a specific group. Further evaluation with cytogenetic or molecular diagnostic tests can, in some cases, facilitate a specific diagnosis.

Fibroblastic-Myofibroblastic Tumors

Mesenchymal tumors with fibroblastic and myofibroblastic components are an important group of neoplasms in childhood and adolescence.[4-12] They account for approximately 12% of soft tissue tumors in the first two decades of life. The histologic similarities, differences in biologic potential, and clinical and molecular variations in this interesting group of lesions create diagnostic challenges. Nonetheless, precise classification is essential for treatment, prognosis, and, in some instances, genetic counseling (Table 4.1).[6,13] Histologically benign lesions are generally classified as fibromas or fibromatoses and malignant lesions as various types of sarcoma. In recent years, the concept of intermediate or "borderline" fibroblastic-myofibroblastic tumors has been refined for lesions with a tendency for local recurrence or very rare metastases,

Table 4.1 Morphologic and Genetic Classification of Fibroblastic-Myofibroblastic Proliferations of Childhood and Adolescence

Type of Lesion	Genetic Properties
Benign Lesions	
Nodular fasciitis	t(7;22)(p13;q13) with *MYH9-USP6* gene fusion
Cranial fasciitis	Insufficient data
Other fasciitis and myositis variants	Insufficient data
Fibromas	
Gardner fibroma	*APC* mutation in patient
Cardiac fibroma	del(9)(q22) or somatic copy number losses involving *PTCH1* gene
Fibromatoses	
Desmoid fibromatosis	Trisomies 8 and 20, *APC* or *CTNNB1* mutation, del(5)(q)
Infantile myofibromatosis	Mutations in *PDGFRB, NDRG4, NOTCH3*
Fibromatosis colli	Insufficient data
Infantile digital fibroma	Insufficient data
Fibrous hamartoma of infancy	*EGFR* mutations
Calcifying aponeurotic fibroma	*FN1-EGF* gene fusion
Lipofibromatosis	Insufficient data
Juvenile nasopharyngeal fibroma	*APC* or *CTNNB1* mutations
Hyaline fibromatosis	*ANTXR2 (CMG2) mutation*
Superficial fibromatosis (plantar, palmar)	Autosomal dominant
Intermediate Neoplasms	
Inflammatory myofibroblastic tumor	*ALK, ROS1, PDGFRB, RET,* or *NTRK3* gene rearrangements
Infantile fibrosarcoma	t(12;15)(p13;q25) with *ETV6-NTRK3* gene fusion; *LMNA-NTRK1* gene fusion; trisomies 8, 11, 17, 20
Primitive myxoid mesenchymal tumor of infancy	*BCOR* internal tandem duplications
Sarcomas	
Low-grade fibromyxoid sarcoma	*FUS-CREB3L2, FUS-CREB3L1,* or *EWSR1-CREB3L1* gene fusion
Myofibrosarcoma	Insufficient data
Infantile rhabdomyofibrosarcoma	Insufficient data

Data from references 6, 10, 12, and 13.

which may not be predictable on clinical or morphologic grounds. Many of these neoplasms of intermediate biologic potential have a predilection for children and young adults.

A summary of fibroblastic-myofibroblastic tumors in the first two decades of life is shown in Table 4.2.[5,8,9,11,13,14]

Table 4.2 Fibroblastic-Myofibroblastic Tumors in Children and Adolescents: Summary of 515 Cases from Six Series

Diagnosis	Number	Percent
Desmoid fibromatosis	151	29
Infantile myofibromatosis	60	12
Fibromatosis colli	49	10
Infantile digital fibroma	18	3
Fibrous hamartoma of infancy	43	8
Calcifying aponeurotic fibroma	11	2
Juvenile nasopharyngeal fibroma	13	3
Superficial (plantar and palmar) fibromatosis	47	9
Hyaline fibromatosis	1	<1
Fibromatosis, not otherwise classified[a]	89	17
Fibrosarcoma	33	6

[a]Category includes congenital keloid and visceral and skeletal fibromatoses that were not otherwise designated.
Data from references 5, 8, 9, 11, and 14.

Benign Tumors That Mimic Sarcomas

Nodular Fasciitis

Nodular fasciitis is a pseudosarcomatous fibroblastic-myofibroblastic proliferation (see also Chapter 3). Both the clinical and pathologic diagnoses present pitfalls in recognition because nodular fasciitis simulates a sarcoma, with its rapid growth and high cellularity.[15-17] In some cases, atypia and mitotic activity further contribute to the difficulty in distinguishing nodular fasciitis from higher-grade neoplasms.

Clinical Features

Up to 20% of cases occur in children and adolescents, with a slight male predominance.[16] Most are solitary. All areas of the body can be affected, including the head and neck, trunk, and extremities.[15,18] In young patients, nodular fasciitis is more frequent in the second decade of life and usually occurs after 5 years of age, although infants and young children are sometimes affected. The rapidly growing, sometimes tender, or painful nodule can occur in subcutaneous or deep soft tissue, including skeletal muscle and fascia. However, approximately 80% are subcutaneous. Unusual sites include upper respiratory tract and oral cavity submucosa and joint spaces.[18,19]

Pathologic Features

Grossly, nodular fasciitis appears as a round or ovoid, unencapsulated variegated soft tissue mass with a rubbery or myxoid cut surface.[15-17,20] Histologically, the cellular phase of nodular fasciitis consists of plump, spindled myofibroblastic and ganglion-like mesenchymal cells in whorls, interlacing fascicles, and sheets (Fig. 4.1A). Clefts or clear slits occur between cells, and the background varies from myxoid or mucoid to collagenous (see Fig. 4.1B). Microcysts with mucoid material in the lumina can be present (see Fig. 4.1C). Sparse chronic inflammation, extravasated erythrocytes, feathery areas of spindle cells in the center of the lesion with a "tissue culture" pattern, and marginal fat necrosis are often seen. In earlier stages, the pattern is predominantly myxoid. Well-developed lesions display osteoclast-like multinucleated giant cells intermingled with spindled and ganglion-like cells (see Fig. 4.1D). In later stages, keloidal collagen and a more fibrous appearance predominate. Histologic variations include cartilaginous metaplasia, calcification, and heterotopic ossification.

Immunohistochemistry

As is the case for most fibroblastic/myofibroblastic lesions, immunohistochemistry plays a minor role in the diagnosis of nodular fasciitis. The fibroblasts and myofibroblasts demonstrate reactivity for vimentin,

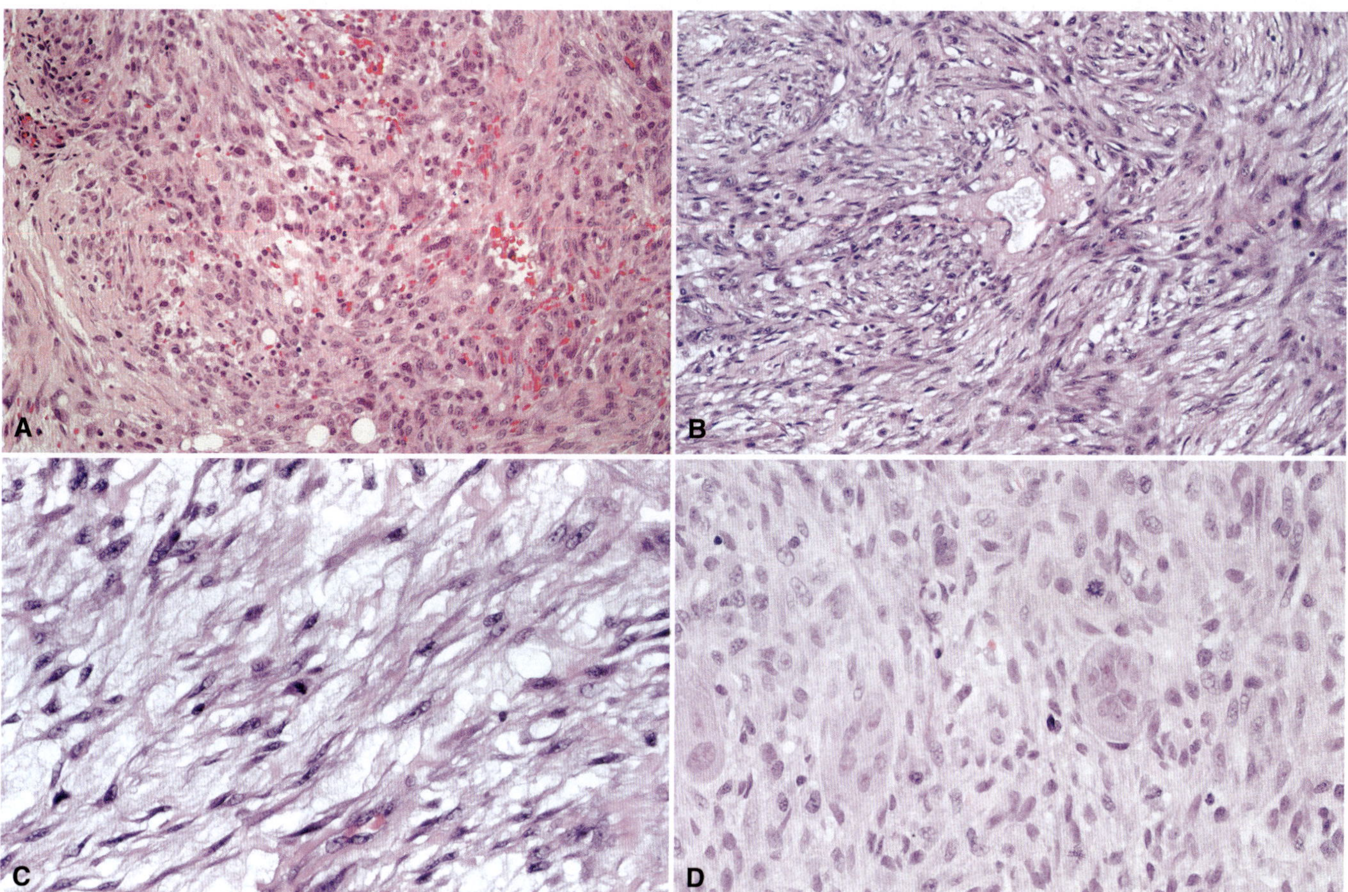

Figure 4.1 Nodular Fasciitis. (A) Nodular fasciitis demonstrates short interlacing bundles of spindle cells with focal extravasation of erythrocytes and scattered multinucleated giant cells. (B) Mucoid microcysts are dispersed between bundles of spindle cells with myxoid background. (C) Spindled myofibroblasts with occasional prominent nucleoli are dispersed in a prominent myxoid matrix with clear clefts between cells. (D) Multinucleated osteoclast-like giant cells intermingle with ganglion-like and spindle cells with sparse chronic inflammation.

smooth muscle actin, muscle-specific actin, and calponin.[20,21] Focal CD68 reactivity is present in histiocytes and osteoclast-like giant cells. Nodular fasciitis is nonreactive for h-caldesmon. Low to moderate proliferative activity is seen with a Ki67 stain and other proliferative markers.[22] Ultrastructural examination reveals myofibroblastic differentiation.[23]

Molecular Genetics

Nodular fasciitis is a clonal lesion.[24] Recent studies have demonstrated an *MYH9-USP6* gene fusion in nodular fasciitis.[25-27] Nearly all cases examined harbor a *USP6* rearrangement, which in 65% of cases is fused to *MYH9*.[28] The gene expression signature of nodular fasciitis is distinct from desmoid-type fibromatosis.[29]

Differential Diagnosis

The differential diagnosis includes desmoid fibromatosis, benign fibrous histiocytoma, infantile myofibromatosis, early fibrodysplasia ossificans progressiva in infancy, low-grade myofibrosarcoma, low-grade malignant peripheral nerve sheath tumor, and low-grade fibromyxoid sarcoma. Desmoid fibromatosis can be a particular challenge in fibrous or late-phase nodular fasciitis, but distinguishing features are aberrant nuclear reactivity for β-catenin; delicate, elongated, thin-walled blood vessels at the edge of spindle cell fascicles; and a mast cell infiltrate. Infantile myofibromatosis lacks the inflammatory infiltrate, mucoid microcysts, extravasation of erythrocytes, and osteoclast-like giant cells of nodular fasciitis. Myofibrosarcoma and other spindle cell sarcomas typically lack the inflammatory infiltrate and zonation pattern of nodular fasciitis, and display more nuclear atypia and pleomorphism.

PRACTICE POINTS: Nodular Fasciitis

- Nodular fasciitis is a rapidly growing, benign lesion that is usually subcutaneous.
- A zonal architectural pattern is typical, and the histologic spectrum ranges from myxoid to cellular or fibrous.
- A rearrangement of the *USP6* gene is frequent.

Prognosis and Treatment

Conservative excision is adequate therapy for nodular fasciitis, which generally does not recur. Regression and involution following biopsy or incomplete resection have been observed.[30] Recurrence has been attributed to persistent growth of an incompletely excised lesion.

Cranial Fasciitis

Cranial fasciitis is similar to nodular fasciitis, except that it is restricted to cranial soft tissue, especially in the temporoparietal region.[20,31,32] In contrast to nodular fasciitis, cranial fasciitis typically affects infants and

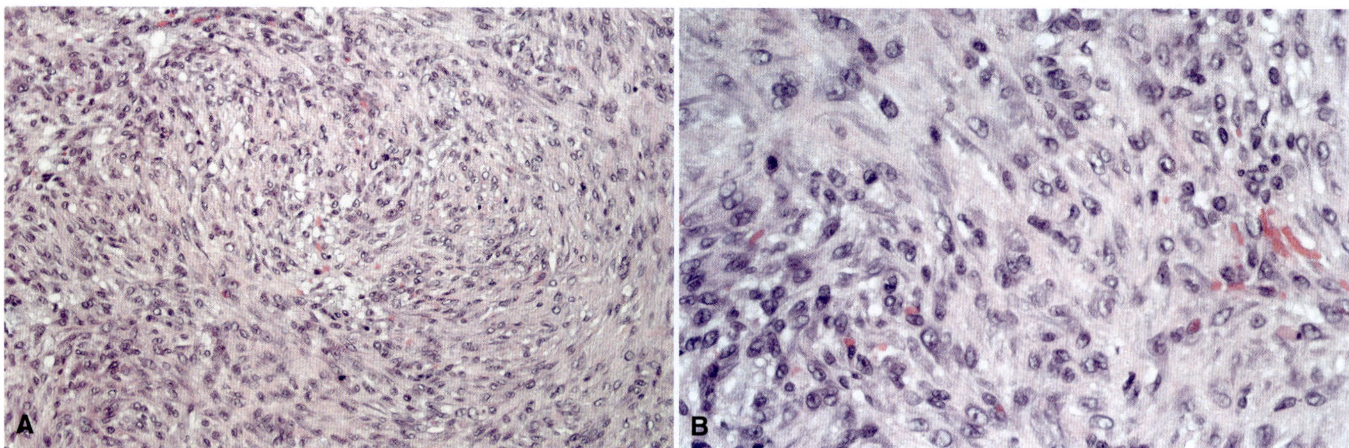

Figure 4.2 Cranial Fasciitis. (A) Bundles of spindle cells with a myxoid background have a uniform appearance. (B) Spindle cells have collagen in the background and sparse chronic inflammation.

children in the first few years of life. Cranial fasciitis is rare in the spectrum of extracranial subcutaneous scalp and skull masses in young children.[33] Like nodular fasciitis, the rapidly growing mass can lead to a clinical concern for malignancy.

Clinical Features

Cranial fasciitis involves the subcutaneous and deep soft tissue of the head, with bone involvement reported in 80% to 90% of cases.[31,34] Children younger than 2 years of age are most often affected, and there is a male predominance. Intracranial extension, rapid growth, and a radiologically aggressive appearance simulate higher-grade lesions.[32,35,28,36]

Pathologic Features

Grossly, cranial fasciitis has a median diameter of 2.5 cm with a range of 1.5 to 9 cm. The gray rubbery mass is usually ovoid and well circumscribed, although occasional examples are multinodular. Histologically, spindled and stellate fibroblastic and myofibroblastic cells are loosely arranged in a myxoid background and have a more uniform appearance than nodular fasciitis (Fig. 4.2A).[32] Patchy hemorrhage, chronic inflammation, occasional osteoclast-like multinucleated giant cells, calcification, osseous metaplasia, and ganglion-like cells are variable. The mitotic rate varies, with up to 10 mitoses per 10 high-power fields. A vague storiform pattern or abundant collagen is sometimes observed (see Fig. 4.2B).

Immunohistochemistry

Similar to nodular fasciitis, immunohistochemical analysis reveals reactivity for vimentin and smooth muscle actin.[32]

Differential Diagnosis

The differential diagnosis of cranial fasciitis is similar to nodular fasciitis, except that cranial fasciitis occurs earlier in childhood, is more restricted in site, and has a more uniform histologic appearance than nodular fasciitis.[32] Differential diagnostic considerations include infantile fibrosarcoma, fibromatoses such as desmoid fibromatosis and infantile myofibromatosis, and low-grade myofibrosarcoma of the head and neck. Infantile fibrosarcoma is larger and more cellular with more nuclear atypia, and can have a hemangiopericytoma-like growth pattern. Infantile myofibromatosis generally lacks inflammation, giant cells, and a prominent myxoid background. Low-grade myofibrosarcoma displays more cellular atypia, lacks inflammation and multinucleated cells, and has an aggressive appearance on imaging studies.

Prognosis and Treatment

Conservative surgical excision is the preferred treatment for cranial fasciitis.[31,34,36] Recurrence is rare. Similar to nodular fasciitis, cranial fasciitis may involute spontaneously.

Fibromas

Gardner Fibroma

Gardner fibroma is a distinctive hypocellular, prominently collagenized growth that is frequently an early manifestation of familial adenomatous polyposis (FAP; Gardner syndrome).[13,37,38] It can be associated with concurrent or subsequent development of desmoid-type fibromatosis.

Clinical Features

Gardner fibroma is soft, poorly demarcated, and slow-growing. It occurs in superficial or deep soft tissue in the paraspinal region, trunk, abdomen, head and neck, or extremities.[13,37-39] Approximately 70% of patients with Gardner fibroma have a history of FAP, and more than 10% have a family history of desmoid-type fibromatosis or soft tissue tumors.[38] Although the age at diagnosis ranges from infancy to adulthood, nearly 80% of Gardner fibromas are recognized in the first decade of life. The clinicopathologic features are summarized in Table 4.3.

Pathologic Features

Grossly, the plaque-like rubbery mass has an infiltrative appearance and a white cut surface speckled with yellow.[37,38] Histologically, the bland hypocellular proliferation consists of haphazardly arranged sheets of coarse collagen fibers separated by clear cracks with intervening small bland spindle cells, small blood vessels, and a sparse mast cell infiltrate (Fig. 4.3). There is no fascicular or bundling architectural pattern. The collagenized proliferation entraps adjacent tissues such as adipose tissue, peripheral nerves, and blood vessels. Gardner fibroma may merge into an adjacent desmoid fibromatosis, which is distinguished by a more compact proliferation of spindle cells arranged in fascicles with more prominent cellularity.

Immunohistochemistry

Immunohistochemical analysis of Gardner fibroma usually reveals diffuse reactivity for CD34 and absence of smooth muscle actin within the lesion.[37] Nuclear β-catenin reactivity is variable and can be positive in up to two-thirds of cases (Fig. 4.4), but it may be nonreactive even in patients with an adenomatous polyposis coli (*APC*) mutation.[38,40,41] Gardner fibroma overexpresses other proteins in the Wnt and β-catenin pathways, such as cyclin D1 and MYC.[38]

Molecular Genetics

Gardner fibroma is associated with *APC* mutation.[42]

Table 4.3 Clinicopathologic Features of Gardner Fibroma

Feature	Specifics
Age at presentation (range, infancy to fourth decade)	
First year	29%
First decade	78%
Second decade	15%
After second decade	7%
Male-to-female ratio	1.3:1
Sites	
Back and paraspinal tissue	61%
Head and neck	14%
Extremities	14%
Chest and abdomen	11%
Genetics	
FAP in patient or family	69%
Family history of soft tissue tumor	4%
Concurrent or subsequent desmoids	19%

FAP, Familial adenomatous polyposis.
Data from references 6, 12, 37, and 38.

Differential Diagnosis

The differential diagnosis for Gardner fibroma includes other types of fibroma, especially nuchal-type fibroma,[37,38,43] and fibromatoses, particularly desmoid fibromatosis with prominent collagen. Table 4.4 compares the pathologic features.[38]

Prognosis and Treatment

Gardner fibroma is a benign lesion with two important caveats. First, it can be the sentinel event in a child for the diagnosis of FAP, Gardner syndrome, familial desmoid-type fibromatosis without other manifestations of FAP, or a new *APC* mutation.[37-39,44,45] Second, it can be associated with concurrent or subsequent desmoid-type fibromatosis, which has been observed in nearly 20% of cases of Gardner fibroma, although this is probably an underestimate based on limited available follow-up.[37-39] Children with Gardner fibroma should have ongoing follow-up and evaluation for development of colorectal tumors and desmoid-type fibromatosis, and their families should be screened for FAP.[38,45]

PRACTICE POINTS: Gardner Fibroma

- Gardner fibroma is a poorly demarcated, plaque-like mass that can be an early manifestation of familial adenomatous polyposis/Gardner syndrome and is associated with *APC* mutation.
- Hypocellular sheets of coarse collagen fibers separated by clear cracks infiltrate and entrap adjacent tissues.
- Gardner fibroma is a desmoid precursor.

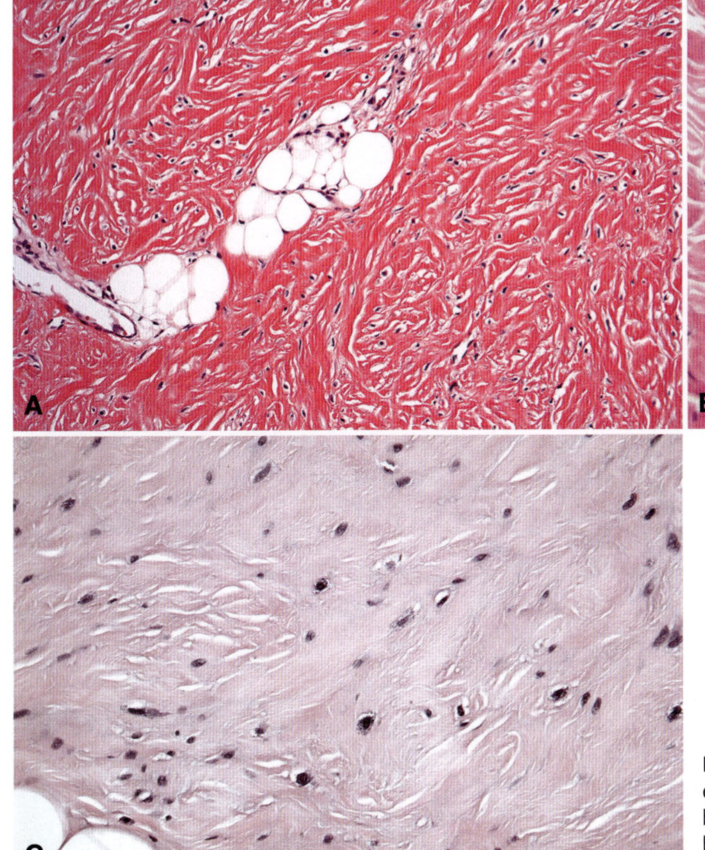
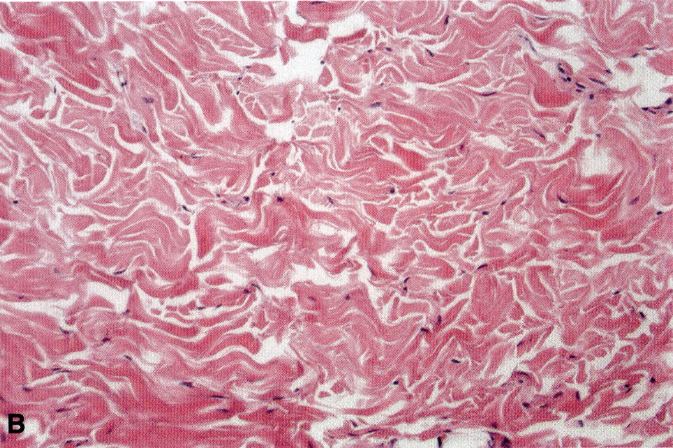

Figure 4.3 Gardner Fibroma. (A) At low power, Gardner fibroma consists of sheets of densely collagenized tissue with entrapment of mature adipose tissue. (B) Indistinct bland spindle cells are dispersed between coarse collagen fibers that are separated by clear clefts. (C) Sparse mast cells are dispersed in the background of Gardner fibroma.

Table 4.4 Comparison of Gardner Fibroma, Nuchal Fibroma, and Desmoid Fibromatosis

Feature	Gardner Fibroma	Nuchal Fibroma	Desmoid Fibromatosis
Gross appearance	Rubbery plaque	Poorly demarcated hard mass	Firm, whorled nodule
Microscopic features	Patternless Hypocellular Hypovascular Matted collagen No mitoses Mast cells	Lobules, criss-crossing areas, neuroma-like areas Hypocellular Hypovascular Thick collagen bundles No mitoses Lymphocytes	Fascicles Moderately cellular Distinctive vessels Fibrillary or keloidal collagen Variable mitoses Mast cells
Clonality	Unknown	Unknown	Yes
Immunohistochemistry	CD34 β-catenin (nuclear)	Unknown	Smooth muscle actin β-catenin (nuclear)

Data from references 6, 12, and 38.

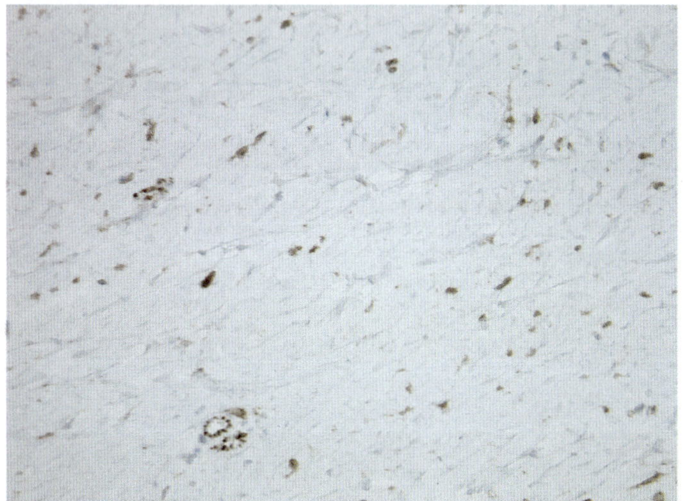

Figure 4.4 Gardner Fibroma. Nuclear reactivity in spindle cells for β-catenin by immunohistochemistry.

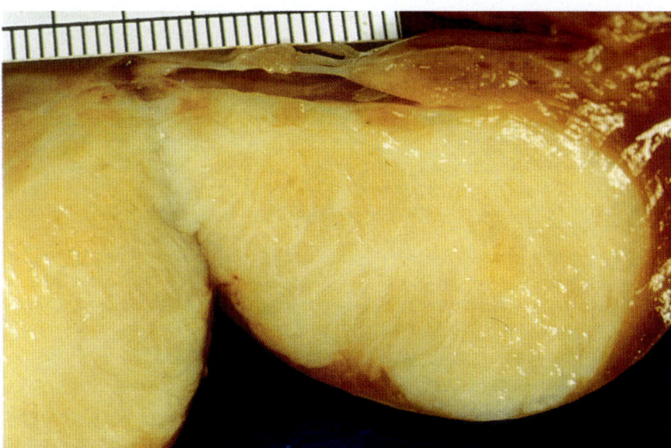

Figure 4.5 Cardiac Fibroma. A cardiac septal fibroma displaces myocardium and has a fleshy yellow and white cut surface.

Cardiac Fibroma

Cardiac tumors are rare in infants and children, and most are benign. After cardiac rhabdomyoma, cardiac fibroma is one of the more common types of this unusual group of lesions.[46,47]

Clinical Features

Cardiac fibroma can be detected antenatally by fetal ultrasound. Initial manifestations in children include unexplained heart failure, arrhythmia, heart murmur, cardiac calcification, or irregular cardiac contours. Most are diagnosed within the first 2 years of life, and nearly all are detected by early adolescence. Males are affected more often than females. Cardiac fibroma can occur anywhere in the heart but most often arises in the left ventricle. The diagnosis can lead to the recognition of the nevoid basal cell carcinoma syndrome (Gorlin syndrome) in the child and the family.[48,49] In addition, cardiac fibroma can be associated with type 1 neurofibromatosis, tuberous sclerosis, familial myxomas, and bilateral cystic renal dysplasia.[48,50]

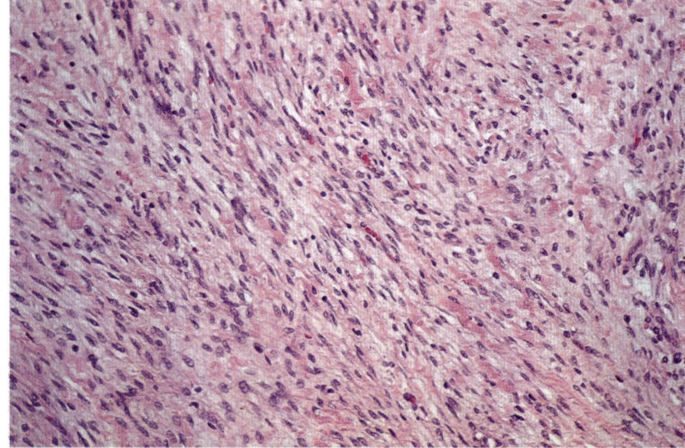

Figure 4.6 Cardiac Fibroma. Bland spindle cells form large fascicles and lack hypercellularity or nuclear atypia.

Pathologic Features

Grossly, cardiac fibroma is a firm, circumscribed, pale tan, intramural, or ventricular cardiac mass (Fig. 4.5). The cut surface displays a firm texture. Satellite nodules may accompany the solitary mass; occasional tumors are multifocal. Histologically, bland fibroblasts intermingle with collagen and elastic fibers (Fig. 4.6). A sparse mast cell infiltrate, prominent vascularity, and variable calcifications may be present. The cellularity ranges from low to moderate.

Immunohistochemistry

Immunohistochemical analysis reveals diffuse reactivity for vimentin and focal reactivity for smooth muscle actin.[48]

Table 4.5 Clinicopathologic Subtypes of Infantile Myofibromatosis

Type	Sites	Age at Onset	Predominant Sex	Natural History
Solitary	Skin, soft tissue	Birth and later	Male	Benign Regression or recurrence
Multiple	Skin, soft tissue, bone	Congenital	Female	Benign Regression
Generalized	Skin, soft tissue, bone, viscera	Congenital	Male	Progression Death in 73% Regression rare

Data from references 6, 54, and 55.

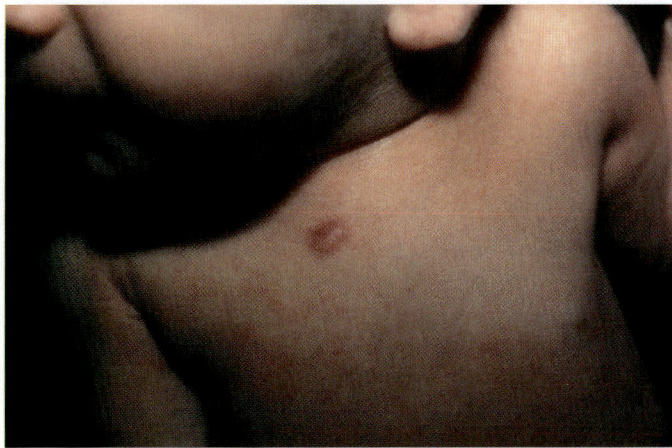

Figure 4.7 Infantile Myofibroma. A cutaneous papular myofibroma has a reddish-blue appearance.

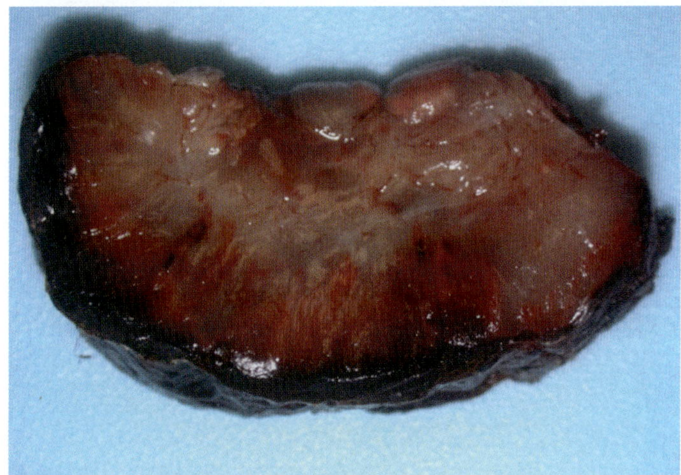

Figure 4.8 Infantile Myofibroma. The cut surface shows a nodular red and tan mass with focal hemorrhage in granular white areas.

Molecular Genetics

Cardiac fibromas may have a rearrangement, deletion, or somatic copy number losses of the *PTCH1* gene at chromosome 9q22.[51,52]

Differential Diagnosis

The differential diagnosis of cardiac fibroma includes other primary cardiac neoplasms such as rhabdomyoma or RMS, cardiac lesions in congenital generalized myofibromatosis (infantile myofibromatosis), and cardiac sarcomas. Cardiac rhabdomyoma is distinguished by the presence of large multivacuolated glycogen-filled cells and "spider" cells. Myofibromatosis is recognized by prominent whorling and an interlacing fascicular architecture with strong reactivity for smooth muscle actin in the clinical setting of congenital generalized myofibromatosis. RMS and other sarcomas are distinguished by a higher-grade appearance with high cellularity, pleomorphism, mitotic activity, and their distinctive immunohistochemical features.

Prognosis and Treatment

Although cardiac fibroma is histologically benign, its location is potentially lethal. Resection or cardiac transplantation may be effective for cases that are detected early.

Fibromatoses

Infantile Myofibroma

Infantile myofibroma or myofibromatosis occurs in three clinicopathologic forms with similar histology but different clinical features and outcome. The three subtypes—solitary, multiple, and congenital generalized myofibromatosis—are summarized in Table 4.5.[53-56]

Clinical Features

The solitary and multiple forms of infantile myofibromatosis involve skin, soft tissue, and bone.[53-57] In contrast, the generalized form also involves these sites and viscera, including the central nervous system, in varying combinations. Lesions can be numerous.[58] The onset is usually in infancy, with a congenital presentation in up to two-thirds of cases, but may be later in childhood, adolescence, or adulthood.[58] Cutaneous lesions have a purplish nodular or papular appearance (Fig. 4.7). Solitary and multiple myofibromas can undergo spontaneous regression with a gangrenous-appearing shrinkage of the mass. Extensive bone involvement can result in multiple fractures as the initial presentation in infants,[59] and rare cases are associated with fetal death.[60] Familial cases have been reported.[55,61] Associated malformations are rare.[62]

Pathologic Features

Grossly, solitary myofibroma is a circumscribed nodular mass with a white to tan firm cut surface. Occasional cases have a soft red central area with variable necrosis and calcification (Fig. 4.8). The multiple and generalized myofibromas form deeper nodules with a white or tan firm cut surface and less extensive necrosis and zonation. Microscopically, short interlacing fascicles of spindled myofibroblastic cells are dispersed in a myxoid and collagenized background with moderate cellularity (Fig. 4.9).[53,54] In sections where adjacent nonlesional tissue is present, peripheral satellite nodules may be seen with a whorled pattern and a focal perivascular and intravascular subendothelial proliferation of immature myofibroblastic and primitive mesenchymal cells. These features suggest a possible origin from perivascular mesenchymal cells and a morphologic continuum with myopericytoma.[53,63] Cellular atypia is absent. Some cases demonstrate a zonal pattern with central primitive round to polygonal cells associated with delicate irregularly branching blood vessels (Fig. 4.10A and B). These areas may merge with more spindled and collagenized whorled myofibroblastic foci (see Fig. 4.10C). In the past, this variant was called "infantile hemangiopericytoma." Increased cellularity, loosely cohesive or absent spindled myofibroblastic nodules, infiltrating borders, and perineural invasion or nerve entrapment may be seen.[64] Prominent apoptosis, necrosis, and dystrophic calcification may be encountered, especially in larger myofibromas (see Fig. 4.10D). Apoptosis has been proposed as a mechanism for spontaneous regression.[65]

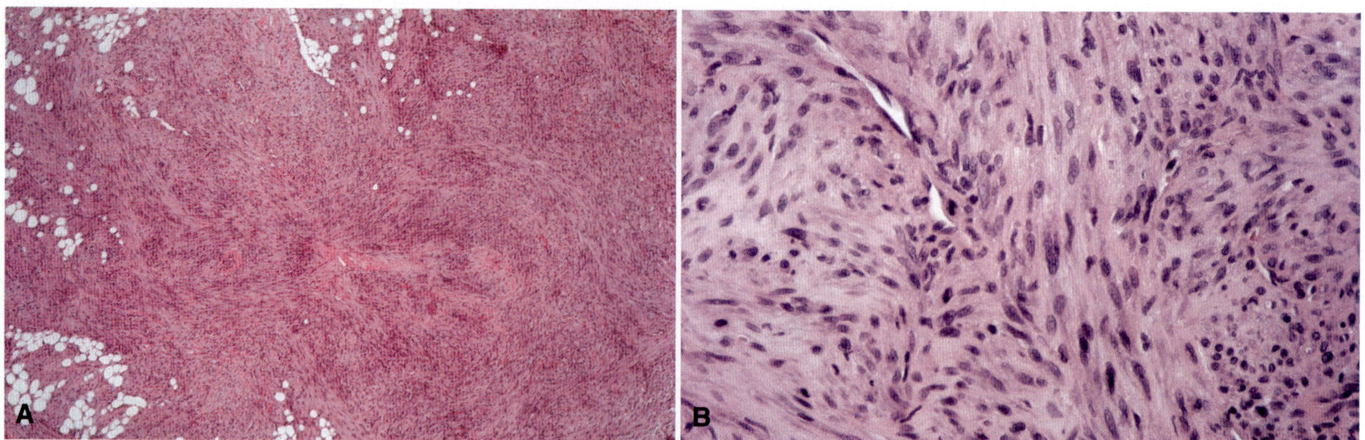

Figure 4.9 **Infantile Myofibroma.** (A) Bands of spindled cells form fascicles and infiltrate adipose tissue. (B) The spindle cells have bland oval nuclei and pale eosinophilic cytoplasm with collagen in the background.

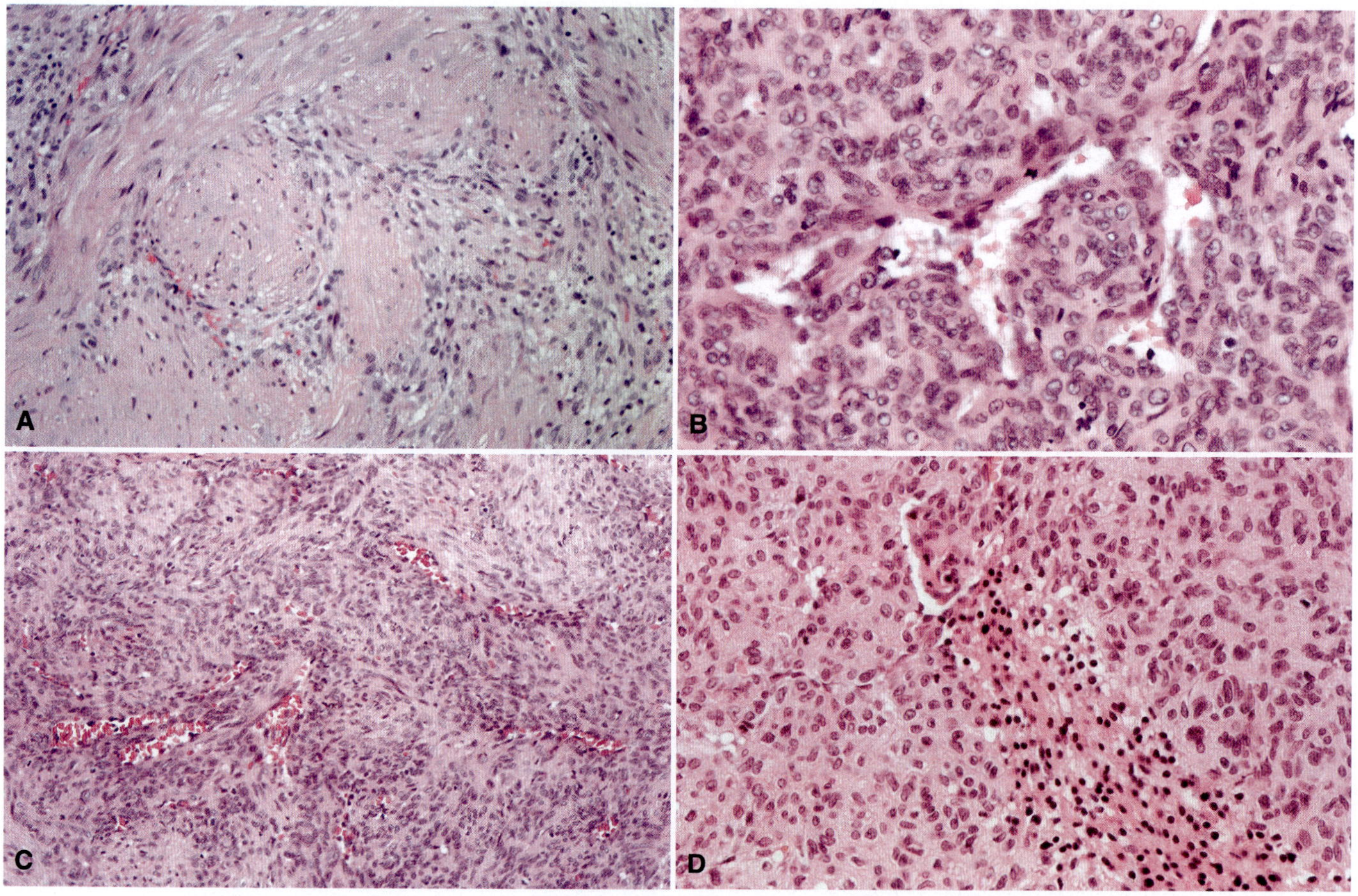

Figure 4.10 **Infantile Myofibroma.** (A) Hemangiopericytoma-like foci are intermingled with small whorled myofibroblastic nodules. (B) Primitive round and polygonal cells with irregular branching blood vessels form hemangiopericytoma-like areas. (C) Spindle cell nodules merge with hemangiopericytoma-like foci. (D) Focal necrosis or apoptosis may be a manifestation of spontaneous regression.

Immunohistochemistry

By immunohistochemistry, the spindled and whorled areas show strong reactivity for smooth muscle actin (Fig. 4.11), and the endothelial cells in the hemangiopericytoma-like areas are reactive for CD34.

Molecular Genetics

A single case has been reported with a chromosome 6 deletion.[66] Autosomal dominant and autosomal recessive patterns of inheritance have been reported in some families.[67-69] Mutations in *PDGFRB*, *NDRG4*, and *NOTCH3* have been identified.[70-73]

Differential Diagnosis

The differential diagnosis includes other fibromatoses, nodular fasciitis, solitary fibrous tumor, fibroblastic-myofibroblastic sarcomas, and pericytic neoplasms such as myopericytoma. It is now recognized that infantile hemangiopericytoma is part of the morphologic spectrum of infantile

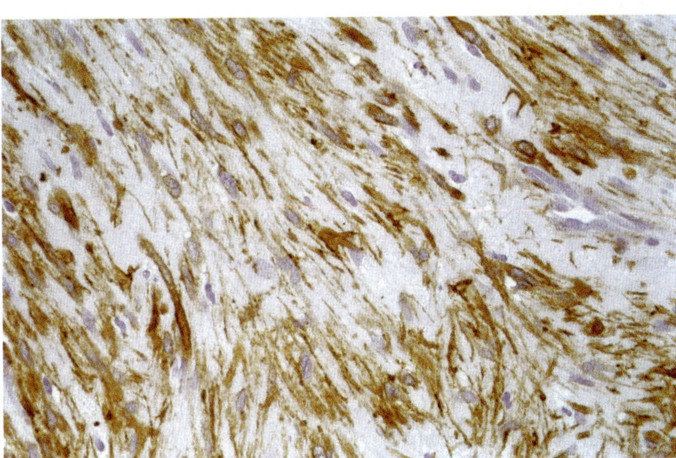

Figure 4.11 **Infantile Myofibroma.** Diffuse cytoplasmic reactivity for smooth muscle actin by immunohistochemistry.

Table 4.6 Desmoid Fibromatosis in Children and Young Adults: Summary of Four Series

Feature	Specifics
Age	
Range	Birth to 28 years
Mean	8 years
Congenital	10%
First year of life	24%
Male-to-female ratio	1.7:1
Sites	
Head and neck	30%
Trunk	45%
Extremities	24%
Multifocal	4%
Outcome	
Recurrence rate	58%
Mortality	6%

Data from references 5, 9, 86, and 87.

myofibroma, and generally these cases are lumped together as infantile myofibroma/myofibromatosis.[53,74] Solitary fibrous tumor in adults is a distinct entity that is unrelated to infantile myofibroma, lacks the fascicular and whorled growth pattern, and usually demonstrates CD34 and STAT6 reactivity in the neoplastic cells. Occasional cases of infantile fibrosarcoma closely resemble myofibroma and are sometimes classified as composite fibromatosis because of the inability to reliably distinguish between the two entities on morphologic features alone.[75,76] In such cases, molecular diagnostic testing for the *ETV6-NTRK3* gene rearrangement associated with infantile fibrosarcoma is very useful. Other neoplasms with myofibroblastic features, a hemangiopericytoma-like vascular pattern, and *NTRK1* gene fusions can resemble highly cellular myofibromas and composite fibromatosis and are discussed with infantile fibrosarcoma. Other fibromatoses, particularly desmoid fibromatosis, and nodular fasciitis can simulate infantile myofibroma and are distinguished by a combination of clinical and morphologic features. Desmoid fibromatosis has a more uniform architecture with long fascicles and usually exhibits nuclear reactivity for β-catenin. Nodular fasciitis shows a zonal architecture with loose fascicles, variably myxoid stroma, extravasated erythrocytes, and focal osteoclast-like giant cells, and it lacks the whorled nodules and perivascular and subendothelial growth of myofibroma.

PRACTICE POINTS: Infantile Myofibroma

- Infantile myofibroma/myofibromatosis can be solitary, multiple, or generalized.
- The histologic spectrum includes a spindled, myofibroblastic fascicular pattern and a hemangiopericytoma-like pattern.
- Mutations in *PDGFRB*, *NDRG4*, or *NOTCH3* may be present.
- Large, cellular infantile myofibroma mimics infantile fibrosarcoma but lacks the *ETV6-NTRK3* gene rearrangement.

Prognosis and Treatment

The prognosis and treatment of infantile myofibroma/myofibromatosis vary according to the clinicopathologic pattern. Solitary myofibroma is frequently self-limited and can undergo spontaneous regression.[65,77,78] In cases that do not regress, excision is effective treatment. Autosomal dominant examples can also regress. Congenital generalized myofibromatosis results in death in up to 70% of patients because of visceral involvement, especially of the lungs, gastrointestinal tract, and genitourinary tract.[53,54,79,80] Limited information suggests that chemotherapy or interferon may be effective in some cases,[81-83] and rare cases may be self-limited.[67,84] Multifocal and generalized types require long-term follow-up.

Desmoid-Type Fibromatosis in Childhood

Desmoid-type fibromatosis accounts for up to 60% of fibrous tumors in childhood (see also Chapter 3).[5,9] In several large series, up to 40% of desmoid fibromatoses were diagnosed in the first two decades of life.[5,9,85-87] Information about desmoid fibromatosis from four series of children and young adults is summarized in Table 4.6.[5,9,86,87] The associations with FAP (Gardner syndrome, with germline *APC* mutation), sporadic *CTNNB1* mutation, and antecedent trauma, surgery, and irradiation are well established.[4,12,88-92] A desmoid in early childhood may be the initial manifestation of an *APC* mutation in the patient or in the family, and desmoid can occur in the same site as a previous or concurrent Gardner fibroma.[37,38,93-96]

Clinical Features

Desmoid fibromatosis in childhood involves superficial or deep soft tissues. It is often extraabdominal; the most common sites are the head and neck region, extremities, shoulder, trunk, and hip.[5,9,86,97] Unusual locations include the abdomen, retroperitoneum, breast, and spermatic cord.[39,98] Some children may have multiple desmoids.[9,99] Most series have demonstrated a male predominance.[86,100,101] The median age for desmoid fibromatosis in the Kiel Pediatric Tumor Registry was 5 years.[9] Up to 30% occur in the first year of life, and congenital examples have been reported.[9]

Although desmoid fibromatosis is occasionally painful, the usual clinical presentation is a slowly growing, hard mass that has been present for weeks to months without tenderness, weight loss, or fever. Desmoids that arise in association with Gardner fibroma may be painful, can grow rapidly, and are firmer and more circumscribed than the adjacent Gardner fibroma.[37,38,96] Desmoid fibromatosis is a locally aggressive tumor that can infiltrate adjacent skeletal muscle, tendons, or periosteum; erode bone; or be associated with osteolysis.[102] Magnetic resonance imaging is useful for detection and monitoring.[103]

Pathologic Features

Grossly, the firm gray-white oval or fusiform mass has a whorled or trabeculated cut surface (Fig. 4.12). The diameter averages 6 to 7 cm but can exceed 15 cm.[5,86] Although the mass may appear to be well circumscribed macroscopically, the margins are often irregular and infiltrative. Histologically, broad sweeping fascicles of spindle cells with an abundantly collagenized background with foci of myxoid change are separated by thin-walled, delicate blood vessels that are aligned along edges of fascicles (Fig. 4.13A–C). Cellularity varies from low to high.[9] The tumor cells are slender and relatively uniform, with a spindled configuration and abundant cytoplasm with indistinct cell borders. The nuclei are oval with fine chromatin and occasional small nucleoli and lack atypia or pleomorphism. Morphologic variations include hyalinized or hypocellular areas, dilated staghorn blood vessels, myxoid change, keloidal collagen bundles, and hypercellular foci.[104] Dystrophic calcification is unusual. Mast cells are scattered throughout the tumor (see Fig. 4.13D) but are more concentrated near blood vessels. A lymphocytic infiltrate may be seen peripherally at the interface between the desmoid and adjacent soft tissue or skeletal muscle. The advancing border infiltrates and entraps muscle fibers or adipose tissue.[87] Atrophic or multinucleated skeletal muscle cells can simulate cellular atypia. Most desmoid tumors have relatively low mitotic rates, but occasional examples may display more than 10 mitoses per 10 high-power fields; this has no prognostic significance.[86] Limited data suggest that foci of myxoid degeneration, abundant plump stellate tumor cells, and a large number of small slit-like blood vessels in the central portions of desmoid may be associated with a higher tendency for recurrence, but in general histology does not correlate with clinical behavior.[105,106] Recurrent desmoids are histologically identical to the primary tumor. In patients who have had previous surgery, it may be difficult to distinguish between a surgical scar and a recurrent desmoid, or to discern the demarcation between the scar and a desmoid fibromatosis. Occasionally, microscopic foci of a previously unrecognized Gardner fibroma can be seen at the periphery of a desmoid. Radiation therapy does not significantly alter the histomorphology, but the presence of zonal necrosis, hypercellularity, severe nuclear atypia,

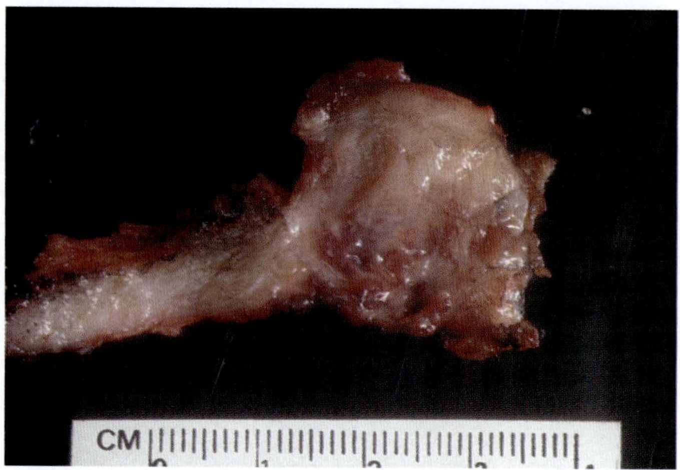

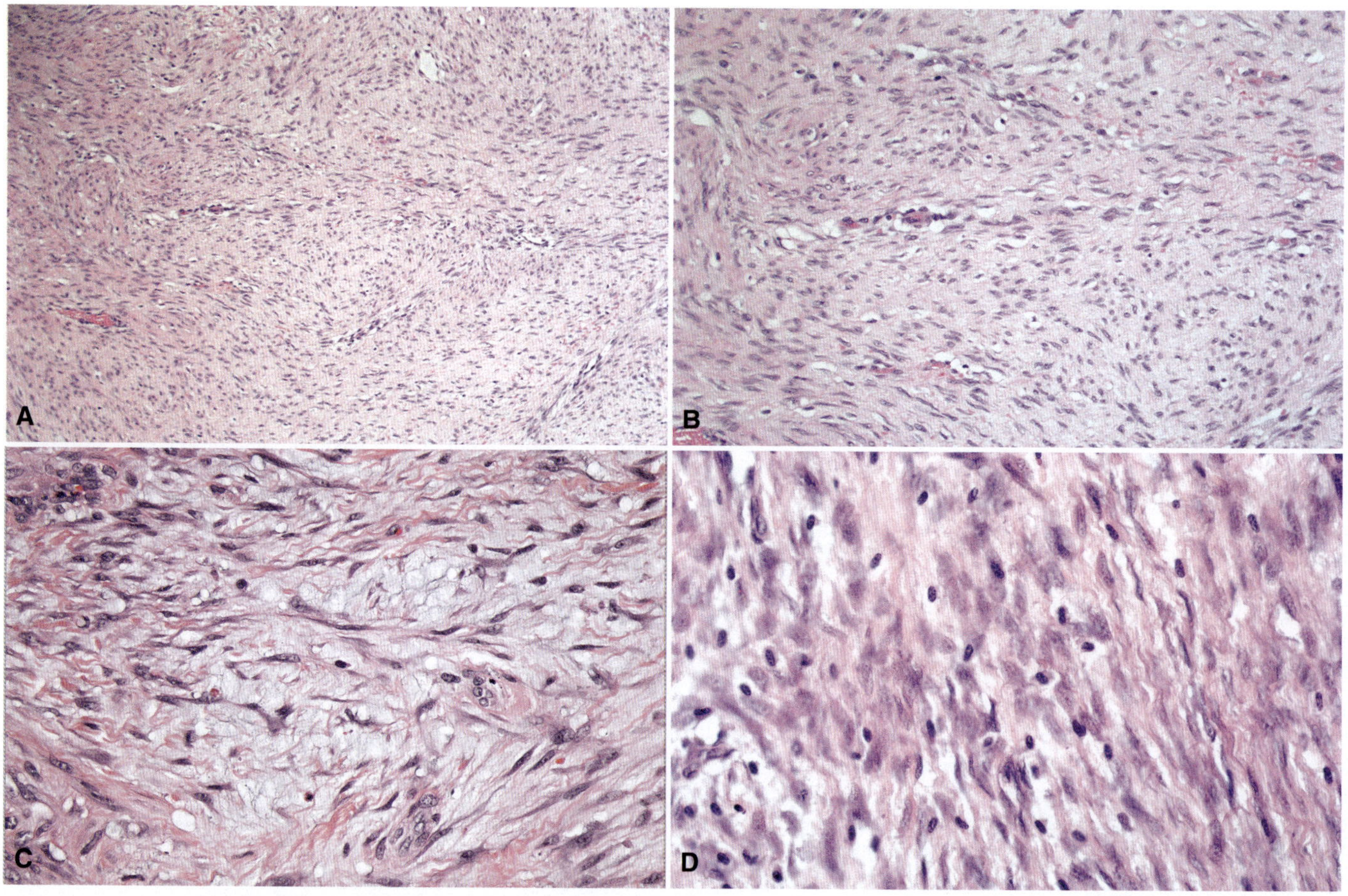

Figure 4.12 Desmoid Fibromatosis Arising in Gardner Fibroma. The round nodular area with a whorled cut surface is a desmoid tumor arising in an adjacent plaque-like area of Gardner fibroma.

Figure 4.13 Desmoid Fibromatosis. (A) Interlacing fascicles of spindle cells are separated by delicate elongated blood vessels at the edges of the fascicles. (B) The spindle cells of desmoid have a bland and relatively uniform appearance. (C) Myxoid and collagenized zones are histologic variations. (D) A mast cell infiltrate is present.

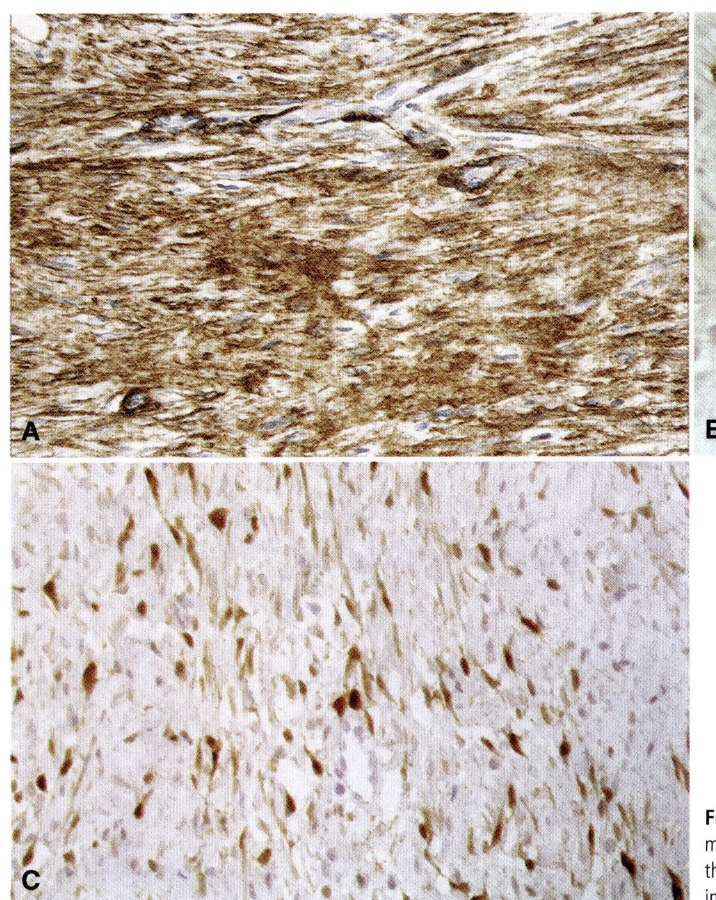

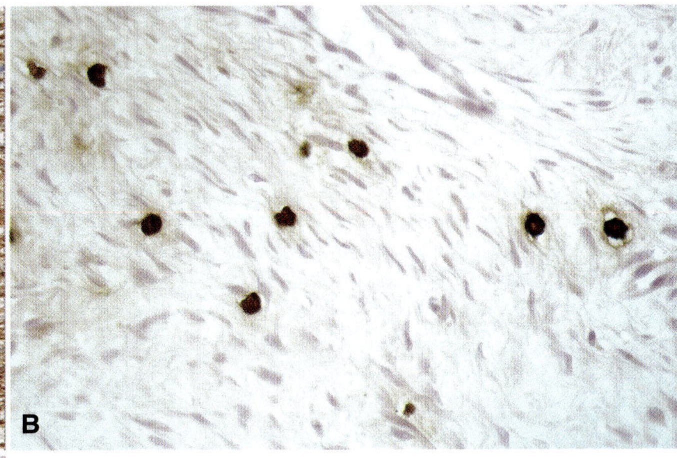

Figure 4.14 Desmoid Fibromatosis. (A) Diffuse cytoplasmic reactivity for smooth muscle actin is evident by immunohistochemistry. (B) Mast cell tryptase highlights the mast cell infiltrate. (C) Nuclear reactivity for β-catenin is apparent by immunohistochemistry.

and increased mitotic activity in a previously irradiated desmoid should prompt consideration of a postradiation sarcoma.[107]

Immunohistochemistry

Immunohistochemical studies of desmoid tumors have demonstrated a fibroblastic-myofibroblastic phenotype. Muscle-specific actin, smooth muscle actin (Fig. 4.14A), and desmin are expressed in varying proportions of cases.[108] The mast cells in desmoid fibromatosis can be highlighted by mast cell tryptase (see Fig. 4.14B) and KIT. Immunohistochemistry for β-catenin with a nuclear pattern of positivity is a helpful confirmatory marker of desmoid fibromatosis (see Fig. 4.14C), but the sensitivity and specificity vary in different studies; overall, approximately 70% of desmoid tumors show nuclear staining for β-catenin.[41,109-111] Coexpression of β-catenin and p53 may be associated with a higher risk of recurrence.[112] Estrogen receptor–β expression is frequent in desmoid fibromatosis.[108,113]

Molecular Genetics

Desmoid fibromatosis is a clonal neoplasm that that can harbor trisomies of chromosomes 8 and 20, 5q deletion, and mutations involving the *APC* or β-catenin (*CTNNB1*) genes.[110,113-116] Desmoids can be associated with many types of *APC* mutations, although mutations that are 3' seem to confer higher incidence and greater severity.[89,96,117,118] A significant proportion of sporadic desmoids in children harbor mutations in *CTNNB1*, including T41A, S45F, and S45P types.[116] Mutations of *AKT1* and *BRAF* have also been detected in pediatric desmoids.[119]

Differential Diagnosis

The differential diagnosis of desmoid fibromatosis includes a wide variety of spindle cell proliferations but especially keloids and hypertrophic scars, nodular fasciitis, Gardner fibroma, other fibromatoses, low-grade fibromyxoid sarcoma, and low-grade myofibrosarcoma.[120] Keloids and hypertrophic scars are usually confined to skin and subcutaneous tissue, which are unusual locations for desmoid tumors, and they lack the fascicular architecture and vascular pattern of desmoids. Gardner fibroma is densely collagenized and contains formless sheets of collagen with indistinct bland spindle cells. Other fibromatoses lack the mast cell infiltrate and vascular pattern of desmoid fibromatosis and lack nuclear β-catenin expression. Low-grade fibromyxoid sarcoma has a well-defined arcading vascular pattern, myxoid zones, and collagen rosettes in some cases; is positive for MUC4 by immunohistochemistry; and has a distinctive t(7;16) translocation with *FUS* gene rearrangement. Myofibrosarcoma demonstrates greater nuclear atypia and clinical and radiologic evidence of very aggressive growth. Other spindle cell neoplasms, such as inflammatory myofibroblastic tumor (IMT) and spindle cell sarcomas, are distinguished by a combination of histologic, immunohistochemical, cytogenetic, and molecular genetic features.

PRACTICE POINTS: Childhood Desmoid Fibromatosis

- Desmoid fibromatosis is a relatively frequent fibrous tumor of childhood and can be an early manifestation of familial adenomatous polyposis/Gardner syndrome or a new *APC* mutation; sporadic desmoids are usually associated with *CTNNB1* mutations.
- A significant proportion of childhood desmoids occur in the first 5 years of life.
- Broad sweeping fascicles of spindle cells are separated by delicate, thin-walled blood vessels and are accompanied by a sparse mast cell infiltrate.
- Mitotic activity has no diagnostic or prognostic significance.
- Nuclear immunoreactivity for β-catenin is observed in approximately 70% of cases.

Prognosis and Treatment
Although surgery has been a standard treatment in the past, other modalities include observation, nonsteroidal antiinflammatory drugs, hormonal therapy, chemotherapy, radiation therapy, and targeted agents. However, responses and outcomes have not been optimal. As a result, the current trend for initial treatment is to observe or manage desmoid-type fibromatosis nonoperatively.[121-123] In children, the recurrence rate is about 20%.[124] Clinical features associated with a higher recurrence risk include young age at diagnosis, intralesional excision, mesenteric location, and associated *APC* mutation and Gardner syndrome.[124] For a child with desmoid-type fibromatosis, the possibility of a new *APC* mutation, FAP, or familial desmoids without colorectal tumors warrants consideration of surveillance and long-term follow-up.[125]

Fibromatosis Colli

Fibromatosis colli, or sternomastoid tumor of infancy, is a neck mass involving the sternocleidomastoid muscle and is associated with torticollis and facial asymmetry.[126,127] It is now seldom encountered as a surgical pathology specimen because it regresses spontaneously and can be treated effectively with physical therapy.[128]

Clinical Features
Fibromatosis colli is the most common type of neonatal neck mass and is usually evident by the first month of life.[128] Males are more often affected than females. The tumor is often right-sided and may be bilateral. After a period of initial rapid growth, the mass stabilizes and then undergoes complete resolution in nearly all patients.

Pathologic Features
Grossly, the firm whorled mass is located within or replaces skeletal muscle (Fig. 4.15). Histologically, bands of fibroblasts with abundant collagen have low to focally increased cellularity and entrap muscle fibers (Fig. 4.16).[129] Fibromatosis colli lacks atypia, inflammation, or significant mitotic activity. Fine needle aspiration is an alternative method of diagnosis.[130]

Differential Diagnosis
The differential diagnosis includes other fibromatoses, especially desmoid fibromatosis, nodular fasciitis, scarring processes, and spindle cell RMS. Desmoid fibromatosis is distinguished by its prominent fascicular architecture with delicate vessels at the edges of fascicles, patchy mast cell infiltrate, and nuclear staining for β-catenin. Nodular fasciitis has a zonal architectural pattern with patchy chronic inflammation, focal osteoclast-like giant cells, extravasation of erythrocytes, and ganglion-like myofibroblasts. Scarring processes are often more diffuse and associated with chronic inflammation and granulation tissue. Spindle cell RMS displays higher cellularity and atypia, fails to regress, and expresses myogenic markers.

Prognosis and Treatment
The treatment is physical therapy. Because more than 90% of patients experience complete resolution, surgery is seldom necessary.[127]

Infantile Digital Fibroma

Infantile digital fibroma is a recurring lesion of the digits that occurs predominantly in infants.[131]

Clinical Features
The mass involves the lateral and dorsal aspects of the fingers and toes, although the great toe or thumb is generally spared. Although most examples of infantile digital fibroma arise in infants, and one-third are congenital, the condition may occur in older children and adults, and at

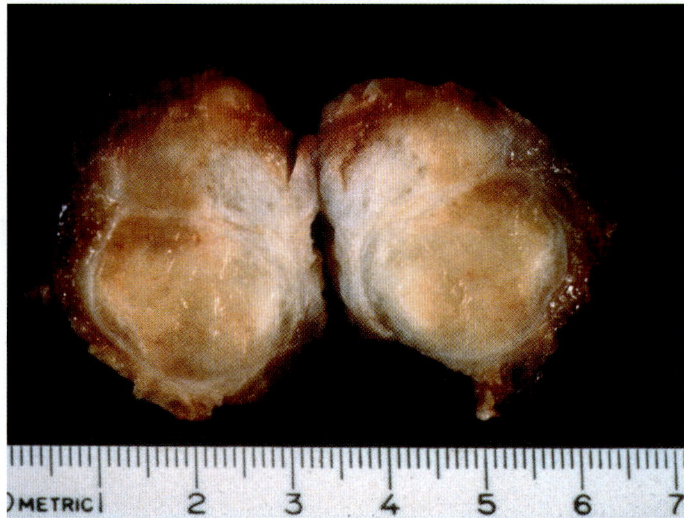

Figure 4.15 Fibromatosis Colli. The cut surface shows a firm whorled mass surrounded by skeletal muscle.

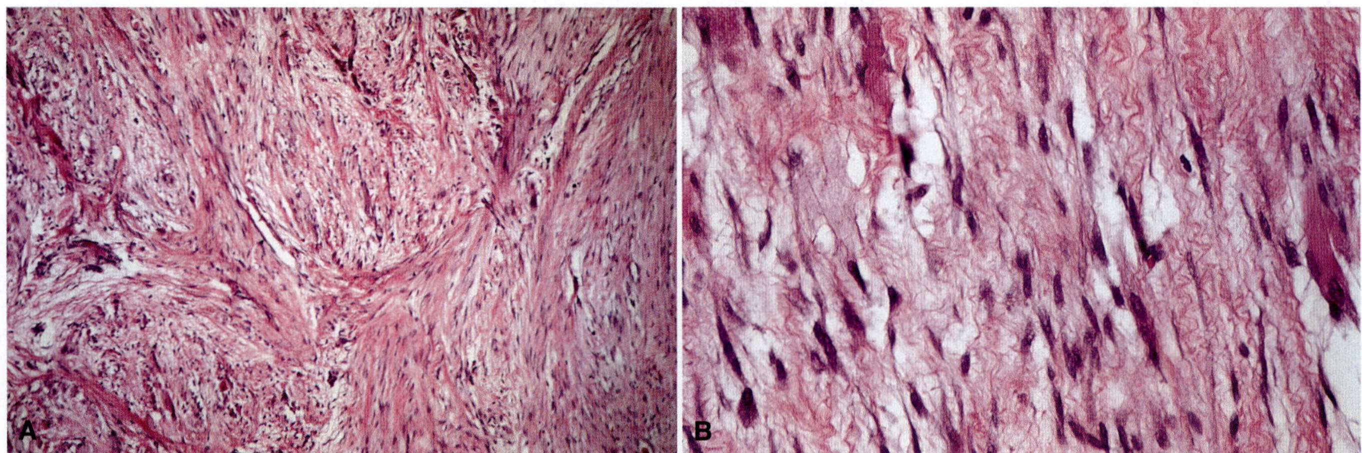

Figure 4.16 Fibromatosis Colli. (A) Irregular interlacing fascicles of spindle cells focally entrap skeletal muscle. (B) The spindle cells are uniform and have oval nuclei, granular chromatin, and indistinct pale eosinophilic cytoplasm.

nondigital sites, where it is designated as "inclusion body fibromatosis."[132] The rapidly growing pink dome-shaped nodule is superficial (Fig. 4.17) but may extend to involve periosteum or rarely invade bone.[131,133,134]

Pathologic Features

The dermal or subcutaneous nodule is covered by smooth skin and has a white firm cut surface. Histologically, whorls and sheets of bland fibroblasts are dispersed in a heavily collagenized background (Fig. 4.18A).[131,135] The tumor cells lack atypia, and the cytoplasm contains variable numbers of round paranuclear eosinophilic inclusions that are often surrounded by a halo (see Fig. 4.18B). Cytoplasmic inclusions decrease with maturation. A lymphocytic infiltrate may be present. The overlying skin is often flattened with loss of rete ridges, hyperkeratosis, and acanthosis, and the spindle cell proliferation entraps cutaneous adnexal structures. With a trichrome stain, the inclusions appear as red globules (see Fig. 4.18C).

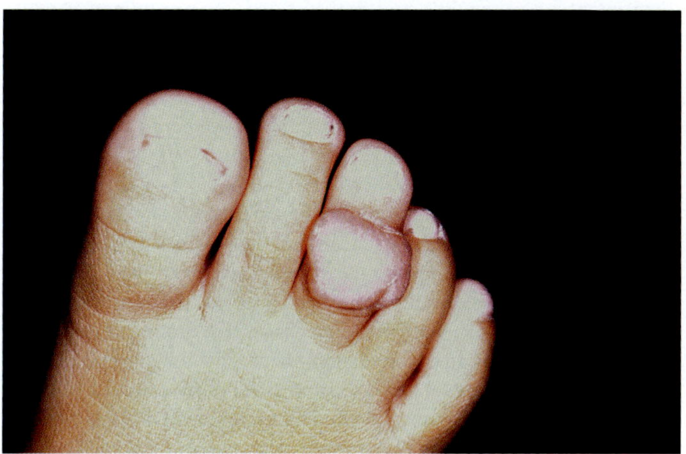

Figure 4.17 Infantile Digital Fibroma. A dome-shaped cutaneous nodule is present on the toe of an infant.

Immunohistochemistry

Reactivity for vimentin, calponin, and smooth muscle actin is typical, and occasional cases are positive for desmin, h-caldesmon, CD34, nuclear β-catenin, and keratin.[136-138] Anticalponin highlights the inclusions.

Differential Diagnosis

The differential diagnosis includes other types of fibromatosis. Palmar or plantar fibromatosis occurs on the hands or feet, and plantar fibromatosis is much more common in children. These types of superficial fibromatosis lack the inclusion bodies and predilection for young infants of digital fibroma. The early phase of calcifying or juvenile aponeurotic fibroma can also occur on the hands and feet of young children, but infantile digital fibroma lacks cartilage or calcification. Desmoid fibromatosis typically occurs in more proximal locations in older children or adults, arises in deep soft tissue, is composed of long sweeping fascicles, and usually demonstrates nuclear staining for β-catenin.[139]

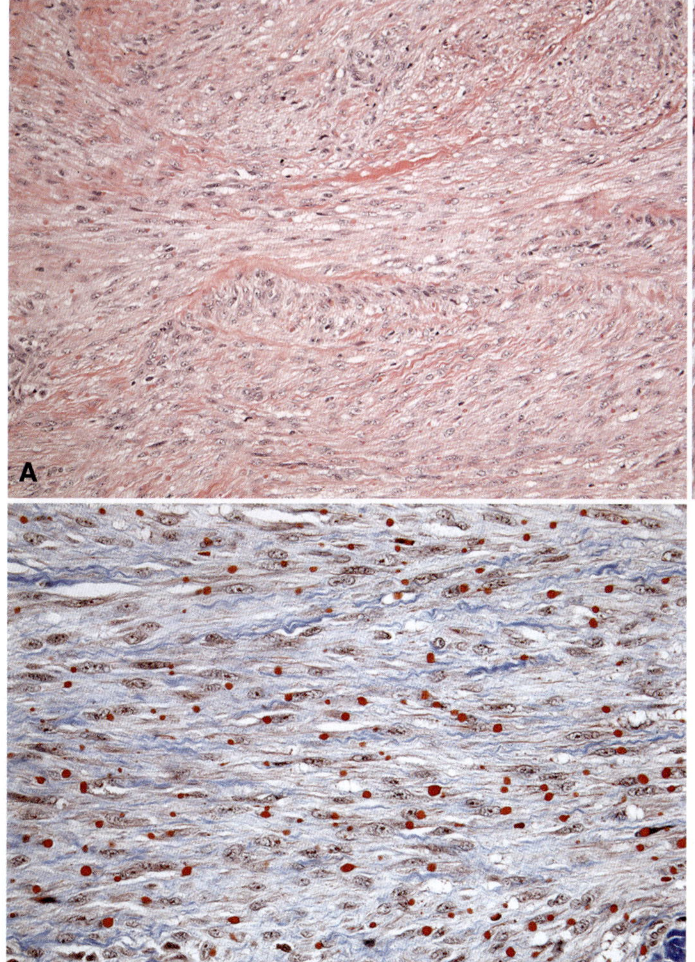

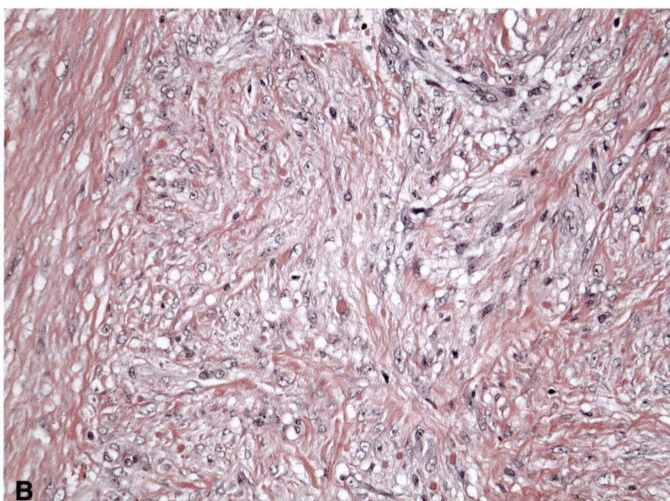

Figure 4.18 Infantile Digital Fibroma. (A) Short interlacing fascicles of spindle cells have a uniform appearance with round to oval nuclei, cytoplasmic vacuoles, and indistinct eosinophilic inclusions. (B) Eosinophilic cytoplasmic inclusions are irregularly dispersed in tumor cells. (C) Trichrome staining highlights the red intracytoplasmic inclusions.

PRACTICE POINTS: Infantile Digital Fibroma

Infantile digital fibroma is most often a dome-shaped mass on the toes and fingers. Cytoplasmic eosinophilic round inclusions are a distinctive histologic feature. Although the condition is benign, the local recurrence rate is high.

Prognosis and Treatment

Infantile digital fibroma is treated with conservative surgical excision.[140] Although it can spontaneously regress, local recurrence has been reported in 60% to 90% of cases.[138,141]

Fibrous Hamartoma of Infancy

Fibrous hamartoma of infancy is a superficial benign tumor that typically occurs in early infancy.[142,143]

Clinical Features

Fibrous hamartoma of infancy shows a marked male predominance and usually appears during the first 2 years of life, with 20% of cases detected at birth and rare cases in older children.[142-147] The rapidly growing tumor is usually solitary but may be multifocal and has a predilection for the trunk, axilla, shoulders, and inguinal region.[147,148] It may rarely involve the head and neck or distal extremities.[145,146]

Pathologic Features

Grossly, fibrous hamartoma of infancy is a poorly demarcated deep dermal or subcutaneous mass that has a pale tan cut surface flecked with soft yellow areas (Fig. 4.19). The characteristic triphasic organoid pattern consists of a combination of mature adipose tissue, mature fibrous tissue, and immature cellular or myxoid mesenchymal tissue with a basophilic or "neural-like" matrix (Fig. 4.20A–C).[142-144,146,147,149] Histologic variations include a central zone with vascular collagenized or hyalinized tissue resembling a vascular neoplasm (see Fig. 4.20D), with organoid triphasic foci detectable at the periphery of the lesion.[142,143,147,149] Electron microscopy reveals a combination of fibroblasts, myofibroblasts, immature mesenchymal tissue, and adipocytes.[150]

Immunohistochemistry

The lesional cells demonstrate reactivity for vimentin and variable positivity for smooth muscle actin and desmin.[144,146,147,150] Vascular foci show CD34 reactivity.

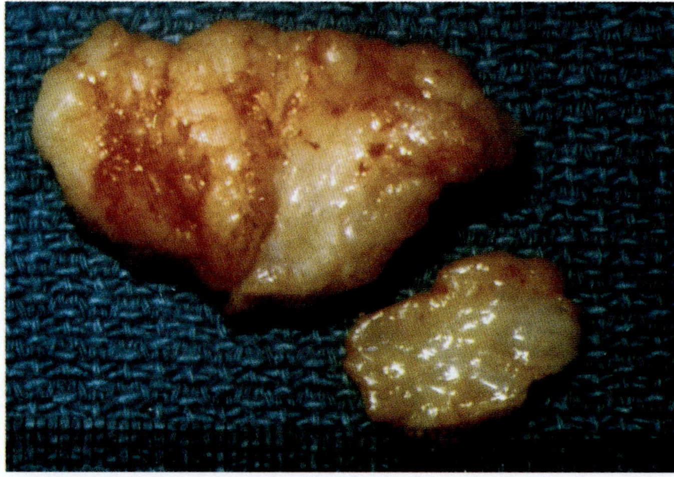

Figure 4.19 Fibrous Hamartoma of Infancy. The fatty mass contains irregular areas of firmer white fibrous tissue.

Molecular Genetics

One case of fibrous hamartoma of infancy with a complex translocation involving chromosomes 6, 8, and 12 and another with a translocation involving chromosomes 2 and 3 have been reported.[151] Recently, insertion/deletion mutations of *EGFR* exon 20 have been identified.[152]

Differential Diagnosis

The differential diagnosis includes fibromatoses, fibrolipoma, lipoblastoma, infantile fibrosarcoma, and, in the lesions with a prominent vascular collagenized central zone, various types of hemangioma or giant cell fibroblastoma. The other fibromatoses are distinguished by their lack of a mature adipocytic component, with the exception of lipofibromatosis, and the absence of the immature basophilic component combined with a well-defined triphasic organoid architecture. Lipofibromatosis is a distinctive type of fibromatosis with two components—mature adipose tissue and delicate interlacing fascicles of fibrous tissue—but it lacks the immature mesenchymal component of fibrous hamartoma of infancy. Lipoblastoma contains lipoblasts in varying proportions and stages of maturation, and may contain prominent myxoid or microcystic areas and fibrolipomatous foci with bands of collagenized tissue that demarcate fat lobules. Infantile fibrosarcoma is a more densely cellular proliferation that can entrap fat but does not contain mature fibrous tissue or mature adipose tissue as an integral component. Occasional cases of juvenile aponeurotic fibroma in the early phase can have immature chondroid tissue that mimics the immature myxoid component of fibrous hamartoma of infancy.

Prognosis and Treatment

Complete local excision is curative. The recurrence rate of less than 15% may be due to incomplete excision, because the borders of the lesion are difficult to identify at the time of surgery.[143,144,152] Fibrous hamartoma of infancy does not regress. Recurrences are histologically similar to the primary lesion.[153]

Calcifying Aponeurotic Fibroma

Calcifying or juvenile aponeurotic fibroma is a type of fibromatosis that has an unusually wide age range. Although it occurs predominantly in children, cases have been reported as late as the sixth decade of life.[154-156]

Clinical Features

The slowly growing painless mass usually involves the hands, wrists, and feet in the first or second decade of life.[154-156] Unusual locations include the back and the proximal upper and lower extremities.[156] It may be attached to fascia, tendons, or aponeuroses. Although most cases are solitary, occasional examples are multiple or involve bone.[157] Most calcifying aponeurotic fibromas are 1 to 3 cm in diameter, but occasional examples grow to a very large size, especially on the proximal extremities.

Pathologic Features

Grossly, calcifying aponeurotic fibroma can demonstrate an irregular contour with a firm fibrous cut surface with gritty areas or small visible calcifications.[156] Three histologic patterns have been observed that reflect different stages in the development of the lesion.[154,158] In the early phase, calcifying aponeurotic fibroma contains fascicles of spindled fibroblasts intermingled with chondroid foci that lack calcification and may display focal palisading of the fibroblasts (Fig. 4.21A). In the middle, fully developed phase, the fibroblasts are arranged in distinct fascicles, chondroid foci are associated with smudgy or granular calcifications, and plump epithelioid giant cells and multinucleated cells are seen adjacent to chondroid foci (see Fig. 4.21B–D). In the late phase,

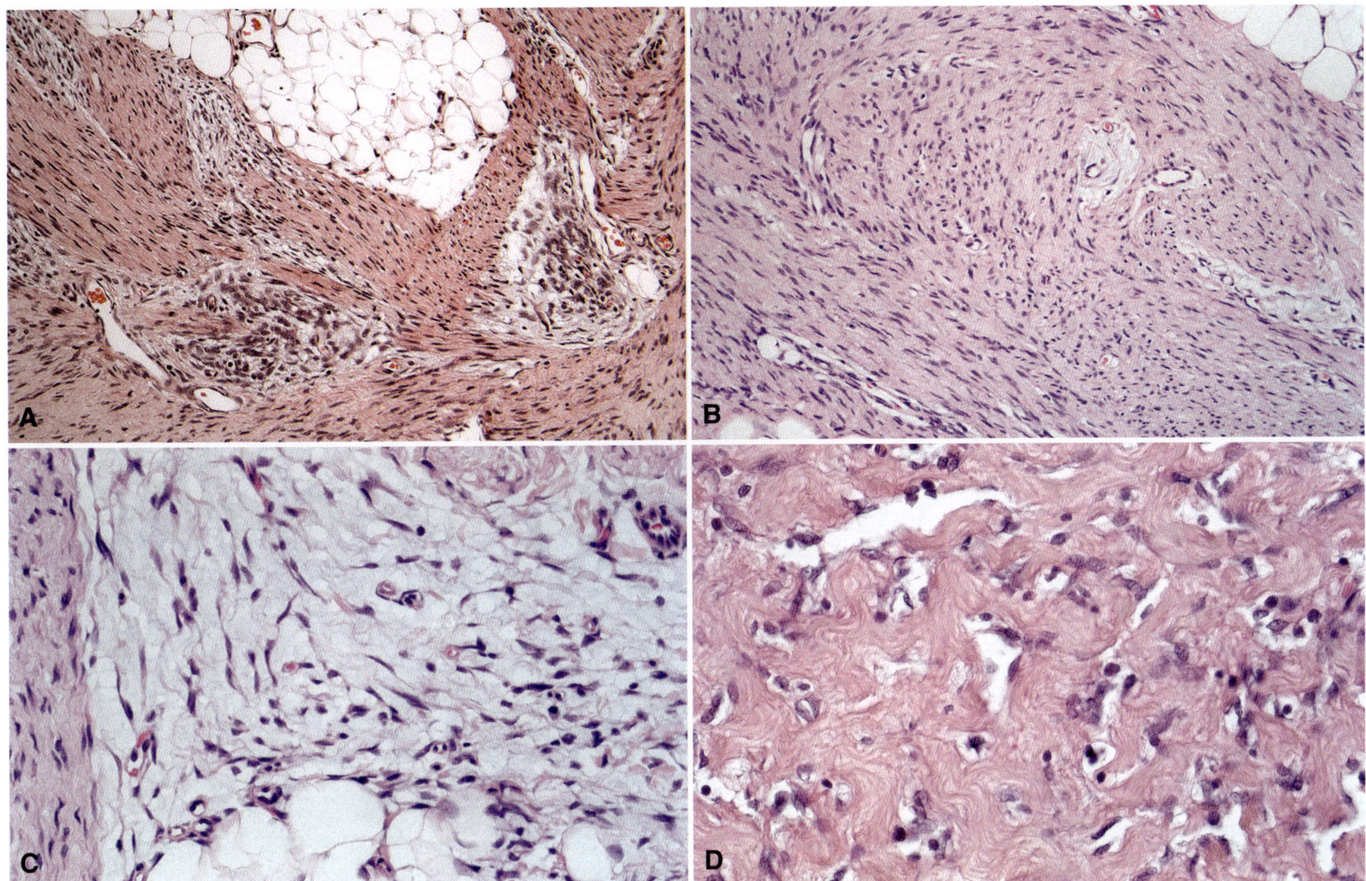

Figure 4.20 Fibrous Hamartoma of Infancy. (A) The triphasic organoid components include mature fibrous tissue, immature basophilic mesenchymal tissue, and mature adipose tissue. (B) The fibrous component forms bundles and fascicles. (C) The immature mesenchymal component in some cases demonstrates a hypocellular myxoid appearance. (D) Collagenized angiectoid foci simulate a vascular neoplasm.

calcification increases, chondroid areas are absent, and cellularity diminishes. Occasional examples demonstrate irregular nuclei and rare mitoses.

Immunohistochemistry

Calcifying aponeurotic fibroma is reactive for vimentin, smooth muscle actin, muscle-specific actin, CD99, and S-100 protein (in the cartilaginous foci).[156]

Molecular Genetics

A gene rearrangement with *FN1-EGF* fusion is present in calcifying aponeurotic fibroma.[159]

Differential Diagnosis

The differential diagnosis includes fibromatoses, soft tissue chondroma, dystrophic calcification, and epithelioid sarcoma. Fibromatoses, such as desmoid fibromatosis or the superficial fibromatoses, typically lack the well-defined chondroid nodules, calcifications, and giant cells of calcifying aponeurotic fibroma. Soft tissue chondroma is a cartilaginous neoplasm that may show calcifications and an associated giant cell reaction, but lacks the fascicular, fibroblastic component of calcifying aponeurotic fibroma. Epithelioid sarcoma can sometimes resemble calcifying aponeurotic fibroma when there are central areas of necrosis and dystrophic calcification, but atypical epithelioid tumor cells with reactivity for keratin and epithelial membrane antigen (EMA) help distinguish epithelioid sarcoma from calcifying aponeurotic fibroma.

PRACTICE POINTS: Calcifying Aponeurotic Fibroma

- Calcifying aponeurotic fibroma is a benign, slowly growing, painless mass.
- In the early phase, cellularity can be high, chondroid foci may be present, and calcifications may be absent.
- *FN1-EGF* gene fusion is present.
- Local recurrence is frequent.

Prognosis and Treatment

Conservative surgical excision is effective treatment. However, the recurrence rate is 50%, and recurrence appears to be more common in young patients.[154,156] Rare cases have been reported with subsequent fibrosarcoma.[160]

Lipofibromatosis

Lipofibromatosis is a locally recurring, nonmetastasizing tumor that has been considered a form of fibromatosis (see also Chapter 12).[161]

Clinical Features

Lipofibromatosis occurs as a poorly demarcated soft tissue mass on the distal extremities, or, less often, on the trunk or head.[161,162] Up to 25% of cases are congenital, and the remainder of cases have been reported in the first two decades of life, with a median age of diagnosis of 1 year. Males are affected more often than females.

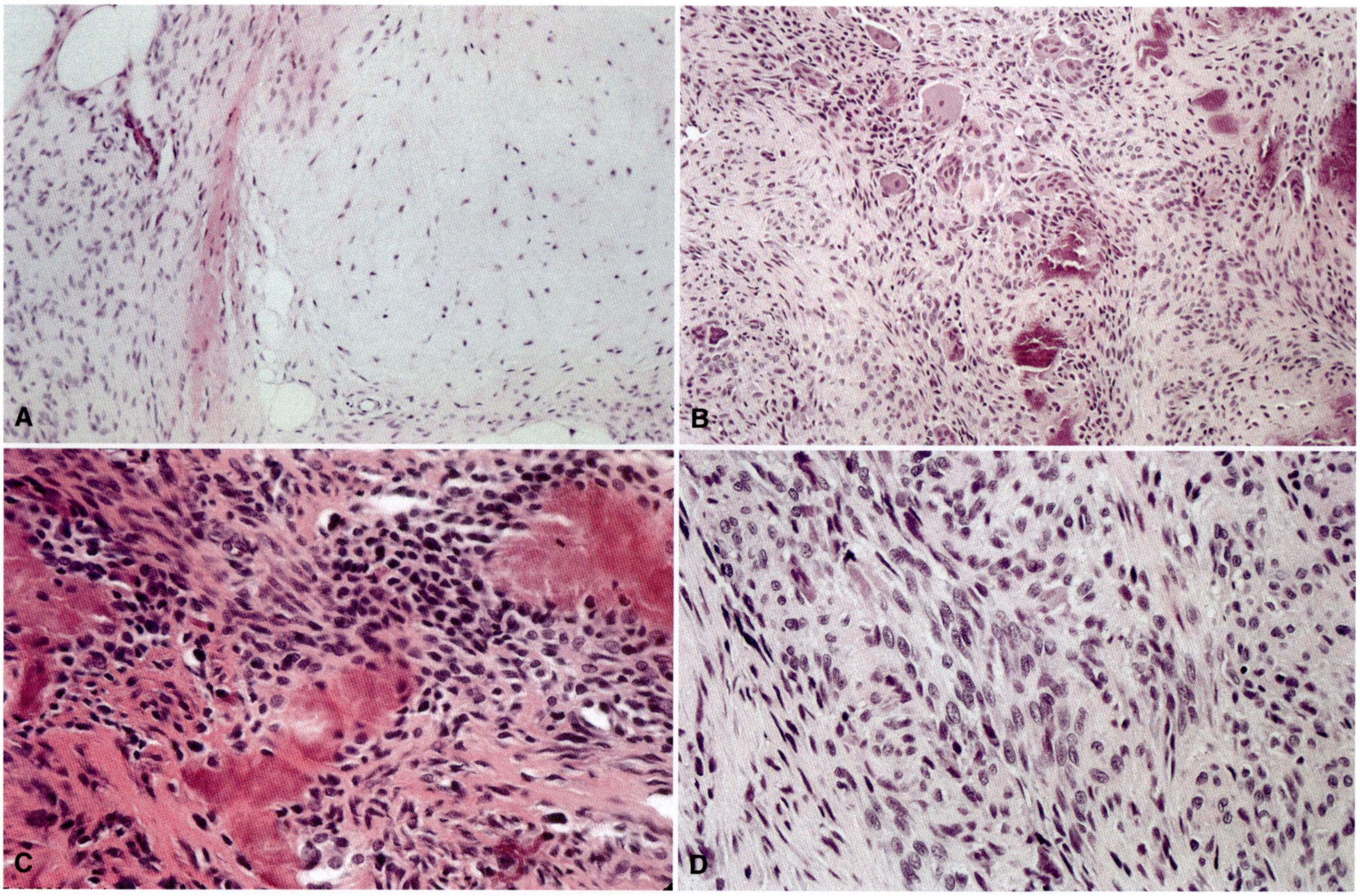

Figure 4.21 Calcifying Aponeurotic Fibroma. (A) A nodule of immature cartilage lies adjacent to fibrous tissue. (B) Fibrous tissue is interspersed with granular amorphous calcifications and multinucleated giant cells. (C) More cellular fibrous tissue is interspersed with granular calcifications. (D) Short interlacing fascicles of spindle cells show higher cellularity.

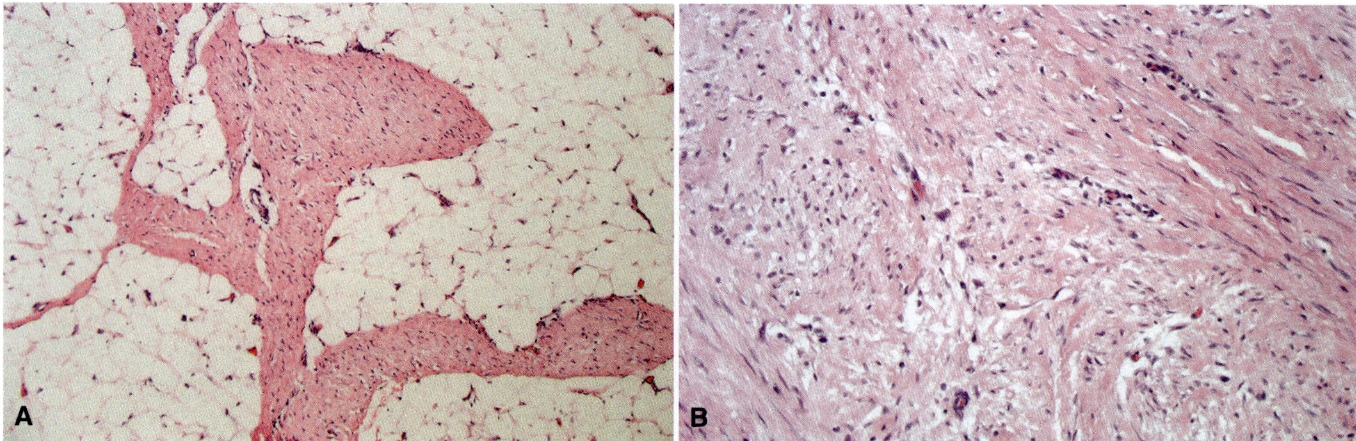

Figure 4.22 Lipofibromatosis. (A) Fascicles of spindle cells are dispersed within mature adipose tissue. (B) The spindle cells form short interlacing fascicles that resemble other fibromatoses.

Pathologic Features

Grossly, lipofibromatosis is a poorly demarcated, white and yellow mass with a variably lobulated or trabeculated cut surface. Disorganized lobules of mature adipose tissue are traversed by bundles of spindled mature fibroblasts (Fig. 4.22).[161,162] In some areas, the fibroblasts form intersecting fascicles similar to other types of fibromatosis. Mitoses are rare, typically less than 1 per 10 high-power fields. The proliferation entraps blood vessels, peripheral nerves, cutaneous adnexal structures, and skeletal muscle fibers. Occasionally, small clusters of univacuolated fat cells are seen at the interface between the fibroblastic fascicles and the mature adipose tissue, but characteristic multivacuolated lipoblasts are not a feature of lipofibromatosis.

Immunohistochemistry

Immunohistochemistry plays a limited role in the diagnosis of lipofibromatosis. Immunohistochemical analysis reveals reactivity for smooth muscle actin, CD34, CD99, BCL2, and muscle-specific actin in variable combinations.[161] Connective tissue growth factor/CCN2 is expressed.[163]

Molecular Genetics

One case has been reported with a complex translocation involving chromosomes 4, 6, and 9.[164]

Differential Diagnosis

The differential diagnosis includes fibromatoses, fibrolipoma, lipoblastoma, and lipofibromatosis-like neural tumors. Lipofibromatosis does not efface adipose tissue, in contrast to other fibromatoses, and instead has fat as an integral component. It lacks the immature mesenchymal component of fibrous hamartoma of infancy. Unlike fibrolipoma, the fibrous component is arranged in well-defined strands and intersecting fascicles instead of perilobular fibrosis. Lipofibromatosis lacks the lobular architecture, myxoid areas, immature lipoblasts, and *PLAG1* gene rearrangement of lipoblastoma. Lipofibromatosis-like neural tumors in young patients are distinguished by cytologic atypia, a neural phenotype with reactivity for CD34 and S100 protein, and a recurrent *NTRK1* gene fusion.[165]

PRACTICE POINTS: Lipofibromatosis

- Lipofibromatosis occurs most often on the distal extremities of young children.
- The two histologic components are disorganized lobules of mature adipose tissue and traversing bundles or fascicles of mature fibroblasts.

Prognosis and Treatment

Surgical resection is effective treatment for lipofibromatosis. Nonetheless, regrowth or persistent growth has been reported in up to 72% of cases.[161] Factors associated with recurrent or persistent disease include congenital onset, location on the hand or foot, mitotic activity in the fibroblastic component, incomplete excision, and male gender.

Juvenile Nasopharyngeal Angiofibroma

Juvenile nasopharyngeal angiofibroma (also known as nasopharyngeal fibroma) is a distinctive tumor that is associated with nasal obstruction, drainage, and epistaxis in adolescent males.[166] This lesion can be associated with *APC* and *CTNNB1* (β-catenin) mutations, and its growth may be stimulated by testosterone.[167]

Clinical Features

Clinically, a sessile or pedunculated mass occurs in the posterior nasal cavity, which can extend into the sinuses and cranial cavity.[168] It can present with life-threatening epistaxis. The median age at diagnosis is 15 years.[169]

Pathologic Features

Grossly, juvenile nasopharyngeal angiofibroma is a lobulated, red and blue tumor with a firm to spongy, focally cystic, and hemorrhagic cut surface.[168] Evenly arranged irregular thin-walled blood vessels with inconspicuous endothelium are dispersed in a loose fibrocollagenous matrix with a patchy mast cell infiltrate (Fig. 4.23).[168] The blood vessels may contain areas of thrombosis or hyalinization. The bland stromal fibroblasts have plump oval nuclei and fine chromatin with stellate cytoplasmic extensions.

Immunohistochemistry

Immunohistochemistry does not contribute to the diagnosis of nasopharyngeal angiofibroma. However, it reveals reactivity for androgen and estrogen receptors and expression of vascular endothelial growth factor receptor 2, high basic fibroblast growth factor, and transforming growth factor β-1.[170-172]

Molecular Genetics

Cytogenetic and molecular genetic analyses have revealed chromosomal gains but no aneuploidy in juvenile nasopharyngeal angiofibroma.[173] The chromosomal gains have been hypothesized to result in activation of oncogenes without loss of tumor suppressor genes.[174] *APC* and *CTNNB1* (β-catenin) mutations have been documented.[175-177]

Differential Diagnosis

The differential diagnosis of juvenile nasopharyngeal angiofibroma includes nasal polyp with prominent blood vessels, lobular capillary hemangioma (pyogenic granuloma), and a variety of other vascular neoplasms, including juvenile hemangioma and cavernous hemangioma. The prominent fibrous stroma and lack of a lobular architectural pattern, combined with the inconspicuous endothelium and delicate thin-walled blood vessels, help establish the diagnosis and distinguish

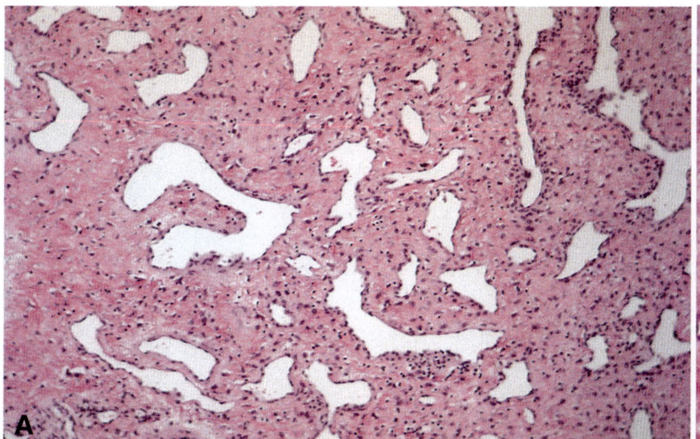

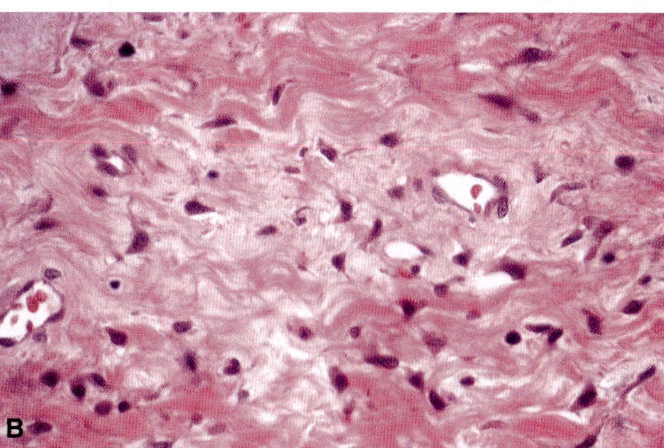

Figure 4.23 Juvenile Nasopharyngeal Angiofibroma. (A) Irregular, delicate, thin-walled blood vessels are dispersed in a hypocellular fibrous stroma. (B) The spindle cells display occasional cytoplasmic extensions and are embedded in a collagenized background.

juvenile nasopharyngeal angiofibroma from lesions with a similar appearance.

Prognosis and Treatment

Surgery and pharmacotherapy with antiandrogens are effective treatments for juvenile nasopharyngeal angiofibroma.[178] Some cases are treated with embolization or chemotherapy. In the past, radiation therapy was used but is associated with an increased risk of postradiation sarcoma.[179,180] A single case of high-grade sarcoma arising in a case without prior irradiation has been reported.[181] The recurrence rate is 68%.

Hyaline Fibromatosis Syndrome

Hyaline fibromatosis syndrome is an autosomal recessive disorder that can affect infants and children. It results in systemic accumulation of hyaline eosinophilic material in the dermis and subcutaneous tissue.[182,183]

Clinical Features

Hyaline fibromatosis demonstrates clinical heterogeneity with juvenile and infantile forms. The infantile form is an autosomal recessive disease with onset at infancy and visceral involvement leading to premature death.[182,184,185] The juvenile form is usually milder.[186] The painful skin as well as the subcutaneous and submucosal lesions can result in gingival hypertrophy, papulonodular skin lesions, bone abnormalities, and joint contractures. Patients ultimately experience impaired movement and disability.

Pathologic Features

Histologically, the nodules of hyaline fibromatosis demonstrate amorphous hyaline or chondroid material with interlacing cords and strands of fibroblasts.[183,187] The earlier lesions display higher cellularity, and the older lesions are more hyalinized.[188] Electron microscopy demonstrates dilated rough endoplasmic reticulum and Golgi filled with granular and fibrillary material.[183,186]

Immunohistochemistry

The immunohistochemical profile of hyaline fibromatosis has not been comprehensively investigated.

Molecular Genetics

Both the infantile and juvenile forms of hyaline fibromatosis result from a mutation in the *ANTXR2* gene (also known as *CMG2*, capillary morphogenesis gene 2) on chromosome 4q21.[182,189]

Differential Diagnosis

The differential diagnosis includes fibrosis, fibromatosis, and gingival fibromatosis. The prominent amorphous hyaline material and demonstration of the *ANTXR2* gene mutation are distinguishing features of hyaline fibromatosis.

Prognosis and Treatment

Interferon 2 alpha has been proposed as a treatment for hyaline fibromatosis.[190] Patients with the infantile type experience failure to thrive and death in childhood.[184] Individuals with the juvenile form live into adulthood.[186]

Intermediate/Rarely Metastasizing Fibroblastic Tumors of Childhood

Inflammatory Myofibroblastic Tumor

IMT is a distinctive neoplasm composed of myofibroblastic spindle cells accompanied by an inflammatory infiltrate of plasma cells, lymphocytes, and eosinophils (see also Chapters 10 and 16).[12,190-196] It is currently regarded as an intermediate rarely metastasizing neoplasm because of its tendency for local recurrence and low risk of metastases. In the past, IMTs have been described under the rubrics of inflammatory pseudotumor, plasma cell granuloma, plasma cell pseudotumor, inflammatory myofibrohistiocytic proliferation, omental mesenteric myxoid hamartoma, and inflammatory fibrosarcoma. The most recent World Health Organization classification of soft tissue and bone tumors has established *inflammatory myofibroblastic tumor* as the preferred term.[12] *Inflammatory pseudotumor* is a more generic term that includes a variety of inflammatory or reactive conditions and neoplasms.[197-199]

Clinical Features

IMT occurs primarily in children and young adults, but it can arise in older adults, with an age range that spans eight decades.[191,197] In up to one-third of patients, a clinical syndrome occurs with fever, growth failure, weight loss, anemia, thrombocytosis, polyclonal hypergammaglobulinemia, and elevated erythrocyte sedimentation rate.[191,196] Resection of the mass leads to resolution of the syndrome, and its reappearance heralds recurrence. The most frequent anatomic sites are the mesentery, omentum, retroperitoneum, abdominal soft tissues, lung, mediastinum, liver, and head and neck. Rare cases have arisen following stem cell transplantation.[191,200] The clinicopathologic features are summarized in Table 4.7.

Pathologic Features

Grossly, IMT is a circumscribed or multinodular firm white or tan mass with a whorled fleshy or myxoid cut surface (Fig. 4.24).[191,193,194,197] In some cases, a zonal appearance with a central scar and softer red or pink periphery is evident. Multinodular separate or contiguous tumors are most frequent in body cavities, especially the abdomen, and are restricted to the same anatomic region. The diameter ranges from several to 20 cm; the mean diameter of extrapulmonary cases is 6 cm.

The spindled myofibroblasts and inflammatory cells form three basic patterns. The first pattern, characterized by loosely arranged plump or spindled myofibroblasts in an edematous myxoid background with abundant blood vessels and an infiltrate of plasma cells, lymphocytes, and eosinophils, mimics granulation tissue, nodular fasciitis, or other reactive processes (Fig. 4.25A). The second pattern is characterized by a compact spindle cell proliferation with a fascicular architecture and

Table 4.7 Clinicopathologic Features of Inflammatory Myofibroblastic Tumor

Feature	Specifics
Age	
Range	Infancy to eighth decade
Peak incidence	Infancy to third decade
Median	9 years
Male-to-female ratio	0.7:1
Sites	
Abdomen and retroperitoneum	73%
Respiratory tract and thorax	11%[a]
Other	16%
Systemic manifestations	15%–30%
ALK gene rearrangements with various partners	50%–60%
Other rearrangements: *ROS1, PDGFRB, RET, NTRK3*	Rare
Outcome	
Recurrence rate	25% (extrapulmonary)
Metastasis	Rare (<2%)
Death	Rare

[a]Incomplete statistical data may result in underrepresentation of respiratory tract tumors.
Data from references 192, 193, 194, 195, 198, and 201-203.

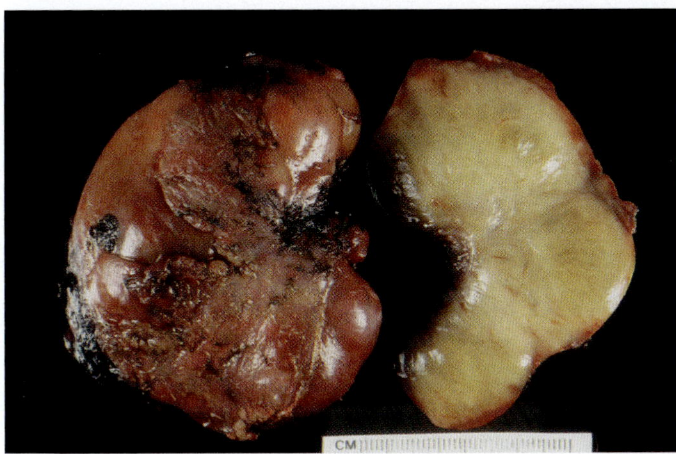

Figure 4.24 Inflammatory Myofibroblastic Tumor. The external surface is red and slightly lobulated, and the cut surface has a firm fleshy and fibrous appearance.

variably myxoid and collagenized regions (see Fig. 4.25B–D). This subtype contains a prominent inflammatory infiltrate with an abundance of plasma cells and variable numbers of eosinophils and lymphocytes. This pattern resembles fibromatosis, fibrous histiocytoma, or other spindle cell neoplasms. Ganglion-like myofibroblasts are seen in both the myxoid vascular pattern and the compact fascicular spindled pattern. Occasionally, spindled myofibroblastic cells surround blood vessels or bulge into vascular spaces. The third pattern is less cellular and resembles a scar or desmoid fibromatosis with plate-like collagen, lower cellularity, and sparse inflammation with plasma cells and eosinophils (see Fig. 4.25E). Occasional examples display coarse calcifications and osseous metaplasia. Rare cases undergo a histologic evolution from a classic appearance to a range of patterns that include highly atypical polygonal cells with oval vesicular nuclei, prominent nucleoli, and variable mitoses; large atypical spindle cells; or rounded histiocytoid cells (Fig. 4.26).[191,193] Although these features have sometimes been associated with aggressive behavior, other identical examples have had a natural history similar to classic examples.

IMT with epithelioid cellular morphology, also known as "epithelioid inflammatory myofibroblastic sarcoma," is a distinctive variant with an aggressive clinical course.[204-207] The plump epithelioid cells are arranged singly or form loose aggregates in a myxoid stroma, often with abundant neutrophils. The eccentric nucleus and prominent large nucleolus of the epithelioid cells resemble malignant rhabdoid tumor.

Immunohistochemistry

Immunohistochemical reactivity for myofibroblastic markers such as smooth muscle actin, muscle-specific actin, and desmin is variable (Fig. 4.27A).[191] Some tumors also demonstrate reactivity for keratin and CD68. Immunohistochemical positivity for ALK (anaplastic lymphoma kinase protein) is usually cytoplasmic and rarely displays a nuclear membrane pattern. It is detected in approximately half of IMTs (see Fig. 4.27B) and indicates the presence of *ALK* gene rearrangements that are detectable by conventional cytogenetics, fluorescence in situ hybridization (FISH), or reverse transcription–polymerase chain reaction (RT-PCR).[208-210] However, not all cases with an *ALK* gene rearrangement are positive by ALK immunohistochemistry using the conventional ALK1 monoclonal antibody; more recently developed highly sensitive antibodies correlate better with *ALK* rearrangement. Epithelioid inflammatory myofibroblastic sarcomas with the *RANBP2-ALK* or *RRBP1-ALK* gene fusions display distinctive patterns of ALK staining characterized by nuclear membranous or perinuclear cytoplasmic reactivity, respectively.[204,205,207]

Molecular Genetics

The *ALK* gene rearrangements on chromosome 2p23 can involve a variety of fusion partners, including *TPM3*, *TPM4*, *CLTC*, *RANBP2*, and other genes (see Chapters 10 and 16).[194,211-215] Recently, a variety of non-*ALK* gene fusions have been discovered in ALK-negative IMTs and involve *ROS1*, *PDGFRB*, *RET*, and *NTRK3*.[201-203,216,217] ALK and ROS1 immunohistochemistry are surrogates for molecular testing in some but not all cases, with the respective gene rearrangements.[201,216] Cases that are negative by ALK immunohistochemistry may require additional testing for the possibility of an *ALK* rearrangement or one of the other gene rearrangements. *TP53* mutations are not found.[218]

Differential Diagnosis

The differential diagnosis is extensive and varies according to the predominant histologic pattern. The principal considerations include myxoid and spindle cell sarcomas, gastrointestinal stromal tumor, malignant peripheral nerve sheath tumor, desmoid fibromatosis, myxoinflammatory fibroblastic sarcoma, mycobacterial spindle cell pseudotumor, follicular dendritic cell sarcoma, and other reactive inflammatory processes, such as sclerosing mesenteritis and retroperitoneal fibrosis (see Chapters 10 and 16). A combination of histologic, immunohistochemical, and cytogenetic or molecular genetic findings helps establish the diagnosis. Significant pleomorphism argues against the diagnosis of IMT and should lead to consideration of a sarcoma. Immunohistochemical reactivity for ALK is useful in the appropriate clinicopathologic context but may also be seen in anaplastic large-cell lymphoma and occasional cases of RMS, neuroblastoma, and other tumors. IgG4-related sclerosing disease, inflammatory pseudotumor of lymph nodes, liver, and spleen, and orbital inflammatory pseudotumor are clinically and pathologically distinct entities.[197-199,219]

PRACTICE POINTS: Inflammatory Myofibroblastic Tumor

- Inflammatory myofibroblastic tumor (IMT) is a neoplasm of intermediate biologic potential with a risk of aggressive local recurrence and very rare incidence of distant metastases.
- Some patients with IMT have an accompanying syndrome of fever, growth failure, weight loss, anemia, thrombocytosis, polyclonal hypergammaglobulinemia, and elevated erythrocyte sedimentation rate.
- IMT simulates sarcoma because of its cellularity, ganglion-like atypical cells, and mitotic activity; it is accompanied by an inflammatory infiltrate with abundant plasma cells.
- Approximately half of IMTs harbor a rearrangement of the *ALK* gene that can be detected by immunohistochemical reactivity for the ALK protein or by genetic tests; other alterations involve *ROS1*, *PDGFRB*, *RET*, and *NTRK3*.

Prognosis and Treatment

Surgery is the most effective treatment. However, regression has been noted in occasional cases. Response to antitumor necrosis factor antibodies and chemotherapy has been reported in individual cases or small series.[220,221] Crizotinib and other small molecule inhibitors of the receptor tyrosine kinase pathway show promise for unresectable or aggressive cases harboring *ALK* or *ROS1* gene rearrangements.[222,223] Extrapulmonary IMTs have a 25% recurrence rate, and metastases are very rare.[191,193,224] Reliable histologic prognostic indicators have been elusive, with the exception of the epithelioid subtype with *RANBP2-ALK* or *RRBP1-ALK* fusion, which is highly aggressive.[193,204,225] Aneuploidy may indicate more aggressive potential, but this is not widely used in clinical practice.[226] Further studies are needed to identify more reliable prognostic indicators for IMT.

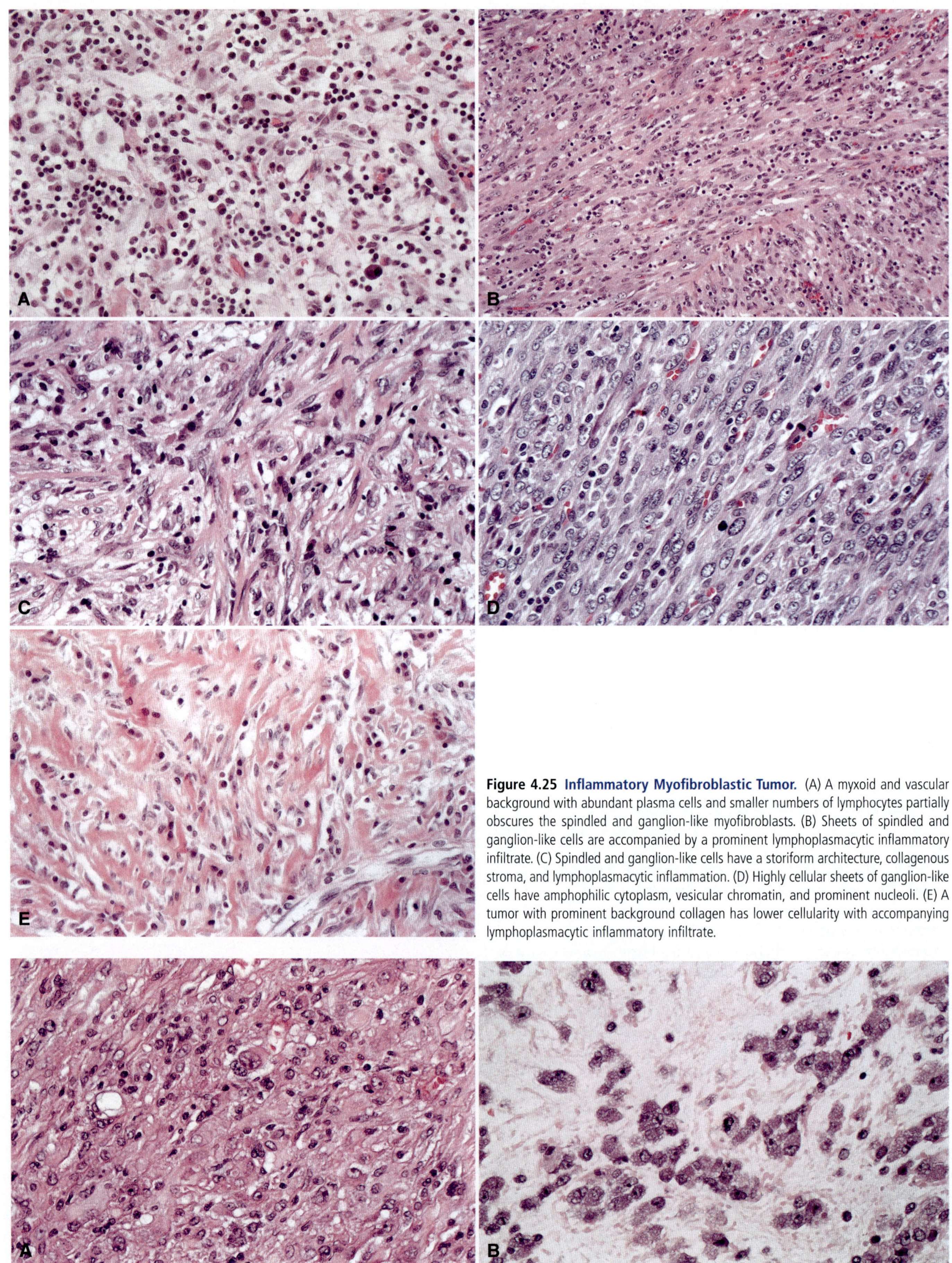

Figure 4.25 Inflammatory Myofibroblastic Tumor. (A) A myxoid and vascular background with abundant plasma cells and smaller numbers of lymphocytes partially obscures the spindled and ganglion-like myofibroblasts. (B) Sheets of spindled and ganglion-like cells are accompanied by a prominent lymphoplasmacytic inflammatory infiltrate. (C) Spindled and ganglion-like cells have a storiform architecture, collagenous stroma, and lymphoplasmacytic inflammation. (D) Highly cellular sheets of ganglion-like cells have amphophilic cytoplasm, vesicular chromatin, and prominent nucleoli. (E) A tumor with prominent background collagen has lower cellularity with accompanying lymphoplasmacytic inflammatory infiltrate.

Figure 4.26 Inflammatory Myofibroblastic Tumor With Histologic Evolution. (A) Large atypical polygonal cells with oval vesicular nuclei and prominent nucleoli simulate a sarcoma. (B) Round histiocytoid cells in a myxoid background simulate a malignant neoplasm.

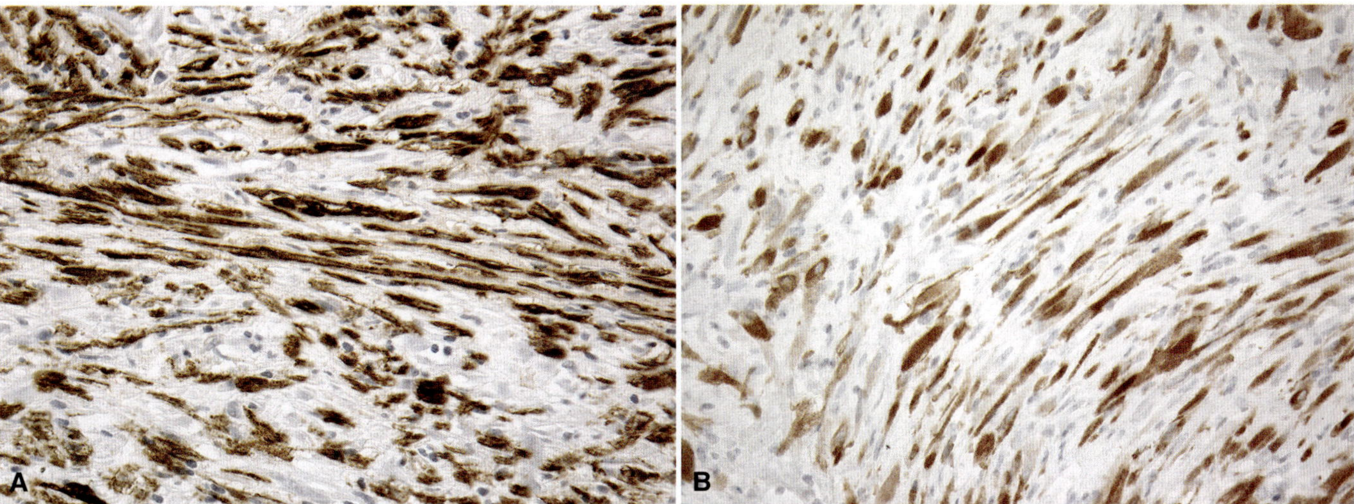

Figure 4.27 Inflammatory Myofibroblastic Tumor. (A) Cytoplasmic reactivity for smooth muscle actin is evident by immunohistochemistry. (B) Cytoplasmic staining for ALK reflects the presence of an *ALK* gene rearrangement.

Infantile Fibrosarcoma

Infantile fibrosarcoma is a cellular, mitotically active, congenital or infantile neoplasm that may histologically resemble adult fibrosarcoma but only rarely metastasizes.[227-231]

Clinical Features

Nearly half of all cases are congenital, and most are diagnosed in the first year of life.[227,228] The most common sites are the distal extremities, head and neck, and trunk. The large, rapidly growing mass can reach a grotesque size relative to the patient, and the clinical appearance may be alarming, with a dark red or purple external surface, prominent areas of vascular dilatation, and surface necrosis. Some resemble an ulcerated hemangioma or vascular malformation.[222,223] Infantile fibrosarcoma has been diagnosed antenatally.[232] Complications vary with anatomic site and include hemorrhage, obstruction of vital organs, bowel perforation with meconium peritonitis, and limitation of mobility or function.[233] Rare cases may be associated with urticaria pigmentosa.[234]

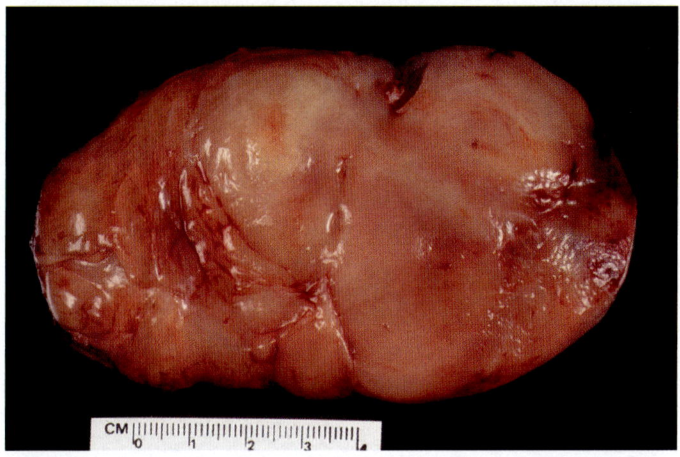

Figure 4.28 Infantile Fibrosarcoma. The lobulated mass has a firm and fleshy cut surface.

Pathologic Features

Grossly, infantile fibrosarcoma is a large solid mass with variable areas of necrosis and a soft to firm cut surface (Fig. 4.28). Histologically, the tumor shows a dense proliferation of spindled and round to plump polygonal cells arranged in sheets, bands, and interlacing fascicles (Fig. 4.29A).[227-230] Foci of necrosis and hemorrhage are common (see Fig. 4.29B). Some cases have a well-developed herringbone pattern similar to adult fibrosarcoma or monophasic synovial sarcoma (see Fig. 4.29C). Dystrophic calcification may be seen. Prominent hemangiopericytoma-like vessels are often present. Histologic variants include a predominantly round cell pattern, a myxoid appearance, extramedullary hematopoiesis with or without patchy chronic inflammation, and widespread necrosis (see Fig. 4.29D and E). In some examples, the spindle cell pattern may be relatively subtle in contrast to the more primitive round and polygonal cell morphology.[235] Histiocytes may be prominent.[236] Infantile fibrosarcoma can regress to a fibrous or hemangiomatous remnant.[237]

Immunohistochemistry

The immunohistochemical profile of infantile fibrosarcoma is nonspecific, with strong diffuse reactivity for vimentin and variable reactivity for CD68 and smooth muscle actin.[228] Consequently, the chief utility of immunohistochemistry is to exclude other cellular spindled, round, or polygonal cell neoplasms of infancy and early childhood. TrkC immunohistochemistry is not specific.[238]

Molecular Genetics

Cytogenetic and molecular genetic abnormalities have been described in detail for infantile fibrosarcoma. Gains of chromosomes 8, 11, 17, and 20 were reported based on early cytogenetic findings.[239,240] Later it was recognized that a translocation between chromosomes 12 and 15 with an *ETV6-NTRK3* gene fusion or *ETV6* rearrangement occurred in nearly all infantile fibrosarcomas.[238,241-245] Recently a gene fusion of *LMNA-NTRK1* has been found in a subset of myofibroblastic tumors of infancy, whose relationship to infantile fibrosarcoma remains to be defined.[246]

Differential Diagnosis

The differential diagnosis of infantile fibrosarcoma includes infantile myofibroma, composite fibromatosis, dermatofibrosarcoma protuberans, spindle cell RMS, infantile rhabdomyofibrosarcoma, and primitive

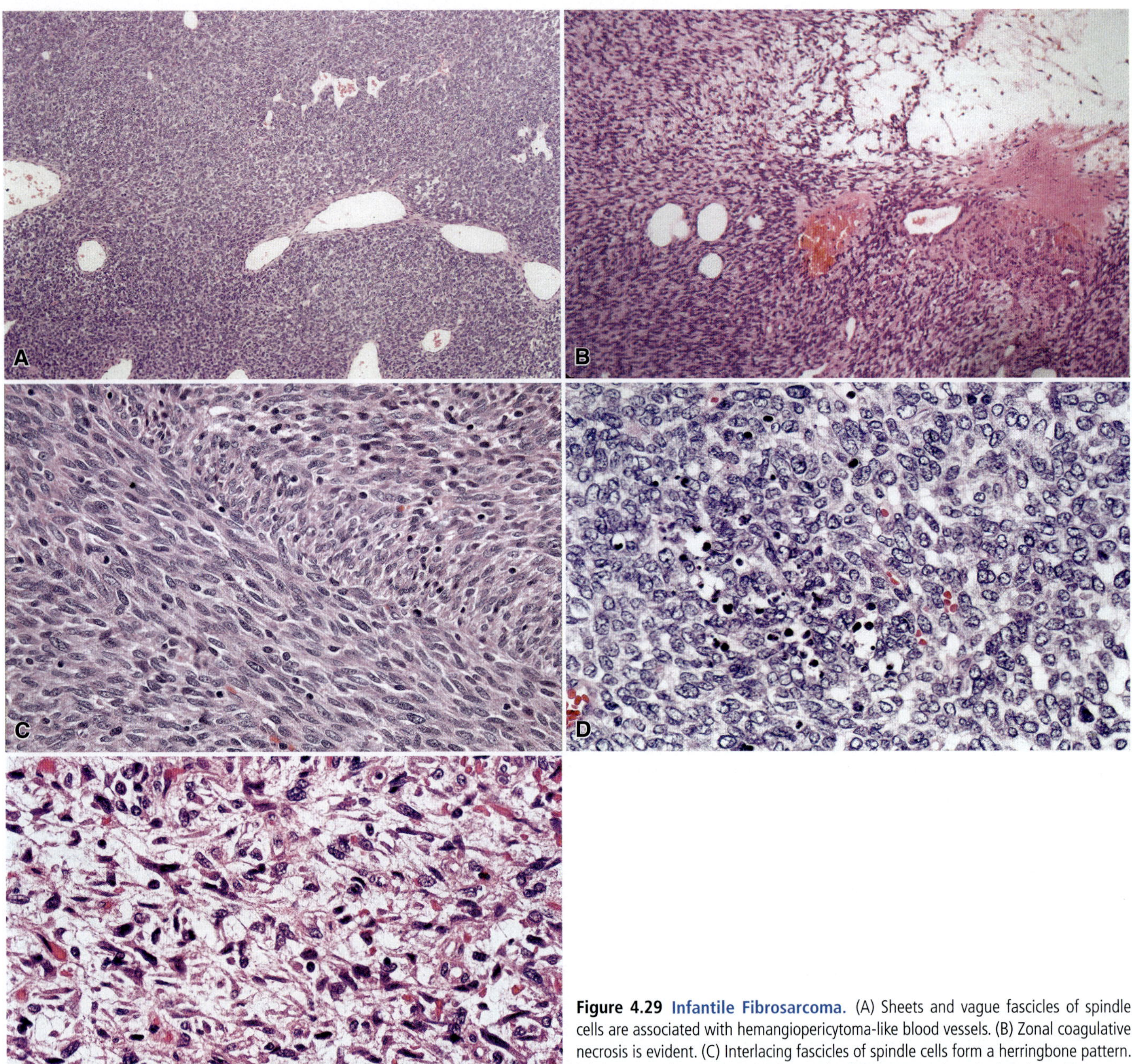

Figure 4.29 Infantile Fibrosarcoma. (A) Sheets and vague fascicles of spindle cells are associated with hemangiopericytoma-like blood vessels. (B) Zonal coagulative necrosis is evident. (C) Interlacing fascicles of spindle cells form a herringbone pattern. (D) Tumors with a predominantly round cell pattern may be mistaken for various types of sarcoma. (E) The myxoid variant is composed of primitive round, spindled, and polygonal cells.

myxoid mesenchymal tumor of infancy. Infantile myofibromas are usually smaller and show prominent smooth muscle actin reactivity and lower cellularity, but examples with features of composite fibromatosis may require cytogenetic or molecular genetic analysis for definitive diagnosis. Dermatofibrosarcoma protuberans is unusual as a congenital neoplasm and is distinguished by its storiform architecture, diffuse reactivity for CD34, and specific gene rearrangement.[247] Spindle cell RMS, especially the infantile form, can bear a striking resemblance to infantile fibrosarcoma and is distinguished by immunohistochemical reactivity for skeletal muscle markers, such as myogenin (MYF4) and desmin. Primitive myxoid mesenchymal tumor of infancy is a less cellular neoplasm with a low-grade appearance, but it can sometimes closely resemble infantile fibrosarcoma in its clinical presentation, site, and morphologic pattern. Whether rare adult sarcomas with an *NTRK1* gene fusion are "infantile fibrosarcomas" outside the expected age group or a separate type of myopericytic sarcoma warrants further study.[248]

PRACTICE POINTS: Infantile Fibrosarcoma

- Infantile fibrosarcoma is a neoplasm of intermediate biologic potential that is frequently congenital; diagnosis after 1 to 2 years of age is very unlikely.
- Genetic abnormalities include t(12;15) with an *ETV6-NTRK3* gene fusion and gains of chromosomes 8, 11, 17, and 20.
- Immunohistochemistry is nonspecific and is most useful for exclusion of other spindle cell neoplasms, such as rhabdomyosarcoma.
- Surgery and chemotherapy are effective treatments.

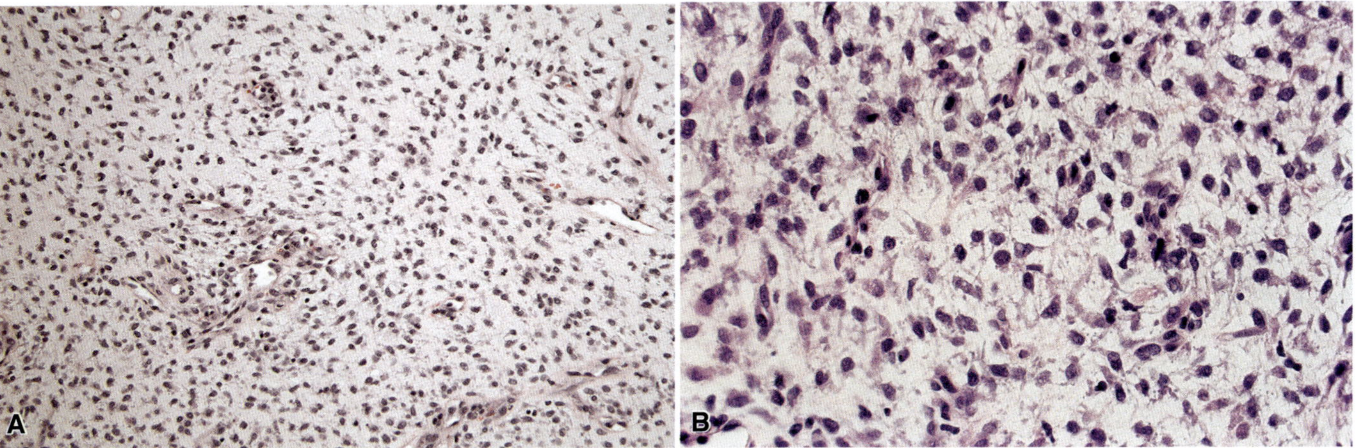

Figure 4.30 Primitive Myxoid Mesenchymal Tumor of Infancy. (A) Polygonal and round cells are dispersed in a myxoid background with variable cellularity and focal condensation around blood vessels. (B) The tumor cells are round to irregular and have a primitive appearance.

Prognosis and Treatment

The treatment of choice for infantile fibrosarcoma is local excision. Chemotherapy is also effective and can also be used as a substitute for surgery or preoperatively to facilitate complete resection.[235,249-255] Recent reports have suggested that tropomyosin-related kinase or vascular endothelial growth factor receptor inhibitor therapy may be effective treatment.[256,257] Biopsies after chemotherapy reveal a hypocellular, bland fibrous proliferation resembling a scar. Occasional cases have regressed spontaneously when incompletely excised. Metastases are rare in infantile fibrosarcoma, although individual case reports have documented metastases in fetuses and children.[232,258-260] Axial tumors may have a worse outcome.[232] The overall 5-year survival is greater than 90%, and the recurrence rate is approximately 30%. The metastatic rate is not well defined because of its rarity and is likely to be much less than 5%.

Primitive Myxoid Mesenchymal Tumor of Infancy

Primitive myxoid mesenchymal tumor of infancy is a rare lesion that overlaps clinically and pathologically with infantile fibrosarcoma, fibromatoses, and undifferentiated sarcoma.[261-264] The soft tissue mass arises in infancy or early childhood and involves the trunk, extremities, or head and neck. The multinodular, focally infiltrative mass has a fleshy white cut surface, and the size ranges from 2 to 15 cm in greatest dimension. A diffuse proliferation of spindled, polygonal, and round cells is dispersed in a myxoid background with a vaguely nodular architecture (Fig. 4.30). Tumor cells are condensed at the periphery of nodules and around blood vessels, and some cases contain rosetted cellular clusters. Condensed areas of tumor cells may be accompanied by increased collagen. Some cells contain cytoplasmic vacuoles with a bubbly appearance. A delicate vascular network is present. Immunohistochemical analysis reveals nonspecific reactivity for vimentin and no reactivity for smooth muscle actin, muscle-specific actin, desmin, S-100 protein, or myogenin. Ultrastructural examination reveals a poorly differentiated fibroblastic proliferation. One reported case had complex structural chromosomal abnormalities.[261] The *ETV6-NTRK3* gene fusion of infantile fibrosarcoma is absent. Cytogenetics and molecular genetic studies of primitive myxoid mesenchymal tumor of infancy have recently revealed *BCOR* internal tandem repeats, which are also found in clear cell sarcoma of the kidney.[264] By immunohistochemistry, both primitive myxoid mesenchymal tumor of infancy (Fig. 4.31) and clear cell sarcoma of the kidney show strong and diffuse nuclear staining

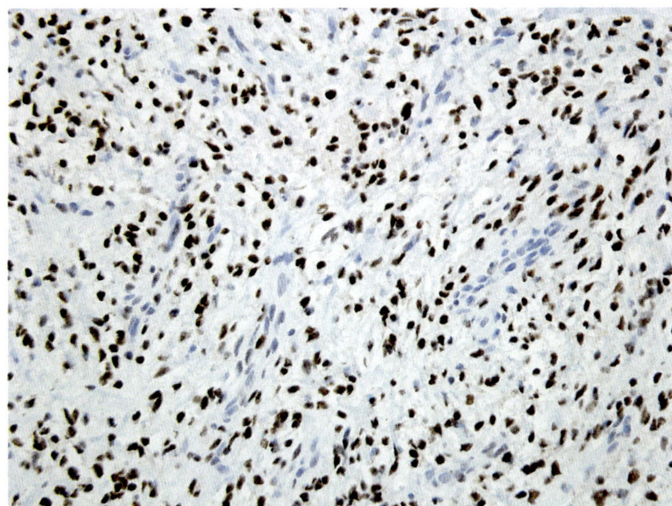

Figure 4.31 Primitive Myxoid Mesenchymal Tumor of Infancy. Diffuse, strong nuclear staining for BCOR is evident by immunohistochemistry.

for BCOR.[265] This suggests that there might be a relationship among primitive myxoid mesenchymal tumor, clear cell sarcoma of kidney, and undifferentiated sarcomas with *BCOR* gene rearrangements. The differential diagnosis includes infantile fibrosarcoma, other types of fibromatosis, low-grade fibromyxoid sarcoma, and undifferentiated sarcoma with *BCOR* genetic abnormalities. A combination of histologic, immunohistochemical, cytogenetic, and molecular genetic features distinguishes these lesions. Primitive myxoid mesenchymal tumor of infancy has been provisionally categorized as an intermediate/rarely metastasizing soft tissue tumor due to the risk of local recurrence and apparently rare episodes of metastasis.[261,266] The current treatment is surgery with or without chemotherapy, although the optimal chemotherapeutic regimen has not been determined. Perhaps in the future primitive myxoid mesenchymal tumor of infancy will be incorporated into the group of undifferentiated sarcomas with *BCOR* abnormalities, or vice versa, or perhaps subgroups of primitive myxoid mesenchymal tumor of infancy will emerge with distinct morphologic, genetic, and prognostic features.

Sarcomas

Low-Grade Fibromyxoid Sarcoma

Low-grade fibromyxoid sarcoma is a rare low-grade sarcoma that includes a morphologic spectrum with hyalinizing spindle cell tumor with giant rosettes at one extreme and a low-grade myxoid sarcoma at the other end of the spectrum (see also Chapters 3 and 5).[267-269] Although this tumor is categorized as a low-grade sarcoma and simulates a variety of benign fibroblastic-myofibroblastic neoplasms, it has a significant potential for late metastases.[270,271]

Clinical Features

The superficial or deep mass occurs in young adults and children, with a predilection for proximal extremities and trunk.[267,269,272-274] Males are affected more often than females. Low-grade fibromyxoid sarcoma can arise at unusual sites, including the head and neck, lung, or spine.[272,275-277] In children, the head and neck are particularly favored sites. Superficial tumors may be more frequent in children.

Pathologic Features

Grossly, the mass is well circumscribed and ranges from 2 to 18 cm in diameter. Histologically, cellular myxoid nodules with perivascular sclerosis mingle with collagenized hypocellular zones (Fig. 4.32).[267,269] The bland spindled fibroblasts rarely display mitoses or atypia. In some cases, collagen rosettes surrounded by a rim of peripheral epithelioid cells (Fig. 4.33A) and areas of ischemic necrosis are seen. Some cases display hypercellularity, cytologic atypia, and increased mitoses, but the significance of these findings is not yet clear. Occasional examples demonstrate some morphologic overlap with sclerosing epithelioid fibrosarcoma (see Chapters 3 and 6).[278]

Immunohistochemistry

The immunohistochemical profile of low-grade fibromyxoid sarcoma includes diffuse (nonspecific) reactivity for vimentin and relatively infrequent focal staining for smooth muscle actin. EMA is at least focally positive in greater than 70% of cases (see Fig. 4.32D).[272,278] Recent studies have shown that MUC4 is nearly always positive in low-grade fibromyxoid sarcoma (Fig. 4.33B).[279] Aberrant DOG1 expression is a potential diagnostic pitfall.[280]

Molecular Genetics

A translocation t(7;16)(q34;p11) with an *FUS-CREB3L2*, or more rarely, t(11;16)(p11;p11) with an *FUS-CREB3L1* gene fusion, is characteristic for low-grade fibromyxoid sarcoma.[273,275,281-284] Rare cases have an *EWSR1-CREB3L1* gene fusion.[285]

Differential Diagnosis

The differential diagnosis includes low-grade myofibrosarcoma, low-grade myxofibrosarcoma, fibromatoses, nodular fasciitis, soft tissue perineurioma, ossifying fibromyxoid tumor, and sclerosing epithelioid

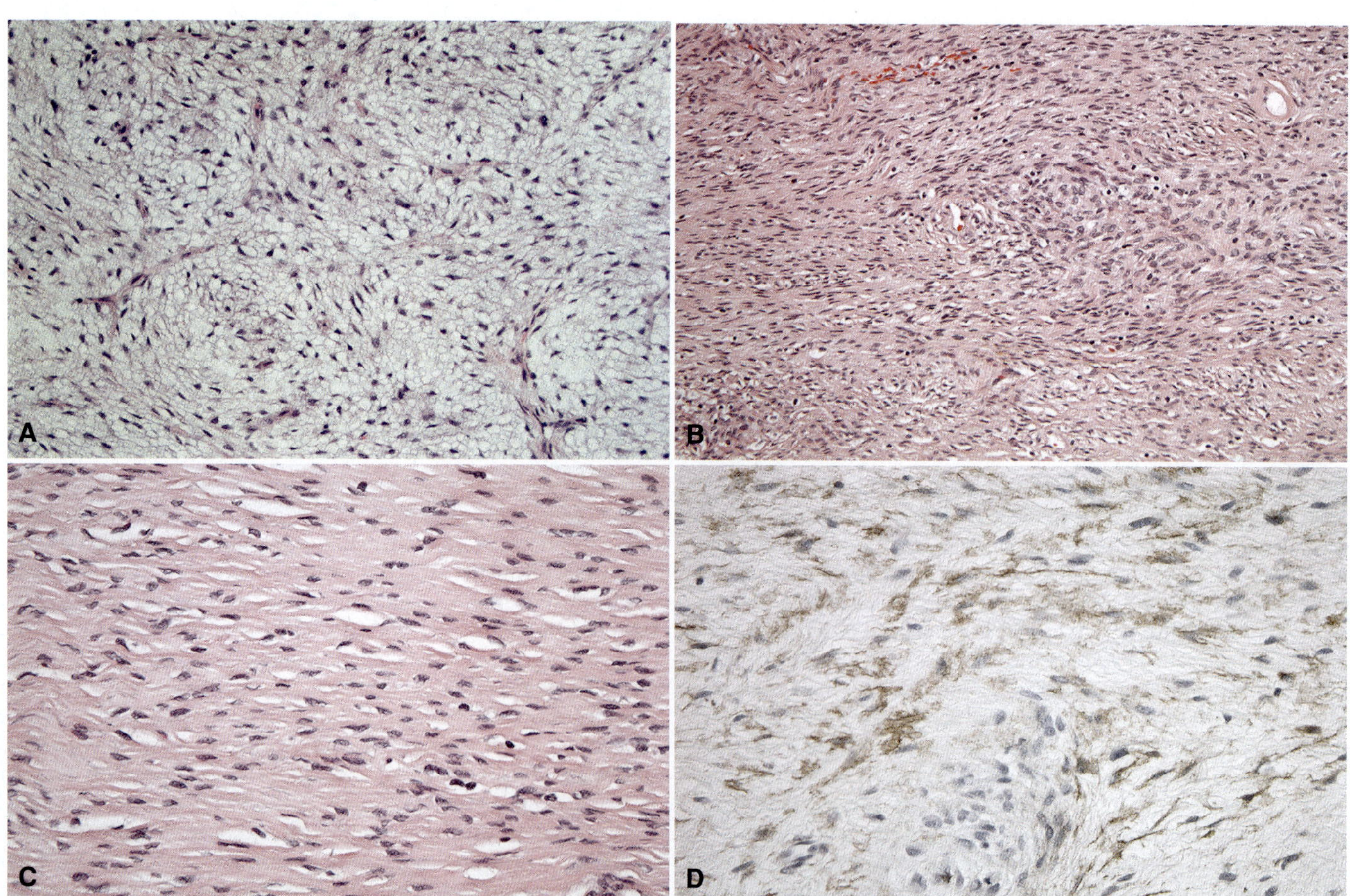

Figure 4.32 Low-grade Fibromyxoid Sarcoma. (A) Short whorling bundles of spindle cells are embedded in a myxoid background and accompanied by an arcading vascular pattern. (B) A collagenized background accompanies the bundles of bland spindle cells without significant atypia. (C) Abundant collagen, bland cytology, and a low mitotic rate are characteristic. (D) Reactivity for epithelial membrane antigen by immunohistochemistry.

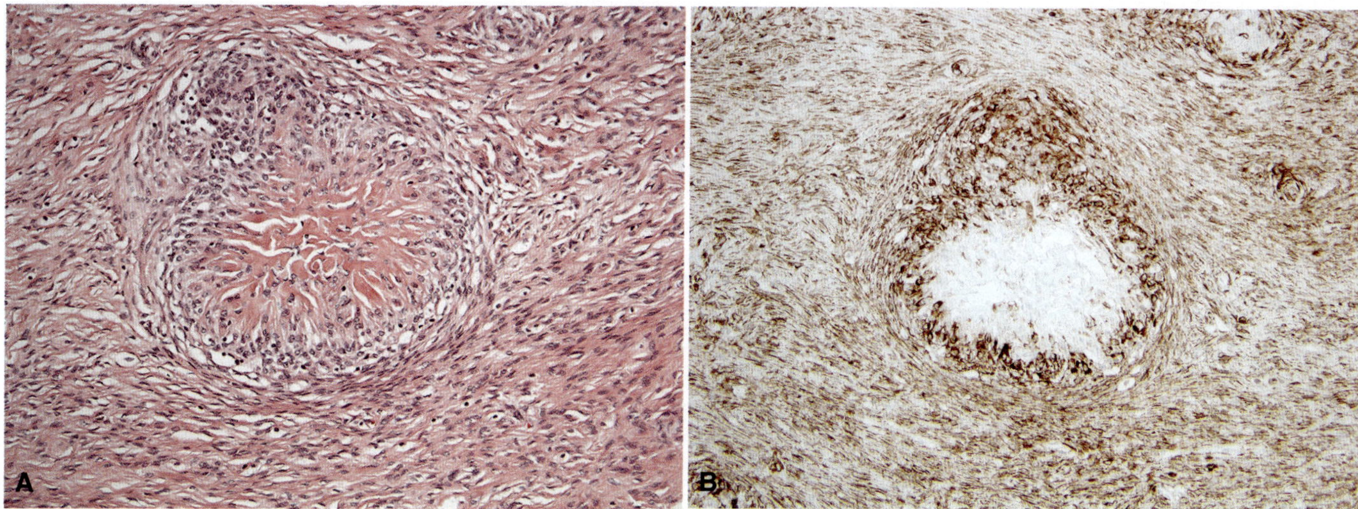

Figure 4.33 Low-grade Fibromyxoid Sarcoma With Giant Collagen Rosette Pattern. (A) Collagen rosettes consisting of a central irregular zone of collagen are surrounded by round to epithelioid cells and accompanied by more conventional spindle cell areas of low-grade fibromyxoid sarcoma. (B) Low-grade fibromyxoid sarcomas show diffuse cytoplasmic staining for MUC4 by immunohistochemistry.

fibrosarcoma. Low-grade myofibrosarcoma is more cellular, fascicular, and uniform, and it typically demonstrates smooth muscle actin and variable desmin reactivity. Low-grade myxofibrosarcoma is distinguished by a prominent myxoid stroma, curvilinear blood vessels, scattered atypical, pleomorphic cells, pseudolipoblasts, and higher mitotic activity.[286] Soft tissue perineurioma shows significant overlap with low-grade fibromyxoid sarcoma, both histologically and immunophenotypically, given its characteristic reactivity for EMA. However, soft tissue perineurioma has a more uniformly whorled and lamellar architecture and generally lacks sharply defined myxoid nodules, MUC4 reactivity, and an *FUS* rearrangement. Rare cases with metaplastic bone mimic ossifying fibromyxoid tumor.[287] Sclerosing epithelioid fibrosarcoma is composed predominantly of epithelioid cells in a densely sclerotic stroma. A gene fusion involving *FUS* and *CREB3L2* has been reported in occasional cases (although *EWSR1* rearrangements predominate),[278,288] and MUC4 is also usually positive in this tumor type.[289] A pathologic continuum may exist that includes low-grade fibromyxoid sarcoma with *FUS-CREB3L1/2* fusions, hybrid tumors with an *FUS-CREB3L2* fusion, and sclerosing epithelioid fibrosarcoma with *EWSR1* gene rearrangements.[288]

PRACTICE POINTS: Low-Grade Fibromyxoid Sarcoma

- In children, the head and neck region is a favored site.
- MUC4 is a sensitive and specific marker.
- *FUS-CREB3L1/2* gene fusions are characteristic.
- Hyalinizing spindle cell tumor with giant collagen rosettes is part of the morphologic spectrum.

Prognosis and Treatment

The preferred treatment is surgical excision with negative margins. Although earlier studies suggested that fewer than 10% of patients have recurrences or metastases, with long follow-up (10 to 20 years), the metastatic rate appears to be much higher—up to 40%.[271] The lung and pleura are the most common metastatic site. The prognosis may depend on the location, with superficial lesions having a more favorable prognosis and deep lesions having a worse outcome.[272]

Low-Grade Myofibrosarcoma

Myofibrosarcoma (myofibroblastic sarcoma) is a usually low-grade sarcoma that overlaps morphologically with low-grade fibromyxoid sarcoma, other subtypes of fibrosarcoma, and other fibroblastic-myofibroblastic lesions.[290-294]

Clinical Features

Low-grade myofibrosarcoma has a predilection for the head and neck in children and can originate in superficial or deep soft tissue and bone. The mass can have an aggressive, destructive appearance on imaging studies.

Pathologic Features

Histologically, the spindled myofibroblastic cells of myofibrosarcoma form large irregular or sinuous fascicles (Fig. 4.34A), occasionally with a myxoid background or a hemangiopericytoma-like vascular pattern. The myofibroblasts demonstrate focal nuclear atypia and occasional ganglion-like cells (see Fig. 4.34B). It is usually low-grade with relatively low mitotic activity. However, a mitotic rate of 6 or more mitoses per 10 high-power fields and/or the presence of necrosis portends higher mortality.[292] High-grade pleomorphic lesions overlap histologically with high-grade undifferentiated pleomorphic sarcoma and are probably more appropriately classified in the category of undifferentiated pleomorphic sarcoma (see Chapter 7).[293,294]

Immunohistochemistry

By immunohistochemistry, low-grade myofibrosarcoma demonstrates variable reactivity for smooth muscle actin, muscle-specific actin, and desmin.[294] Absence of h-caldesmon expression helps distinguish the tumor from a smooth muscle neoplasm.

Differential Diagnosis

The differential diagnosis includes desmoid fibromatosis, nodular fasciitis, low-grade fibromyxoid sarcoma, other types of fibrosarcoma, spindle cell RMS, and leiomyosarcoma. The degree of nuclear atypia and strikingly infiltrative growth distinguish low-grade myofibrosarcoma from desmoid fibromatosis. The other lesions are distinguished on the basis of their clinicopathologic and histologic features. Immunohistochemistry to

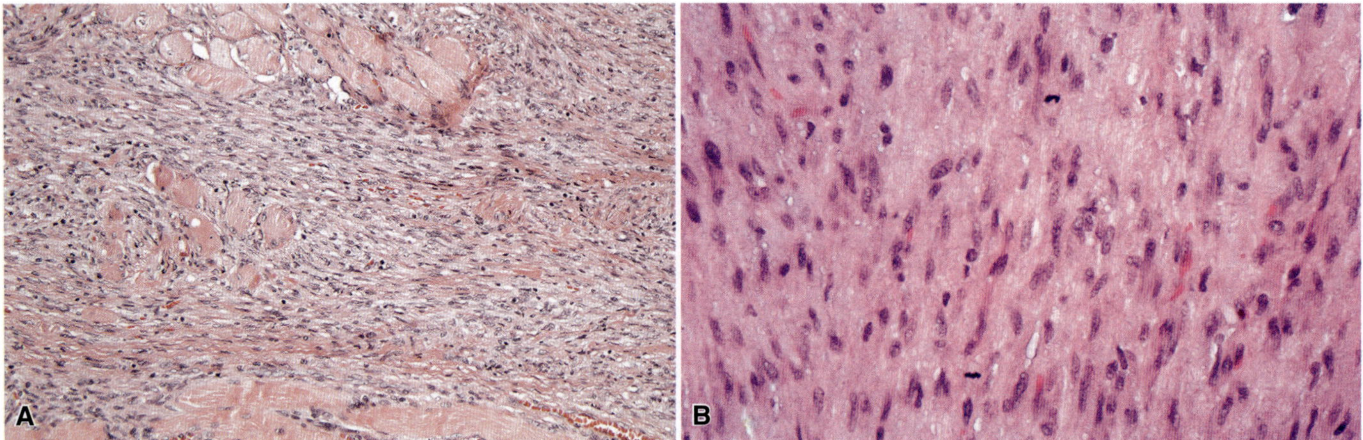

Figure 4.34 **Low-grade Myofibrosarcoma.** (A) Bundles of spindle cells have slightly irregular, atypical nuclei and variable collagen. Note the diffuse infiltration of skeletal muscle. (B) Mitoses and mild nuclear atypia are present.

exclude a skeletal muscle or a smooth muscle phenotype is useful in selected cases.

PRACTICE POINTS: Low-Grade Myofibrosarcoma

- Low-grade myofibrosarcoma in children has a predilection for the head and neck.
- The myofibroblastic tumor cells display more prominent nuclear atypia, pleomorphism, and mitoses than benign myofibroblastic proliferations such as desmoid fibromatosis.
- Radiologic evidence of aggressive, destructive growth can be a helpful distinguishing feature.

Prognosis and Treatment

Low-grade myofibrosarcoma has a favorable prognosis if completely resected.[294,295] Local recurrence and metastases can arise late after initial treatment, although in general, metastases are rare. Low-grade myofibrosarcoma has been included in the intermediate (rarely metastasizing) category of soft tissue neoplasms.

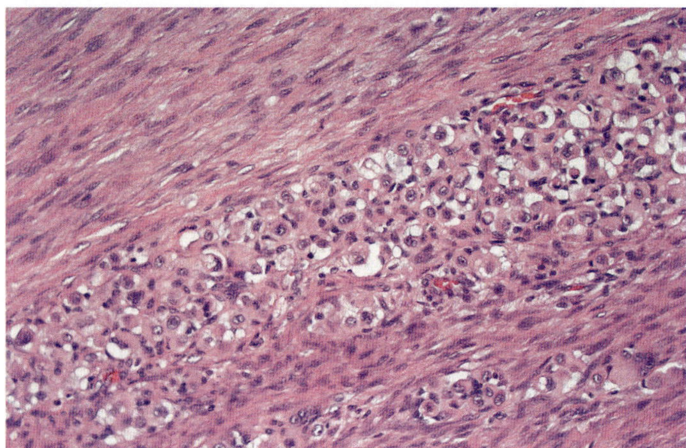

Figure 4.35 **Infantile Rhabdomyofibrosarcoma.** Two components are present, one resembling infantile fibrosarcoma and the other with features of rhabdomyosarcoma.

Infantile Rhabdomyofibrosarcoma

Infantile rhabdomyofibrosarcoma is a rare high-grade sarcoma of infancy and early childhood. It mimics infantile fibrosarcoma and RMS and is a poorly understood, rather controversial lesion because of its incomplete pathologic and molecular genetic characterization.[296-299] It is included here with the recognition that further study of this extremely rare neoplasm may eventually lead to its reclassification as a variant of spindle cell RMS. There is a male predominance. Sites include soft tissue and thoracic cavity. The spindle cell neoplasm resembles infantile fibrosarcoma with a focal component of polygonal cells, with intracytoplasmic eosinophilic globoid inclusions resembling rhabdomyoblasts and elongated eosinophilic cytoplasmic extensions resembling strap cells (Fig. 4.35). Immunohistochemical analysis demonstrates a combination of fibroblastic-myofibroblastic and rhabdomyoblastic differentiation with reactivity for vimentin, desmin, smooth muscle actin, muscle-specific actin, and focal myogenin and MYOD1. Ultrastructural reports emphasized a predominance of fibroblasts and myofibroblasts but also noted cells with sarcomeric structures. Rare cases have been reported with monosomy 19, monosomy 22, or complex structural cytogenetic changes, including a translocation between chromosomes 2 and 11. In contrast to embryonal RMS, there is no loss of heterozygosity at chromosome 11p15.5. The differential diagnosis includes infantile fibrosarcoma, RMS, and myofibrosarcoma. This highly aggressive tumor is often fatal, with local recurrences and metastases to the lung and mediastinum. The optimal treatment is unclear, but the aggressiveness of infantile rhabdomyofibrosarcoma suggests that it is more similar to RMS than to infantile fibrosarcoma.

Other Spindle Cell Tumors of Childhood and Adolescence

Other spindle cell tumors of childhood and adolescence are shown in Table 4.8. With the exception of the fibroblastic-myofibroblastic tumors discussed previously and fetal rhabdomyoma, spindle cell RMS, and undifferentiated sarcoma, other spindle cell neoplasms are quite uncommon in childhood. Angiomatoid fibrous histiocytoma and plexiform fibrohistiocytic tumor can occur in both children and adults and are discussed in Chapters 3, 10, and 11. Kaposiform hemangioendothelioma, an early childhood vascular neoplasm, is discussed in Chapter 13.

Fetal Rhabdomyoma

Fetal rhabdomyoma is a rare tumor that usually occurs in the first 3 years of life, may be congenital, and has a male predilection.[300,301] The postauricular region in the head and neck is the most frequent site; unusual locations include the trunk, extremities, and submucosa of larynx and anus. Some cases are associated with the Gorlin-Goltz nevoid basal cell carcinoma syndrome, and some have mutations in the Hedgehog pathway gene *PTCH1*.[302] Grossly, the mass is circumscribed and soft.

The histologic spectrum recapitulates fetal skeletal muscle, with varying proportions of immature mesenchymal cells, myotubes, eosinophilic myocytes, and strap cells with cross-striations. "Classic" fetal rhabdomyoma contains abundant myxoid stroma and is dominated by immature spindled mesenchymal cells (Fig. 4.36A), whereas "intermediate" ("cellular") fetal rhabdomyoma is more cellular and fascicular, and contains more differentiated rhabdomyoblasts (see Fig. 4.36B). Regardless of immaturity or cellularity, the nuclei are bland and lack atypia, pleomorphism, and anaplasia, and most cases lack mitoses; these features distinguish fetal rhabdomyoma from RMS. Immunohistochemistry is seldom necessary because of the recognizable skeletal muscle differentiation; the tumor cells show strong, diffuse reactivity for desmin and muscle-specific actin, and scattered cells are positive for myogenin. With conservative excision, recurrence is rare.

Table 4.8 Nonfibroblastic-Myofibroblastic Spindle Cell Tumors of Childhood

Tumor Type	Comment
Fetal rhabdomyoma	Infants and young children
Spindle cell/sclerosing rhabdomyosarcoma	Often paratesticular, favorable prognosis
Undifferentiated sarcoma	Uncommon, several subtypes
Giant cell fibroblastoma	Children and adolescents
Dermatofibrosarcoma protuberans	Rare in children, may be plaque-like, congenital
Angiomatoid fibrous histiocytoma	Children, adolescents, and adults
Plexiform fibrohistiocytic tumor	Children, adolescents, and adults
Kaposiform hemangioendothelioma	Infants and young children
Synovial sarcoma	Adolescents and adults
Sclerosing epithelioid fibrosarcoma	Older children and adults
Myxoinflammatory fibroblastic sarcoma	Rare in children
Malignant peripheral nerve sheath tumor	May be associated with NF1 in children
Ectomesenchymoma	Children and adolescents, may be a rhabdomyosarcoma variant
Leiomyosarcoma	Uncommon in children
Gastrointestinal stromal tumor	Rare in children, may be associated with NF1

NF1, Neurofibromatosis type 1.

Spindle Cell Rhabdomyosarcoma

The 2013 WHO classification of soft tissue tumors designates spindle cell/sclerosing RMS as a separate type of RMS, in contrast to past classifications in which it was included in the category of embryonal RMS.[12,303-306] It accounts for less than 5% of RMSs in childhood.[304,305] Spindle cell RMS has been regarded as a favorable subtype of childhood RMS, while sclerosing RMS was initially regarded as a subtype of RMS with a predilection for adults.[12,303-308] More recently, the clinical and genetic heterogeneity of childhood spindle cell/sclerosing RMSs has become evident, and concepts about classification continue to evolve (see also Chapter 3).[309]

Clinical Features

The most common sites for spindle cell RMS are the paratesticular soft tissue and the head and neck region; other sites include the urinary bladder, abdomen, retroperitoneum, trunk, and extremities.[303,310] There is a male predilection.[303,311,312]

Pathologic Features

Grossly, the nodular or lobulated mass has a solid, fleshy, variably whorled cut surface. Histologically, a predominant population of spindle cells is arranged in bundles and fascicles with variable collagen in the background, in a pattern that simulates leiomyosarcoma (Fig. 4.37A). The tumor cells are elongated and may be strap-like, with abundant eosinophilic cytoplasm and occasionally visible cross-striations. Mitotic activity, nuclear atypia, and pleomorphism vary (see Fig. 4.37B), and some examples have anaplastic features. Necrosis is uncommon. Hyaline sclerosis is focal to widespread. Predominantly sclerosing tumors display small round to polygonal cells with a subtle rim of cytoplasm, coarse chromatin, and occasional cytoplasmic vacuoles that may impart a chondrocytic appearance. The tumor cells form nests, cords, or strands in a stroma with a myxoid, basophilic chondroid, or hyalinized eosinophilic matrix that may resemble osteoid.[12,309] Some examples have a microalveolar or solid pattern that simulates alveolar RMS.[313]

Immunohistochemistry

The immunohistochemical profile of spindle cell RMS is identical to other RMS subtypes, with reactivity for muscle-specific actin, desmin, myogenin (MYF4), and MYOD1.[303,311,314]

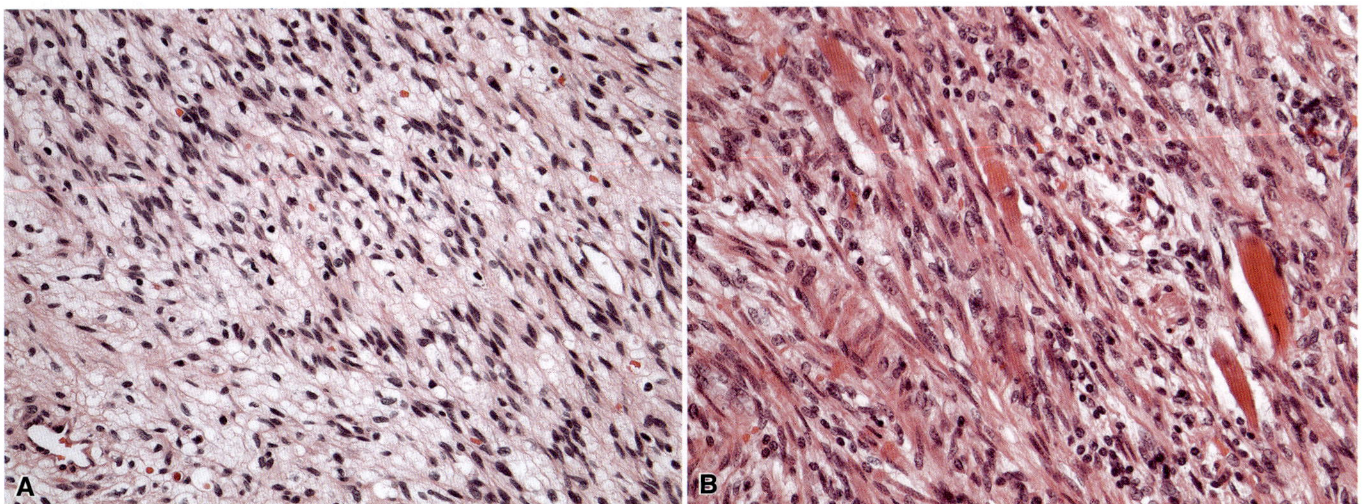

Figure 4.36 Fetal Rhabdomyoma. (A) Classic fetal rhabdomyoma is composed of bland primitive spindle cells in a myxoid stroma. (B) Cellular ("intermediate") fetal rhabdomyoma is composed of cellular fascicles of spindle cells with eosinophilic cytoplasm, including scattered differentiated rhabdomyoblasts.

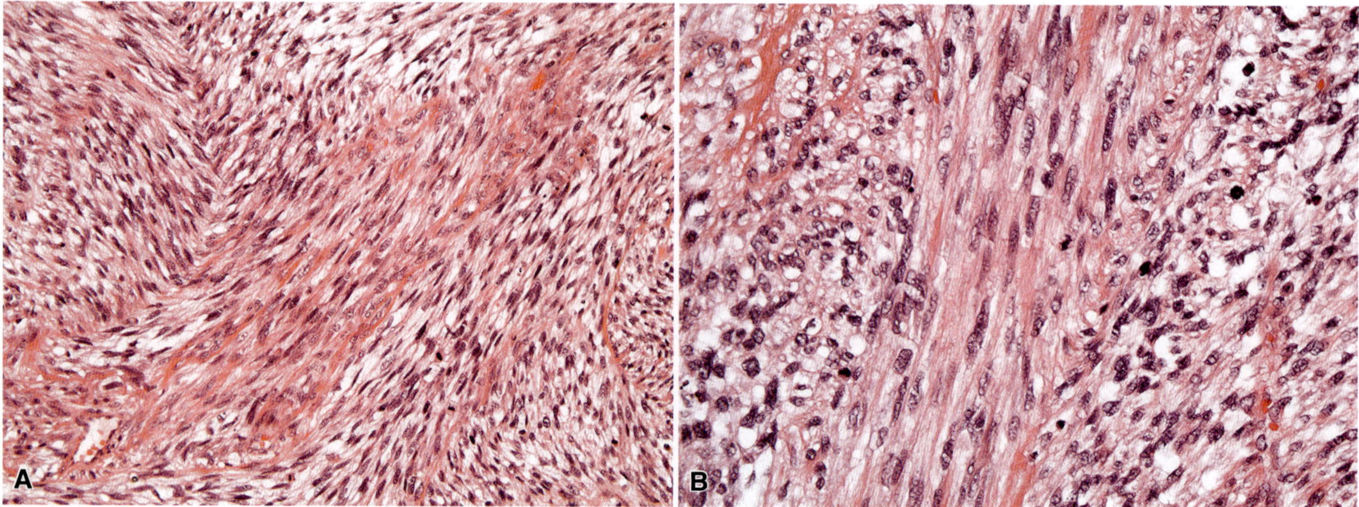

Figure 4.37 Spindle Cell Rhabdomyosarcoma. (A) Intersecting fascicles of spindle cells with brightly eosinophilic cytoplasm are present. (B) Mitoses and nuclear atypia are present.

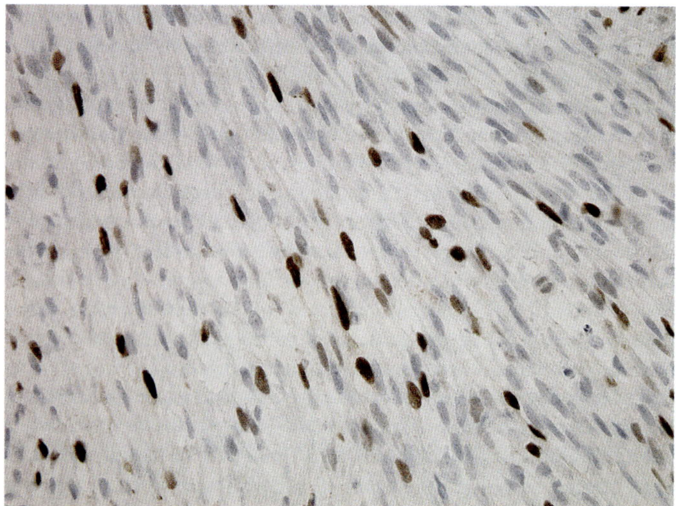

Figure 4.38 Spindle Cell Rhabdomyosarcoma. Nuclear staining for myogenin by immunohistochemistry.

The extent of nuclear reactivity for myogenin can range from focal to diffuse (Fig. 4.38). MYOD1 is often more diffusely positive than myogenin. Some examples also express myoglobin and other less sensitive markers of skeletal muscle differentiation.

Molecular Genetics

Genetic heterogeneity is a feature of spindle cell/sclerosing RMS in children, with several emerging subtypes. Many infantile spindle cell RMSs harbor a recurrent *VGLL2-CITED2* or *NCOA2* gene rearrangement, with various partner genes for *NCOA2*, including *SRF* and *TEAD1*.[309,315] Spindle cell RMSs in older children, generally after 10 years of age, can have mutations in *MYOD1*, sometimes accompanied by *PIK3CA* or *FGFR4* mutations.[309,315-317]

Differential Diagnosis

Leiomyosarcoma, classical embryonal RMS, fetal rhabdomyoma, genital rhabdomyoma, and infantile fibrosarcoma are the principal differential diagnostic considerations. Leiomyosarcoma is relatively uncommon in young patients, lacks cytoplasmic cross-striations, and has a distinctive immunohistochemical profile, with reactivity for smooth muscle actin and h-caldesmon. Fetal rhabdomyoma displays less cellular atypia and also has myoblasts intermingled with primitive mesenchymal cells. Genital rhabdomyoma typically occurs in middle adulthood and lacks immaturity and atypia. Infantile fibrosarcoma and infantile spindle cell RMS with *VGLL2* or *NCOA2* gene rearrangements resemble each other closely, so immunohistochemistry and molecular tests can be very useful for their distinction.[309]

PRACTICE POINTS: Spindle Cell Rhabdomyosarcoma

- Pediatric spindle cell rhabdomyosarcoma (RMS) is a favorable histologic-prognostic subtype of RMS.
- The most frequent sites are the paratesticular soft tissue in two-thirds of cases and the head and neck, particularly the periorbital region.
- The histologic pattern simulates leiomyosarcoma, and immunohistochemical expression of skeletal muscle markers is useful for differential diagnosis.
- Emerging molecular genetic subtypes include infantile spindle cell RMS with *NCOA2* or *VGLL2* gene rearrangement and spindle cell RMS in older children with *MYOD1* and other mutations.

Prognosis and Treatment

The prognosis varies. Although COG studies indicated that the outcome of spindle cell RMS was favorable and similar to embryonal RMS, except for the more aggressive parameningeal tumors, recent data have demonstrated prognostically significant clinical and molecular genetic subsets.[313] The infantile spindle cell RMSs with *VGLL2* or *NCOA2* rearrangements have a favorable prognosis, while the spindle cell RMSs with *MYOD1* mutations in older children are highly aggressive.[309,313,315-317] Surgery is the initial treatment, with chemotherapy and/or radiation therapy according to childhood cancer protocols.

Undifferentiated Sarcoma in Childhood

The 2013 WHO classification of soft tissue tumors included the specific category of undifferentiated sarcoma for the first time and subdivided them into round cell, spindle cell, epithelioid, and pleomorphic subtypes.[12,318] According to the WHO classification, undifferentiated sarcoma has no definable line of differentiation using "currently available technologies."[12] For decades, the presence of a significant group of childhood sarcomas with an undifferentiated appearance has been recognized, despite the availability of electron microscopy, immunohistochemistry, and molecular genetic tests as adjuncts to diagnosis.[319-322] This discussion focuses on the spindle cell subset of undifferentiated sarcomas in children; other subtypes are discussed in Chapters 3, 7, and 8.

In a recent Children's Oncology Group (COG) study of nonrhabdomyosarcomatous soft tissue sarcomas, COG ARST0332, 12% of the tumors were undifferentiated sarcomas.[323] These tumors in COG ARST0332 were divided into the same subtypes as defined in the WHO classification, and one quarter had a predominantly spindle cell appearance, although combined pattern tumors were not unusual. The clinical presentation is similar to other types of soft tissue sarcomas, and undifferentiated sarcoma can occur as a second malignant neoplasm. Knowledge about clinical-morphologic-genetic subtypes continues to evolve from the 2013 WHO classification. Spindle cell or combined spindle and round cell undifferentiated sarcomas can harbor a *BCOR-CCNB3* or *MLL4-GPS2* gene fusion.[12,324,325,247] *BCOR* internal tandem duplications and *YWHAE-NUTM2B* fusions have also been identified in undifferentiated sarcomas and cases of primitive myxoid mesenchymal tumors of infancy.[264] Whether primitive myxoid mesenchymal tumor of infancy (discussed previously), particularly the group with *BCOR* genetic alterations, will eventually be reclassified as undifferentiated sarcomas or will be given a more specific designation is a consideration for the future.

The differential diagnosis of spindle cell undifferentiated sarcoma includes a wide range of soft tissue neoplasms, so careful selection of diagnostic adjuncts is essential. RMS, synovial sarcoma, malignant peripheral nerve sheath tumor, infantile fibrosarcoma, liposarcoma, myoepithelial neoplasms, lipoblastoma with a predominantly myxoid appearance, solitary fibrous tumor, and many benign, intermediate, and malignant fibroblastic-myofibroblastic tumors can mimic undifferentiated sarcoma, especially in a small biopsy.

Although undifferentiated sarcomas are considered high grade at present, the biologic behavior and prognosis may vary according to age, morphology, and molecular genetic features, and data are limited. According to recent past studies, the overall survival for childhood undifferentiated sarcoma is 70% to 75%.[321,322]

References

1. Harms D: Soft tissue sarcomas in the Kiel Pediatric Tumor Registry, *Curr Top Pathol* 89:31–45, 1995.
2. Gurney JG, Young JL, Jr, Roffers SD, et al: Soft tissue sarcomas. InRies LAG, Smith LA, Gurney JG, et al, editors: *Cancer incidence and survival among children and adolescents: U.S. SEER Program, 1975–1995*, National Cancer Institute, SEER Program, NIH Pub. No. 99-4969. Bethesda, 1999, National Institutes of Health, pp 111–123.
3. Coffin CM, Dehner LP: Pathologic evaluation of pediatric soft tissue tumors, *Am J Clin Pathol* 109:S38–S52, 1998.
4. Coffin CM, O'Shea PA, Dehner LP: *Pediatric soft tissue tumors: a clinical, pathological, and therapeutic approach*, Philadelphia, 1997, Lippincott Williams & Wilkins.
5. Coffin CM, Dehner LP: Fibroblastic-myofibroblastic tumors in children and adolescents: a clinicopathologic study of 108 examples in 103 patients, *Pediatr Pathol* 11:569–588, 1991.
6. Coffin CM, Alaggio R: Fibroblastic and myofibroblastic tumors in children and adolescents, *Pediatr Dev Pathol* 15(Suppl 1):127–180, 2012.
7. Sargar KM, Sheybani EF, Shenoy A, et al: Pediatric fibroblastic and myofibroblastic tumors; a pictorial review, *Radiographics* 36:1195–1214, 2016.
8. Dehner LP, Askin FB: Tumors of fibrous tissue origin in childhood. A clinicopathologic study of cutaneous and soft tissue neoplasms in 66 children, *Cancer* 38:888–900, 1976.
9. Schmidt D: Fibrous tumors and tumor-like lesions of childhood: diagnosis, differential diagnosis, and prognosis, *Curr Top Pathol* 89:175–191, 1995.
10. Coffin C, Boccon-Gibod L: Fibroblastic-myofibroblastic proliferations of childhood and adolescents, *Ann Pathol* 24:605–620, 2004.
11. Rosenberg HS, Stenback WA, Spjut HJ: The fibromatoses of infancy and childhood, *Perspect Pediatr Pathol* 4:269–348, 1978.
12. Fletcher CDM, Bridge JA, Hogendoorn PCW, et al, editors: *WHO classification of tumours of soft tissue and bone*, Lyon, France, 2013, IARC.
13. Coffin CM, Davis JL, Borinstein SC: Syndrome-associated soft tissue tumours, *Histopathology* 64:68–87, 2014.
14. Schmidt D, Harms D: Fibromatosis of infancy and childhood. Histology, ultrastructure and clinicopathologic correlation, *Z Kinderchir* 40:40–46, 1985.
15. Allen PW: Nodular fasciitis, *Pathology* 4:9–26, 1972.
16. Stout AP: Pseudosarcomatous fascitis in children, *Cancer* 14:1216–1222, 1961.
17. Price EB, Jr, Sillliphant WM, Shuman R: Nodular fasciitis: a clinicopathologic analysis of 65 cases, *Am J Clin Pathol* 35:122–136, 1961.
18. Coffin CM, Randall RL: Nodular fasciitis: clinicopathologic and differential diagnostic features, *Pathol Case Rev* 5:71–76, 2000.
19. Hornick JL, Fletcher CD: Intraarticular nodular fasciitis—a rare lesion: clinicopathologic analysis of a series, *Am J Surg Pathol* 30:237–241, 2006.
20. Montgomery EA, Meis JM: Nodular fasciitis. Its morphologic spectrum and immunohistochemical profile, *Am J Surg Pathol* 15:942–948, 1991.
21. Perez-Montiel MD, Plaza JA, Dominguez-Malagon H, et al: Differential expression of smooth muscle myosin, smooth muscle actin, h-caldesmon, and calponin in the diagnosis of myofibroblastic and smooth muscle lesions of skin and soft tissue, *Am J Dermatopathol* 28:105–111, 2006.
22. Oshiro Y, Fukuda T, Tsuneyoshi M: Fibrosarcoma versus fibromatoses and cellular nodular fasciitis. A comparative study of their proliferative activity using proliferating cell nuclear antigen, DNA flow cytometry, and p53, *Am J Surg Pathol* 18:712–719, 1994.
23. Wirman JA: Nodular fasciitis, a lesion of myofibroblasts: an ultrastructural study, *Cancer* 38:2378–2389, 1976.
24. Koizumi H, Mikami M, Doi M, et al: Clonality analysis of nodular fasciitis by HUMARA-methylation-specific PCR, *Histopathology* 47:320–321, 2005.
25. Oliveira AM, Chou MM: USP6-induced neoplasms: the biologic spectrum of aneurysmal bone cyst and nodular fasciitis, *Hum Pathol* 45:1–11, 2014.
26. Shin C, Low I, Ng D, et al: USP6 gene rearrangement in nodular fasciitis and histologic mimics, *Histopathology* 69:784–791, 2016.
27. Erickson-Johnson MR, Chou MM, Evers BR, et al: Nodular fasciitis: a novel model of transient neoplasia induced by MYH9-USP6 gene fusion, *Lab Invest* 91:1427–1433, 2011.
28. Hussein MR: Cranial fasciitis of childhood: a case report and review of literature, *J Cutan Pathol* 35:212–214, 2008.
29. Bacac M, Migliavacca E, Stehle JC, et al: A gene expression signature that distinguishes desmoid tumours from nodular fasciitis, *J Pathol* 208:543–553, 2006.
30. Stanley MW, Skoog L, Tani EM, et al: Nodular fasciitis: spontaneous resolution following diagnosis by fine-needle aspiration, *Diagn Cytopathol* 9:322–324, 1993.
31. Lauer DH, Enzinger FM: Cranial fasciitis of childhood, *Cancer* 45:401–406, 1980.
32. Sarangarajan R, Dehner LP: Cranial and extracranial fasciitis of childhood: a clinicopathologic and immunohistochemical study, *Hum Pathol* 30:87–92, 1999.
33. Cummings TJ, George TM, Fuchs HE, et al: The pathology of extracranial scalp and skull masses in young children, *Clin Neuropathol* 23:34–43, 2004.
34. Sato Y, Kitamura T, Suganuma Y, et al: Cranial fasciitis of childhood: a case report, *Eur J Pediatr Surg* 3:107–109, 1993.
35. Agozzino M, Cavallero A, Inzani F, et al: Cranial fasciitis with exclusive intracranial extension in an 8-year-old girl, *Acta Neuropathol* 111:286–288, 2006.
36. Oh CK, Whang SM, Kim BG, et al: Congenital cranial fasciitis—"watch and wait" or early intervention, *Pediatr Dermatol* 24:263–266, 2007.
37. Wehrli BM, Weiss SW, Yandow S, et al: Gardner-associated fibromas (GAF) in young patients: a distinct fibrous lesion that identifies unsuspected Gardner syndrome and risk for fibromatosis, *Am J Surg Pathol* 25:645–651, 2001.
38. Coffin CM, Hornick JL, Zhou H, et al: Gardner fibroma: a clinicopathologic and immunohistochemical analysis of 45 patients with 57 fibromas, *Am J Surg Pathol* 31:410–416, 2007.
39. Pho LN, Coffin CM, Burt RW: Abdominal desmoid in familial adenomatous polyposis presenting as a pancreatic cystic lesion, *Fam Cancer* 4:135–138, 2005.
40. Dahl NA, Sheil A, Knapke S, et al: Gardner fibroma; clinical and histopathologic implications of germline APC mutation association, *J Pediatr Hematol Oncol* 38:e154–e157, 2016.
41. Carlson JW, Fletcher CD: Immunohistochemistry for beta-catenin in the differential diagnosis of spindle cell lesions: analysis of a series and review of the literature, *Histopathology* 51:509–514, 2007.
42. Vieira J, Pinto C, Alfonso M, et al: Identification of previously unrecognized FAP in children with Gardner fibroma, *Eur J Hum Genet* 23:715–718, 2015.
43. Michal M: Non-nuchal-type fibroma associated with Gardner's syndrome. A hitherto-unreported mesenchymal tumor different from fibromatosis and nuchal-type fibroma, *Pathol Res Pract* 196:857–860, 2000.
44. Levesque S, Ahmed N, Nguyen VH, et al: Neonatal Gardner fibroma: a sentinel presentation of severe familial adenomatous polyposis, *Pediatrics* 126:e1599–e1602, 2010.
45. Lanckohr C, Debiec-Rychter M, Muller O, et al: Gardner fibroma: case report and discussion of a new soft tissue tumor, *Pathologe* 31:97–105, 2010.
46. Isaacs H, Jr: Fetal and neonatal cardiac tumors, *Pediatr Cardiol* 25:252–273, 2004.
47. Uzun O, Wilson DG, Vujanic GM, et al: Cardiac tumours in children, *Orphanet J Rare Dis* 2:11, 2007.
48. Coffin CM: Congenital cardiac fibroma associated with Gorlin syndrome, *Pediatr Pathol* 12:255–262, 1992.
49. Bossert T, Walther T, Vondrys D, et al: Cardiac fibroma as an inherited manifestation of nevoid basal-cell carcinoma syndrome, *Tex Heart Inst J* 33:88–90, 2006.
50. Jones KL, Wolf PL, Jensen P, et al: The Gorlin syndrome: a genetically determined disorder associated with cardiac tumor, *Am Heart J* 111:1013–1015, 1986.

51. Ferguson HL, Hawkins EP, Cooley LD: Infant cardiac fibroma with clonal t(1;9)(q32;q22) and review of benign fibrous tissue cytogenetics, *Cancer Genet Cytogenet* 87:34–37, 1996.
52. Zhang Q, Wang T, Wang D, et al: Somatic copy number losses on chromosome 9q21.333q22.33 encompassing the PTCH1 loci associated with cardiac fibroma, *Cancer Genet* 208:615–620, 2015.
53. Coffin CM, Neilson KA, Ingels S, et al: Congenital generalized myofibromatosis: a disseminated angiocentric myofibromatosis, *Pediatr Pathol Lab Med* 15:571–587, 1995.
54. Chung EB, Enzinger FM: Infantile myofibromatosis, *Cancer* 48:1807–1818, 1981.
55. Oudjik L, den Bakker MA, Hop WC, et al: Solitary, multifocal and generalized myofibromas: clinicopathological and immunohistochemical features of 114 cases, *Histopathology* 60:E1–E11, 2012.
56. Mashiah J, Hadj-Rabia S, Dompmartin A, et al: Infantile myofibromatosis: a series of 28 cases, *J Am Acad Dermatol* 71:264–270, 2014.
57. Stanford D, Rogers M: Dermatological presentations of infantile myofibromatosis: a review of 27 cases, *Australas J Dermatol* 41:156–161, 2000.
58. Daimaru Y, Hashimoto H, Enjoji M: Myofibromatosis in adults (adult counterpart of infantile myofibromatosis), *Am J Surg Pathol* 13:859–865, 1989.
59. Greeley CS: Re: a newborn with multiple fractures as first presentation of infantile myofibromatosis, *J Perinatol* 27:136, 2007, author reply 137.
60. Pelluard-Nehme F, Coatleven F, Carles D, et al: Multicentric infantile myofibromatosis: two perinatal cases, *Eur J Pediatr* 166:997–1001, 2007.
61. Arcangeli F, Calista D: Congenital myofibromatosis in two siblings, *Eur J Dermatol* 16:181–183, 2006.
62. Michel M, Ninane J, Claus D, et al: Major malformations in a case of infantile myofibromatosis, *Eur J Pediatr* 149:251–252, 1990.
63. Granter SR, Badizadegan K, Fletcher CD: Myofibromatosis in adults, glomangiopericytoma, and myopericytoma: a spectrum of tumors showing perivascular myoid differentiation, *Am J Surg Pathol* 22:513–525, 1998.
64. Linos K, Carter JM, Gardner JM, et al: Myofibromas with atypical features: expanding the morphologic spectrum of a benign entity, *Am J Surg Pathol* 38:1649–1654, 2014.
65. Fukasawa Y, Ishikura H, Takada A, et al: Massive apoptosis in infantile myofibromatosis. A putative mechanism of tumor regression, *Am J Pathol* 144:480–485, 1994.
66. Stenman G, Nadal N, Persson S, et al: del(6)(q12q15) as the sole cytogenetic anomaly in a case of solitary infantile myofibromatosis, *Oncol Rep* 6:1101–1104, 1999.
67. Zand DJ, Huff D, Everman D, et al: Autosomal dominant inheritance of infantile myofibromatosis, *Am J Med Genet* 126A:261–266, 2004.
68. Ikediobi NI, Iyengar V, Hwang L, et al: Infantile myofibromatosis: support for autosomal dominant inheritance, *J Am Acad Dermatol* 49:S148–S150, 2003.
69. Narchi H: Four half-siblings with infantile myofibromatosis: a case for autosomal-recessive inheritance, *Clin Genet* 59:134–135, 2001.
70. Cheung YH, Gayden T, Campeau PM, et al: A recurrent PDGFRB mutation causes familial infantile myofibromatosis, *Am J Hum Genet* 92:996–1000, 2013.
71. Arts FA, Chand D, Pecquet C, et al: PDGFRB mutants found in patients with familial infantile myofibromatosis or overgrowth syndrome are oncogenic and sensitive to Imatinib, *Oncogene* 35:3239–3248, 2016.
72. Linhares ND, Freire MC, Cardenas RG, et al: Exome sequencing identifies a novel homozygous variant in NDRG4 in a family with infantile myofibromatosis, *Eur J Med Genet* 57:643–648, 2014.
73. Martignetti JA, Tian L, Li D, et al: Mutations in PDGFRB cause autosomal dominant infantile myofibromatosis, *Am J Hum Genet* 92:1001–1007, 2013.
74. Mentzel T, Calonje E, Nascimento AG, et al: Infantile hemangiopericytoma versus infantile myofibromatosis. Study of a series suggesting a continuous spectrum of infantile myofibroblastic lesions, *Am J Surg Pathol* 18:922–930, 1994.
75. Variend S, Bax NM, van Gorp J: Are infantile myofibromatosis, congenital fibrosarcoma and congenital haemangiopericytoma histogenetically related?, *Histopathology* 26:57–62, 1995.
76. Alaggio R, Barisani D, Ninfo V, et al: Morphologic overlap between infantile myofibromatosis and infantile fibrosarcoma: a pitfall in diagnosis, *Pediatr Dev Pathol* 11:355–362, 2008.
77. Rossbach C, Tannapfel A, Troebs RB, et al: Successful treatment of relapsed multifocal nonvisceral infantile myofibromatosis, *Pediatr Hematol Oncol* 22:695–698, 2005.
78. Hatzidaki E, Korakaki E, Voloudaki A, et al: Infantile myofibromatosis with visceral involvement and complete spontaneous regression, *J Dermatol* 28:379–382, 2001.
79. Kauffman SL, Stout AP: Congenital mesenchymal tumors, *Cancer* 18:460–476, 1965.
80. Molnar P, Olah E, Miko TL, et al: Aggressive infantile myofibromatosis: report of a case of a clinically progressive congenital multiple fibromatosis, *Med Pediatr Oncol* 14:332–337, 1986.
81. Day M, Edwards AO, Weinberg A, et al: Brief report: successful therapy of a patient with infantile generalized myofibromatosis, *Med Pediatr Oncol* 38:371–373, 2002.
82. Gandhi MM, Nathan PC, Weitzman S, et al: Successful treatment of life-threatening generalized infantile myofibromatosis using low-dose chemotherapy, *J Pediatr Hematol Oncol* 25:750–754, 2003.
83. Savasan S, Fulgenzi LA, Rabah R, et al: Generalized infantile myofibromatosis in a patient with Turner's syndrome: a trial of interferon-alpha, *J Pediatr* 133:694–696, 1998.
84. Martin JM, Jorda E, Calduch L, et al: Self-healing generalized infantile myofibromatosis, *J Eur Acad Dermatol Venereol* 22:236–238, 2008.
85. Dormans JP, Spiegel D, Meyer J, et al: Fibromatoses in childhood: the desmoid/fibromatosis complex, *Med Pediatr Oncol* 37:126–131, 2001.
86. Ayala AG, Ro JY, Goepfert H, et al: Desmoid fibromatosis: a clinicopathologic study of 25 children, *Semin Diagn Pathol* 3:138–150, 1986.
87. Stout AP: Juvenile fibromatoses, *Cancer* 7:953–978, 1954.
88. Naylor EW, Gardner EJ, Richards RC: Desmoid tumors and mesenteric fibromatosis in Gardner's syndrome: report of kindred 109, *Arch Surg* 114:1181–1185, 1979.
89. Scott RJ, Froggatt NJ, Trembath RC, et al: Familial infiltrative fibromatosis (desmoid tumours) (MIM135290) caused by a recurrent 3' APC gene mutation, *Hum Mol Genet* 5:1921–1924, 1996.
90. Soravia C, Berk T, McLeod RS, et al: Desmoid disease in patients with familial adenomatous polyposis, *Dis Colon Rectum* 43:363–369, 2000.
91. Gardner EJ: Follow-up study of a family group exhibiting dominant inheritance for a syndrome including intestinal polyps, osteomas, fibromas and epidermal cysts, *Am J Hum Genet* 14:376–390, 1962.
92. Gardner EJ, Richards RC: Multiple cutaneous and subcutaneous lesions occurring simultaneously with hereditary polyposis and osteomatosis, *Am J Hum Genet* 5:139–147, 1953.
93. Halata MS, Miller J, Stone RK: Gardner syndrome. Early presentation with a desmoid tumor. Discovery of multiple colonic polyps, *Clin Pediatr* 28:538–540, 1989.
94. de Silva DC, Wright MF, Stevenson DA, et al: Cranial desmoid tumor associated with homozygous inactivation of the adenomatous polyposis coli gene in a 2-year-old girl with familial adenomatous polyposis, *Cancer* 77:972–976, 1996.
95. Clark SK, Smith TG, Katz DE, et al: Identification and progression of a desmoid precursor lesion in patients with familial adenomatous polyposis, *Br J Surg* 85:970–973, 1998.
96. Clark SK, Pack K, Pritchard J, et al: Familial adenomatous polyposis presenting with childhood desmoids, *Lancet* 349:471–472, 1997.
97. Faulkner LB, Hajdu SI, Kher U, et al: Pediatric desmoid tumor: retrospective analysis of 63 cases, *J Clin Oncol* 13:2813–2818, 1995.
98. Richards RC, Rogers SW, Gardner EJ: Spontaneous mesenteric fibromatosis in Gardner's syndrome, *Cancer* 47:597–601, 1981.
99. Weyl Ben Arush M, Meller I, Moses M, et al: Multifocal desmoid tumor in childhood: report of two cases and review of the literature, *Pediatr Hematol Oncol* 15:55–61, 1998.
100. Reitamo JJ, Scheinin TM, Hayry P: The desmoid syndrome. New aspects in the cause, pathogenesis and treatment of the desmoid tumor, *Am J Surg* 151:230–237, 1986.
101. Reitamo JJ, Hayry P, Nykyri E, et al: The desmoid tumor. I. Incidence, sex-, age- and anatomical distribution in the Finnish population, *Am J Clin Pathol* 77:665–673, 1982.
102. Sahn EE, Cook WJ, Gross RH, et al: Musculoaponeurotic fibromatosis (extraabdominal desmoid tumor) in a child with idiopathic multicentric osteolysis, *Pediatr Dermatol* 10:49–53, 1993.
103. McCarville MB, Hoffer FA, Adelman CS, et al: MRI and biologic behavior of desmoid tumors in children, *AJR Am J Roentgenol* 189:633–640, 2007.
104. Zreik RT, Fritchie KJ: Morphologic spectrum of desmoid-type fibromatosis, *Am J Clin Pathol* 145:332–340, 2016.
105. Schmidt D, Klinge P, Leuschner I, et al: Infantile desmoid-type fibromatosis. Morphological features correlate with biological behaviour, *J Pathol* 164:315–319, 1991.
106. Yokoyama R, Tsuneyoshi M, Enjoji M, et al: Extra-abdominal desmoid tumors: correlations between histologic features and biologic behavior, *Surg Pathol* 2:29–42, 1989.
107. Cates JM, Black J, Wolfe CC, et al: Morphologic and immunohistochemical analysis of desmoid-type fibromatosis after radiation therapy, *Hum Pathol* 43:1418–1424, 2012.
108. Leithner A, Gapp M, Radl R, et al: Immunohistochemical analysis of desmoid tumours, *J Clin Pathol* 58:1152–1156, 2005.
109. Bhattacharya B, Dilworth HP, Iacobuzio-Donahue C, et al: Nuclear beta-catenin expression distinguishes deep fibromatosis from other benign and malignant fibroblastic and myofibroblastic lesions, *Am J Surg Pathol* 29:653–659, 2005.
110. Amary MF, Pauwels P, Meulemans E, et al: Detection of beta-catenin mutations in paraffin-embedded sporadic desmoid-type fibromatosis by mutation-specific restriction enzyme digestion (MSRED): an ancillary diagnostic tool, *Am J Surg Pathol* 31:1299–1309, 2007.
111. Thway K, Gibson S, Ramsey A, et al: Beta-catenin expression in pediatric fibroblastic and myofibroblastic lesions: a study of 100 cases, *Pediatr Dev Pathol* 12:292–296, 2009.
112. Gebert C, Hardes J, Kersting C, et al: Expression of beta-catenin and p53 are prognostic factors in deep aggressive fibromatosis, *Histopathology* 50:491–497, 2007.
113. Deyrup AT, Tretiakova M, Montag AG: Estrogen receptor-beta expression in extraabdominal fibromatoses: an analysis of 40 cases, *Cancer* 106:208–213, 2006.
114. Li M, Cordon-Cardo C, Gerald WL, et al: Desmoid fibromatosis is a clonal process, *Hum Pathol* 27:939–943, 1996.
115. Kouho H, Aoki T, Hisaoka M, et al: Clinicopathological and interphase cytogenetic analysis of desmoid tumours, *Histopathology* 31:336–341, 1997.
116. Wang WL, Nero C, Pappo A, et al: CTNNB1 genotyping and APC screening in pediatric desmoid tumors: a proposed algorithm, *Pediatr Dev Pathol* 15:361–367, 2012.
117. Nieuwenhuis MH, De Vos Tot Nederveen Cappel W, Botma A, et al: Desmoid tumors in a Dutch cohort of patients with familial adenomatous polyposis, *Clin Gastroenterol Hepatol* 6:215–219, 2008.
118. Church J, Xhaja X, LaGuardia L, et al: Desmoids and genotype in familial adenomatous polyposis, *Dis Colon Rectum* 58:444–448, 2015.
119. Meazza C, Belfiore A, Busica A, et al: AKT1 and BRAF mutations in pediatric aggressive fibromatosis, *Cancer Med* 5:1204–1213, 2016.
120. Goldstein JA, Cates JMM: Differential diagnostic considerations of desmoid-type fibromatosis, *Adv Anat Pathol* 22:260–266, 2015.

121. Burtenshaw SM, Cannell AJ, McAlister ED, et al: Toward observation as first line management in abdominal desmoid tumors, *Ann Surg Oncol* 23:2212–2219, 2016.
122. Eastley N, McCulloch T, Esler C, et al: Extra-abdominal desmoid fibromatosis: a review of management, current guidance and unanswered questions, *Eur J Surg Oncol* 42:1071–1083, 2016.
123. Fiore M, MacNeill A, Gronchi A, et al: Desmoid-type fibromatosis: evolving treatment strategies, *Surg Oncol Clin N Am* 25:803–826, 2016.
124. Woltsche N, Glig MM, Fraissler L, et al: Is wide resection obsolete for desmoid tumors in children and adolescents? Evaluation of histological margins, immunohistochemical markers and review of literature, *Pediatr Hematol Oncol* 32:60–69, 2015.
125. Septer S, Lawson CE, Anant S, et al: Familial adenomatous polyposis in pediatrics: natural history, emerging surveillance ad management protocols, chemopreventive strategies and areas of ongoing debate, *Fam Cancer* 15:477–485, 2016.
126. Reye RD: Sterno-mastoid tumour and congenital muscular torticollis, *Med J Aust* 1:867–870, 1951.
127. Lowry KC, Estriff JA, Rahbar R: The presentation and management of fibromatosis colli, *Ear Nose Throat J* 89:e4–e8, 2010.
128. MacDonald D: Sternomastoid tumour and muscular torticollis, *J Bone Joint Surg Br* 51:432–443, 1969.
129. Lawrence WT, Azizkhan RG: Congenital muscular torticollis: a spectrum of pathology, *Ann Plast Surg* 23:523–530, 1989.
130. Sharma S, Mishra K, Khanna G: Fibromatosis colli in infants. A cytologic study of eight cases, *Acta Cytol* 47:359–362, 2003.
131. Reye RD: Recurring digital fibrous tumors of childhood, *Arch Pathol* 80:228–231, 1965.
132. Purdy LJ, Colby TV: Infantile digital fibromatosis occurring outside the digit, *Am J Surg Pathol* 8:787–790, 1984.
133. Allen PW: Recurring digital fibrous tumours of childhood, *Pathology* 4:215–223, 1972.
134. Craver RD, Heinrich S: Bone invasion by a recurrent digital fibroma of infancy in a child with Beckwith-Wiedemann syndrome, *Pediatr Pathol Lab Med* 15:147–151, 1995.
135. Grenier N, Liang C, Capaldi L, et al: A range of histologic findings in infantile digital fibromatosis, *Pediatr Dermatol* 25:72–75, 2008.
136. Henderson H, Peng YJ, Salter DM: Anti-calponin 1 antibodies highlight intracytoplasmic inclusions of infantile digital fibromatosis, *Histopathology* 64:752–755, 2014.
137. Mukai M, Torikata C, Iri H, et al: Immunohistochemical identification of aggregated actin filaments in formalin-fixed, paraffin-embedded sections. I. A study of infantile digital fibromatosis by a new pretreatment, *Am J Surg Pathol* 16:110–115, 1992.
138. Laskin WB, Miettinen M, Fetsch JF: Infantile digital fibroma/fibromatosis: a clinicopathologic and immunohistochemical study of 69 tumors from 57 patients with long-term follow-up, *Am J Surg Pathol* 33:1–13, 2009.
139. Montgomery E, Lee JH, Abraham SC, et al: Superficial fibromatoses are genetically distinct from deep fibromatoses, *Mod Pathol* 14:695–701, 2001.
140. Talbot C, Khan T, Smith M: Infantile digital fibromatosis, *J Pediatr Orthop B* 16:110–112, 2007.
141. Niamba P, Leaute-Labreze C, Boralevi F, et al: Further documentation of spontaneous regression of infantile digital fibromatosis, *Pediatr Dermatol* 24:280–284, 2007.
142. Reye RD: A consideration of certain subdermal fibromatous tumours of infancy, *J Pathol Bacteriol* 72:149–154, 1956.
143. Enzinger FM: Fibrous hamartoma of infancy, *Cancer* 18:241–248, 1965.
144. Fletcher CD, Powell G, van Noorden S, et al: Fibrous hamartoma of infancy: a histochemical and immunohistochemical study, *Histopathology* 12:65–74, 1988.
145. Kirby W, Coffin CM, Dehner LP: Fibrous hamartoma of infancy: a clinicopathologic study of 19 cases emphasizing unusual sites and an expanded age range, *Pediatr Pathol* 14:547–548, 1994.
146. Sotelo-Avila C, Bale PM: Subdermal fibrous hamartoma of infancy: pathology of 40 cases and differential diagnosis, *Pediatr Pathol* 14:39–52, 1994.
147. Saab ST, McClain CM, Coffin CM: Fibrous hamartoma of infancy: a clinicopathologic analysis of 60 cases, *Am J Surg Pathol* 38:394–401, 2014.
148. Popek EJ, Montgomery EA, Fourcroy JL: Fibrous hamartoma of infancy in the genital region: findings in 15 cases, *J Urol* 152:990–993, 1994.
149. Dickey GE, Sotelo-Avila C: Fibrous hamartoma of infancy: current review, *Pediatr Dev Pathol* 2:236–243, 1999.
150. Groisman G, Lichtig C: Fibrous hamartoma of infancy: an immunohistochemical and ultrastructural study, *Hum Pathol* 22:914–918, 1991.
151. Rougemont AL, Fetni R, Murthy S, et al: A complex translocation (6;12;8)(q25;q24.3;q13) in a fibrous hamartoma of infancy, *Cancer Genet Cytogenet* 171:115–118, 2006.
152. Park JY, Cohen C, Lopez D, et al: EGFR exon 20 insertion/duplication mutations characterize fibrous hamartoma of infancy, *Am J Surg Pathol* 40:1713–1718, 2016.
153. Imaji R, Goto T, Takahashi Y, et al: A case of recurrent and synchronous fibrous hamartoma of infancy, *Pediatr Surg Int* 21:119–120, 2005.
154. Keasbey LE: Juvenile aponeurotic fibroma (calcifying fibroma); a distinctive tumor arising in the palms and soles of young children, *Cancer* 6:338–346, 1953.
155. Allen PW, Enzinger FM: Juvenile aponeurotic fibroma, *Cancer* 26:857–867, 1970.
156. Fetsch JF, Miettinen M: Calcifying aponeurotic fibroma: a clinicopathologic study of 22 cases arising in uncommon sites, *Hum Pathol* 29:1504–1510, 1998.
157. Hassel B: Calcifying aponeurotic fibroma. A case of multiple primary tumours. Case report, *Scand J Plast Reconstr Surg Hand Surg* 26:115–116, 1992.
158. Sferopoulos NK, Kotakidou R: Calcifying aponeurotic fibroma: a report of three cases, *Acta Orthop Belg* 67:412–416, 2001.
159. Puls F, Hofvander J, Magnusson L, et al: FN1-EGF gene fusions are recurrent in calcifying aponeurotic fibroma, *J Pathol* 238:502–507, 2016.
160. Lafferty KA, Nelson EL, Demuth RJ, et al: Juvenile aponeurotic fibroma with disseminated fibrosarcoma, *J Hand Surg Am* 11:737–740, 1986.
161. Fetsch JF, Miettinen M, Laskin WB, et al: A clinicopathologic study of 45 pediatric soft tissue tumors with an admixture of adipose tissue and fibroblastic elements, and a proposal for classification as lipofibromatosis, *Am J Surg Pathol* 24:1491–1500, 2000.
162. Herrmann BW, Dehner LP, Forsen JW, Jr: Lipofibromatosis presenting as a pediatric neck mass, *Int J Pediatr Otorhinolaryngol* 68:1545–1549, 2004.
163. Kabasawa Y, Katsube K, Harada H, et al: A male infant case of lipofibromatosis in the submental region exhibited the expression of the connective tissue growth factor, *Oral Surg Oral Med Oral Pathol Oral Radiol Endod* 103:677–682, 2007.
164. Kenney B, Richkind KE, Friedlaender G, et al: Chromosomal rearrangements in lipofibromatosis, *Cancer Genet Cytogenet* 179:136–139, 2007.
165. Agaram NP, Zhang L, Sung YS, et al: Recurrent NTRK1 gene fusions define a novel subset of locally aggressive lipofibromatosis-like neural tumors, *Am J Surg Pathol* 40:1407–1416, 2016.
166. Neel HB, Whicker JH, Devine KD, et al: Juvenile angiofibroma. Review of 120 cases, *Am J Surg* 126:547–556, 1973.
167. Ponti G, Losi L, Pellacani G, et al: Wnt pathway, angiogenetic and hormonal markers in sporadic and familial adenomatous polyposis–associated juvenile nasopharyngeal angiofibromas (JNA), *Appl Immunohistochem Mol Morphol* 16:173–178, 2008.
168. Sternberg SS: Pathology of juvenile nasopharyngeal angiofibroma; a lesion of adolescent males, *Cancer* 7:15–28, 1954.
169. Glad H, Vainer B, Buchwald C, et al: Juvenile nasopharyngeal angiofibromas in Denmark 1981–2003: diagnosis, incidence, and treatment, *Acta Otolaryngol* 127:292–299, 2007.
170. Montag AG, Tretiakova M, Richardson M: Steroid hormone receptor expression in nasopharyngeal angiofibromas. Consistent expression of estrogen receptor beta, *Am J Clin Pathol* 125:832–837, 2006.
171. Pauli J, Gundelach R, Vanelli-Rees A, et al: Juvenile nasopharyngeal angiofibroma: an immunohistochemical characterisation of the stromal cell, *Pathology* 40:396–400, 2008.
172. Schuon R, Brieger J, Heinrich UR, et al: Immunohistochemical analysis of growth mechanisms in juvenile nasopharyngeal angiofibroma, *Eur Arch Otorhinolaryngol* 264:389–394, 2007.
173. Heinrich UR, Brieger J, Gosepath J, et al: Frequent chromosomal gains in recurrent juvenile nasopharyngeal angiofibroma, *Cancer Genet Cytogenet* 175:138–143, 2007.
174. Coutinho-Camillo CM, Brentani MM, Nagai MA: Genetic alterations in juvenile nasopharyngeal angiofibromas, *Head Neck* 30:390–400, 2008.
175. Abraham SC, Montgomery EA, Giardiello FM, et al: Frequent beta-catenin mutations in juvenile nasopharyngeal angiofibromas, *Am J Pathol* 158:1073–1078, 2001.
176. Guertl B, Beham A, Zechner R, et al: Nasopharyngeal angiofibroma: an APC-gene-associated tumor?, *Hum Pathol* 31:1411–1413, 2000.
177. Giardiello FM, Hamilton SR, Krush AJ, et al: Nasopharyngeal angiofibroma in patients with familial adenomatous polyposis, *Gastroenterology* 105:1550–1552, 1993.
178. Goepfert H, Cangir A, Ayala AG, et al: Chemotherapy of locally aggressive head and neck tumors in the pediatric age group. Desmoid fibromatosis and nasopharyngeal angiofibroma, *Am J Surg* 144:437–444, 1982.
179. Chen KT, Bauer FW: Sarcomatous transformation of nasopharyngeal angiofibroma, *Cancer* 49:369–371, 1982.
180. Spagnolo DV, Papadimitriou JM, Archer M: Postirradiation malignant fibrous histiocytoma arising in juvenile nasopharyngeal angiofibroma and producing alpha-1-antitrypsin, *Histopathology* 8:339–352, 1984.
181. Allensworth JJ, Troob SH, Lanciault C, et al: high-grade malignant transformation of a radiation-naïve nasopharyngeal angiofibroma, *Head Neck* 38(Suppl 1):e2425–e2427, 2016.
182. Antaya RJ, Cajaiba MM, Madri J, et al: Juvenile hyaline fibromatosis and infantile systemic hyalinosis overlap associated with a novel mutation in capillary morphogenesis protein-2 gene, *Am J Dermatopathol* 29:99–103, 2007.
183. Remberger K, Krieg T, Kunze D, et al: Fibromatosis hyalinica multiplex (juvenile hyalin fibromatosis). Light microscopic, electron microscopic, immunohistochemical, and biochemical findings, *Cancer* 56:614–624, 1985.
184. Landing BH: Nadorra R. Infantile systemic hyalinosis: report of four cases of a disease, fatal in infancy, apparently different from juvenile systemic hyalinosis, *Pediatr Pathol* 6:55–79, 1986.
185. Muniz ML, Lobo AZ, Machado MC, et al: Exuberant juvenile hyaline fibromatosis in two patients, *Pediatr Dermatol* 23:458–464, 2006.
186. Woyke S, Domagala W, Markiewicz C: A 19-year follow-up of multiple juvenile hyaline fibromatosis, *J Pediatr Surg* 19:302–304, 1984.
187. Castro DJ, Hoover L, Lufkin RB, et al: Multicentric fibromatosis of familial inheritance, *Arch Pathol Lab Med* 111:867–869, 1987.
188. Finlay AY, Ferguson SD, Holt PJ: Juvenile hyaline fibromatosis, *Br J Dermatol* 108:609–616, 1983.
189. Youssefian L, Vahidnezhad H, Aghigi Y, et al: Hyaline fibromatosis syndrome: a novel mutation and recurrent founder mutation in the CMG2/ANTXR2 gene, *Acta Derm Venereol* 97:108–109, 2017.
190. Ruiz-Maldonado R, Duran-McKinster C, Saez-de-Ocariz M, et al: Interferon alpha-2B in juvenile hyaline fibromatosis, *Clin Exp Dermatol* 31:478–479, 2006.

191. Coffin CM, Watterson J, Priest JR, et al: Extrapulmonary inflammatory myofibroblastic tumor (inflammatory pseudotumor). A clinicopathologic and immunohistochemical study of 84 cases, *Am J Surg Pathol* 19:859–872, 1995.
192. Coffin CM, Humphrey PA, Dehner LP: Extrapulmonary inflammatory myofibroblastic tumor: a clinical and pathological survey, *Semin Diagn Pathol* 15:85–101, 1998.
193. Coffin CM, Hornick JL, Fletcher CD: Inflammatory myofibroblastic tumor: comparison of clinicopathologic, histologic, and immunohistochemical features including ALK expression in atypical and aggressive cases, *Am J Surg Pathol* 31:509–520, 2007.
194. Gleason BC, Hornick JL: Inflammatory myofibroblastic tumours: where are we now?, *J Clin Pathol* 61:428–437, 2008.
195. Lai LM, McCarville MB, Kirby P, et al: Shedding light on inflammatory pseudotumor in children: spotlight on inflammatory myofibroblastic tumor, *Pediatr Radiol* 45:1738–1752, 2015.
196. Souid AK, Ziemba MC, Dubansky AS, et al: Inflammatory myofibroblastic tumor in children, *Cancer* 72:2042–2048, 1993.
197. Coffin CM, Dehner LP, Meis-Kindblom JM: Inflammatory myofibroblastic tumor, inflammatory fibrosarcoma, and related lesions: an historical review with differential diagnostic considerations, *Semin Diagn Pathol* 15:102–110, 1998.
198. Dehner LP, Coffin CM: Idiopathic fibrosclerotic disorders and other inflammatory pseudotumors, *Semin Diagn Pathol* 15:161–173, 1998.
199. Dehner LP: Inflammatory myofibroblastic tumor: the continued definition of one type of so-called inflammatory pseudotumor, *Am J Surg Pathol* 28:1652–1654, 2004.
200. Vroobel K, Judson I, Dainton M, et al: ALK-positive inflammatory myofibroblastic tumor harboring ALK gene rearrangement, occurring after allogeneic stem cell transplant in an adult male, *Pathol Res Pract* 212:743–746, 2016.
201. Hornick JL, Sholl LM, Dal Cin P, et al: Expression of ROS1 predicts ROS1 gene rearrangement in inflammatory myofibroblastic tumors, *Mod Pathol* 28:732–739, 2015.
202. Yamamoto H, Yoshida A, Taguchi K, et al: ALK, ROS1 and NTRK3 gene rearrangements in inflammatory myofibroblastic tumours, *Histopathology* 69:72–83, 2016.
203. Alassiri AH, Ali RH, Shen Y, et al: ETV6-NTRK3 is expressed in a subset of ALK-negative inflammatory myofibroblastic tumors, *Am J Surg Pathol* 40:1051–1061, 2016.
204. Mariño-Enríquez A, Wang WL, Roy A, et al: Epithelioid inflammatory myofibroblastic sarcoma: an aggressive intra-abdominal variant of inflammatory myofibroblastic tumor with nuclear membrane or perinuclear ALK, *Am J Surg Pathol* 35:135–144, 2011.
205. Lee JC, Wu JM, Liau JY, et al: Cytopathologic features of epithelioid inflammatory myofibroblastic sarcoma with correlation of histopathology, immunohistochemistry and molecular cytogenetic analysis, *Cancer Cytopathol* 123:495–504, 2015.
206. Liu Q, Kan Y, Zhao Y, et al: Epithelioid inflammatory myofibroblastic sarcoma treated with ALK inhibitor: a case report and review of the literature, *Int Clin Exp Pathol* 8:15328–15332, 2015.
207. Yu L, Liu J, Lao IW, et al: Epithelioid inflammatory myofibroblastic sarcoma: a clinicopathological, immunohistochemical, and molecular cytogenetic analysis of five additional cases and review of the literature, *Diagn Pathol* 11:67–75, 2016.
208. Cessna MH, Zhou H, Sanger WG, et al: Expression of ALK1 and p80 in inflammatory myofibroblastic tumor and its mesenchymal mimics: a study of 135 cases, *Mod Pathol* 15:931–938, 2002.
209. Coffin CM, Patel A, Perkins S, et al: ALK1 and p80 expression and chromosomal rearrangements involving 2p23 in inflammatory myofibroblastic tumor, *Mod Pathol* 14:569–576, 2001.
210. Cook JR, Dehner LP, Collins MH, et al: Anaplastic lymphoma kinase (ALK) expression in the inflammatory myofibroblastic tumor: a comparative immunohistochemical study, *Am J Surg Pathol* 25:1364–1371, 2001.
211. Griffin CA, Hawkins AL, Dvorak C, et al: Recurrent involvement of 2p23 in inflammatory myofibroblastic tumors, *Cancer Res* 59:2776–2780, 1999.
212. Tavora F, Shilo K, Ozbudak IH, et al: Absence of human herpesvirus-8 in pulmonary inflammatory myofibroblastic tumor: immunohistochemical and molecular analysis of 20 cases, *Mod Pathol* 20:995–999, 2007.
213. Debelenko LV, Arthur DC, Pack SD, et al: Identification of CARS-ALK fusion in primary and metastatic lesions of an inflammatory myofibroblastic tumor, *Lab Invest* 83:1255–1265, 2003.
214. Cole B, Zhou H, McAllister N, et al: Inflammatory myofibroblastic tumor with thrombocytosis and a unique chromosomal translocation with ALK rearrangement, *Arch Pathol Lab Med* 130:1042–1045, 2006.
215. Lawrence B, Perez-Atayde A, Hibbard MK, et al: TPM3-ALK and TPM4-ALK oncogenes in inflammatory myofibroblastic tumors, *Am J Pathol* 157:377–384, 2000.
216. Lovly CM, Gupta A, Lipson D, et al: Inflammatory myofibroblastic tumors harbor multiple potentially actionable kinase fusions, *Cancer Discov* 4:889–895, 2014.
217. Antonescu CR, Suurmeijer AJH, Zhang L, et al: Molecular characterization of inflammatory myofibroblastic tumors with frequent ALK and ROS1 fusions and rare novel RET gene rearrangement, *Am J Surg Pathol* 39:957–967, 2015.
218. Yamamoto H, Oda Y, Saito T, et al: p53 Mutation and MDM2 amplification in inflammatory myofibroblastic tumours, *Histopathology* 42:431–439, 2003.
219. Saab ST, Hornick JL, Fletcher CD, et al: IgG4 plasma cells in inflammatory myofibroblastic tumor: inflammatory marker or pathogenic link?, *Mod Pathol* 24:606–612, 2011.
220. Dishop MK, Warner BW, Dehner LP, et al: Successful treatment of inflammatory myofibroblastic tumor with malignant transformation by surgical resection and chemotherapy, *J Pediatr Hematol Oncol* 25:153–158, 2003.
221. Germanidis G, Xanthakis I, Tsitouridis I, et al: Regression of inflammatory myofibroblastic tumor of the gastrointestinal tract under infliximab treatment, *Dig Dis Sci* 50:262–265, 2005.
222. Butrynski JE, D'Adamo DR, Hornick JL, et al: Crizotinib in ALK-rearranged inflammatory myofibroblastic tumor, *N Engl J Med* 363:1727–1733, 2010.
223. Mansfield AS, Murphy SJ, Harris FR, et al: Chromoplectic TPM3-ALK rearrangement in a patient with inflammatory myofibroblastic tumor who responded to ceritinib after progression on crizotinib, *Ann Oncol* 27:2111–2117, 2016.
224. Morotti RA, Legman MD, Kerkar N, et al: Pediatric inflammatory myofibroblastic tumor with late metastasis to the lung: case report and review of the literature, *Pediatr Dev Pathol* 8:224–229, 2005.
225. Hussong JW, Brown M, Perkins SL, et al: Comparison of DNA ploidy, histologic, and immunohistochemical findings with clinical outcome in inflammatory myofibroblastic tumors, *Mod Pathol* 12:279–286, 1999.
226. Biselli R, Ferlini C, Fattorossi A, et al: Inflammatory myofibroblastic tumor (inflammatory pseudotumor): DNA flow cytometric analysis of nine pediatric cases, *Cancer* 77:778–784, 1996.
227. Chung EB, Enzinger FM: Infantile fibrosarcoma, *Cancer* 38:729–739, 1976.
228. Coffin CM, Jaszcz W, O'Shea PA, et al: So-called congenital-infantile fibrosarcoma: does it exist and what is it?, *Pediatr Pathol* 14:133–150, 1994.
229. Soule EH, Pritchard DJ: Fibrosarcoma in infants and children: a review of 110 cases, *Cancer* 40:1711–1721, 1977.
230. Stout AP: Fibrosarcoma in infants and children, *Cancer* 15:1028–1040, 1962.
231. Van Grotel M, Blanco E, Sebire NJ, et al: Distant metastatic spread of molecularly proven infantile fibrosarcoma of the chest in a 2-month old girl: case report and review of the literature, *J Pediatr Hematol Oncol* 36:231–233, 2014.
232. Huang SY, Wang CW, Wang CJ, et al: Combined prenatal ultrasound and magnetic resonance imaging in an extensive congenital fibrosarcoma: a case report and review of the literature, *Fetal Diagn Ther* 20:266–271, 2005.
233. Islam S, Soldes OS, Ruiz R, et al: Primary colonic congenital infantile fibrosarcoma presenting as meconium peritonitis, *Pediatr Surg Int* 24:621–623, 2008.
234. Bakhshi S, Savasan S, Abella E: Infantile fibrosarcoma associated with urticaria pigmentosa, *Pediatr Hematol Oncol* 19:445–447, 2002.
235. Ramphal R, Manson D, Viero S, et al: Retroperitoneal infantile fibrosarcoma: clinical, molecular, and therapeutic aspects of an unusual tumor, *Pediatr Hematol Oncol* 20:635–642, 2003.
236. Gonzalez-Crussi F, Wiederhold MD, Sotelo-Avila C: Congenital fibrosarcoma: presence of a histiocytic component, *Cancer* 46:77–86, 1980.
237. Miura K, Han G, Sano M, et al: Regression of congenital fibrosarcoma to hemangiomatous remnant with histological and genetic findings, *Pathol Int* 52:612–618, 2002.
238. Dubus P, Coindre JM, Groppi A, et al: The detection of Tel-TrkC chimeric transcripts is more specific than TrkC immunoreactivity for the diagnosis of congenital fibrosarcoma, *J Pathol* 193:88–94, 2001.
239. Schofield DE, Fletcher JA, Grier HE, et al: Fibrosarcoma in infants and children. Application of new technique, *Am J Surg Pathol* 18:14–24, 1994.
240. Sankary S, Dickman PS, Wiener E, et al: Consistent numerical chromosome aberrations in congenital fibrosarcoma, *Cancer Genet Cytogenet* 65:152–156, 1993.
241. Knezevich SR, McFadden DE, Tao W, et al: A novel ETV6-NTRK3 gene fusion in congenital fibrosarcoma, *Nat Genet* 18:184–187, 1998.
242. Adem C, Gisselsson D, Dal Cin P, et al: ETV6 rearrangements in patients with infantile fibrosarcomas and congenital mesoblastic nephromas by fluorescence in situ hybridization, *Mod Pathol* 14:1246–1251, 2001.
243. Argani P, Fritsch MK, Shuster AE, et al: Reduced sensitivity of paraffin-based RT-PCR assays for ETV6-NTRK3 fusion transcripts in morphologically defined infantile fibrosarcoma, *Am J Surg Pathol* 25:1461–1464, 2001.
244. Bourgeois JM, Knezevich SR, Mathers JA, et al: Molecular detection of the ETV6-NTRK3 gene fusion differentiates congenital fibrosarcoma from other childhood spindle cell tumors, *Am J Surg Pathol* 24:937–946, 2000.
245. Sheng WQ, Hisaoka M, Okamoto S, et al: Congenital-infantile fibrosarcoma. A clinicopathologic study of 10 cases and molecular detection of the ETV6-NTRK3 fusion transcripts using paraffin-embedded tissues, *Am J Clin Pathol* 115:348–355, 2001.
246. Wong V, Pavlick D, Brennan T, et al: Evaluation of a congenital infantile fibrosarcoma by comprehensive genomic profiling reveals and LMNA-NTRK1 gene fusion responsive to crizotinib, *J Natl Cancer Inst* 108(1):pii: djv307, 2015, doi:10.1093/jnci/djv307. PMID: 26563356.
247. O'Meara E, Stack D, Phelan S, et al: Identification of an MLL4-GPS2 fusion as an oncogenic driver of undifferentiated spindle cell sarcoma in a child, *Genes Chromosomes Cancer* 53:991–998, 2014.
248. Haller F, Knopf J, Ackermann A, et al: Paediatric and adult soft tissue sarcomas with NTRK1 gene fusions: a subset of spindle cell sarcomas unified by a prominent myopericytic/haemangiopericytic pattern, *J Pathol* 238:700–710, 2016.
249. Orbach D, Brennan B, De Paoli A, et al: Conservative strategy in infantile fibrosarcoma is possible: the European paediatric soft tissue sarcoma study group experience, *Eur J Cancer* 57:1–9, 2016.
250. Kynaston JA, Malcolm AJ, Craft AW, et al: Chemotherapy in the management of infantile fibrosarcoma, *Med Pediatr Oncol* 21:488–493, 1993.
251. Shetty AK, Yu LC, Gardner RV, et al: Role of chemotherapy in the treatment of infantile fibrosarcoma, *Med Pediatr Oncol* 33:425–427, 1999.
252. Cecchetto G, Carli M, Alaggio R, et al: Fibrosarcoma in pediatric patients: results of the Italian Cooperative Group studies (1979–1995), *J Surg Oncol* 78:225–231, 2001.

253. Loh ML, Ahn P, Perez-Atayde AR, et al: Treatment of infantile fibrosarcoma with chemotherapy and surgery: results from the Dana-Farber Cancer Institute and Children's Hospital, Boston, *J Pediatr Hematol Oncol* 24:722–726, 2002.
254. McCahon E, Sorensen PH, Davis JH, et al: Non-resectable congenital tumors with the ETV6-NTRK3 gene fusion are highly responsive to chemotherapy, *Med Pediatr Oncol* 40:288–292, 2003.
255. Grier HE, Perez-Atayde AR, Weinstein HJ: Chemotherapy for inoperable infantile fibrosarcoma, *Cancer* 56:1507–1510, 1985.
256. Nagasubramanian R, Wei J, Gordon P, et al: Infantile fibrosarcoma with NTRK3-RETV6 fusion successfully treated with the tropomyosin-related kinase inhibitor LOXO-101, *Pediatr Blood Cancer* 63:1468–1470, 2016.
257. Yanagisawa R, Noguchi M, Fujita K, et al: Preoperative treatment with pazopanib in a case of chemotherapy-resistant infantile fibrosarcoma, *Pediatr Blood Cancer* 63:348–351, 2016.
258. Nonaka D, Sun CC: Congenital fibrosarcoma with metastasis in a fetus, *Pediatr Dev Pathol* 7:187–191, 2004.
259. Punnett HH, Tomczak EZ, Pawel BR, et al: ETV6-NTRK3 gene fusion in metastasizing congenital fibrosarcoma, *Med Pediatr Oncol* 35:137–139, 2000.
260. Rootman J, Carvounis EP, Dolman CL, et al: Congenital fibrosarcoma metastatic to the choroid, *Am J Ophthalmol* 87:632–638, 1979.
261. Alaggio R, Ninfo V, Rosolen A, et al: Primitive myxoid mesenchymal tumor of infancy: a clinicopathologic report of 6 cases, *Am J Surg Pathol* 30:388–394, 2006.
262. Foster JH, Vasudevan SA, Hicks JM, et al: primitive myxoid mesenchymal tumor of infancy involving the chest wall in an infant: a case report and clinicopathologic correlation, *Pediar Dev Pathol* 19:244–248, 2016.
263. Cipriani NA, Ryan DP, Nielsen GP: Primitive myxoid mesenchymal tumor of infancy with rosettes: a new finding and literature review, *Int J Surg Pathol* 22:647–651, 2014.
264. Kao YC, Sung YS, Zhang L, et al: Recurrent BCOR internal tandem duplication and YWHAE-NUTM2B fusions in soft tissue undifferentiated round cell sarcoma of infancy: overlapping genetic features with clear cell sarcoma of kidney, *Am J Surg Pathol* 40:1009–1020, 2016.
265. Kao YC, Sung YS, Zhang L, et al: BCOR overexpression is a highly sensitive marker in round cell sarcomas with BCOR genetic abnormalities, *Am J Surg Pathol* 40:1670–1678, 2016.
266. Guilbert MC, Rougemont AL, Samson Y, et al: Transformation of a primitive myxoid mesenchymal tumor of infancy to an undifferentiated sarcoma: a first reported case, *J Pediatr Hematol Oncol* 37:e118–e120, 2015.
267. Evans HL: Low-grade fibromyxoid sarcoma. A report of 12 cases, *Am J Surg Pathol* 17:595–600, 1993.
268. Lane KL, Shannon RJ, Weiss SW: Hyalinizing spindle cell tumor with giant rosettes: a distinctive tumor closely resembling low-grade fibromyxoid sarcoma, *Am J Surg Pathol* 21:1481–1488, 1997.
269. Folpe AL, Lane KL, Paull G, et al: Low-grade fibromyxoid sarcoma and hyalinizing spindle cell tumor with giant rosettes: a clinicopathologic study of 73 cases supporting their identity and assessing the impact of high-grade areas, *Am J Surg Pathol* 24:1353–1360, 2000.
270. Evans HL: Low-grade fibromyxoid sarcoma. A report of two metastasizing neoplasms having a deceptively benign appearance, *Am J Clin Pathol* 88:615–619, 1987.
271. Evans HL: Low-grade fibromyxoid sarcoma: a clinicopathologic study of 33 cases with long-term follow-up, *Am J Surg Pathol* 35:1450–1462, 2011.
272. Billings SD, Giblen G, Fanburg-Smith JC: Superficial low-grade fibromyxoid sarcoma (Evans tumor): a clinicopathologic analysis of 19 cases with a unique observation in the pediatric population, *Am J Surg Pathol* 29:204–210, 2005.
273. Mertens F, Fletcher CD, Antonescu CR, et al: Clinicopathologic and molecular genetic characterization of low-grade fibromyxoid sarcoma, and cloning of a novel FUS/CREB3L1 fusion gene, *Lab Invest* 85:408–415, 2005.
274. Sargar K, Kao SC, Spunt SL, et al: MRI and CT of low-grade fibromyxoid sarcoma in children: a report from Children's Oncology Group Study ARST0332, *AJR Am J Roentgenol* 205:414–420, 2015.
275. Kim L, Yoon YH, Choi SJ, et al: Hyalinizing spindle cell tumor with giant rosettes arising in the lung: report of a case with FUS-CREB3L2 fusion transcripts, *Pathol Int* 57:153–157, 2007.
276. Canpolat C, Evans HL, Corpron C, et al: Fibromyxoid sarcoma in a four-year-old child: case report and review of the literature, *Med Pediatr Oncol* 27:561–564, 1996.
277. Rando G, Buonuomo V, D'Urzo C, et al: Fibromyxoid sarcoma in a 4-year-old boy: case report and review of the literature, *Pediatr Surg Int* 21:311–312, 2005.
278. Guillou L, Benhattar J, Gengler C, et al: Translocation-positive low-grade fibromyxoid sarcoma: clinicopathologic and molecular analysis of a series expanding the morphologic spectrum and suggesting potential relationship to sclerosing epithelioid fibrosarcoma: a study from the French Sarcoma Group, *Am J Surg Pathol* 31:1387–1402, 2007.
279. Doyle LA, Möller E, Dal Cin P, et al: MUC4 is a highly sensitive and specific marker for low-grade fibromyxoid sarcoma, *Am J Surg Pathol* 35:733–741, 2011.
280. Thway K, Ng W, Benson C, et al: DOG1 expression in low-grade fibromyxoid sarcoma: a study of 11 cases, with molecular characterization, *Int J Surg Pathol* 23:454–460, 2015.
281. Reid R, de Silva MV, Paterson L, et al: Low-grade fibromyxoid sarcoma and yalinizing spindle cell tumor with giant rosettes share a common t(7;16)(q34;p11) translocation, *Am J Surg Pathol* 27:1229–1236, 2003.
282. Matsuyama A, Hisaoka M, Shimajiri S, et al: Molecular detection of FUS-CREB3L2 fusion transcripts in low-grade fibromyxoid sarcoma using formalin-fixed, paraffin-embedded tissue specimens, *Am J Surg Pathol* 30:1077–1084, 2006.
283. Panagopoulos I, Moller E, Dahlen A, et al: Characterization of the native CREB3L2 transcription factor and the FUS/CREB3L2 chimera, *Genes Chromosomes Cancer* 46:181–191, 2007.
284. Downs-Kelly E, Goldblum JR, Patel RM, et al: The utility of fluorescence in situ hybridization (FISH) in the diagnosis of myxoid soft tissue neoplasms, *Am J Surg Pathol* 32:8–13, 2008.
285. Lau PP, Lui PC, Lau GT, et al: EWSR1-CREB3L1 gene fusion: a novel alternative molecular aberration of low-grade fibromyxoid sarcoma, *Am J Surg Pathol* 37:734–738, 2013.
286. Oda Y, Takahira T, Kawaguchi K, et al: Low-grade fibromyxoid sarcoma versus low-grade myxofibrosarcoma in the extremities and trunk. A comparison of clinicopathological and immunohistochemical features, *Histopathology* 45:29–38, 2004.
287. Thway K, Chisholm J, Hayes A, et al: Pediatric low-grade fibromyxoid sarcoma mimicking ossifying fibromyxoid tumor: adding to the diagnostic spectrum of soft tissue tumors with a bony shell, *Hum Pathol* 46:461–466, 2015.
288. Prieto Granada C, Zhang L, Chen HW, et al: A genetic dichotomy between pure sclerosing epithelioid fibrosarcoma (SEF) and hybrid SEF/low-grade fibromyxoid sarcoma: a pathologic and molecular study of 18 cases, *Genes Chromosomes Cancer* 54:28–38, 2015.
289. Doyle LA, Wang WL, Dal Cin P, et al: MUC4 is a sensitive and extremely useful marker for sclerosing epithelioid fibrosarcoma: association with FUS gene rearrangement, *Am J Surg Pathol* 36:1444–1451, 2012.
290. Smith DM, Mahmoud HH, Jenkins JJ, et al: Myofibrosarcoma of the head and neck in children, *Pediatr Pathol Lab Med* 15:403–418, 1995.
291. Mentzel T, Dry S, Katenkamp D, et al: Low-grade myofibroblastic sarcoma: analysis of 18 cases in the spectrum of myofibroblastic tumors, *Am J Surg Pathol* 22:1228–1238, 1998.
292. Cai C, Dehner LP, El-Mofty SK: In myofibroblastic sarcomas of the head and neck, mitotic activity and necrosis define grade: a case study and literature review, *Virchows Arch* 463:827–836, 2013.
293. Montgomery E, Fisher C: Myofibroblastic differentiation in malignant fibrous histiocytoma (pleomorphic myofibrosarcoma): a clinicopathological study, *Histopathology* 38:499–509, 2001.
294. Fisher C: Myofibrosarcoma, *Virchows Arch* 445:215–223, 2004.
295. Keller C, Gibbs CN, Kelly SM, et al: Low-grade myofibrosarcoma of the head and neck: importance of surgical therapy, *J Pediatr Hematol Oncol* 26:119–120, 2004.
296. Lundgren L, Angervall L, Stenman G, et al: Infantile rhabdomyofibrosarcoma: a high-grade sarcoma distinguishable from infantile fibrosarcoma and rhabdomyosarcoma, *Hum Pathol* 24:785–795, 1993.
297. Miki H, Kobayashi S, Kushida Y, et al: A case of infantile rhabdomyofibrosarcoma with immunohistochemical, electron microscopical, and genetic analyses, *Hum Pathol* 30:1519–1522, 1999.
298. Mentzel T, Mentzel HJ, Katenkamp D: Infantile rhabdomyofibrosarcoma. An aggressive tumor in the spectrum of spindle cell tumors in childhood, *Pathologe* 17:296–300, 1996.
299. Rao SI, Uppin SG, Ratnakar KS, et al: Infantile rhabdomyofibrosarcoma: a distinct variant or a missing link between fibrosarcoma and rhabdomyosarcoma?, *Indian J Cancer* 43:39–42, 2006.
300. Dehner LP, Enzinger FM, Font RL: Fetal rhabdomyoma. An analysis of nine cases, *Cancer* 30:160–166, 1972.
301. Willis J, Abdul-Karim FW, di Sant'Agnese PA: Extracardiac rhabdomyomas, *Semin Diagn Pathol* 11:15–25, 1994.
302. Hettmer S, Teot LA, van Hummelen P, et al: Mutations in Hedgehog pathway genes in fetal rhabdomyomas, *J Pathol* 231:44–53, 2013.
303. Cavazzana AO, Schmidt D, Ninfo V, et al: Spindle cell rhabdomyosarcoma. A prognostically favorable variant of rhabdomyosarcoma, *Am J Surg Pathol* 16:229–235, 1992.
304. Newton WA, Gehan EA, Webber BL, et al: Classification of rhabdomyosarcomas and related sarcomas. Pathologic aspects and proposal for a new classification—an Intergroup Rhabdomyosarcoma Study, *Cancer* 76:1073–1085, 1995.
305. Asmar L, Gehan EA, Newton WA, et al: Agreement among and within groups of pathologists in the classification of rhabdomyosarcoma and related childhood sarcomas. Report of an international study of four pathology classifications, *Cancer* 74:2579–2588, 1994.
306. Qualman SJ, Coffin CM, Newton WA, et al: Intergroup Rhabdomyosarcoma Study: update for pathologists, *Pediatr Dev Pathol* 1:550–561, 1998.
307. Mentzel T, Katenkamp D: Sclerosing pseudovascular rhabdomyosarcoma in adults. Clinicopathological and immunohistochemical analysis of three cases, *Virchows Arch* 436:305–311, 2000.
308. Folpe AL, McKenney JK, Bridge JA, et al: Sclerosing rhabdomyosarcoma in adults: report of four cases of a hyalinizing, matrix-rich variant of rhabdomyosarcoma that may be confused with osteosarcoma, chondrosarcoma, or angiosarcoma, *Am J Surg Pathol* 26:1175–1183, 2002.
309. Alaggio R, Zhang L, Sung YS, et al: A molecular study of pediatric spindle and sclerosing rhabdomyosarcoma: identification of novel and recurrent VGLL2-related fusions in infantile cases, *Am J Surg Pathol* 40:224–235, 2016.
310. Gulbahce HE, Manivel JC: Congenital spindle cell rhabdomyosarcoma of the urinary bladder, *Pediatr Pathol Mol Med* 18:207–212, 1998.
311. Leuschner I, Newton WA, Schmidt D, et al: Spindle cell variants of embryonal rhabdomyosarcoma in the paratesticular region. A report of the Intergroup Rhabdomyosarcoma Study, *Am J Surg Pathol* 17:221–230, 1993.
312. Gupta A, Maddalozzo J, Win Htin T, et al: Spindle cell rhabdomyosarcoma of the tongue in an infant: a case report with emphasis on differential diagnosis of childhood spindle cell lesions, *Pathol Res Pract* 200:537–543, 2004.

313. Rudzinski ER, Anderson JR, Hawkins DS, et al: The World Health Organization classification of skeletal muscle tumors in pediatric rhabdomyosarcoma: a report from the Children's Oncology Group, *Arch Pathol Lab Med* 139:1281–1287, 2015.
314. Cessna MH, Zhou H, Perkins SL, et al: Are myogenin and myoD1 expression specific for rhabdomyosarcoma? A study of 150 cases, with emphasis on spindle cell mimics, *Am J Surg Pathol* 25:1150–1157, 2001.
315. Mosquera JM, Sboner A, Zhang L, et al: Recurrent NCOA2 gene rearrangements in congenital/infantile spindle cell rhabdomyosarcoma, *Genes Chromosomes Cancer* 52:538–550, 2013.
316. Agaram NP, Chen CL, Zhang L, et al: Recurrent MYOD1 mutations in pediatric and adult sclerosing and spindle cell rhabdomyosarcomas: evidence for a common pathogenesis, *Genes Chromosomes Cancer* 53:779–787, 2014.
317. Kohsaka S, Shukla N, Ameur N, et al: A recurrent neomorphic mutation in MYOD1 defines a clinically aggressive subset of embryonal rhabdomyosarcoma associated with PI3K-AKT pathway mutations, *Nat Genet* 46:595–600, 2014.
318. Fletcher CDM: The evolving classification of soft tissue tumours—an update based on the new 2013 WHO classification, *Histopathology* 64:2–11, 2014.
319. Alaggio R, Bisogno G, Rosato A, et al: Undifferentiated sarcoma: does it exist? A clinicopathologic study of 7 pediatric cases and review of literature, *Hum Pathol* 40:1600–1610, 2009.
320. Harms D: Soft tissue sarcomas in the Kiel Pediatric Tumor Registry, *Curr Top Pathol* 89:31–45, 1995.
321. Pawel BR, Hamoudi AB, Asmar L, et al: Undifferentiated sarcomas of children: pathology and clinical behavior. An Intergroup Rhabdomyosarcoma Study, *Med Pediatr Oncol* 29:170–180, 1997.
322. Somers GR, Gupta AA, Doria AS, et al: Pediatric undifferentiated sarcoma of the soft tissues: a clinicopathologic study, *Pediatr Dev Pathol* 9:132–142, 2006.
323. Black JO, Coffin CM, Parham DM, et al: Opportunities for improvement in pathology reporting of childhood nonrhabdomyosarcoma soft tissue sarcomas: a report from Children's Oncology Group (COG) Study ARST0332, *Am J Clin Pathol* 146:323–338, 2016.
324. Pierron G, Tirode F, Lucchesi C, et al: A new subtype of bone sarcoma defined by BCOR-CCNB3 gene fusion, *Nat Genet* 44:461–466, 2012.
325. Peters TL, Kumar K, Polikepehad S, et al: BCOR-CCNB3 fusions are frequent in undifferentiated sarcomas of male children, *Mod Pathol* 28:575–586, 2015.

5

Tumors With Myxoid Stroma

Vickie Y. Jo, MD, and Jason L. Hornick, MD, PhD

Myxoid tumors of soft tissue are remarkable for their characteristic abundant extracellular matrix material. This heterogeneous group of lesions includes benign (and self-limited) tumors, those with a significant potential for local recurrence, and sarcomas. Because there is considerable clinical and histologic overlap, myxoid soft tissue tumors can pose problems in differential diagnosis. Immunohistochemistry is of limited help in distinguishing among the fibroblastic/myofibroblastic lesions in this group, although it can be very helpful to confirm the line of differentiation for other tumors with myxoid stroma. Other ancillary tools such as cytogenetics and molecular genetics can also corroborate the diagnosis of several lesions in this category (Box 5.1).

It is helpful to pay attention to several key features when encountering a myxoid soft tissue tumor, including depth (dermal, subcutaneous, or subfascial), the extent of myxoid stroma (abundant or limited; diffuse or focal), the presence (or absence) of nuclear pleomorphism, and the presence of distinctive vasculature. For example, intramuscular/cellular myxoma lacks nuclear atypia, in contrast to myxofibrosarcoma, which contains pleomorphic cells, even in low-grade examples. Myxoid liposarcoma is characterized by thin-walled, branching ("crow's feet") blood vessels, whereas low-grade fibromyxoid sarcoma (LGFMS) contains arcades of thin-walled vessels. Therefore extensive sampling of these tumors, with attention to such morphologic cues, is critical for the proper analysis of these neoplasms (Boxes 5.2–5.5).

The differential diagnosis of myxoid mesenchymal tumors also includes select soft tissue neoplasms that only occasionally display prominent myxoid stroma, such as peripheral nerve sheath tumors, dermatofibrosarcoma protuberans (DFSP), synovial sarcoma, and solitary fibrous tumor (SFT). Although immunohistochemistry can aid in the proper diagnosis of several of these tumor types (such as S-100 protein for nerve sheath tumors and epithelial membrane antigen [EMA], keratins, and TLE1 for synovial sarcoma), proper diagnosis often relies on identifying areas with conventional histologic features. Nonmesenchymal tumors, such as carcinoma and melanoma, very rarely show significant myxoid stroma.

Ganglion Cyst

Ganglion cyst is a common reactive lesion of soft tissue that appears to result from myxoid degeneration of connective tissue as a result of trauma.[1] It is commonly identified on imaging studies; on computed tomography scan, it appears as an oval or round lesion with uniform low signal intensity on T1-weighted images and high signal on T2-weighted images.[1,2]

Clinical Features

Ganglion cyst is one of the most common soft tissue lesions of the hands and wrists.[1-3] It can also affect other joints, such as the knee, ankle, and foot.[4-6] Men are affected slightly more often than women.[3,5,6] Most patients are between the fourth and sixth decades of life.[3-6]

Although patients are often asymptomatic, pain or a palpable lesion is occasionally present.

Box 5.1 Myxoid Tumors of Soft Tissue

Benign

Ganglion cyst
Intramuscular/cellular myxoma
Juxtaarticular myxoma
Dermal nerve sheath myxoma
Superficial acral fibromyxoma (digital fibromyxoma)
Superficial angiomyxoma
Deep ("aggressive") angiomyxoma
Myoepithelioma
Ossifying fibromyxoid tumor (usually)

Intermediate

Myxoinflammatory fibroblastic sarcoma

Malignant

Myoepithelial carcinoma
Ossifying fibromyxoid tumor (rarely)
Myxofibrosarcoma
Myxoid liposarcoma
Extraskeletal myxoid chondrosarcoma
Low-grade fibromyxoid sarcoma

Box 5.2 Usual Anatomic Depth of Myxoid Tumors of Soft Tissue

Superficial (Dermal or Subcutaneous)

Ganglion cyst
Dermal nerve sheath myxoma
Superficial acral fibromyxoma (digital fibromyxoma)
Superficial angiomyxoma
Juxtaarticular myxoma
Soft tissue myoepithelioma
Ossifying fibromyxoid tumor
Myxofibrosarcoma (two thirds of cases)
Myxoinflammatory fibroblastic sarcoma

Deep or Subfascial

Intramuscular/cellular myxoma
Deep angiomyxoma
Soft tissue myoepithelioma and myoepithelial carcinoma
Myxoid liposarcoma
Myxofibrosarcoma (one third of cases)
Extraskeletal myxoid chondrosarcoma
Low-grade fibromyxoid sarcoma

Box 5.3 Extent of Myxoid Stroma

Limited

Superficial acral fibromyxoma (digital fibromyxoma)
Ossifying fibromyxoid tumor
Low-grade fibromyxoid sarcoma

Extensive

Intramuscular/cellular myxoma
Juxtaarticular myxoma
Dermal nerve sheath myxoma
Superficial angiomyxoma
Deep angiomyxoma
Myxoinflammatory fibroblastic sarcoma
Myxofibrosarcoma (especially low-grade tumors)
Myxoid liposarcoma
Extraskeletal myxoid chondrosarcoma

Variable

Ganglion cyst
Myoepithelioma and myoepithelial carcinoma

Box 5.4 Myxoid Tumors With Pleomorphism

Myxoinflammatory fibroblastic sarcoma
Myoepithelial carcinoma
Myxofibrosarcoma

Box 5.5 Myxoid Tumors With Distinctive Vascular Patterns

Deep angiomyxoma: perivascular hyalinization with smooth muscle cells spinning off of vessels
Myxofibrosarcoma: curvilinear vessels
Myxoid liposarcoma: thin-walled, branching capillaries ("crow's feet" or "chicken-wire" pattern)
Low-grade fibromyxoid sarcoma: arcades of blood vessels

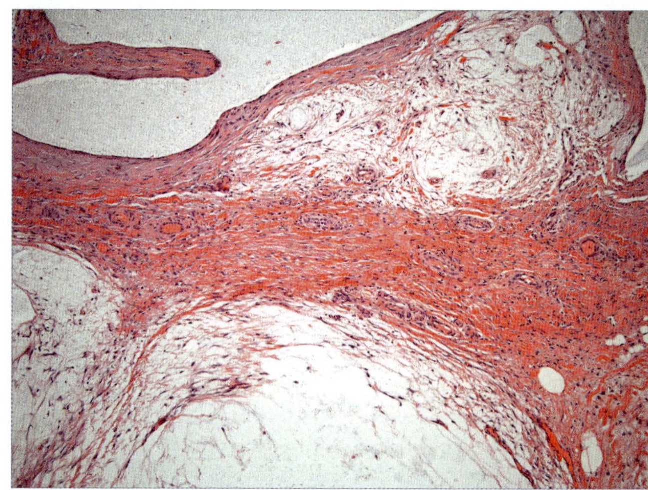

Figure 5.1 **Ganglion Cyst.** A ruptured ganglion cyst with extravasated fluid dissecting connective tissue, mimicking a myxoid soft tissue tumor.

Pathologic Features

Grossly, ganglion cysts are small, well-circumscribed lesions, with a thick fibrous pseudocapsule, attached to tendons or bursae. Occasionally, there may be communication with the underlying joint space.

Histologically, cysts may be uni- or multiloculated; filled with clear, acellular, viscous fluid; and lined by flat cells, which are likely fibroblastic/myofibroblastic in origin. Not uncommonly, ganglion cysts may rupture and extravasated fluid dissects into adjacent connective tissues (Fig. 5.1). Ruptured ganglion cysts may be mistaken for other myxoid lesions of soft tissue.

Differential Diagnosis

Ganglion cyst should be distinguished from juxtaarticular myxoma and myxoinflammatory fibroblastic sarcoma. Juxtaarticular myxoma often affects larger joints, such as the knee, as well as the elbow, shoulder, ankle, and hip.[7] Histologically, juxtaarticular myxoma is a variably cellular spindle cell lesion with prominent myxoid stroma and ill-defined borders, more cellular than ganglion cyst. Myxoinflammatory fibroblastic sarcoma shows a predilection for the distal extremities. It is a low-grade sarcoma characterized by alternating hypo- and hypercellular areas and containing a prominent chronic inflammatory infiltrate and scattered large atypical pleomorphic cells with prominent nucleoli. In contrast, ganglion cysts typically lack an inflammatory component and do not contain atypical cells.

Prognosis and Treatment

Symptomatic ganglion cysts can be treated by simple excision or aspiration. Recurrences are uncommon.

Intramuscular/Cellular Myxoma

The term *intramuscular myxoma* was coined by Stout; in 1965 Enzinger reported the first large series of intramuscular myxomas, a group of deep-seated, benign-appearing soft tissue tumors showing abundant myxoid stroma.[8] Tumors showing higher cellularity and more collagenous stroma are designated "cellular myxoma." Intramuscular/cellular myxoma may occur sporadically or in association with fibrous dysplasia (also known as *Mazabraud syndrome*).[9]

Clinical Features

Intramuscular myxoma affects middle-aged adults (median age, 50 to 60 years) with a female predominance (female-to-male ratio, 3:1).[8-16] Most patients present with a painless, slowly growing mass.[8-16] Tumors most frequently arise in the lower extremities, especially the thigh.[8-16] The vast majority of lesions are intramuscular, and a smaller subset arise in subcutaneous tissue.[8-16]

Pathologic Features

Grossly, intramuscular myxomas are usually between 5 and 10 cm and appear well circumscribed, with a thin fibrous pseudocapsule. The cut surface is usually gelatinous and may show areas of cystic change.

Histologically, classic intramuscular myxoma is uniformly hypocellular and composed of small, bland spindle and stellate-shaped cells, with oval nuclei, inconspicuous nucleoli, and small amounts of palely eosinophilic cytoplasm, embedded in an abundant myxoid matrix (Fig. 5.2). Scattered small blood vessels are often present. Tumors frequently infiltrate adjacent muscle and adipose tissue. Mitoses are rare, and necrosis is absent.

A subset of intramuscular myxomas show hypercellular areas that may be focal or diffuse.[15] Such tumors are referred to as "cellular myxomas" (Fig. 5.3A).[15] These neoplasms are composed of cells with cytologic features similar to those of intramuscular myxoma. No atypia, nuclear pleomorphism, or mitotic activity is observed in cellular myxoma (see Fig. 5.3B). In addition, the stroma in cellular myxoma is more collagenous than in conventional intramuscular myxoma.

Immunohistochemistry

Intramuscular and cellular myxomas are often positive for CD34 and are negative for smooth muscle actin (SMA), desmin, and S-100 protein; EMA may be focally positive, most often in core needle biopsy specimens, a potential diagnostic pitfall.[12,13,15,17]

Molecular Genetics

Both intramuscular and cellular myxomas, whether sporadic or associated with Mazabraud syndrome, often harbor activating mutations in codon 201 of the *GNAS* gene, which encodes for the α subunit of the G protein that stimulates cyclic adenosine monophosphate formation.[18-20] A recent study found no *GNAS* mutations in juxtaarticular myxomas, which suggests that intramuscular/cellular myxomas are distinct from juxta-articular myxomas (discussed later).[21]

Differential Diagnosis

The differential diagnosis of intramuscular/cellular myxoma includes low-grade myxofibrosarcoma, LGFMS, and myxoid nerve sheath tumors, in particular myxoid neurofibroma and soft tissue perineurioma.

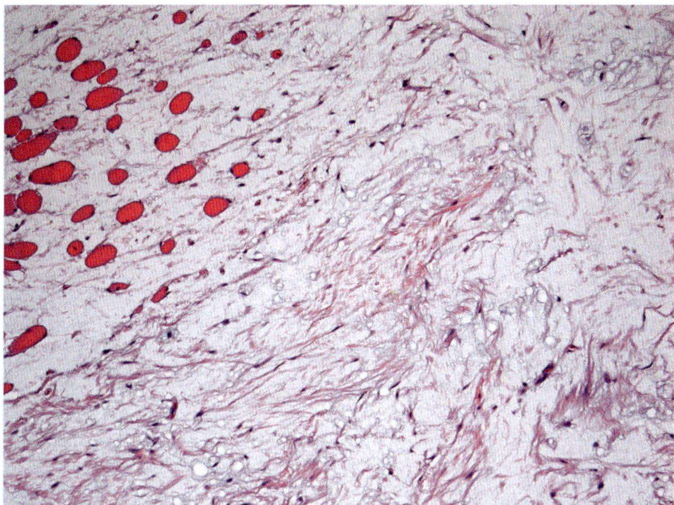

Figure 5.2 Intramuscular Myxoma. Intramuscular myxoma is a hypocellular lesion with abundant myxoid stroma. Note the entrapment of adjacent skeletal muscle fibers.

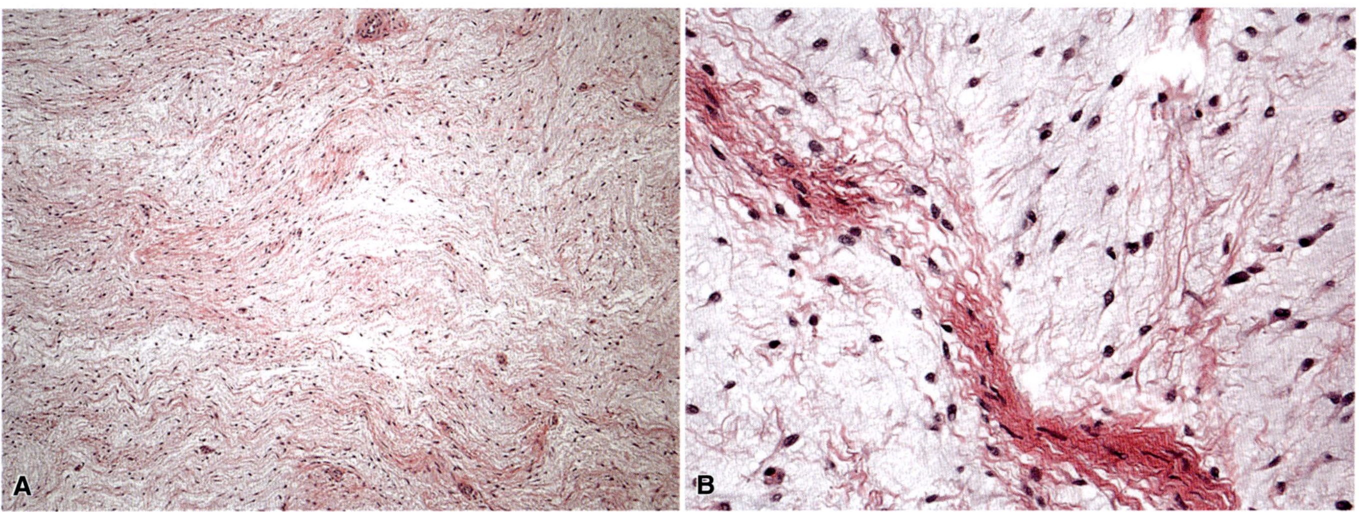

Figure 5.3 Cellular Myxoma. (A) Cellular myxoma is more cellular and more collagenous than conventional intramuscular myxoma. (B) The lesional cells are uniform and bland, with no nuclear pleomorphism.

Similar to intramuscular/cellular myxoma, low-grade myxofibrosarcoma affects older adults and often arises in the thigh. However, myxofibrosarcoma usually occurs in subcutaneous tissue and involves the skin, which is rarely the case in intramuscular/cellular myxoma. Low-grade myxofibrosarcoma can be distinguished from intramuscular myxoma based on the presence of distinctive curvilinear blood vessels and scattered atypical pleomorphic cells.

Typically, LGFMS affects younger patients than intramuscular/cellular myxoma. Morphologically, it shows alternating myxoid and collagenous areas, with arcades of thin-walled blood vessels. LGFMS can be distinguished from intramuscular/cellular myxoma by a more uniformly cellular appearance, expression of MUC4 and often EMA, and the characteristic t(7;16) translocation involving the *FUS* gene, which can be detected by conventional cytogenetics or fluorescence in situ hybridization (FISH) studies.

Myxoid neurofibroma contains cells with wavy, tapering nuclei and shows positive staining for S-100 protein. Soft tissue perineurioma may have variably myxoid stroma, but usually shows a whorled architecture and contains slender cells with elongated bipolar cytoplasmic processes, which are positive for EMA and often for claudin-1. As intramuscular/cellular myxoma often shows staining for EMA in core needle biopsy specimens, it is not always possible to distinguish between perineurioma and intramuscular/cellular myxoma in limited samples[17]; in such cases, an interim diagnosis of "benign myxoid spindle cell neoplasm" is appropriate.

Prognosis and Treatment

Intramuscular and cellular myxomas have a low risk of local recurrence if incompletely excised; therefore, simple surgical excision is adequate therapy.[8-16]

PRACTICE POINTS: Intramuscular/Cellular Myxoma

- Occurs sporadically or as part of Mazabraud syndrome.
- Affects middle-aged adults, with female predominance.
- Arises most frequently in the lower extremity and is often intramuscular.
- Intramuscular myxoma is a hypocellular myxoid lesion with bland cytology, inconspicuous vessels, and nondestructive infiltration of adjacent tissues.
- Cellular myxoma is more cellular, more collagenous, and more vascular than conventional intramuscular myxoma.
- Lesions are negative for S-100 protein; EMA may be positive in core needle biopsies.
- Contains activating mutations in codon 201 of the *GNAS* gene.

Juxtaarticular Myxoma

Juxtaarticular myxoma is a benign myxoid lesion that morphologically resembles intramuscular/cellular myxoma; however, these lesions appear to be distinct, based on recent genetic analysis.[18,21]

Clinical Features

Men are affected more often than women (male-to-female ratio, 2.6 : 1).[22] The age range is wide, but most patients are between the fifth and sixth decades.[22] Juxtaarticular myxoma usually arises adjacent to large joints, with the knee the most commonly affected site (>85% of cases), followed by the shoulder, elbow, hip, and ankle.[22] Patients come to medical attention because of a mass lesion with occasional pain or tenderness.[22] Rarely, patients report a history of trauma or osteoarthritis at the involved site.[22]

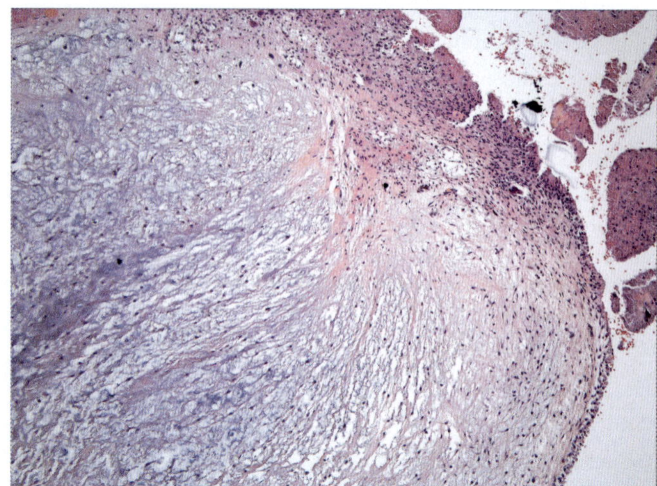

Figure 5.4 Juxtaarticular Myxoma. Juxtaarticular myxoma histologically resembles cellular myxoma, but is located adjacent to the synovium *(right)*.

Pathologic Features

Grossly, most tumors are between 2 and 6 cm, with a mucoid or gelatinous cut surface and a soft consistency. Areas of cystic degeneration are often present.

Histologically, juxtaarticular myxoma shows an infiltrative growth pattern with entrapment of adjacent subcutaneous adipose or tendinous tissue. The cells are uniform, with small, ovoid nuclei and inconspicuous nucleoli, embedded in a myxoid stroma. Most lesions are hypocellular; however, areas of increased cellularity (resembling cellular myxoma, discussed earlier) are common (Fig. 5.4). Most lesions (90%) show areas of ganglion cyst-like features with a fibrous pseudocapsule and accumulation of acellular myxoid matrix. In addition, foci of hemorrhage, chronic inflammation, and fibrin deposition may be seen in a subset of cases, likely secondary to trauma.

Immunohistochemistry

The immunophenotype is nonspecific, with variable positivity for CD34 and SMA, and negativity for S-100 protein.[7]

Molecular Genetics

It appears that juxtaarticular myxoma lacks the activating *GNAS* gene mutations characteristic of intramuscular and cellular myxomas, suggesting that intramuscular/cellular myxoma and juxtaarticular myxoma are unrelated, despite their histologic similarities.[21]

Differential Diagnosis

The differential diagnosis for juxtaarticular myxoma includes ganglion cyst, intramuscular myxoma, and low-grade myxofibrosarcoma.

In contrast to juxtaarticular myxoma, ganglion cysts mainly affect the small joints of the hands and feet and are characterized by the accumulation of acellular mucin surrounded by a dense fibrous pseudocapsule. When the capsule is disrupted, mucin can dissect through adjacent tissues with a pseudoinfiltrative growth pattern that is reminiscent of juxtaarticular myxoma.

The histologic features are essentially identical to those of intramuscular/cellular myxoma, and the two conditions can be distinguished only by anatomic location (adjacent to joints, in contrast to within large muscles).

Myxofibrosarcoma usually arises in superficial soft tissues of the extremities; joints are rarely involved. Histologically, myxofibrosarcoma can be distinguished from juxtaarticular myxoma by the presence of nuclear atypia and characteristic curvilinear blood vessels.

Prognosis and Treatment

In approximately 35% of cases, juxtaarticular myxoma recurs locally but does not metastasize.[22] Complete surgical excision is adequate treatment.

PRACTICE POINTS: Juxtaarticular Myxoma

- Predilection for men between fifth and sixth decades
- Juxtaarticular myxoma occurs in the large joints; the knee is involved in more than 85% of cases.
- Hypocellular myxoid lesion with bland cytology (similar to intramuscular myxoma) and infiltrative growth pattern.
- Lacks activating mutations of *GNAS* gene.
- Recurs in approximately 35% of cases, but shows no metastatic potential.

Dermal Nerve Sheath Myxoma

Until recently, dermal nerve sheath myxoma (formerly also referred to as *myxoid neurothekeoma*) was believed to be related to cellular neurothekeoma because the latter lesion may show myxoid stromal change.[23,24] However, it is now clear that these two lesions are unrelated and show distinct clinical and immunohistochemical features (nerve sheath myxoma is an S-100 protein-positive true Schwann cell neoplasm, whereas cellular neurothekeoma shows no specific immunophenotype), as well as differences in recurrent potential. Dermal nerve sheath myxoma is also discussed in Chapter 15.

Clinical Features

Dermal nerve sheath myxoma affects men and women equally, with a predilection for younger adults (mean age, 35 years).[25-27] Patients typically present with small, painless nodules on the distal extremities.

Pathologic Features

Dermal nerve sheath myxoma is a well-circumscribed small nodule, usually between 0.5 and 2 cm, primarily involving the dermis, with frequent extension into subcutaneous tissue. These tumors show a lobulated growth pattern, with sharply demarcated lobules separated by fibrous tissue (Fig. 5.5A). The lobules contain abundant myxoid matrix, with tumor cells growing in a reticular pattern; tumor cells may be arranged in circular, ring-like structures at the periphery of lobules (see Fig. 5.5B). Neoplastic cells are spindled to stellate, with hyperchromatic nuclei and scant cytoplasm (see Fig. 5.5C). Mitoses are scarce and nuclear pleomorphism is minimal.

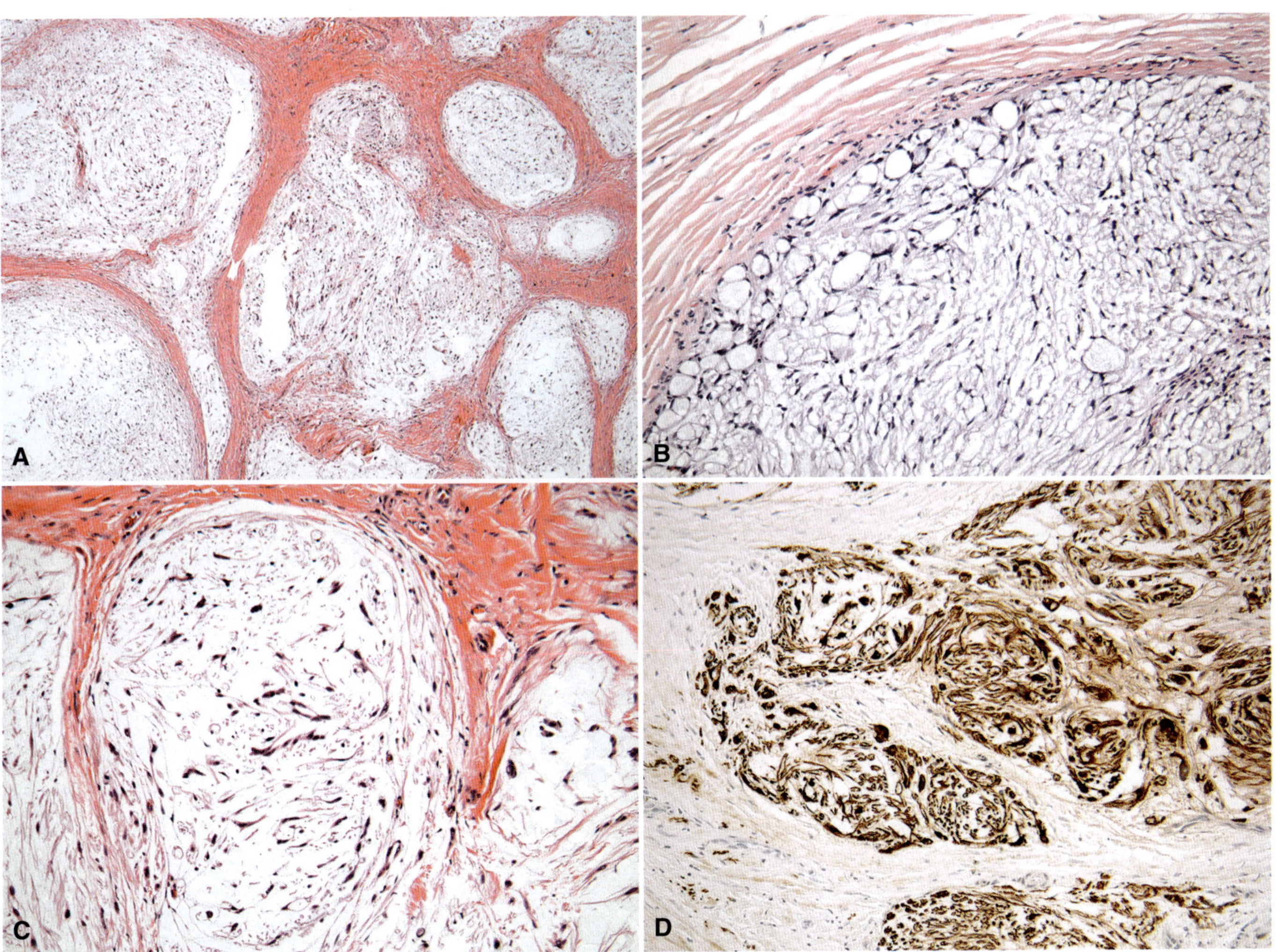

Figure 5.5 Dermal Nerve Sheath Myxoma. (A) Dermal nerve sheath myxoma shows a lobulated growth pattern. (B) At the periphery of the lobules, the neoplastic cells often form ring-like structures. (C) The spindled to stellate cells contain hyperchromatic nuclei. (D) Tumor cells are strongly positive for S-100 protein.

Immunohistochemistry

Dermal nerve sheath myxoma diffusely expresses S-100 protein (see Fig. 5.5D) as well as glial fibrillary acidic protein (GFAP) in most cases, confirming the Schwann cell nature of this tumor type.[26,27]

Differential Diagnosis

The differential diagnoses include cellular neurothekeoma, plexiform neurofibroma, superficial angiomyxoma, and low-grade myxofibrosarcoma. Immunohistochemical studies are helpful in this distinction.

Cellular neurothekeoma shows a predilection for the head and neck and upper extremities, and rarely affects the fingers and toes (see Chapter 15). In contrast to dermal nerve sheath myxoma, cellular neurothekeoma is poorly circumscribed with a micronodular architecture and is composed of nests of predominantly epithelioid cells with abundant pale cytoplasm. Myxoid stroma may be present, but it rarely predominates. Cellular neurothekeoma is positive for NKI-C3 and negative for S-100 protein.[28-30]

Plexiform neurofibroma is essentially pathognomonic of neurofibromatosis type 1 (von Recklinghausen disease).[31] This neurofibroma variant often occurs in superficial locations and shows a multinodular (or plexiform) growth pattern. However, in contrast to dermal nerve sheath myxoma, tumor nodules in plexiform neurofibroma are not surrounded by a thick, fibrous capsule. Occasional cases may show stromal myxoid changes, but unlike dermal nerve sheath myxoma, these lesions are not uniformly myxoid. Neurofibromas are usually less diffusely positive for S-100 protein and may show patchy expression of EMA; neurofilament protein highlights scattered axons.

Superficial angiomyxoma shows a predilection for the trunk and head and neck, and is rare in the distal extremities.[32,33] The tumor is poorly circumscribed, with ill-defined lobules that lack the sharp circumscription of dermal nerve sheath myxoma. Stromal neutrophils are seen in half of cases.[32,33] In contrast to dermal nerve sheath myxoma, neoplastic cells are negative for S-100 protein.[32,33]

Myxofibrosarcoma is often superficial and primarily affects the extremities of elderly patients. It is an infiltrative neoplasm with a lobulated growth pattern. In contrast to dermal nerve sheath myxoma, low-grade myxofibrosarcoma contains distinctive curvilinear blood vessels and scattered atypical hyperchromatic cells and is negative for S-100 protein.

Prognosis and Treatment

Dermal nerve sheath myxoma shows a relatively high rate of nondestructive local recurrence (up to 45%) after simple excision.[27] There is no metastatic potential.

Superficial Acral Fibromyxoma (Digital Fibromyxoma)

Although superficial acral fibromyxoma (also known as digital fibromyxoma) is a relatively common lesion, it remains underrecognized. This tumor type is also discussed in Chapter 15.

Clinical Features

Superficial acral fibromyxoma affects adults and shows a slight male predominance, with the majority arising as painless nodules on the fingers and toes, usually in the periungual regions.[34,35]

Pathologic Features

Superficial acral fibromyxoma is usually a small polypoid or dome-shaped skin lesion, without ulceration of the overlying epidermis. It is a poorly circumscribed and unencapsulated, predominantly dermal cellular proliferation of elongated or stellate, cytologically uniform bland fibroblasts, arranged in a haphazard pattern (Fig. 5.6A). Tumor cells are embedded in a variably collagenous or myxoid stroma and show no nuclear atypia (see Fig. 5.6B). Mitoses are rare, and necrosis is not observed.

Immunohistochemistry

Immunohistochemistry is of limited value in the diagnosis of superficial acral fibromyxoma. Neoplastic cells are usually diffusely positive for CD34 and may occasionally show reactivity for EMA, whereas S-100 protein is negative.[34,35] Loss of RB1 (retinoblastoma) expression appears to be common in this tumor type.[36]

Molecular Genetics

Recent studies have demonstrated monoallelic deletions of 13q12, including the tumor suppressor gene *RB1*[36].

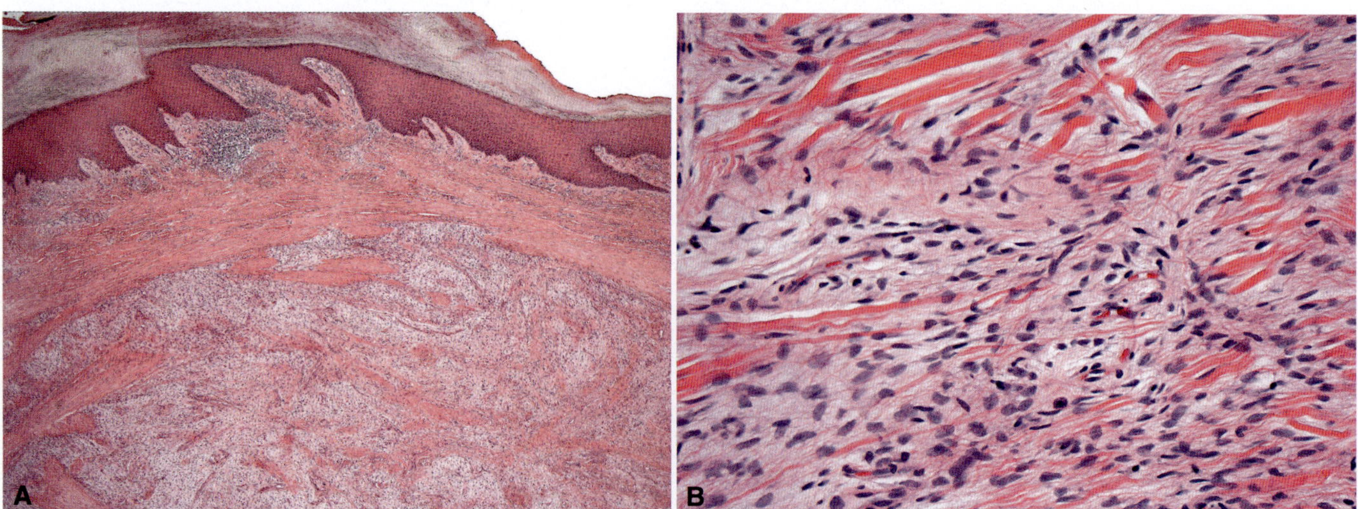

Figure 5.6 Superficial Acral (Digital) Fibromyxoma. (A) Digital fibromyxoma is situated in the dermis and is composed of short spindle cells embedded in a variably collagenous and myxoid stroma. (B) Bland spindle cells arranged in a haphazard growth pattern.

Differential Diagnosis

The differential diagnosis of superficial acral fibromyxoma mainly includes superficial angiomyxoma, the myxoid variant of benign fibrous histiocytoma, the myxoid variant of DFSP, and soft tissue perineurioma.

Superficial angiomyxoma arises primarily on the trunk and head and neck, unlike digital fibromyxoma. Morphologically, it contains more abundant myxoid stroma, shows a lobulated growth pattern, and often contains scattered neutrophils, which are not a feature of superficial acral fibromyxoma.[32,33]

Benign fibrous histiocytoma very rarely contains myxoid stroma. Recognizing typical areas of benign fibrous histiocytoma with lateral entrapment of hyaline dermal collagen is helpful in correctly diagnosing this entity. In contrast to superficial acral fibromyxoma, the vast majority of benign fibrous histiocytomas are negative for CD34.

The myxoid variant of DFSP is rare.[37,38] As with conventional DFSP, this variant rarely arises on the digits. In the majority of cases, myxoid DFSP can be recognized by the presence of foci with the typical morphologic features of DFSP, a storiform architecture, and a diffusely infiltrative growth pattern.[37,38] Immunohistochemistry is not helpful in the differential diagnosis because both entities are positive for CD34.[34,37,38]

Soft tissue perineurioma usually affects subcutaneous tissue, but approximately 10% of cases arise in the dermis.[39] Unlike superficial acral fibromyxoma, it is usually well circumscribed and shows variably myxoid and collagenous stroma, with cells arranged in storiform, whorled, and lamellar growth patterns.[39] In addition to CD34, soft tissue perineurioma is consistently positive for EMA; claudin-1 is positive in a subset of cases.[39,40]

Prognosis and Treatment

Superficial acral fibromyxoma is benign, recurs locally in up to 25% of cases (especially periungual lesions), but does not metastasize.[34,35]

PRACTICE POINTS: Superficial Acral Fibromyxoma (Digital Fibromyxoma)

- Affects adults, with a slight male predominance
- Painless nodule in the periungual region of fingers and toes
- Poorly circumscribed, unencapsulated dermal lesion composed of bland fibroblasts embedded in variably collagenous or myxoid stroma
- Deletions of 13q12 resulting in loss of RB1 expression
- Local recurrence in up to 25%

Superficial Angiomyxoma

Superficial angiomyxoma is a distinctive cutaneous mesenchymal lesion with a propensity for local recurrence (see Chapter 15 for additional discussion).

Clinical Features

Superficial angiomyxoma predominantly affects middle-aged adults, with a slight male predominance (male-to-female ratio, 1.5:1). This tumor type typically presents as a painless, slowly growing nodule. The most common sites are the trunk and head and neck.[32,33] The external genital area may also be affected; women are more often affected at this location (see also Chapter 17 for the differential diagnosis at this site).[41] A small subset of superficial angiomyxomas are associated with Carney complex, especially those arising in the external ear and breast.[32,33,41]

Pathologic Features

Superficial angiomyxoma is a hypocellular dermal lesion with abundant myxoid stroma (Fig. 5.7A), composed of ill-defined lobules, which often infiltrate into subcutaneous tissue (see Fig. 7.7B). Superficial angiomyxoma is composed of small spindled or stellate cells with ovoid, vesicular nuclei, inconspicuous nucleoli, and scant cytoplasm; small blood vessels are often prominent (see Fig. 5.7C). Scattered neutrophils are observed in approximately half of cases (see Fig. 5.7D), unassociated with necrosis or ulceration of the overlying skin. In approximately 20% of cases, entrapped epithelial structures, including epidermoid cysts and strands of squamous epithelium, are found within the lesion. Nuclear atypia and pleomorphism are not observed.

Immunohistochemistry

The tumor cells are usually positive for CD34 and negative for S-100 protein, desmin, and keratins.[32,33,41] Loss of PRKAR1A expression is detected in up to two thirds of tumors.[42]

Molecular Genetics

Superficial angiomyxomas arising both sporadically and in the setting of Carney complex are associated with inactivating mutations in *PRKAR1A*, which encodes protein kinase A regulatory subunit 1-alpha.[42-44]

Differential Diagnosis

The differential diagnosis for superficial angiomyxoma includes dermal nerve sheath myxoma, deep (aggressive) angiomyxoma, and low-grade myxofibrosarcoma.

Dermal nerve sheath myxoma has a predilection for the digits and is composed of lobules sharply demarcated from the surrounding tissues, unlike the ill-defined lobules of superficial angiomyxoma (see also Chapter 15).[27] Tumor cells are strongly positive for S-100 protein, which is also helpful in this distinction.[27]

Similar to a subset of superficial angiomyxomas, deep (aggressive) angiomyxoma characteristically affects the genital area (see also Chapter 17) but arises in deeper soft tissue, shows a diffusely infiltrative growth pattern, and contains a characteristic vascular pattern, with bundles of smooth muscle cells spinning off of medium-sized blood vessels.[45]

Myxofibrosarcoma more commonly affects elderly patients and usually arises on the extremities. The presence of distinctive curvilinear vessels and scattered atypical pleomorphic cells are helpful distinguishing features.

Prognosis and Treatment

Superficial angiomyxoma has a high rate of nondestructive local recurrence (30%) but has no potential to metastasize.[32,33,41] Complete surgical excision is curative.

Deep Angiomyxoma

Deep ("aggressive") angiomyxoma is a distinctive gynecologic soft tissue neoplasm that occasionally also affects males.[46-49] Given its predilection for the lower genital tract, this tumor type is discussed in detail in Chapter 17.

Clinical Features

Deep angiomyxoma is a disease of young to middle-aged adults, with a marked female predominance, although men are affected in a minority of cases. The tumor occurs as a mass or swelling in the pelvic/perineal or scrotal areas.[45-52] Common sites include the vulva, vagina, inguinal area, and pelvis.[45-52]

Pathologic Features

Grossly, deep angiomyxoma is a large, deep-seated mass with infiltrative margins.[45-47,50-52] Histologically, deep angiomyxoma is a hypocellular neoplasm (Fig. 5.8A) composed of small monomorphic spindle cells, embedded in a myxoid or edematous stroma (see Fig. 5.8B). In addition, small- to medium-sized blood vessels with perivascular hyalinization

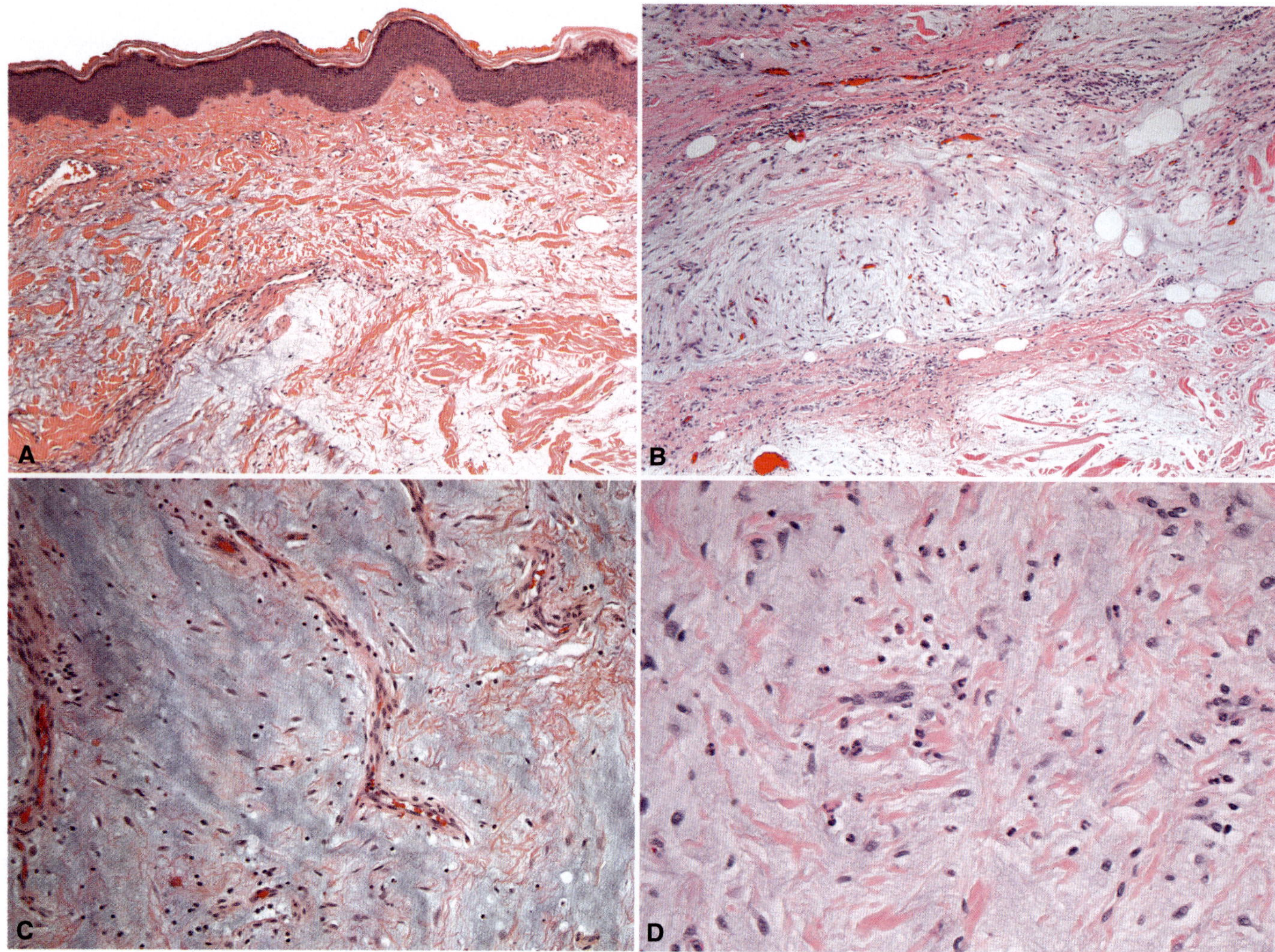

Figure 5.7 Superficial Angiomyxoma. (A) Superficial angiomyxoma is a dermal neoplasm with a lobulated growth pattern and irregular margins. (B) Lobules of tumor often extend into subcutaneous tissue. (C) Abundant myxoid stroma and scattered thin-walled blood vessels are typical features. (D) The tumor contains short spindle cells with bland nuclei. Note the prominent stromal neutrophils.

and smooth muscle cells spinning off of vessel walls are characteristic features (see Fig. 5.8C).

Immunohistochemistry

Deep angiomyxoma shows overexpression of HMGA2 by immunohistochemistry (see Fig. 5.8D).[53-55]

Molecular Genetics

Translocations involving 12q15, leading to rearrangement of *HMGA2*, have been reported in a subset of deep angiomyxomas.[56-60]

Differential Diagnosis

The main differential diagnosis includes cellular angiofibroma, angiomyofibroblastoma, superficial angiomyxoma, fibroepithelial stromal polyp, myxoid variant of DFSP, and botryoid rhabdomyosarcoma. The differential diagnosis with other lower genital tumors is discussed in more detail in Chapter 17.

Cellular angiofibroma is a benign tumor that arises in the vulvovaginal and inguinoscrotal regions of middle-aged men and women in equal proportions.[61] This tumor is composed of short spindle cells with delicate collagen and numerous small, round, often hyalinized vessels. Loss of nuclear RB1 expression distinguishes cellular angiofibroma from deep angiomyxoma. In contrast to deep angiomyxoma, superficial angiomyxoma involves the skin and subcutaneous tissue of the trunk, extremities, and head and neck regions.[32] Tumor nodules are hypocellular with small, bland-appearing cells embedded in a myxoid stroma. Fibroepithelial stromal polyps are relatively common in the vulvovaginal area of adult women.[62] These lesions typically extend to the epidermis, with ill-defined margins. The myxoid variant of DFSP rarely affects the vulvovaginal or scrotal region. It is a poorly circumscribed lesion that is very difficult to recognize in the absence of typical areas of DFSP.[37] Embryonal rhabdomyosarcoma often arises at mucosal sites. In the botryoid variant, neoplastic cells form a tight band known as the "cambium layer" underneath the epithelial surface, which is a key finding for the diagnosis. Immunohistochemistry for myogenin confirms the diagnosis of rhabdomyosarcoma.

Prognosis and Treatment

Although early studies suggested a high rate of local recurrence (often multiple), more recent data indicated that deep angiomyxoma is rarely aggressive and can usually be cured by simple (but complete) local excision. There is no potential for distant metastasis.[45-47,50-52]

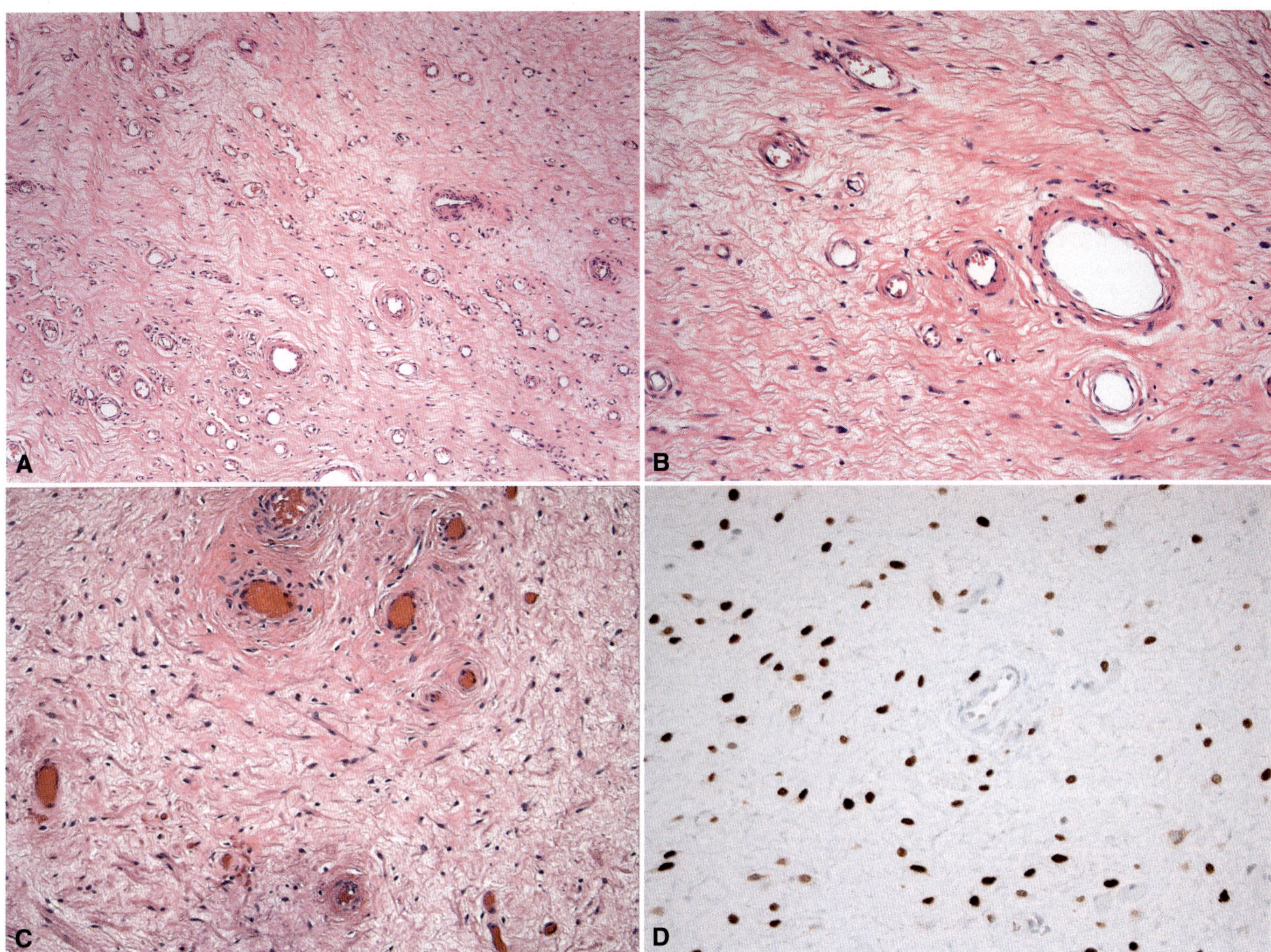

Figure 5.8 Deep ("Aggressive") Angiomyxoma. (A) Deep angiomyxoma is a hypocellular neoplasm with abundant edematous or myxoid stroma. (B) The uniform short spindle cells contain bland, hyperchromatic nuclei. (C) Smooth muscle cells characteristically spin off of medium-sized blood vessels. (D) Nuclear expression of HMGA2 is typical of deep angiomyxoma.

PRACTICE POINTS: Deep ("Aggressive") Angiomyxoma

- Affects predominantly young to middle-aged adult women
- Common sites include the vulva, vagina, inguinal area, and pelvis
- Deep-seated, infiltrative mass with monomorphic spindle cells in myxoid stroma, and small to medium-sized blood vessels
- Smooth muscle cells spin off of blood vessels
- Expression of HMGA2 protein
- Abnormalities in 12q15 with rearrangement of the *HMGA2* gene
- May recur locally, but shows no metastatic potential

Ossifying Fibromyxoid Tumor

Ossifying fibromyxoid tumor (OFMT) is a tumor of uncertain differentiation that was first described by Enzinger and colleagues in 1989.[63] It is usually benign, although a small subset of tumors show atypical or malignant histologic features and follow an aggressive clinical course.[64] OFMT is also discussed in Chapter 6.

Clinical Features

Adults are predominantly affected, and the median age is 50 years.[63-65] OFMT occurs more often in men (male-to-female ratio, 1.5 to 2 : 1).[63-65] The most common sites are the upper and lower extremities, followed by the trunk and head and neck.[63-65] Patients usually seek medical attention for a slowly growing, long-standing painless subcutaneous or intramuscular mass.[63-65]

Pathologic Features

Grossly, OFMT is well circumscribed and multinodular, with an average size of 4 to 5 cm.[63-65] The tumor usually involves subcutaneous tissues, is often attached to underlying tendons or fascia, and contains a fibrous or fibro-osseous pseudocapsule.

Histologically, in more than 80% of cases, OFMT is a lobulated mass surrounded by an incomplete shell of lamellar bone (Fig. 5.9A); nonossifying examples are uncommon. In approximately 15% of cases, the tumor invades through the pseudocapsule and forms satellite nodules (see Fig. 5.9B), with an appearance similar to that of pleomorphic adenoma of salivary glands. These nodules are also usually surrounded

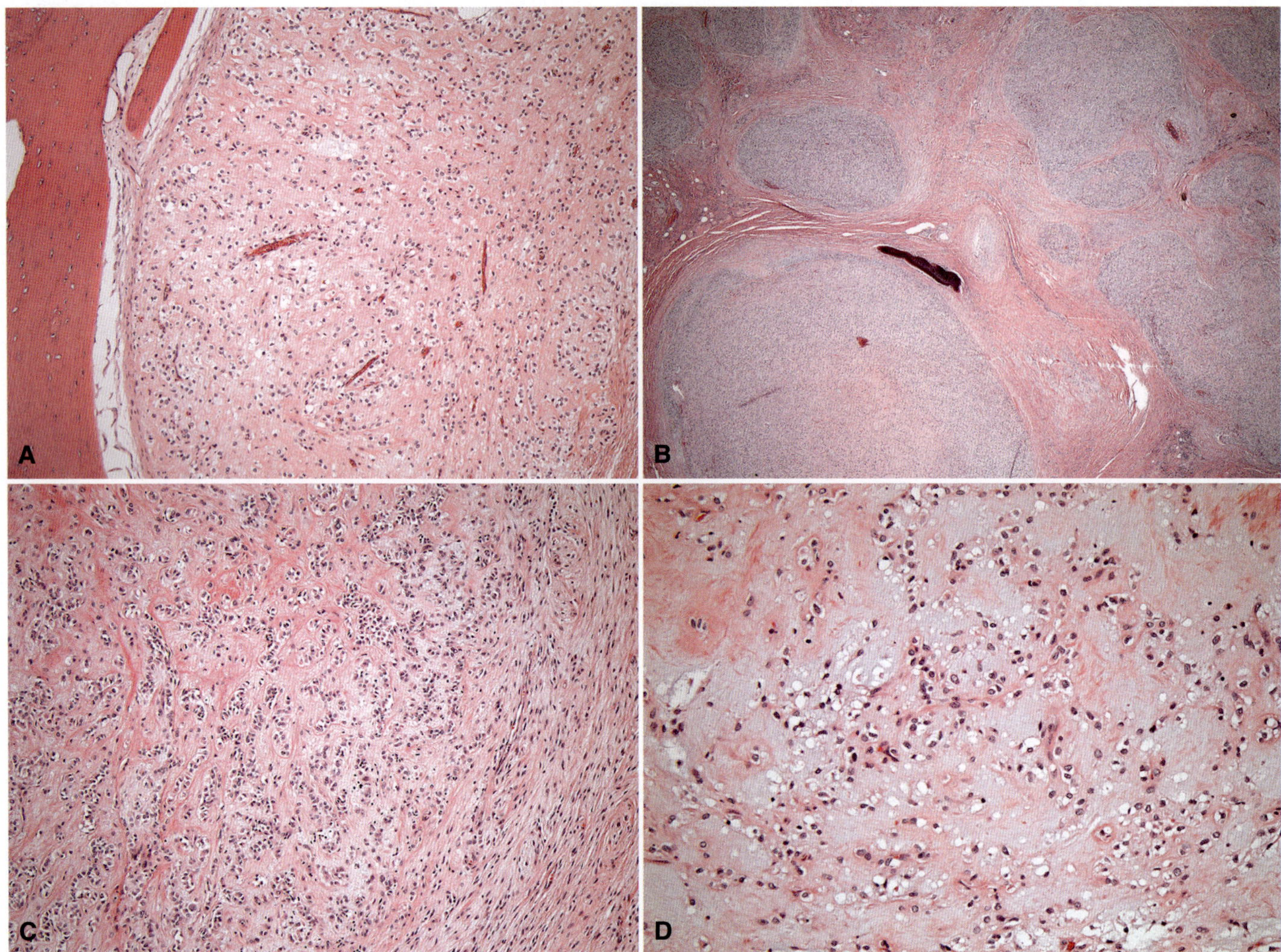

Figure 5.9 Ossifying Fibromyxoid Tumor. (A) Ossifying fibromyxoid tumor is usually surrounded by an incomplete shell of lamellar bone. (B) The tumor shows a multinodular growth pattern with satellite nodules infiltrating adjacent tissues. (C) Neoplastic cells are arranged in cords and trabeculae. (D) Cords of bland ovoid cells in a variably fibromyxoid stroma.

by a fibrous pseudocapsule. The tumor is composed of monomorphic round to ovoid cells arranged in cords and trabeculae (see Fig. 5.9C) within a variably fibromyxoid stroma (see Fig. 5.9D). Mitoses are generally scarce.

A small proportion of cases (<10%) shows histologic features that have been variably associated with more aggressive behavior. Such tumors are accordingly designated "atypical" or "malignant" OFMT.[64,66-68] These features include hypercellularity, greater than 2 mitoses per 50 high-power fields, necrosis, vascular invasion, moderate or severe nuclear atypia, and bone centrally located or randomly distributed throughout the tumor. When nuclear atypia is associated with osteoid (which is more often seen in recurrences), the tumor may mimic osteosarcoma.[64,66,67] Folpe and Weiss proposed categories that apply these criteria: the presence of either high nuclear grade or high cellularity and greater than 2 mitoses per 50 high-power fields warrants a malignant diagnosis.[64] Tumors may be classified as "atypical" when the other features described earlier are present without high nuclear grade or a high mitotic rate.[64]

Immunohistochemistry

In most cases (70% to 90%), OFMT is positive for S-100 protein, although expression may be focal (Fig. 5.10A).[69-72] OFMT is positive for desmin in up to 50% of cases (see Fig. 5.10B), and tumor cells occasionally show focal staining for keratins or EMA (<10%).[69-72] MUC4 may be positive in a small subset of cases.[68]

Molecular Genetics

Recurrent rearrangements of the *PHF1* gene are characteristic of OFMT, found in typical, atypical, and malignant variants; the diagnosis can be confirmed by FISH for *PHF1*.[73,74] A subset of tumors harbor *PHF1-EP400* fusion.[75,76] Other fusions have been identified in small numbers of OFMT cases, including *ZC3H7B-BCOR*, *CREBBP-BCORL1*, and *KDM2A-WWTR1*.[76,77]

Differential Diagnosis

Primarily, OFMT should be distinguished from soft tissue myoepithelioma and extraskeletal myxoid chondrosarcoma (EMC). Immunohistochemistry is useful in differential diagnosis (Table 5.1).

Soft tissue myoepithelioma usually shows more intratumoral heterogeneity than OFMT, with a range of cell types and varying growth patterns, including solid areas. Myoepithelial neoplasms are usually positive for S-100 protein, keratins, and EMA, and 50% are positive for GFAP. They are negative for desmin.[78] Approximately 50% of myoepithelial tumors of soft tissue harbor *EWSR1* gene rearrangements.[79]

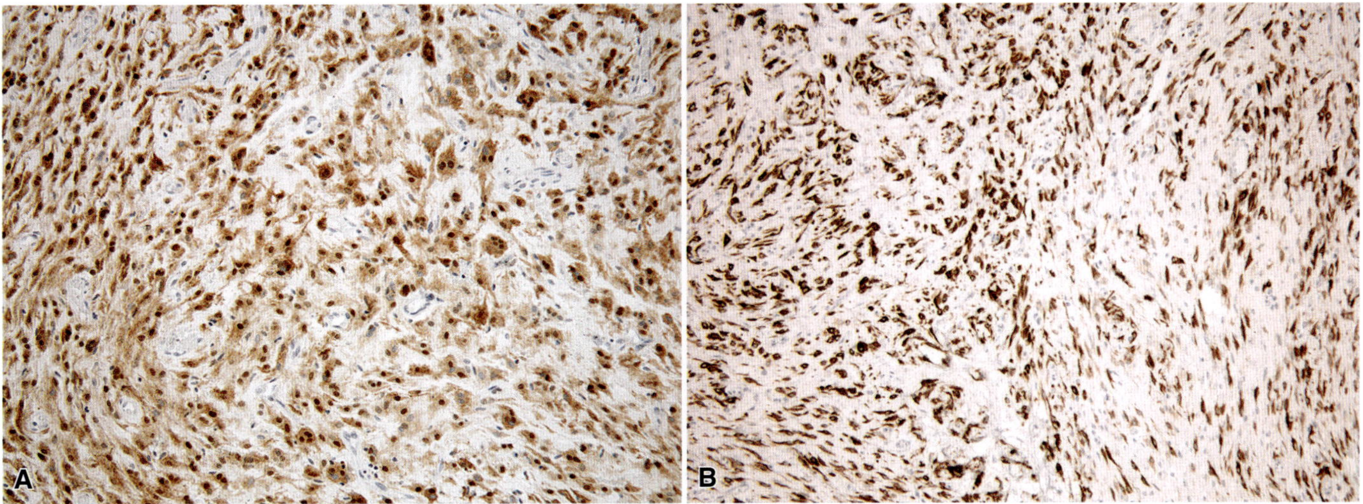

Figure 5.10 Ossifying Fibromyxoid Tumor. Coexpression of S-100 protein (A) and desmin (B) is commonly observed.

Table 5.1 Immunohistochemistry in the Differential Diagnosis of Ossifying Fibromyxoid Tumor, Soft Tissue Myoepithelioma, and Extraskeletal Myxoid Chondrosarcoma

	S-100 Protein	Keratins	Epithelial Membrane Antigen	Desmin
Ossifying fibromyxoid tumor	++	rare	rare	+
Soft tissue myoepithelioma	+++	+++	+++	−
Extraskeletal myxoid chondrosarcoma	±	−	rare	−

EMC contains more abundant myxoid stroma than OFMT and is usually composed of larger spindled to epithelioid cells with a uniformly reticular architecture. Positivity for S-100 protein is found in only a small subset of cases (<20%), and desmin is consistently negative.[80] EMC can be confirmed by the characteristic t(9;22) translocation involving the *EWSR1* and *NR4A3* genes or other variants involving *NR4A3*.

Prognosis and Treatment

Surgery is the treatment of choice for OFMT. The recurrence rate for typical OFMT is approximately 10% to 20%. Metastases are rare, occurring in fewer than 2% of cases.[63-65,68] In the largest series examining atypical and malignant examples of OFMT, tumors considered atypical resembled benign tumors in rates of recurrence and metastatic potential. Tumors meeting the criteria for malignancy showed a 60% rate of local recurrence and metastasis.[64]

PRACTICE POINTS: Ossifying Fibromyxoid Tumor

- Affects adults, with a male predominance
- Common sites include the extremities, trunk, head, and neck
- Lobulated mass with incomplete shell of bone composed of monomorphic ovoid cells arranged in cords and trabeculae, and variable fibromyxoid stroma
- Criteria for malignancy: (1) high nuclear grade or (2) high cellularity and mitotic activity (>2 per 50 high-power fields)
- Neoplastic cells are usually positive for S-100 protein and often express desmin
- *PHF1* gene rearrangements are frequent
- Recurrence rate of 10% to 20% and rare metastases in benign cases; recurrence and metastasis in up to 60% of malignant cases

Myoepithelioma and Myoepithelial Carcinoma

Mixed tumor and myoepithelioma/myoepithelial carcinoma are considered related neoplasms that lie along a morphologic continuum.[7] Myoepithelial neoplasms of soft tissue are histologically analogous to those arising in the salivary glands. Malignant examples (myoepithelial carcinoma), defined by the presence of nuclear atypia (discussed later), often pursue an aggressive clinical course.[81] These tumors are also discussed in Chapters 6 and 9.

Clinical Features

Myoepithelial tumors of soft tissue have a peak incidence in adults in the third to fifth decades, with an equal gender distribution.[78,82-84] A subset of these tumors occur in children.[81] Within the pediatric population, myoepithelial carcinomas are more common than myoepitheliomas. Most patients have a palpable mass with or without pain. The most common sites are the limbs and limb girdles (75% of cases), followed by the head and neck and trunk.[78,82-84] Myoepithelial tumors arise in subcutaneous tissue and deep soft tissue in similar proportions.[78,82-84]

Pathologic Features

Soft tissue myoepithelioma averages 3.5 to 4 cm in greatest dimension and is usually grossly well circumscribed, with a lobulated growth pattern and a thin pseudocapsule.[78,82,83] The tumor is usually firm, often with a myxoid or glistening cut surface. Myoepithelial carcinomas are usually larger than myoepitheliomas.[78,81] The cut surface is firm or fleshy, sometimes with focal areas of calcification and necrosis.[78,81]

Histologically, myoepithelioma of soft tissue most often shows a reticular growth pattern, with prominent chondromyxoid or hyalinized stroma (Fig. 5.11A). Less frequently, tumors may be composed of sheets of cells embedded in less prominent stroma, and intratumoral heterogeneity and mixed patterns are common. Neoplastic cells are arranged in cords, sheets, or nests, and are epithelioid or spindled, with eosinophilic cytoplasm (see Fig. 5.11B). Occasionally, epithelioid cells with eccentrically placed nuclei and hyaline cytoplasmic inclusions ("plasmacytoid" cells) are focally or extensively present (see Fig. 5.11C). Other features that may be seen in a subset of cases include focal clear cell areas; ductal (in mixed tumor; see Fig. 5.11D), squamous, or adipocytic differentiation; and metaplastic cartilage or bone.

The single most important criterion for malignancy in a myoepithelial tumor of soft tissue is the presence of at least moderate nuclear atypia,

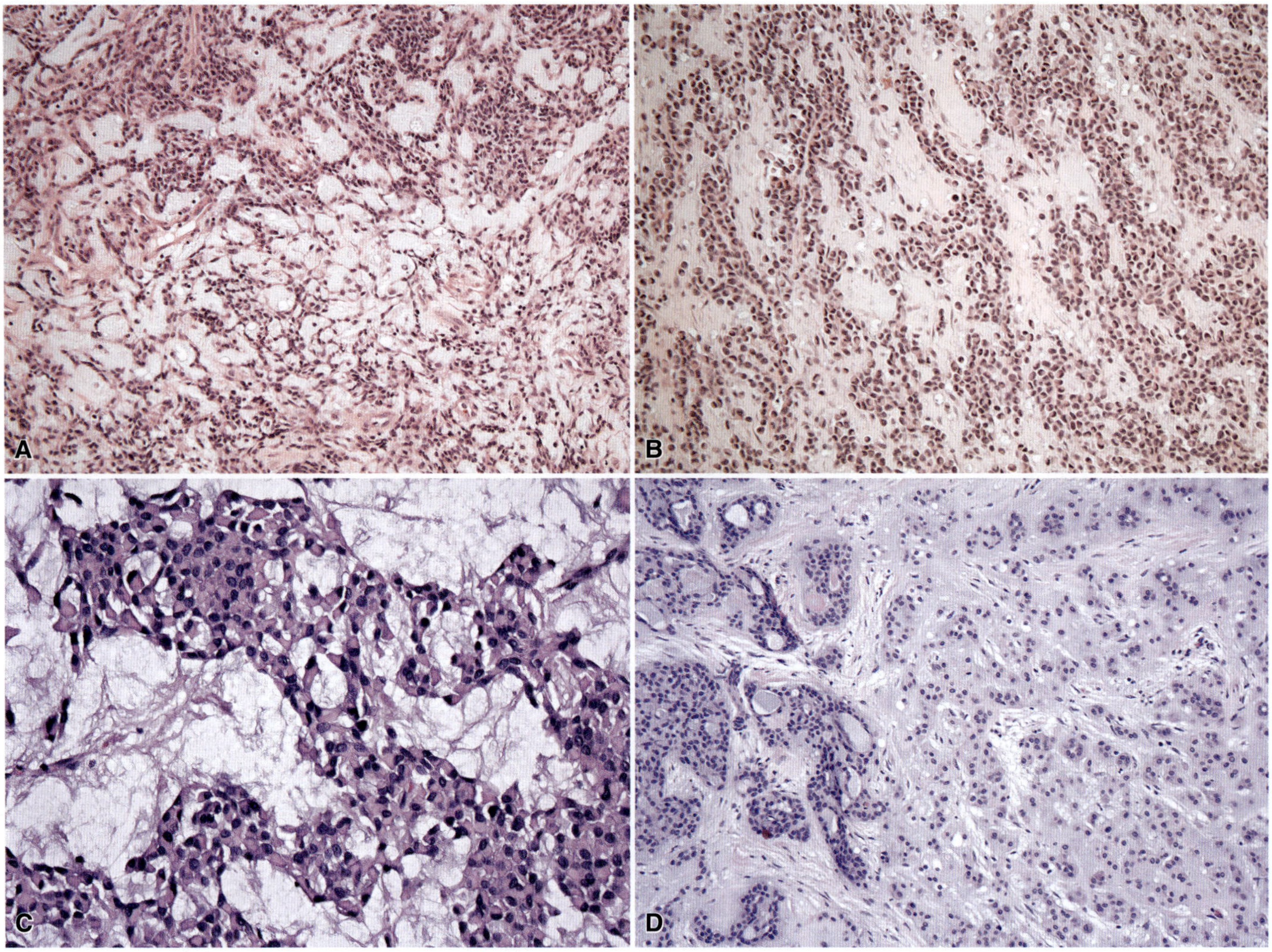

Figure 5.11 Myoepithelioma. (A) Soft tissue myoepithelioma composed of spindle cells with a reticular growth pattern in a myxoid stroma. (B) Cords of epithelioid cells with eosinophilic cytoplasm in a chondromyxoid stroma. (C) Plasmacytoid myoepithelial cells with eccentric nuclei. (D) Soft tissue myoepithelioma with focal ductal differentiation ("mixed tumor").

which is defined by enlarged nuclei, vesicular or coarse chromatin, and prominent nucleoli (Fig. 5.12).[78,81] Although myoepithelial carcinoma may show infiltrative margins, a high mitotic rate, or necrosis, these features alone are insufficient to establish a malignant diagnosis, and tumors with marked nuclear atypia that lack these other features may also behave aggressively.[78,81]

Immunohistochemistry

Myoepithelial tumors are almost always positive for at least one broad-spectrum keratin or EMA (Fig. 5.13A). It is sometimes necessary to perform more than one keratin immunostain.[78] In addition, most cases are positive for S-100 protein (see Fig. 5.13B), and approximately half are positive for GFAP.[78] Myogenic markers generally are not helpful, although the tumors are often positive for calponin, and reactivity for SMA is seen in approximately 30% of cases. The tumors are usually negative for desmin. p63 is positive in up to 45% of myoepitheliomas and 40% of myoepithelial carcinomas and may be a useful marker in some cases.[85] Myoepithelioma shows frequent expression of SOX10 (80%), although SOX10 positivity is seen in only a third of myoepithelial carcinomas.[86] Mixed tumors of soft tissue often show nuclear staining for PLAG1, reflecting gene rearrangement (discussed later).[87] A subset

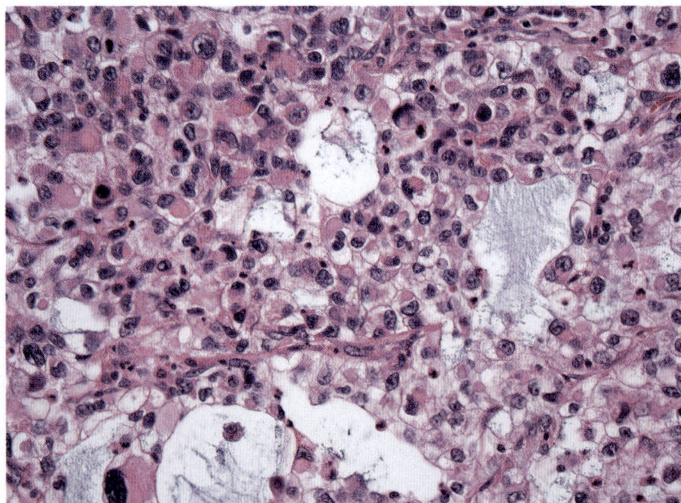

Figure 5.12 Myoepithelial Carcinoma. Myoepithelial carcinoma composed of epithelioid cells with coarse chromatin and prominent nucleoli. Note the focal myxoid stroma.

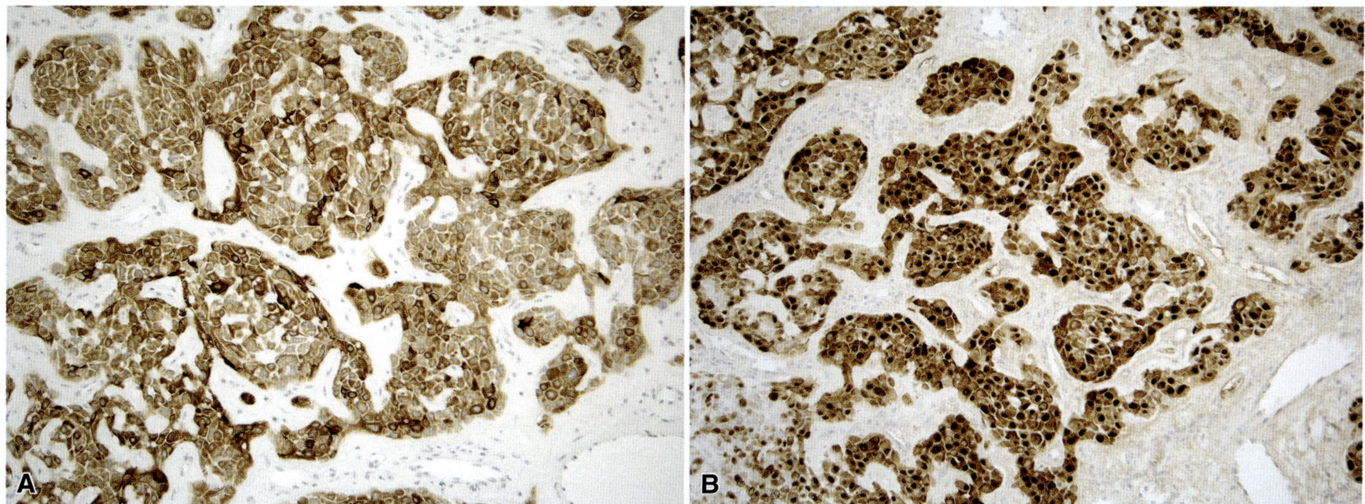

Figure 5.13 Myoepithelioma. Neoplastic cells in soft tissue myoepithelioma are usually positive for keratins (A) and S-100 protein (B).

of myoepithelial carcinomas show loss of expression of SMARCB1 (INI1; 10% in adults; 40% in children).[81,88,89]

Molecular Genetics

EWSR1 gene rearrangements have been identified in approximately 50% of myoepithelial tumors of skin and soft tissue, with different fusion partners than other mesenchymal tumors.[79,90-94] The reported translocations include *EWSR1-PBX1*, *EWSR1-ZNF444*, *EWSR1-POU5F1*, and *EWSR1-KLF17*.[79,90-92] However, these fusion partners appear to account for fewer than 50% of the *EWSR1* rearrangements; the other involved genes remain to be determined. Some of these fusion partners may be associated with distinct histologic patterns.[79] Variant *FUS* rearrangement instead of *EWSR1* also occurs in myoepithelial tumors.[90,95] Similar to its salivary counterpart, mixed tumors of soft tissue often harbor *PLAG1* gene rearrangements.[87,96,97]

Differential Diagnosis

The differential diagnosis for myoepithelial tumors can be broad, depending on the histologic pattern and whether the tumor is morphologically benign or malignant (see also Chapters 6 and 9). This discussion focuses on the examples with myxoid stroma.

Soft tissue myoepithelioma with myxoid stroma and the characteristic reticular growth pattern should be differentiated from OFMT, EMC, and epithelioid schwannoma (see Table 5.1). Myoepithelial carcinoma of soft tissue should be distinguished from metastatic carcinoma, metastatic melanoma, and proximal-type epithelioid sarcoma (Table 5.2).

Both OFMT and EMC can be differentiated from myoepithelial tumors with immunohistochemical stains (see Table 5.1 and the differential diagnosis of OFMT). Epithelioid schwannoma contains epithelioid cells arranged in cords and nests, often with a lobulated growth pattern and sometimes with prominent myxoid stroma.[98-100] It is strongly and diffusely positive for S-100 protein and GFAP, and the capsule is often positive for EMA.[98-100] A subset of epithelioid schwannoma also shows loss of SMARCB1 (INI1).[101] However, these tumors are negative for keratins.

Metastatic carcinoma very rarely shows myxoid stroma. Similar to primary soft tissue myoepithelial carcinoma, metastatic carcinoma is positive for keratins; however, it is usually negative for S-100 protein

Table 5.2 Immunohistochemistry in the Differential Diagnosis of Myoepithelial Carcinoma

	Keratin	Epithelial Membrane Antigen	S-100 Protein	CD34	Loss of INI1
Myoepithelial carcinoma	+++	++	+++	–	±
Metastatic carcinoma	+++	+	–	–	–
Malignant melanoma	–	–	+++	–	–
Proximal-type epithelioid sarcoma	+++	+++	–	±	+++

(except for a subset of breast carcinomas), GFAP, and myogenic markers. Malignant melanoma also rarely shows myxoid stroma and can be distinguished from myoepithelial carcinoma with immunohistochemistry, because melanoma is often positive for HMB-45 and melan A and negative for keratins and EMA. Finally, proximal-type epithelioid sarcoma is characterized by large epithelioid cells, with prominent nuclei and amphophilic cytoplasm, occasionally embedded in a somewhat myxoid background. Similar to myoepithelial carcinoma, epithelioid sarcoma is positive for keratins and EMA, but unlike myoepithelial tumors, it is positive for CD34 in approximately 50% of cases and negative for S-100 protein and GFAP. In addition, SMARCB1 (INI1) expression is absent in nearly all epithelioid sarcomas but in only a subset of myoepithelial carcinomas.[81,88,89]

Prognosis and Treatment

Complete surgical excision with negative margins is the treatment of choice for myoepithelioma and myoepithelial carcinoma. Histologically benign myoepitheliomas recur in approximately 20% of cases and very rarely metastasize.[78,82,83] In contrast, myoepithelial carcinomas have a local recurrence rate of approximately 40% and a metastatic rate of at least 30%.[78] In children, myoepithelial carcinomas are even more aggressive, with rates of recurrence, metastasis, and mortality of approximately 50%.[81] The most common sites of metastasis include lung, lymph nodes, and soft tissues.[78,81] Metastatic myoepithelial carcinomas appear to be sensitive to carboplatin and paclitaxel.[102]

PRACTICE POINTS: Myoepithelioma

- Peak incidence in adults in the third to fifth decades
- Arise most commonly in the limbs and limb girdles
- Often characterized by a reticular growth pattern with chondromyxoid or hyalinized stroma, and shows prominent intratumoral heterogeneity
- Neoplastic cells are arranged in cords, sheets, or nests, and are epithelioid or spindled with eosinophilic cytoplasm
- Most cases are positive for keratins, epithelial membrane antigen, and S-100 protein. p63 and SOX10 are often positive
- Rearrangements of the *EWSR1* gene are common
- Recurrence rate of 20%; metastases are rare

PRACTICE POINTS: Myoepithelial Carcinoma

- Criterion for malignancy: moderate or severe nuclear atypia (enlarged nuclei with coarse chromatin and prominent nucleoli)
- Histologic features insufficient for the diagnosis of myoepithelial carcinoma: infiltrative margins, high mitotic rate, and necrosis
- Rearrangements of the *EWSR1* gene are common
- Recurrence rate of 40% to 50%; metastatic rate of 30% to 50%
- Sites of metastasis: lung, lymph nodes, and soft tissues

Myxofibrosarcoma

Myxofibrosarcoma was first described in 1977 by Angervall and colleagues, who reported a series of 30 patients with a myxoid soft tissue tumor affecting primarily the extremities in older patients.[103] Almost simultaneously, Weiss and Enzinger described 78 cases of a myxoid variant of "malignant fibrous histiocytoma" with similar clinicopathologic characteristics.[104] Over the next few years, several authors showed that many of the tumors classified under the "malignant fibrous histiocytoma" rubric could by reclassified into more specific categories of neoplasms with reproducible clinical and morphologic features (see Chapter 7).[105-107] Myxofibrosarcoma is currently the preferred nomenclature, because this designation better describes this fibroblastic sarcoma with variably prominent myxoid stroma (depending on the histologic grade; discussed later). High-grade myxofibrosarcoma can be difficult to distinguish from other pleomorphic sarcomas and is also discussed in Chapter 7.

Clinical Features

Myxofibrosarcoma is the most common sarcoma of the elderly, with a slight male predominance.[103,104,108-110] The majority of tumors arise in the lower limbs (especially the thigh) and limb girdles, followed by the upper extremities.[103,104,108-110] Most cases reported in the retroperitoneum and other body cavities represent dedifferentiated liposarcoma.[111-113] Myxofibrosarcoma is usually superficial, involving the subcutis and dermis, whereas deep-seated (subfascial) tumors occur in approximately one third of cases. The most common presentation is a painless mass.

Pathologic Features

Grossly, myxofibrosarcoma is usually a large multinodular mass with infiltrative margins. The cut surface is variably myxoid and firm, with gross areas of hemorrhage and necrosis. Histologically, myxofibrosarcoma is lobulated (Fig. 5.14A) and often contains alternating hypocellular myxoid areas and hypercellular areas. In low-grade tumors, there is abundant myxoid stroma, with occasional pleomorphic cells and characteristic curvilinear blood vessels (see Fig. 5.14B). The presence of these distinctive vessels is a very helpful diagnostic clue.

The tumor cells range from spindled to pleomorphic, with hyperchromatic nuclei, variably prominent nucleoli, and moderate amounts of cytoplasm (see Fig. 5.14C). Within the myxoid areas, pseudolipoblasts may be seen. These are neoplastic cells containing cytoplasmic mucin, pushing the nuclei to the periphery and creating a vacuolated, lipoblast-like appearance. Mitoses, including atypical forms, may be numerous, and necrosis and hemorrhage are often present in high-grade tumors.

Rarely, myxofibrosarcoma may contain epithelioid tumor cells and therefore mimic nonmesenchymal neoplasms (such as melanoma and carcinoma).[114] These may be focal or diffuse, but are usually admixed with areas of conventional myxofibrosarcoma.[114]

Myxofibrosarcoma is graded using a three-tier system (i.e., low, intermediate, and high grades), based predominantly on the degree of cellularity (and the presence of a nonmyxoid component). Low-grade tumors are predominantly hypocellular and myxoid, with scattered atypical cells and prominent curvilinear vessels (see Fig. 5.14B). In contrast, high-grade myxofibrosarcoma is characteristically predominantly hypercellular (see Fig. 5.14D), with a more prominent fibrous stroma and prominent nuclear atypia, and may be indistinguishable from undifferentiated pleomorphic sarcoma (see Chapter 7). In such tumors, a careful search for the myxoid areas leads to the correct diagnosis. The extent of hypercellular areas required to reach intermediate or high grade is not firmly established; however, the presence of any hypercellular (nonmyxoid) areas should probably be regarded as at least intermediate grade.

Immunohistochemistry

Immunohistochemistry plays a limited role in the diagnosis of myxofibrosarcoma, except to exclude other tumor types in the differential diagnosis. Focal reactivity for CD34 or SMA may be seen in a subset of cells, whereas these tumors are usually negative for desmin, S-100 protein, and keratins.

Molecular Genetics

Myxofibrosarcoma shows a nondistinctive complex karyotype, with numerical and structural chromosomal abnormalities.[115] Interestingly, recurrent cases often show increasingly complex karyotypic alterations.[115]

Differential Diagnosis

The differential diagnosis for myxofibrosarcoma depends on the tumor grade. Low-grade tumors should be distinguished from intramuscular/cellular myxoma, myxoid neurofibroma, low-grade malignant peripheral nerve sheath tumor (MPNST), and LGFMS, whereas high-grade tumors must be differentiated from other high-grade pleomorphic sarcomas. The differential diagnosis of pleomorphic sarcomas is discussed in Chapter 7.

Cellular myxomas are usually large intramuscular myxoid tumors that, in contrast to low-grade myxofibrosarcoma, have no nuclear pleomorphism despite being relatively hypercellular. Low-grade MPNST does not contain curvilinear blood vessels and shows less nuclear pleomorphism than would be expected for a myxofibrosarcoma with a similar degree of cellularity. Neurofibromas are consistently positive for S-100 protein, as are approximately 40% of MPNSTs; low-grade examples (particularly those arising from neurofibromas) are more often positive. LGFMS affects mainly younger patients. Similar to low-grade myxofibrosarcoma, LGFMS is characterized by alternating hypo- and hypercellular areas; however, in contrast to myxofibrosarcoma, there is no nuclear pleomorphism and the vessels form arcades in LGFMS. MUC4 is specific for LGFMS in this differential diagnosis.

Prognosis and Treatment

The prognosis depends on the histologic grade and tumor depth. Because of the characteristically infiltrative borders along connective tissue planes,

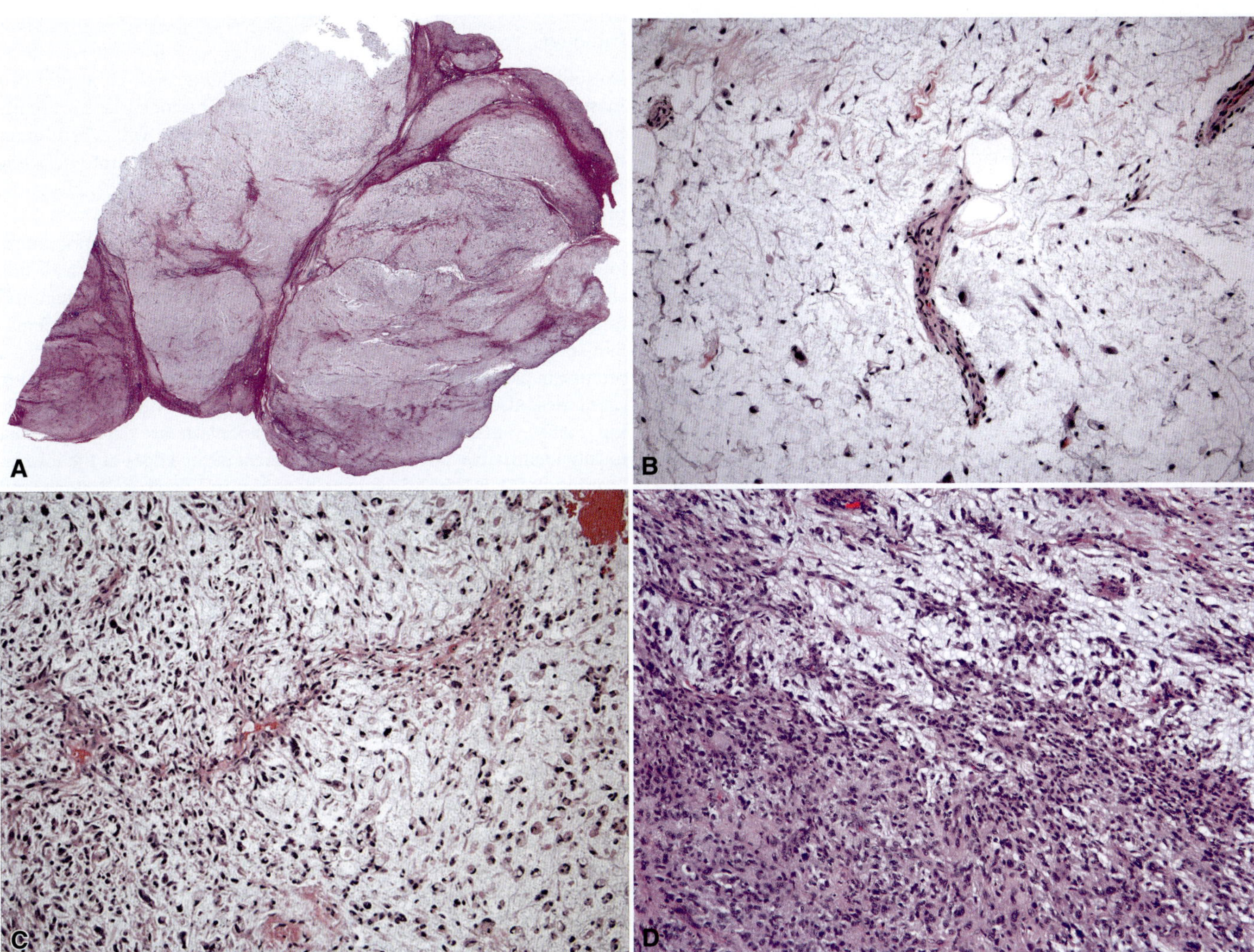

Figure 5.14 Myxofibrosarcoma. (A) Myxofibrosarcoma shows a lobulated appearance. (B) A low-grade tumor with abundant myxoid stroma containing curvilinear blood vessels and occasional pleomorphic cells. (C) An intermediate-grade tumor with increased cellularity and pleomorphism. Note the curvilinear blood vessel. (D) High-grade myxofibrosarcoma shows a transition from typical myxoid foci to solidly cellular areas with a pleomorphic appearance.

often much farther than is clinically suspected, positive margins are common, and the overall rate of local recurrence is 50% to 60%, which appears to be independent of grade.[103,104,108,109] Interestingly, tumor grade shows a tendency to increase with recurrences. The metastatic rate, on the other hand, is directly linked to grade and ranges from less than 5% for low-grade myxofibrosarcoma to approximately 35% for high-grade tumors.[103,104,108,109] The most common sites of metastasis are the lung, intraabdominal organs, and retroperitoneum.[103,104,108,109] Myxofibrosarcoma is one of the few adult spindle cell and pleomorphic sarcomas that may also metastasize to lymph nodes. The overall mortality rate is approximately 50%.

The cornerstone of treatment for myxofibrosarcoma is complete surgical excision, with negative margins, optimally with at least 2 cm of surrounding normal tissue or an intact anatomic barrier, such as a fascial plane or periosteum. As mentioned earlier, this may be difficult to achieve. Adjuvant radiation therapy may decrease the likelihood of local recurrence, in particular in cases where the margins are close or compromised. Myxofibrosarcoma is one of the few soft tissue sarcomas that still occasionally results in amputations, typically following multiple surgical resections and eventual uncontrolled local recurrences. Chemotherapy does not currently play a role in the treatment of myxofibrosarcoma.

PRACTICE POINTS: Myxofibrosarcoma

- Affects elderly patients, with a slight male predominance
- Most often occurs in the lower limbs and limb girdles, followed by the upper extremities
- Most tumors arise in subcutaneous tissue
- Characterized by alternating hypocellular, myxoid areas with hypercellular, fibrous areas; presence of curvilinear vessels and variable degree of pleomorphism
- Rarely, myxofibrosarcoma may have epithelioid morphology
- Tumor may be graded as low, intermediate, or high grade; cellularity is the most important criterion
- Local recurrence rate of 50% to 60%, independent of grade
- Metastatic rate varies from less than 5% in low-grade tumors to 35% in high-grade lesions

Myxoid Liposarcoma

Myxoid and round cell liposarcomas represent morphologic variants of the same tumor type. These entities were initially believed to be two distinct neoplasms; however, cytogenetic evidence has shown them to be identical at the molecular level. High-grade areas in myxoid liposarcoma are not exclusively round cell in appearance but may instead show spindle cell morphology. This tumor type is discussed in more detail in Chapter 12.

Clinical Features

Myxoid liposarcoma is the second most common type of liposarcoma in adults and the most common variant in children and adolescents.[7,116] Younger adults are more often affected, with a peak incidence in the fifth decade and a slight male predominance.[7,117-121] Patients usually present with a slowly growing painless mass.[7,117-121] The lower extremity, in particular the thigh, is the most commonly affected site.[7,117-121] The vast majority of lesions are subfascial, with a small minority located in subcutaneous tissue.[7,117-121] The retroperitoneum, abdomen, pelvis, and mediastinum are very rarely involved, and suspected myxoid liposarcomas at these locations likely represent either metastatic disease or other types of tumors mimicking myxoid liposarcoma (in particular well-differentiated liposarcoma; discussed later).[7,117-121]

Pathologic Features

Myxoid liposarcoma usually presents as a large, well-circumscribed mass, with a median size of 10 to 12 cm.[117-121] The cut surface is usually homogeneous and gelatinous. Tumors with tan to white firm areas usually show higher histologic grade and may demonstrate necrosis; such areas must be thoroughly sampled because the grade affects the prognosis (discussed later).

Histologically, low-grade myxoid liposarcoma is a hypocellular, lobulated lesion composed of monotonous small ovoid cells with fine chromatin, inconspicuous nucleoli, and scant cytoplasm. The background is myxoid, and areas of mucin pooling, imparting a "pulmonary edema-like" pattern, may be present (Fig. 5.15A). In addition, there is a prominent plexiform vascular pattern composed of thin-walled, branching capillaries, also known as "chicken-wire" or "crow's feet" vessels (see Fig. 5.15B). Small uni- or bivacuolated lipoblasts are usually at least focally identifiable and are most prominent at the edges of the lobules (see Fig. 5.15C). Necrosis is usually absent in low-grade lesions, and the mitotic rate is usually low (<1 mitosis per 10 high-power fields). Importantly, nuclear pleomorphism is not a feature of myxoid liposarcoma.

High-grade myxoid liposarcoma ("round cell" liposarcoma) is composed of monomorphic rounded or ovoid cells with scattered small lipoblasts and the characteristic vascular pattern. High-grade myxoid

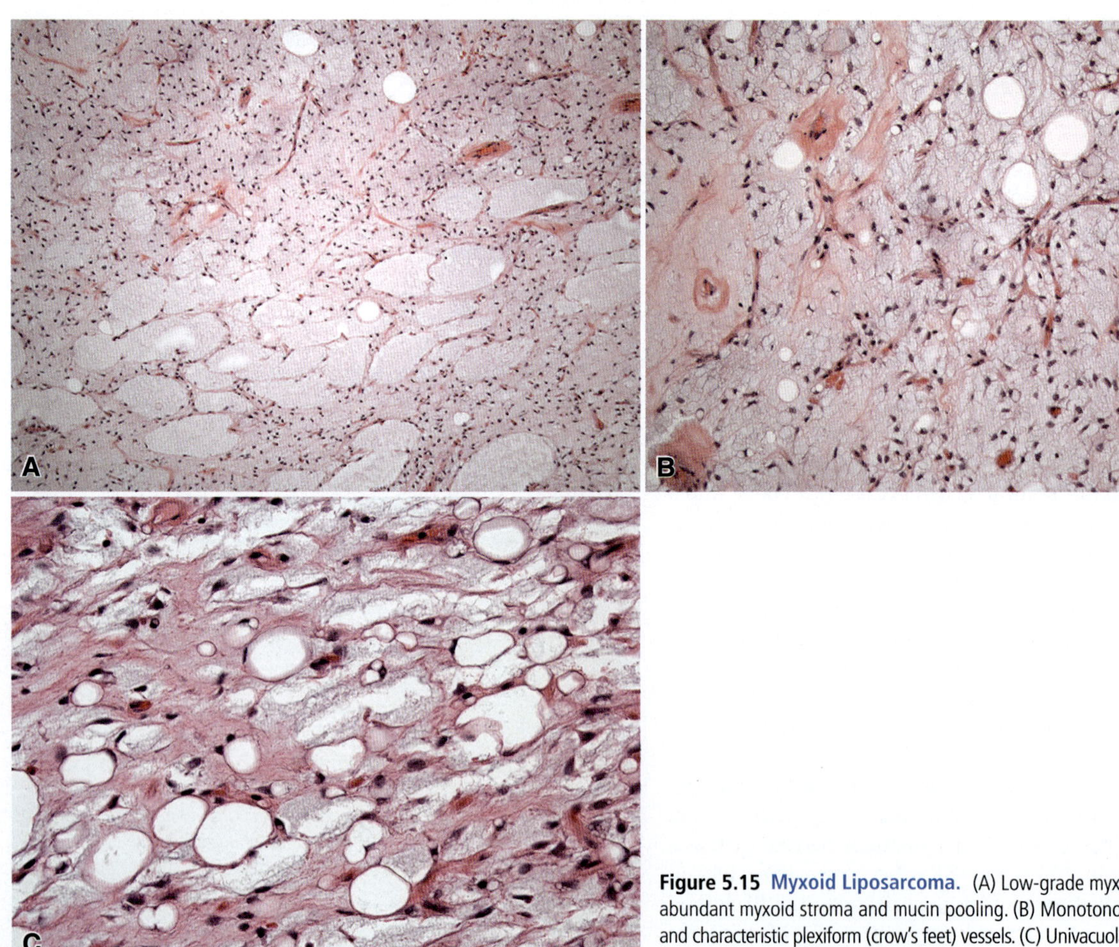

Figure 5.15 Myxoid Liposarcoma. (A) Low-grade myxoid liposarcoma with abundant myxoid stroma and mucin pooling. (B) Monotonous short spindle cells and characteristic plexiform (crow's feet) vessels. (C) Univacuolated and bivacuolated lipoblasts are often focally present.

liposarcoma is discussed in more detail in Chapter 12 and mentioned briefly in the context of round cell sarcomas in Chapter 8.

Immunohistochemistry

Immunohistochemistry does not play a role in the diagnosis of myxoid liposarcoma, although these tumors are often positive for S-100 protein.[7,122] Myxoid liposarcoma is rarely positive (<5%) for MDM2 and CDK4, which are nearly always overexpressed in well-differentiated and dedifferentiated liposarcomas.[123]

Molecular Genetics

Myxoid liposarcoma most often harbors the balanced translocation t(12;16)(q13;p11),[124-128] which juxtaposes the *DDIT3* gene on chromosome 12 and *FUS* on chromosome 16.[129,130] In addition, a variant translocation t(12;22)(q13;q12) is present in approximately 10% of cases.[131] In this translocation, *DDIT3* is fused with *EWSR1* on chromosome 22.[132]

Differential Diagnosis

The differential diagnosis for myxoid liposarcoma includes cellular myxoma, well-differentiated liposarcoma with myxoid change, EMC, and low-grade myxofibrosarcoma. Most cases of myxoid liposarcoma can be diagnosed based on careful attention to histologic features; however, in difficult cases, conventional cytogenetics or FISH for the detection of *FUS* or *DDIT3* gene rearrangement can be used to confirm the diagnosis.

Cellular myxoma shows bland cytomorphologic features with small spindled cells embedded in a myxoid background. Lobular architecture, lipoblasts, and "crow's feet" vessels are not features of cellular myxoma.

Well-differentiated liposarcoma may occasionally show focal or extensive areas of myxoid change that may mimic myxoid liposarcoma.[113] The presence of scattered hyperchromatic atypical cells distinguishes well-differentiated liposarcoma from myxoid liposarcoma. Immunohistochemical stains for MDM2 and CDK4, which are positive in more than 95% of well-differentiated liposarcomas, are rarely positive in myxoid liposarcoma.[123]

EMC has a prominent myxoid matrix, with neoplastic cells arranged in cords with no lipoblasts and inconspicuous vascularity. In low-grade myxofibrosarcoma, the vessels are prominent and curvilinear, and there are no true lipoblasts. Furthermore, even low-grade myxofibrosarcoma contains scattered pleomorphic cells, which are not seen in myxoid liposarcoma.

Prognosis and Treatment

Myxoid liposarcoma has overall rates of local recurrence and distant metastasis of 30% and 40%, respectively, and the latter is directly related to histologic grade.[118] Neoplasms showing more than 5% round cell morphology have significantly worse outcome compared with low-grade myxoid liposarcoma.[118] The overall mortality rate is approximately 25% to 40%.[98] The most common sites for metastasis include soft tissues (such as the contralateral extremity and retroperitoneum), bone, and lungs; metastatic myxoid liposarcoma has an unusual predilection for the spine.[118,133]

The treatment of choice for myxoid liposarcoma is surgery. Radiation therapy can be used to decrease the risk of local recurrence in cases with close or positive surgical margins; however, the role of chemotherapy remains unclear.[134] Trabectedin (ecteinascidin-743) is effective systemic therapy for this tumor type, with 3- and 6-month progression-free survival rates of 56% and 36%, respectively.[135-137] Tumors that undergo radiation therapy may show cytodifferentiation, appearing hypocellular with prominent stromal hyalinization and extensive adipocytic differentiation.[138]

Predictors of poor outcome in localized myxoid liposarcoma include age older than 45 years, a round cell component (variably defined as >5% or >25% of tumor volume), and necrosis.[117,118]

PRACTICE POINTS: Myxoid Liposarcoma

- Affects predominantly younger patients (<40 years); most common type of liposarcoma in children and adolescents
- Presents as a slow-growing, deep-seated mass with a predilection for the lower extremities
- Characterized by a uniform myxoid background, with monotonous cells and thin-walled, branching capillaries and small uni- and bivacuolated lipoblasts
- High-grade myxoid (or "round cell") liposarcoma is characterized by high cellularity and often contains sheets of round cells
- Harbors t(12;16)(q13;p11) or t(12;22)(q13;q12)
- Recurrence rate of 30%, overall metastatic rate of 40%, and mortality rate of 25% to 40%
- Sites of metastasis include soft tissues, spine, bone, and lungs
- Poor prognostic features include patient age older than 45 years, grade (presence of round cell component), and necrosis

Extraskeletal Myxoid Chondrosarcoma

EMC was first described by Stout and Verner in 1953 under the name *chondrosarcoma of the extraskeletal soft tissues.*[139] The term *extraskeletal myxoid chondrosarcoma* was subsequently coined in 1972 by Enzinger and Shiraki.[140] Despite its name, there is no convincing evidence of cartilaginous differentiation in this tumor type.

Clinical Features

A rare tumor, EMC represents approximately 3% of all soft tissue sarcomas.[141] Most patients affected are adults, with a peak in the sixth decade.[7,140-146] EMC occurs more often in males (male-to-female ratio, 1.5 to 2 : 1).[7,140-146] Limbs and limb girdles are the most commonly affected sites, in particular the thigh and buttocks, followed by the upper extremities and head and neck.[7,140-146] In fewer than 10% of cases, the retroperitoneum, abdominal cavity, or pelvis is affected.[146]

The majority of patients present with a slowly growing painless mass.[7,140-146] Tumors are most often located in subfascial locations, frequently associated with fascia or tendons.[7,140-146]

Pathologic Features

Grossly, EMC is a multinodular, well-circumscribed mass, with a thin pseudocapsule and a myxoid, soft cut surface. Most tumors are large, with an average size of 7 cm. Areas of cystic degeneration and hemorrhage are common.

Histologically, EMC is lobulated, with the tumor lobules separated by fibrous septa (Fig. 5.16A). Tumor cells are epithelioid to spindled; usually arranged in cords, strands, or clusters (see Fig. 5.16B); and tend to accumulate at the periphery of individual lobules. Neoplastic cells are embedded in abundant myxoid stroma and have round or elongated nuclei, fine chromatin, small nucleoli, and moderate amounts of eosinophilic cytoplasm (see Fig. 5.16C). Mitoses are infrequent and necrosis is uncommon. Cartilaginous differentiation is absent.

Occasionally, EMC may show areas with increased cellularity and even solid areas (high-grade EMC). Hypercellularity is often associated with a high mitotic rate and necrosis. In addition, high-grade tumor cells are often large and epithelioid, with prominent nucleoli (see Fig. 5.16D). Some tumors show rhabdoid features with prominent eosinophilic cytoplasmic inclusions (Fig. 5.17).

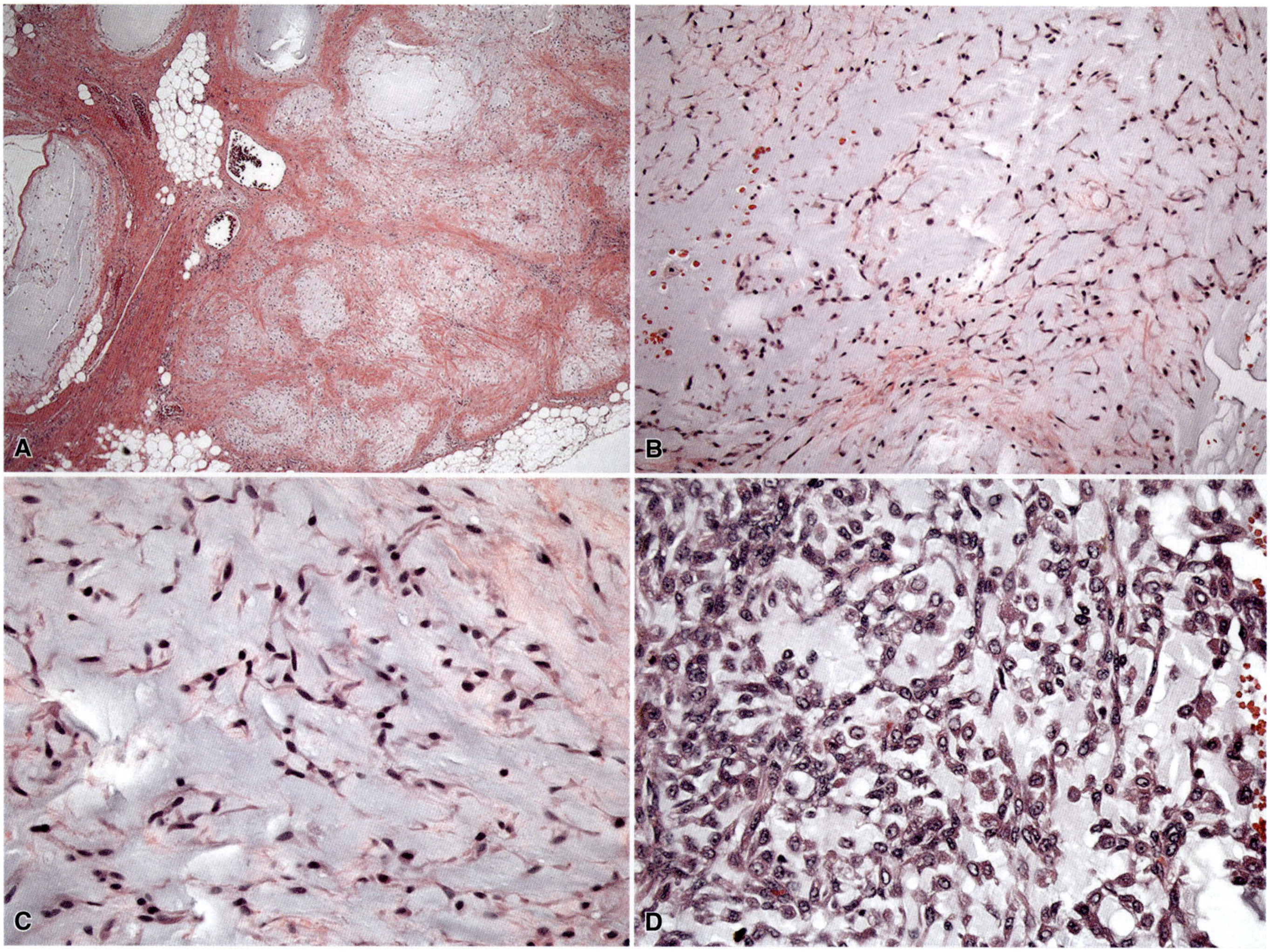

Figure 5.16 Extraskeletal Myxoid Chondrosarcoma. (A) Extraskeletal myxoid chondrosarcoma shows a lobulated growth pattern. (B) Tumor cells are arranged in a reticular architecture in a prominent myxoid stroma. (C) Bland, uniform spindle cells with eosinophilic cytoplasm. (D) High-grade extraskeletal myxoid chondrosarcoma composed of large atypical epithelioid to spindled cells with coarse chromatin and visible nucleoli.

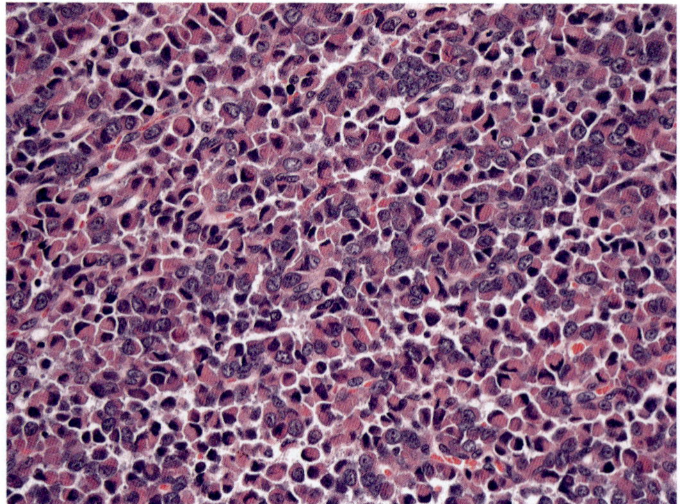

Figure 5.17 Extraskeletal Myxoid Chondrosarcoma. Some high-grade examples show rhabdoid morphology.

Immunohistochemistry

In 15% to 20% of cases, EMC is positive for S-100 protein.[143,144,147-149] It is rarely positive for EMA and keratins. Although some studies have reported that synaptophysin and neuron-specific enolase are positive in some cases,[80,143,144,149] this has not been our experience. Loss of SMARCB1 (INI1) expression is seen in a small subset of tumors, which tend to show rhabdoid features.[150]

Molecular Genetics

Four balanced chromosomal translocations have been reported in EMC, namely t(9;22)(q22;q12), t(9;17)(q22;q11), t(9;15)(q22;q21), and t(3;9)(q11-q12;q22).[144,147,151-155] The first translocation is the most common, found in 50% to 70% of cases, which juxtaposes the *EWSR1* gene on chromosome 22 and the *NR4A3* gene located at 9q22.[151,152] In the t(9;17) translocation, the *NR4A3* gene is fused with the *TAF15* gene, located at 17q11.[152-154] The other translocations are rare and result in the fusion of the *TCF12* or *TFG* and *NR4A3* genes.[155] FISH for *EWSR1* is often used to confirm the diagnosis, although probes directed against *NR4A3* are more sensitive and specific for EMC and may also be used.[156] Variant *FUS-NR4A3* fusion resulting from t(9;16)(q22;p11.2) has also been identified in EMC.[157] Most recently, a *HSPA8-NR4A3* fusion has been reported.[158] Deletions or mutations involving the *SMARCB1* gene have been identified in a small subset of EMC cases, particularly with rhabdoid morphology.[150]

Differential Diagnosis

Conventional EMC should be differentiated from myoepithelial neoplasms, OFMT, myxoid liposarcoma, and low-grade myxofibrosarcoma (see Table 5.1). The differential diagnosis for high-grade (hypercellular) EMC includes myoepithelial carcinoma, malignant melanoma, metastatic carcinoma, and proximal-type epithelioid sarcoma. Ancillary studies, especially immunohistochemistry and cytogenetics or FISH, are helpful in the differential diagnosis.

Similar to EMC, soft tissue myoepithelioma frequently shows a lobulated architecture, with cords of epithelioid or spindled cells embedded in a myxoid stroma. However, myoepithelial tumors often show intratumoral architectural and cytologic heterogeneity, whereas EMC is usually very uniform. By immunohistochemistry, myoepitheliomas are nearly always positive for keratins, EMA, and S-100 protein, and 50% are positive for GFAP.[78,81] EMC is less often positive for S-100 protein and is usually negative for the other markers. Because *EWSR1* gene rearrangements are detected in both EMC and myoepithelial tumors of soft tissue,[79] FISH for *EWSR1* cannot be used to distinguish between these tumor types. However, FISH for *NR4A3* is specific for EMC in this differential diagnosis.[159]

Similarly, OFMT is lobulated and is composed of cords of uniform small ovoid cells in a variably fibromyxoid stroma. However, OFMT generally lacks the abundant myxoid matrix of EMC. The shell of lamellar bone that is seen in the majority of cases of OFMT is not a feature of EMC.[63-65] In contrast to EMC, OFMT is usually positive for S-100 protein, and up to 50% of tumors are positive for desmin.[63-65] Identification of *PHF1* gene rearrangement can also confirm the diagnosis of OFMT.

Myxoid liposarcoma is composed of monomorphic small spindled cells, also embedded in a prominent myxoid stroma. Distinctive features include thin-walled branching ("crow's feet") capillaries, uni- or bivacuolated lipoblasts, and mucin pooling, which are not seen in EMC. Although immunohistochemistry is not helpful, cytogenetics or molecular studies can usually distinguish between these tumor types, because myxoid liposarcoma is characterized by t(12;16) involving the *FUS* and *DDIT3* genes in most cases.

Myxofibrosarcoma most often arises in subcutaneous tissue, in contrast to the subfascial location of EMC. Similar to EMC, low-grade myxofibrosarcoma is lobulated, with abundant myxoid stroma. In contrast to EMC, however, myxofibrosarcoma contains characteristic curvilinear blood vessels and scattered pleomorphic cells.

Distinction between high-grade EMC and other epithelioid malignant neoplasms, namely metastatic melanoma, metastatic carcinoma, and proximal-type epithelioid sarcoma, relies heavily on immunohistochemistry because EMC is usually negative for all lineage markers. Melanoma is positive for S-100 protein and SOX10 in the vast majority of cases and also often expresses melanocytic markers, such as melan A and HMB-45. EMC is negative for melanocytic markers. Metastatic carcinoma is positive for keratins. Proximal-type epithelioid sarcoma consistently expresses keratins and EMA and is positive for CD34 in 50% of cases.[160]

Prognosis and Treatment

Wide surgical excision with negative margins is the cornerstone of treatment for EMC. Radiation therapy may help prevent local recurrence.

The rate of both local recurrence (35% to 50%) and distant metastasis (25% to 50%) is high in EMC, although metastases often occur late.[7,140,142-147] The most common sites of metastasis are the lung, lymph nodes, bone, and other soft tissue sites.[7,140,142-147] The 5- and 10-year overall survival rates are approximately 90% and 70%, respectively.[7,140,142-147]

Older age, proximal extremity location, and large tumor size (>10 cm) confer a worse prognosis.[80,143] High-grade EMC pursues a more aggressive clinical course than conventional EMC, with a higher metastatic rate.[148]

PRACTICE POINTS: Extraskeletal Myxoid Chondrosarcoma

- Affects mostly adults, with a slight male predominance
- Limbs and limb girdles are the most common sites, followed by head and neck
- Most common in subfascial location; multinodular, well-circumscribed mass
- Characterized by uniform epithelioid or spindled cells arranged in cords or strands, embedded in an abundant myxoid background
- Areas of increased cellularity, solid growth pattern, and larger cell size characterize high-grade extraskeletal myxoid chondrosarcomas
- Consistent rearrangements of *NR4A3* (*EWSR1-NR4A3* fusion most common)
- FISH for *NR4A3* can confirm diagnosis
- High rates of local recurrence (35% to 50%) and metastasis (25% to 50%), with metastases often occurring late
- Poor prognostic factors include older age, proximal location, large tumor size, and high-grade features

Low-Grade Fibromyxoid Sarcoma

LGFMS was first described by Evans in 1987 and further characterized in a larger series in 1993 as a deceptively bland-appearing neoplasm with a significant potential for local recurrence and metastasis.[161,162] A decade later, Lane and colleagues described a series of tumors as "hyalinizing spindle cell tumor with giant rosettes," which shared many histologic features with LGFMS in addition to distinctive rosette-like structures.[163] Subsequent studies showed that these two entities harbor the same distinctive chromosomal translocations and lie along a morphologic spectrum.[164,165] LGFMS is also discussed in Chapter 3.

Clinical Features

A tumor of young to middle-aged adults, LGFMS has an equal gender distribution. Most patients are between the third and fifth decades; a subset of tumors occurs in children (see Chapter 4).[161-167] Most patients present with a long-standing painless, large, deep-seated (subfascial) mass, although some cases arise in the subcutis and may extend into the dermis. The tumor affects predominantly the extremities, with the thigh the most common site.[161-168] Other sites include the trunk, head and neck, and retroperitoneum.

Pathologic Features

Although LGFMS is usually grossly well circumscribed, occasional tumors may show infiltration of adjacent tissues. The cut surface is tan, firm, and homogeneous, usually without necrosis or hemorrhage.

Histologically, LGFMS is characterized by alternating fibrous and myxoid areas, with a whorled growth pattern (Fig. 5.18A). Arcades of thin-walled blood vessels, occasionally with perivascular hyalinization, are a typical feature in the myxoid areas (see Fig. 5.18B). The tumors are composed of bland, short spindle cells with ovoid nuclei, fine chromatin, inconspicuous nucleoli, and scant cytoplasm (see Fig. 5.18C). Nuclear atypia is rarely observed. Mitoses are usually scarce, and necrosis is rare.

In approximately one third of cases, "giant rosettes" are present (see Fig. 5.18D).[164] These structures are characterized by dense, hyalinized collagen surrounded by palisaded epithelioid tumor cells.

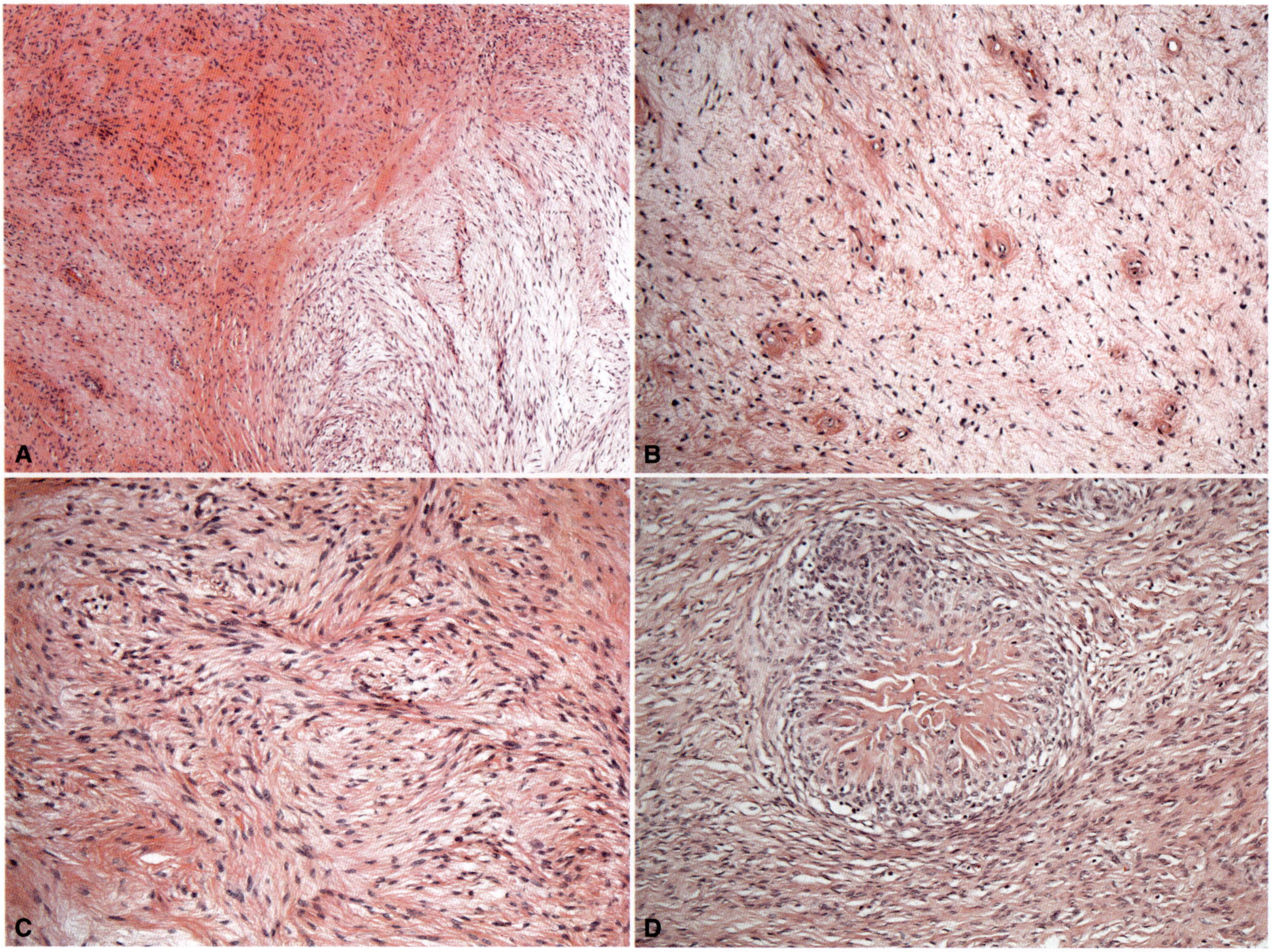

Figure 5.18 Low-grade Fibromyxoid Sarcoma. (A) Low-grade fibromyxoid sarcoma is characterized by alternating fibrous and myxoid areas and shows a whorled growth pattern. (B) Arcades of small vessels are often observed in the myxoid areas. (C) The tumor is composed of uniform small bland spindle cells arranged in whorls. (D) A subset of tumors contains giant collagen pseudorosettes.

Although LGFMS is usually uniform, the morphologic spectrum also includes lesions with higher cellularity and more nuclear atypia than is seen in the classic examples.[169] Rarely, recurrent LGFMS may show histologic "dedifferentiation" to a high-grade round cell sarcoma.[170] Occasional cases show hybrid features of LGFMS and sclerosing epithelioid fibrosarcoma (see Chapter 6).[169,171]

Immunohistochemistry

By immunohistochemistry, LGFMS is occasionally positive for CD34, SMA, or desmin. More than 60% of tumors show reactivity for EMA. Tumor cells are negative for keratins and S-100 protein. MUC4 is a highly sensitive and specific marker for LGFMS (Fig. 5.19).[171]

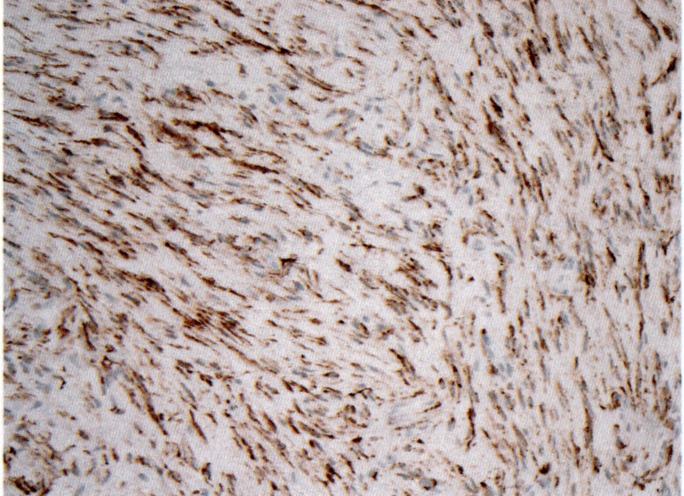

Figure 5.19 Low-Grade Fibromyxoid Sarcoma. MUC4 is a useful diagnostic marker for this tumor type.

Molecular Genetics

Distinctive chromosomal translocations associated with LGFMS include t(7;16)(q34;p11) and t(11;16)(p11;p11), which juxtapose the *FUS* gene located at 16p11 with either the *CREB3L2* or (more rarely) *CREB3L1* gene on 7q34 or 11p11, respectively.[172] The former translocation is identified in up to 95% of cases, including tumors with hybrid features of both LGFMS and sclerosing epithelioid fibrosarcoma.[172] Rare examples may harbor alternate fusions with *EWSR1* instead of *FUS*; in such instances *CREB3L1* is usually the fusion partner.[169,173-175]

Differential Diagnosis

With the high specificity of MUC4 and the t(7;16) translocation, the diagnosis of LGFMS can be confirmed quite easily with the use of immunohistochemistry or FISH.[176] The differential diagnosis for LGFMS includes solitary fibrous tumor (SFT), soft tissue perineurioma, desmoid fibromatosis, low-grade MPNST, and low-grade myxofibrosarcoma.

Characteristic features of SFT include alternating hypocellular and hypercellular areas containing small, nondescript spindle cells arranged in a "patternless" architecture, with a distinctive "hemangiopericytoma"-like branching vascular pattern. SFT rarely shows myxoid stroma and lacks the whorled architecture of LGFMS. SFT may also show reactivity for EMA in approximately 20% of cases. In contrast to LGFMS, SFT is usually diffusely positive for CD34 and STAT6 and is negative for MUC4.[177-179]

Soft tissue perineurioma shows significant histologic overlap with LGFMS, including a storiform to whorled growth pattern and collagenous stroma, and a subset of tumors contain myxoid stroma. However, soft tissue perineurioma lacks the sharply demarcated fibrous and myxoid areas and arcades of blood vessels characteristic of LGFMS.[39] Both tumor types are often positive for EMA, but MUC4 is specific for LGFMS in this differential diagnosis.

Desmoid fibromatosis contains bland spindle cells similar to those seen in LGFMS. However, desmoid tumors are composed of long fascicles with more plump, elongated spindle cells and show more infiltrative margins than are generally seen in LGFMS. In contrast to LGFMS, desmoid tumors are negative for MUC4 and EMA. In addition, a large proportion (~70%) of desmoid tumors show aberrant nuclear immunopositivity for β-catenin, whereas this staining pattern is uncommon in LGFMS.[180]

Low-grade MPNST is usually more infiltrative and often shows alternating hypocellular and hypercellular areas, and condensation of neoplastic cells around blood vessels. The tumor cells are generally longer spindled cells with tapering nuclei, and scattered atypia and mitotic figures are usually present. Unlike LGFMS, MPNST is at least focally positive for S-100 protein, GFAP, or SOX10 in 40% to 50% of cases.[86] Although myxofibrosarcoma has a similar name as LGFMS (which may lead to diagnostic confusion), these tumor types differ significantly. Myxofibrosarcoma is a disease of older adults that most often arises in superficial soft tissues. Low-grade myxofibrosarcoma is more hypocellular, with more uniformly myxoid stroma, and it contains characteristic curvilinear blood vessels. Unlike LGFMS, which is uniformly bland, myxofibrosarcoma contains scattered atypical pleomorphic cells. When myxofibrosarcoma is as cellular as LGFMS, it shows more notable nuclear atypia, with the appearance of a high-grade spindle cell or pleomorphic sarcoma. Myxofibrosarcoma is negative for MUC4 and is characterized by a nondistinctive complex karyotype, in contrast to the simple karyotype of LGFMS with t(7;16).

Prognosis and Treatment

LGFMS is associated with significant potential for local recurrence and distant metastasis, the latter often after a long tumor-free interval (even decades).[170] Although the 5-year metastatic rate is less than 10%, the long-term risk is 30% to 40% after 10 to 20 years.[170] Superficial tumors may have a more favorable prognosis.[167] The preferential sites of metastasis are the lungs and pleura. Patients should be treated by wide local excision, and long-term follow-up is required.

PRACTICE POINTS: Low-Grade Fibromyxoid Sarcoma

- Predilection for young adults, with equal gender distribution
- Tumor arises mainly in deep location and is usually well circumscribed
- Shows alternating fibrous and myxoid areas, with bland cytology and arcades of small blood vessels
- Occasionally "giant rosette" structures may be present
- Nuclear pleomorphism is not a feature
- MUC4 is a sensitive and specific marker
- Characterized by t(7;16)(q34;p11) with *FUS* rearrangement in more than 95% of cases
- Significant potential for local recurrence and metastasis (especially to lung), particularly late (10 to 20 years); long-term follow-up is required.

Myxoinflammatory Fibroblastic Sarcoma

Myxoinflammatory fibroblastic sarcoma was first described in 1998 almost simultaneously by two groups under the names "inflammatory myxohyaline tumor of distal extremities with virocyte or Reed-Sternberg–like cells" and "acral myxoinflammatory fibroblastic sarcoma."[181,182] Currently, the term "acral" is no longer used because this neoplasm may occasionally arise at anatomic locations other than the distal extremities.[183] Myxoinflammatory fibroblastic sarcoma is also discussed in Chapter 7 in the context of pleomorphic tumors.

Clinical Features

Myxoinflammatory fibroblastic sarcoma affects mainly adults, with an equal gender distribution and a median age in the fifth to sixth decades.[181,182] The vast majority of lesions arise in the subcutaneous tissue of the fingers, hands, ankles, and feet (upper limb more often than lower limb).[181,182] Less commonly, proximal extremities, including the upper arm and thigh, are affected.[183]

Pathologic Features

Tumors are infiltrative, with ill-defined margins, and contain variably myxoid and fibrous (or inflammatory) stroma (Fig. 5.20A and B). In the myxoid areas, pseudolipoblasts may be numerous (see Fig. 5.20C), similar to myxofibrosarcoma. Occasional distinctive large pleomorphic cells with vesicular nuclei, prominent inclusion-like nucleoli, and moderate amounts of palely eosinophilic cytoplasm are present (see Fig. 5.20D). These cells often resemble virally infected cells or Reed-Sternberg cells of Hodgkin lymphoma. A blander spindle cell component is also often present (see Fig. 5.20B).

In addition, the neoplastic cells are usually accompanied and obscured by a variably prominent mixed inflammatory infiltrate composed of small lymphocytes, plasma cells, and eosinophils. Some examples may show atypical features, including hypercellular foci, increased mitotic activity or atypical mitotic figures, and a vascular pattern mimicking the curvilinear vessels of myxofibrosarcoma; however, the presence of these features alone is not predictive of overall outcome (although some correlation between atypical features and increased recurrence has been suggested).[184]

Immunohistochemistry

Immunohistochemistry does not help with the diagnosis of myxoinflammatory fibroblastic sarcoma. The large neoplastic cells may be positive for such nonspecific markers as vimentin, CD68, and CD34, but are negative for keratins, S-100 protein, and the Hodgkin lymphoma–associated markers CD30, PAX5, and CD15.

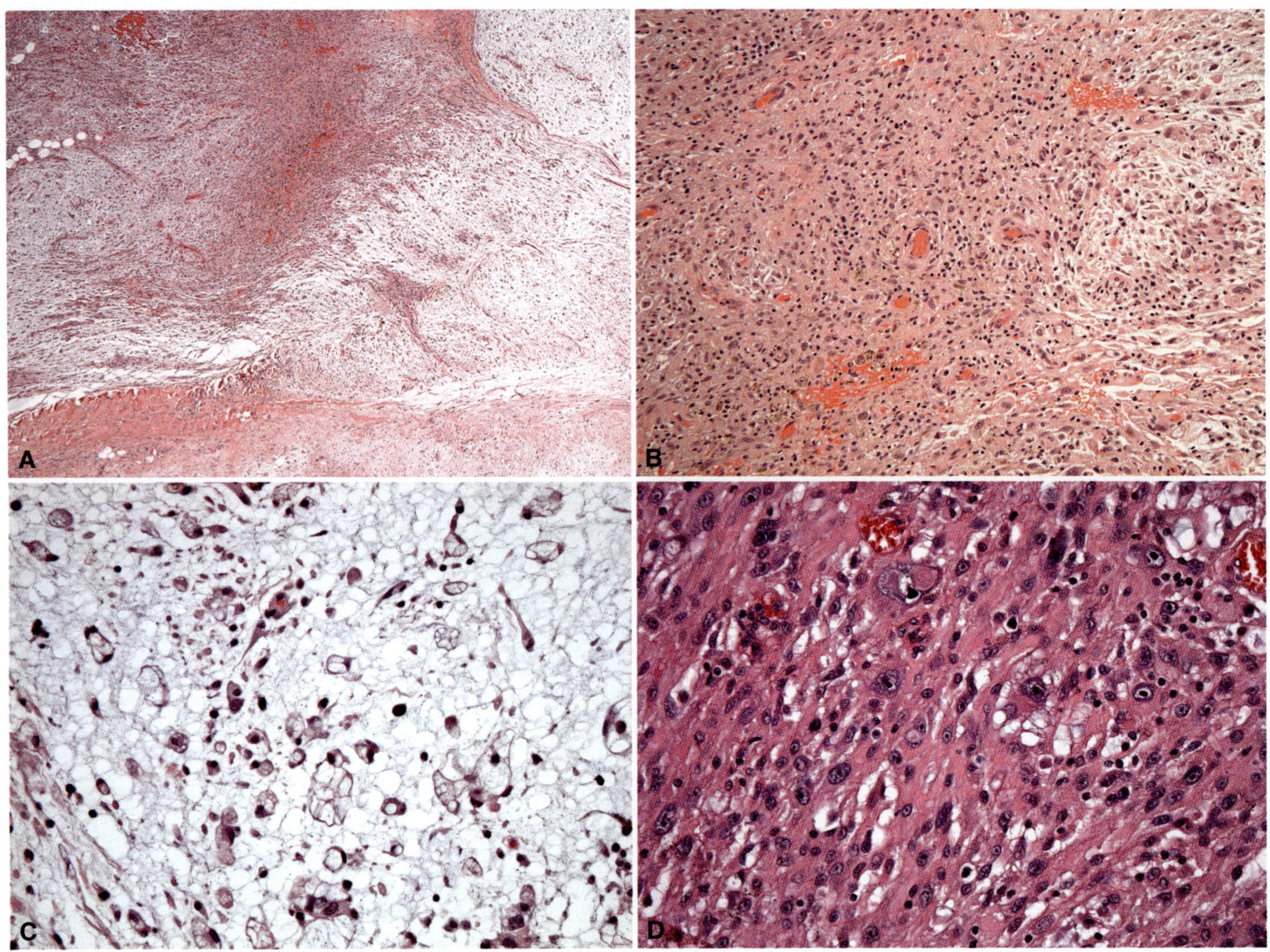

Figure 5.20 Myxoinflammatory Fibroblastic Sarcoma. (A) Myxoinflammatory fibroblastic sarcoma shows variably myxoid and cellular fibroinflammatory areas. (B) The cellular areas contain bland spindle cells and prominent chronic inflammation. (C) In the myxoid areas, pseudolipoblasts may be numerous. (D) Occasional pleomorphic (Reed-Sternberg–like) cells with large nucleoli are usually present.

Molecular Genetics

Myxoinflammatory fibroblastic sarcoma harbors the translocation t(1;10)(p22;q24), involving *TGFBR3* and *MGEA5*, in the majority of cases, often along with amplification of chromosome 3p11-12, sometimes in the form of ring chromosomes.[185-189] Interestingly, recent studies have reported the presence of t(1;10) in hemosiderotic fibrolipomatous tumor as well.[188-190] This finding, as well as the existence of tumors showing hybrid features of myxoinflammatory fibroblastic sarcoma and hemosiderotic fibrolipomatous tumor, suggests that these tumor types may be morphologic variants of the same entity (see Chapter 12).[188,189]

Differential Diagnosis

Because of prominent inflammation, a bland spindle cell component, and ill-defined margins, myxoinflammatory fibroblastic sarcoma is often mistaken for an inflammatory or reactive lesion, until the pleomorphic cells and myxoid component are identified. Myxoinflammatory fibroblastic sarcoma should be distinguished from myxofibrosarcoma and Hodgkin lymphoma, although the latter is not a realistic diagnostic option in superficial soft tissues of the extremities.

Myxofibrosarcoma also typically involves superficial soft tissues of the extremities of older adults, but more commonly arises in proximal locations. Myxofibrosarcoma also shows similar scattered pleomorphic cells. However, myxofibrosarcoma contains characteristic prominent curvilinear blood vessels, has more extensive myxoid stroma, and generally lacks inflammation.

Hodgkin lymphoma is positive for CD30, CD15, and PAX5, whereas myxoinflammatory fibroblastic sarcoma is negative for these markers. Hodgkin lymphoma does not arise on the extremities.

Prognosis and Treatment

Myxoinflammatory fibroblastic sarcoma recurs frequently, with reported rates ranging from 20% to 70%; however, only very rarely has metastatic disease been reported, mainly to lymph nodes and lung.[181,182,184,191] Wide local excision with negative margins should be attempted whenever possible.

PRACTICE POINTS: Myxoinflammatory Fibroblastic Sarcoma

- Occurs mainly in adults in the fifth and sixth decades, with equal gender distribution
- Affects mainly the subcutaneous tissues of hands and feet
- Characterized by variably myxoid and fibrous stroma, with scattered Reed-Sternberg–like cells and prominent inflammatory infiltrate
- Consistent t(1;10) translocation
- Recurs frequently, but rarely metastasizes

Myxoid Nerve Sheath Tumors

Although most nerve sheath neoplasms do not characteristically show a myxoid stroma, in approximately 10% of cases, benign and malignant nerve sheath neoplasms may show focal or extensive myxoid stromal change. The myxoid matrix may make recognition of these neoplasms difficult without appropriate immunohistochemical studies. Conventional examples of these tumors are discussed in more detail in Chapter 3.

Myxoid Neurofibroma

Neurofibroma with myxoid stroma is an uncommon histologic variant (approximately 10% of cases). Myxoid neurofibroma shows no increased association with type 1 neurofibromatosis. Histologically, like conventional neurofibromas, these tumors are composed of small spindle cells with variably tapering nuclei, condensed chromatin, inconspicuous nucleoli, and scant cytoplasm. However, instead of collagenous stroma, they are embedded in abundant myxoid matrix (Fig. 5.21A).[192] Confirmation of the diagnosis is straightforward with immunohistochemical studies. The majority of tumor cells are positive for S-100 protein; a subset may be positive for EMA. Scattered neurofilament protein–positive axons are usually identified. Simple excision is curative.

Reticular and Myxoid Soft Tissue Perineurioma

Soft tissue perineurioma is an uncommon benign lesion with an equal gender predilection. Soft tissue perineurioma may arise in the subcutis or deep soft tissues in a wide anatomic distribution, whereas reticular perineurioma most commonly arises in the subcutaneous tissue of the

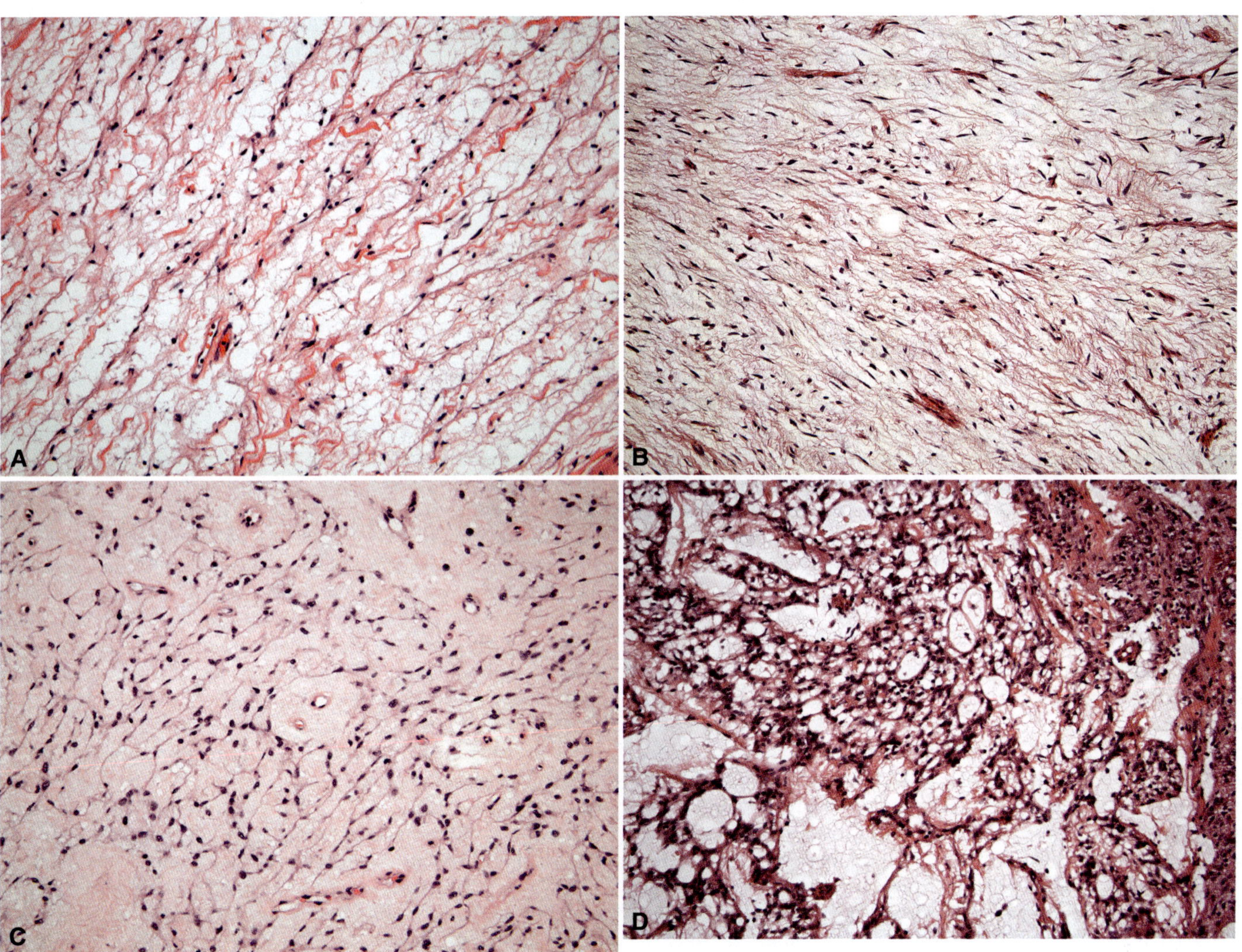

Figure 5.21 Myxoid Nerve Sheath Tumors. (A) Myxoid neurofibroma is characterized by small spindle cells with tapering nuclei and scant pale cytoplasm, embedded in a myxoid stroma. (B) A subset of soft tissue perineuriomas contains prominent myxoid stroma. Note the slender spindle cells with elongated cytoplasmic processes. (C) Reticular perineurioma shows a net-like architecture. The tumor cells are connected by bipolar cytoplasmic processes. (D) A microcystic schwannoma contains spindle cells arranged in a reticular and microcystic growth pattern.

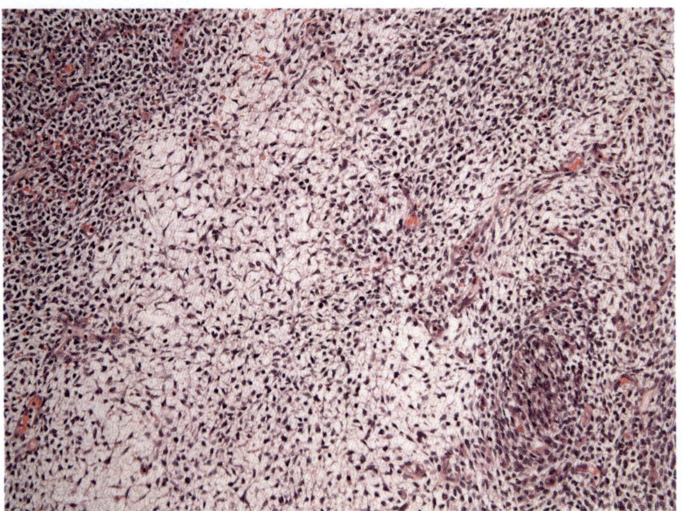

Figure 5.22 Myxoid Malignant Peripheral Nerve Sheath Tumor. Malignant peripheral nerve sheath tumors may show areas with prominent myxoid stroma. Note the varying cellularity and hyperchromatic, tapering nuclei.

distal extremities.[39,193] Soft tissue perineurioma shows a storiform, whorled, or lamellar architecture and is composed of bland ovoid to spindle cells with slender nuclei. In approximately one third of soft tissue perineuriomas, the matrix is partially or predominantly myxoid (see Fig. 5.21B). Reticular perineurioma is a distinctive variant characterized by a net-like proliferation of elongated spindle cells with bipolar cytoplasmic processes embedded in a variably myxoid stroma (see Fig. 5.21C). Both reticular and myxoid soft tissue perineuriomas are positive for EMA (often highlighting the delicate cytoplasmic processes), although staining may be focal or weak. Perineuriomas rarely recur.[39,193]

Microcystic/Reticular (Myxoid) Schwannoma

Microcystic schwannoma is an unusual variant that occurs preferentially in visceral locations (especially the gastrointestinal tract; see Chapter 16) of older adults.[194] The tumor is composed of spindle cells with elongated, tapering nuclei and a small amount of eosinophilic cytoplasm, arranged in a reticular growth pattern and often forming small cystic spaces (see Fig. 5.21D). As with conventional schwannomas, microcystic schwannoma is diffusely and strongly positive for S-100 protein. Although focal infiltration of surrounding tissues may be identified, excision is curative and recurrences have not been reported.[194]

Myxoid Malignant Peripheral Nerve Sheath Tumor

MPNST may arise sporadically, in the setting of type 1 neurofibromatosis, or after radiation therapy, most often in the deep soft tissues of adults. In approximately 10% of cases, tumors may show focal or extensive myxoid stromal change (Fig. 5.22).[192] Characteristic features include a fascicular growth pattern, varying cellularity, tapering nuclei, and perivascular increased cellularity. These tumors are positive for S-100 protein, GFAP, or SOX10 in 40% to 50% of cases; staining is often focal.[86] Up to half of MPNSTs overall (over 90% of high grade tumors) show loss of nuclear staining for H3K27me3 (histone H3 with lysine 27 trimethylation), a surrogate marker for polycomb repressive complex 2 (PRC2) dysfunction, secondary to loss-of-function mutations in *EED* or *SUZ12*.[195-197]

Other Tumors With Myxoid Stroma

Other soft tissue tumors may also occasionally show prominent myxoid stroma. In myxoid areas, histologic overlap among these diverse tumor types can be considerable. Proper diagnosis of such tumors may be very difficult without identification of areas with conventional histology. The most common examples are discussed briefly.

Myxoid Nodular Fasciitis

Nodular fasciitis is a benign fibroblastic/myofibroblastic neoplasm that usually arises in subcutaneous tissue and follows a self-limited course (see Chapters 3 and 4 for detailed discussion). Occasional examples contain abundant myxoid stroma and may therefore be mistaken for other myxoid soft tissue tumors. The discussion here is limited to this subset.

Nodular fasciitis affects males and females equally. Most patients are young to middle-aged adults. Myxoid examples of nodular fasciitis constitute approximately 5% of cases. This subset is more common in children and often occurs in the head and neck area (see Chapter 4).[192,198]

Histologically, myxoid nodular fasciitis contains bland-appearing fibroblasts and myofibroblasts that form short fascicles and are embedded in an abundant myxoid matrix, with extravasated red blood cells (Fig. 5.23A).

Although previously considered a reactive or non-neoplastic process, nodular fasciitis is now known to be characterized by a recurrent *MYH9-USP6* gene fusion resulting from translocation t(17;22)(p13;q13.1).[199]

Myxoid Dermatofibrosarcoma Protuberans

Myxoid DFSP is a rare variant, accounting for approximately 5% of cases.[37,38] The clinical features of this variant are similar to those of conventional DFSP (see Chapter 15).[37,38] Myxoid DFSP affects the dermis and subcutaneous tissue and is characterized by a monomorphic proliferation of small spindle cells embedded in a myxoid matrix. Because examples with abundant myxoid stroma typically lack the tight storiform architecture that is critical to the diagnosis of DFSP, histologic recognition is challenging (see Fig. 5.23B). Identification of areas of conventional DFSP is crucial for the correct diagnosis of the myxoid variant. Diffuse infiltration of subcutaneous adipose tissue (with a "honeycomb" pattern) is a helpful diagnostic clue. Neoplastic cells are positive for CD34, similar to conventional DFSP. DFSP harbors the recurrent translocation t(17;22)(q21;q13), resulting in *COL1A1-PDGFB* fusion;[200,201] the diagnosis can be confirmed in challenging cases using FISH to detect *PDGFB* rearrangement.

Myxoid Solitary Fibrous Tumor

SFT is an anatomically ubiquitous mesenchymal neoplasm with an equal gender distribution that often presents as a large, deep-seated soft tissue or visceral mass (see Chapter 3). Histologically, SFT is characterized by alternating hypo- and hypercellular areas with prominent stromal collagen and branching hemangiopericytoma-like vessels. By immunohistochemistry, greater than 95% of tumors are positive for CD34. STAT6 is a highly sensitive and specific marker for SFT.[177,202] STAT6 overexpression in SFT is secondary to the characteristic *NAB2-STAT6* fusion oncogene that results from inversion of the two genes located on chromosome 12q13.[203,204] Myxoid examples of SFT are uncommon and are composed of short neoplastic spindle cells arranged in a somewhat reticular growth pattern embedded in an abundant myxoid matrix (see Fig. 5.23C).[205] The patternless architecture and hemangiopericytoma-like vessels are diagnostic clues, but recognition of conventional areas is critical for proper diagnosis.

Myxoid Synovial Sarcoma

Myxoid stromal change in synovial sarcoma is often focal; however, rarely, myxoid stroma may predominate, in which case recognizing this tumor type is challenging. Myxoid synovial sarcoma is a rare variant

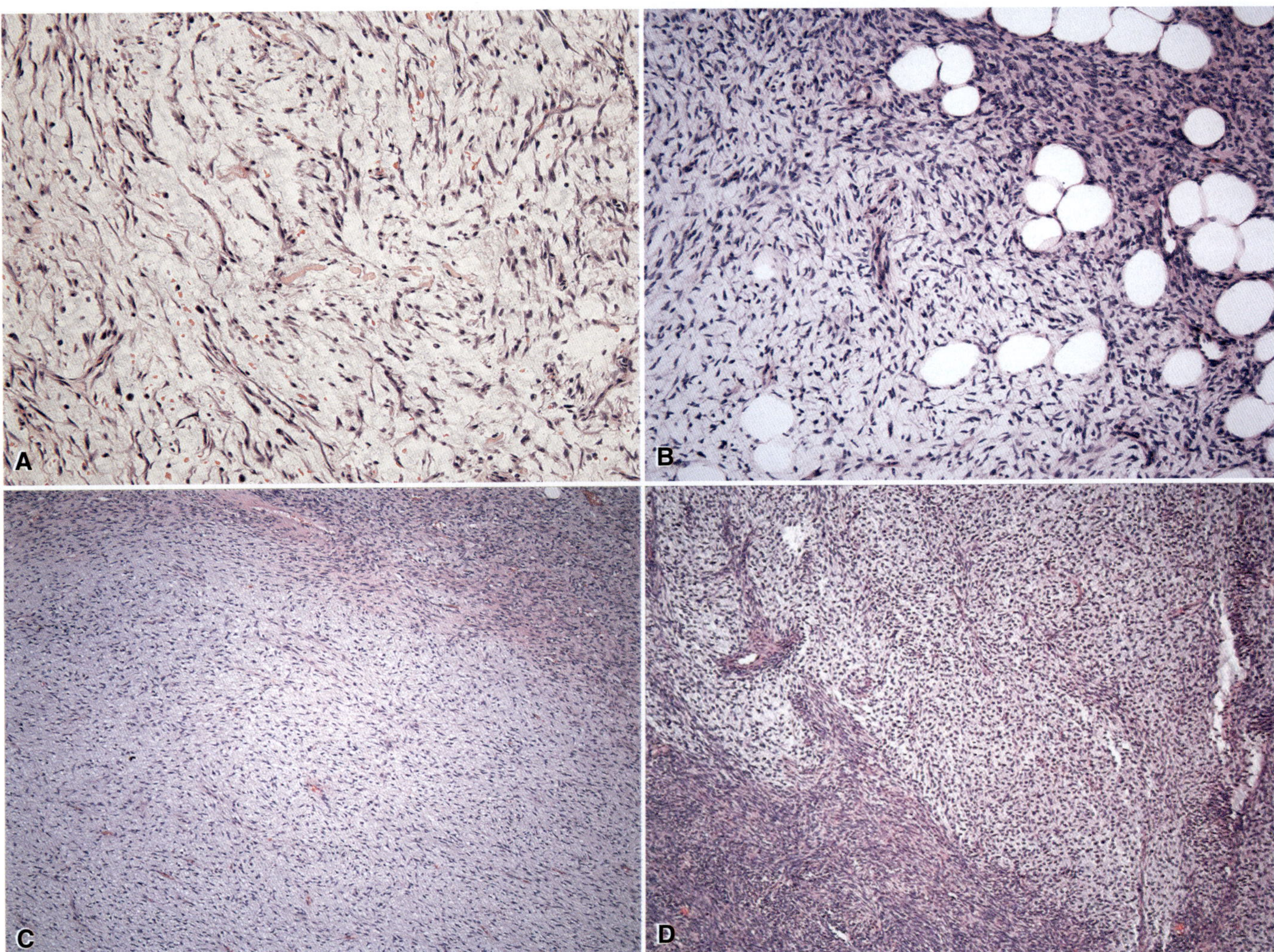

Figure 5.23 **Other Tumors With Myxoid Stroma.** (A) Nodular fasciitis occasionally shows prominent myxoid stroma. Note the loose fascicular architecture and extravasated red blood cells. (B) The myxoid variant of dermatofibrosarcoma protuberans can be recognized by identifying conventional cellular storiform areas. Note the diffuse infiltration through subcutaneous adipose tissue. (C) Myxoid variant of solitary fibrous tumor. (D) Myxoid synovial sarcoma.

that has demographic features similar to those of conventional synovial sarcoma (see Chapter 3).[206] Patients are usually young adults, and the extremities are most often involved. Histologically, neoplastic cells are embedded in a prominent myxoid stroma and arranged in a lacy, reticular growth pattern (see Fig. 5.23D). Identification of areas of conventional monophasic or biphasic synovial sarcoma is pivotal for the correct diagnosis of this variant. Immunohistochemistry for EMA, keratins, and TLE1 is useful, but FISH for *SS18* rearrangement may be required to confirm the diagnosis.

References

1. Lowden CM, Attiah M, Garvin G, et al: The prevalence of wrist ganglia in an asymptomatic population: magnetic resonance evaluation, *J Hand Surg [Br]* 30:302–306, 2005.
2. Capelastegui A, Astigarraga E, Fernandez-Canton G, et al: Masses and pseudomasses of the hand and wrist: MR findings in 134 cases, *Skeletal Radiol* 28:498–507, 1999.
3. Nahra ME, Bucchieri JS: Ganglion cysts and other tumor related conditions of the hand and wrist, *Hand Clin* 20:249–260, v, 2004.
4. Rozbruch SR, Chang V, Bohne WH, et al: Ganglion cysts of the lower extremity: an analysis of 54 cases and review of the literature, *Orthopedics* 21:141–148, 1998.
5. Krudwig WK, Schulte KK, Heinemann C: Intra-articular ganglion cysts of the knee joint: a report of 85 cases and review of the literature, *Knee Surg Sports Traumatol Arthrosc* 12: 123–129, 2004.
6. James SL, Connell DA, Bell J, et al: Ganglion cysts at the gastrocnemius origin: a series of ten cases, *Skeletal Radiol* 36:139–143, 2007.
7. Fletcher CDM, Bridge JA, Hogendoorn PCW, et al, editors: *WHO classification of tumours of soft tissue and bone*, Lyon, France, 2013, IARC Press.
8. Enzinger FM: Intramuscular myxoma; a review and follow-up study of 34 cases, *Am J Clin Pathol* 43:104–113, 1965.
9. Ireland DC, Soule EH, Ivins JC: Myxoma of somatic soft tissues. A report of 58 patients, 3 with musltiple tumors and fibrous dysplasia of bone, *Mayo Clin Proc* 48:401–410, 1973.
10. Rosin RD: Intramuscular myxomas, *Br J Surg* 60:122–124, 1973.
11. Kindblom LG, Stener B, Angervall L: Intramuscular myxoma, *Cancer* 34:1737–1744, 1974.
12. Miettinen M, Hockerstedt K, Reitamo J, et al: Intramuscular myxoma–a clinicopathological study of twenty-three cases, *Am J Clin Pathol* 84:265–272, 1985.
13. Hashimoto H, Tsuneyoshi M, Daimaru Y, et al: Intramuscular myxoma. A clinicopathologic, immunohistochemical, and electron microscopic study, *Cancer* 58:740–747, 1986.
14. Nielsen GP, O'Connell JX, Rosenberg AE: Intramuscular myxoma: a clinicopathologic study of 51 cases with emphasis on hypercellular and hypervascular variants, *Am J Surg Pathol* 22: 1222–1227, 1998.
15. van Roggen JF, McMenamin ME, Fletcher CD: Cellular myxoma of soft tissue: a clinicopathological study of 38 cases confirming indolent clinical behaviour, *Histopathology* 39:287–297, 2001.
16. Silver WP, Harrelson JM, Scully SP: Intramuscular myxoma: a clinicopathologic study of 17 patients, *Clin Orthop Relat Res* 403:191–197, 2002.
17. Yang EJ, Hornick JL, Qian X: Fine-needle aspiration of soft tissue perineurioma: a comparative analysis of cytomorphology and immunohistochemistry with benign and malignant mimics, *Cancer Cytopathol* 124:651–658, 2016.
18. Okamoto S, Hisaoka M, Ushijima M, et al: Activating Gs(alpha) mutation in intramuscular myxomas with and without fibrous dysplasia of bone, *Virchows Arch* 437:133–137, 2000.
19. Delaney D, Diss TC, Presneau N, et al: GNAS1 mutations occur more commonly than previously thought in intramuscular myxoma, *Mod Pathol* 22:718–724, 2009.

20. Willems SM, Mohseny AB, Balog C, et al: Cellular/intramuscular myxoma and grade I myxofibrosarcoma are characterized by distinct genetic alterations and specific composition of their extracellular matrix, *J Cell Mol Med* 13:1291–1301, 2009.
21. Okamoto S, Hisaoka M, Meis-Kindblom JM, et al: Juxta-articular myxoma and intramuscular myxoma are two distinct entities. activating gs alpha mutation at arg 201 codon does not occur in juxta-articular myxoma, *Virchows Arch* 440:12–15, 2002.
22. Meis JM, Enzinger FM: Juxta-articular myxoma: a clinical and pathologic study of 65 cases, *Hum Pathol* 23:639–646, 1992.
23. Gallager RL, Helwig EB: Neurothekeoma–a benign cutaneous tumor of neural origin, *Am J Clin Pathol* 74:759–764, 1980.
24. Pulitzer DR, Reed RJ: Nerve-sheath myxoma (perineurial myxoma), *Am J Dermatopathol* 7:409–421, 1985.
25. Angervall L, Kindblom LG, Haglid K: Dermal nerve sheath myxoma. A light and electron microscopic, histochemical and immunohistochemical study, *Cancer* 53:1752–1759, 1984.
26. Fletcher CD, Chan JK, McKee PH: Dermal nerve sheath myxoma: a study of three cases, *Histopathology* 10:135–145, 1986.
27. Fetsch JF, Laskin WB, Miettinen M: Nerve sheath myxoma: a clinicopathologic and immunohistochemical analysis of 57 morphologically distinctive, S-100 protein- and GFAP-positive, myxoid peripheral nerve sheath tumors with a predilection for the extremities and a high local recurrence rate, *Am J Surg Pathol* 29:1615–1624, 2005.
28. Hornick JL, Fletcher CD: Cellular neurothekeoma: detailed characterization in a series of 133 cases, *Am J Surg Pathol* 31:329–340, 2007.
29. Fetsch JF, Laskin WB, Hallman JR, et al: Neurothekeoma: an analysis of 178 tumors with detailed immunohistochemical data and long-term patient follow-up information, *Am J Surg Pathol* 31:1103–1114, 2007.
30. Laskin WB, Fetsch JF, Miettinen M: The "neurothekeoma": immunohistochemical analysis distinguishes the true nerve sheath myxoma from its mimics, *Hum Pathol* 31:1230–1241, 2000.
31. McCarron KF, Goldblum JR: Plexiform neurofibroma with and without associated malignant peripheral nerve sheath tumor: a clinicopathologic and immunohistochemical analysis of 54 cases, *Mod Pathol* 11:612–617, 1998.
32. Allen PW, Dymock RB, MacCormac LB: Superficial angiomyxomas with and without epithelial components. report of 30 tumors in 28 patients, *Am J Surg Pathol* 12:519–530, 1988.
33. Calonje E, Guerin D, McCormick D, et al: Superficial angiomyxoma: clinicopathologic analysis of a series of distinctive but poorly recognized cutaneous tumors with tendency for recurrence, *Am J Surg Pathol* 23:910–917, 1999.
34. Fetsch JF, Laskin WB, Miettinen M: Superficial acral fibromyxoma: a clinicopathologic and immunohistochemical analysis of 37 cases of a distinctive soft tissue tumor with a predilection for the fingers and toes, *Hum Pathol* 32:704–714, 2001.
35. Hollmann TJ, Bovee JV, Fletcher CD: Digital fibromyxoma (superficial acral fibromyxoma): a detailed characterization of 124 cases, *Am J Surg Pathol* 36:789–798, 2012.
36. Agaimy A, Michal M, Giedl J, et al: Superficial acral fibromyxoma: clinicopathologic, immunohistochemical and molecular study of 11 cases highlighting frequent Rb1 loss/deletions, *Hum Pathol* 60:192–198, 2017.
37. Reimann JD, Fletcher CD: Myxoid dermatofibrosarcoma protuberans: a rare variant analyzed in a series of 23 cases, *Am J Surg Pathol* 31:1371–1377, 2007.
38. Mentzel T, Scharer L, Kazakov DV, et al: Myxoid dermatofibrosarcoma protuberans: clinicopathologic, immunohistochemical, and molecular analysis of eight cases, *Am J Dermatopathol* 29:443–448, 2007.
39. Hornick JL, Fletcher CD: Soft tissue perineurioma: clinicopathologic analysis of 81 cases including those with atypical histologic features, *Am J Surg Pathol* 29:845–858, 2005.
40. Fetsch JF, Miettinen M: Sclerosing perineurioma: a clinicopathologic study of 19 cases of a distinctive soft tissue lesion with a predilection for the fingers and palms of young adults, *Am J Surg Pathol* 21:1433–1442, 1997.
41. Fetsch JF, Laskin WB, Tavassoli FA: Superficial angiomyxoma (cutaneous myxoma): a clinicopathologic study of 17 cases arising in the genital region, *Int J Gynecol Pathol* 16:325–334, 1997.
42. Marino-Enriquez A, Fletcher C, Doyle LA: Superficial angiomyxoma is characterized by loss of PRKAR1A expression [abstract], *Mod Pathol* 29:77A, 2016.
43. Kirschner LS, Carney JA, Pack SD, et al: Mutations of the gene encoding the protein kinase A type I-alpha regulatory subunit in patients with the carney complex, *Nat Genet* 26:89–92, 2000.
44. Park KU, Kim HS, Lee SK, et al: Novel mutation in PRKAR1A in carney complex, *Korean J Pathol* 46:595–600, 2012.
45. Fetsch JF, Laskin WB, Lefkowitz M, et al: Aggressive angiomyxoma: a clinicopathologic study of 29 female patients, *Cancer* 78:79–90, 1996.
46. Begin LR, Clement PB, Kirk ME, et al: Aggressive angiomyxoma of pelvic soft parts: a clinicopathologic study of nine cases, *Hum Pathol* 16:621–628, 1985.
47. Tsang WY, Chan JK, Lee KC, et al: Aggressive angiomyxoma. A report of four cases occurring in men, *Am J Surg Pathol* 16:1059–1065, 1992.
48. Iezzoni JC, Fechner RE, Wong LS, et al: Aggressive angiomyxoma in males. A report of four cases, *Am J Clin Pathol* 104:391–396, 1995.
49. van Roggen JF, van Unnik JA, Briaire-de Bruijn IH, et al: Aggressive angiomyxoma: a clinicopathological and immunohistochemical study of 11 cases with long-term follow-up, *Virchows Arch* 446:157–163, 2005.
50. Granter SR, Nucci MR, Fletcher CD: Aggressive angiomyxoma: reappraisal of its relationship to angiomyofibroblastoma in a series of 16 cases, *Histopathology* 30:3–10, 1997.
51. Amezcua CA, Begley SJ, Mata N, et al: Aggressive angiomyxoma of the female genital tract: a clinicopathologic and immunohistochemical study of 12 cases, *Int J Gynecol Cancer* 15:140–145, 2005.
52. Magtibay PM, Salmon Z, Keeney GL, et al: Aggressive angiomyxoma of the female pelvis and perineum: a case series, *Int J Gynecol Cancer* 16:396–401, 2006.
53. Dreux N, Marty M, Chibon F, et al: Value and limitation of immunohistochemical expression of HMGA2 in mesenchymal tumors: about a series of 1052 cases, *Mod Pathol* 23:1657–1666, 2010.
54. McCluggage WG, Connolly L, McBride HA: HMGA2 is a sensitive but not specific immunohistochemical marker of vulvovaginal aggressive angiomyxoma, *Am J Surg Pathol* 34:1037–1042, 2010.
55. Bigby SM, Symmans PJ, Miller MV, et al: Aggressive angiomyxoma [corrected] of the female genital tract and pelvis–clinicopathologic features with immunohistochemical analysis, *Int J Gynecol Pathol* 30:505–513, 2011.
56. Kazmierczak B, Wanschura S, Meyer-Bolte K, et al: Cytogenic and molecular analysis of an aggressive angiomyxoma, *Am J Pathol* 147:580–585, 1995.
57. Nucci MR, Weremowicz S, Neskey DM, et al: Chromosomal translocation t(8;12) induces aberrant HMGIC expression in aggressive angiomyxoma of the vulva, *Genes Chromosomes Cancer* 32:172–176, 2001.
58. Micci F, Panagopoulos I, Bjerkehagen B, et al: Deregulation of HMGA2 in an aggressive angiomyxoma with t(11;12)(q23;q15), *Virchows Arch* 448:838–842, 2006.
59. Rabban JT, Dal Cin P, Oliva E: HMGA2 rearrangement in a case of vulvar aggressive angiomyxoma, *Int J Gynecol Pathol* 25:403–407, 2006.
60. Medeiros F, Erickson-Johnson MR, Keeney GL, et al: Frequency and characterization of HMGA2 and HMGA1 rearrangements in mesenchymal tumors of the lower genital tract, *Genes Chromosomes Cancer* 46:981–990, 2007.
61. Iwasa Y, Fletcher CD: Cellular angiofibroma: clinicopathologic and immunohistochemical analysis of 51 cases, *Am J Surg Pathol* 28:1426–1435, 2004.
62. Chirayil SJ, Tobon H: Polyps of the vagina: a clinicopathologic study of 18 cases, *Cancer* 47:2904–2907, 1981.
63. Enzinger FM, Weiss SW, Liang CY: Ossifying fibromyxoid tumor of soft parts. A clinicopathological analysis of 59 cases, *Am J Surg Pathol* 13:817–827, 1989.
64. Folpe AL, Weiss SW: Ossifying fibromyxoid tumor of soft parts: a clinicopathologic study of 70 cases with emphasis on atypical and malignant variants, *Am J Surg Pathol* 27:421–431, 2003.
65. Miettinen M, Finnell V, Fetsch JF: Ossifying fibromyxoid tumor of soft parts–a clinicopathologic and immunohistochemical study of 104 cases with long-term follow-up and a critical review of the literature, *Am J Surg Pathol* 32:996–1005, 2008.
66. Kilpatrick SE, Ward WG, Mozes M, et al: Atypical and malignant variants of ossifying fibromyxoid tumor. clinicopathologic analysis of six cases, *Am J Surg Pathol* 19:1039–1046, 1995.
67. Zamecnik M, Michal M, Simpson RH, et al: Ossifying fibromyxoid tumor of soft parts: a report of 17 cases with emphasis on unusual histological features, *Ann Diagn Pathol* 1:73–81, 1997.
68. Graham RP, Dry S, Li X, et al: Ossifying fibromyxoid tumor of soft parts: a clinicopathologic, proteomic, and genomic study, *Am J Surg Pathol* 35:1615–1625, 2011.
69. Miettinen M: Ossifying fibromyxoid tumor of soft parts. Additional observations of a distinctive soft tissue tumor, *Am J Clin Pathol* 95:142–149, 1991.
70. Schofield JB, Krausz T, Stamp GW, et al: Ossifying fibromyxoid tumour of soft parts: immunohistochemical and ultrastructural analysis, *Histopathology* 22:101–112, 1993.
71. Williams SB, Ellis GL, Meis JM, et al: Ossifying fibromyxoid tumour (of soft parts) of the head and neck: a clinicopathological and immunohistochemical study of nine cases, *J Laryngol Otol* 107:75–80, 1993.
72. Matsumoto K, Yamamoto T, Min W, et al: Ossifying fibromyxoid tumor of soft parts: clinicopathologic, immunohistochemical and ultrastructural study of four cases, *Pathol Int* 49:742–746, 1999.
73. Gebre-Medhin S, Nord KH, Moller E, et al: Recurrent rearrangement of the PHF1 gene in ossifying fibromyxoid tumors, *Am J Pathol* 181:1069–1077, 2012.
74. Graham RP, Weiss SW, Sukov WR, et al: PHF1 rearrangements in ossifying fibromyxoid tumors of soft parts: a fluorescence in situ hybridization study of 41 cases with emphasis on the malignant variant, *Am J Surg Pathol* 37:1751–1755, 2013.
75. Endo M, Kohashi K, Yamamoto H, et al: Ossifying fibromyxoid tumor presenting EP400-PHF1 fusion gene, *Hum Pathol* 44:2603–2608, 2013.
76. Kao YC, Sung YS, Zhang L, et al: Expanding the molecular signature of ossifying fibromyxoid tumors with two novel gene fusions: CREBBP-BCORL1 and KDM2A-WWTR1, *Genes Chromosomes Cancer* 56:42–50, 2017.
77. Antonescu CR, Sung YS, Chen CL, et al: Novel ZC3H7B-BCOR, MEAF6-PHF1, and EPC1-PHF1 fusions in ossifying fibromyxoid tumors–molecular characterization shows genetic overlap with endometrial stromal sarcoma, *Genes Chromosomes Cancer* 53:183–193, 2014.
78. Hornick JL, Fletcher CD: Myoepithelial tumors of soft tissue: a clinicopathologic and immunohistochemical study of 101 cases with evaluation of prognostic parameters, *Am J Surg Pathol* 27:1183–1196, 2003.
79. Antonescu CR, Zhang L, Chang NE, et al: EWSR1-POU5F1 fusion in soft tissue myoepithelial tumors. A molecular analysis of sixty-six cases, including soft tissue, bone, and visceral lesions,

showing common involvement of the EWSR1 gene, *Genes Chromosomes Cancer* 49:1114–1124, 2010.

80. Meis-Kindblom JM, Bergh P, Gunterberg B, et al: Extraskeletal myxoid chondrosarcoma: a reappraisal of its morphologic spectrum and prognostic factors based on 117 cases, *Am J Surg Pathol* 23:636–650, 1999.
81. Gleason BC, Fletcher CD: Myoepithelial carcinoma of soft tissue in children: an aggressive neoplasm analyzed in a series of 29 cases, *Am J Surg Pathol* 31:1813–1824, 2007.
82. Michal M, Miettinen M: Myoepitheliomas of the skin and soft tissues. report of 12 cases, *Virchows Arch* 434:393–400, 1999.
83. Kilpatrick SE, Hitchcock MG, Kraus MD, et al: Mixed tumors and myoepitheliomas of soft tissue: a clinicopathologic study of 19 cases with a unifying concept, *Am J Surg Pathol* 21:13–22, 1997.
84. Mentzel T, Requena L, Kaddu S, et al: Cutaneous myoepithelial neoplasms: clinicopathologic and immunohistochemical study of 20 cases suggesting a continuous spectrum ranging from benign mixed tumor of the skin to cutaneous myoepithelioma and myoepithelial carcinoma, *J Cutan Pathol* 30:294–302, 2003.
85. Jo VY, Fletcher CD: p63 immunohistochemical staining is limited in soft tissue tumors, *Am J Clin Pathol* 136:762–766, 2011.
86. Miettinen M, McCue PA, Sarlomo-Rikala M, et al: Sox10-A marker for not only schwannian and melanocytic neoplasms but also myoepithelial cell tumors of soft tissue: a systematic analysis of 5134 tumors, *Am J Surg Pathol* 39:826, 2015.
87. Bahrami A, Dalton JD, Krane JF, et al: A subset of cutaneous and soft tissue mixed tumors are genetically linked to their salivary gland counterpart, *Genes Chromosomes Cancer* 51:140–148, 2012.
88. Hornick JL, Dal Cin P, Fletcher CD: Loss of INI1 expression is characteristic of both conventional and proximal-type epithelioid sarcoma, *Am J Surg Pathol* 33:542–550, 2009.
89. Hollmann TJ, Hornick JL: INI1-deficient tumors: diagnostic features and molecular genetics, *Am J Surg Pathol* 35:e47–e63, 2011.
90. Huang SC, Chen HW, Zhang L, et al: Novel FUS-KLF17 and EWSR1-KLF17 fusions in myoepithelial tumors, *Genes Chromosomes Cancer* 54:267–275, 2015.
91. Brandal P, Panagopoulos I, Bjerkehagen B, et al: Detection of a t(1;22)(q23;q12) translocation leading to an EWSR1-PBX1 fusion gene in a myoepithelioma, *Genes Chromosomes Cancer* 47:558–564, 2008.
92. Brandal P, Panagopoulos I, Bjerkehagen B, et al: t(19;22)(q13;q12) translocation leading to the novel fusion gene EWSR1-ZNF444 in soft tissue myoepithelial carcinoma, *Genes Chromosomes Cancer* 48:1051–1056, 2009.
93. Flucke U, Palmedo G, Blankenhorn N, et al: EWSR1 gene rearrangement occurs in a subset of cutaneous myoepithelial tumors: a study of 18 cases, *Mod Pathol* 24:1444–1450, 2011.
94. Jo VY, Antonescu CR, Zhang L, et al: Cutaneous syncytial myoepithelioma: clinicopathologic characterization in a series of 38 cases, *Am J Surg Pathol* 37:710–718, 2013.
95. Puls F, Arbajian E, Magnusson L, et al: Myoepithelioma of bone with a novel FUS-POU5F1 fusion gene, *Histopathology* 65:917–922, 2014.
96. Matsuyama A, Hisaoka M, Hashimoto H: PLAG1 expression in mesenchymal tumors: an immunohistochemical study with special emphasis on the pathogenetical distinction between soft tissue myoepithelioma and pleomorphic adenoma of the salivary gland, *Pathol Int* 62:1–7, 2012.
97. Antonescu CR, Zhang L, Shao SY, et al: Frequent PLAG1 gene rearrangements in skin and soft tissue myoepithelioma with ductal differentiation, *Genes Chromosomes Cancer* 52:675–682, 2013.
98. Kindblom LG, Meis-Kindblom JM, Havel G, et al: Benign epithelioid schwannoma, *Am J Surg Pathol* 22:762–770, 1998.
99. Hart J, Gardner JM, Edgar M, et al: Epithelioid schwannomas: an analysis of 58 cases including atypical variants, *Am J Surg Pathol* 40:704–713, 2016.
100. Laskin WB, Fetsch JF, Lasota J, et al: Benign epithelioid peripheral nerve sheath tumors of the soft tissues: clinicopathologic spectrum of 33 cases, *Am J Surg Pathol* 29:39–51, 2005.
101. Jo VY, Fletcher CD: SMARCB1/INI1 loss in epithelioid schwannoma: A clinicopathologic and immunohistochemical study of 65 cases, *Am J Surg Pathol* 41:1013–1022, 2017.
102. Noronha V, Cooper DL, Higgins SA, et al: Metastatic myoepithelial carcinoma of the vulva treated with carboplatin and paclitaxel, *Lancet Oncol* 7:270–271, 2006.
103. Angervall L, Kindblom LG, Merck C: Myxofibrosarcoma. A study of 30 cases, *Acta Pathol Microbiol Scand [A]* 85A:127–140, 1977.
104. Weiss SW, Enzinger FM: Myxoid variant of malignant fibrous histiocytoma, *Cancer* 39:1672–1685, 1977.
105. Fletcher CD: Pleomorphic malignant fibrous histiocytoma: fact or fiction? A critical reappraisal based on 159 tumors diagnosed as pleomorphic sarcoma, *Am J Surg Pathol* 16:213–228, 1992.
106. Hollowood K, Fletcher CD: Malignant fibrous histiocytoma: morphologic pattern or pathologic entity?, *Semin Diagn Pathol* 12:210–220, 1995.
107. Fletcher CD, Gustafson P, Rydholm A, et al: Clinicopathologic re-evaluation of 100 malignant fibrous histiocytomas: prognostic relevance of subclassification, *J Clin Oncol* 19:3045–3050, 2001.
108. Merck C, Angervall L, Kindblom LG, et al: Myxofibrosarcoma. A malignant soft tissue tumor of fibroblastic-histiocytic origin. A clinicopathologic and prognostic study of 110 cases using multivariate analysis, *Acta Pathol Microbiol Immunol Scand Suppl* 282:1–40, 1983.
109. Mentzel T, Calonje E, Wadden C, et al: Myxofibrosarcoma. Clinicopathologic analysis of 75 cases with emphasis on the low-grade variant, *Am J Surg Pathol* 20:391–405, 1996.
110. Huang HY, Lal P, Qin J, et al: Low-grade myxofibrosarcoma: a clinicopathologic analysis of 49 cases treated at a single institution with simultaneous assessment of the efficacy of 3-tier and 4-tier grading systems, *Hum Pathol* 35:612–621, 2004.
111. McCormick D, Mentzel T, Beham A, et al: Dedifferentiated liposarcoma. Clinicopathologic analysis of 32 cases suggesting a better prognostic subgroup among pleomorphic sarcomas, *Am J Surg Pathol* 18:1213–1223, 1994.
112. Henricks WH, Chu YC, Goldblum JR, et al: Dedifferentiated liposarcoma: a clinicopathological analysis of 155 cases with a proposal for an expanded definition of dedifferentiation, *Am J Surg Pathol* 21:271–281, 1997.
113. Sioletic S, Dal Cin P, Fletcher CD, et al: Well-differentiated and dedifferentiated liposarcomas with prominent myxoid stroma: analysis of 56 cases, *Histopathology* 62:287–293, 2013.
114. Nascimento AF, Bertoni F, Fletcher CD: Epithelioid variant of myxofibrosarcoma: expanding the clinicomorphologic spectrum of myxofibrosarcoma in a series of 17 cases, *Am J Surg Pathol* 31:99–105, 2007.
115. Willems SM, Debiec-Rychter M, Szuhai K, et al: Local recurrence of myxofibrosarcoma is associated with increase in tumour grade and cytogenetic aberrations, suggesting a multistep tumour progression model, *Mod Pathol* 19:407–416, 2006.
116. Shmookler BM, Enzinger FM: Liposarcoma occurring in children: an analysis of 17 cases and review of the literature, *Cancer* 52:567–574, 1983.
117. Smith TA, Easley KA, Goldblum JR: Myxoid/round cell liposarcoma of the extremities. A clinicopathologic study of 29 cases with particular attention to extent of round cell liposarcoma, *Am J Surg Pathol* 20:171–180, 1996.
118. Kilpatrick SE, Doyon J, Choong PF, et al: The clinicopathologic spectrum of myxoid and round cell liposarcoma. A study of 95 cases, *Cancer* 77:1450–1458, 1996.
119. Antonescu CR, Tschernyavsky SJ, Decuseara R, et al: Prognostic impact of P53 status, TLS-CHOP fusion transcript structure, and histological grade in myxoid liposarcoma: a molecular and clinicopathologic study of 82 cases, *Clin Cancer Res* 7:3977–3987, 2001.
120. Tateishi U, Hasegawa T, Beppu Y, et al: Prognostic significance of grading (MIB-1 system) in patients with myxoid liposarcoma, *J Clin Pathol* 56:579–582, 2003.
121. ten Heuvel SE, Hoekstra HJ, van Ginkel RJ, et al: Clinicopathologic prognostic factors in myxoid liposarcoma: a retrospective study of 49 patients with long-term follow-up, *Ann Surg Oncol* 14:222–229, 2007.
122. Hashimoto H, Daimaru Y, Enjoji M: S-100 protein distribution in liposarcoma. an immunoperoxidase study with special reference to the distinction of liposarcoma from myxoid malignant fibrous histiocytoma, *Virchows Arch A Pathol Anat Histopathol* 405:1–10, 1984.
123. Binh MB, Sastre-Garau X, Guillou L, et al: MDM2 and CDK4 immunostainings are useful adjuncts in diagnosing well-differentiated and dedifferentiated liposarcoma subtypes: a comparative analysis of 559 soft tissue neoplasms with genetic data, *Am J Surg Pathol* 29:1340–1347, 2005.
124. Limon J, Turc-Carel C, Dal Cin P, et al: Recurrent chromosome translocations in liposarcoma, *Cancer Genet Cytogenet* 22:93–94, 1986.
125. Turc-Carel C, Limon J, Dal Cin P, et al: Cytogenetic studies of adipose tissue tumors. II. Recurrent reciprocal translocation t(12;16)(q13;p11) in myxoid liposarcomas, *Cancer Genet Cytogenet* 23:291–299, 1986.
126. Sreekantaiah C, Karakousis CP, Leong SP, et al: Cytogenetic findings in liposarcoma correlate with histopathologic subtypes, *Cancer* 69:2484–2495, 1992.
127. Sreekantaiah C, Karakousis CP, Leong SP, et al: Trisomy 8 as a nonrandom secondary change in myxoid liposarcoma, *Cancer Genet Cytogenet* 51:195–205, 1991.
128. Tallini G, Akerman M, Dal Cin P, et al: Combined morphologic and karyotypic study of 28 myxoid liposarcomas. implications for a revised morphologic typing (a report from the CHAMP group), *Am J Surg Pathol* 20:1047–1055, 1996.
129. Aman P, Ron D, Mandahl N, et al: Rearrangement of the transcription factor gene CHOP in myxoid liposarcomas with t(12;16)(q13;p11), *Genes Chromosomes Cancer* 5:278–285, 1992.
130. Crozat A, Aman P, Mandahl N, et al: Fusion of CHOP to a novel RNA-binding protein in human myxoid liposarcoma, *Nature* 363:640–644, 1993.
131. Dal Cin P, Sciot R, Panagopoulos I, et al: Additional evidence of a variant translocation t(12;22) with EWS/CHOP fusion in myxoid liposarcoma: clinicopathological features, *J Pathol* 182:437–441, 1997.
132. Panagopoulos I, Hoglund M, Mertens F, et al: Fusion of the EWS and CHOP genes in myxoid liposarcoma, *Oncogene* 12:489–494, 1996.
133. Schwab JH, Boland PJ, Antonescu C, et al: Spinal metastases from myxoid liposarcoma warrant screening with magnetic resonance imaging, *Cancer* 110:1815–1822, 2007.
134. Fiore M, Grosso F, Lo Vullo S, et al: Myxoid/round cell and pleomorphic liposarcomas: prognostic factors and survival in a series of patients treated at a single institution, *Cancer* 109:2522–2531, 2007.
135. Grosso F, Jones RL, Demetri GD, et al: Efficacy of trabectedin (ecteinascidin-743) in advanced pretreated myxoid liposarcomas: a retrospective study, *Lancet Oncol* 8:595–602, 2007.
136. Cesne AL, Judson I, Maki R, et al: Trabectedin is a feasible treatment for soft tissue sarcoma patients regardless of patient age: a retrospective pooled analysis of five phase II trials, *Br J Cancer* 109:1717–1724, 2013.
137. Demetri GD, von Mehren M, Jones RL, et al: Efficacy and safety of trabectedin or dacarbazine for metastatic liposarcoma or leiomyosarcoma after failure of conventional chemotherapy: results of a phase III randomized multicenter clinical trial, *J Clin Oncol* 34:786–793, 2016.

138. Wortman JR, Tirumani SH, Tirumani H, et al: Neoadjuvant radiation in primary extremity liposarcoma: correlation of MRI features with histopathology, *Eur Radiol* 26:1226–1234, 2016.
139. Stout AP, Verner EW: Chondrosarcoma of the extraskeletal soft tissues, *Cancer* 6:581–590, 1953.
140. Enzinger FM, Shiraki M: Extraskeletal myxoid chondrosarcoma. an analysis of 34 cases, *Hum Pathol* 3:421–435, 1972.
141. Tsuneyoshi M, Enjoji M, Iwasaki H, et al: Extraskeletal myxoid chondrosarcoma–a clinicopathologic and electron microscopic study, *Acta Pathol Jpn* 31:439–447, 1981.
142. Saleh G, Evans HL, Ro JY, et al: Extraskeletal myxoid chondrosarcoma. A clinicopathologic study of ten patients with long-term follow-up, *Cancer* 70:2827–2830, 1992.
143. Oliveira AM, Sebo TJ, McGrory JE, et al: Extraskeletal myxoid chondrosarcoma: a clinicopathologic, immunohistochemical, and ploidy analysis of 23 cases, *Mod Pathol* 13:900–908, 2000.
144. Okamoto S, Hisaoka M, Ishida T, et al: Extraskeletal myxoid chondrosarcoma: a clinicopathologic, immunohistochemical, and molecular analysis of 18 cases, *Hum Pathol* 32:1116–1124, 2001.
145. Kawaguchi S, Wada T, Nagoya S, et al: Extraskeletal myxoid chondrosarcoma: a multi-institutional study of 42 cases in Japan, *Cancer* 97:1285–1292, 2003.
146. Drilon AD, Popat S, Bhuchar G, et al: Extraskeletal myxoid chondrosarcoma: a retrospective review from 2 referral centers emphasizing long-term outcomes with surgery and chemotherapy, *Cancer* 113:3364–3371, 2008.
147. Antonescu CR, Argani P, Erlandson RA, et al: Skeletal and extraskeletal myxoid chondrosarcoma: a comparative clinicopathologic, ultrastructural, and molecular study, *Cancer* 83:1504–1521, 1998.
148. Lucas DR, Fletcher CD, Adsay NV, et al: High-grade extraskeletal myxoid chondrosarcoma: a high-grade epithelioid malignancy, *Histopathology* 35:201–208, 1999.
149. Goh YW, Spagnolo DV, Platten M, et al: Extraskeletal myxoid chondrosarcoma: a light microscopic, immunohistochemical, ultrastructural and immuno-ultrastructural study indicating neuroendocrine differentiation, *Histopathology* 39:514–524, 2001.
150. Kohashi K, Oda Y, Yamamoto H, et al: SMARCB1/INI1 protein expression in round cell soft tissue sarcomas associated with chromosomal translocations involving EWS: a special reference to SMARCB1/INI1 negative variant extraskeletal myxoid chondrosarcoma, *Am J Surg Pathol* 32:1168–1174, 2008.
151. Clark J, Benjamin H, Gill S, et al: Fusion of the EWS gene to CHN, a member of the steroid/thyroid receptor gene superfamily, in a human myxoid chondrosarcoma, *Oncogene* 12:229–235, 1996.
152. Sjogren H, Meis-Kindblom J, Kindblom LG, et al: Fusion of the EWS-related gene TAF2N to TEC in extraskeletal myxoid chondrosarcoma, *Cancer Res* 59:5064–5067, 1999.
153. Sjogren H, Wedell B, Meis-Kindblom JM, et al: Fusion of the NH2-terminal domain of the basic helix-loop-helix protein TCF12 to TEC in extraskeletal myxoid chondrosarcoma with translocation t(9;15)(q22;q21), *Cancer Res* 60:6832–6835, 2000.
154. Panagopoulos I, Mertens F, Isaksson M, et al: Molecular genetic characterization of the EWS/CHN and RBP56/CHN fusion genes in extraskeletal myxoid chondrosarcoma, *Genes Chromosomes Cancer* 35:340–352, 2002.
155. Sjogren H, Meis-Kindblom JM, Orndal C, et al: Studies on the molecular pathogenesis of extraskeletal myxoid chondrosarcoma-cytogenetic, molecular genetic, and cDNA microarray analyses, *Am J Pathol* 162:781–792, 2003.
156. Noguchi H, Mitsuhashi T, Seki K, et al: Fluorescence in situ hybridization analysis of extraskeletal myxoid chondrosarcomas using EWSR1 and NR4A3 probes, *Hum Pathol* 41:336–342, 2010.
157. Broehm CJ, Wu J, Gullapalli RR, et al: Extraskeletal myxoid chondrosarcoma with a t(9;16)(q22;p11.2) resulting in a NR4A3-FUS fusion, *Cancer Genet* 207:276–280, 2014.
158. Urbini M, Astolfi A, Pantaleo MA, et al: HSPA8 as a novel fusion partner of NR4A3 in extraskeletal myxoid chondrosarcoma, *Genes Chromosomes Cancer* 56:582–586, 2017.
159. Flucke U, Tops BB, Verdijk MA, et al: NR4A3 rearrangement reliably distinguishes between the clinicopathologically overlapping entities myoepithelial carcinoma of soft tissue and cellular extraskeletal myxoid chondrosarcoma, *Virchows Arch* 460:621–628, 2012.
160. Chbani L, Guillou L, Terrier P, et al: Epithelioid sarcoma: a clinicopathologic and immunohistochemical analysis of 106 cases from the French sarcoma group, *Am J Clin Pathol* 131:222–227, 2009.
161. Evans HL: Low-grade fibromyxoid sarcoma. A report of two metastasizing neoplasms having a deceptively benign appearance, *Am J Clin Pathol* 88:615–619, 1987.
162. Evans HL: Low-grade fibromyxoid sarcoma. A report of 12 cases, *Am J Surg Pathol* 17:595–600, 1993.
163. Lane KL, Shannon RJ, Weiss SW: Hyalinizing spindle cell tumor with giant rosettes: a distinctive tumor closely resembling low-grade fibromyxoid sarcoma, *Am J Surg Pathol* 21:1481–1488, 1997.
164. Folpe AL, Lane KL, Paull G, et al: Low-grade fibromyxoid sarcoma and hyalinizing spindle cell tumor with giant rosettes: a clinicopathologic study of 73 cases supporting their identity and assessing the impact of high-grade areas, *Am J Surg Pathol* 24:1353–1360, 2000.
165. Reid R, de Silva MV, Paterson L, et al: Low-grade fibromyxoid sarcoma and hyalinizing spindle cell tumor with giant rosettes share a common t(7;16)(q34;p11) translocation, *Am J Surg Pathol* 27:1229–1236, 2003.
166. Goodlad JR, Mentzel T, Fletcher CD: Low grade fibromyxoid sarcoma: clinicopathological analysis of eleven new cases in support of a distinct entity, *Histopathology* 26:229–237, 1995.
167. Billings SD, Giblen G, Fanburg-Smith JC: Superficial low-grade fibromyxoid sarcoma (Evans tumor): a clinicopathologic analysis of 19 cases with a unique observation in the pediatric population, *Am J Surg Pathol* 29:204–210, 2005.
168. Zamecnik M, Michal M: Low-grade fibromyxoid sarcoma: a report of eight cases with histologic, immunohistochemical, and ultrastructural study, *Ann Diagn Pathol* 4:207–217, 2000.
169. Guillou L, Benhattar J, Gengler C, et al: Translocation-positive low-grade fibromyxoid sarcoma: clinicopathologic and molecular analysis of a series expanding the morphologic spectrum and suggesting potential relationship to sclerosing epithelioid fibrosarcoma: a study from the French sarcoma group, *Am J Surg Pathol* 31:1387–1402, 2007.
170. Evans HL: Low-grade fibromyxoid sarcoma: a clinicopathologic study of 33 cases with long-term follow-up, *Am J Surg Pathol* 35:1450–1462, 2011.
171. Doyle LA, Moller E, Dal Cin P, et al: MUC4 is a highly sensitive and specific marker for low-grade fibromyxoid sarcoma, *Am J Surg Pathol* 35:733–741, 2011.
172. Mertens F, Fletcher CD, Antonescu CR, et al: Clinicopathologic and molecular genetic characterization of low-grade fibromyxoid sarcoma, and cloning of a novel FUS/CREB3L1 fusion gene, *Lab Invest* 85:408–415, 2005.
173. Doyle LA, Wang WL, Dal Cin P, et al: MUC4 is a sensitive and extremely useful marker for sclerosing epithelioid fibrosarcoma: association with FUS gene rearrangement, *Am J Surg Pathol* 36:1444–1451, 2012.
174. Lau PP, Lui PC, Lau GT, et al: EWSR1-CREB3L1 gene fusion: a novel alternative molecular aberration of low-grade fibromyxoid sarcoma, *Am J Surg Pathol* 37:734–738, 2013.
175. Arbajian E, Puls F, Magnusson L, et al: Recurrent EWSR1-CREB3L1 gene fusions in sclerosing epithelioid fibrosarcoma, *Am J Surg Pathol* 38:801–808, 2014.
176. Panagopoulos I, Storlazzi CT, Fletcher CD, et al: The chimeric FUS/CREB3l2 gene is specific for low-grade fibromyxoid sarcoma, *Genes Chromosomes Cancer* 40:218–228, 2004.
177. Doyle LA, Vivero M, Fletcher CD, et al: Nuclear expression of STAT6 distinguishes solitary fibrous tumor from histologic mimics, *Mod Pathol* 27:390–395, 2014.
178. Yoshida A, Tsuta K, Ohno M, et al: STAT6 immunohistochemistry is helpful in the diagnosis of solitary fibrous tumors, *Am J Surg Pathol* 38:552–559, 2014.
179. Cheah AL, Billings SD, Goldblum JR, et al: STAT6 rabbit monoclonal antibody is a robust diagnostic tool for the distinction of solitary fibrous tumour from its mimics, *Pathology* 46:389–395, 2014.
180. Carlson JW, Fletcher CD: Immunohistochemistry for beta-catenin in the differential diagnosis of spindle cell lesions: analysis of a series and review of the literature, *Histopathology* 51:509–514, 2007.
181. Montgomery EA, Devaney KO, Giordano TJ, et al: Inflammatory myxohyaline tumor of distal extremities with virocyte or reed-sternberg-like cells: a distinctive lesion with features simulating inflammatory conditions, hodgkin's disease, and various sarcomas, *Mod Pathol* 11:384–391, 1998.
182. Meis-Kindblom JM, Kindblom LG: Acral myxoinflammatory fibroblastic sarcoma: a low-grade tumor of the hands and feet, *Am J Surg Pathol* 22:911–924, 1998.
183. Jurcic V, Zidar A, Montiel MD, et al: Myxoinflammatory fibroblastic sarcoma: a tumor not restricted to acral sites, *Ann Diagn Pathol* 6:272–280, 2002.
184. Laskin WB, Fetsch JF, Miettinen M: Myxoinflammatory fibroblastic sarcoma: a clinicopathologic analysis of 104 cases, with emphasis on predictors of outcome, *Am J Surg Pathol* 38:1–12, 2014.
185. Lambert I, Debiec-Rychter M, Guelinckx P, et al: Acral myxoinflammatory fibroblastic sarcoma with unique clonal chromosomal changes, *Virchows Arch* 438:509–512, 2001.
186. Mansoor A, Fidda N, Himoe E, et al: Myxoinflammatory fibroblastic sarcoma with complex supernumerary ring chromosomes composed of chromosome 3 segments, *Cancer Genet Cytogenet* 152:61–65, 2004.
187. Hallor KH, Sciot R, Staaf J, et al: Two genetic pathways, t(1;10) and amplification of 3p11-12, in myxoinflammatory fibroblastic sarcoma, haemosiderotic fibrolipomatous tumour, and morphologically similar lesions, *J Pathol* 217:716–727, 2009.
188. Elco CP, Marino-Enriquez A, Abraham JA, et al: Hybrid myxoinflammatory fibroblastic sarcoma/hemosiderotic fibrolipomatous tumor: report of a case providing further evidence for a pathogenetic link, *Am J Surg Pathol* 34:1723–1727, 2010.
189. Antonescu CR, Zhang L, Nielsen GP, et al: Consistent t(1;10) with rearrangements of TGFBR3 and MGEA5 in both myxoinflammatory fibroblastic sarcoma and hemosiderotic fibrolipomatous tumor, *Genes Chromosomes Cancer* 50:757–764, 2011.
190. Wettach GR, Boyd LJ, Lawce HJ, et al: Cytogenetic analysis of a hemosiderotic fibrolipomatous tumor, *Cancer Genet Cytogenet* 182:140–143, 2008.
191. Sakaki M, Hirokawa M, Wakatsuki S, et al: Acral myxoinflammatory fibroblastic sarcoma: a report of five cases and review of the literature, *Virchows Arch* 442:25–30, 2003.
192. Graadt van Roggen JF, Hogendoorn PC, Fletcher CD: Myxoid tumours of soft tissue, *Histopathology* 35:291–312, 1999.
193. Graadt van Roggen JF, McMenamin ME, Belchis DA, et al: Reticular perineurioma: a distinctive variant of soft tissue perineurioma, *Am J Surg Pathol* 25:485–493, 2001.
194. Liegl B, Bennett MW, Fletcher CD: Microcystic/reticular schwannoma: a distinct variant with predilection for visceral locations, *Am J Surg Pathol* 32:1080–1087, 2008.
195. Schaefer IM, Fletcher CD, Hornick JL: Loss of H3K27 trimethylation distinguishes malignant peripheral nerve sheath tumors from histologic mimics, *Mod Pathol* 29:4–13, 2016.
196. Cleven AH, Sannaa GA, Briaire-de Bruijn I, et al: Loss of H3K27 tri-methylation is a diagnostic marker for malignant peripheral nerve sheath tumors and an indicator for an inferior survival, *Mod Pathol* 29:582–590, 2016.

197. Prieto-Granada CN, Wiesner T, Messina JL, et al: Loss of H3K27me3 expression is a highly sensitive marker for sporadic and radiation-induced MPNST, *Am J Surg Pathol* 40:479–489, 2016.
198. Shimizu S, Hashimoto H, Enjoji M: Nodular fasciitis: an analysis of 250 patients, *Pathology* 16:161–166, 1984.
199. Erickson-Johnson MR, Chou MM, Evers BR, et al: Nodular fasciitis: a novel model of transient neoplasia induced by MYH9-USP6 gene fusion, *Lab Invest* 91:1427–1433, 2011.
200. Pedeutour F, Simon MP, Minoletti F, et al: Translocation, t(17;22)(q22;q13), in dermatofibrosarcoma protuberans: a new tumor-associated chromosome rearrangement, *Cytogenet Cell Genet* 72:171–174, 1996.
201. Patel KU, Szabo SS, Hernandez VS, et al: Dermatofibrosarcoma protuberans COL1A1-PDGFB fusion is identified in virtually all dermatofibrosarcoma protuberans cases when investigated by newly developed multiplex reverse transcription polymerase chain reaction and fluorescence in situ hybridization assays, *Hum Pathol* 39:184–193, 2008.
202. Schweizer L, Koelsche C, Sahm F, et al: Meningeal hemangiopericytoma and solitary fibrous tumors carry the NAB2-STAT6 fusion and can be diagnosed by nuclear expression of STAT6 protein, *Acta Neuropathol* 125:651–658, 2013.
203. Mohajeri A, Tayebwa J, Collin A, et al: Comprehensive genetic analysis identifies a pathognomonic NAB2/STAT6 fusion gene, nonrandom secondary genomic imbalances, and a characteristic gene expression profile in solitary fibrous tumor, *Genes Chromosomes Cancer* 52:873–886, 2013.
204. Robinson DR, Wu YM, Kalyana-Sundaram S, et al: Identification of recurrent NAB2-STAT6 gene fusions in solitary fibrous tumor by integrative sequencing, *Nat Genet* 45:180–185, 2013.
205. de Saint Aubain Somerhausen N, Rubin BP, Fletcher CD: Myxoid solitary fibrous tumor: a study of seven cases with emphasis on differential diagnosis, *Mod Pathol* 12:463–471, 1999.
206. Krane JF, Bertoni F, Fletcher CD: Myxoid synovial sarcoma: an underappreciated morphologic subset, *Mod Pathol* 12:456–462, 1999.

6

Epithelioid and Epithelial-Like Tumors

Leona A. Doyle, MD, and Jason L. Hornick, MD, PhD

The group of epithelioid mesenchymal tumors encompasses neoplasms that are composed, partly or extensively, of rounded or polygonal cells, at least somewhat resembling epithelial cells (Boxes 6.1 to 6.3). These tumors show variable, sometimes misleading growth patterns, including nested, sheetlike, strandlike, cordlike, or glandular-like architecture. In this chapter, only those tumors occurring in deep soft tissue and subcutis are examined in detail. Dermal lesions showing epithelioid cytology (e.g., epithelioid fibrous histiocytoma, myoepithelioma/mixed tumor/chondroid syringoma of the skin, cellular neurothekeoma) are discussed in Chapter 15, although these lesions are briefly discussed in the differential diagnosis sections and in boxes and tables when appropriate. Epithelioid mesenchymal tumors of soft tissue are rare, and many are malignant. Between 5% and 10% of soft tissue sarcomas exhibit at least focally epithelioid features.

Approach to the Diagnosis of Epithelioid Tumors of Soft Tissue

Before a diagnosis of an epithelioid mesenchymal tumor is considered, it is important to exclude histologic mimics. These include metastatic carcinomas (e.g., from lung, breast, or gastrointestinal tract), metastatic melanoma, malignant mesothelioma, and hematologic malignancies (especially diffuse large B-cell lymphoma, plasmacytoma, and anaplastic large-cell lymphoma), which can occasionally be found in soft tissue (Box 6.4). In this context, the previous medical history is crucial. Any history of a malignancy should prompt a review of the pathologic material for comparison.

Clinical Presentation

When dealing with an epithelioid mesenchymal lesion, the pathologist should first pay attention to the clinical setting. Patient age and sex, tumor location, tumor size, and medical history (e.g., history of soft tissue sarcoma, history of radiation therapy, or personal or familial history of tuberous sclerosis or type 1 neurofibromatosis) are important data to be taken into consideration. For instance, some tumors arise almost exclusively in infants or children, whereas others are predominantly observed in middle-aged or elderly adults (Box 6.5).

Anatomic location and tumor depth are also helpful for differential diagnosis. Some tumors are most likely to be found in the distal extremities (Box 6.6) or skin and subcutaneous tissues (Box 6.7), whereas others show limited anatomic distribution (Box 6.8).

Box 6.1 Benign Lesions of Soft Tissue With Epithelioid/Epithelial-Like Appearances

Most Frequent

Glomus tumor
Epithelioid fibrous histiocytoma
Epithelioid hemangioma
Granular cell tumor
Localized tenosynovial giant cell tumor (giant cell tumor of tendon sheath)
Diffuse-type tenosynovial giant cell tumor

Rare or Exceptional

Perivascular epithelioid cell tumor (PEComa)
Rhabdomyoma (adult type)
Epithelioid leiomyoma
Myxopapillary ependymoma of soft tissues
Myoepithelioma/mixed tumor
Epithelioid schwannoma
Chondroid lipoma
Extracranial meningioma
Histiocytic lesions (Rosai-Dorfman disease, reticulohistiocytoma)
Polyvinylpyrrolidone granuloma
Sclerosing perineurioma
Ossifying fibromyxoid tumor
Cellular neurothekeoma

Box 6.2 Soft Tissue Sarcomas With Predominantly Epithelioid/Epithelial-Like Appearances

Cytomorphology

Epithelioid sarcoma (including proximal type)
Epithelioid malignant peripheral nerve sheath tumor
Epithelioid hemangioendothelioma
Epithelioid angiosarcoma
Alveolar soft part sarcoma
Malignant perivascular epithelioid cell tumor (PEComa)
Extrarenal malignant rhabdoid tumor
Myoepithelial carcinoma
Chordoma
Malignant granular cell tumor
Sclerosing epithelioid fibrosarcoma
Gastrointestinal stromal tumor (epithelioid type)
Histiocytic sarcoma

Box 6.3 Soft Tissue Sarcomas Occasionally With Epithelioid/Epithelial-Like Appearances

Cytomorphology

Synovial sarcoma (glandular variant)
Malignant peripheral nerve sheath tumor (glandular variant)
Myxofibrosarcoma (epithelioid variant)
Pleomorphic liposarcoma (epithelioid variant)
Dedifferentiated liposarcoma with epithelioid features
Desmoplastic small round cell tumor
Clear cell sarcoma
Leiomyosarcoma (epithelioid variant)
Extraskeletal myxoid chondrosarcoma (epithelioid/rhabdoid variant)
Undifferentiated pleomorphic sarcoma
Rhabdomyosarcoma
Myxoinflammatory fibroblastic sarcoma
Intimal sarcoma
Inflammatory myofibroblastic tumor (epithelioid inflammatory myofibroblastic sarcoma)

Box 6.4 Nonmesenchymal Epithelioid Tumors That May Be Encountered in Soft Tissue

Frequent

Carcinoma (metastases)
Melanoma (metastases)
Hematologic malignancies (diffuse large B-cell lymphoma, anaplastic large-cell lymphoma, plasmacytoma/plasma cell myeloma)

Rare or Exceptional

Extragonadal primary and metastatic germ cell tumors
Paraganglioma
Adenomatoid tumor
Malignant mesothelioma (epithelioid and deciduoid variants)
Leydig/Sertoli cell tumor (metastases)
Myeloid sarcoma
Histiocytic lesions (e.g., Rosai-Dorfman disease)

Box 6.5 Epithelioid Soft Tissue Tumors: Distribution According to Age

Mostly in Infants and Children

Extrarenal malignant rhabdoid tumor
Extracranial meningioma
Congenital granular cell tumor

Mostly in Adolescents and Young Adults

Synovial sarcoma (biphasic and glandular variants)
Epithelioid sarcoma
Alveolar soft part sarcoma
Desmoplastic small round cell tumor
Extracranial meningioma
Clear cell sarcoma
Epithelioid malignant peripheral nerve sheath tumor

Mostly in Middle-Aged and Elderly Adults

Pleomorphic liposarcoma (epithelioid variant)
Myxofibrosarcoma (epithelioid variant)
Dedifferentiated liposarcoma (with epithelioid features)
Epithelioid hemangioendothelioma
Epithelioid angiosarcoma
Extraskeletal myxoid chondrosarcoma (epithelioid/rhabdoid variant)
Chordoma
Epithelioid leiomyosarcoma
Malignant peripheral nerve sheath tumor (glandular variant)
Undifferentiated pleomorphic sarcoma
Malignant granular cell tumor

Box 6.6 Epithelioid Soft Tissue Tumors of the Distal Extremities (Hands and Feet)

Glomus tumor
Sclerosing perineurioma
Myoepithelioma/mixed tumor
Ossifying fibromyxoid tumor
Giant cell tumor of tendon sheath (localized tenosynovial giant cell tumor)
Synovial sarcoma (biphasic and predominantly glandular variants)
Epithelioid sarcoma
Clear cell sarcoma

Box 6.7 Epithelioid Soft Tissue Tumors of the Skin and Subcutaneous Tissues[a]

Epithelioid fibrous histiocytoma
Epithelioid hemangioma
Cellular neurothekeoma
Reticulohistiocytoma
Juvenile xanthogranuloma
Glomus tumor
Granular cell tumor
Ectopic meningioma
Ectopic myxopapillary ependymoma
Myoepithelioma/mixed tumor (chondroid syringoma)
Ossifying fibromyxoid tumor
Sclerosing perineurioma
Epithelioid sarcoma
Epithelioid hemangioendothelioma
Epithelioid angiosarcoma

[a]See also Chapter 15.

Box 6.8 Epithelioid Soft Tissue Tumors Occurring at Specific Sites

Chordoma (sacrum, occiput, sphenoidal region)
Gastrointestinal stromal tumor (gastrointestinal tract, mesentery, omentum, retroperitoneum)
Desmoplastic small round cell tumor (peritoneum, paratesticular region)
Adult rhabdomyoma (head and neck region, upper aerodigestive tract)
Extracranial meningioma (scalp, head and neck region)
Myxopapillary ependymoma of soft tissue (subcutis, dorsal to sacrococcygeal area)

Microscopic Examination

Histologic examination alone can help limit the differential diagnosis. Features to evaluate on hematoxylin and eosin–stained slides are: (1) cell arrangement (growth pattern), (2) cytomorphologic appearance, and (3) quality of the extracellular matrix.

Some sarcomas can be easily recognized at low-power magnification, simply on the basis of their growth pattern (e.g., alveolar soft part sarcoma [ASPS]) or the mere presence of glandular structures (Box 6.9 and Fig. 6.1), whereas others usually display more complex and variable growth patterns, as exemplified by epithelioid sarcoma or epithelioid angiosarcoma.

Cytomorphologic features that should be taken into consideration when evaluating epithelioid soft tissue tumors include: (1) the appearance of the nuclei and (2) the quality of the cytoplasm.

Many epithelioid soft tissue neoplasms exhibit vesicular nuclei with a single central prominent nucleolus (Box 6.10 and Fig. 6.2). Conversely, perivascular epithelioid cell tumors (PEComas) and gastrointestinal stromal tumors, for instance, tend to show nuclei with fine chromatin and indistinct nucleoli.

Tumor cell cytoplasm can be copious or minimal and may show an eosinophilic or clear appearance. In some tumor types, the cytoplasm is often vacuolated (e.g., chordoma, epithelioid hemangioendothelioma [EHE], epithelioid angiosarcoma), or may contain rhabdoid inclusions (e.g., malignant rhabdoid tumor (MRT), epithelioid sarcoma, myoepithelioma/myoepithelial carcinoma), or occasionally melanin pigment (e.g., clear cell sarcoma, PEComa).

The distinctive tumor stroma is sometimes very helpful in pointing to a specific diagnosis. The extracellular matrix is usually poorly developed or virtually absent in some tumor types, such as extrarenal MRT or epithelioid malignant peripheral nerve sheath tumor (MPNST). In contrast, some other neoplasms are characterized by a prominent collagenous stroma (e.g., undifferentiated pleomorphic sarcoma, epithelioid sarcoma), myxoid stroma (e.g., extraskeletal myxoid chondrosarcoma

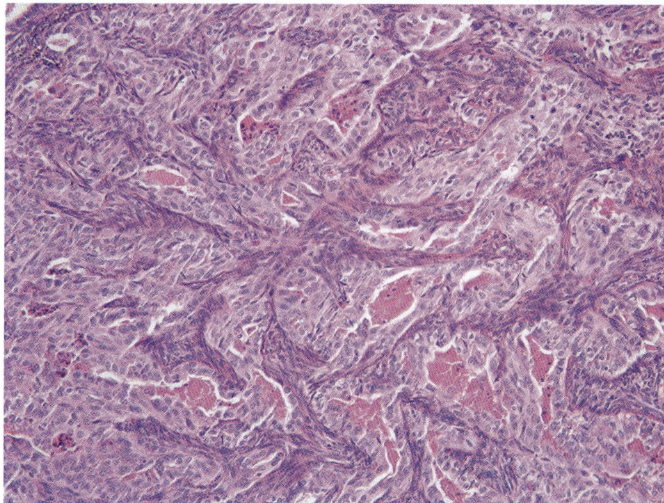

Figure 6.1 **Biphasic Synovial Sarcoma.** The tumor contains numerous glandular structures, resembling metastatic adenocarcinoma. The presence of the spindle cell component between the glands is a diagnostic clue.

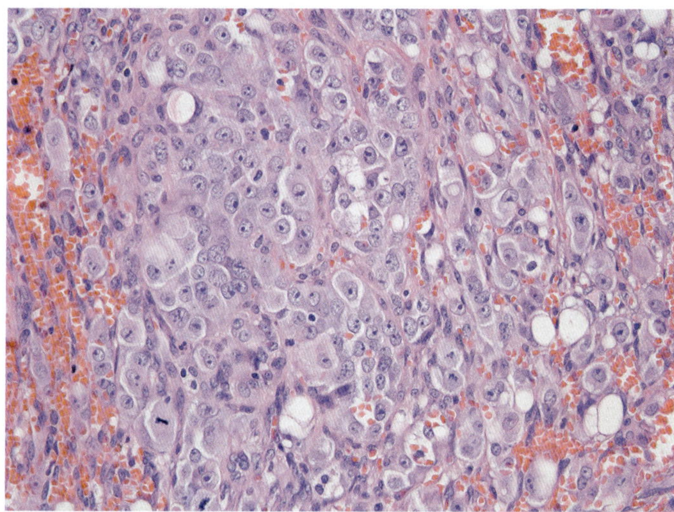

Figure 6.2 **Epithelioid Angiosarcoma.** Tumor cell nuclei are typically vesicular with a single prominent central nucleolus.

Box 6.9 Epithelioid Tumors That May Show Glandular, Pseudoglandular, or Tubular Structures

Myoepithelioma/mixed tumor
Synovial sarcoma (biphasic and glandular variants)
Malignant peripheral nerve sheath tumor (glandular variant)
Epithelioid angiosarcoma
Epithelioid sarcoma

Box 6.10 Epithelioid Soft Tissue Sarcomas Usually Displaying Vesicular Nuclei With a Single Central Prominent Nucleolus

Extrarenal malignant rhabdoid tumor
Epithelioid sarcoma
Epithelioid angiosarcoma
Epithelioid malignant peripheral nerve sheath tumor
Alveolar soft part sarcoma
Rhabdomyosarcoma (epithelioid variant)
Clear cell sarcoma
Epithelioid leiomyosarcoma

Table 6.1 Immunohistochemistry in Epithelioid Tumors of Soft Tissue

	KRT	EMA	S-100	HMB-45	SMA	Des	Myog	CD34	CD31	INI1
Carcinoma	+	+	±	–	–	–	–	–	–	+
Melanoma	–	–	+	+	–	–	–	–	–	+
Mesothelioma	+	+	–	–	–	±	–	–	–	+
Chordoma	+	+	+	–	–	–	–	–	–	+
Myoepithelioma	+	+	+	–	±	–	–	–	–	±
Synovial sarcoma	+	+	±	–	–	–	–	–	–	+
Epithelioid sarcoma	+	+	–	–	±	–	–	±	–	–
Clear cell sarcoma	–	–	+	+	–	–	–	–	–	+
Alveolar soft part sarcoma	–	–	–	–	–	–	–	–	–	+
Extraskeletal myxoid chondrosarcoma	–	–	±	–	±	–	–	–	–	+
Rhabdomyosarcoma	–	–	±	–	±	+	+	–	–	+
Epithelioid hemangioendothelioma	±	–	–	–	±	–	–	+	+	+
Epithelioid angiosarcoma	±	–	–	–	–	–	–	+	+	+
Epithelioid malignant peripheral nerve sheath tumor	–	–	+	–	–	–	–	–	–	±
Desmoplastic small round cell tumor	+	+	±	–	–	+	–	–	–	+
Malignant rhabdoid tumor	+	+	±	–	±	–	–	–	–	–

Des, Desmin; *EMA*, epithelial membrane antigen; *KRT*, keratins; *Myog*, myogenin; *SMA*, smooth muscle actin.

(EMC), myoepithelioma, chordoma), or hyalinized to chondromyxoid stroma (e.g., chondroid lipoma, myoepithelioma, EHE).

Immunohistochemistry

Immunohistochemistry is required for the evaluation of most epithelioid mesenchymal tumors, not only for tumor typing and subtyping but also to exclude nonmesenchymal tumors, such as metastatic carcinoma, metastatic melanoma, lymphoma, paraganglioma, and malignant mesothelioma.

The immunoprofiles of the most common epithelioid tumors of soft tissue are summarized in Table 6.1.

Cytogenetics

Some sarcomas that show an epithelioid appearance bear specific translocations (see also Chapter 18), which can be detected with conventional karyotyping, fluorescence in situ hybridization (FISH), or reverse transcriptase-polymerase chain reaction (RT-PCR) (Table 6.2).

Epithelioid Hemangioma

Originally described as *angiolymphoid hyperplasia with eosinophilia*, epithelioid hemangioma is an unusual benign vascular neoplasm occurring mostly in the skin but also occasionally in deep soft tissue, bone, and viscera.[1,2] It is unrelated to Kimura disease, with which it has previously been confused.[3–5] Epithelioid hemangioma is also discussed in Chapter 13.

Clinical Features

Epithelioid hemangioma mostly affects adults 20 to 40 years of age, who are predominantly women. This tumor type has a predilection for the head and neck region, especially around the ear. Lesions are superficial, may be solitary or multiple (20% of cases), and present clinically as small (≤1 cm), sometimes ulcerated, bluish nodules.[1,2]

Table 6.2 Chromosomal Abnormalities of Diagnostic Relevance in Epithelioid Tumors of Soft Tissue

Sarcoma Type	Main Chromosomal or Molecular Abnormalities	Genes Involved
Synovial sarcoma	t(X;18)(p11;q11)	*SS18-SSX1/SSX2*
Extraskeletal myxoid chondrosarcoma	t(9;22)(q22;q12) t(9;17)(q22;q11) t(9;15)(q22;q21)	*EWSR1-NR4A3* *RBP56-NR4A3* *TCF12-NR4A3*
Myoepithelial tumors	t(1;22)(q23;q12) t(19;22)(q13;q12) t(6;22)(p21;q12)	*EWSR1-PBX1* *EWSR1-ZNF444* *EWSR1-POU5F1*
Clear cell sarcoma	t(12;22)(q13;q12) t(2;22)(q32.3;q12)	*ATF1-EWSR1* *CREB1-EWSR1*
Malignant rhabdoid tumor	Mutations, deletions	*SMARCB1 (INI1)*
Alveolar soft part sarcoma	t(X;17)(p11.2;q25)	*ASPSCR1-TFE3*
Desmoplastic small round cell tumor	t(11;22)(p13;q12)	*WT1-EWSR1*
Dedifferentiated liposarcoma	Ring and giant marker chromosomes (amplification of 12q13-15)	*MDM2, CDK4*
Gastrointestinal stromal tumor	Mutations, deletions	*KIT, PDGFRA*
Sclerosing epithelioid fibrosarcoma	t(11;22)(p11.2;q12.2) t(7;22)(q33;q12.2) t(7;16)(q33;p11)	*EWSR1-CREB3L1* *EWSR1-CREB3L2* *FUS-CREB3L1*
Proximal-type epithelioid sarcoma	Deletions, mutations	*SMARCB1 (INI1)* Rarely *SMARCA4*
Epithelioid hemangioendothelioma	t(1;3)(p36;q25) t(X;11)(p11;q22)	*WWTR1-CAMTA1* *YAP1-TFE3*

Pathologic Features

Epithelioid hemangioma is a circumscribed lesion of the dermis and subcutis. It is rarely found in deep soft tissue. In this situation, it tends to be larger, shows a more infiltrative growth pattern, and frequently develops around a large vein.

Histologically, epithelioid hemangioma is a lobulated lesion composed of a variable admixture of small capillary-sized vessels, bland epithelioid cells, and inflammatory cells (Figs. 6.3 and 6.4). Small vessels tend to aggregate around a central larger parent vessel, similar to pyogenic granuloma. Endothelial cells that line the vessels have prominent epithelioid cytology and tend to protrude into the lumina in a hobnail fashion, resembling tombstones (Fig. 6.5). The cytoplasm is copious, eosinophilic to amphophilic, and sometimes vacuolated. Nuclei are small and vesicular, often with small central nucleoli. There is no significant cytologic atypia or necrosis, and mitotic figures are scarce. Some epithelioid hemangiomas are densely cellular, and the underlying vascular architecture may be difficult to appreciate (Figs. 6.6 and 6.7A). Many epithelioid hemangiomas are associated with a prominent inflammatory component composed predominantly of eosinophils, but also of lymphocytes, mast cells, and plasma cells. Lymphoid aggregates may be observed in long-standing lesions.

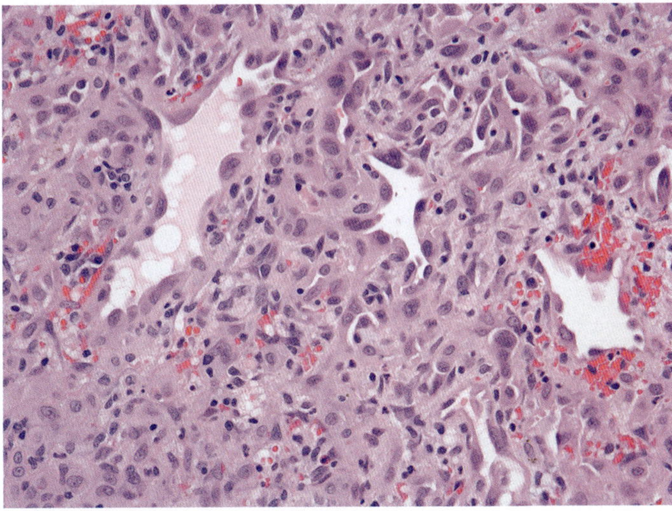

Figure 6.5 Epithelioid Hemangioma. Epithelioid endothelial cells with eosinophilic cytoplasm protrude into the vessel lumina.

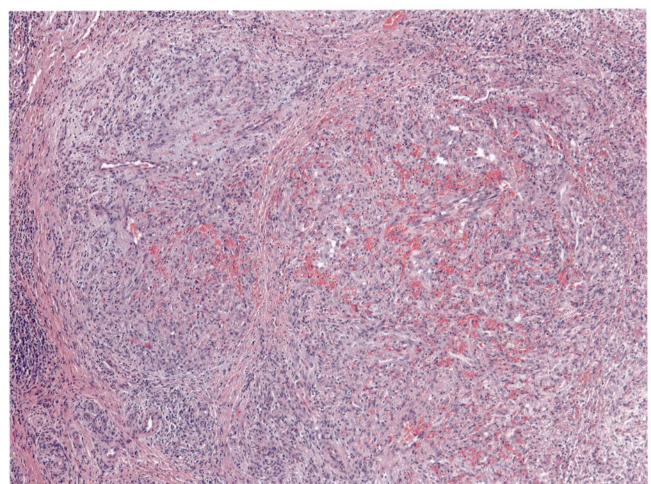

Figure 6.3 Epithelioid Hemangioma. The tumor typically shows a multinodular appearance.

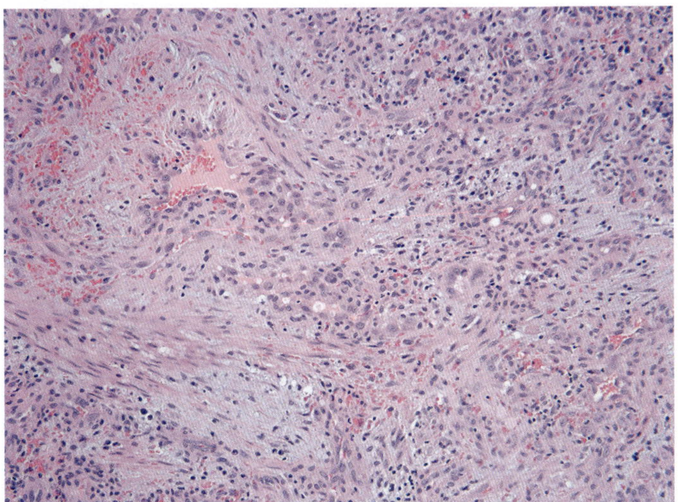

Figure 6.4 Epithelioid Hemangioma. Small- to medium-sized blood vessels are lined by epithelioid endothelial cells. Note the scattered lymphocytes.

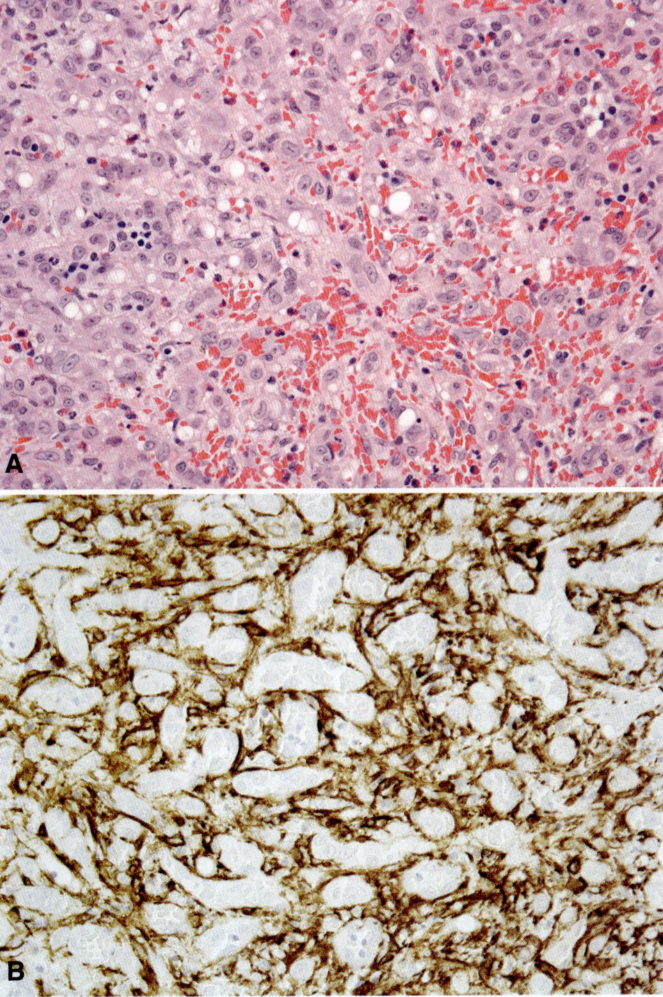

Figure 6.6 Cellular Epithelioid Hemangioma. (A) The tumor is composed of epithelioid endothelial cells. The architecture is difficult to appreciate. Note the scattered lymphocytes and eosinophils. (B) Smooth muscle actin stains the pericytic component and highlights the well-formed blood vessels.

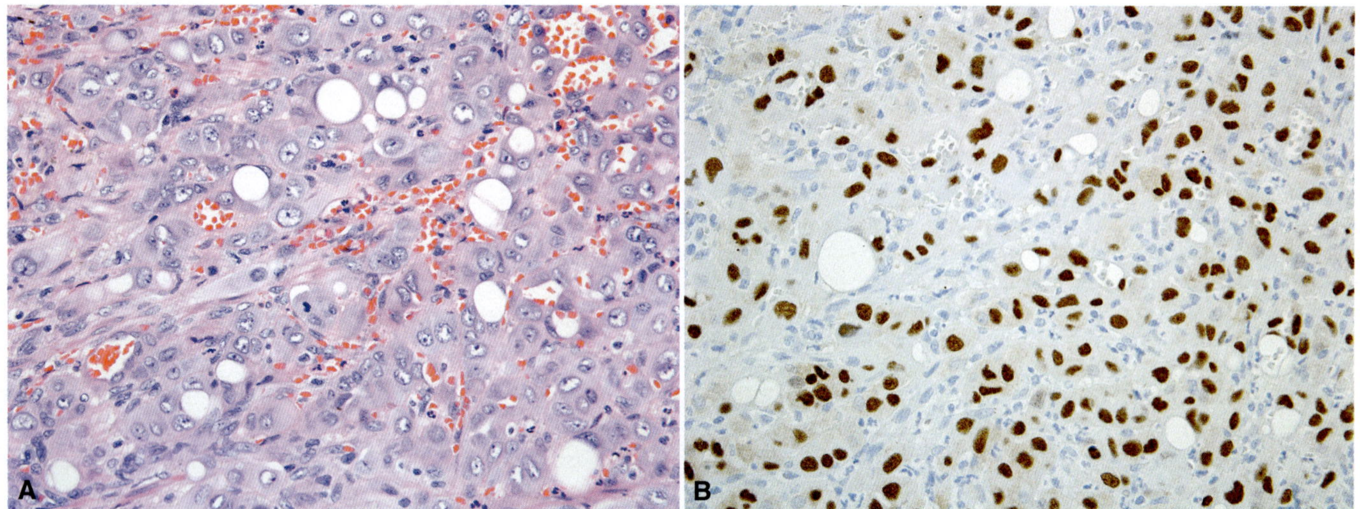

Figure 6.7 Cellular Epithelioid Hemangioma. (A) The tumor is composed of large epithelioid cells with glassy eosinophilic cytoplasm. Note the scattered cytoplasmic vacuoles. (B) Strong nuclear expression of FOSB is observed in more than 50% of cases. This finding can help distinguish epithelioid hemangioma from malignant epithelioid endothelial neoplasms.

Occasionally, larger blood vessels with muscular walls showing myxoid change are observed within the lesion. Origin from a muscular artery or a vein is sometimes evident.

Intravascular epithelioid hemangioma is a rare variant of epithelioid hemangioma in which endothelial cells proliferate within a large vein. This lesion was originally called *intravenous atypical vascular proliferation*.[6] Epithelioid angiomatous nodule is a benign cutaneous lesion that shows some morphologic overlap with epithelioid hemangioma (see Chapter 13).[7] It develops mostly on the trunk (50% of cases) and extremities (30%). Morphologically, it differs from conventional epithelioid hemangioma in that it has a more solid growth pattern, and prominent nucleoli are often seen (Fig. 6.8). At the periphery of the lesion, well-formed blood vessels and hemosiderin deposition may be present. Mitotic activity may be identified. Despite these worrisome features, the behavior is entirely benign.

Immunohistochemistry

Epithelioid cells in epithelioid hemangioma react with vascular markers, namely CD31, CD34, ERG, and FLI1. CD31 is more sensitive than CD34. On occasion, epithelioid cells may focally express keratins (10% of cases).[1,2] Overexpression of FOSB is seen in approximately 50% of epithelioid hemangiomas, reflecting the presence of *FOSB* rearrangements (see Fig. 6.7B).[8,9] Reactivity for FOSB is also observed in pseudomyogenic hemangioendothelioma, due to the presence of a *SERPINE1-FOSB* fusion gene,[10] but not in other epithelioid vascular tumors; therefore, FOSB may be helpful in distinguishing epithelioid hemangioma from EHE.

Molecular Genetics

Recently, *FOSB* gene rearrangements have been identified in approximately 20% of epithelioid hemangiomas across different anatomic locations and histologic variants; however, the highest prevalence is seen in cellular and intraosseous lesions.[9] Fusion partners identified to date include *ZFP36* and *LMNA*. The recurrent fusion *ZFP36-FOSB* is seen in cases with increased cellularity, necrosis, and cytologic atypia; these lesions are often penile in location. To date, *FOSB* gene rearrangements have not been identified in the subset of epithelioid hemangiomas with features of angiolymphoid hyperplasia with eosinophilia, suggesting a distinct pathogenesis for this particular subtype (although immunohistochemistry for FOSB is positive in such lesions). Another 30% of epithelioid hemangiomas harbor *FOS* gene rearrangements (with a range of fusion partners), most often in soft tissue and bone lesions.[11,12]

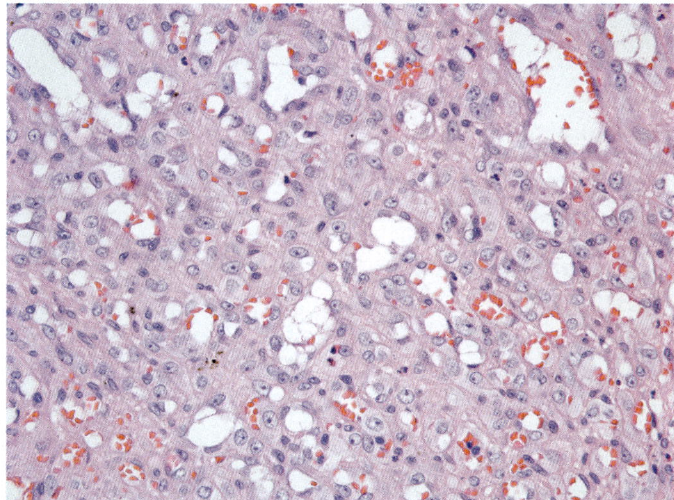

Figure 6.8 Epithelioid Angiomatous Nodule. The lesion is composed of sheets of uniform epithelioid endothelial cells with prominent nucleoli.

Differential Diagnosis

Refer to Box 6.11 for the differential diagnosis of epithelioid hemangioma.

Bacillary angiomatosis is composed of epithelioid cells and blood vessels, bearing some resemblance to pyogenic granuloma. The lesion contains numerous neutrophils and easily overlooked clusters of bacteria.

EHE is larger and more atypical cytologically than epithelioid hemangioma. Capillary-sized vessels and a prominent inflammatory infiltrate are not features of EHE. In contrast to epithelioid hemangioma, tumor cells in EHE are arranged in cords and nests and are characteristically set in a distinctive chondroid-to-myxohyaline matrix. Around 90% of EHE cases show nuclear expression of CAMTA1, due to the

Box 6.11 Differential Diagnosis of Epithelioid Hemangioma

Bacillary angiomatosis
Epithelioid fibrous histiocytoma
Epithelioid schwannoma
Epithelioid hemangioendothelioma
Epithelioid angiosarcoma
Myoepithelioma
Carcinoma
Melanoma

presence of the *WWTR1-CAMTA1* fusion gene; CAMTA1 expression is not seen in epithelioid hemangioma.[13,14]

Solid forms of epithelioid hemangioma may be confused with epithelioid angiosarcoma, epithelioid sarcoma, and myoepithelioma with plasmacytoid (hyaline cell) features. Epithelioid angiosarcoma is composed of large epithelioid cells with prominent nucleoli. The presence of marked nuclear atypia and sheetlike growth distinguishes epithelioid angiosarcoma from epithelioid hemangioma. Foci of necrosis and a high mitotic rate are common in epithelioid angiosarcoma.

Epithelioid sarcoma is composed of epithelioid and occasionally spindle cells in varying proportions. In contrast to epithelioid hemangioma, epithelioid sarcoma is often necrotic and infiltrative. In addition, tumor cells in epithelioid sarcoma are usually diffusely positive for keratins and epithelial membrane antigen (EMA). They can express CD34 but not CD31. Loss of INI1 (SMARCB1) expression is helpful to confirm the diagnosis of epithelioid sarcoma.

Myoepithelioma with hyaline cell (plasmacytoid) features may mimic epithelioid hemangioma. This lesion, however, expresses epithelial markers, S-100 protein, and often SOX10 and is negative for CD31 and CD34.

Kimura disease has been confused with epithelioid hemangioma, although these lesions are histologically dissimilar and unrelated.[3–5] Kimura disease affects mainly young Asian men and presents as a combination of a soft tissue mass, lymphadenopathy, systemic eosinophilia, elevated serum immunoglobulin E, and various other immunologic disorders. This lesion, which often involves the skin and deep soft tissues of the head and neck region, is a pseudotumor composed of an admixture of dense lymphoid aggregates with prominent germinal centers, an eosinophilic infiltrate including eosinophilic microabscesses, small blood vessels, and fibrosis. As opposed to epithelioid hemangioma, there are no vessels lined by epithelioid endothelial cells in Kimura disease.

Prognosis and Treatment

Epithelioid hemangioma may recur locally (in 30% of cases) but does not metastasize. Complete surgical excision is the treatment of choice.

Glomus Tumor

Accounting for approximately 0.5% to 1.5% of soft tissue tumors, glomus tumors may present in two different forms: a sporadic form, where the lesion is usually solitary, and a familial form, which tends to occur in children as multifocal lesions associated with dilated veins (*glomuvenous malformation*; see Chapter 13).[1]

Clinical Features

In the sporadic form, glomus tumors present as solitary lesions of the distal extremities of middle-aged adults. There is a female predominance (female-to-male ratio, 3 : 1) in patients with subungual lesions. Glomus tumors are often exquisitely painful and are sensitive to cold and tactile stimuli. They are usually found in subungual locations, although they can also be observed in the deep dermis or subcutis of the hands, wrists, forearms, and feet. Glomus tumors are rare in deep soft tissues. Rarely, they are observed at other sites, such as the nasal cavity, trachea, stomach, and bone.

In the familial form, glomus tumors and glomangiomas (also known as *glomuvenous malformations*) are multifocal and may be diffusely infiltrative (glomangiomatosis); such lesions occur predominantly in children. These tumors are sometimes painful and rarely subungual. They can be congenital and are usually seen in the superficial soft tissues of the arms and legs.

Pathologic Features

Glomus tumors often develop as small blue-red nodules measuring less than 1 cm when superficially located. Histologically, they are composed of a variable admixture of three components: small, rounded, uniform epithelioid cells, often with punched-out nuclei and sharply defined cytoplasmic borders; small, capillary-sized vessels, surrounded by the glomus cells; and smooth muscle bundles sometimes associated with thick-walled blood vessels (Fig. 6.9). Hyaline or myxoid stroma is relatively common (Fig. 6.10). Cytologic atypia and mitotic activity are not observed in benign glomus tumors.

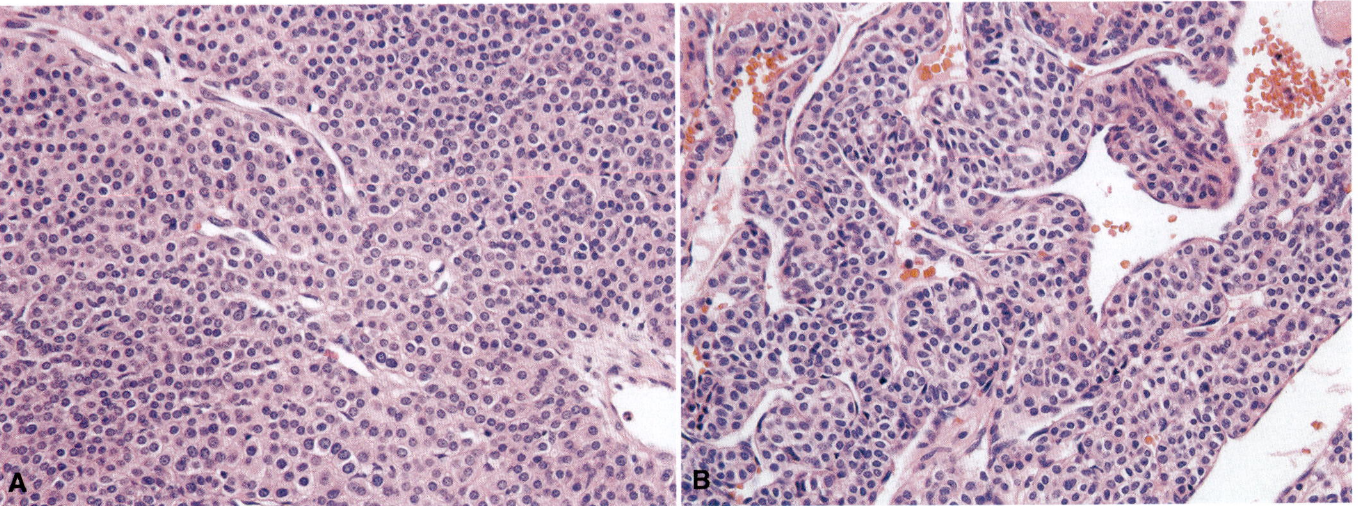

Figure 6.9 Glomus Tumor. (A) The tumor is composed of rounded cells with sharply defined cell borders. (B) Glomus tumor with prominent branching thin-walled vessels. The tumor cells are situated beneath the endothelium.

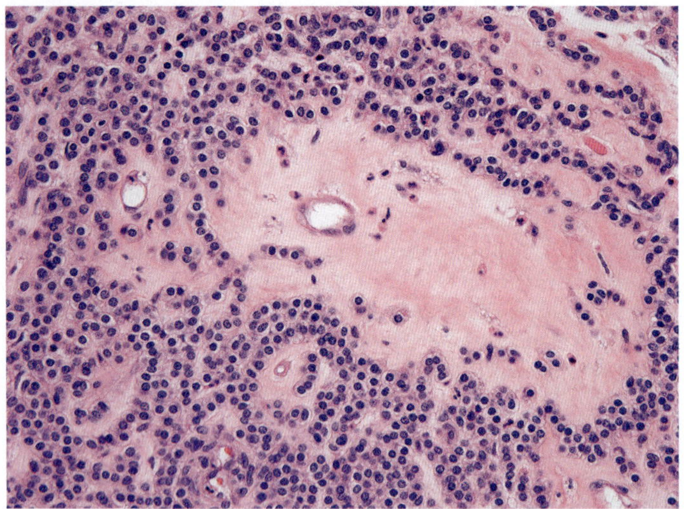

Figure 6.10 Glomus Tumor. This tumor contains hyalinized stroma. Note the uniform cytology and clear cytoplasm.

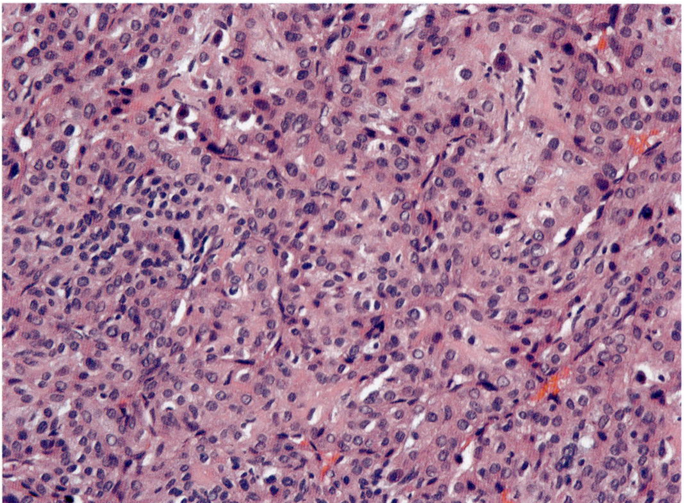

Figure 6.11 Epithelioid (Oncocytic) Glomus Tumor. The tumor cells contain brightly eosinophilic cytoplasm.

Some variants of glomus tumor with unusual histologic features are recognized. Epithelioid (oncocytic) glomus tumor is a variant characterized by large polygonal epithelioid cells with abundant eosinophilic cytoplasm and large nuclei, sometimes admixed with spindle cell areas (Fig. 6.11).[15]

Symplastic glomus tumor shows degenerative nuclear atypia (analogous to symplastic leiomyoma).

The rare malignant glomus tumors may be composed of sheets of round cells with marked nuclear atypia and mitotic activity (see "Prognosis and Treatment") or fascicles of atypical spindle cells, sometimes mimicking leiomyosarcoma; the latter group of tumors is difficult to recognize unless there is a conventional glomus tumor component.

Glomangioma is a lesion characterized by dilated cavernous venous structures (resembling those of a cavernous hemangioma), surrounded by a thin rim of glomus cells (also known as *glomuvenous malformation*) (Fig. 6.12). This form is predominantly observed in familial glomus tumors.

Glomangiomyoma has morphologic features identical to those of conventional glomus tumor or glomangioma, in addition to the presence of well-developed smooth muscle and large vessel components (Fig. 6.13). The elongated smooth muscle cells appear to arise from large vessel walls and may show a gradual transition to conventional small round glomus cells.

Glomangiopericytoma (also called *myopericytoma* or *perivascular myoma*) shares features of conventional glomus tumor, glomangiomyoma, and vascular leiomyoma (angioleiomyoma) (Fig. 6.14). It belongs to the spectrum of lesions showing perivascular myoid differentiation along with myofibroma.[16] Glomangiopericytoma occurs predominantly in the superficial soft tissues of the distal extremities, often the wrist and ankle (see Chapter 3).[16,17]

Glomus coccygeum corresponds to a prominent or hyperplastic glomus structure located at the ventral tip of the coccyx. Rarely, a true glomus tumor may develop from this structure.[18]

Immunohistochemistry

Glomus cells show strong reactivity for smooth muscle actin (Fig. 6.15), muscle-specific actin, and h-caldesmon. Desmin is occasionally positive (up to 20% of cases), usually only focally. Glomus cells can also be focally CD34 positive. S-100 protein, CD31, and epithelial markers are negative. Tumor cells are surrounded by pericellular basement membrane

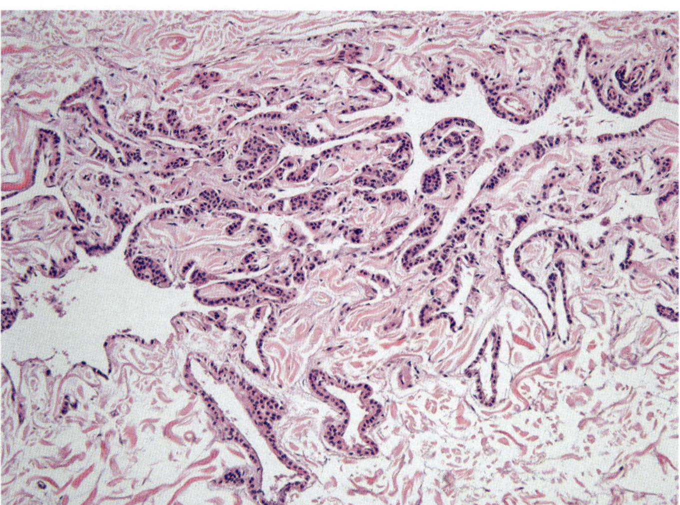

Figure 6.12 Glomangioma (Glomuvenous Malformation). The lesion is composed of dilated cavernous venous structures surrounded by glomus cells.

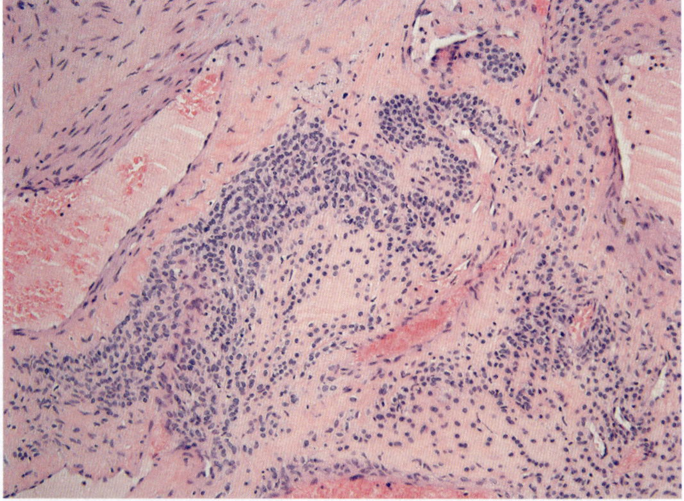

Figure 6.13 Glomangiomyoma. Glomus cells between thick-walled blood vessels with a prominent smooth muscle component.

material, which can be visualized with antibodies against collagen IV and laminin, although these are rarely used for diagnosis.

Molecular Genetics

NOTCH gene rearrangements occur in approximately 60% of glomus tumors. *NOTCH2* rearrangements predominate and are identified in most malignant glomus tumors, whereas *NOTCH1* and *NOTCH3* rearrangements are found in a small subset of predominantly benign glomus tumors.[19] *MIR143* has been identified as a fusion partner with *NOTCH* in some cases. *BRAF* V600E and *KRAS* mutations have been reported in a few glomus tumor cases.[20]

Differential Diagnosis

A cellular, epithelioid glomus tumor may occasionally be confused with a solid variant of nodular hidradenoma (Fig. 6.16). In contrast to a glomus tumor, nodular hidradenoma is positive for keratins, EMA, and carcinoembryonic antigen.

Unlike glomus tumors, intradermal melanocytic nevus (including the pseudovascular variant) is composed of S-100 protein–positive cells.

A carcinoma can be excluded based on clinical findings, reactivity for keratin and EMA, and negativity for smooth muscle actin.

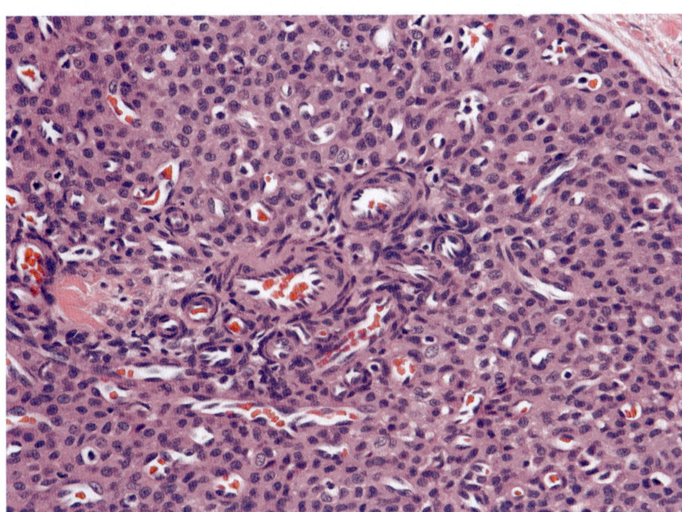

Figure 6.14 Glomangiopericytoma. In this myopericytoma, many perivascular cells show glomoid morphologic features.

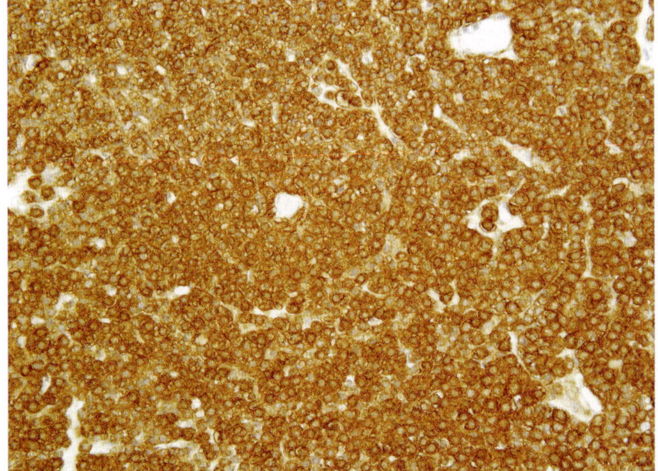

Figure 6.15 Glomus Tumor. Strong and diffuse expression of smooth muscle actin by tumor cells.

Conventional cavernous hemangioma may superficially resemble glomangioma. However, unlike conventional cavernous hemangioma, glomangioma shows a thin rim of glomus cells situated around the vascular spaces.

Glomus tumors showing a well-developed smooth muscle component or prominent hemangiopericytoma-like features may be confused with myofibroma, infantile myofibromatosis, or myopericytoma. This distinction is of little importance, however, because these entities are related, benign lesions that lie on a morphologic continuum (Box 6.12).[16,17]

Prognosis and Treatment

Glomus tumors may recur locally (10% of cases, especially infiltrative lesions). Malignant glomus tumors are exceptional and include (1) glomus tumors showing marked nuclear atypia along with any mitotic activity and (2) those containing atypical mitotic figures.[1,21] In a study by Folpe and colleagues, metastases developed in 38% of patients with malignant glomus tumors (defined by these criteria).[21]

Glomus tumors of "uncertain malignant potential" have been defined as superficial lesions lacking nuclear atypia but containing numerous mitoses (>5 per 50 high-power fields), large (>2 cm) glomus tumors, and deep-seated glomus tumors. Glomus tumors with these features usually behave in a benign fashion.

Myoepithelioma/Mixed Tumor/Myoepithelial Carcinoma of Soft Tissue

Well known in salivary glands, mixed tumors (pleomorphic adenomas), myoepitheliomas, and myoepithelial carcinomas can also arise primarily

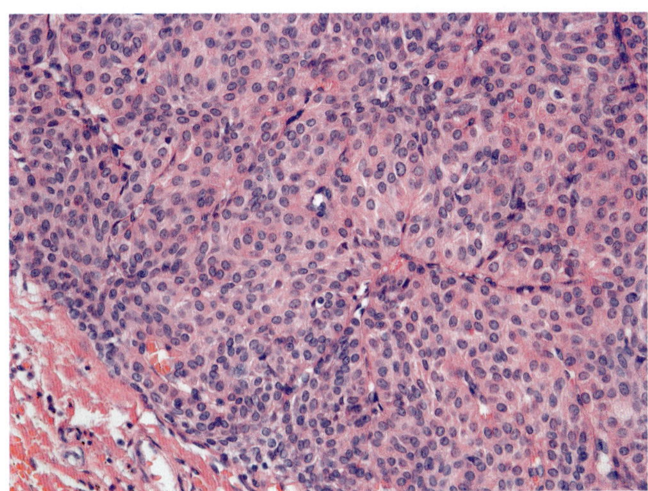

Figure 6.16 Nodular Hidradenoma. This tumor may be confused with a glomus tumor.

Box 6.12 Differential Diagnosis of Glomus Tumor

Conventional Solid Glomus Tumor

Adnexal tumor (hidradenoma [solid form], eccrine spiradenoma)
Carcinoma (metastasis)
Meningioma (cutaneous)
Intradermal nevus (pseudovascular nevus)
Epithelioid leiomyoma

Glomangioma

Cavernous hemangioma

Glomangiomyoma/Glomangiopericytoma

Myofibroma/myofibromatosis
Leiomyoma and vascular leiomyoma (angioleiomyoma)

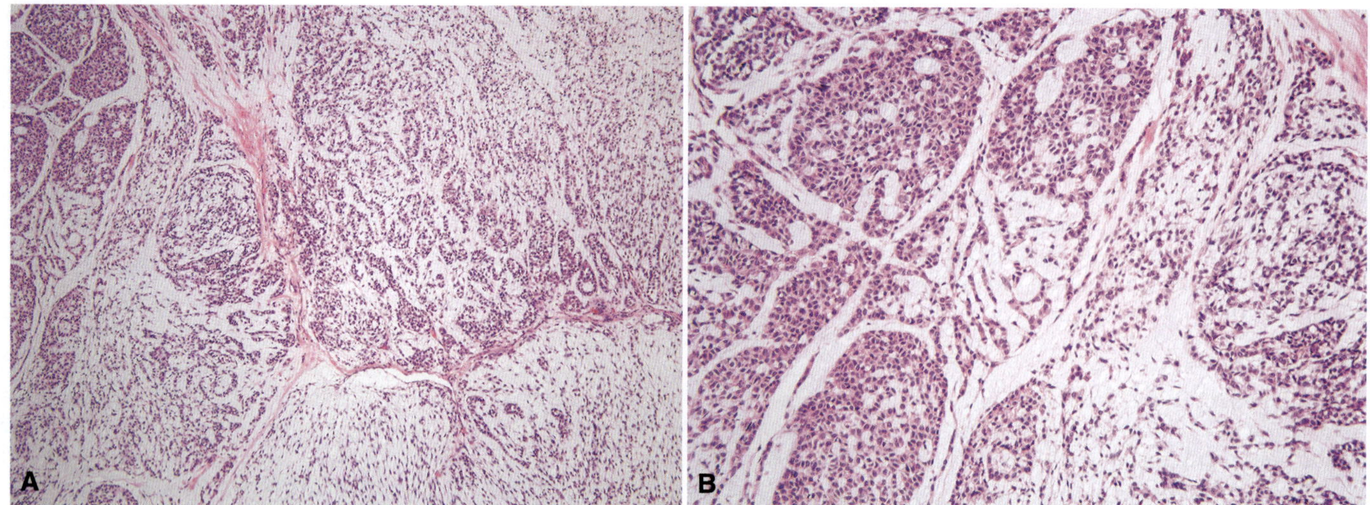

Figure 6.17 Myoepithelioma of Soft Tissue. (A) The tumor shows a lobulated architecture. Note the prominent myxoid stroma. (B) The tumor cells contain eosinophilic cytoplasm and show a reticular to trabecular architecture.

in soft tissue and bone.[22–26] Chondroid syringoma, a mixed tumor of the skin, has been incorporated into the spectrum of cutaneous neoplasms that show myoepithelial differentiation (see Chapter 15). Parachordoma, a rare soft tissue tumor described by Dabska in 1977, is a morphologic variant of soft tissue myoepithelioma.[1] Myoepithelial neoplasms of soft tissue range from benign to aggressive malignant tumors. Several criteria have been proposed to assess their malignant potential (see the discussion of prognosis). Myoepithelial tumors are also discussed in Chapters 5 and 9.

Clinical Features

Myoepitheliomas of soft tissue develop predominantly in the limbs (65% of cases) and limb girdles (shoulder, thigh, inguinal region) of middle-aged adults (median age, 40 to 50 years), with a slight male predominance (male-to-female ratio, 1.3 : 1). The trunk, head and neck, and visceral soft tissue are less frequently involved.[22–25] Myoepithelial tumors are most often located in the subcutis (60%); a minority arise in deep soft tissue (intramuscular or subfascial). Most patients present with a painless mass.

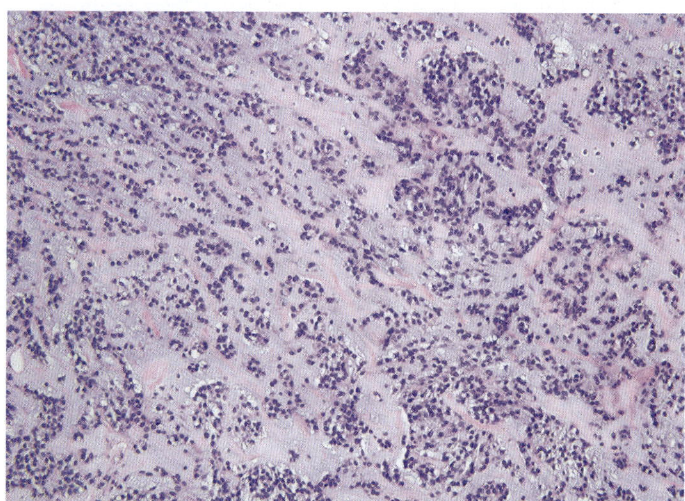

Figure 6.18 Myoepithelioma of Soft Tissue. The tumor is composed of epithelioid cells with a trabecular architecture in a chondromyxoid stroma.

Pathologic Features

Grossly, most myoepithelial neoplasms of soft tissue are well circumscribed and nodular, although a subset of tumors show infiltrative borders or satellite nodules. The mean size of benign tumors is 4 cm, compared with 6 cm for malignant lesions, with a wide range in size (1 to 20 cm).[22] Gelatinous/myxoid areas are common. Areas of calcification or ossification may be seen. Necrosis is rare.

Histologically, myoepithelial tumors of soft tissue are heterogeneous, paralleling mixed tumors of salivary glands. Characteristically, they show a lobulated architecture (Fig. 6.17), and are composed of a variable admixture of cords, strands, and nests of epithelioid to spindled cells, set in a hyalinized to chondromyxoid matrix (Fig. 6.18; see also Fig. 6.17). Some tumors are composed predominantly of spindle cells, whereas others are epithelioid in appearance. Epithelioid myoepithelial cells may be large, with abundant clear to eosinophilic cytoplasm (Figs. 6.19 and 6.20). Occasionally, tumor cells may have a plasmacytoid appearance, with prominent hyaline cytoplasmic inclusions (Fig. 6.21). Metaplastic cartilage or bone is detected in 10% to 15% of cases. Approximately 10% of myoepitheliomas show ductal differentiation; such tumors can alternatively be referred to as *mixed tumors of soft tissue* (see also Chapter 9). An adipocytic component, squamous differentiation, osteoclastic giant cells, amianthoid collagen fibers, and tyrosine crystals are additional uncommon morphologic features.

Myoepithelial carcinomas of soft tissue are usually larger than benign lesions and show a variable degree of nuclear atypia (see Figs. 6.19 and 6.20), along with mitotic activity and tumor necrosis (40% of cases; see "Prognosis and Treatment").[22,25,26] Myoepithelial carcinomas may contain an undifferentiated round cell component, particularly in children. In a small number of cases, a malignant heterologous mesenchymal component (osteosarcoma or chondrosarcoma) may be present (*malignant mixed tumor*). Unlike myoepithelial carcinomas of the salivary glands, a benign precursor lesion is rarely identified in myoepithelial carcinomas of soft tissue.

Immunohistochemistry

By immunohistochemistry, tumor cells of myoepitheliomas of soft tissue usually express epithelial markers, such as broad-spectrum keratins (90% to 95% of cases), EMA (60%), and S-100 protein (80% to 90%) (Fig. 6.22).[22–25] Calponin (80% to 90%), glial fibrillary acidic protein (GFAP) (40% to 50%), smooth muscle actin (35% to 40%), and desmin (10% to 15%) can also be expressed.[22,25] p63 is positive in 20% to 40%

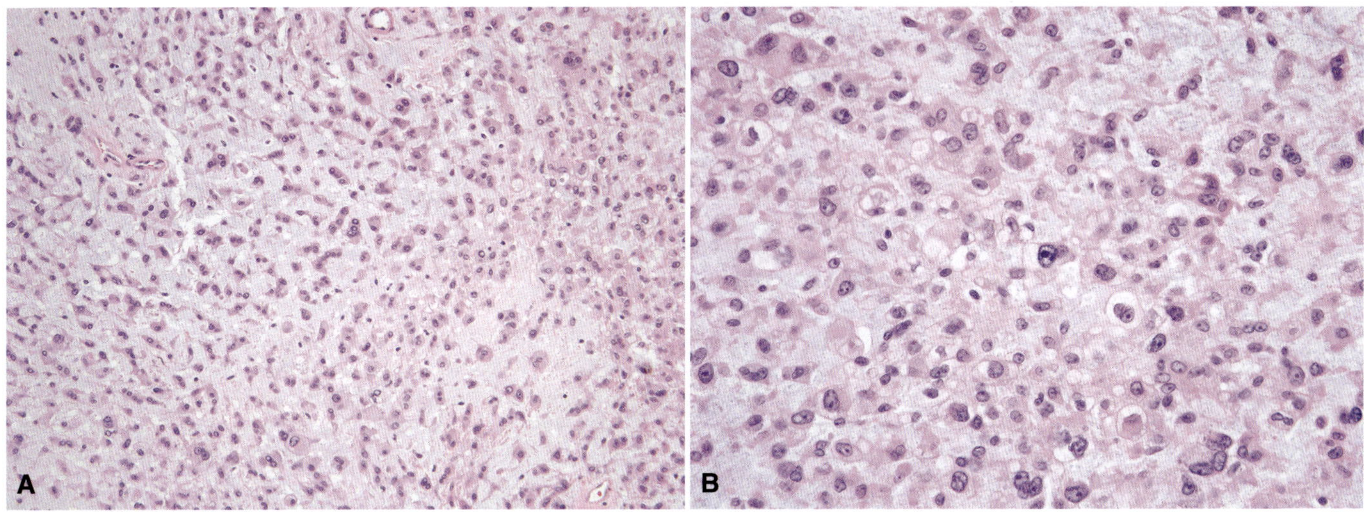

Figure 6.19 Myoepithelial Carcinoma of Soft Tissue. (A) The tumor is composed of cords and nests of large epithelioid cells in a myxoid stroma. (B) The epithelioid tumor cells have abundant eosinophilic cytoplasm. Note the prominent nucleoli.

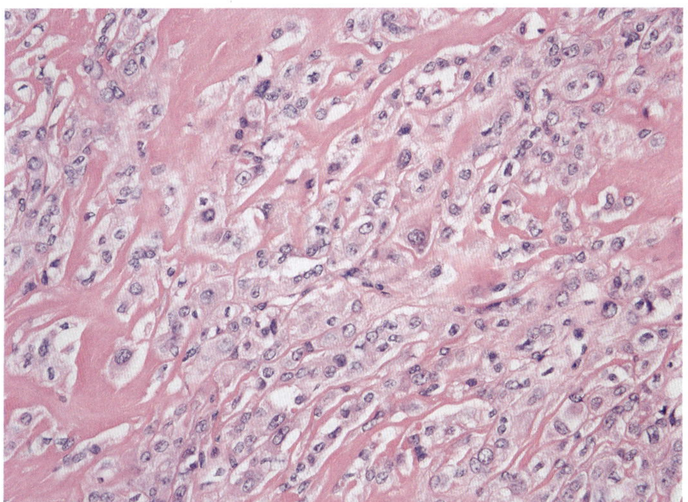

Figure 6.20 Myoepithelial Carcinoma of Soft Tissue. This tumor is composed of nests of epithelioid cells with abundant palely eosinophilic cytoplasm in a hyalinized stroma.

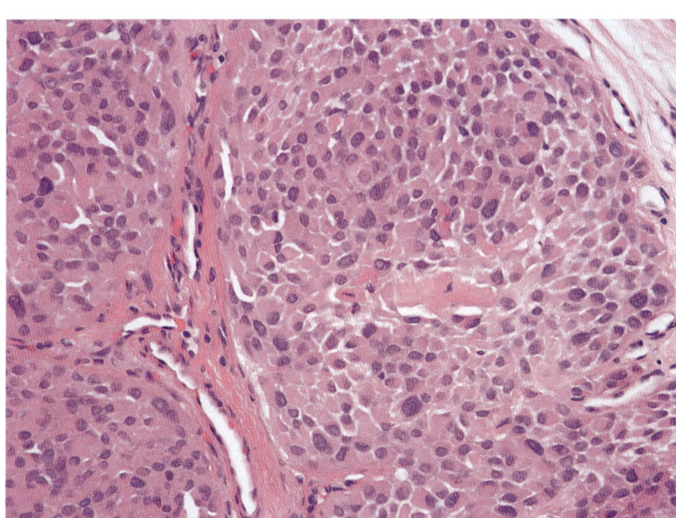

Figure 6.21 Myoepithelioma. This tumor shows plasmacytoid morphology with hyaline cytoplasmic inclusions.

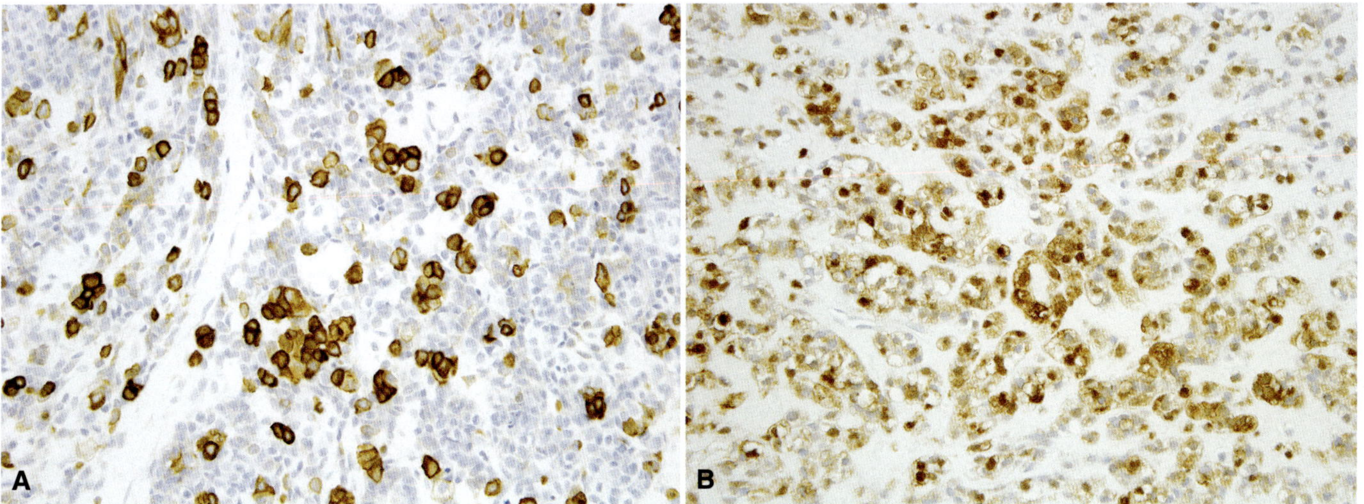

Figure 6.22 Myoepithelioma of Soft Tissue. Tumor cells are usually positive for both keratins (A) and S-100 protein (B).

of cases.[22,25] SOX10 is positive in most soft tissue myoepitheliomas, but less often in myoepithelial carcinomas.[27] A subset of myoepithelial carcinomas of soft tissue shows loss of expression of INI1 (SMARCB1), most often in pediatric cases (up to 40%).[26]

Molecular Genetics

The genetic profile of soft tissue myoepitheliomas appears heterogeneous.[28,29] Rearrangements of the *EWSR1* gene have been detected in approximately 50% of myoepithelial tumors of skin and soft tissue, involving diverse fusion partners: *POU5F1* (6p21), *PBX1* (1q23), *ZNF444* (19q23), *ATF1* (12q13), *PBX3* (9q33), and *KLF17* (1p34); these genes only account for a subset of tumors with *EWSR1* rearrangement.[29–32] A subset of myoepithelial tumors that lack *EWSR1* rearrangement instead have alternative *FUS* rearrangement.[31,33] Similar to their salivary gland counterparts, mixed tumors of skin and soft tissue often harbor *PLAG1* rearrangements.[34] *EWSR1* and *PLAG1* rearrangements are mutually exclusive.

Differential Diagnosis

In deep soft tissues, myoepithelioma should be differentiated primarily from EMC, metastatic chordoma, ossifying fibromyxoid tumor (OFMT), epithelioid schwannoma, and chondroid lipoma. Tumors predominantly composed of myoepithelial cells that display a plasmacytoid or rhabdoid appearance may be confused with metastatic carcinoma, metastatic melanoma, or sarcomas with epithelioid morphology (e.g., epithelioid sarcoma, epithelioid MPNST, EHE, or epithelioid angiosarcoma) (Box 6.13).

Box 6.13 Differential Diagnosis of Myoepithelioma of Soft Tissue

- Extraskeletal myxoid chondrosarcoma
- Ossifying fibromyxoid tumor
- Epithelioid schwannoma
- Chondroid lipoma
- Chondroma of soft tissue
- Chordoma
- Epithelioid sarcoma
- Epithelioid hemangioendothelioma and angiosarcoma
- Epithelioid malignant peripheral nerve sheath tumor
- Carcinoma (metastasis)
- Melanoma (metastasis)

EMC is a lobulated neoplasm composed of cords and strands of small epithelioid cells in an abundant myxoid matrix. Tumor cells, which are arranged in a reticular or sometimes pseudoacinar pattern (Fig. 6.23A) and tend to accumulate at the periphery of tumor lobules, can be epithelioid or rhabdoid, particularly in high-grade cases (see Fig. 6.23B). By immunohistochemistry, a subset of EMCs express S-100 protein (20% of cases) less consistently than myoepithelioma, and S-100 protein expression is usually only focal. Most EMCs are negative for epithelial markers, although occasional cases can show scattered cells positive for EMA and smooth muscle actin or GFAP. EMC bears specific reciprocal translocations, most commonly the t(9;22)(q22;q12) translocation involving *NR4A3* and *EWSR1*, less often t(9;17)(q22;q11) involving *NR4A3* and *TAF2N*, and rarely other translocations involving *NR4A3*, chromosomal abnormalities that are not observed in myoepithelioma. However, because some myoepithelial tumors harbor *EWSR1* rearrangements, FISH for *EWSR1* cannot distinguish between these tumor types.

Metastatic chordoma may closely resemble soft tissue myoepitheliomas, with epithelioid cells that have abundant cytoplasm (Fig. 6.24) and usually express epithelial markers and S-100 protein. However, chordomas are uniform, whereas myoepithelial tumors characteristically show considerable intratumoral heterogeneity with reticular and solid areas as well as mixed epithelioid and spindle cell components. Chordomas are consistently positive for brachyury. Very rarely, chordoma can arise primarily at extraaxial sites, exceptionally in soft tissue ("chordoma periphericum").[35,36] Such tumors are indistinguishable from metastatic chordoma; the clinical history is therefore essential.

In OFMT, the tumor cells are uniform and bland, with round to ovoid nuclei, arranged in cords within a variably fibromyxoid matrix. Most lesions (80%) are surrounded by a characteristic rim of mature lamellar bone. Tumor cells in OFMT usually express S-100 protein (70% of cases), and in 50% of cases desmin is positive. Occasionally, GFAP and smooth muscle actin may be focally positive. In contrast to myoepithelioma, OFMT is generally negative for keratins and EMA.

Epithelioid schwannoma is a well-circumscribed lobulated neoplasm, composed of nests and trabeculae of bland, small, rounded Schwann cells with abundant eosinophilic cytoplasm.[37,38] The extracellular matrix may be myxoid or fibrillary. Tumor cells are strikingly positive for S-100 protein but negative for epithelial markers, in contrast to myoepitheliomas.

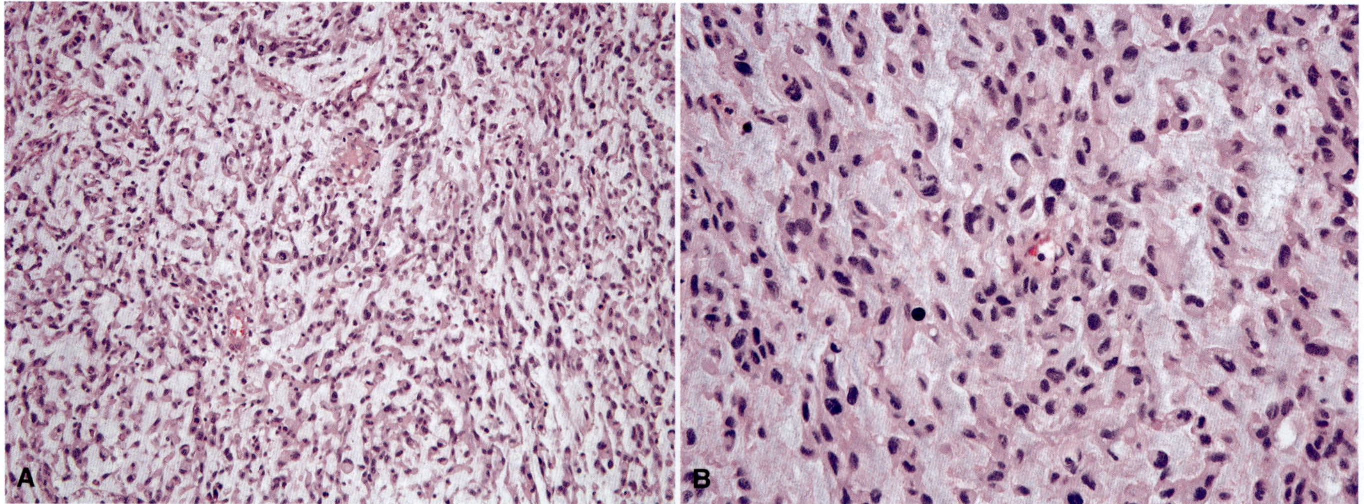

Figure 6.23 High-Grade Extraskeletal Myxoid Chondrosarcoma. (A) The tumor shows a trabecular architecture with abundant myxoid stroma. (B) In cases with high-grade features, the tumor cells may show epithelioid morphology with eosinophilic cytoplasm.

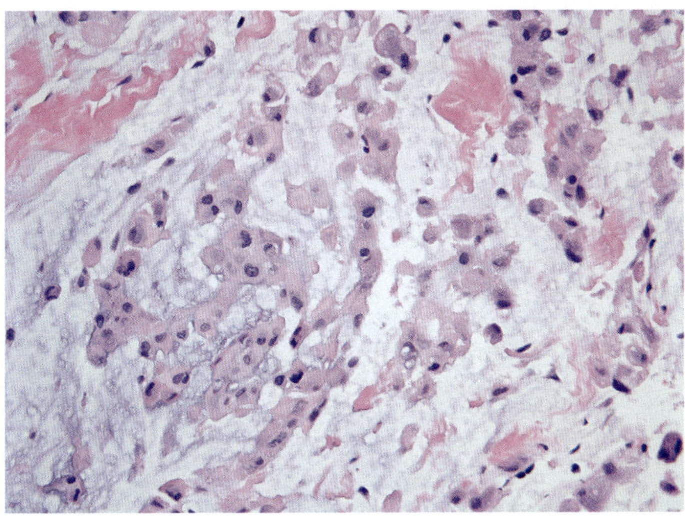

Figure 6.24 Chordoma. The tumor is composed of cords of large epithelioid cells with abundant eosinophilic cytoplasm in a prominent myxoid matrix.

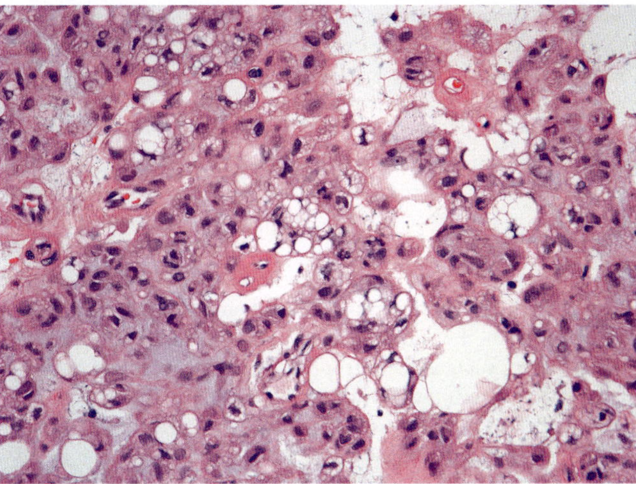

Figure 6.25 Chondroid Lipoma. Cords and sheets of large epithelioid cells and multivacuolated cells, embedded in a chondromyxoid matrix, admixed with mature adipocytes. This tumor type may resemble myoepithelioma or extraskeletal myxoid chondrosarcoma.

Chondroid lipoma is a benign adipocytic neoplasm that typically presents as a painless nodule in the subcutis or skeletal muscle of middle-aged adults, mostly women.[39] It usually involves the proximal extremities or limb girdles. Histologically, chondroid lipoma shows a lobulated growth pattern and is composed of a variable admixture of large uni- or multivacuolated lipoblast-like cells, cords and strands of finely vacuolated cells resembling hibernoma cells or chondroblasts, and mature adipocytes, set in a myxoid to hyalinized or chondroid matrix (Fig. 6.25). Tumor cells in chondroid lipoma are consistently immunoreactive for S-100 protein but negative for smooth muscle actin and EMA. Occasionally, keratins may be focally positive.

Myoepitheliomas showing prominent cartilaginous differentiation should be differentiated from soft tissue chondroma, which is composed solely of cartilaginous cells that are negative for epithelial markers.

Solid spindle cell myoepitheliomas may be confused with schwannomas or smooth muscle tumors of deep soft tissue.

Myoepithelial carcinomas of soft tissue should be differentiated primarily from epithelioid MPNST, high-grade EMC, sclerosing epithelioid fibrosarcoma (SEF), proximal-type epithelioid sarcoma, metastatic carcinoma, and metastatic melanoma (see Chapter 5).

Prognosis and Treatment

Myoepithelial tumors of soft tissue have the potential to recur and metastasize. Unlike myoepithelial tumors of salivary glands, infiltrative margins do not correlate with malignancy in myoepithelial neoplasms of soft tissue.[22] Myoepithelial tumors with moderate or severe nuclear atypia in the form of nuclear pleomorphism, vesicular or coarse chromatin, and prominent nucleoli should be classified as myoepithelial carcinomas.[17] Mitotic activity and tumor necrosis do not correlate with outcome.

Soft tissue myoepithelial carcinomas have a 35% to 40% local recurrence rate and a 30% to 40% metastatic rate.[22,25,26] The most common metastatic sites are the lungs, lymph nodes, bone, and soft tissue. Myoepithelial carcinomas of deep soft tissue and those at visceral sites have a worse prognosis than superficial lesions.[25,26] Myoepithelial tumors of soft tissue in children are much more likely to be malignant than those in adults.[26] Cytologically benign or low-grade lesions (myoepitheliomas) may recur locally (15% to 20% of cases), but do not metastasize, with rare exceptions.[22,25] All myoepithelial neoplasms should be completely excised with negative margins. The role of adjuvant chemotherapy or radiation therapy remains to be determined, although combination chemotherapy with carboplatin and paclitaxel shows promise for patients with metastatic disease.[40]

PEComa of Soft Tissue

The concept of neoplasms with perivascular epithelioid cell (PEC) differentiation was developed in 1992 by Bonetti and colleagues.[41,42] These authors observed that a group of neoplasms found at various locations were composed of cells that seemed to originate from the walls of blood vessels and showed distinctive morphologic, immunohistochemical, and ultrastructural characteristics, namely, features of both smooth muscle and melanocytic differentiation. They proposed the descriptive term PEC to describe these cells and proposed grouping the neoplasms composed of these cells under the term *PEComa*. Gradually, this family of tumors gained wide acceptance and now includes renal and extrarenal angiomyolipoma (AML), lymphangio(leio)myoma and lymphangio(leio)myomatosis (LAM), clear cell ("sugar") tumor (CCST) of the lungs and extrapulmonary sites, clear cell myomelanocytic tumor of the falciform ligament/ligamentum teres, and abdominopelvic sarcoma of PECs.[41–46] An association between the tuberous sclerosis complex (TSC) and some PEC neoplasms (e.g., AML, LAM) has also been recognized. PEComas are now increasingly recognized at diverse anatomic locations, including soft tissues, skin, bone, and visceral organs.[43–46] Monotypic epithelioid AML, extrapulmonary "sugar" tumor, and PEC tumor are all synonyms for the term PEComa. In this section, only renal AMLs and PEComas of soft tissue showing predominantly epithelioid features are specifically discussed. Pulmonary and extrapulmonary LAMs,[43–45] which are usually composed predominantly of spindle cells, are not discussed in this chapter (see Chapter 3).

Clinical Features

PEComas are rare neoplasms, occurring mostly in women. In addition to the kidney (renal AML), the lungs (CCST and LAM), and the liver (epithelioid AML), rare cases have been described at diverse anatomic sites, such as the retroperitoneum, uterus, vulva, falciform ligament/ligamentum teres, large and small bowel, pancreas, mesentery, omentum, pelvis, heart, and bone.[43–48] Clinical features depend mainly on the size and location of the neoplasm. The term *PEComa not otherwise specified* (PEComa NOS), or simply *PEComa*, refers to all PEComas other than AML and LAM.

Renal and Extrarenal Angiomyolipoma

AML occurs most commonly in middle-aged patients (median age, 40 to 50 years), with a female predominance (female-to-male ratio, 4:1 for sporadic AML, whereas this sex predilection is not found in AML associated with TSC). Fewer than half of cases are associated with TSC.[44,47,49] This lesion, which has long been considered a hamartoma, is now recognized as a clonal mesenchymal neoplasm. The most common presenting symptoms include pain, hematuria, and fever. AML may also present as an incidental finding on computed tomography scan, at the time of surgery, or at autopsy. Rarely, tumor rupture leads to massive, life-threatening retroperitoneal hemorrhage.[49] Most cases of AML develop in the kidneys, but some are occasionally found at extrarenal sites, such as the retroperitoneum, pelvis, liver, oral cavity, or lungs.[49] Some retroperitoneal tumors are attached to the kidney by a small pedicle. The radiologic (computed tomography and magnetic resonance imaging scans) appearance is characteristic, allowing preoperative diagnosis in many cases. Outside of TSC, AML usually presents as a solitary mass, measuring 1 to 20 cm (median, 9 cm). Patients with TSC usually have AMLs in both kidneys; these tumors are often multiple, of varying size (often small), and asymptomatic.[43–49]

PEComa

PEComas other than AML and LAM are rare neoplasms that have been described under different names, including primary extrapulmonary "sugar" tumor, clear cell myomelanocytic tumor, and abdominopelvic sarcoma of PECs.[1,43–47] PEComas tend to occur in middle-aged patients, mostly women (female-to-male ratio, 7:1). Up to 40% of these tumors occur in the gynecologic tract, mostly in the uterus but also in the vagina and vulva. An additional 40% are found in the retroperitoneum, soft tissues, and skin, with the remaining cases found mainly in the gastrointestinal tract.[43–47] However, nearly any anatomic site may be involved. Presenting symptoms depend on the location and size of the tumor.

Pathologic Features

Renal and Extrarenal Angiomyolipoma

Grossly, AMLs present as a yellow to gray unencapsulated mass, but the color varies according to the proportions of each component: adipocytes, smooth muscle, and blood vessels. In some cases, especially in the retroperitoneum, the neoplasm may show infiltrative margins and may contain hemorrhagic or necrotic areas. Some tumors may extend into the renal vein and inferior vena cava. AMLs may also involve regional lymph nodes and, more rarely, the spleen; these foci should not be misinterpreted as metastatic deposits of a sarcoma.[1,43–47,49]

Histologically, although a conventional AML is typically composed of mature fat, thick-walled blood vessels, and smooth muscle in varying proportions, an epithelioid AML is composed predominantly or exclusively of epithelioid cells. Pure epithelioid ("monotypic") AMLs are identical to (and synonymous with) PEComa (discussed later). Tumor cells are large and polygonal, with abundant palely eosinophilic granular to clear cytoplasm (Fig. 6.26). Blood vessels and a mature adipocytic component are focal or absent. When present, blood vessels are usually muscular and thick walled, with hyalinization of the media. Epithelioid cells are less frequently arranged around blood vessels than in conventional AMLs. Nests of tumor cells are often surrounded by delicate capillary vessels (Fig. 6.27), similar to renal cell carcinoma. Nuclear atypia is common, and multinucleated tumor giant cells may be seen. Areas of hemorrhage or tumor necrosis may also be observed. Mitotic activity is usually minimal, except in frankly malignant cases (discussed later).[1,43–47,49]

PEComa

The morphologic features of PEComa are broad.[43–47] Many of these neoplasms are indistinguishable from epithelioid (monotypic) AML.

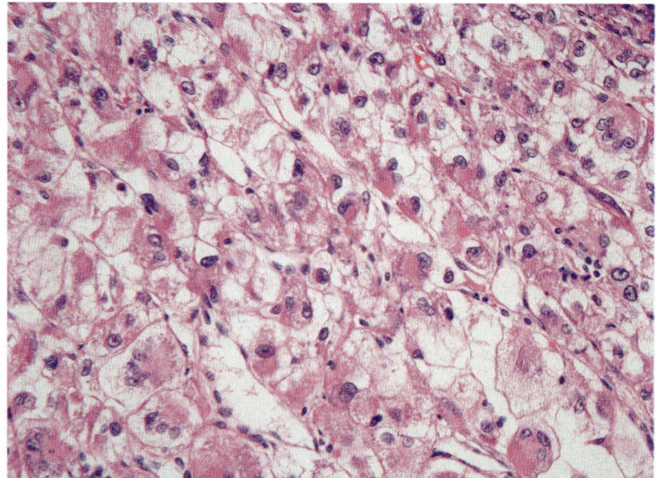

Figure 6.26 Epithelioid Angiomyolipoma (Perivascular Epithelioid Cell Tumor). The tumor is composed of nests of large polygonal epithelioid cells with voluminous granular eosinophilic to clear cytoplasm.

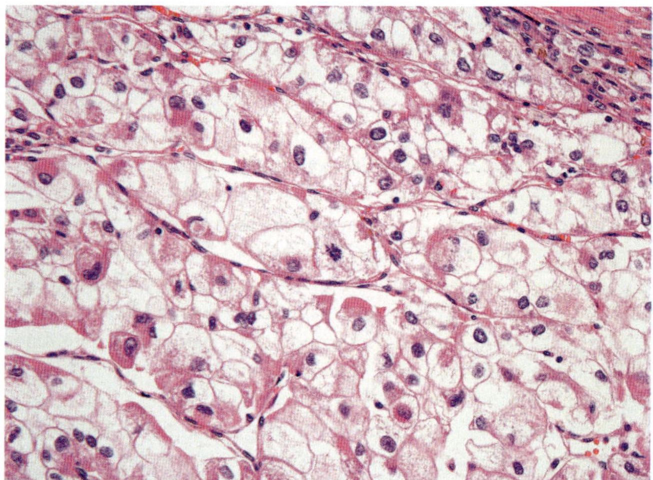

Figure 6.27 Epithelioid Angiomyolipoma (Perivascular Epithelioid Cell Tumor). Nests of epithelioid tumor cells are surrounded by delicate capillary vessels.

They are predominantly or exclusively composed of large polygonal epithelioid cells, with abundant granular eosinophilic to clear cytoplasm (Fig. 6.28), often arranged in nests surrounded by delicate capillary vessels. The tumor cells often show focal association with the walls of blood vessels (Fig. 6.29). Some tumors contain multinucleated giant cells (Fig. 6.30). In other cases, the tumor cells are more spindled, with clear cytoplasm, resembling CCST of the lung (Fig. 6.31). Clear cell morphologic features often predominate in tumors of the falciform ligament/ligamentum teres[50] and cutaneous PEComas.[51,52] A distinctive subset of PEComas (most arising in the retroperitoneum) shows marked stromal hyalinization and a trabecular architecture ("sclerosing PEComa") (Fig. 6.32).[53] PEComas of the uterus may be difficult to distinguish from epithelioid smooth muscle neoplasms (discussed later).[44,54,55] Occasionally, PEComas contain melanin pigment.

Immunohistochemistry

PEComas are characteristically reactive for both smooth muscle markers, most often smooth muscle actin (in ~80% of cases), and melanocytic markers, most often HMB-45 (in ~90% of cases) (Fig. 6.33), but also melan A (~70%) and microphthalmia transcription factor (MITF).[43–47] The cytoplasmic positivity for HMB-45 is typically finely granular.

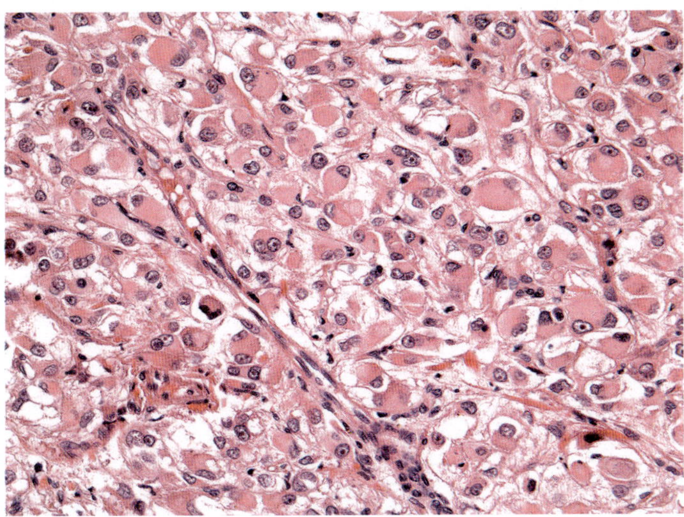

Figure 6.28 **Perivascular Epithelioid Cell Tumor.** The tumor is composed of epithelioid cells with eosinophilic cytoplasm.

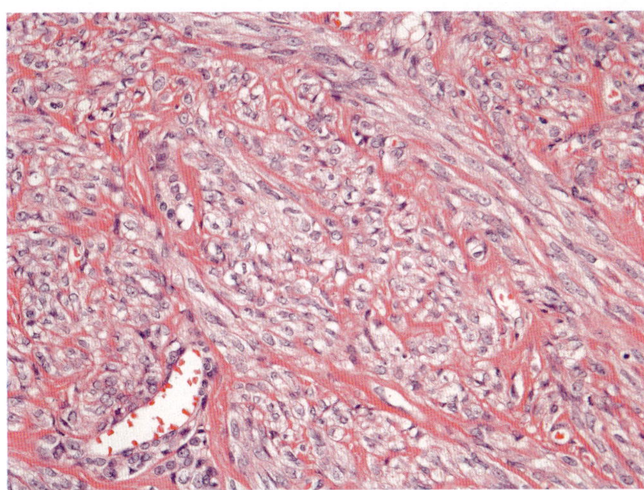

Figure 6.31 **Perivascular Epithelioid Cell Tumor.** The tumor is composed of spindled to epithelioid cells with predominantly clear cytoplasm.

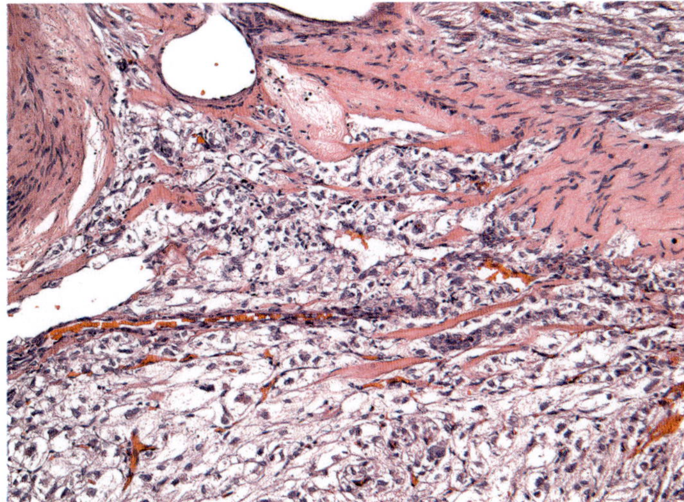

Figure 6.29 **Perivascular Epithelioid Cell Tumor.** The tumor cells contain finely granular to clear cytoplasm and are associated with the walls of dilated blood vessels.

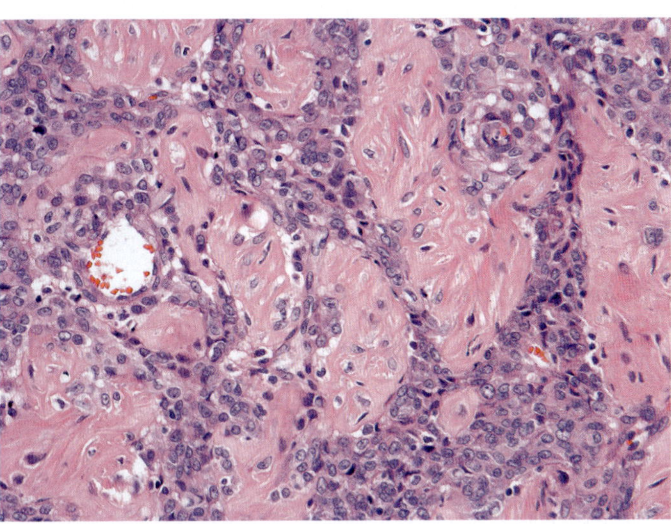

Figure 6.32 **Sclerosing Perivascular Epithelioid Cell Tumor.** The tumor is composed of cords of epithelioid cells in a densely hyalinized stroma. Note the association with vessel walls. Such tumors usually arise in the retroperitoneum.

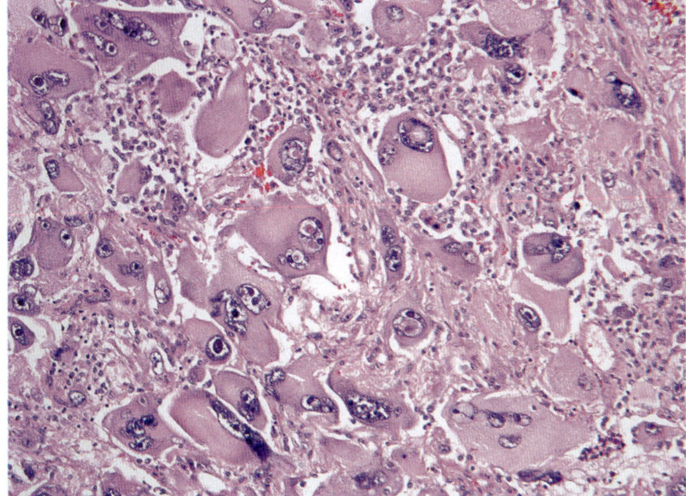

Figure 6.30 **Malignant Perivascular Epithelioid Cell Tumor.** The tumor is composed of pleomorphic epithelioid and multinucleated cells with eosinophilic cytoplasm. Such tumors may mimic pleomorphic rhabdomyosarcoma.

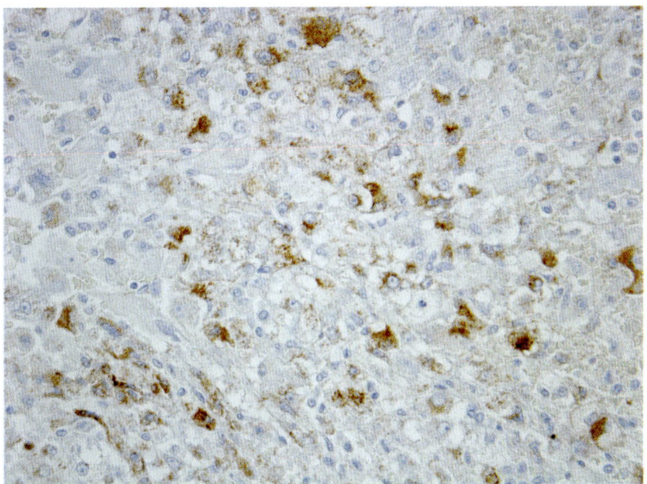

Figure 6.33 **Perivascular Epithelioid Cell Tumor.** In most cases, scattered tumor cells express HMB-45.

Approximately 80% of cases coexpress smooth muscle actin and HMB-45 or melan A. Predominantly epithelioid tumors tend to express melanocytic markers more strongly than myogenic markers, whereas the opposite is seen in predominantly spindled PEComas.[44] Desmin (~30%) and S-100 protein (10%) are less often expressed. Occasional PEComas (especially those with clear-cell features) express melanocytic markers without smooth muscle actin (SMA) and desmin. Keratins, EMA, KIT, and CD34 are rarely expressed. Estrogen and progesterone receptors are frequently expressed in AML but less often in other PEComas.[44] Approximately 20% of PEComas show nuclear staining for TFE3,[46] many of which harbor *TFE3* gene rearrangements.[56] Cathepsin K has been reported to be a useful marker for PEComa,[57,58] but in our experience it is relatively nonspecific; expression is also seen in many other mesenchymal tumor types.

Molecular Genetics

PEComas, including AMLs, LAM, and CCSTs, often bear genetic alterations of the *TSC* genes. TSC is a genetic disorder caused by mutations of the *TSC1* (9q34) or *TSC2* (16p13.3) gene (reviewed in references 43 and 44). Manifestations of TSC include intellectual disability, seizures, renal cysts, AML, LAM, subependymal giant cell astrocytoma, hyperpigmented spots, periungual fibromas, cutaneous angiofibromas, cardiac rhabdomyoma, gliosis, and calcification of the cerebral cortex. TSC genes play an important role in the regulation of the mammalian target of rapamycin (mTOR) pathway, and this signaling pathway has been found to be deregulated (leading to mTORC1 hyperactivation) in a subset of renal AMLs and extrarenal PEComas.[43,44] Between 30% and 50% of AMLs occur in patients with TSC, and approximately half of patients with TSC have multiple AMLs. Mutations in *TSC1* and *TSC2* genes, with loss of expression of the protein products hamartin and tuberin, respectively, have been documented in AMLs. The prevalence of LAM in women with TSC is approximately 35%. In the context of TSC, LAM sometimes occurs in association with multiple AMLs (approximately 25% of patients with LAM have AMLs). Although less than 10% of patients with non-AML, non-LAM PEComa show signs of TSC,[46] deletions of 16p (bearing the *TSC2* gene) or allelic losses of *TSC2* are the most common genetic changes in both TSC-associated and sporadic PEComas,[59] and lead to activation of the mTOR pathway.[60] In addition, *TP53* mutations are also present in most malignant PEComas with *TSC2* mutations.[61] The most common alternative pathway of tumorigenesis in PEComa involves *TFE3* alterations. Approximately 20% of PEComas (of soft tissue or visceral sites) harbor *TFE3* gene rearrangements, which often correlates with a nested or pseudoalveolar growth pattern and overexpression of the TFE3 protein.[56,61] Fusions involving *RAD51L1* (*RAD51B*) with either *RRAGB* or *OPHN1* have been described in a small subset of uterine PEComas.[61]

Differential Diagnosis

Renal and Extrarenal Epithelioid Angiomyolipoma

Immunohistochemistry plays a critical role in differential diagnosis. Predominantly epithelioid AML should be differentiated from carcinoma, especially renal cell carcinoma (positivity for keratins and EMA, negativity for melanocytic markers except in renal cell carcinomas with *TFEB* rearrangement), epithelioid metastatic melanoma (strong and diffuse S-100 reactivity, negativity for smooth muscle actin and desmin), rhabdomyosarcoma (strong and diffuse positivity for desmin and myogenin), epithelioid leiomyosarcoma (negativity for melanocytic markers), epithelioid sarcoma (reactivity for epithelial markers and CD34 in 50% of cases, loss of expression of INI1, negativity for melanocytic markers), MRT (loss of expression of INI1), and epithelioid gastrointestinal stromal tumor (GIST; reactivity for KIT, CD34, and DOG1; only focal positivity for smooth muscle actin; negativity for desmin and melanocytic markers; mutations in the *KIT* or *PDGFRA* gene). Making the distinction between ASPS and PEComa may be difficult because both neoplasms show a nested growth pattern and may show nuclear staining for TFE3, although unlike PEComa, ASPS is consistently negative for HMB-45 (Box 6.14).

PEComa

Again, immunohistochemistry is helpful in distinguishing PEComa from other tumors. PEComas composed predominantly of epithelioid cells should be differentiated primarily from metastatic carcinoma, metastatic melanoma, mesothelioma, epithelioid GIST, sarcomas displaying epithelioid cytomorphology, and large cell lymphomas (Box 6.15).

Metastases from hepatocellular carcinoma (positivity for keratins, especially CAM5.2, HepPar1, ARG1, and cytoplasmic TTF-1), adrenal cortical carcinoma (positivity for melan A, inhibin, and SF1), and renal cell carcinoma (positivity for keratins, EMA, and PAX8) may easily be confused with PEComa. Epithelioid melanomas are usually strongly positive for S-100 protein and SOX10, often in addition to melan A, HMB-45, and MITF, whereas PEComas are generally negative for the S-100 protein (or show at most focal cytoplasmic staining) and SOX10.

Epithelioid mesothelioma, including the deciduoid variant, is generally positive for keratins, EMA, calretinin, and WT1, and negative for melanocytic markers. Both PEComa and mesothelioma can express desmin.

Myoepitheliomas composed predominantly of plasmacytoid (hyaline) cells usually react with epithelial markers, smooth muscle actin, calponin, S-100 protein, and 50% for GFAP, and they are negative for melanocytic markers.

Box 6.14 Differential Diagnosis of Renal and Extrarenal Epithelioid Angiomyolipoma

Carcinoma (especially renal cell carcinoma)
Metastatic melanoma
Rhabdomyosarcoma
Epithelioid leiomyosarcoma
Epithelioid sarcoma
Malignant rhabdoid tumor
Alveolar soft part sarcoma
Epithelioid gastrointestinal stromal tumor

Box 6.15 Differential Diagnosis of Perivascular Epithelioid Cell Tumors Other Than Angiomyolipoma and Lymphangio(leio)myomatosis

If an Epithelioid Component Predominates

Metastatic carcinoma
Metastatic melanoma
Epithelioid (deciduoid) malignant mesothelioma
Large cell lymphoma and plasma cell neoplasms
Rhabdomyosarcoma
Alveolar soft part sarcoma
Epithelioid leiomyosarcoma
Epithelioid sarcoma (especially proximal type)
Epithelioid myoepithelioma
Epithelioid angiosarcoma
Malignant rhabdoid tumor
Epithelioid gastrointestinal stromal tumor

If a Spindle Cell Component Predominates

Leiomyoma, leiomyosarcoma
Gastrointestinal stromal tumor

If a Clear Cell Component Predominates

Clear cell carcinoma
Clear cell sarcoma

Sarcomas resembling epithelioid PEComas include epithelioid leiomyosarcoma (positivity for smooth muscle actin and desmin, negativity for melanocytic markers), rhabdomyosarcoma (desmin and myogenin reactivity), ASPS (reactivity for TFE3, negative for HMB-45), epithelioid angiosarcoma (positivity for CD31 and ERG and often CD34, negativity for melanocytic markers), epithelioid sarcoma (reactivity for keratin, EMA, and CD34; loss of INI1 expression; negativity for melanocytic markers), epithelioid GIST (reactivity for KIT, DOG1, and CD34; negativity for melanocytic markers; mutations in the *KIT* or *PDGFRA* gene), predominantly epithelioid clear cell sarcoma (reactivity for S-100 protein in addition to melanocytic markers, t(12;22) or t(2;22) translocation), epithelioid MPNST (diffuse positivity for S-100 protein and SOX10, negativity for melanocytic markers, often loss of INI1 expression), and MRT (loss of INI1 expression). Among lymphomas, diffuse large B-cell lymphoma (reactivity for CD20, CD45, and PAX5; negativity for melanocytic and muscle markers), T-cell lymphomas (reactivity for CD45 and CD3), anaplastic large-cell lymphoma (positivity for CD30, EMA, and often ALK), and plasma cell neoplasms (positivity for EMA, CD138, and MUM1; negativity for melanocytic markers) are most likely to be confused with epithelioid PEComas.

PEComas composed predominantly of clear cells should be differentiated primarily from clear cell renal cell carcinoma and clear cell sarcoma, as described earlier.

Prognosis and Treatment

Renal and Extrarenal Epithelioid Angiomyolipoma

Conventional AMLs are usually benign. Development of a sarcoma within a conventional AML is extremely rare.[49] In contrast, a significant subset of epithelioid AMLs behave in an aggressive fashion, and these are characterized by local recurrences and metastatic dissemination, especially to the lungs, bone, and liver. Factors that are predictive of aggressive behavior for epithelioid AMLs appear similar to those for other PEComas (discussed later), and include marked nuclear atypia, pleomorphism, a high mitotic rate, and for renal primary tumors, extrarenal extension or renal vein involvement.[62,63]

PEComa

The behavior of PEComas is difficult to predict. Although many PEComas behave in a benign fashion, a significant proportion of these tumors behave aggressively. Local recurrence occurs in 10% to 15% of patients, and distant metastases (most frequently to liver, lungs, and bone) occur in 20%.[46] Overall, 10% of patients with PEComa die of disease. Large size and histologic features such as high nuclear grade, mitotic activity, and tumor necrosis, have been shown to correlate with aggressive behavior in small studies. Based on the examination of 26 PEComas of soft tissue and gynecologic origin as well as 45 well-documented cases from the literature, Folpe and colleagues found that the development of aggressive local recurrence or distant metastases was associated with tumor size greater than 5 cm, infiltrative growth pattern, high cellularity, high nuclear grade, mitotic activity greater than one per 50 high-power fields, and necrosis.[46] Mitotic activity showed the highest predictive value, and tumor necrosis ranked second in their statistical analysis. The authors proposed classifying PEComas into three risk categories: benign, uncertain malignant potential, and malignant.[46] A more recent study of PEComas arising in the gastrointestinal tract found that mitotic activity ≥2 per 10 high-power fields and the presence of diffuse cytologic pleomorphism and marked nuclear atypia were significantly associated with the development of metastasis; tumor size did not correlate with outcome.[64] Given the relatively small cohort size in these studies, firm minimal criteria for malignancy are uncertain; in our practice, we consider PEComas with any mitotic activity, along with marked nuclear atypia or diffuse pleomorphism, to be malignant.

Recently, it has been shown that sirolimus (and the derivatives temsirolimus and everolimus), a specific inhibitor of the mTOR pathway, has efficacy in renal AMLs and pulmonary LAM. Some patients with metastatic malignant PEComas have benefited from treatment with sirolimus, but larger clinical trials are ongoing to evaluate the efficacy of this therapeutic approach for PEComas.[44,65,66]

PRACTICE POINTS: Perivascular Epithelioid Cell Tumor

- Marked female predominance
- Most common in the retroperitoneum, uterus, and abdomen/pelvis
- Large epithelioid cells, with clear to granular eosinophilic cytoplasm
- Arranged in nests surrounded by delicate capillary vessels
- Focally associated with blood vessel walls
- "Sclerosing PEComa" is a distinctive variant in the retroperitoneum, with marked stromal hyalinization and trabecular architecture.
- Characteristically coexpress melanocytic markers (especially HMB-45) and smooth muscle markers (smooth muscle actin or desmin)
- Most PEComas are benign
- Malignant PEComas have a highly aggressive clinical course with metastases to the liver and lungs.

Adult-Type Rhabdomyoma

Extracardiac rhabdomyomas segregate into three main clinical and morphologic forms: adult-type, fetal (juvenile), and genital rhabdomyomas. Because the adult-type rhabdomyoma is composed mainly of large, epithelioid cells, this variant is discussed in this section.

Clinical Features

Adult-type rhabdomyomas usually occur in the head and neck region as a small, slow-growing, painless mass. Middle-aged and elderly adults (mean age, 60 years) are most commonly affected, especially men (male-to-female ratio, 3:1). The oral cavity (floor of the mouth), base of the tongue, larynx, pharynx, and soft tissues of the neck are common tumor locations; patients sometimes present with hoarseness or difficulties in breathing or swallowing. In 20% to 30% of cases, multiple rhabdomyomas develop in the same patient, usually in the same area of the head and neck. There is no association with tuberous sclerosis.[67]

Pathologic Features

Adult-type rhabdomyomas usually present as a solitary, well-demarcated, sometimes polypoid, submucosal nodule, with a mean size of 3 cm. Histologically, adult rhabdomyoma is composed of tightly apposed rounded to polygonal cells, with abundant granular eosinophilic cytoplasm (Fig. 6.34) and small vesicular nuclei containing small nucleoli (Fig. 6.35). Tumor cells are separated by a delicate stroma containing small vessels. Cytoplasmic vacuolization is a common finding in adult rhabdomyomas, resulting in a clear cell appearance or the formation of "spider cells," where some delicate strands of cytoplasm remain attached to the cell membrane. Intracytoplasmic crystalloid structures, resembling those observed in ASPS, are occasionally seen. Mitotic activity and necrosis are not observed in adult rhabdomyomas.

Immunohistochemistry

Because tumor cells display skeletal muscle differentiation, they are reactive for desmin, myoglobin, muscle-specific actin (HHF35), and skeletal fast myosin. S-100 protein reactivity and, less frequently, smooth muscle actin expression can be observed. There is no expression of myogenin, unless the lesion has been traumatized.

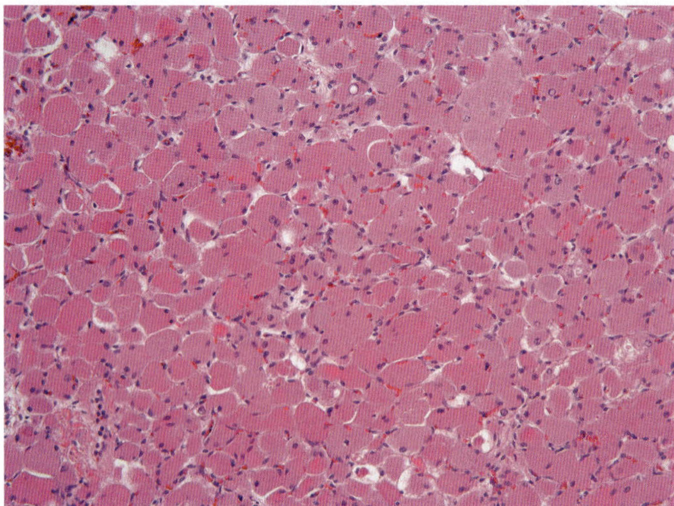

Figure 6.34 Adult-Type Rhabdomyoma. The tumor is composed of uniform large epithelioid cells with brightly eosinophilic cytoplasm.

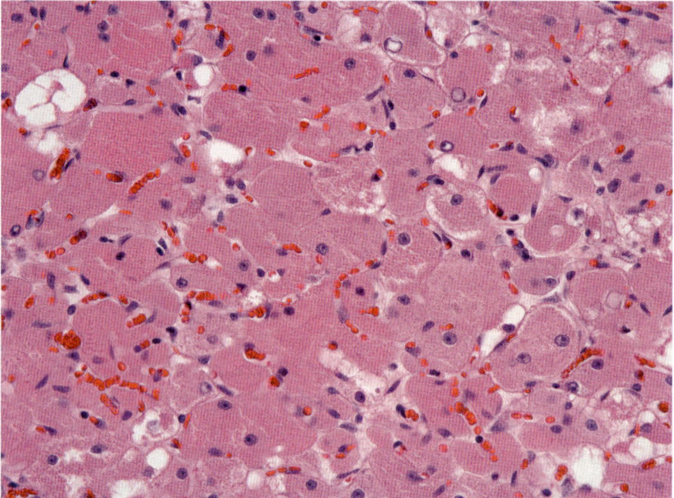

Figure 6.35 Adult-Type Rhabdomyoma. Tumor cells contain abundant granular eosinophilic cytoplasm, vesicular nuclei, and small central nucleoli.

Differential Diagnosis

Adult rhabdomyoma should be differentiated from well-differentiated forms of embryonal rhabdomyosarcoma, including recurrent or metastatic well-differentiated embryonal rhabdomyosarcoma after prolonged chemotherapy, pleomorphic rhabdomyosarcoma, a rhabdomyoblastic component in another sarcoma type (dedifferentiated liposarcoma, MPNST), ASPS, and metastatic melanoma. Crystal-storing histiocytosis, granular cell tumor, hibernoma, oncocytoma, paraganglioma, and extranodal Rosai-Dorfman disease might also enter the differential diagnosis.

Pleomorphic rhabdomyosarcoma is easily distinguished from adult rhabdomyoma because of the presence of mitoses, necrosis, and marked nuclear pleomorphism. The head and neck region is a site of predilection for both adult rhabdomyoma and embryonal rhabdomyosarcoma. Unlike adult rhabdomyoma, however, embryonal rhabdomyosarcoma is usually observed in children or young adults and not in the elderly. In addition, even in the most differentiated forms of embryonal rhabdomyosarcoma, there is invariably some degree of nuclear pleomorphism coexisting with an admixture of mature and immature (or less mature) rhabdomyoblasts, at least focally. Rhabdomyosarcomas often show more infiltrative margins, and contain mitotic figures or tumor necrosis. Rhabdomyosarcomas following chemotherapy may occasionally show a highly differentiated, rhabdomyoma-like appearance (Fig. 6.36).[68,69] In this situation, a previous medical history of rhabdomyosarcoma along with young patient age should alert the pathologist. By immunohistochemistry, in addition to desmin and other skeletal muscle markers, embryonal rhabdomyosarcoma cells usually express myogenin (usually in <50% of cells) and MYOD1, a feature not observed in adult rhabdomyomas.

ASPS, which is also composed of large cells with abundant eosinophilic cytoplasm, can occur in the head and neck area. Tumor cells, however, are more atypical than those of adult rhabdomyoma. Tumor cells grow in an alveolar pattern, nuclei are larger with more vesicular chromatin, and nucleoli are more prominent. The intratumoral vascular network is well developed in ASPS, and tumor emboli are frequently observed. As opposed to adult rhabdomyoma, ASPS bears a t(X;17) unbalanced translocation that involves the *TFE3* gene. The fusion product that accumulates in the nucleus can be detected using anti-TFE3 antibodies.

Granular cell tumors and hibernomas lack features of skeletal muscle differentiation. Instead, granular cell tumor is strongly and diffusely positive for S-100 protein. Hibernoma is usually found in the interscapular region in young to middle-aged adults. Crystal-storing histiocytosis is a condition associated with lymphoplasmacytic neoplasms and monoclonal immunoglobulin production.[70] The histiocytes, which have phagocytized crystallized immunoglobulins, stain for CD68 and CD163 and are negative for skeletal muscle markers.

Prognosis and Treatment

Adult rhabdomyoma is benign; simple excision is curative. Adult rhabdomyoma may recur if incompletely excised (15% to 40% of cases), sometimes many years after initial surgery.[67] Recurrences are best treated by complete reexcision.

Epithelioid Schwannoma

Epithelioid schwannoma is discussed in Chapter 15.

Granular Cell Tumor

Granular cell tumors are most common in the tongue, skin, and subcutaneous tissue. A small proportion of these tumors are observed in the breast and visceral organs (e.g., esophagus, pharynx, larynx, bronchi,

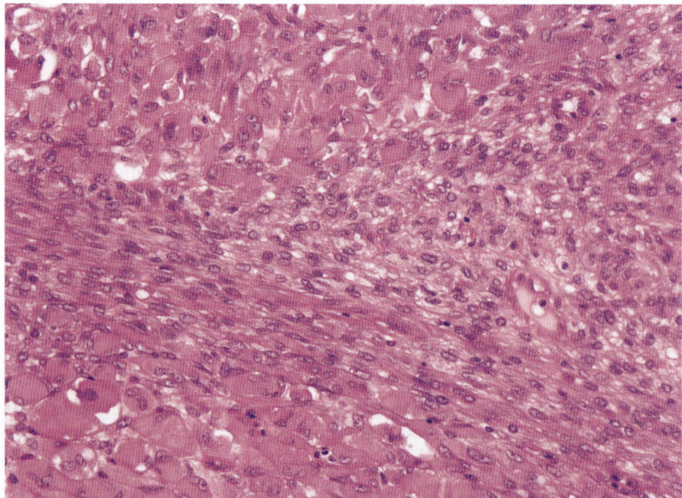

Figure 6.36 Embryonal Rhabdomyosarcoma. This tumor shows cytodifferentiation after chemotherapy. The tumor contains numerous well-differentiated rhabdomyoblasts and can be confused with adult-type rhabdomyoma.

stomach, and colon), as well as in deep soft tissue. Only granular cell tumors of deep soft tissue are discussed in this section. Granular cell tumors are also discussed in Chapters 15 and 16.

Clinical Features

Granular cell tumors are rarely observed in deep soft tissue.[71] They usually occur in middle-aged adults, with a predilection for women. Proximal extremities and trunk are predominantly affected. Up to 10% of patients (especially African Americans) with granular cell tumors display multiple lesions. Approximately 2% of granular cell tumors are clinically malignant.

Pathologic Features

Granular cell tumors of soft tissue tend to be larger (5 to 7 cm on average) than lesions of skin and subcutis (2 cm on average). A cut section shows a gray to whitish appearance. On low-power examination, the lesion is ill defined with infiltrative borders. Tumor cells are arranged in sheets, cords, ribbons, or nests separated by dense collagenous stroma (Fig. 6.37). Older lesions tend to be more collagenized. Tumor cells are typically rounded to polygonal and, characteristically, contain abundant, eosinophilic, finely granular cytoplasm with ill-defined borders (Fig. 6.38). The cytoplasm often contains small ovoid structures corresponding to dilated lysosomes (phagolysosomes) (see Fig. 6.38). Nuclei are either small and dark with inconspicuous nucleoli or large and vesicular with small nucleoli. In benign lesions, mitotic figures and tumor necrosis are absent. Nests of tumor cells are commonly observed surrounding peritumoral or intratumoral nerves (Fig. 6.39).

Malignant granular cell tumors show marked nuclear atypia, vesicular nuclei with large nucleoli, cell spindling, mitotic activity, and/or areas of tumor necrosis (see "Treatment and Prognosis"; Fig. 6.40).

Immunohistochemistry

Granular cell tumors show strong and diffuse reactivity for S-100 protein (Fig. 6.41) and SOX10, reflecting their schwannian differentiation, as well as for calretinin and inhibin.[72] They are also variably positive for CD68, CD57, and PGP9.5 (protein gene product 9.5); these markers are generally not useful for diagnosing mesenchymal neoplasms. Nuclear expression of TFE3 is seen in approximately 90% of granular cell tumors, but does not seem to correlate with the presence of *TFE3* gene rearrangement.[73] Tumor cells are negative for neurofilament protein and GFAP. Staining for collagen IV and laminin is frequently seen around nests of tumor cells. In practice, S-100 protein staining alone is sufficient to confirm the diagnosis. Strong staining for p53 and a high MIB1 (Ki-67) index (>10%) are often detected in malignant granular cell tumors.[71,74]

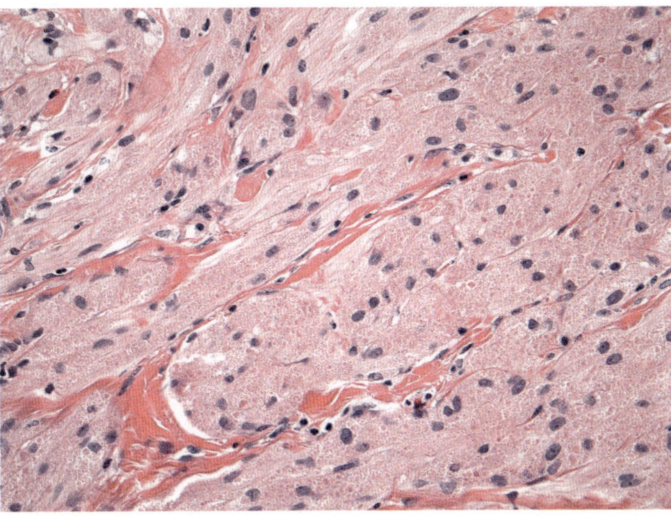

Figure 6.38 Granular Cell Tumor. The tumor cells contain abundant palely eosinophilic granular cytoplasm with ill-defined cell borders. Intracytoplasmic small rounded structures correspond to dilated lysosomes. Note the uniform bland nuclei.

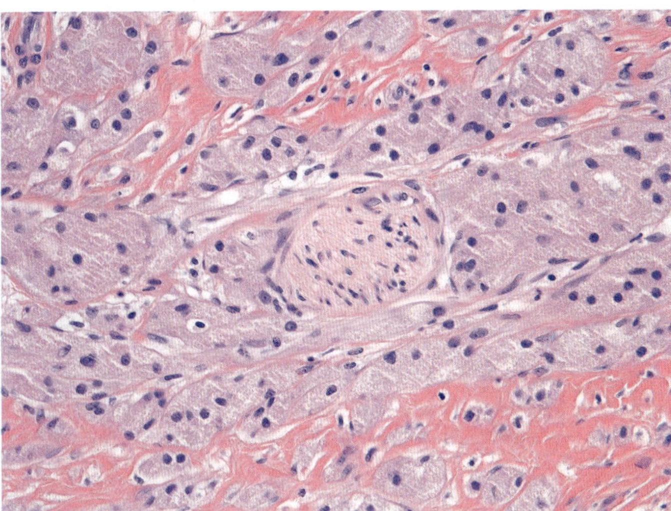

Figure 6.39 Granular Cell Tumor. The tumor surrounds a small nerve. This finding is of no clinical consequence.

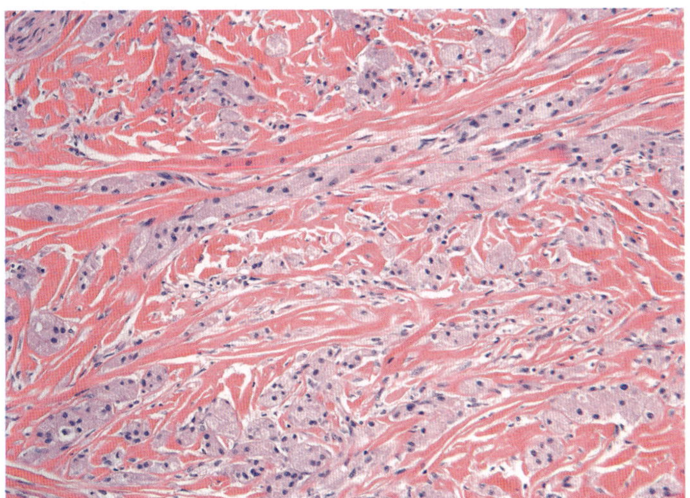

Figure 6.37 Granular Cell Tumor. Cords and nests of epithelioid cells with granular cytoplasm are separated by dense collagenous stroma.

Differential Diagnosis

The diagnosis of granular cell tumors is usually straightforward. On occasion, granular cell tumors may be confused with lesions that contain a significant proportion of tumor cells with a granular appearance: adult rhabdomyoma; hibernoma (Fig. 6.42); dermatofibrosarcoma with granular cells; leiomyoma and leiomyosarcoma with granular cell change;[71,75] angiosarcoma with granular cells; MPNST; undifferentiated pleomorphic sarcoma with granular cells;[71] melanoma; metastatic histiocytoid carcinoma (e.g., from the breast); and histiocytic pseudotumors secondary to surgery, prosthetic joint replacement, or previous trauma. By immunohistochemistry, granular cell tumor can be easily distinguished from these other lesions, due to strong and diffuse S-100 protein expression. Unlike melanoma, granular cell tumors are negative for HMB-45 and melan A.

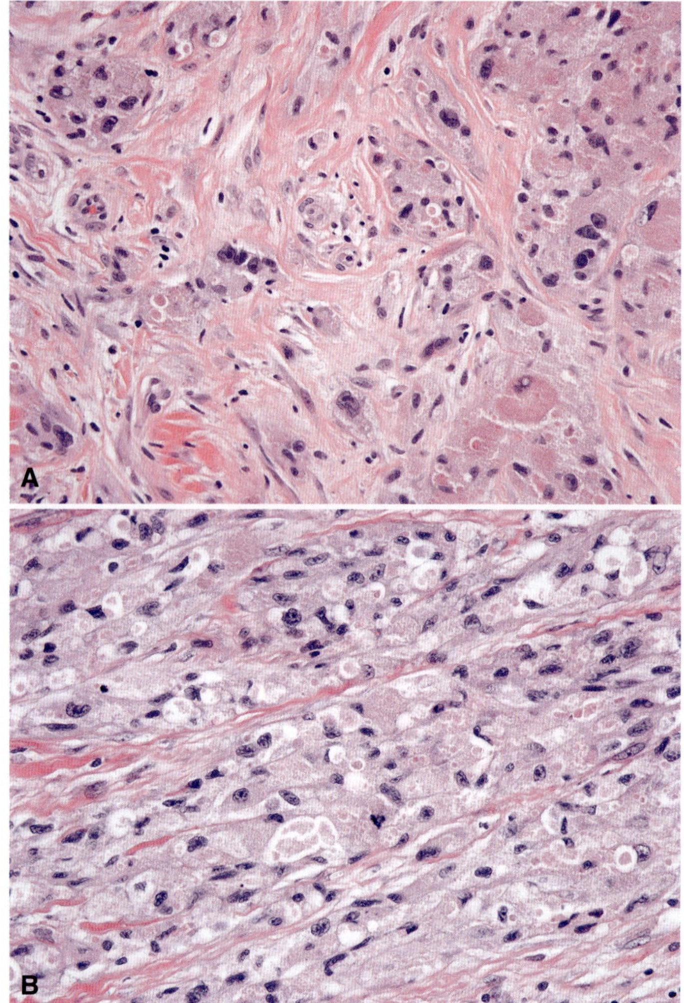

Figure 6.40 Malignant Granular Cell Tumor. (A) Nests of tumor cells show nuclear atypia with large nucleoli. (B) Epithelioid to spindled cells show coarse chromatin and mitotic activity.

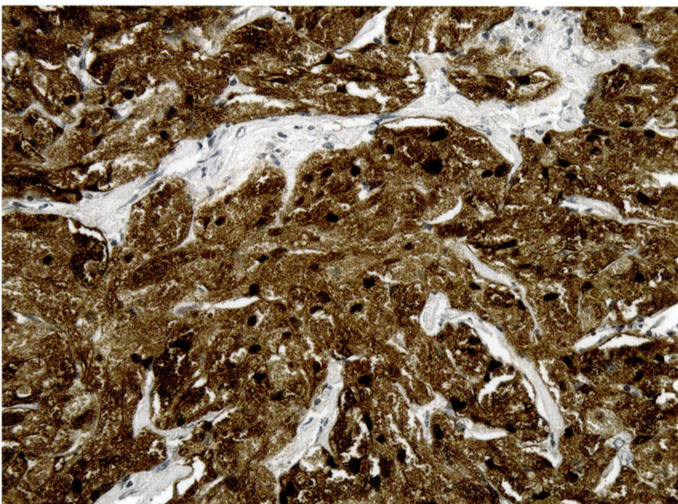

Figure 6.41 Granular Cell Tumor. Tumor cells strongly express S-100 protein.

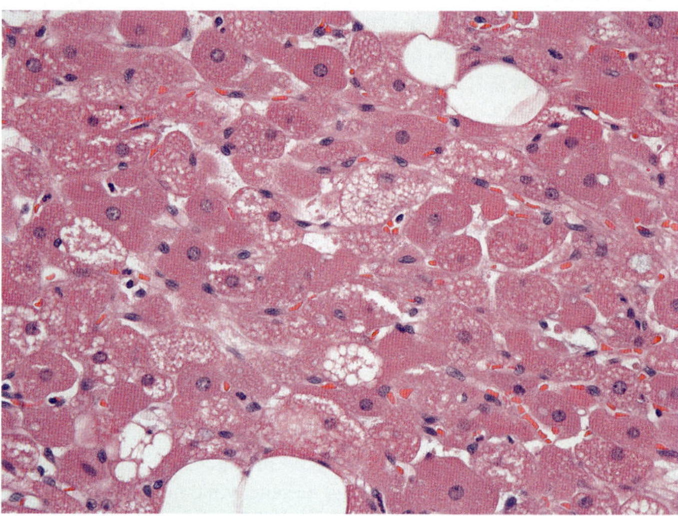

Figure 6.42 Hibernoma. Many tumor cells show abundant granular eosinophilic cytoplasm, resembling granular cell tumor. Multivacuolated cells and mature adipocytes are also characteristic.

Prognosis and Treatment

Most granular cell tumors are superficial and benign; simple excision is curative. The local recurrence rate for benign lesions is less than 5%. Malignant granular cell tumors are rare, accounting for approximately 2% of cases. Criteria for malignancy in granular cell tumors include at least three of the following features: pleomorphism, high nuclear-to-cytoplasmic ratio, vesicular nuclei with large nucleoli, cell spindling, more than two mitoses per 10 high-power fields, and tumor necrosis.[71] Tumors with only one or two of these features do not metastasize and can be classified as "atypical granular cell tumor." Multicentric granular cell tumors are generally benign. The local recurrence and metastatic rates for malignant granular cell tumors in one study were 32% and 50%, respectively.[71] Between 40% and 50% of patients with malignant granular cell tumors die of disease at a median interval of 3 years.[71,73] The most common sites of metastases are lymph nodes, lung, and bone.[71,73] Malignant granular cell tumors should be treated as aggressive neoplasms. Wide excision is the treatment of choice. Adjuvant radiation therapy should be considered in individual cases for local control. Even cytologically bland granular cell tumors have the capacity to metastasize, although this is an exceedingly rare event.[74]

Sclerosing Perineurioma

Sclerosing perineurioma is discussed in Chapters 3 and 15.

Extracranial Meningioma

This lesion typically arises in the skin and soft tissues of the scalp, or close to the vertebral column. Extracranial meningiomas usually develop in children and young adults, and may be discovered at birth. Some tumors result from abnormalities of neural tube closure (similar to meningocele). Histologically, this lesion resembles classical intracranial meningioma, but it often shows an infiltrative growth pattern (Fig. 6.43). Ectopic meningothelial hamartoma is a distinctive variant of extracranial meningioma involving the skin and subcutaneous tissue of the scalp with a microcystic and infiltrative (angiosarcoma-like) appearance (see also Chapter 15).[76] By immunohistochemistry, meningioma cells express EMA, SSTR2, and progesterone receptor; they are rarely positive for keratins. Before contemplating a diagnosis of extracranial meningioma, extracranial extension of an intracranial tumor should be carefully excluded.

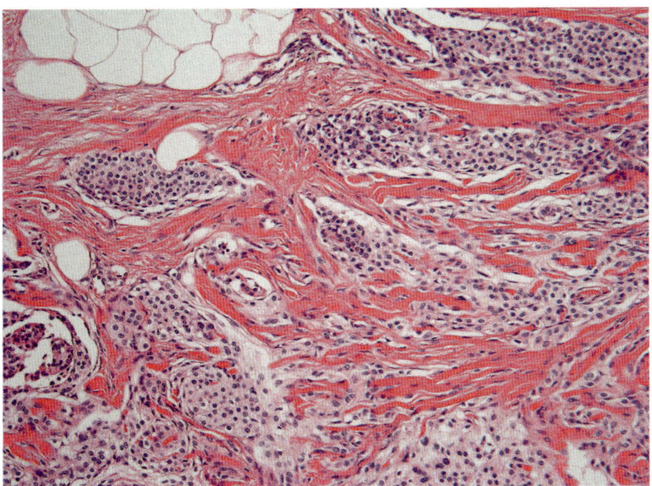

Figure 6.43 **Extracranial Meningioma.** Nests of bland epithelioid cells infiltrate the deep soft tissue of the scalp.

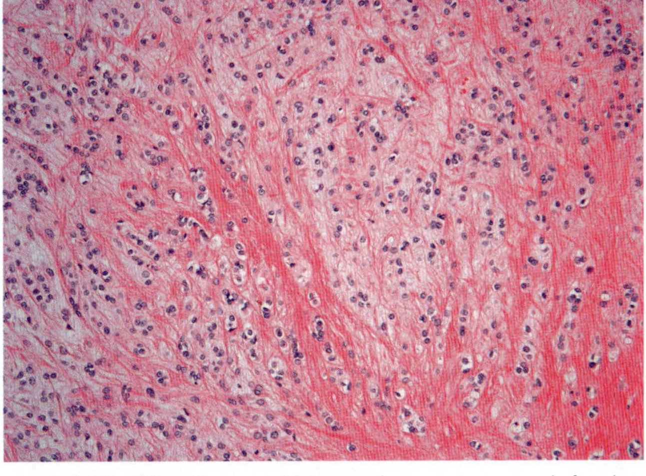

Figure 6.44 **Ossifying Fibromyxoid Tumor.** The tumor is composed of cords and strands of bland ovoid cells set in a fibromyxoid stroma.

Ossifying Fibromyxoid Tumor

OFMT of soft parts is discussed in detail in Chapter 5. Some cases of OFMT show prominent epithelioid cytology and may therefore be confused with other epithelioid lesions.

Clinical Features

OFMT occurs in middle-aged adults with a male predominance. The extremities (70%) are mainly affected, although the trunk (20%) and head and neck regions (10%) can also be involved. Most lesions develop in the deep subcutis; they are rare in deep soft tissues.[77–80]

Pathologic Features

In its conventional form, OFMT is composed of rounded to ovoid or short spindle cells arranged in cords or strands, set in a well-developed fibromyxoid to hyalinized collagenous stroma (Fig. 6.44). Some OFMT are predominantly composed of bland epithelioid cells with eosinophilic or clear cytoplasm, somewhat mimicking an epithelial neoplasm (Fig. 6.45).[77–80] Tumor cell nuclei are round, small, and often vesicular, with small nucleoli. Cytoplasmic borders are ill defined. Mitoses are very rare. A helpful diagnostic feature of OFMT is the presence of an incomplete rim of mature lamellar bone at the periphery of the lesion, although foci of bone can be observed within the lesion, and some tumors may lack this shell of bone (up to 20%).

Immunohistochemistry

By immunohistochemistry, tumors cells in OFMT characteristically express S-100 protein (70% of cases) and desmin (up to 50% of cases). Neuron-specific enolase and GFAP may also occasionally be detected. They are usually negative for epithelial markers.[77–80]

Molecular Genetics

Gene fusions involving *PHF1* and *BCOR* have been identified in 85% of OFMT, both benign and malignant forms, with fusion partners including *EP400* (*PHF-EP400* is the most common fusion gene overall, found in approximately 40% of OFMT), *MEAF6, ZC3H7B* and *EPC*.[81,82] Recently, alternate fusion genes have been identified in a small subset of OFMTs, including *CREBBP-BCORL1* and *KDM2A-WWTR1*.[83] Because most of these genes play a role in histone modification, epigenetic dysregulation has been proposed as a significant pathogenetic mechanism in OFMTs. FISH analysis for rearrangement of the *PHF1* locus may be a helpful diagnostic tool to confirm a diagnosis of OFMT, particularly in examples with atypical morphologic features.

Differential Diagnosis

An OFMT exhibiting prominent epithelioid cytomorphology should be differentiated from other benign and malignant epithelioid neoplasms, as summarized in Box 6.16 (see Chapter 5 for additional comments).

Myoepithelioma of soft tissue is usually composed of a variable combination of epithelioid and spindle cells. There is no peripheral shell of bone, and the extracellular matrix is more often myxoid or chondromyxoid than fibromyxoid or hyalinized. Tumor cells are usually reactive for epithelial markers (keratins or EMA) and S-100 protein in myoepithelioma of soft tissue; 50% of tumors are positive for GFAP. EMA-positive ductal structures may occasionally be present.

There is some histologic overlap between nerve sheath tumors and OFMTs. Both lesions are S-100 protein positive, and both malignant OFMTs and MPNSTs may contain benign- or malignant-appearing bone. However, unlike OFMTs, nerve sheath tumors generally lack the distinctive uniform architecture with cords of cells and are not surrounded by a rim of bone.

EMC usually arises in deep soft tissues and not in the subcutis. It typically shows a multinodular growth pattern and contains abundant myxoid extracellular matrix. In contrast to most OFMTs, there is neither a peripheral shell of bone nor fibromyxoid to collagenous background in EMC. Tumor cells express S-100 protein in only 20% of cases (usually focally) and are negative for desmin.

Prognosis and Treatment

OFMTs may recur locally (10% to 20% of cases). Occasionally, tumors behave in a malignant fashion.[77–80] These neoplasms are characteristically large, tend to be deep-seated, and are highly cellular with nuclear atypia and easily identified mitotic figures. In addition, malignant OFMTs often contain foci of bone within (as opposed to around) the tumors.

Ependymoma of Soft Tissue

Ependymomas of soft tissue are rare neoplasms that occur either in the subcutaneous tissue dorsal to the sacrum and coccyx, or less frequently, anteriorly in the presacral deep soft tissue. Some patients who develop ependymoma of the dorsal coccygeal region have developmental abnormalities, such as spina bifida. These neoplasms present as

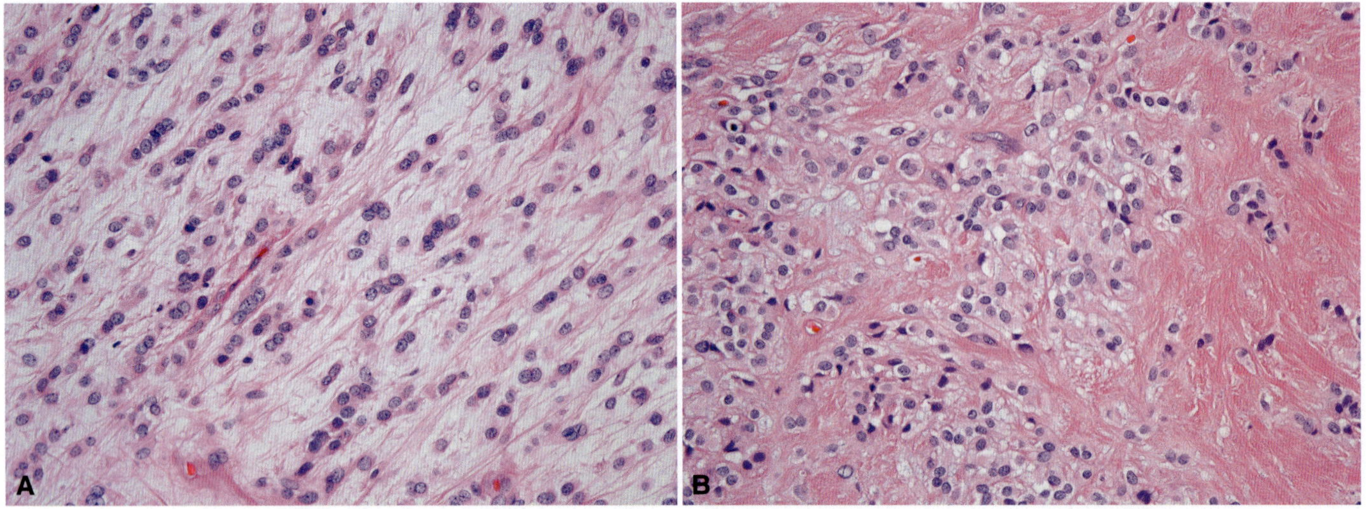

Figure 6.45 **Ossifying Fibromyxoid Tumor.** (A) Cords of uniform rounded cells with scant eosinophilic cytoplasm. Note the fibromyxoid stroma. (B) In this example, the tumor cells show an epithelioid appearance with more abundant cytoplasm.

Box 6.16 Differential Diagnosis of Epithelioid Ossifying Fibromyxoid Tumor

Myoepithelioma of soft tissue
Sclerosing perineurioma (epithelioid variant)
Epithelioid schwannoma
Chordoma
Extraskeletal myxoid chondrosarcoma
Osteosarcoma (epithelioid variant)
Malignant peripheral nerve sheath tumor
Sclerosing epithelioid fibrosarcoma

well-demarcated subcutaneous masses, clinically suggestive of teratomas or sweat gland tumors. Histologically, they are often lobulated and myxoid, composed of epithelioid cells (sometimes resembling those of a carcinoid tumor), papillary structures, and perivascular rosettes in varying proportions. Many resemble myxopapillary ependymomas of the cauda equina (Fig. 6.46). Tumor cells express GFAP and often keratins (a potential diagnostic pitfall) but are negative for EMA. Complete surgical excision is the treatment of choice. Dorsal coccygeal ependymomas have the capacity to metastasize to regional lymph nodes or lungs (20% to 30% of cases), often late in the course of the disease.

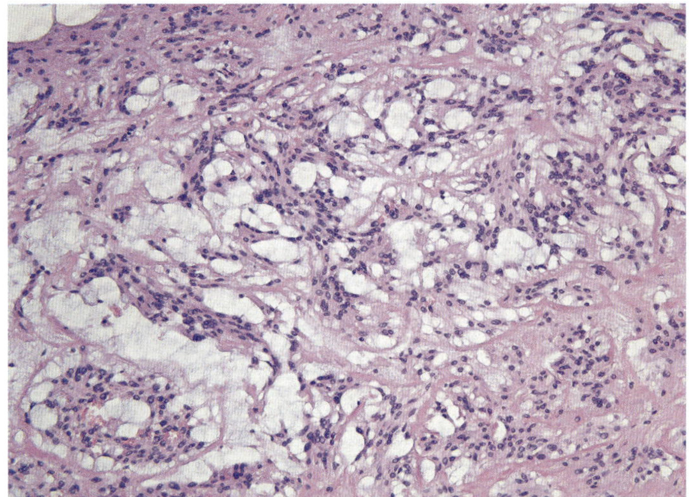

Figure 6.46 **Myxopapillary Ependymoma of Soft Tissue.** Epithelioid and spindle cells show a nested and microcystic architecture. Note the focally myxoid stroma.

Alveolar Soft Part Sarcoma

Described in 1952 by Christopherson and colleagues,[84] ASPS is an uncommon neoplasm of uncertain lineage, which has a high propensity for metastatic dissemination, especially to the lungs.

Clinical Features

ASPS occurs preferentially in adolescents and young adults (15 to 35 years of age), mostly in females. It usually presents as a deep-seated, often intramuscular or extracompartmental mass, located predominantly in the lower extremities (especially the thigh) in adults, and in the head and neck region (periorbital region, tongue) in children. Clinically, this neoplasm tends to remain asymptomatic for years, and distant metastases to lungs, brain, or bone may be the first presenting sign.[85–89]

Pathologic Features

On gross examination, ASPS is usually an ill-defined, soft, grayish tumor, ranging from 1 and 20 cm in size (median, 6 cm). Necrosis and hemorrhage are common.[85–89]

Histologically, this tumor type is often lobulated and shows a characteristic monotonous nested, alveolar, or pseudoalveolar growth pattern as a result of loss of cell cohesion within tumor nests (Fig. 6.47). Alveolar structures contain epithelioid cells with abundant granular eosinophilic, sometimes focally clear cytoplasm (Fig. 6.48). Characteristic periodic acid–Schiff (PAS)-positive, diastase-resistant crystals and granules may be observed in the cytoplasm of neoplastic cells in some cases, although demonstration of this feature is not required for diagnosis. Tumor cell nuclei are large and vesicular, and they contain prominent central nucleoli (see Fig. 6.48). A delicate, sinusoidal vascular stroma surrounds tumor nests. Tumor cell emboli are frequently observed within intratumoral or peritumoral dilated veins (Fig. 6.49). Mitotic figures are rare.

In the solid variant of ASPS, the alveolar growth pattern is not apparent and the tumor presents as a compact proliferation of large epithelioid cells with copious eosinophilic cytoplasm (Fig. 6.50). This solid or compact variant of ASPS tends to predominate in children, often involving the tongue, and is associated with a better prognosis.[89,90]

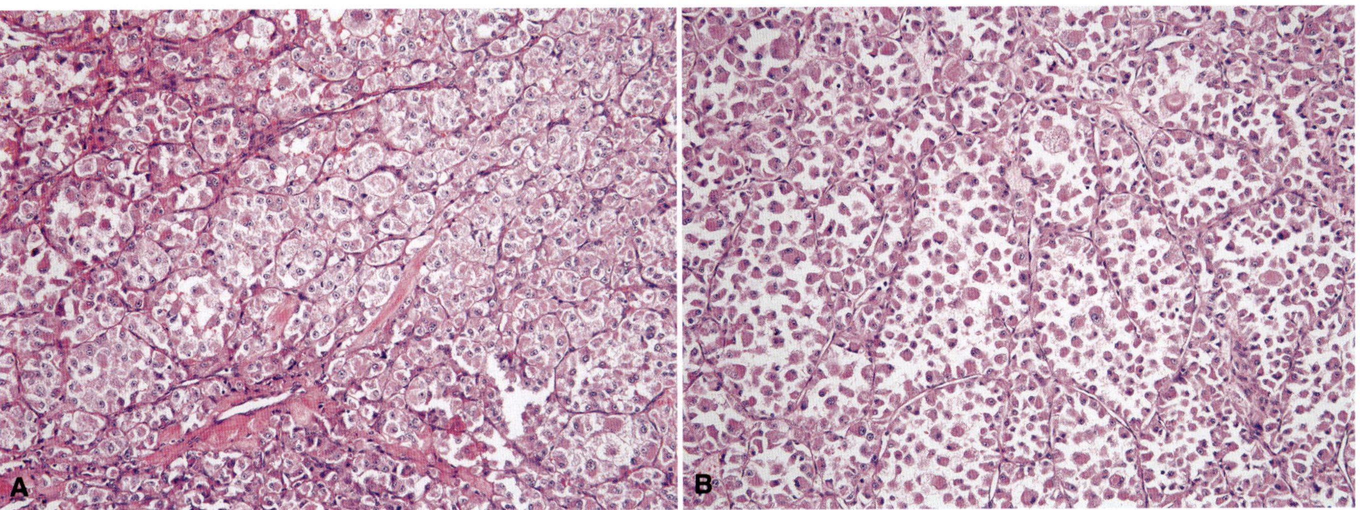

Figure 6.47 **Alveolar Soft Part Sarcoma.** The tumor shows a uniform nested (A) or pseudoalveolar architecture (B).

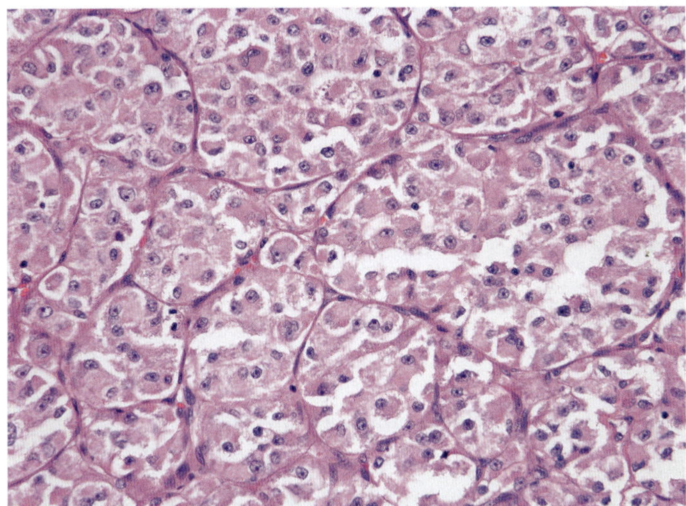

Figure 6.48 **Alveolar Soft Part Sarcoma.** Alveolar structures contain epithelioid cells with abundant eosinophilic cytoplasm, vesicular nuclei, and prominent central nucleoli.

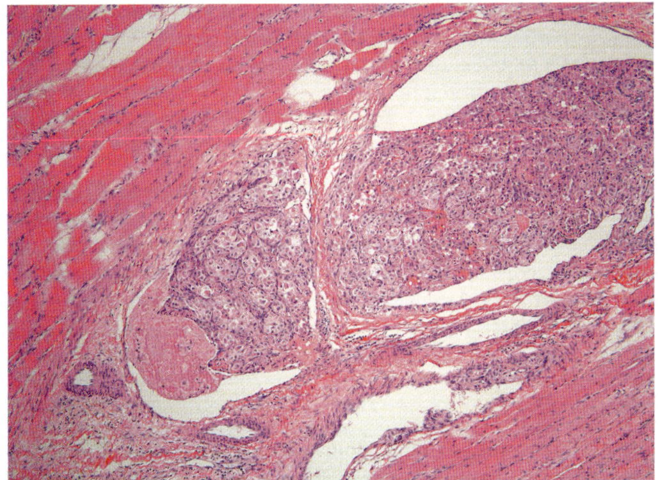

Figure 6.49 **Alveolar Soft Part Sarcoma.** Large vessel invasion is common.

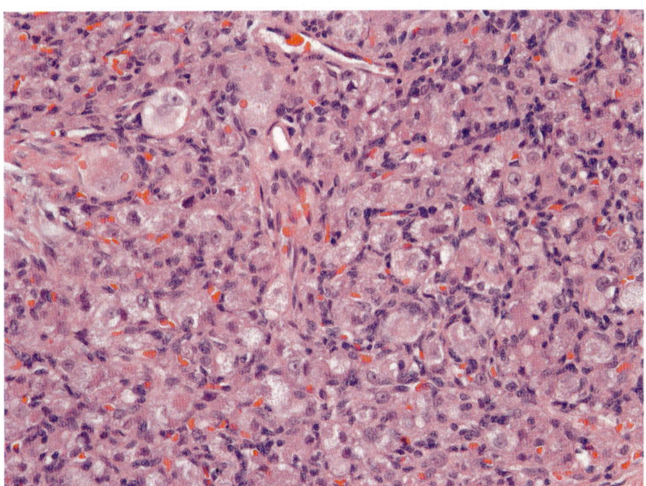

Figure 6.50 **Solid Variant of Alveolar Soft Part Sarcoma.** The tongue is a relatively common anatomic site.

Immunohistochemistry

Many markers have been tested in ASPS, with conflicting results. In general, ASPS is negative for neuroendocrine and epithelial markers but may be positive for muscle-specific actin; desmin expression is rare. Anti-TFE3 antibodies are of value to confirm the diagnosis of ASPS (especially the solid variant), as well as other neoplasms bearing a t(X;17) translocation (see "Molecular Genetics"). Positive staining is nuclear (Fig. 6.51).[91]

Molecular Genetics

Nearly all cases of ASPS bear an unbalanced (nonreciprocal) der(17) t(X;17)(p11;q25) translocation.[92,93] This translocation is highly specific for ASPS but can also be encountered in a variant of renal cell carcinoma that predominantly affects children.[93] The two genes involved in this translocation are *TFE3* on Xp11.2 and *ASPSCR1* on 17q25. The fusion protein localizes to the nucleus and functions as an aberrant transcription factor (see Chapter 18 for additional comments). The gene fusion can be detected in paraffin-embedded tissue by FISH.[94]

Differential Diagnosis

See Box 6.17 for the differential diagnosis of ASPS.

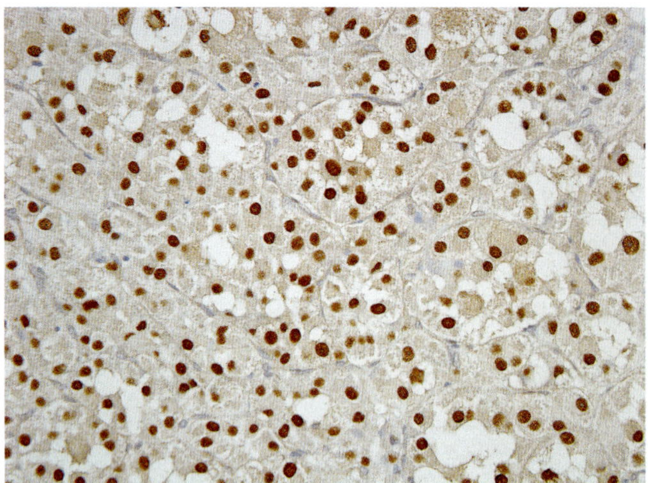

Figure 6.51 **Alveolar Soft Part Sarcoma.** The tumor cells show nuclear reactivity for TFE3.

Box 6.17 Differential Diagnosis of Alveolar Soft Part Sarcoma

- Renal cell carcinoma (metastasis)
- Paraganglioma (primary or metastasis)
- Malignant granular cell tumor (primary or metastasis)
- Melanoma (metastasis)
- Epithelioid leiomyosarcoma
- Epithelioid angiosarcoma
- Rhabdomyosarcoma (especially pleomorphic)
- Extrarenal malignant rhabdoid tumor
- Perivascular epithelioid cell tumor

Metastatic renal cell carcinoma, especially the eosinophilic variant of clear cell carcinoma, may mimic ASPS. It is important to exclude this possibility before diagnosing ASPS, especially in middle-aged adults. Tumor cells in renal cell carcinoma are usually immunoreactive for keratins, EMA, and PAX8, whereas tumor cells in ASPS are negative for these markers. In children and young adults, it is important to exclude metastatic Xp11 translocation renal cell carcinoma. Both ASPS and this subtype of renal cell carcinoma are positive for TFE3.

Malignant granular cell tumor, extrarenal MRT, and rhabdomyosarcoma lack the delicate vascular stroma of ASPS. Tumor cells in the former are strongly and diffusely positive for S-100 protein and SOX10, whereas rhabdomyosarcoma cells react with muscle markers (desmin and myogenin). In contrast to ASPS, tumor cells in extrarenal MRT are often positive for epithelial markers (keratin, EMA), and occasionally for desmin, and they show loss of expression of INI1.

Metastatic melanoma may sometimes display morphologic features almost identical to those of ASPS. However, a predominantly epithelioid metastatic melanoma is generally positive for S-100 protein and SOX10 but can be negative for HMB-45 and melan A, whereas ASPS is consistently negative for S-100 protein.

Distinguishing paraganglioma from ASPS is straightforward using immunohistochemistry, because the former is diffusely positive for neuroendocrine markers (chromogranin and synaptophysin). In addition, paraganglioma almost never arises in the limbs.

Some cases of ASPS may closely resemble PEComas. To complicate the issue, some PEComas express TFE3 (and harbor *TFE3* gene rearrangements). However, as opposed to ASPS, PEComas are usually positive for smooth muscle actin and melanocytic markers (HMB-45 or melan A), and often also for desmin; HMB-45 is the best marker to distinguish between these tumor types.

Epithelioid angiosarcoma almost never shows a uniform alveolar growth pattern, although pseudoglandular structures may occasionally be present. Reactivity for the endothelial markers CD31, CD34, and ERG is not a feature of ASPS. Finally, with the exception of Xp11 translocation renal cell carcinomas and a small subset of PEComas, the previously mentioned neoplasms are negative for TFE3.

Prognosis and Treatment

ASPS has a high tendency to develop metastases, especially to the brain, lungs, and bone, either at an early stage of the disease or late in the disease course. Lymph node metastases are rare. Five-year overall and median survival are 87% and 11 years, respectively, for patients with localized disease at diagnosis; however, only 15% to 20% of such patients remain disease-free at 20 years.[87,88] Five-year overall and median survival for patients with metastases at the time of diagnosis (25% of cases) are 20% and 3 years, respectively.[87] Local recurrence is observed in 20% to 30% of cases. Localized disease at presentation, small tumor size (<5 cm), and young age (children and adolescents) are the most important favorable prognostic factors.[86–89] The prognosis is notably better for childhood cases, especially for those arising in the head and neck, with up to 100% 5-year survival.[89]

PRACTICE POINTS: Alveolar Soft Part Sarcoma

- Marked predilection for the thighs of young women
- May present with lung, brain, or soft tissue metastases
- Uniform nested or alveolar growth pattern
- Large epithelioid cells, with abundant eosinophilic cytoplasm, vesicular nuclei, and prominent central nucleoli
- Solid variant lacking nested architecture predominates in the tongue of children
- t(X;17) and nuclear staining for TFE3 are characteristic findings
- High rate of metastasis; may occur late in the course of disease

Epithelioid Hemangioendothelioma

EHE is a vascular tumor that can arise in deep soft tissues but also in other locations such as lungs, liver, and bones.[95–98] Some patients present with EHE in several different organs simultaneously (e.g., in liver and lungs); in this situation, it is sometimes difficult, if not impossible, to determine the source of the primary tumor. Initially considered a vascular neoplasm of intermediate biologic potential, EHE is now classified as a sarcoma, because metastasis and tumor-related death occur in 25% and 15% of cases, respectively.[1,95–99] EHE has been molecularly characterized over the last few years as a translocation-associated sarcoma; the majority of tumors harbor a *WWTR1-CAMTA1* fusion gene,[100,101] and less than 5% a *YAP1-TFE3* fusion.[102] EHE is also discussed in Chapter 13.

Clinical Features

EHE of soft tissue mainly affects adult patients (median age, 50 years), without a sex predilection. It may occur anywhere in the body, involving superficial or deep (60% of cases) soft tissue. The extremities are most often affected (two-thirds of cases), followed by the head and neck region (10% to 15%), trunk and mediastinum (15%), and other sites (5% to 10%).[95–98] The lesions can be multicentric, sometimes coexisting with pulmonary, liver, or bone lesions. The median size varies between 1 and 3 cm (range, 0.5 to 18 cm).

Pathologic Features

Most EHEs present as solitary tumor nodules, in up to 50% of cases developing around or from a large vein. Vein lumina are often obstructed by the tumor cells, and concomitant thrombosis is frequent.

Conventional EHE is an infiltrative lesion composed of cords, strands, or nests of epithelioid cells in a characteristic myxohyaline stroma (Fig. 6.52). The tumor cells contain abundant glassy eosinophilic cytoplasm with well-defined cell borders, and round to ovoid, bland, often vesicular nuclei with small central nucleoli (Fig. 6.53). Cytoplasmic vacuoles are often seen in occasional tumor cells (Fig. 6.54). There are few mitoses and limited cytologic atypia. Tumor necrosis is uncommon in conventional EHE.

The "aggressive" variant of EHE, also referred to as *malignant EHE,* differs morphologically from conventional EHE by showing a more compact/solid growth pattern, marked cytologic atypia, nuclear pleomorphism and hyperchromasia, spindle cell areas, foci of tumor necrosis, and a high mitotic rate (Fig. 6.55).[97,98] In some areas, the morphologic features are almost identical to epithelioid angiosarcoma. Areas of both conventional and aggressive EHE may coexist within the same neoplasm.

Immunohistochemistry

By immunohistochemistry, tumor cells in EHE are positive for vascular markers (CD31, CD34, ERG, and sometimes D2-40).[96–98] ERG and CD31 (Fig. 6.56A) are the most sensitive markers for EHE. CD34 often

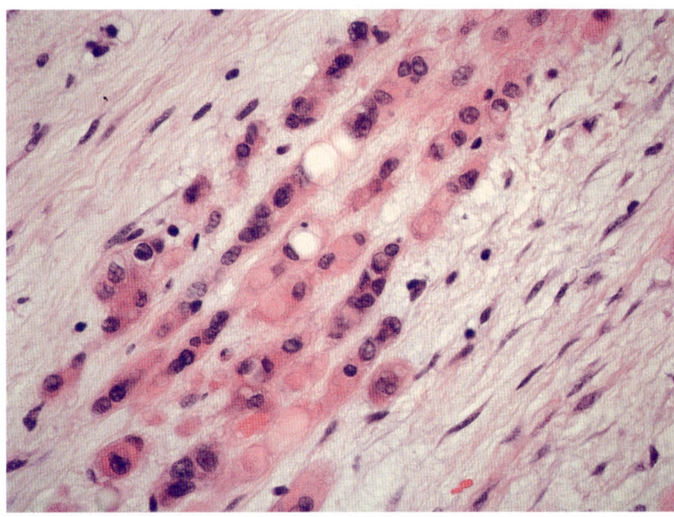

Figure 6.54 Epithelioid Hemangioendothelioma. Cytoplasmic vacuolation is seen in occasional tumor cells. Note the eosinophilic cytoplasm and mild nuclear atypia.

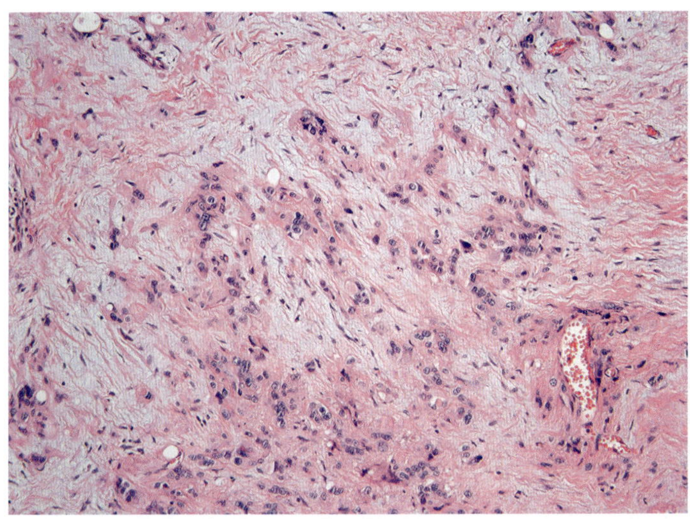

Figure 6.52 Epithelioid Hemangioendothelioma. The tumor is composed of cords of epithelioid cells in a myxohyaline stroma.

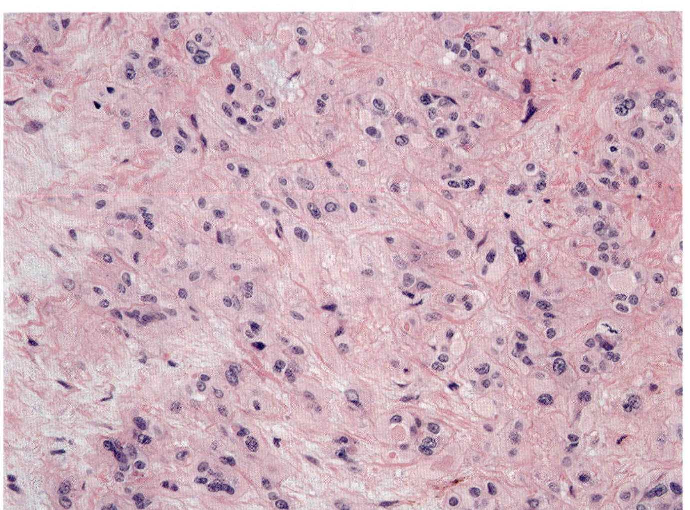

Figure 6.53 Epithelioid Hemangioendothelioma. The epithelioid tumor cells contain abundant glassy eosinophilic cytoplasm.

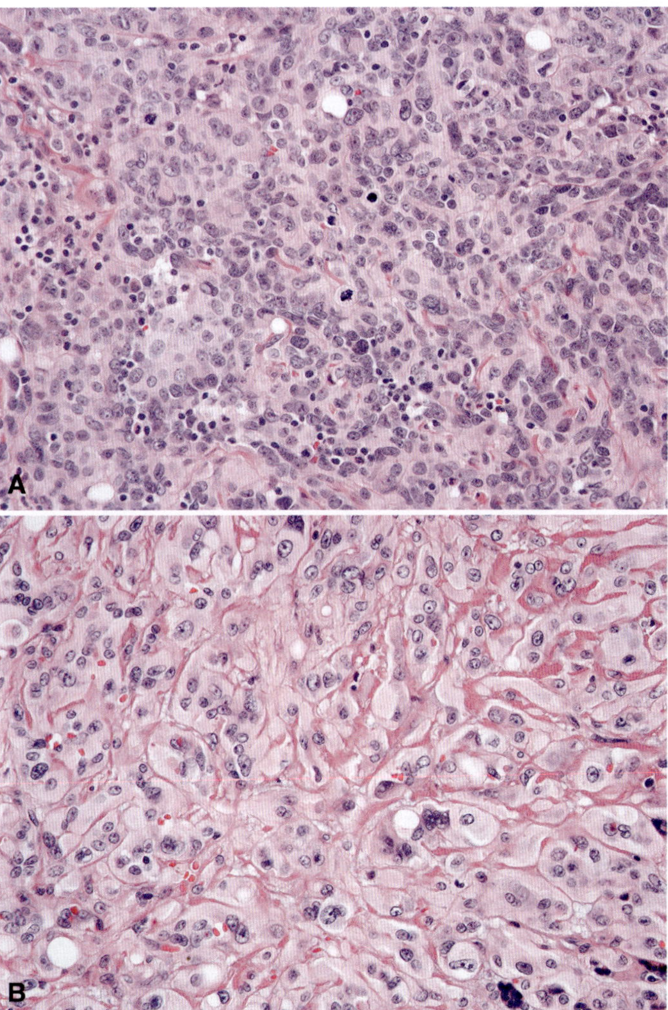

Figure 6.55 "Malignant" Epithelioid Hemangioendothelioma. The tumor shows a solid growth pattern, a high mitotic rate (A), and marked cytologic atypia and focal pleomorphism (B). Note the glassy eosinophilic cytoplasm.

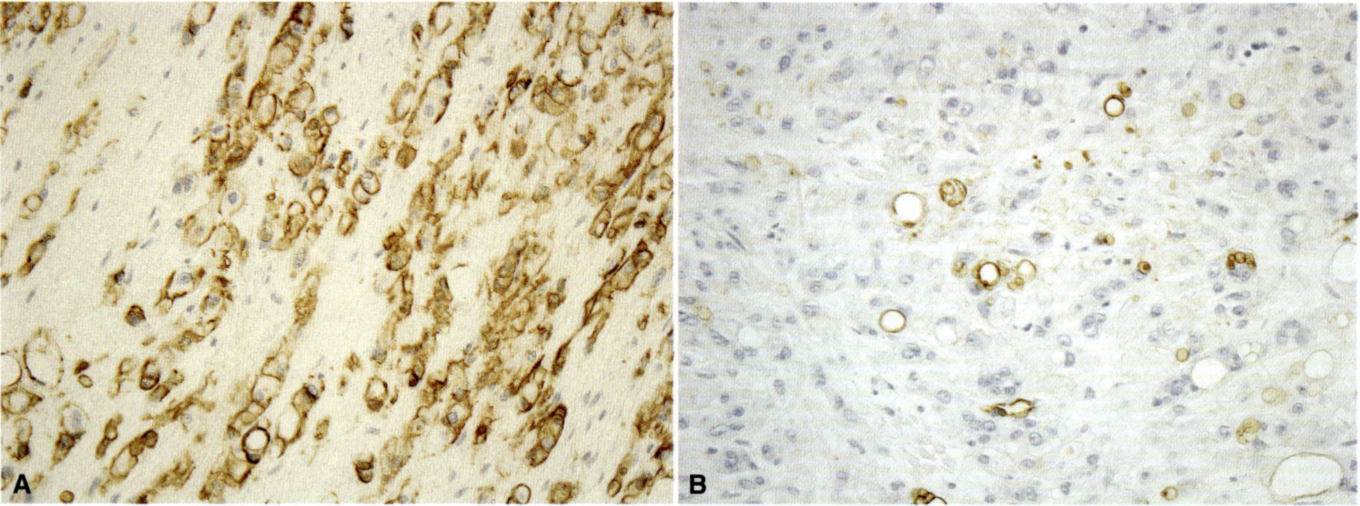

Figure 6.56 Epithelioid Hemangioendothelioma. (A) CD31 is usually positive in tumor cells. (B) CD34 may highlight cytoplasmic vacuoles.

highlights cytoplasmic vacuoles (see Fig. 6.56B). EHE can also be focally positive for keratins (20% to 30% of cases) and smooth muscle actin.[97] EHE is consistently negative for EMA, and expression of INI1 is retained. The discovery of *WWTR1-CAMTA1* and *YAP1-TFE3* fusion genes in EHE (see later) has resulted in the development of immunohistochemical correlates for these genetic changes as diagnostic tools. Nuclear expression of CAMTA1 is a sensitive and specific surrogate marker for the fusion gene; nuclear expression is seen in around 90% of EHE cases (Fig. 6.57).[13,14] Expression of CAMTA1 is not seen in epithelioid angiosarcoma, epithelioid hemangioma, or soft tissue tumors of other types. CAMTA1 expression is particularly useful for distinguishing those examples of EHE with marked cytologic or architectural atypia ("malignant" EHE) from angiosarcoma. Of those EHE cases negative for CAMTA1, the majority will show nuclear expression of TFE3; however, TFE3 is a less specific surrogate marker for the *YAP1-TFE3* gene fusion: only strong diffuse staining appears to correlate with the presence of the fusion gene.

Molecular Genetics

Recent studies have identified a *WWTR1-CAMTA1* gene fusion, resulting from the t(1;3)(p36;q25) chromosomal translocation, in EHE of soft tissue, bone, and visceral sites.[100,101] This gene fusion is a consistent feature of EHE and has not been identified in other vascular neoplasms. WWTR1 is involved in transcription factor signaling in the Hippo pathway and is normally expressed in endothelial cells,[103] whereas CAMTA1 belongs to a family of calmodulin-binding transcription activators and has been implicated as a tumor suppressor gene.[104,105] The *WWTR1-CAMTA1* fusion gene has been identified in approximately 90% of EHE cases with classic morphology. A subset of EHE that is negative for the *WWTR1-CAMTA1* fusion gene harbors a *YAP1-TFE3* fusion gene. This latter subtype occurs mainly in soft tissues of young adults and often shows distinctive morphology, including large epithelioid cells with abundant eosinophilic cytoplasm and focally well-formed vascular channels.[102] YAP1 is also associated with the Hippo pathway and shows significant functional and sequence homology with WWTR1.

Differential Diagnosis

Carcinoma, melanoma, and malignant mesothelioma should be excluded before the diagnosis of EHE is considered (Box 6.18). Carcinoma and malignant mesothelioma react for keratins and EMA; EHE may be positive for keratins but generally not for EMA. Carcinomas and melanomas do not react with vascular markers. Malignant mesothelioma is negative for CD34 and CD31 but is reactive for podoplanin (D2-40), in addition to keratins, EMA, calretinin, and WT1.

Epithelioid hemangiomas and cutaneous epithelioid angiomatous nodules are small cutaneous neoplasms (described in Chapter 13). Both show features of vascular differentiation. However, in contrast to EHE, epithelioid hemangiomas contain well-formed vascular channels surrounded by pericytes (although in cellular examples the architecture may be difficult to appreciate), as well as a mixed inflammatory infiltrate composed of eosinophils and lymphocytes in many cases. Epithelioid angiomatous nodules show a solid growth pattern, similar to some cases of EHE. CAMTA1 expression is specific for EHE in this differential diagnosis.

Myoepitheliomas, especially those composed predominantly of epithelioid or plasmacytoid cells and those exhibiting a prominent chondromyxoid extracellular matrix, may be confused with EHE. Although both tumor types may be positive for keratins, in contrast to EHE, myoepitheliomas also express EMA and S-100 protein, and often GFAP and SOX10, and are negative for vascular markers.

Epithelioid sarcomas may mimic EHE. Both lesions may be strongly positive for keratins, but EMA is only detected in epithelioid sarcomas. CD34 expression can be observed in both EHE and epithelioid sarcoma (50% of epithelioid sarcomas express CD34), but CD31 expression is restricted to EHE, with rare exceptions. Variable staining for ERG is observed in epithelioid sarcoma, depending on the antibody used. Antibodies against the N-terminus show expression of ERG in around two-thirds of cases, whereas antibodies against the C-terminus are rarely positive (<5% of cases).[106,107] EHE retains expression of INI1, unlike epithelioid sarcoma.

Pseudomyogenic hemangioendothelioma (also known as *epithelioid sarcoma–like hemangioendothelioma*) is composed of sheets and loose fascicles of plump spindle cells with abundant brightly eosinophilic cytoplasm that may mimic rhabdomyoblasts (see Chapters 3 and 15) (Fig. 6.58).[108,109] A minor epithelioid component is often present and may occasionally be prominent, in which case EHE may be a diagnostic consideration. Pseudomyogenic hemangioendothelioma typically presents in young adult male patients as multifocal disease in a limb, often within different tissue planes (skin, subcutis, skeletal muscle, and bone). This tumor type lacks the myxohyaline stroma and cords of cells characteristic of EHE. In contrast to EHE, pseudomyogenic hemangioendothelioma shows strong and diffuse expression of broad-spectrum keratins

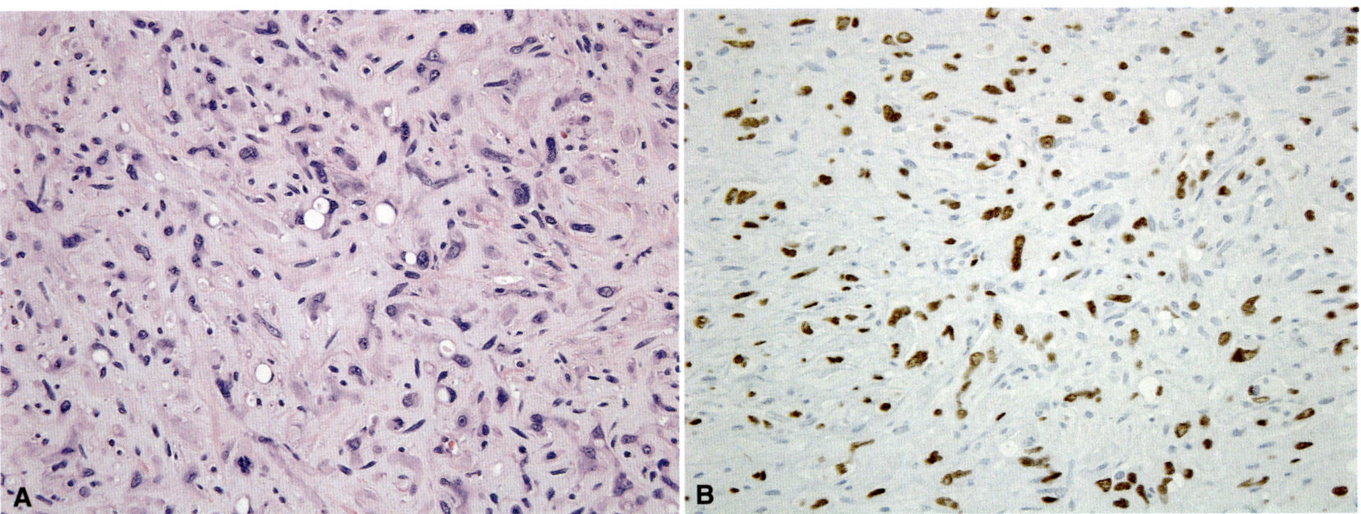

Figure 6.57 Epithelioid Hemangioendothelioma. (A) Cords of epithelioid cells with moderate nuclear atypia and eosinophilic cytoplasm embedded in a myxohyaline stroma. Note the cytoplasmic vacuoles. (B) Nuclear expression of CAMTA1 is a characteristic feature.

Box 6.18 Differential Diagnosis of Epithelioid Hemangioendothelioma

First Line

Epithelioid hemangioma
Carcinoma (especially signet-ring-cell carcinoma)
Melanoma
Malignant mesothelioma (epithelioid and deciduoid variants)
Epithelioid angiosarcoma
Epithelioid sarcoma
Pseudomyogenic hemangioendothelioma
Epithelioid malignant peripheral nerve sheath tumor

Second Line

Large cell lymphoma
Myoepithelioma of soft tissue/plasmacytoid chondroid syringoma
Epithelioid schwannoma
Epithelioid (Spitz) nevus, reticulohistiocytoma, and epithelioid fibrous histiocytoma
Epithelioid skin adnexal tumors

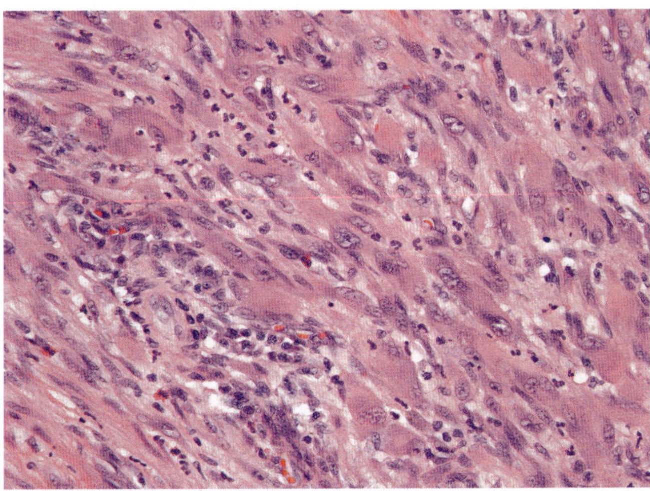

Figure 6.58 Pseudomyogenic Hemangioendothelioma. The tumor is composed of loose fascicles of plump spindled to epithelioid cells with brightly eosinophilic cytoplasm.

(especially AE1/AE3), whereas CD34 is negative. Similar to EHE, nuclear staining for ERG is observed, but CD31 is only positive in around 50% of cases of pseudomyogenic hemangioendothelioma. FOSB expression is a consistent finding in pseudomyogenic hemangioendothelioma and reflects the presence of a *SERPINE1-FOSB* fusion gene.[8] Pseudomyogenic hemangioendothelioma is negative for CAMTA1.

Epithelioid angiosarcoma shows more cytologic atypia and mitotic activity than conventional EHE. Tumor cells often contain amphophilic cytoplasm and are arranged in solid sheets. Vasoformative areas may be seen, and necrosis is common. Epithelioid angiosarcomas generally lack the myxohyaline background typical of EHE. In contrast to EHE, many epithelioid angiosarcomas are negative for CD34 but are also positive for CD31. In addition, CAMTA1 is negative in epithelioid angiosarcoma and is helpful to distinguish epithelioid angiosarcoma from "malignant" EHE.

Prognosis and Treatment

The clinical course of EHE is highly variable, ranging from indolent to highly aggressive; it is often difficult to estimate the biologic potential of a given tumor.[95–97] Mentzel and colleagues observed that marked cytologic atypia, tumor cell spindling, tumor necrosis, increased mitotic activity (>2 mitoses per 10 high-power fields), and solid, angiosarcoma-like foci were associated with poor outcome, although the correlation between outcome and histologic features was not statistically significant.[97] They proposed the term *malignant EHE* to designate this variant of EHE showing worrisome histologic features. They also observed that the interval between diagnosis and metastasis was shorter in "atypical" or "malignant" EHE compared with conventional EHE. Using a combination of mitotic rate and tumor size, Deyrup and coworkers were able to segregate patients with EHE into two groups, low risk and high risk.[98] In the low-risk category, which included EHEs measuring 3 cm or less, with three or fewer mitoses per 50 high-power fields, the metastatic rate was 15%, and there were no tumor-related deaths. In contrast, in the high-risk category, which included EHEs larger than 3 cm or with more than 3 mitoses per 50 high-power fields, the 5-year disease-specific survival was 59% and the metastatic rate was 32%.[98] In their study, Deyrup and coworkers found no correlation between disease-specific survival and cytologic atypia, tumor cell spindling, and tumor necrosis, suggesting that, with the exception of mitotic rate, histology may not be a reliable predictor of outcome in EHE.

EHE metastasizes mainly to regional lymph nodes, but also to lungs, liver, and bone. A combination of wide excision with tumor-free margins and consideration for regional lymph node dissection is the treatment of choice for EHE. Thus far, chemotherapy has not been shown to be effective treatment for metastatic EHE.

Epithelioid Sarcoma

Described by Enzinger in 1970,[110] epithelioid sarcoma is a distinctive sarcoma type that typically involves the distal extremities, shows epithelioid cytomorphology, expresses epithelial markers, and can be confused with a benign granulomatous process or a carcinoma.[110–112] More recently, a proximal (large cell) variant of epithelioid sarcoma has been described.[113,114] This variant shows clinical and morphologic differences from conventional ("distal-type") epithelioid sarcoma and pursues a more aggressive clinical course. Inactivation of the *SMARCB1* (*INI1*) gene at 22q11 has been identified in both tumor types (discussed later) and is a characteristic feature of epithelioid sarcoma. A very small subset of epithelioid sarcomas with intact INI1 instead show *SMARCA4* (*BRG1*) inactivation (see following section).[115–117]

Clinical Features

Epithelioid sarcoma typically involves the distal extremities (especially forearm, wrist, and hand) of young adults (median age, 30 years), with a male gender predilection (male-to-female ratio, 2:1). Epithelioid sarcoma presents as a firm, slow-growing nodule, multiple nodules, or a plaque-like lesion in the skin, subcutis, tendon, or fascia.[110–112] Tumors tend to develop on the flexor surfaces of the limbs and are often mistaken clinically for an inflammatory process. The trunk (including genital region) and head and neck are occasionally involved. The overlying skin may be ulcerated.

Proximal-type epithelioid sarcoma usually arises in the pelvis, perineum, axilla, mediastinum, or genital tract (pubis, vulva, penis) and rarely in the distal extremities.[111,113,114,118] This variant tends to occur in somewhat older adults (median age, 40 years) than the conventional (i.e., distal) variant of epithelioid sarcoma. Patients often present with a large infiltrative mass in the deep soft tissue.

Pathologic Features

In the classic form of epithelioid sarcoma, patients present with small indurated, ill-defined dermal and subcutaneous nodules, or larger, variably necrotic masses involving tendons or fascia. On cut section, the tumor is often white, with a yellow to brown center as a result of necrosis or hemorrhage. The size of the superficial nodules varies from a few millimeters to 5 cm; deep-seated tumors tend to be larger (up to 15 cm).[110–112]

Histologically, conventional epithelioid sarcoma is characterized by a proliferation of predominantly epithelioid to occasionally spindled cells with mild nuclear atypia, vesicular nuclei, and small nucleoli (Figs. 6.59 and 6.60). There is often abundant intercellular collagen deposition. Tumor cells aggregate in nodules that frequently undergo central necrosis, resulting in a pseudogranulomatous appearance simulating (at least on low power) a benign necrobiotic process such as a rheumatoid nodule or granuloma annulare (Fig. 6.61). Mitotic activity is usually low, often less than 5 per 10 high-power fields. Perineural and vascular infiltration are commonly seen. Dystrophic calcification, bone formation, and accompanying chronic inflammation may also be present.[111,112]

Proximal-type epithelioid sarcoma often shows a multinodular growth pattern and is composed of large epithelioid cells with eosinophilic to amphophilic cytoplasm, marked nuclear atypia, vesicular nuclei, and prominent nucleoli (Fig. 6.62).[113,114] Rhabdoid features are common and may even predominate in some lesions (Fig. 6.63), mimicking MRT.[118–121] Tumor necrosis is common, but the granuloma-like pattern observed

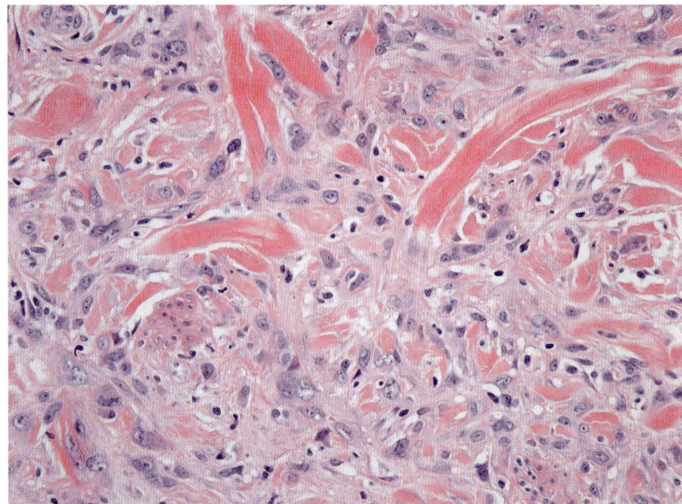

Figure 6.59 Epithelioid Sarcoma. Epithelioid tumor cells with pale eosinophilic cytoplasm, indistinct cell borders, and mild nuclear atypia infiltrate through the dermal collagen.

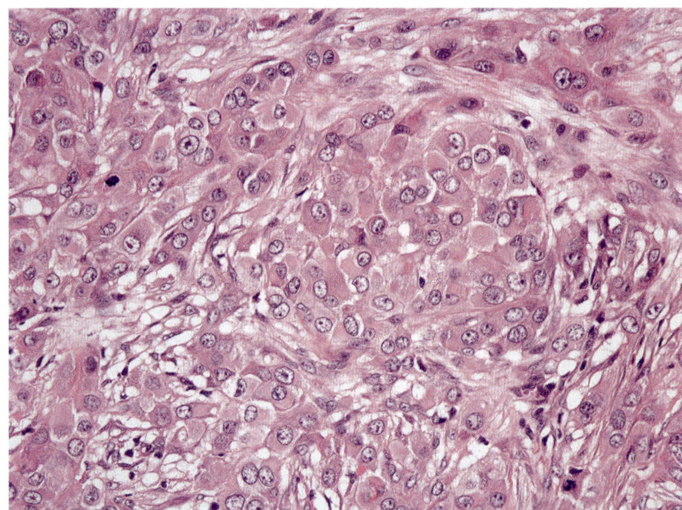

Figure 6.60 Epithelioid Sarcoma. The tumor is composed of epithelioid cells with abundant eosinophilic cytoplasm, vesicular chromatin, and small nucleoli.

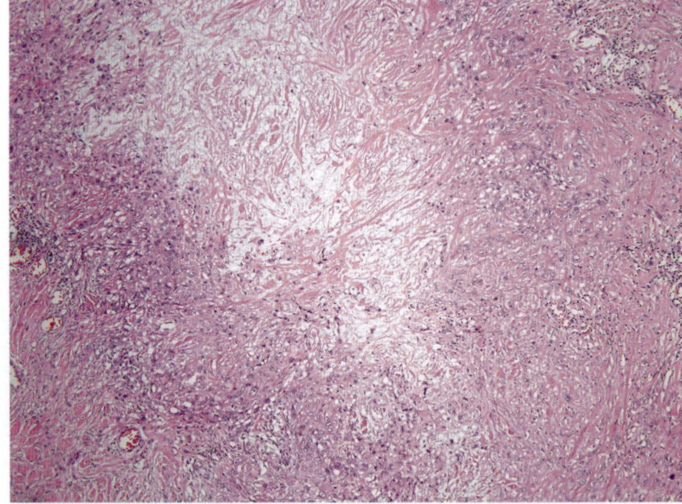

Figure 6.61 Epithelioid Sarcoma. A large nodule of tumor cells shows central necrosis. This feature may superficially mimic a necrobiotic process.

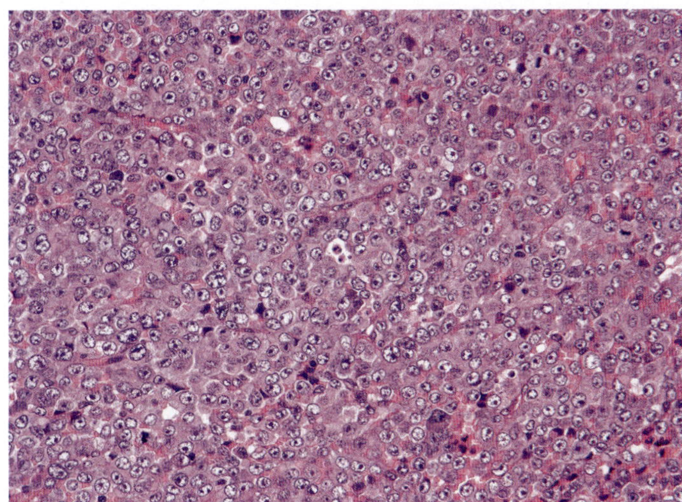

Figure 6.62 Proximal-Type Epithelioid Sarcoma. This variant is composed of sheets of large epithelioid cells with amphophilic cytoplasm, marked nuclear atypia, vesicular chromatin, and prominent nucleoli.

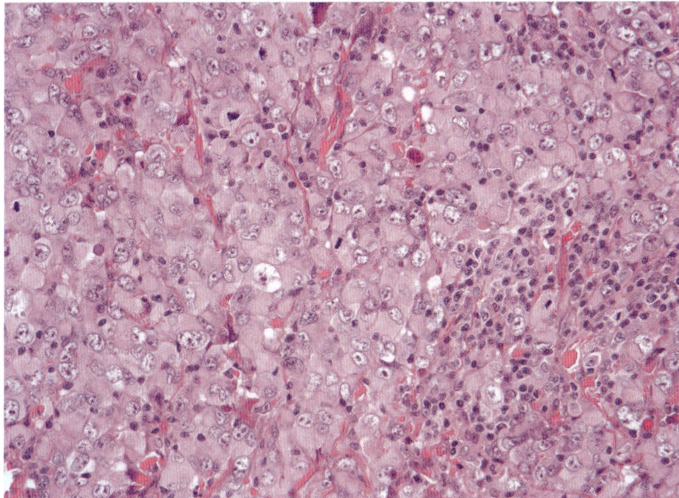

Figure 6.63 Proximal-Type Epithelioid Sarcoma. The cells in this tumor contain eosinophilic hyaline (rhabdoid) cytoplasmic inclusions.

in conventional epithelioid sarcoma is not seen. The "fibroma-like" variant of epithelioid sarcoma was the original designation for a distinctive tumor type now recognized to be endothelial in nature and unrelated to epithelioid sarcoma.[122] Now known as *pseudomyogenic hemangioendothelioma* (also referred to as *epithelioid sarcoma-like hemangioendothelioma*), this tumor type, which is composed of plump spindle cells with abundant brightly eosinophilic cytoplasm and minimal cytologic atypia, often presents as multiple discontiguous lesions in different tissue planes.[108,109] Pseudomyogenic hemangioendothelioma is discussed in more detail in Chapters 3 and 15. The "angiomatoid" variant of epithelioid sarcoma is similar to conventional epithelioid sarcoma except for the presence of hemorrhagic spaces surrounded by tumor cells, mimicking a vascular neoplasm, especially epithelioid angiosarcoma.[111,118]

Immunohistochemistry

By immunohistochemistry, tumor cells in epithelioid sarcoma show consistent diffuse reactivity for EMA and keratins (both low and high molecular weight) (Fig. 6.64), as well as the nonspecific marker vimentin; 50% of cases are also positive for CD34.[111,112,118,123,124] Proximal-type epithelioid sarcoma is somewhat more often positive for CD34 than conventional epithelioid sarcoma.[124] Occasional reactivity for smooth muscle actin, muscle-specific actin (HHF35), and S-100 protein has also been reported.[118,124] Epithelioid sarcoma is usually negative for desmin and CD31, and expression of p63 and keratin 5/6 is infrequent, distinguishing epithelioid sarcoma from cutaneous squamous cell carcinoma.[118,123,125] Similar to MRT, loss of INI1 expression is seen in approximately 90% of conventional and 95% of proximal-type epithelioid sarcomas (Fig. 6.65).[124,126,127]

Molecular Genetics

Abnormalities of 8q, 18q, and 22q have been identified in epithelioid sarcoma, including loss of heterozygosity on 22q, t(8;22)(q22;q11), and t(10;22).[111,127–132] The *SMARCB1* (*INI1*) tumor suppressor gene located at 22q11 is inactivated in both proximal-type and conventional epithelioid sarcoma (which correlates with the loss of protein expression by immunohistochemistry).[124,127] Monoallelic deletion of *SMARCB1*, along with epigenetic silencing by particular miRNAs, is a common mechanism of *SMARCB1* inactivation in epithelioid sarcoma; a small subset of cases show biallelic *SMARCB1* deletion.[133–136] This contrasts with MRT, in which biallelic *SMARCB1* gene deletions and point mutations are common. Comparative genomic hybridization studies have also reported gains at chromosomes 11q, 1q, 6p, and 9q in epithelioid sarcoma.[137]

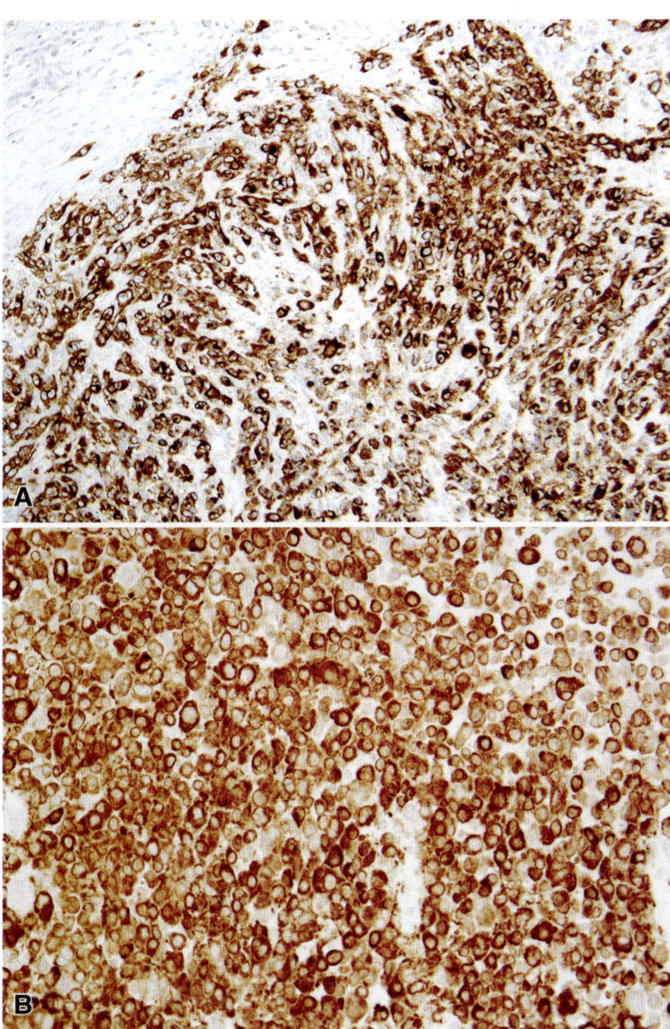

Figure 6.64 Epithelioid Sarcoma. This tumor type is nearly always positive for both epithelial membrane antigen (A) and keratins (B).

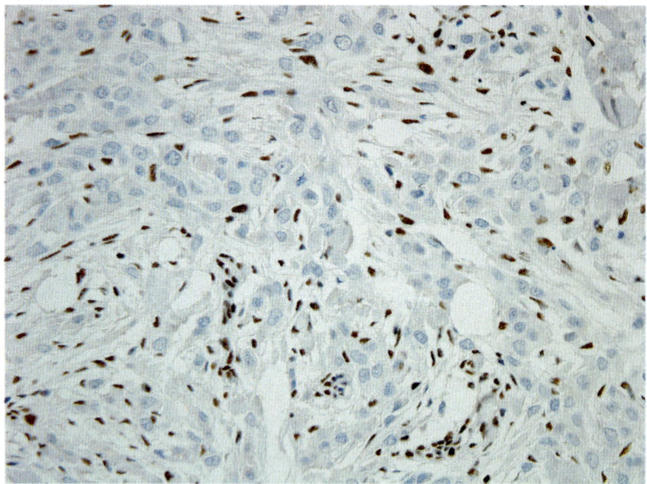

Figure 6.65 **Epithelioid Sarcoma.** Loss of INI1 protein expression is a characteristic feature. Note the nuclear staining in lymphocytes and stromal cells, which serve as an internal control.

Box 6.19 Differential Diagnosis of Epithelioid Sarcoma

If a Granuloma-Like Appearance Predominates

Granuloma annulare
Rheumatoid nodule

If an Epithelioid Appearance Predominates

Carcinoma (squamous cell carcinoma)
Melanoma
Malignant mesothelioma
Epithelioid hemangioendothelioma
Epithelioid angiosarcoma
Pseudomyogenic hemangioendothelioma
Epithelioid malignant peripheral nerve sheath tumor
Extrarenal malignant rhabdoid tumor
Myoepithelioma/myoepithelial carcinoma of soft tissue

If a Spindle Cell Appearance Predominates

Clear cell sarcoma
Myofibroblastic sarcoma
Pseudomyogenic hemangioendothelioma

Differential Diagnosis

Many entities should be considered in the differential diagnosis of epithelioid sarcoma (Box 6.19). Conventional epithelioid sarcoma should primarily be differentiated from carcinoma (especially ulcerating squamous cell carcinoma), EHE, epithelioid angiosarcoma, pseudomyogenic hemangioendothelioma, melanoma, and epithelioid MPNST, as well as benign conditions such as rheumatoid nodule and (deep) granuloma annulare.[109,111,112,118] Unlike epithelioid sarcoma, squamous cell carcinoma is usually diffusely positive for p63 and keratin 5/6, retains expression of INI1, and is negative for CD34.[118,123,125] Unlike epithelioid sarcoma, epithelioid melanomas show diffuse expression of S-100 protein and SOX10, often in addition to HMB-45 and melan A, whereas INI1 expression is retained. Some rhabdoid melanomas may express keratins, which can be a diagnostic pitfall; expression of melanocytic markers and INI1 is helpful in this context.[127] Epithelioid MPNST is strongly positive for S-100 protein and SOX10 and is usually negative for epithelial markers, although two-thirds of epithelioid MPNST cases show loss of INI1 expression, similar to epithelioid sarcoma.[127] Epithelioid sarcoma composed predominantly of spindle cells may be confused with a myofibroblastic sarcoma because both lesions may be positive for muscle-specific actin (HHF35) and smooth muscle actin. However, myofibroblastic sarcomas are negative for EMA, usually negative for keratins, and often positive for desmin. Finally, benign conditions such as rheumatoid nodule and (deep) granuloma annulare might also be included in the differential diagnosis of conventional epithelioid sarcoma, if a granulomatous pattern is evident. However, on close examination, granulomatous conditions lack the cytologic atypia of epithelioid sarcoma, and immunohistochemistry for EMA and keratins can easily confirm the diagnosis of epithelioid sarcoma.

The angiomatoid variant of epithelioid sarcoma (as well as conventional epithelioid sarcoma) should be distinguished from epithelioid angiosarcoma. Epithelioid angiosarcoma may express keratins (in up to 50% of cases), but EMA is negative. Unlike epithelioid sarcoma, epithelioid angiosarcoma is consistently positive for CD31 and shows retained expression of INI1. Pseudomyogenic hemangioendothelioma shows clinical similarities to epithelioid sarcoma (young adults, soft tissues of distal extremities) and also strongly expresses keratins. However, the morphologic features (plump spindle cell morphology and bright cytoplasmic eosinophilia) more closely resemble a myogenic neoplasm, and expression of ERG, CD31, and INI1 as well as lack of staining for EMA and CD34 allow for the distinction between these tumor types.

Proximal-type epithelioid sarcoma can be confused with metastatic melanoma and extrarenal MRT.[138] Indeed, there is considerable overlap between MRT and proximal-type epithelioid sarcoma in terms of morphologic features (both tumor types may contain rhabdoid cells) and immunoprofile (both tumor types express vimentin, keratins, and EMA, and they show loss of INI1 expression). There are, however, significant differences between the two neoplasms (reviewed in reference 127). MRT occurs in infants and young children and pursues a more rapidly aggressive clinical course than epithelioid sarcoma. Morphologically, MRT is often dominated by rhabdoid cells, whereas epithelioid sarcoma usually shows at most a limited rhabdoid component. The two neoplasms also show genetic differences. Although both tumor types often show deletions of *SMARCB1*, mutations in this gene are consistently observed in MRT, but are rare in epithelioid sarcoma.[133,134]

Prognosis and Treatment

Epithelioid sarcoma is characterized by a protracted clinical course. It tends to propagate along fascial planes, tendons, and nerve sheaths. Local recurrence, metastasis, and death can occur 20 years or longer after the initial diagnosis; long-term follow-up is therefore mandatory. The prognosis chiefly depends on the initial tumor stage at presentation (localized versus disseminated disease) and resectability.[126,139–142] In a study by Jawad and colleagues of 441 cases, the disease-specific survival was 68% at 5 years and 61% at 10 years.[142] Patients with localized disease had a better 5-year survival (75%) than patients with regional spread, who had a 5-year survival rate of 49%.[142] The recurrence rate, which depends mainly on the adequacy of the initial surgical excision, varies between 30% and 85%.[112,124,139,142] Metastases develop in 20% to 60% of patients, usually after repeated local recurrences, primarily to lungs, but also to regional lymph nodes (20% to 40% of cases), bone, and scalp (20% of cases).[111,112,124,139,142] Because positive margins are associated with an increased recurrence rate and reduced survival, radical surgery (wide excision or amputation) is advocated as the primary treatment of epithelioid sarcoma,[139] although encouraging results were recently obtained using a combination of conservative surgery and radiation therapy.[141] In a study by Chbani and colleagues, 39 of 48 patients (81%) who underwent initial complete resection were free from local recurrence at last examination with a median follow-up of 4 years.[124] Lymph node dissection is indicated only if clinically apparent lymph node metastases are present. Potential adverse prognostic factors in epithelioid sarcoma include male sex, advanced age (>75 years), large tumor size (>5 cm), deep or proximal location, the presence of tumor necrosis, nuclear pleomorphism, high mitotic activity, vascular or nerve invasion, inadequate excision, multiple local recurrences, and regional lymph node metastases at diagnosis.[111,112,124,139–142]

Proximal-type epithelioid sarcoma is associated with a more aggressive clinical course and earlier tumor-related deaths compared to the more indolent behavior and protracted course of conventional epithelioid sarcoma.[112,113]

PRACTICE POINTS: Epithelioid Sarcoma

- Predilection for the distal extremities of young adults
- Nodular growth pattern with central necrosis may superficially mimic a granulomatous process
- Uniform epithelioid cells with mild nuclear atypia and eosinophilic cytoplasm
- Proximal-type epithelioid sarcoma arises in the pelvis, perineum, and axilla and shows large cell morphology with marked cytologic atypia
- Diffusely positive for epithelial membrane antigen (EMA) and keratins; 50% positive for CD34
- Loss of INI1 expression is a characteristic finding
- Protracted clinical course, with late recurrences and metastases
- Proximal-type epithelioid sarcoma has a more aggressive course

SMARCA4-Deficient Thoracic Sarcoma

SMARCA4 is the ATPase subunit of the SWI/SNF chromatin-remodeling complex. Recently, *SMARCA4* mutations were identified in ovarian small cell carcinoma of hypercalcemic type,[143,144] a small subset of MRTs (with intact INI1 expression),[145] and some undifferentiated thoracic sarcomas with epithelioid features.[115,116] This group of thoracic sarcomas arises in the chest wall, pleura, or mediastinum, usually in male smokers, and includes tumors that are morphologically and immunohistochemically similar to proximal-type epithelioid sarcoma but show intact INI1 expression.[115,116] Others may resemble poorly differentiated carcinomas but show expression of CD34,[115,116] a finding that generally argues against carcinoma, and lack expression of TTF-1 or other lineage-specific markers. Similar to proximal-type epithelioid sarcomas, these tumors often have a multinodular growth pattern and are composed of monomorphic large epithelioid tumor cells with moderate amounts of amphophilic or palely eosinophilic cytoplasm and round to oval nuclei with prominent nucleoli (Fig. 6.66A). Tumor cells often have rhabdoid features, and geographic tumor necrosis is common. Expression of EMA, keratins, and CD34 is observed in most cases and INI1 is intact. However, loss of SMARCA4 protein expression (see Fig. 6.66B) and concomitant loss of SMARCA2 (another member of the SWI/SNF complex) are also seen, which correspond to the presence of *SMARCA4* mutations; strong SOX2 expression is another characteristic finding. These tumors pursue an aggressive clinical course; metastases are often detected at the time of presentation.[115,116]

Extrarenal Malignant Rhabdoid Tumor

Extrarenal MRT is a malignant neoplasm of infants and children that is composed of epithelioid cells with large eccentric nuclei with vesicular chromatin and prominent nucleoli and abundant cytoplasm with variably prominent eosinophilic hyaline inclusions, which are composed of whorls of intermediate filaments.[1] MRTs typically arise in the kidney, brain (atypical teratoid/rhabdoid tumor), and soft tissue, pursue a highly aggressive clinical course, and show biallelic inactivation of the *SMARCB1* (*INI1*) tumor suppressor gene in the vast majority of cases; a small subset instead have mutations in *SMARCA4* (*BRG1*).[126,144,146–148] Morphologically similar tumors have been reported in adults, either as pure or composite rhabdoid neoplasms.[148–151] Over time, it has become clear that in adults, the rhabdoid phenotype is a nonspecific pattern that can be observed in many unrelated neoplasms, including carcinomas (e.g., kidney, lung, stomach, endometrium, bladder, liver), melanoma, large cell lymphoma, malignant mesothelioma, meningioma, glioma, and various sarcoma subtypes (Box 6.20).[1,99,148,152] SMARCB1 or SMARCA4 deficiency due to mutations with loss of corresponding protein expression has now been described in a subset of endometrial, renal, gastrointestinal, and lung carcinomas, as well as some gliomas, most of which (but not all) show rhabdoid morphology or are morphologically undifferentiated.[153–162]

Clinical Features

MRTs of soft tissue are rare, accounting for less than 1% of all soft tissue sarcomas.[1,142,146–148,163,164] They develop most frequently in the deep soft

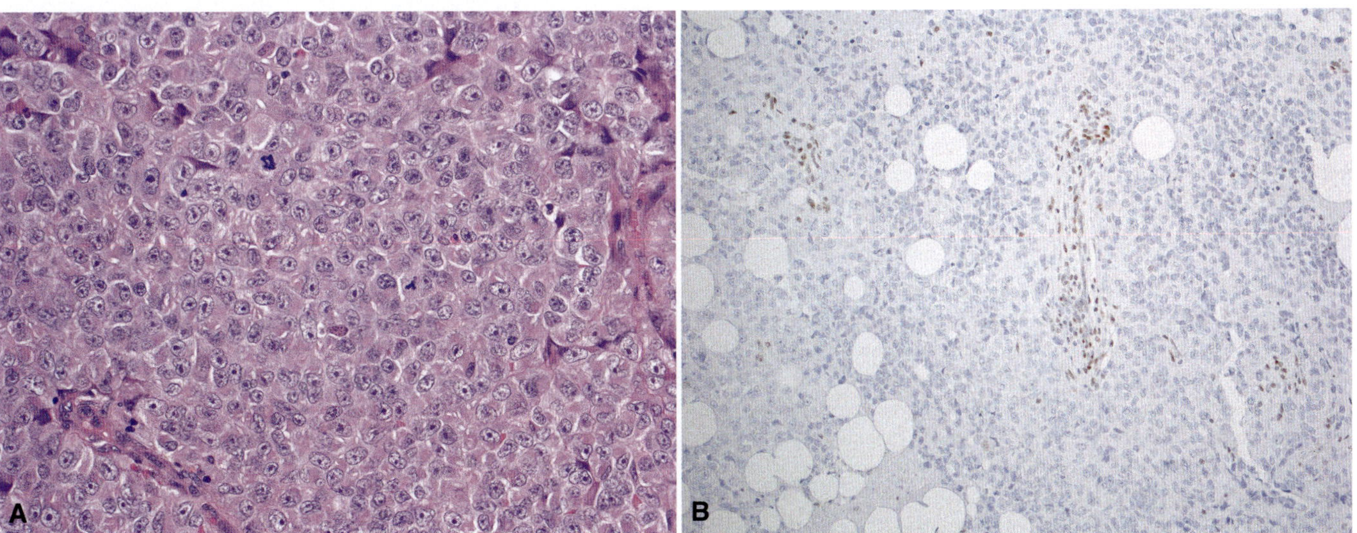

Figure 6.66 SMARCA4-Deficient Thoracic Sarcoma. (A) The tumor is composed of sheets of large epithelioid cells with vesicular chromatin, prominent nucleoli, and eosinophilic cytoplasm. (B) Loss of SMARCA4 protein expression is a defining feature.

Box 6.20 Rhabdoid Phenotype in Mesenchymal Lesions

Mesenchymal Lesions That Frequently Display a Rhabdoid Phenotype
Malignant rhabdoid tumor (renal and extrarenal)
Epithelioid sarcoma (conventional and proximal-type)
SMARCA4-deficient thoracic sarcoma
Epithelioid angiosarcoma
Perivascular epithelioid cell tumor/epithelioid angiomyolipoma

Mesenchymal Lesions That Occasionally Display a Rhabdoid Phenotype
Rhabdomyosarcoma
Myoepithelioma/myoepithelial carcinoma
Epithelioid malignant peripheral nerve sheath tumor
Desmoplastic small round cell tumor
Extraskeletal myxoid chondrosarcoma
Synovial sarcoma
Alveolar soft part sarcoma
Epithelioid hemangioendothelioma
Leiomyosarcoma (epithelioid variant)
Endometrial stromal sarcoma

tissues of the proximal extremities and limb girdles, but may also occur in the pelvis, perineum, abdomen, retroperitoneum, and neck, and tend to localize along the vertebral axis. Infants and young children are predominantly affected, without gender predilection. Almost all cases affect children who are younger than 10 years of age.[146-148,163,164]

Pathologic Features

Tumors present as unencapsulated masses that measure between 2 and 25 cm (median size, 5 to 7 cm). On sectioning, the lesions are often fleshy and gray or tan, with variable areas of necrosis and hemorrhage.

Histologically, MRTs are predominantly or exclusively composed of rhabdoid cells, with eccentric vesicular nuclei; prominent nucleoli; and glassy, eosinophilic, inclusion-like cytoplasm (Fig. 6.67).[148,163,164] Inclusion-like structures correspond to paranuclear aggregates of intermediate filaments on ultrastructural examination. Tumor cells are usually arranged in solid sheets or trabeculae separated by fibrous septa, or occasionally in an alveolar growth pattern. Mitoses are usually numerous, and necrosis is common. Some cases may be dominated by primitive undifferentiated round cells with few cells showing the classic rhabdoid phenotype (Fig. 6.68).[148,163,164]

Immunohistochemistry

Classically, MRTs express vimentin, keratins, and EMA. Overall, 80% of cases are positive for at least one epithelial marker, and two-thirds express CD99.[148,163,164] Keratin positivity is most common with CK8 and CK18 and it is often confined to globoid paranuclear inclusions. Expression of neural markers is also common. More than 50% of cases expressed synaptophysin, CD57, and neuron-specific enolase (NSE).[164] Smooth muscle actin and S-100 protein are expressed in a small subset of cases, usually only focally. MRTs are usually negative for HMB-45, melan A, chromogranin, GFAP, CD34, and desmin. Nearly all cases of MRT show loss of INI1 protein expression by immunohistochemistry (Fig. 6.69).[146-148,165] Nuclear staining for INI1 is seen in normal cells such as endothelial cells and lymphocytes, which serve as internal positive controls. Although initially considered relatively specific for MRT, loss of INI1 expression has also been observed in the majority (>95%) of epithelioid sarcomas (both conventional and proximal-type), two-thirds of epithelioid MPNSTs, and a subset of myoepithelial carcinomas (10% to 40% of cases).[26,124,127,130] In addition, among nonmesenchymal neoplasms, a small subset of carcinomas, melanomas, and meningiomas occurring in adults show a secondary rhabdoid phenotype (sometimes

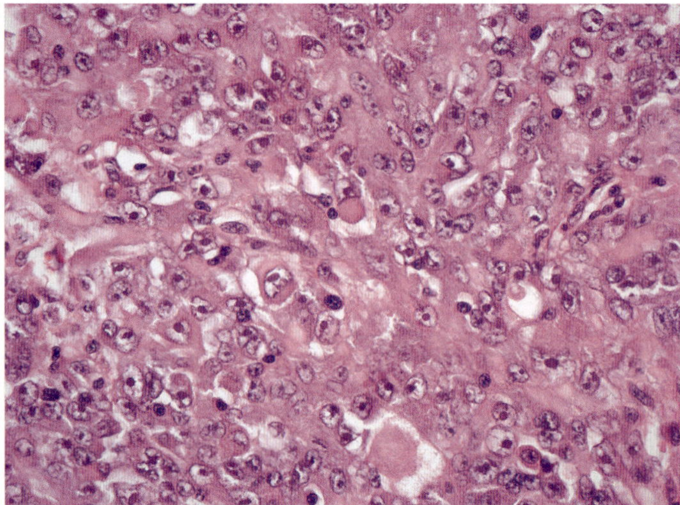

Figure 6.67 Malignant Rhabdoid Tumor. Large epithelioid tumor cells contain vesicular nuclei, large nucleoli, and eosinophilic hyaline cytoplasmic inclusions.

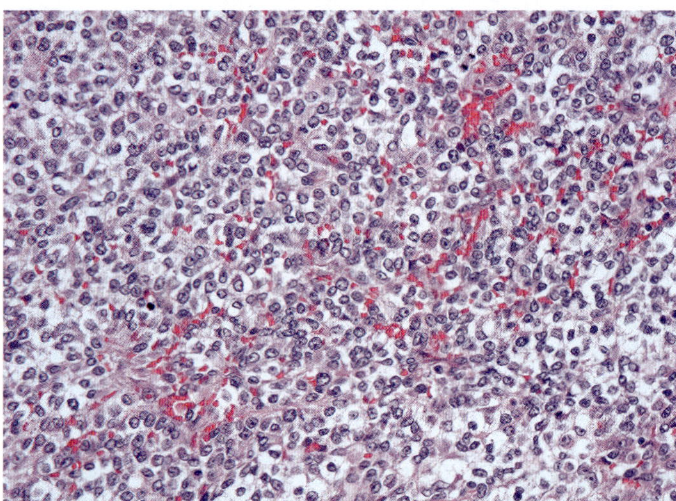

Figure 6.68 Malignant Rhabdoid Tumor. Some cases are dominated by undifferentiated cells, with only limited areas showing the characteristic rhabdoid morphology.

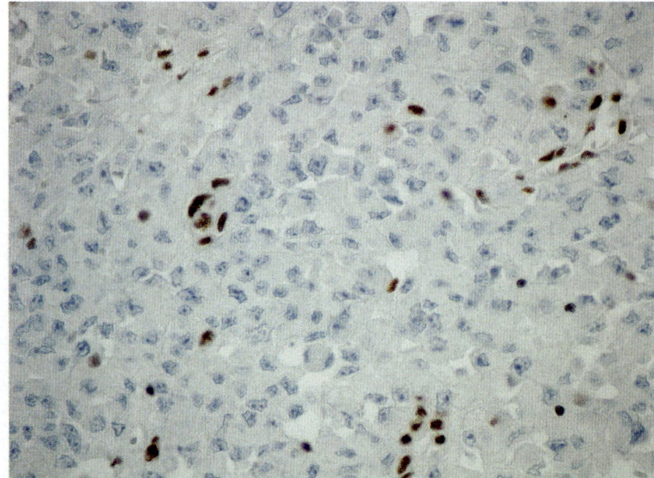

Figure 6.69 Malignant Rhabdoid Tumor. The tumor cells show loss of INI1 expression. Note the nuclear staining in endothelial cells and lymphocytes.

referred to as "composite rhabdoid tumors") and may have loss of INI1 or SMARCA4 expression, reflecting dysfunction of the SWI/SNF complex.[153-162,166] For such cases, evaluation of additional immunohistochemical stains in conjunction with clinical history is needed.

Molecular Genetics

Nearly all MRTs show biallelic inactivation of the *SMARCB1* (*INI1*) tumor suppressor gene on 22q11.2, resulting in loss of protein expression (as detected by immunohistochemistry).[146,147] The *SMARCB1* gene, a member of the SWI/SNF complex, plays a critical role in adenosine triphosphate (ATP)-dependent chromatin remodeling, and the regulation of cell cycle and cytoskeletal dynamics. Chromosomal alterations involving the *SMARCB1* gene include deletions or translocations involving 22q, monosomy 22, and inactivating mutations.[146,147] Mutations and monosomy 22 are predominantly observed in MRTs of the central nervous system and kidney, whereas homozygous deletions and translocations are more common in MRTs of soft tissues.[146,147,159] Patients with multiple MRTs often show germline mutations of the *SMARCB1* gene.[146,147] The *TP53* gene is also often mutated in renal and extrarenal MRTs.[148]

It has recently been shown that the small subset of MRTs that show retained INI1 expression instead have mutations in *SMARCA4* (*BRG1*), another member of the SWI/SNF chromatin-remodeling complex. Corresponding loss of protein expression of SMARCA4 can be identified by immunohistochemistry in these rare tumors, most of which have been reported in the brain (atypical teratoid/rhabdoid tumor).

Differential Diagnosis

In adult patients, MRTs are exceptionally rare, and other tumor types with rhabdoid morphology must be considered, including metastatic carcinoma, metastatic melanoma, malignant mesothelioma, and lymphoma (especially diffuse large B-cell lymphoma, anaplastic large-cell lymphoma, and plasmacytoma). Soft tissue tumors that can be confused with MRTs are listed in Box 6.20.

In contrast to MRT, tumor cells in rhabdomyosarcomas express desmin, myogenin, and INI1, and are usually negative for epithelial markers, although a subset of alveolar rhabdomyosarcomas may express keratins. Epithelioid angiosarcoma and EHE are positive for CD31 and less often for CD34 and podoplanin (D2-40). Approximately 50% of epithelioid angiosarcomas express keratins, but they are negative for EMA and show intact expression of INI1. PEComas usually express HMB-45 or melan A and are negative for keratins and EMA. Myoepithelial tumors may overlap morphologically and immunophenotypically with MRTs, although they are more consistently positive for S-100 protein, GFAP, and smooth muscle actin than MRT. Of note, myoepithelial carcinomas of soft tissue may show loss of expression of INI1, especially in children.[26,127] Epithelioid MPNST may be confused with MRT, inasmuch as epithelioid MPNST shows loss of INI1 expression in up to two-thirds of cases.[127,167] However, as opposed to MRTs, epithelioid MPNSTs are strongly and diffusely positive for S-100 protein and negative for keratins. Desmoplastic small round cell tumors may occasionally contain rhabdoid cell–rich areas. However, they also usually contain more typical areas composed of sheets and nests of small cells separated by an abundant, myofibroblast-rich, collagenous stroma, a feature not observed in MRTs. In addition to expressing epithelial markers and desmin, in contrast to MRTs, desmoplastic small round cell tumors retain expression of INI1. Some cellular and poorly differentiated variants of EMC may focally contain rhabdoid cells. As opposed to MRTs, most EMCs express INI1 and are negative for keratins. In difficult cases, the detection of the characteristic fusion transcripts (*NR4A3-EWSR1* or variants) can aid in this distinction. Some exceptional cases of EMC with prominent rhabdoid features may lack these fusion transcripts and may show loss of INI1; the significance of this unusual finding is uncertain.[153] In ASPS, tumor cells are usually larger with more abundant eosinophilic cytoplasm than in MRT. In contrast with MRTs, the cells of ASPS typically show a pseudoalveolar growth pattern, retain INI1 staining, and express the TFE3 protein, as a consequence of the t(X;17) translocation.

Although there is morphologic and immunophenotypic overlap between MRT and proximal-type epithelioid sarcoma, there are also significant differences between these tumor types.[120,127,149-151] In contrast to MRT, proximal-type epithelioid sarcoma affects young to middle-aged adults, tends to show a multinodular growth pattern, and is usually dominated by large epithelioid cells with eosinophilic to amphophilic cytoplasm. Although proximal-type epithelioid sarcoma has a high rate of metastasis, it does not have the rapidly progressive clinical course typical of MRT. Although both tumors show loss of INI1 expression by immunohistochemistry, only MRTs often harbor *SMARCB1* mutations. *TP53* mutations are also more common in MRTs than in epithelioid sarcomas.

Prognosis and Treatment

MRTs are malignant neoplasms characterized by highly aggressive behavior and early death. For MRTs of soft tissue, the local recurrence rate is 20% to 25%, and the metastatic rate is 50% to 80%; nearly two-thirds of patients are dead of disease within 2 years of diagnosis.[163,164] The 5-year survival rate is only 15% to 20%.[148,163,164] The most common sites of metastasis are the lungs, pleura, lymph nodes, liver, and bone.

Optimal treatment consists of combinations of multiagent neoadjuvant chemotherapy and radiation therapy, followed by complete excision of the tumor with tumor-free margins, although responses to chemotherapy are often short-lived.

PRACTICE POINTS: Malignant Rhabdoid Tumor

- Affects infants and young children
- Arises in the kidney and brain ("atypical teratoid/rhabdoid tumor"), with wide anatomic distribution in deep soft tissue
- Rhabdoid cytology: eccentric vesicular nuclei with prominent nucleoli and hyaline eosinophilic cytoplasmic inclusions
- Rhabdoid features are also seen in adult tumor types (melanoma, mesothelioma, carcinoma)—no relationship to malignant rhabdoid tumor of infancy
- Positive for epithelial membrane antigen (EMA) and keratins; loss of INI1 expression is a characteristic finding; rare cases instead show loss of SMARCA4 expression
- Highly aggressive behavior, with disseminated metastases and early death

Sclerosing Epithelioid Fibrosarcoma

Described in 1995 by Meis-Kindblom and colleagues, SEF is a rare aggressive variant of fibrosarcoma that can easily be confused with metastatic carcinoma.[168] Recent studies have demonstrated that a subset of SEFs are associated with, and share the genetic signature of, low-grade fibromyxoid sarcoma.

Clinical Features

SEF occurs in adults (median age, 45 years) with an equal gender distribution. Tumors are often painful and develop predominantly in the deep soft tissue of the limbs (especially lower limbs) and limb girdles.[168-172] Rarely, SEF arises in bone.[173] Radiologically, SEF is usually a well-circumscribed and rarely calcified mass.

Pathologic Features

SEF measures 5 to 10 cm in maximal diameter. It is a well-circumscribed, lobulated tumor that may show calcifications, cystic areas, or myxoid change on sectioning. Necrosis is uncommon.

Histologically, SEF is characterized by epithelioid or clear tumor cells, arranged in strands (mimicking signet-ring-cell carcinoma), nests, or acini (mimicking paraganglioma), embedded in a densely hyalinized collagenous matrix (Fig. 6.70).[168–173] Nuclei are round and relatively bland, and mitotic activity is usually minimal (Fig. 6.71). Sclerotic hypocellular areas sometimes coexist with more cellular zones containing fascicles of spindle cells, resembling conventional fibrosarcoma (Fig. 6.72). Focal myxoid change, metaplastic cartilage or bone, slitlike pseudovascular spaces, and calcified foci may also be observed. Rare hybrid tumors are composed of both SEF and low-grade fibromyxoid sarcoma, the latter component showing characteristic sharply demarcated myxoid and fibrous areas, a whorling growth pattern, arcades of thin-walled blood vessels, and bland spindle cell morphology. The tumor often shows infiltrative margins into surrounding tissues and may invade periosteum and bone.

Immunohistochemistry

Tumor cells in SEF show variable staining for EMA (in ~50% of cases); expression of S-100 protein and keratins is uncommon. CD34, desmin, smooth muscle actin, and HMB-45 are consistently negative.[168–173] MUC4, a marker of low-grade fibromyxoid sarcoma identified by gene expression profiling (see Chapter 3), is positive in the majority of SEF cases, including tumors with hybrid features of both SEF and low-grade fibromyxoid sarcoma.[174,175]

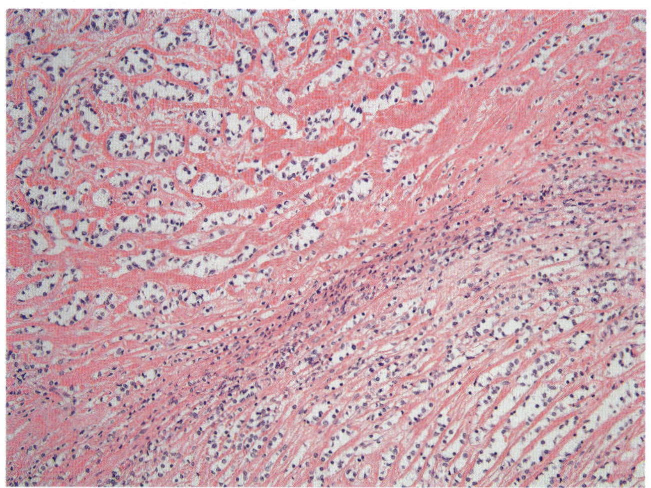

Figure 6.70 **Sclerosing Epithelioid Fibrosarcoma.** Cords and trabeculae of epithelioid cells in a densely hyalinized stroma.

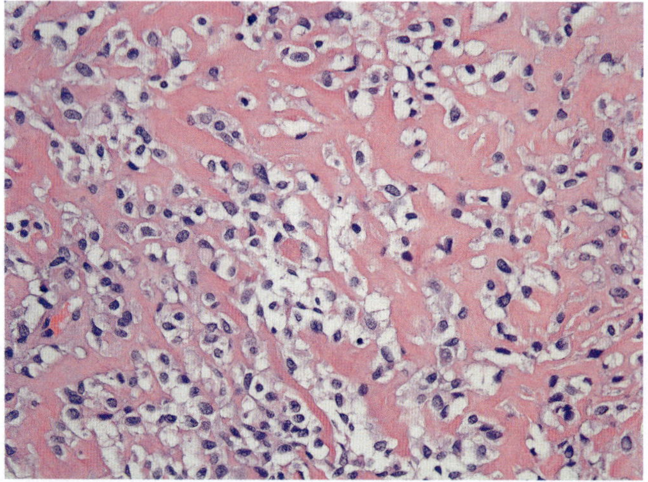

Figure 6.71 **Sclerosing Epithelioid Fibrosarcoma.** Bland uniform epithelioid cells have clear cytoplasm. The sclerotic stroma may mimic osteoid.

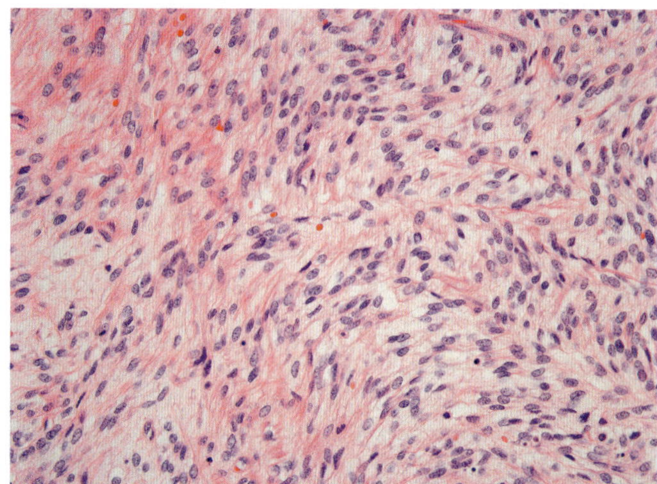

Figure 6.72 **Sclerosing Epithelioid Fibrosarcoma.** A fascicular, fibroblastic spindle cell component is sometimes also present.

Molecular Genetics

Most SEFs contain an *EWSR1-CREB3L1* or less often *EWSR1-CREB3L2* fusion gene,[175–178] whereas the hybrid tumors with areas of both SEF and low-grade fibromyxoid sarcoma harbor the *FUS-CREB3L2* fusion, resulting from the t(7;16) translocation characteristic of low-grade fibromyxoid sarcoma; a small subset of "pure" SEF cases also harbor *FUS* rearrangements.[175,179,180]

Differential Diagnosis

The differential diagnosis of SEF is wide (summarized in Box 6.21). This tumor should be differentiated primarily from metastatic carcinoma, especially signet-ring-cell carcinoma and lobular breast carcinoma, sclerosing lymphoma, and extraskeletal osteosarcoma. In this context, previous medical history, clinical presentation, immunohistochemical features, and molecular data should all be taken into consideration.

SEFs often express EMA, but most cases are negative for keratins, which allows for the distinction from metastatic carcinoma. Expression of CK20 and CDX-2 would support metastatic gastric carcinoma, whereas GATA3, estrogen receptor, and progesterone receptor expression would favor lobular breast carcinoma. The rare epithelioid (nonglandular) variant of synovial sarcoma may resemble SEF, although the trabecular growth pattern and dense sclerotic stroma would favor SEF. Synovial sarcoma is usually positive for EMA, keratins, and TLE1, and, in contrast to SEF, bears the t(X;18) translocation. Myoepithelial carcinomas are usually more highly cellular, with areas of myxoid stroma, and show more intratumoral heterogeneity than SEF. Although some myoepithelial carcinomas show expression of MUC4, which may be a diagnostic pitfall, in most cases expression in such tumors is focal, in contrast to the diffuse expression typical of SEF.[175] Coexpression of keratins, EMA, and S-100 protein is characteristic of myoepithelial carcinoma. Both tumor types may have *EWSR1* gene rearrangement; therefore, FISH for *EWSR1* is not useful in this differential diagnosis. Sclerosing rhabdomyosarcoma is positive for desmin and myogenin, and negative for EMA. Making the distinction between extraskeletal osteosarcoma and SEF may be very difficult. Both neoplasms exhibit a prominent densely hyalinized, osteoid-like collagenous matrix, in addition to epithelioid cells. However, most osteosarcomas show more significant nuclear atypia

Box 6.21 Differential Diagnosis of Sclerosing Epithelioid Fibrosarcoma

Nonmesenchymal Lesions

Metastatic carcinoma (signet-ring-cell carcinoma or lobular carcinoma of breast)
Metastatic melanoma
Malignant mesothelioma (epithelioid variant)
Paraganglioma
Lymphoma (sclerosing variant)

Mesenchymal Lesions

Hyalinizing plexiform leiomyoma
Ossifying fibromyxoid tumor
Epithelioid synovial sarcoma
Epithelioid sarcoma
Clear cell sarcoma
Epithelioid malignant peripheral nerve sheath tumor
Extraskeletal osteosarcoma
Spindle cell/sclerosing rhabdomyosarcoma
Myoepithelial carcinoma of soft tissue

than SEF, and the characteristic lacy osteoid matrix surrounding tumor cells is diagnostic of osteosarcoma. MUC4 is helpful in this setting, because osteosarcomas usually lack expression.

Prognosis and Treatment

SEFs are aggressive neoplasms. Between 30% and 50% of patients develop local recurrences, and more than 50% metastases, mainly to the lungs, bone, pleura, and soft tissues; approximately 15% of patients have distant metastases at presentation.[168–172] A literature review of 67 cases of SEF showed that 23 patients (34%) died of disease after a mean of 46 months, 24 (35%) were alive with disease, and 20 (31%) were alive without evidence of disease.[172] Proximal location, large tumor size, and male sex appear to be adverse prognostic factors. Tumors developing in the spine or head and neck seem to have the worst prognosis.[171,172] Optimal treatment consists of a combination of wide resection and preoperative or postoperative radiation therapy. Responses to conventional chemotherapy thus far have been poor.

Epithelioid and Epithelial-Like Variants of Other Sarcomas

See Boxes 6.22 to 6.24.

Box 6.22 Epithelioid Variants of Other Sarcomas

Epithelioid angiosarcoma (including the glandular variant)
Epithelioid malignant peripheral nerve sheath tumor
Epithelioid gastrointestinal stromal tumor
Epithelioid myxofibrosarcoma
Epithelioid pleomorphic liposarcoma
Epithelioid inflammatory myofibroblastic sarcoma

Box 6.23 Sarcomas Occasionally Showing Epithelioid Features

Cellular/poorly differentiated extraskeletal myxoid chondrosarcoma
Desmoplastic small round cell tumor
Dedifferentiated liposarcoma
Leiomyosarcoma
Clear cell sarcoma (especially in metastases)
Myxoinflammatory fibroblastic sarcoma

Box 6.24 Epithelial (Glandular) Variants of Other Sarcomas

Predominantly epithelial (glandular) synovial sarcoma
Glandular malignant peripheral nerve sheath tumor

Epithelioid Angiosarcoma

Angiosarcomas are malignant neoplasms showing endothelial differentiation. Several distinct clinicopathologic forms have been described, including cutaneous angiosarcoma of the head and neck, angiosarcoma arising in the setting of lymphedema (i.e., Stewart-Treves syndrome), postradiation angiosarcoma, mammary angiosarcoma, angiosarcoma of visceral organs, and angiosarcoma of soft tissue. Morphologically, the neoplasms vary in appearance from vasoformative to spindle cell or epithelioid. Angiosarcomas are discussed in detail in Chapter 13. This section discusses epithelioid angiosarcoma of soft tissue.

Clinical Features

Epithelioid angiosarcomas are rare, accounting for less than 1% of soft tissue sarcomas. This variant most often arises in the deep soft tissues of the lower extremities (especially thigh), retroperitoneum, or abdominal cavity of middle-aged to elderly adults, predominantly men.[1,181,182]

Pathologic Features

On gross examination, epithelioid angiosarcoma often presents as a large hemorrhagic and necrotic mass with a median size of 5 cm. Histologically, epithelioid angiosarcoma is composed of solid sheets of large epithelioid cells, set in a variably collagenous stroma (Fig. 6.73). The tumor often exhibits a multinodular growth pattern and infiltrative margins. The tumor cells contain abundant eosinophilic to amphophilic cytoplasm, with well-defined cell borders, and large vesicular nuclei with prominent central nucleoli (Fig. 6.74). Some epithelioid cells may be vacuolated. Occasionally, slit-like, papillary, or pseudoglandular structures may be present (Fig. 6.75). Tumor necrosis and hemorrhage are very common and may be so prominent as to obscure the tumor cells. Mitoses are often numerous. Some epithelioid angiosarcomas contain a prominent inflammatory infiltrate composed of lymphocytes, plasma cells, and less often neutrophils and eosinophils, which can also obscure the neoplastic cells.

Immunohistochemistry

Similar to conventional angiosarcomas, tumor cells in epithelioid angiosarcoma usually show reactivity for endothelial markers, including CD31, CD34, FLI1, ERG, and podoplanin (D2-40).[1,181–183] CD31 and ERG are more sensitive than CD34 and D2-40; some epithelioid angiosarcomas can be entirely negative for CD34. Approximately 30% to 50% of epithelioid angiosarcomas are positive for keratins, rarely diffusely, but they are negative for EMA.[181,182] Focal staining for smooth muscle actin may also be detected. INI1 expression is retained.[127]

Differential Diagnosis

Before epithelioid angiosarcoma can be diagnosed, it is important to exclude nonmesenchymal epithelioid mimics, namely carcinoma, melanoma, epithelioid malignant mesothelioma, and large cell non-Hodgkin lymphomas (Box 6.25). The fact that a significant subset of epithelioid angiosarcomas is positive for keratins increases the risk of confusion with carcinoma or malignant mesothelioma. Predominantly or exclusively epithelioid angiosarcomas can also be confused with other epithelioid mesenchymal tumors (see Box 6.25), especially the cellular (solid) variant of epithelioid hemangioma, epithelioid angiomatous nodule, EHE, proximal-type epithelioid sarcoma, epithelioid MPNST, and extrarenal MRT.

Epithelioid hemangiomas and epithelioid angiomatous nodules are small cutaneous or subcutaneous lesions. In epithelioid angiomatous nodules, bland epithelioid endothelial cells are arranged in sheets, whereas well-formed vessels lined by epithelioid ("hobnail") endothelial cells

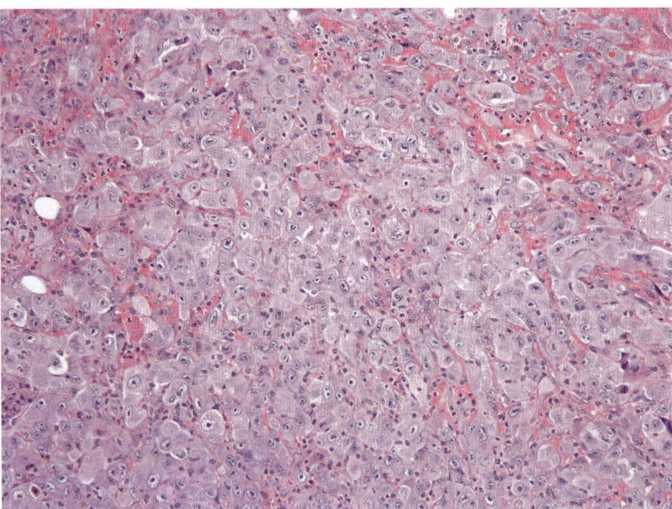

Figure 6.73 Epithelioid Angiosarcoma. The tumor is composed of sheets of large epithelioid cells.

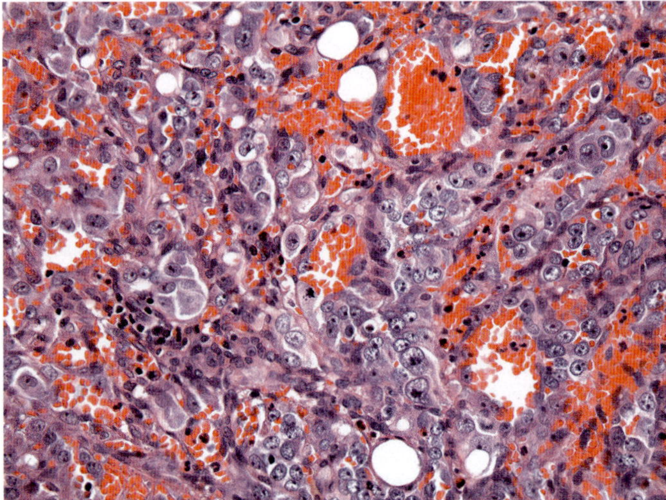

Figure 6.74 Epithelioid Angiosarcoma. The epithelioid tumor cells contain vesicular nuclei with prominent nucleoli.

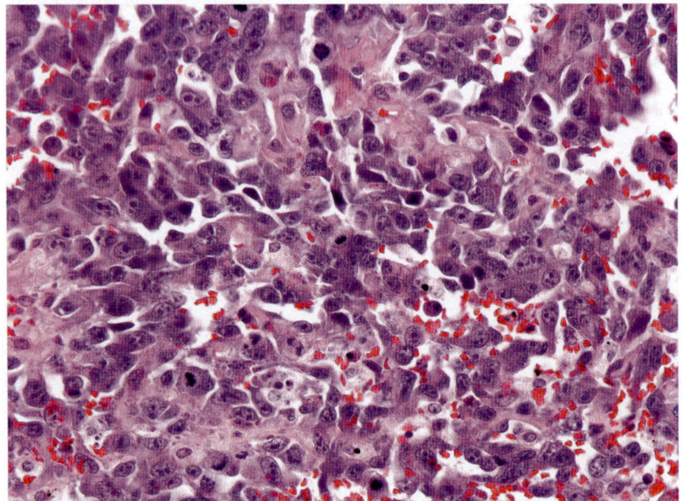

Figure 6.75 Epithelioid Angiosarcoma. The tumor cells contain amphophilic cytoplasm. Note the slit-like spaces and frequent mitotic figures.

Box 6.25 Differential Diagnosis of Epithelioid Angiosarcoma

Nonmesenchymal Lesions

Metastatic carcinoma
Metastatic melanoma
Malignant mesothelioma (epithelioid and deciduoid variants)
Lymphoma (diffuse large B-cell lymphoma and anaplastic large-cell lymphoma)
Plasma cell neoplasms

Mesenchymal Lesions

Epithelioid hemangioma
Epithelioid angiomatous nodule
Bacillary angiomatosis
Epithelioid schwannoma
Epithelioid hemangioendothelioma
Epithelioid sarcoma (especially angiomatoid variant)
Epithelioid malignant peripheral nerve sheath tumor
Epithelioid leiomyosarcoma
Epithelioid gastrointestinal stromal tumor
Extrarenal malignant rhabdoid tumor
Myoepithelial carcinoma of soft tissue
Malignant perivascular epithelioid cell tumor

are seen in epithelioid hemangioma; both lesions may contain a prominent inflammatory infiltrate. Involvement of deep soft tissue is rare. Necrosis is absent, and mitotic figures are scarce. Tumor cell nuclei and nucleoli are much smaller than in epithelioid angiosarcoma. FOSB expression can help distinguish epithelioid hemangioma from epithelioid angiosarcoma.

Conventional EHE differs significantly from epithelioid angiosarcoma. Tumors cells in EHE are less cytologically atypical than in epithelioid angiosarcoma and are arranged in cords set in a myxohyaline stroma, in contrast to the solid sheet-like growth of epithelioid angiosarcoma. "Malignant EHE" shows histologic features intermediate between conventional EHE and epithelioid angiosarcoma.[78,79] A uniformly solid growth pattern favors epithelioid angiosarcoma, whereas glassy cytoplasm and focally myxohyaline stroma favor EHE. The recent identification of the *WWTR1-CAMTA1* fusion gene and corresponding overexpression of CAMTA1 in EHE has provided a helpful diagnostic tool to distinguish malignant EHE from epithelioid angiosarcoma, the latter having a more aggressive clinical course.

Epithelioid sarcoma may show pseudovascular features due to cell disaggregation and the occasional presence of large hemorrhagic lakes, leading to potential confusion with epithelioid angiosarcoma.[87,91] Proximal-type epithelioid sarcoma also commonly arises in deep soft tissue and shows a nodular growth pattern and relatively uniform cytomorphology, features that are also shared with epithelioid angiosarcoma. Both neoplasms can be positive for keratins and CD34, but epithelioid sarcoma is positive for EMA and negative for CD31. INI1 expression is lost in epithelioid sarcoma (>90% of cases), but not in epithelioid angiosarcoma.

In contrast to epithelioid angiosarcomas, epithelioid MPNSTs usually arise in subcutaneous tissue and are strongly and diffusely positive for S-100 protein and negative for CD31; two-thirds of tumors show loss of INI1 expression. Extrarenal MRTs often coexpress keratin and EMA, whereas CD31 and CD34 are consistently negative; loss of INI1 expression is characteristic of MRTs.

Prognosis and Treatment

Angiosarcoma of soft tissue, including the epithelioid variant, is an aggressive neoplasm.[1,181,182] In one study, 20% of patients experienced local recurrences, 50% developed distant metastases (to the lung, lymph nodes, bone, and soft tissue), and 50% died of disease within 1 year.[182]

Poor prognostic indicators include older age, retroperitoneal location, and large tumor size.[1,182] Standard treatment of angiosarcoma of soft tissue consists of wide excision (if possible), combined with radiation therapy and chemotherapy. For patients with unresectable tumors and those with metastases, anthracycline or taxane-based (docetaxel, paclitaxel) chemotherapeutic regimens show clinical benefit.[184]

Epithelioid Malignant Peripheral Nerve Sheath Tumor

Epithelioid MPNST is rare, accounting for only 5% of all cases of MPNST.

Clinical Features

Epithelioid MPNSTs most often arise in the subcutaneous tissue of young to middle-aged adults (mean age, 35 to 45 years), and less frequently in the deep soft tissues.[167,185–187] The extremities are most commonly affected. This tumor is rarely observed in the trunk and almost never in the head and neck region. As opposed to conventional (i.e., spindle cell) MPNSTs, epithelioid MPNSTs do not occur in the context of type 1 neurofibromatosis.[167,185–187] Between 30% and 50% of cases develop in association with a large nerve or in a preexisting benign nerve sheath tumor (especially schwannoma).[167,185,186,188] Median tumor size varies from 3.5 cm (superficial lesions) to 5 cm (deep-seated tumors).[185,186]

Pathologic Features

Histologically, epithelioid MPNSTs are usually well circumscribed (especially if superficial), and often show a multinodular growth pattern (Fig. 6.76). Some tumors show a variable admixture of epithelioid and spindle cells (although this is uncommon), with a predominance of the epithelioid component.[167,185–187] Epithelioid cells usually grow in sheets but may also be arranged in nests, cords, or strands separated by hyalinized collagen bundles or within a myxoid stroma (Fig. 6.77). Characteristically, the tumor cells are relatively uniform with abundant eosinophilic cytoplasm, rounded nuclei with vesicular chromatin, and a single prominent central nucleolus (Fig. 6.78). Despite the resemblance to melanoma cells, there is no evidence of melanogenesis. Mitoses are readily found, and tumor necrosis may occasionally be present.

Immunohistochemistry

By immunohistochemistry, in contrast to conventional spindle cell MPNSTs, tumor cells in epithelioid MPNSTs are strongly and diffusely positive for S-100 protein (Fig. 6.79A) and SOX10. They are negative for melanocytic (HMB-45, melan A, MiTF), vascular (CD34, CD31), and myogenic markers (smooth muscle actin, desmin).[167,185–187] Occasional cases may show focal reactivity for epithelial markers (keratins, EMA). Approximately two-thirds of epithelioid MPNSTs show loss of INI1 expression (see Fig. 6.79B).[99,167]

Differential Diagnosis

The differential diagnosis of epithelioid MPNSTs is roughly similar to that of epithelioid angiosarcoma (see Box 6.25). Epithelioid MPNSTs may be confused with many epithelioid neoplasms, including metastatic melanoma, metastatic carcinoma, large cell lymphomas, myoepithelial carcinoma, epithelioid schwannoma, and other soft tissue sarcomas with epithelioid features (e.g., epithelioid angiosarcoma, epithelioid sarcoma, clear cell sarcoma, PEComa, rhabdomyosarcoma, extrarenal MRTs).

Metastatic melanomas usually shows more nuclear atypia and pleomorphism and a higher mitotic rate than epithelioid MPNSTs, and the tumor cells are typically not only positive for S-100 protein and SOX10 but also for other melanocytic markers, including HMB-45, melan A, and MITF. Loss of INI1 expression is not seen in melanoma. Unlike epithelioid MPNSTs, clear cell sarcoma also shows reactivity for melanocytic markers; loss of INI1 expression is specific for epithelioid MPNSTs in

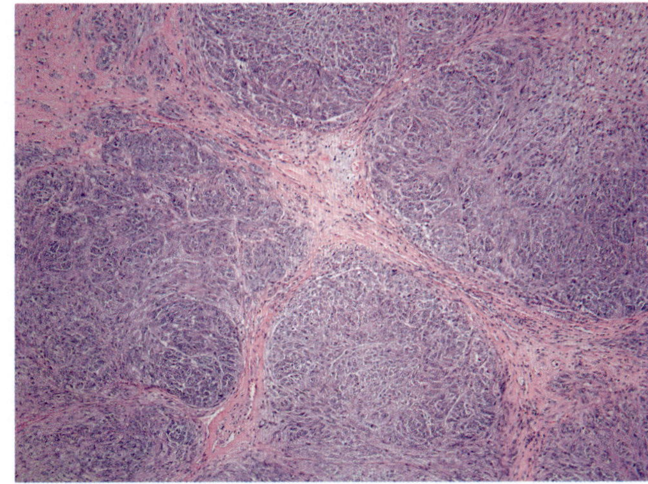

Figure 6.76 Epithelioid Malignant Peripheral Nerve Sheath Tumor. The tumor shows a multinodular growth pattern.

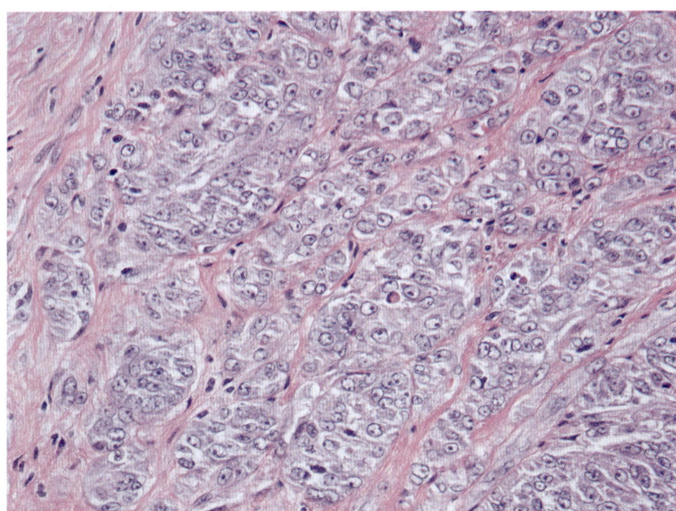

Figure 6.77 Epithelioid Malignant Peripheral Nerve Sheath Tumor. Nests of uniform epithelioid cells are seen within a collagenous stroma.

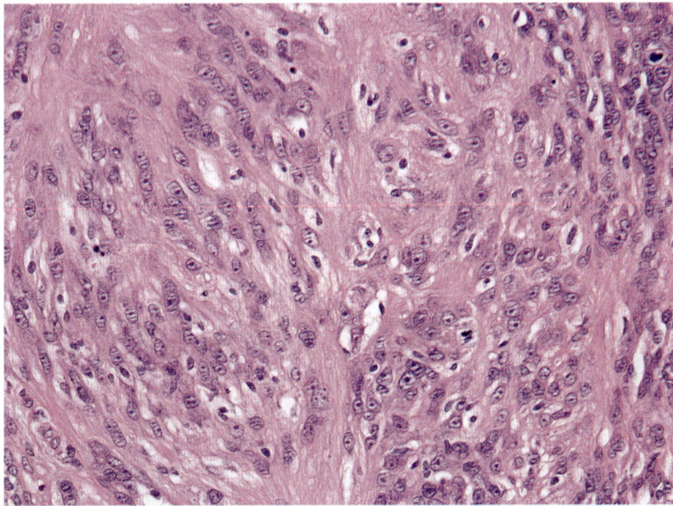

Figure 6.78 Epithelioid Malignant Peripheral Nerve Sheath Tumor. Sheets of epithelioid cells have vesicular nuclei and prominent nucleoli. Note the eosinophilic cytoplasm.

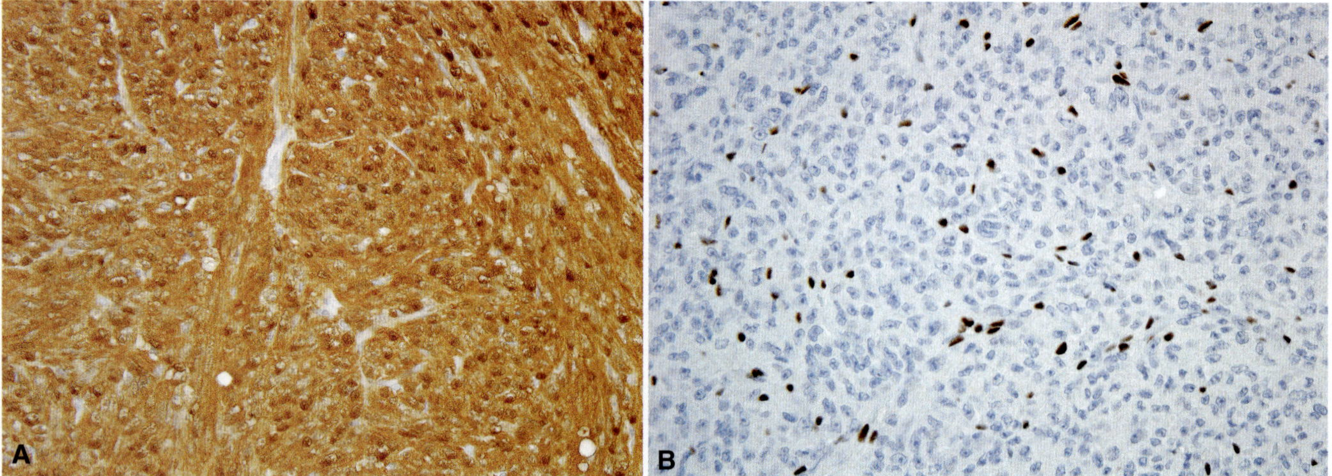

Figure 6.79 Epithelioid Malignant Peripheral Nerve Sheath Tumor. (A) Tumor cells are strongly and diffusely positive for S-100 protein. (B) Around two-thirds of tumors show loss of INI1 expression.

this differential diagnosis. Carcinomas and lymphomas can be excluded on the basis of negativity for epithelial (EMA, keratins) and lymphoid (CD45, CD20, CD3, CD30) markers. In addition to other distinctive immunophenotypic features, epithelioid sarcoma, epithelioid angiosarcoma, rhabdomyosarcoma, and extrarenal MRTs never show strong and diffuse staining for S-100 protein. In contrast to the uniformity of epithelioid MPNSTs, myoepithelial carcinoma characteristically shows intratumoral heterogeneity in both architecture and cytomorphology, and expresses epithelial markers as well as S-100 protein. Loss of INI1 expression may be seen in both tumor types. *EWSR1* gene rearrangement supports myoepithelial carcinoma in this differential diagnosis. Superficial examples of epithelioid MPNSTs may be confused with epithelioid schwannoma, inasmuch as both tumor types are strongly positive for S-100 protein and SOX10. However, tumor cells in epithelioid schwannoma are smaller than those of epithelioid MPNST, display small, usually indistinct nucleoli, and are often arranged in well-formed nests and trabeculae set in a myxoid matrix. Mitoses are rare in epithelioid schwannoma, and necrosis is absent.[37,38]

Prognosis and Treatment

The prognosis of epithelioid MPNSTs varies according to the size and depth of the lesion. Superficial lesions that are small (<5 cm) and more easily amenable to complete surgical excision have the best outcome. Large, deep-seated tumors may be more aggressive. Early studies suggested an overall 5-year survival of approximately 50%, with 30% to 50% of patients developing distant metastases. A recent study suggested a lower rate of metastasis of around 15% (median follow-up, 3 years) and a local recurrence rate of 30%, independent of depth.[167] The most common sites of metastasis are the lungs and pleura; liver and regional lymph nodes are less common.[167,185–187]

PRACTICE POINTS: Epithelioid Malignant Peripheral Nerve Sheath Tumor

- Often arises in the superficial soft tissues of the extremities of young adults
- Well circumscribed with a multinodular growth pattern
- Sheets, nests, or cords of uniform epithelioid cells, with eosinophilic cytoplasm, vesicular chromatin, and prominent central nucleoli (melanoma-like)
- Strong, diffuse staining for S-100 protein; two-thirds show loss of INI1 expression
- Less aggressive behavior than conventional malignant peripheral nerve sheath tumor

Epithelioid Gastrointestinal Stromal Tumor

GIST is discussed in Chapter 16.

Epithelioid Myxofibrosarcoma

Myxofibrosarcoma, previously also designated myxoid malignant fibrous histiocytoma, usually arises in the subcutaneous tissue or deep soft tissue of the limbs (especially lower limbs) and limb girdles of older patients (median age, 60 years).[1] This tumor type is discussed in detail in Chapters 5 and 7.

Histologically, myxofibrosarcoma is composed of myxoid areas juxtaposed with cellular zones resembling undifferentiated pleomorphic sarcoma, in variable proportions. Myxofibrosarcoma can be graded depending on the extent of cytologic atypia and the proportions of myxoid and nonmyxoid components, which correlate with metastatic potential. The epithelioid variant of myxofibrosarcoma accounts for less than 5% of all myxofibrosarcomas.[189] Gender distribution, tumor location, and size parallel those of conventional myxofibrosarcoma. Histologically, epithelioid myxofibrosarcoma is a high-grade neoplasm displaying a prominent carcinoma-like appearance. At low power, the tumor is often multinodular (Fig. 6.80), and epithelioid areas may be admixed with areas of more conventional histology. The tumor cells have round nuclei with vesicular chromatin, prominent nucleoli, and abundant eosinophilic cytoplasm (Fig. 6.81). Mitoses are usually numerous in cellular areas, and tumor necrosis may be present. By immunohistochemistry, tumor cells are generally negative for epithelial markers (keratins, EMA), desmin, and S-100 protein. The differential diagnosis includes metastatic poorly differentiated carcinoma and melanoma, myoepithelial carcinoma, pleomorphic liposarcoma (PLPS), pleomorphic rhabdomyosarcoma, and myxoinflammatory fibroblastic sarcoma. Identification of areas of conventional myxofibrosarcoma is critical to confirm the diagnosis. Epithelioid myxofibrosarcoma pursues a more aggressive course than conventional high-grade myxofibrosarcoma, with a higher metastatic rate (at least 50%).[189]

Pleomorphic Liposarcoma, Epithelioid Variant

PLPS is an uncommon variant of liposarcoma that accounts for less than 5% of all liposarcomas (see also Chapters 7 and 12). It occurs predominantly in the deep soft tissues (75% of cases) of the lower extremities, especially the thigh, of elderly patients (median age, 55 to 65 years).[190–193] Limb girdles and the trunk (including the retroperitoneum) are each

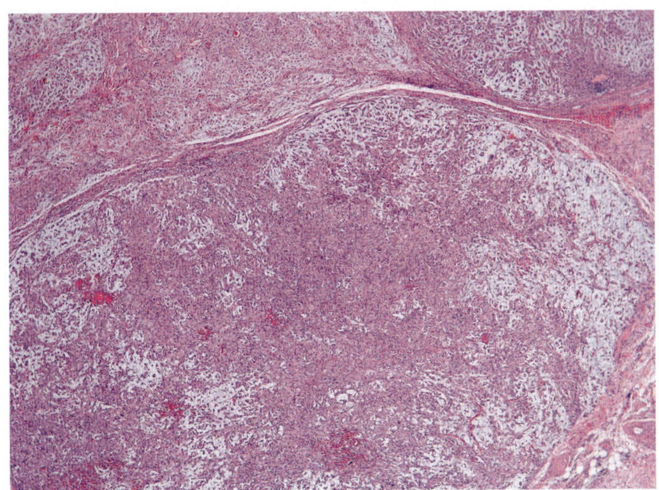

Figure 6.80 Epithelioid Variant of Myxofibrosarcoma. The tumor shows a multinodular growth pattern. Note the focal areas with myxoid stroma.

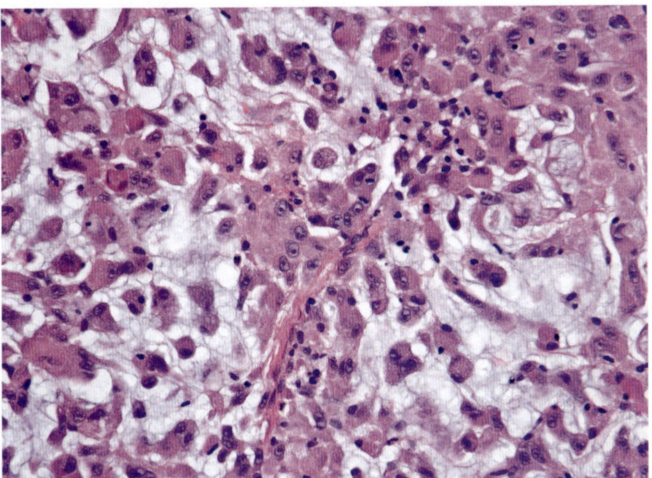

Figure 6.81 Epithelioid Variant of Myxofibrosarcoma. The tumor cells contain abundant eosinophilic cytoplasm and rounded nuclei with vesicular chromatin and prominent nucleoli.

involved in approximately 20% of cases. Histologically, PLPS is composed of a variable combination of lipogenic and nonlipogenic areas. Lipogenic areas are composed of pleomorphic, often multivacuolated lipoblasts with scalloped hyperchromatic nuclei. Nonlipogenic areas may show a highly variable appearance, with undifferentiated pleomorphic, spindle cell, round cell, and epithelioid features. Between 15% and 30% of PLPSs contain areas with prominent epithelioid features, resembling carcinoma or melanoma (Fig. 6.82).[190,191] The epithelioid variant of PLPS should be distinguished primarily from metastatic renal cell carcinoma and adrenal cortical carcinoma, with which it can easily be confused.[190–192] Epithelioid tumor cells may show focal staining for keratins or EMA in a minority of cases.[190–192] Identification of lipoblasts is critical to make the diagnosis. PLPS is a high-grade sarcoma that recurs locally in 35% to 50% and metastasizes in 50% of cases. Five-year overall, metastasis-free, and local recurrence-free survival rates are 40% to 60%, 30% to 60%, and 25% to 75%, respectively.[190,191,193] In two studies of PLPS, epithelioid cytomorphology was associated with aggressive behavior.[191,192]

Synovial Sarcoma, Epithelial/Glandular Variant

Synovial sarcoma accounts for 5% to 10% of adult soft tissue sarcomas. Several histologic variants have been described, including biphasic

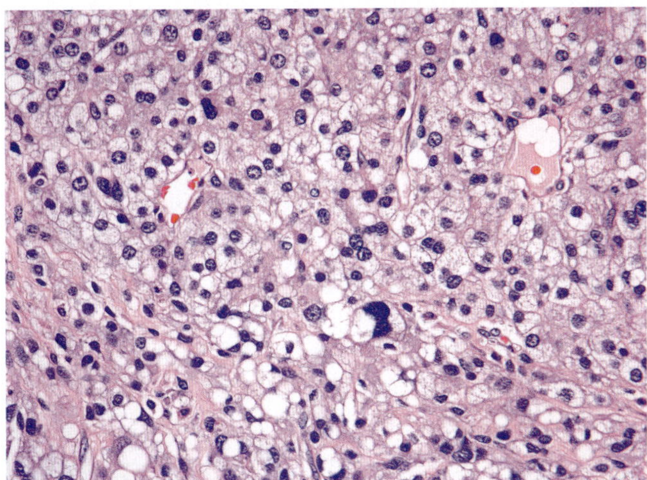

Figure 6.82 Epithelioid Variant of Pleomorphic Liposarcoma. Sheets of epithelioid cells have microvesicular cytoplasm. Such tumors may be mistaken for metastatic carcinoma, especially adrenal cortical or renal cell carcinoma.

synovial sarcoma, monophasic spindle cell synovial sarcoma, poorly differentiated synovial sarcoma, cystic synovial sarcoma, synovial sarcoma with bone and calcification (calcifying synovial sarcoma), and myxoid synovial sarcoma. Synovial sarcoma is discussed in detail in Chapter 3, and biphasic synovial sarcoma is covered in Chapter 9. This section discusses only the rare, predominantly glandular variant of synovial sarcoma, which can easily be confused with an epithelial neoplasm.

Synovial sarcoma, including the glandular variant, usually develops in the deep soft tissues of the limbs and limb girdles of adolescents and young adults, especially adjacent to large joints.[194] A palpable mass, pain or tenderness, paresthesia, and limitation of motion may be presenting symptoms.

Histologically, predominantly epithelial synovial sarcoma is simply a variant of biphasic synovial sarcoma in which the spindle cell component is scant and, as a consequence, easily overlooked. The epithelial component forms solid nests, tubular/glandular structures, or less commonly, pseudopapillary structures (Fig. 6.83).[194–196] The epithelial cells are characteristically large with round, vesicular nuclei, pale cytoplasm, and easily discernible cell borders. Glandular lumina often contain eosinophilic material with staining characteristics of epithelial mucin. Squamous differentiation may rarely be seen. As in conventional biphasic synovial sarcoma, predominantly epithelial synovial sarcoma nearly always contains a spindle cell component, which may be minimal, but identification of that component is critical for diagnosis. Thick collagen bundles and calcifications are also seen. Purely epithelioid synovial sarcoma composed of plump epithelioid cells without glandular structures is exceedingly rare. Synovial sarcoma containing prominent rhabdoid cells is better classified as poorly differentiated synovial sarcoma.

By immunohistochemistry, predominantly epithelial synovial sarcoma is positive for keratins and EMA. Carcinoembryonic antigen can be focally expressed, whereas reactivity for CD99 and S-100 protein is sometimes observed in the minor spindle cell component.[194] Similar to other variants, predominantly epithelial synovial sarcoma is usually positive for TLE1 and negative for CD34.[197,198]

The molecular biology of synovial sarcoma is discussed in detail in Chapters 3 and 18. Like other variants, the predominantly epithelial variant of synovial sarcoma bears the t(X;18) translocation involving the *SS18* (*SYT*) gene on chromosome 18 (18q11) and either the *SSX1* or the *SSX2* gene on chromosome X (Xp11.23).[199] The t(X;18) translocation, which can be detected by FISH or RT-PCR, is entirely specific for synovial sarcoma. Biphasic synovial sarcoma, including predominantly

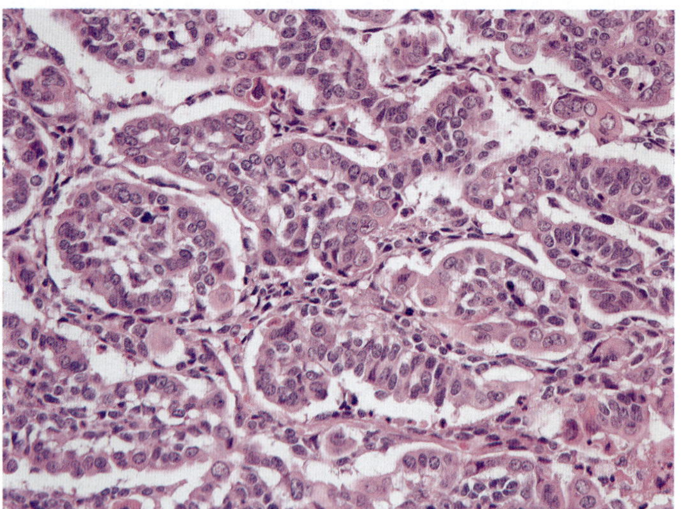

Figure 6.83 Predominantly Glandular Synovial Sarcoma. The tumor is dominated by tubular and papillary structures lined by cuboidal to columnar epithelial cells with eosinophilic cytoplasm. The inconspicuous spindle cell component can easily be overlooked.

epithelial synovial sarcoma, is rarely associated with *SS18-SSX2* fusion transcripts, suggesting a relationship between morphology and genetics.[200,201]

Predominantly epithelial biphasic synovial sarcoma should be differentiated from tumors showing an admixture of glandular structures and spindle cells, including metastatic adenocarcinoma, carcinosarcoma, glandular malignant peripheral nerve sheath tumors, endometriosis, and mixed tumor/myoepithelioma of soft tissue.

Purely glandular synovial sarcoma may easily be confused with adenocarcinoma, especially metastatic endometrial adenocarcinoma or Müllerian carcinosarcoma (malignant mixed Müllerian tumor). Identification of the spindle cell component, even if minimal, is helpful to diagnose synovial sarcoma. Both synovial sarcoma and adenocarcinoma are positive for epithelial markers and negative for CD34. In this situation, clinical presentation and detection of the t(X;18) translocation are critical.

Mixed tumors and myoepitheliomas of soft tissue are more heterogeneous in composition than synovial sarcoma. The epithelioid cells usually contain abundant eosinophilic or clear cytoplasm, arranged in nests, cords, or trabeculae, often embedded in a myxoid stroma. The spindle cells in myoepitheliomas are plumper and contain more abundant eosinophilic cytoplasm than those of synovial sarcoma. Mixed tumors contain occasional ducts and may contain foci of cartilaginous differentiation.

In the glandular variant of the MPNST, the glands often contain goblet cells and chromogranin-positive neuroendocrine cells, features not observed in synovial sarcoma. In addition, glands are usually few in number, sharply demarcated from the spindle cell component, and frequently found very focally within the spindle cell neoplasm. In contrast, glands in predominantly epithelial synovial sarcoma tend to be grouped and tightly apposed, and the transition between the glandular and spindle cell components is more gradual. MPNSTs and synovial sarcomas may both develop within a large nerve.[196,202] Only synovial sarcomas contain the t(X;18) translocation. Glandular MPNSTs are almost exclusively found in patients with neurofibromatosis type 1, and often contain other heterologous elements, including rhabdomyosarcomatous and osteochondrosarcomatous areas.

The prognosis and treatment of predominantly epithelial synovial sarcoma is the same as for other variants of synovial sarcoma (see Chapter 3 for details).

Glandular Malignant Peripheral Nerve Sheath Tumor

The glandular variant of MPNST is discussed in Chapter 9.

Other Epithelioid Variants of Specific Sarcomas

In addition to those entities previously described, several other specific sarcomas (see Box 6.22) may, on occasion, show prominent epithelioid features, including dedifferentiated liposarcomas (Fig. 6.84), clear cell sarcomas (especially in metastatic deposits, such as lymph node) (Fig. 6.85), myxoinflammatory fibroblastic sarcomas, EMC,[203] leiomyosarcomas, desmoplastic small round cell tumors, and inflammatory myofibroblastic tumors ("epithelioid inflammatory myofibroblastic sarcoma").[204] Adjacent to epithelioid areas, most of these tumors usually display more conventional histologic features, allowing for proper recognition. Details about these tumor types can be found in other chapters.

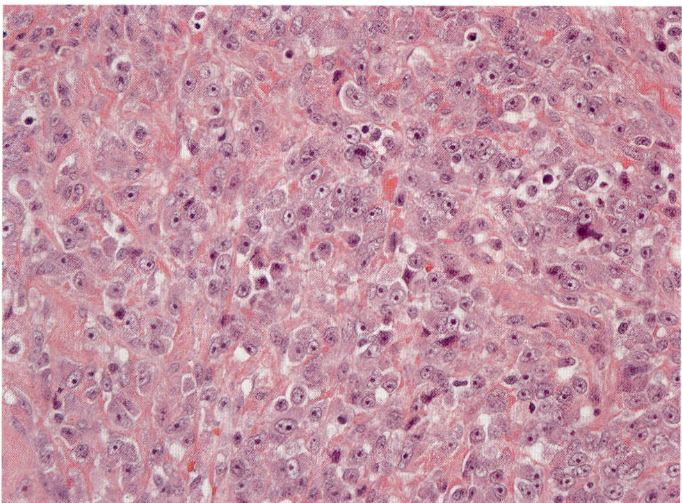

Figure 6.84 Dedifferentiated Liposarcoma With Epithelioid Features. Tumors with such morphologic features may be mistaken for carcinoma. The presence of striking intratumoral heterogeneity with pleomorphic and spindle cell components is a clue to the diagnosis.

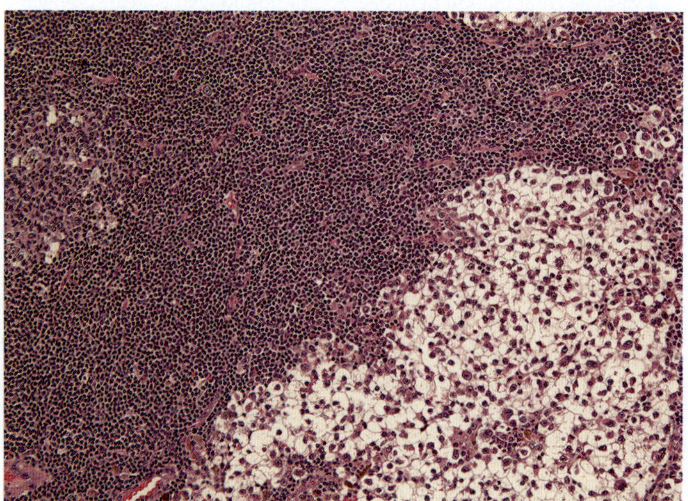

Figure 6.85 Clear Cell Sarcoma. Some cases show prominent epithelioid morphology, especially in lymph node metastases. Note the abundant clear cytoplasm.

References

1. Fletcher CDM, Bridge JA, Hogendoorn PCW, et al, editors: *WHO classification of tumours of soft tissue and bone*, ed 4, Lyon, 2013, IARC Press.
2. Olsen TG, Helwig EB: Angiolymphoid hyperplasia with eosinophilia: a clinicopathologic study of 116 patients, *J Am Acad Dermatol* 12:781–796, 1985.
3. Chan JKC, Hui PK, Ng CS, et al: Epithelioid hemangioma (angiolymphoid hyperplasia with eosinophilia) and Kimura's disease in Chinese, *Histopathology* 15:557–574, 1989.
4. Kuo TT, Shih LY, Chan HL: Kimura's disease: involvement of regional lymph nodes and distinction from angiolymphoid hyperplasia with eosinophilia, *Am J Surg Pathol* 12:843–854, 1988.
5. Urabe A, Tsuneyoshi M, Enjoji M: Epithelioid hemangioma versus Kimura's disease. A comparative clinicopathologic study, *Am J Surg Pathol* 11:758–766, 1987.
6. Rosai J, Ackerman LR: Intravenous atypical vascular proliferation. A cutaneous lesion simulating a malignant blood vessel tumor, *Arch Dermatol* 109:714–717, 1974.
7. Brenn T, Fletcher CDM: Cutaneous epithelioid angiomatous nodule: a distinct lesion in the morphologic spectrum of epithelioid vascular tumors, *Am J Dermatopathol* 26:14–21, 2004.
8. Hung YP, Fletcher CD, Hornick JL: FOSB is a useful diagnostic marker for pseudomyogenic hemangioendothelioma, *Am J Surg Pathol* 41:596–606, 2017.
9. Antonescu CR, Chen HW, Zhang L, et al: ZFP36-FOSB fusion defines a subset of epithelioid hemangioma with atypical features, *Genes Chromosomes Cancer* 53:951–959, 2014.
10. Walther C, Tayebwa J, Lilljebjorn H, et al: A novel SERPINE1-FOSB fusion gene results in transcriptional up-regulation of FOSB in pseudomyogenic haemangioendothelioma, *J Pathol* 232:534–540, 2014.
11. Huang SC, Zhang L, Sung YS, et al: Frequent FOS gene rearrangements in epithelioid hemangioma: a molecular study of 58 cases with morphologic reappraisal, *Am J Surg Pathol* 39:1313–1321, 2015.
12. van IJzendoorn DG, de Jong D, Romagosa C, et al: Fusion events lead to truncation of FOS in epithelioid hemangioma of bone, *Genes Chromosomes Cancer* 54:565–574, 2015.
13. Shibuya R, Matsuyama A, Shiba E, et al: CAMTA1 is a useful immunohistochemical marker for diagnosing epithelioid haemangioendothelioma, *Histopathology* 67:827–835, 2015.
14. Doyle LA, Fletcher CD, Hornick JL: Nuclear expression of CAMTA1 distinguishes epithelioid hemangioendothelioma from histologic mimics, *Am J Surg Pathol* 40:94–102, 2016.
15. Pulitzer DR, Martin PC, Reed RJ: Epithelioid glomus tumor, *Hum Pathol* 26:1022–1027, 1995.
16. Granter SR, Badizadegan K, Fletcher CDM: Myofibromatosis in adults, glomangiopericytoma, and myopericytoma. A spectrum of tumors showing perivascular myoid differentiation, *Am J Surg Pathol* 22:513–525, 1998.
17. Mentzel T, Tos AP, Sapi Z, et al: Myopericytoma of skin and soft tissue. Clinicopathologic and immunohistochemical study of 54 cases, *Am J Surg Pathol* 30:104–113, 2006.
18. Albrecht S, Zbieranowski J: Incidental glomus coccygeum. When a normal structure looks like a tumor, *Am J Surg Pathol* 14:922–924, 1990.
19. Mosquera JM, Sboner A, Zhang L, et al: Novel MIR143-NOTCH fusions in benign and malignant glomus tumors, *Genes Chromosomes Cancer* 52:1075–1087, 2013.
20. Chakrapani A, Warrick A, Nelson D, et al: BRAF and KRAS mutations in sporadic glomus tumors, *Am J Dermatopathol* 34:533–535, 2012.
21. Folpe AL, Fanburg-Smith JC, Miettinen M, et al: Atypical and malignant glomus tumors. Analysis of 53 cases with a proposal for the reclassification of glomus tumors, *Am J Surg Pathol* 25:1–12, 2001.
22. Gleason BC, Hornick JL: Myoepithelial tumours of skin and soft tissue: an update, *Diagn Histopathol* 14:552–562, 2008.
23. Kilpatrick SE, Hitchkock MG, Kraus MD, et al: Mixed tumors and myoepitheliomas of soft tissue: a clinicopathologic study of 19 cases with a unifying concept, *Am J Surg Pathol* 21:13–22, 1997.
24. Michal M, Miettinen M: Myoepitheliomas of the skin and soft tissues. Report of 12 cases, *Virchows Arch* 434:393–400, 1999.
25. Hornick JL, Fletcher CD: Myoepithelial tumors of soft tissue: a clinicopathologic and immunohistochemical study of 101 cases with evaluation of prognostic parameters, *Am J Surg Pathol* 27:1183–1196, 2003.
26. Gleason BC, Fletcher CDM: Myoepithelial carcinoma of soft tissue in children: an aggressive neoplasm analyzed in a series of 29 cases, *Am J Surg Pathol* 31:1813–1824, 2007.
27. Miettinen M, McCue PA, Sarlomo-Rikala M, et al: Sox10–a marker for not only schwannian and melanocytic neoplasms but also myoepithelial cell tumors of soft tissue: A systematic analysis of 5134 tumors, *Am J Surg Pathol* 39:826–835, 2015.
28. Hallor KH, Teixeira MR, Fletcher CDM, et al: Heterogeneous genetic profiles in soft tissue myoepitheliomas, *Mod Pathol* 21:1311–1319, 2008.
29. Antonescu CR, Zhang L, Chang NE, et al: EWSR1-POU5F1 fusion in soft tissue myoepithelial tumors. A molecular analysis of sixty-six cases, including soft tissue, bone, and visceral lesions, showing common involvement of the EWSR1 gene, *Genes Chromosomes Cancer* 49:1114–1124, 2010.
30. Flucke U, Palmedo G, Blankenhorn N, et al: EWSR1 gene rearrangement occurs in a subset of cutaneous myoepithelial tumors: a study of 18 cases, *Mod Pathol* 24:1444–1450, 2011.
31. Huang SC, Chen HW, Zhang L, et al: Novel FUS-KLF17 and EWSR1-KLF17 fusions in myoepithelial tumors, *Genes Chromosomes Cancer* 54:267–275, 2015.
32. Agaram NP, Chen HW, Zhang L, et al: EWSR1-PBX3: A novel gene fusion in myoepithelial tumors, *Genes Chromosomes Cancer* 54:63–71, 2015.
33. Leduc C, Zhang L, Oz B, et al: Thoracic myoepithelial tumors: a pathologic and molecular study of 8 cases with review of the literature, *Am J Surg Pathol* 40:212–223, 2016.
34. Bahrami A, Dalton JD, Krane JF, et al: A subset of cutaneous and soft tissue mixed tumors are genetically linked to their salivary gland counterpart, *Genes Chromosomes Cancer* 51:140–148, 2012.
35. Nielsen GP, Mangham DC, Grimer RJ, et al: Chordoma periphericum: a case report, *Am J Surg Pathol* 25:263–267, 2001.
36. Tirabosco R, Mangham DC, Rosenberg AE, et al: Brachyury expression in extra-axial skeletal and soft tissue chordomas: a marker that distinguishes chordoma from mixed tumor/myoepithelioma/parachordoma in soft tissue, *Am J Surg Pathol* 32:572–580, 2008.
37. Kindblom LG, Meis-Kindblom JM, Havel G, et al: Benign epithelioid schwannoma, *Am J Surg Pathol* 22:762–770, 1998.
38. Laskin WB, Fetsch JF, Lasota J, et al: Benign epithelioid peripheral nerve sheath tumors of the soft tissues. Clinicopathologic spectrum of 33 cases, *Am J Surg Pathol* 29:39–51, 2005.
39. Meis JM, Enzinger FM: Chondroid lipoma: a unique tumor simulating liposarcoma and myxoid chondrosarcoma, *Am J Surg Pathol* 17:1103–1112, 1993.
40. Noronha V, Cooper DL, Higgins SA, et al: Metastatic myoepithelial carcinoma of the vulva treated with carboplatin and paclitaxel, *Lancet Oncol* 7:270–271, 2006.
41. Bonetti F, Pea M, Martignoni G, et al: PEC and sugar, *Am J Surg Pathol* 16:307–308, 1992.
42. Bonetti F, Pea M, Martignoni G, et al: Clear cell ("sugar") tumor of the lung is a lesion strictly related to angiomyolipoma—the concept of a family of lesions characterized by the presence of the perivascular epithelioid cells (PEC), *Pathology* 26:230–236, 1994.
43. Martignoni G, Pea M, Reghellin D, et al: PEComas: the past, the present, and the future, *Virchows Arch* 452:119–132, 2008.
44. Folpe AL, Kwiatkowski DJ: Perivascular epithelioid cell neoplasms: pathology and pathogenesis, *Hum Pathol* 41:1–15, 2010.
45. Hornick JL, Fletcher CDM: PEComa: what do we know so far?, *Histopathology* 48:75–82, 2006.
46. Folpe AL, Mentzel T, Lehr HA, et al: Perivascular epithelioid cell neoplasms of soft tissue and gynecologic origin. A clinicopathologic study of 26 cases and review of the literature, *Am J Surg Pathol* 29:1558–1575, 2005.
47. Martignoni G, Pea M, Reghellin D, et al: Perivascular epithelioid cell tumor (PEComa) in the genitourinary tract, *Adv Anat Pathol* 14:36–41, 2007.
48. Yamashita K, Fletcher CD: PEComa presenting in bone: clinicopathologic analysis of 6 cases and literature review, *Am J Surg Pathol* 34:1622–1629, 2010.
49. Eble JN: Angiomyolipoma of kidney, *Semin Diagn Pathol* 15:21–40, 1998.
50. Folpe AL, Goodman ZD, Ishak KG, et al: Clear cell myomelanocytic tumor of the falciform ligament/ligamentum teres: a novel member of the perivascular epithelioid clear cell family of tumors with a predilection for children and young adults, *Am J Surg Pathol* 24:1239–1246, 2000.
51. Mentzel T, Reisshauer S, Rütten A, et al: Cutaneous clear cell myomelanocytic tumour: a new member of the growing family of perivascular epithelioid cell tumours (PEComas). Clinicopathologic and immunohistochemical analysis of seven cases, *Histopathology* 46:498–504, 2005.
52. Liegl B, Hornick JL, Fletcher CDM: Primary cutaneous PEComa: distinctive clear cell lesions of skin, *Am J Surg Pathol* 32:608–614, 2008.
53. Hornick JL, Fletcher CDM: Sclerosing PEComa: clinicopathologic analysis of a distinctive variant with a predilection for the retroperitoneum, *Am J Surg Pathol* 32:493–501, 2008.
54. Vang R, Kempson RL: Perivascular epithelioid cell tumor (PEComa) of the uterus. A subset of HMB-45-positive epithelioid mesenchymal neoplasms with an uncertain relationship to pure smooth muscle tumors, *Am J Surg Pathol* 26:1–13, 2002.
55. Fadare O: Perivascular epithelioid cell tumor (PEComa) of the uterus. An outcome-based clinicopathologic analysis of 41 reported cases, *Adv Anat Pathol* 15:63–75, 2008.
56. Argani P, Aulmann S, Illei PB, et al: A distinctive subset of PEComas harbors TFE3 gene fusions, *Am J Surg Pathol* 34:1395–1406, 2010.
57. Martignoni G, Bonetti F, Chilosi M, et al: Cathepsin K expression in the spectrum of perivascular epithelioid cell (PEC) lesions of the kidney, *Mod Pathol* 25:100–111, 2012.
58. Rao Q, Cheng L, Xia QY, et al: Cathepsin K expression in a wide spectrum of perivascular epithelioid cell neoplasms (PEComas): a clinicopathological study emphasizing extrarenal PEComas, *Histopathology* 62:642–650, 2013.
59. Pan CC, Chung MY, Ng KF, et al: Constant allelic alteration on chromosome 16p (TSC2 gene) in perivascular epithelioid cell tumour (PEComa): genetic evidence for the relationship of PEComa with angiomyolipoma, *J Pathol* 214:387–393, 2008.
60. Kenerson H, Folpe AL, Takayama TK, et al: Activation of the mTOR pathway in sporadic angiomyolipoma and other perivascular epithelioid cell neoplasms, *Hum Pathol* 38:1361–1371, 2007.
61. Agaram NP, Sung YS, Zhang L, et al: Dichotomy of genetic abnormalities in PEComas with therapeutic implications, *Am J Surg Pathol* 39:813–825, 2015.
62. Brimo F, Robinson B, Guo C, et al: Renal epithelioid angiomyolipoma with atypia: a series of 40 cases with emphasis on clinicopathologic prognostic indicators of malignancy, *Am J Surg Pathol* 34:715–722, 2010.
63. Nese N, Martignoni G, Fletcher CD, et al: Pure epithelioid PEComas (so-called epithelioid angiomyolipoma) of the kidney: a clinicopathologic study of 41 cases: detailed assessment of morphology and risk stratification, *Am J Surg Pathol* 35:161–176, 2011.
64. Doyle LA, Hornick JL, Fletcher CD: PEComa of the gastrointestinal tract: clinicopathologic study of 35 cases with evaluation of prognostic parameters, *Am J Surg Pathol* 37:1769–1782, 2013.

65. Martignoni G, Bissler JJ, McCormack FX, et al: Sirolimus for angiomyolipoma in tuberous sclerosis complex or lymphangioleiomyomatosis, *N Engl J Med* 358:140–151, 2008.
66. Wagner AJ, Malinowska-Kolodziej I, Morgan JA, et al: Clinical activity of mTOR inhibition with sirolimus in malignant perivascular epithelioid cell tumors: targeting the pathogenic activation of mTORC1 in tumors, *J Clin Oncol* 28:835–840, 2010.
67. Kapadia SB, Meis JM, Frisman DM, et al: Adult rhabdomyoma of the head and neck: a clinicopathologic and immunophenotypic study, *Hum Pathol* 24:608–617, 1993.
68. D'Amore ES, Tollot M, Stracca-Pansa V, et al: Therapy associated differentiation in rhabdomyosarcomas, *Mod Pathol* 7:69–75, 1994.
69. Smith LM, Anderson JR, Coffin CM: Cytodifferentiation and clinical outcome after chemotherapy and radiation therapy for rhabdomyosarcoma (RMS), *Med Pediatr Oncol* 38:398–404, 2002.
70. Kapadia SB, Enzinger FM, Heffner DK, et al: Crystal-storing histiocytosis associated with lymphoplasmacytic neoplasms. Report of three cases mimicking adult rhabdomyoma, *Am J Surg Pathol* 17:461–467, 1993.
71. Fanburg-Smith JC, Meis-Kindblom JM, Fante R, et al: Malignant granular cell tumor of soft tissue. Diagnostic criteria and clinicopathologic correlation, *Am J Surg Pathol* 22:779–794, 1998.
72. Fine SW, Li M: Expression of calretinin and the alpha-subunit of inhibin in granular cell tumors, *Am J Clin Pathol* 119:259–264, 2003.
73. Schoolmeester JK, Lastra RR: Granular cell tumors overexpress TFE3 without corollary gene rearrangement, *Hum Pathol* 46:1242–1243, 2015.
74. Ordonez NG: Granular cell tumor: a review and update, *Adv Anat Pathol* 6:186–203, 1999.
75. Mentzel T, Wadden C, Fletcher CDM: Granular cell change in smooth muscle tumours of skin and soft tissue, *Histopathology* 24:223–231, 1994.
76. Suster S, Rosai J: Hamartoma of the scalp with ectopic meningothelial elements. A distinctive benign soft tissue lesion that may simulate angiosarcoma, *Am J Surg Pathol* 14:1–11, 1990.
77. Enzinger FM, Weiss SW, Liang CY: Ossifying fibromyxoid tumor of soft parts. A clinicopathological analysis of 59 cases, *Am J Surg Pathol* 13:817–827, 1989.
78. Folpe AL, Weiss SW: Ossifying fibromyxoid tumor of soft parts: a clinicopathologic study of 70 cases with emphasis on atypical and malignant variants, *Am J Surg Pathol* 27:421–431, 2003.
79. Zamecnik M, Michal M, Simpson RH, et al: Ossifying fibromyxoid tumor of soft parts: a report of 17 cases with emphasis on unusual histological features, *Ann Diagn Pathol* 1:73–81, 1997.
80. Kilpatrick SE, Ward WG, Mozes M, et al: Atypical and malignant variants of ossifying fibromyxoid tumor. Clinicopathologic analysis of six cases, *Am J Surg Pathol* 19:1039–1046, 1995.
81. Gebre-Medhin S, Nord KH, Moller E, et al: Recurrent rearrangement of the PHF1 gene in ossifying fibromyxoid tumors, *Am J Pathol* 181:1069–1077, 2012.
82. Graham RP, Weiss SW, Sukov WR, et al: PHF1 rearrangements in ossifying fibromyxoid tumors of soft parts: a fluorescence in situ hybridization study of 41 cases with emphasis on the malignant variant, *Am J Surg Pathol* 37:1751–1755, 2013.
83. Kao YC, Sung YS, Zhang L, et al: Expanding the molecular signature of ossifying fibromyxoid tumors with two novel gene fusions: CREBBP-BCORL1 and KDM2A-WWTR1, *Genes Chromosomes Cancer* 56:42–50, 2017.
84. Christopherson WM, Foote FW, Jr, Stewart FW: Alveolar soft-part sarcomas; structurally characteristic tumors of uncertain histogenesis, *Cancer* 5:100–111, 1952.
85. Folpe AL, Deyrup AT: Alveolar soft-part sarcoma: a review and update, *J Clin Pathol* 59:1127–1132, 2006.
86. Lieberman PH, Brennan MF, Kimmel M, et al: Alveolar soft part sarcoma. A clinico-pathologic study of half a century, *Cancer* 63:1–13, 1989.
87. Portera CA, Jr, Ho V, Patel SR, et al: Alveolar soft part sarcoma: clinical course and patterns of metastasis in 70 patients treated at a single institution, *Cancer* 91:585–591, 2001.
88. Ogose A, Yazawa Y, Ueda T, et al: Alveolar soft part sarcoma in Japan: multi-institutional study of 57 patients from the Japanese Musculoskeletal Oncology Group, *Oncology* 65:7–13, 2003.
89. Casanova M, Ferrari A, Bisogno G, et al: Alveolar soft part sarcoma in children and adolescents: a report from the Soft-Tissue Sarcoma Italian Cooperative Group, *Ann Oncol* 11:1445–1449, 2000.
90. Fanburg-Smith JC, Miettinen M, Folpe AL, et al: Lingual alveolar soft part sarcoma; 14 cases: novel clinical and morphological observations, *Histopathology* 45:526–537, 2004.
91. Argani P, Lal P, Hutchinson B, et al: Aberrant nuclear immunoreactivity for TFE3 in neoplasms with TFE3 gene fusions: a sensitive and specific immunohistochemical assay, *Am J Surg Pathol* 27:750–761, 2003.
92. Ladanyi M, Lui MY, Antonescu CR, et al: The der(17) t(X;17)(p11;q25) of human alveolar soft part sarcoma fuses the TFE3 transcription factor gene to ASPL, a novel gene at 17q25, *Oncogene* 20:48–57, 2001.
93. Fisher C: Soft tissue sarcomas with non-EWS translocations: molecular genetic features and pathologic and clinical correlations, *Virchows Arch* 456:153–166, 2010.
94. Aulmann S, Longerich T, Schirmacher P, et al: Detection of the ASPSCR1-TFE3 gene fusion in paraffin-embedded alveolar soft part sarcomas, *Histopathology* 50:881–886, 2007.
95. Weiss SW, Enzinger FM: Epithelioid hemangioendothelioma:a vascular tumor often mistaken for a carcinoma, *Cancer* 50:970–981, 1982.
96. Weiss SW, Ishak KG, Dail DH, et al: Epithelioid hemangioendothelioma and related lesions, *Semin Diagn Pathol* 3:259–287, 1986.
97. Mentzel T, Beham A, Calonje E, et al: Epithelioid hemangioendothelioma of skin and soft tissues: clinicopathologic and immunohistochemical study of 30 cases, *Am J Surg Pathol* 21:363–374, 1997.
98. Deyrup AT, Tighiouart M, Montag AG, et al: Epithelioid hemangioendothelioma of soft tissue: a proposal for risk stratification based on 49 cases, *Am J Surg Pathol* 32:924–927, 2008.
99. Fletcher CDM: The evolving classification of soft tissue tumours: an update based on the new WHO classification, *Histopathology* 48:3–12, 2006.
100. Tanas MR, Sboner A, Oliveira AM, et al: Identification of a disease-defining gene fusion in epithelioid hemangioendothelioma, *Sci Transl Med* 3:98ra82, 2011.
101. Errani C, Zhang L, Sung YS, et al: A novel WWTR1-CAMTA1 gene fusion is a consistent abnormality in epithelioid hemangioendothelioma of different anatomic sites, *Genes Chromosomes Cancer* 50:644–653, 2011.
102. Antonescu CR, Le Loarer F, Mosquera JM, et al: Novel YAP1-TFE3 fusion defines a distinct subset of epithelioid hemangioendothelioma, *Genes Chromosomes Cancer* 52:775–784, 2013.
103. Chan SW, Lim CJ, Chen L, et al: The hippo pathway in biological control and cancer development, *J Cell Physiol* 226:928–939, 2011.
104. Barbashina V, Salazar P, Holland EC, et al: Allelic losses at 1p36 and 19q13 in gliomas: Correlation with histologic classification, definition of a 150-kb minimal deleted region on 1p36, and evaluation of CAMTA1 as a candidate tumor suppressor gene, *Clin Cancer Res* 11:1119–1128, 2005.
105. Attiyeh EF, London WB, Mosse YP, et al: Chromosome 1p and 11q deletions and outcome in neuroblastoma, *N Engl J Med* 353:2243–2253, 2005.
106. Miettinen M, Wang Z, Sarlomo-Rikala M, et al: ERG expression in epithelioid sarcoma: A diagnostic pitfall, *Am J Surg Pathol* 37:1580–1585, 2013.
107. Stockman DL, Hornick JL, Deavers MT, et al: ERG and FLI1 protein expression in epithelioid sarcoma, *Mod Pathol* 27:496–501, 2014.
108. Billings SD, Folpe AL, Weiss SW: Epithelioid sarcoma-like hemangioendothelioma, *Am J Surg Pathol* 27:48–57, 2003.
109. Hornick JL, Fletcher CD: Pseudomyogenic hemangioendothelioma: a distinctive, often multicentric tumor with indolent behavior, *Am J Surg Pathol* 35:190–201, 2011.
110. Enzinger FM: Epithelioid sarcoma. A sarcoma simulating a granuloma or a carcinoma, *Cancer* 26:1029–1041, 1970.
111. Fisher C: Epithelioid sarcoma of Enzinger, *Adv Anat Pathol* 13:114–121, 2006.
112. Chase DR, Enzinger FM: Epithelioid sarcoma: diagnosis, prognostic indicators and treatment, *Am J Surg Pathol* 9:241–263, 1985.
113. Guillou L, Wadden C, Coindre JM, et al: "Proximal-type" epithelioid sarcoma, a distinctive aggressive neoplasm showing rhabdoid features. Clinicopathologic, immunohistochemical, and ultrastructural study of a series, *Am J Surg Pathol* 21:130–146, 1997.
114. Hasegawa T, Matsuno Y, Shimoda T, et al: Proximal-type epithelioid sarcoma: a clinicopathologic study of 20 cases, *Mod Pathol* 14:655–663, 2001.
115. Le Loarer F, Watson S, Pierron G, et al: SMARCA4 inactivation defines a group of undifferentiated thoracic malignancies transcriptionally related to BAF-deficient sarcomas, *Nat Genet* 47:1200–1205, 2015.
116. Doyle LA, Fletcher CDM, Hornick JL: A subset of epithelioid sarcomas with intact INI1 (SMARCB1) is deficient for SMARCA4 and SMARCA2, *Mod Pathol* 29:17A, 2016.
117. Kohashi K, Yamamoto H, Yamada Y, et al: SWI/SNF chromatin remodeling complex status in SMARCB1/INI1-preserved epithelioid sarcoma cases, *Mod Pathol* 29:21A, 2016.
118. Miettinen M, Fanburg-Smith JC, Virolainen M, et al: Epithelioid sarcoma: an immunohistochemical analysis of 112 classical and variant cases and a discussion on the differential diagnosis, *Hum Pathol* 30:934–942, 1999.
119. Molenaar WM, DeJong B, Dam-Meiring A, et al: Epithelioid sarcoma or malignant rhabdoid tumor of soft tissue. Epithelioid immunophenotype and rhabdoid karyotype, *Hum Pathol* 20:347–351, 1989.
120. Chase DR: Rhabdoid versus epithelioid sarcoma, *Am J Surg Pathol* 14:792–794, 1990.
121. Perrone T, Swanson PE, Twiggs L, et al: Malignant rhabdoid tumor of the vulva: is distinction from epithelioid sarcoma possible, *Am J Surg Pathol* 13:848–858, 1989.
122. Mirra JM, Kessler S, Bhuta S, et al: The fibroma-like variant of epithelioid sarcoma: a fibrohistiocytic/myoid cell lesion often confused with benign and malignant spindle cell tumors, *Cancer* 69:1382–1395, 1992.
123. Laskin WB, Miettinen M: Epithelioid sarcoma: new insights based on an extended immunohistochemical analysis, *Arch Pathol Lab Med* 127:1161–1168, 2003.
124. Chbani L, Guillou L, Terrier P, et al: Epithelioid sarcoma: a clinicopathologic and immunohistochemical analysis of 106 cases from the French sarcoma Group, *Am J Clin Pathol* 131:222–227, 2009.
125. Lin L, Skacel M, Sigel JE, et al: Epithelioid sarcoma: an immunohistochemical analysis evaluating the utility of cytokeratin 5/6 in distinguishing superficial epithelioid sarcoma from spindled squamous cell carcinoma, *J Cutan Pathol* 30:114–117, 2003.
126. Sigauke E, Rakheja D, Maddox D, et al: Absence of expression of SMARCB1/INI1 in malignant rhabdoid tumors of the central nervous system, kidneys and soft tissue: an immunohistochemical study with implications for diagnosis, *Mod Pathol* 19:717–725, 2006.
127. Hornick JL, Dal Cin P, Fletcher CDM: Loss of INI1 expression is characteristic of both conventional and proximal-type epithelioid sarcoma, *Am J Surg Pathol* 33:542–550, 2009.
128. Quezado MM, Middleton LP, Bryant B, et al: Allelic loss on chromosome 22q in epithelioid sarcomas, *Hum Pathol* 29:604–608, 1998.
129. Lualdi E, Modena P, Debiec-Rychter M, et al: Molecular cytogenetic characterization of proximal-type epithelioid sarcoma, *Genes Chromosomes Cancer* 41:283–290, 2004.
130. Modena P, Lualdi E, Facchinetti F, et al: SMARCB1/INI1 tumor suppressor gene is frequently inactivated in epithelioid sarcomas, *Cancer Res* 65:4012–4019, 2005.

131. Cordoba JC, Parham DM, Meyer WH, et al: A new cytogenetic finding in a epithelioid sarcoma, t(8;22)(q22;q11), *Cancer Genet Cytogenet* 72:151–154, 1994.
132. Sonobe H, Ohtsuki Y, Sugimoto T, et al: Involvement of 8q, 22q, and monosomy 21 in an epithelioid sarcoma, *Cancer Genet Cytogenet* 96:178–180, 1997.
133. Kohashi K, Izumi T, Oda Y, et al: Infrequent SMARCB1/INI1 gene alteration in epithelioid sarcoma: a useful tool in distinguishing epithelioid sarcoma from malignant rhabdoid tumor, *Hum Pathol* 40:349–355, 2009.
134. Flucke U, Slootweg PJ, Mentzel T, et al: Infrequent SMARCB1/INI1 gene alteration in epithelioid sarcoma: a useful tool in distinguishing epithelioid sarcoma from malignant rhabdoid tumor: direct evidence of mutational inactivation of SMARCB1/INI1 in epithelioid sarcoma, *Hum Pathol* 40:1361–1362, 2009.
135. Le Loarer F, Zhang L, Fletcher CD, et al: Consistent SMARCB1 homozygous deletions in epithelioid sarcoma and in a subset of myoepithelial carcinomas can be reliably detected by FISH in archival material, *Genes Chromosomes Cancer* 53:475–486, 2014.
136. Sapi Z, Papp G, Szendroi M, et al: Epigenetic regulation of SMARCB1 by miR-206, -381 and -671-5p is evident in a variety of SMARCB1 immunonegative soft tissue sarcomas, while miR-765 appears specific for epithelioid sarcoma. A miRNA study of 223 soft tissue sarcomas, *Genes Chromosomes Cancer* 55:786–802, 2016.
137. Lushnikova T, Knuutila S, Miettinen M: DNA copy number changes in epithelioid sarcoma and its variants: a comparative genomic hybridization study, *Mod Pathol* 13:1092–1096, 2000.
138. Banerjee SS, Harris M: Morphological and immunophenotypic variations in malignant melanoma, *Histopathology* 36:387–402, 2000.
139. de Visscher SAHJ, van Ginkel RJ, Wobbes T, et al: Epithelioid sarcoma: still an only surgically curable disease, *Cancer* 107:606–612, 2006.
140. Baratti D, Pennacchioli E, Casali PG, et al: Epithelioid sarcoma: prognostic factors and survival in a series of patients treated at a single institution, *Ann Surg Oncol* 14:3542–3551, 2007.
141. Callister MD, Ballo MT, Pisters PW, et al: Epithelioid sarcoma: results of conservative surgery and radiotherapy, *Int J Radiat Oncol Biol Phys* 51:384–391, 2001.
142. Jawad MU, Extein J, Min ES, et al: Prognostic factors for survival in patients with epithelioid sarcoma: 441 cases from the SEER database, *Clin Orthop Relat Res* 467:2939–2948, 2009.
143. Ramos P, Karnezis AN, Craig DW, et al: Small cell carcinoma of the ovary, hypercalcemic type, displays frequent inactivating germline and somatic mutations in SMARCA4, *Nat Genet* 46:427–429, 2014.
144. Witkowski L, Carrot-Zhang J, Albrecht S, et al: Germline and somatic SMARCA4 mutations characterize small cell carcinoma of the ovary, hypercalcemic type, *Nat Genet* 46:438–443, 2014.
145. Schneppenheim R, Fruhwald MC, Gesk S, et al: Germline nonsense mutation and somatic inactivation of SMARCA4/BRG1 in a family with rhabdoid tumor predisposition syndrome, *Am J Hum Genet* 86:279–284, 2010.
146. Biegel JA, Tan L, Zhang F, et al: Alterations of the hSNF5/INI1 gene in central nervous system atypical teratoid/rhabdoid tumors and renal and extrarenal rhabdoid tumors, *Clin Cancer Res* 8:3461–3467, 2002.
147. Bourdeaut F, Fréneaux P, Thuille B, et al: hSNF5/INI1-deficient tumours and rhabdoid tumours are convergent but not fully overlapping entities, *J Pathol* 211:323–330, 2007.
148. Oda Y, Tsuneyoshi M: Extrarenal rhabdoid tumors of soft tissue: clinicopathological and molecular genetic review and distinction from other soft-tissue sarcomas with rhabdoid features, *Pathol Int* 56:287–295, 2006.
149. Parham DM, Weeks DA, Beckwith JB: The clinicopathologic spectrum of putative extrarenal rhabdoid tumors. An analysis of 42 cases studied with immunohistochemistry or electron microscopy, *Am J Surg Pathol* 18:1010–1029, 1994.
150. Wick MR, Ritter JH, Dehner LP: Malignant rhabdoid tumors: a clinicopathologic review and conceptual discussion, *Semin Diagn Pathol* 12:233–248, 1995.
151. Ogino S, Ro JY, Redline RW: Malignant rhabdoid tumor: a phenotype? An entity? A controversy revisited, *Adv Anat Pathol* 7:181–190, 2000.
152. Tsuneyoshi M, Daimaru Y, Hashimoto H, et al: The existence of rhabdoid cells in specified soft tissue sarcomas. Histopathological, ultrastructural and immunohistochemical evidence, *Virchows Arch A Pathol Anat Histopathol* 411:509–514, 1987.
153. Kohashi K, Oda Y, Yamamoto H, et al: SMARCB1/INI1 protein expression in round cell soft tissue sarcomas associated with chromosomal translocations involving EWS: a special reference to SMARCB1/INI1 negative variant extraskeletal myxoid chondrosarcoma, *Am J Surg Pathol* 32:1168–1174, 2008.
154. Cheng JX, Tretiakova M, Gong C, et al: Renal medullary carcinoma: rhabdoid features and the absence of INI1 expression as markers of aggressive behavior, *Mod Pathol* 21:647–652, 2008.
155. Agaimy A, Cheng L, Egevad L, et al: Rhabdoid and undifferentiated phenotype in renal cell carcinoma: analysis of 32 cases indicating a distinctive common pathway of dedifferentiation frequently associated with SWI/SNF complex deficiency, *Am J Surg Pathol* 41:253–262, 2017.
156. Donner LR, Wainwright LM, Zhang F, et al: Mutation of the INI1 gene in composite rhabdoid tumor of the endometrium, *Hum Pathol* 38:935–939, 2007.
157. Strehl JD, Wachter DL, Fiedler J, et al: Pattern of SMARCB1 (INI1) and SMARCA4 (BRG1) in poorly differentiated endometrioid adenocarcinoma of the uterus: analysis of a series with emphasis on a novel SMARCA4-deficient dedifferentiated rhabdoid variant, *Ann Diagn Pathol* 19:198–202, 2015.
158. Ramalingam P, Croce S, McCluggage WG: Loss of expression of SMARCA4 (BRG1), SMARCA2 (BRM) and SMARCB1 (INI1) in undifferentiated carcinoma of the endometrium is not uncommon and is not always associated with rhabdoid morphology, *Histopathology* 70:359–366, 2017.
159. Judkins AR: Immunohistochemistry of INI1 expression: a new tool for old challenges in CNS and soft tissue pathology, *Adv Anat Pathol* 14:335–339, 2007.
160. Cho YM, Choi J, Lee OJ, et al: SMARCB1/INI1 missense mutation in mucinous carcinoma with rhabdoid features, *Pathol Int* 56:702–706, 2006.
161. Agaimy A, Daum O, Markl B, et al: SWI/SNF complex-deficient undifferentiated/rhabdoid carcinomas of the gastrointestinal tract: a series of 13 cases highlighting mutually exclusive loss of SMARCA4 and SMARCA2 and frequent co-inactivation of SMARCB1 and SMARCA2, *Am J Surg Pathol* 40:544–553, 2016.
162. Herpel E, Rieker RJ, Dienemann H, et al: SMARCA4 and SMARCA2 deficiency in non-small cell lung cancer: immunohistochemical survey of 316 consecutive specimens, *Ann Diagn Pathol* 26:47–51, 2017.
163. Kodet R, Newton WA, Sachs N, et al: Rhabdoid tumors of soft tissues: a clinicopathologic study of 26 cases enrolled on the Intergroup Rhabdomyosarcoma Study, *Hum Pathol* 22:674–684, 1991.
164. Fanburg-Smith JC, Hengge M, Hengge U, et al: Extrarenal rhabdoid tumors of soft tissue: a clinicopathologic and immunohistochemical study of 18 cases, *Ann Diagn Pathol* 2:351–362, 1998.
165. Hoot AC, Russo P, Judkins AR, et al: Immunohistochemical analysis of hSNF5/INI1 distinguishes renal and extra-renal malignant rhabdoid tumors from other pediatric soft tissue tumors, *Am J Surg Pathol* 28:1485–1491, 2004.
166. Perry A, Fuller CE, Judkins AR, et al: INI1 expression is retained in composite rhabdoid tumors, including rhabdoid meningiomas, *Mod Pathol* 18:951–958, 2005.
167. Jo VY, Fletcher CD: Epithelioid malignant peripheral nerve sheath tumor: clinicopathologic analysis of 63 cases, *Am J Surg Pathol* 39:673–682, 2015.
168. Meis-Kindblom JM, Kindblom LG, Enzinger FM: Sclerosing epithelioid fibrosarcoma. A variant of fibrosarcoma simulating carcinoma, *Am J Surg Pathol* 19:979–993, 1995.
169. Eyden BP, Manson C, Banerjee SS, et al: Sclerosing epithelioid fibrosarcoma: a study of five cases emphasizing diagnostic criteria, *Histopathology* 33:354–360, 1998.
170. Antonescu CR, Rosenblum MK, Pereira P, et al: Sclerosing epithelioid fibrosarcoma: a study of 16 cases and confirmation of a clinicopathologically distinct tumor, *Am J Surg Pathol* 25:699–709, 2001.
171. Bilsky MH, Schefler AM, Sandberg DI: Sclerosing epithelioid fibrosarcomas involving the neuraxis: report of three cases, *Neurosurgery* 47:956–960, 2000.
172. Ossendorf C, Studer GM, Bode B, et al: Sclerosing epithelioid fibrosarcoma: case presentation and a systematic review, *Clin Orthop Relat Res* 466:1485–1491, 2008.
173. Wojcik JB, Bellizzi AM, Dal Cin P, et al: Primary sclerosing epithelioid fibrosarcoma of bone: analysis of a series, *Am J Surg Pathol* 38:1538–1544, 2014.
174. Doyle LA, Möller E, Dal Cin P, et al: MUC4 is a highly sensitive and specific marker for low-grade fibromyxoid sarcoma, *Am J Surg Pathol* 35:733–741, 2011.
175. Doyle LA, Wang WL, Dal Cin P, et al: MUC4 is a sensitive and extremely useful marker for sclerosing epithelioid fibrosarcoma: association with FUS gene rearrangement, *Am J Surg Pathol* 36:1444–1451, 2012.
176. Lau PP, Lui PC, Lau GT, et al: EWSR1-CREB3L1 gene fusion: a novel alternative molecular aberration of low-grade fibromyxoid sarcoma, *Am J Surg Pathol* 37:734–738, 2013.
177. Doyle LA, Hornick JL: EWSR1 rearrangements in sclerosing epithelioid fibrosarcoma, *Am J Surg Pathol* 37:1630–1631, 2013.
178. Arbajian E, Puls F, Magnusson L, et al: Recurrent EWSR1-CREB3L1 gene fusions in sclerosing epithelioid fibrosarcoma, *Am J Surg Pathol* 38:801–808, 2014.
179. Guillou L, Benhattar J, Gengler C, et al: Translocation-positive low-grade fibromyxoid sarcoma: clinicopathologic and molecular analysis of a series expanding the morphologic spectrum and suggesting potential relationship to sclerosing epithelioid fibrosarcoma: a study from the French Sarcoma Group, *Am J Surg Pathol* 31:1387–1402, 2007.
180. Rekhi B, Folpe AL, Deshmukh M, et al: Sclerosing epithelioid fibrosarcoma—a report of two cases with cytogenetic analysis of FUS gene rearrangement by FISH technique, *Pathol Oncol Res* 17:145–148, 2011.
181. Fletcher CD, Beham A, Bekir S, et al: Epithelioid angiosarcoma of deep soft tissue: a distinctive tumor readily mistaken for an epithelial neoplasm, *Am J Surg Pathol* 15:915–924, 1991.
182. Meis-Kindblom JM, Kindblom LG: Angiosarcoma of soft tissue: a study of 80 cases, *Am J Surg Pathol* 22:683–697, 1998.
183. Miettinen M, Wang ZF, Paetau A, et al: ERG transcription factor as an immunohistochemical marker for vascular endothelial tumors and prostatic carcinoma, *Am J Surg Pathol* 35:432–441, 2011.
184. Penel N, Bui BN, Bay JO, et al: Phase II trial of weekly paclitaxel for unresectable angiosarcoma: the ANGIOTAX study, *J Clin Oncol* 26:5269–5274, 2008.
185. Lodding P, Kindblom LG, Angervall L: Epithelioid malignant schwannoma. A study of 14 cases, *Virchows Arch A Pathol Anat Histopathol* 409:433–451, 1986.
186. Laskin WB, Weiss SW, Bratthauer GL: Epithelioid variant of malignant peripheral nerve sheath tumor (malignant epithelioid schwannoma), *Am J Surg Pathol* 15:1136–1145, 1991.
187. Allison K, Patel R, Goldblum J, et al: Superficial malignant peripheral nerve sheath tumor: a rare and challenging diagnosis, *J Clin Pathol* 124:685–692, 2005.

188. McMenamin ME, Fletcher CD: Expanding the spectrum of malignant change in schwannomas: epithelioid malignant change, epithelioid malignant peripheral nerve sheath tumor, and epithelioid angiosarcoma: a study of 17 cases, *Am J Surg Pathol* 25:13–25, 2001.
189. Nascimento AF, Bertoni F, Fletcher CDM: Epithelioid variant of myxofibrosarcoma: expanding the clinicomorphologic spectrum of myxofibrosarcoma in a series of 17 cases, *Am J Surg Pathol* 31:99–105, 2007.
190. Gebhard S, Coindre JM, Michels JJ, et al: Pleomorphic liposarcoma: clinicopathologic, immunohistochemical, and follow-up analysis of 63 cases: a study from the French Federation of Cancer Centers Sarcoma Group, *Am J Surg Pathol* 26:601–616, 2002.
191. Hornick JL, Bosenberg MW, Mentzel T, et al: Pleomorphic liposarcoma: clinicopathologic analysis of 57 cases, *Am J Surg Pathol* 28:1257–1267, 2004.
192. Miettinen M, Enzinger FM: Epithelioid variant of pleomorphic liposarcoma: a study of 12 cases of a distinctive variant of high-grade liposarcoma, *Mod Pathol* 12:722–728, 1999.
193. Ghadimi MP, Liu P, Peng T, et al: Pleomorphic liposarcoma: clinical observations and molecular variables, *Cancer* 117:5359–5369, 2011.
194. Fisher C: Synovial sarcoma, *Ann Diagn Pathol* 2:401–421, 1998.
195. Majeste RM, Beckman EN: Synovial sarcoma with an overwhelming epithelial component, *Cancer* 61:2527–2531, 1988.
196. Weinreb I, Perez-Ordoñez B, Guha A, et al: Mucinous, gland predominant synovial sarcoma of a large peripheral nerve: a rare case closely mimicking metastatic mucinous carcinoma, *J Clin Pathol* 61:672–676, 2008.
197. Terry J, Saito T, Subramanian S, et al: TLE1 as a diagnostic immunohistochemical marker for synovial sarcoma emerging from gene expression profiling studies, *Am J Surg Pathol* 31:240–246, 2007.
198. Foo WC, Cruise MW, Wick MR, et al: Immunohistochemical staining for TLE1 distinguishes synovial sarcoma from histologic mimics, *Am J Clin Pathol* 135:839–844, 2011.
199. Sandberg AA, Bridge JA: Updates on the cytogenetics and molecular genetics of bone and soft tissue tumors. Synovial sarcoma, *Cancer Genet Cytogenet* 133:1–23, 2002.
200. Ladanyi M, Antonescu CR, Leung DH, et al: Impact of SYT-SSX fusion type on the clinical behavior of synovial sarcoma: a multi-institutional retrospective study of 243 patients, *Cancer Res* 62:135–140, 2002.
201. Guillou L, Benhattar J, Bonichon F, et al: Histologic grade, but not SYT-SSX fusion type, is an important prognostic factor in patients with synovial sarcoma: a multicenter, retrospective analysis, *J Clin Oncol* 22:4040–4050, 2004.
202. Scheithauer BW, Amrami KK, Folpe AL, et al: Synovial sarcoma of nerve, *Hum Pathol* 42:568–577, 2011.
203. Lucas DR, Fletcher CD, Adsay NV, et al: High-grade extraskeletal myxoid chondrosarcoma: a high-grade epithelioid malignancy, *Histopathology* 35:201–208, 1999.
204. Mariño-Enríquez A, Wang WL, Roy A, et al: Epithelioid inflammatory myofibroblastic sarcoma: an aggressive intra-abdominal variant of inflammatory myofibroblastic tumor with nuclear membrane or perinuclear ALK, *Am J Surg Pathol* 35:135–144, 2011.

7

Pleomorphic Sarcomas

J. Frans Graadt van Roggen, MB ChB, BSc Hons, PhD, and Pancras C.W. Hogendoorn, MD, PhD

Pleomorphic sarcomas are defined as malignant mesenchymal neoplasms characterized at a histologic level by prominent cellular pleomorphism and often brisk mitotic activity, with or without a readily identifiable line of differentiation.

Cellular pleomorphism in mesenchymal neoplasms is probably best defined as a significant variation in the size and shape of individual cells within a lesion, primarily as a result of striking alterations in nuclear and cytoplasmic morphology. It may either be a consistent and defining feature of a particular neoplasm (e.g., pleomorphic fibroma of the skin, atypical fibrous histiocytoma, symplastic ["bizarre"] leiomyoma of the uterus, pleomorphic hyalinizing angiectatic tumor [PHAT], pleomorphic myogenic sarcomas) or fall within the accepted histologic spectrum of certain well-defined soft tissue tumors (e.g., schwannoma with degenerative atypia, pleomorphic, and spindle cell lipoma). It may also involve a lesion diffusely (e.g., pleomorphic fibroma of the skin) or be present only focally (e.g., schwannoma, pleomorphic lipoma). From the previously mentioned examples, and Boxes 7.1 and 7.2, it becomes apparent that cellular pleomorphism may be present in lesions encompassing a broad spectrum of biologic behavior, ranging from those that are completely harmless to those with a malignant and extremely aggressive clinical course. Pleomorphism is therefore not in itself an indicator of aggressive behavior.

Mitotic activity is a separate histologic feature, independent of the presence or absence of cellular pleomorphism. Mitotic activity (as for cellular pleomorphism) is not per se an indicator of aggressive behavior (e.g., brisk mitotic activity in benign lesions such as nodular fasciitis and giant cell tumor of tendon sheath).

However, the combination of cellular pleomorphism *and* mitotic activity is generally a more ominous finding and is often associated with malignancy in soft tissue neoplasms. Rare exceptions to this rule exist: atypical fibroxanthoma (AFX), a neoplasm with significant cellular pleomorphism and brisk mitotic activity, when strictly defined, is generally accepted as being a benign non-metastasizing lesion.

PRACTICE POINTS: Pleomorphism and Mitotic Activity

- Benign and malignant mesenchymal neoplasms may exhibit cellular pleomorphism, either diffusely or focally.
- Benign and malignant neoplasms may exhibit mitotic activity.
- Cellular pleomorphism together with mitotic activity in a mesenchymal neoplasm is highly suggestive of malignancy.

Consequently, when confronted with a pleomorphic "sarcomatoid" neoplasm, the principal issues are the following:

1. To exclude nonsarcomatous lesions (e.g., pleomorphic/anaplastic carcinoma as typically seen in the thyroid gland, lung, and pancreas; melanoma; large cell lymphoma), which may mimic high-grade sarcomas. This is readily achieved with an appropriate panel of immunohistochemical markers (Table 7.1).
2. To avoid classifying a benign lesion as malignant. This requires a familiarity with benign mimics of pleomorphic sarcomas (see Box 7.1).
3. To maximize efforts in subclassifying the lesion, including the use of ancillary techniques such as immunohistochemistry, various (cyto) genetic modalities (including fluorescence in situ hybridization), and (rarely) electron microscopy. This is important for the selection of appropriate treatment strategies and inclusion in relevant and meaningful clinical trials.
4. To minimize classification as an undifferentiated pleomorphic sarcoma. This is a "wastebasket" label for a heterogeneous group

Box 7.1 Benign Mesenchymal Tumors With Substantial Cellular Pleomorphism

Pleomorphic fibroma of skin
Atypical (pseudosarcomatous) fibrous histiocytoma
Atypical fibroxanthoma
Pleomorphic lipoma
Symplastic (bizarre) leiomyoma of the uterus
Schwannoma with degenerative atypia ("ancient" schwannoma)
Pleomorphic hyalinizing angiectatic tumor (probably benign and characterized by repeated local recurrences but long-term biologic behavior uncertain)

Box 7.2 Malignant Mesenchymal Tumors With Substantial Cellular Pleomorphism

Myxoinflammatory fibroblastic sarcoma (probably of low-grade malignancy with rare distant metastases but long-term biologic behavior is uncertain)
Myxofibrosarcoma, high-grade
Pleomorphic leiomyosarcoma
Pleomorphic rhabdomyosarcoma
Pleomorphic liposarcoma
Dedifferentiated liposarcoma, morphologically high-grade
Extraskeletal osteosarcoma
Malignant mesenchymoma
Undifferentiated pleomorphic sarcoma

of tumors that remain unclassifiable despite the use of currently available ancillary diagnostic techniques.

Accurate classification of pleomorphic soft tissue tumors is therefore best regarded as a "gestalt" based on a summation of the clinical setting, histologic features (including results of ancillary techniques), and clinicopathologic experience.

PRACTICE POINTS: Mimics of Pleomorphic Sarcoma

Pleomorphic/anaplastic carcinoma, melanoma, and anaplastic large cell lymphoma are notorious mimics of pleomorphic sarcoma.
Benign mesenchymal lesions may mimic pleomorphic sarcoma.

A host of benign mesenchymal lesions may exhibit pleomorphic features (see Box 7.1 and discussion in the relevant chapters elsewhere in this book). This chapter primarily addresses malignant mesenchymal lesions with a pleomorphic phenotype, ranging from pleomorphic sarcomas readily classifiable on the basis of recognizable histologic features (with or without the aid of ancillary techniques) to those lesions that remain unclassifiable with currently available techniques, previously categorized under the nosologically meaningless rubric *malignant fibrous histiocytoma (MFH)*. Now, in keeping with the most recent World Health Organization (WHO) consensus classification, these latter lesions are designated as undifferentiated (high-grade) pleomorphic sarcoma (see Box 7.2).[1]

Atypical Fibroxanthoma

When strictly defined, AFX, also discussed in Chapter 15, is no longer regarded as a malignant neoplasm, but it is nevertheless briefly covered in this section because it is histologically and immunohistochemically indistinguishable from undifferentiated pleomorphic sarcoma. AFX is an intradermal tumor, probably of fibroblastic origin, arising almost exclusively in actinically damaged skin of the head and neck area of older adults, with pleomorphic and/or spindle-cell features, usually with an expansile growth pattern, and without invasion into subcutaneous tissue, vascular invasion, or necrosis.[2–9] Cases of so-called AFX described at sites without actinic damage and in younger patients are possibly examples of atypical (pseudosarcomatous) fibrous histiocytoma, although

Table 7.1 Immunohistochemical Panel to Exclude Nonsarcomatous Mimics of Pleomorphic Sarcoma

	Pleomorphic Carcinoma	Melanoma	ALCL	DLBCL
Keratins	+	−	−	−
S-100 protein	−	+	−	−
HMB45	−	±	−	−
Melan A	−	±	−	−
CD45	−	−	±	+
CD20/CD79a/PAX5	−	−	−	+
CD2/CD3	−	−	±	−
CD30	−	−	+	−
ALK	−	−	±	−

ALCL, Anaplastic large-cell lymphoma; *DLBCL*, diffuse large B-cell lymphoma.

convincing clinicopathologic studies supporting this hypothesis are as yet not available.[2]

Clinical Features

AFX presents as a skin-colored nodular lesion in the head and neck area of older patients. The nodule is usually less than 2 cm in diameter, and frequently there is a history of rapid growth. Ulceration may be present, but is, in our experience, relatively uncommon.

Pathologic Features

Histologically, all cases of AFX are centered in the dermis, generally abutting the epidermis, although occasionally a grenz zone may be present. The lesion is usually well circumscribed, often polypoid, and the overlying epidermis may form a collarette around the tumor (Fig. 7.1A and B). AFX is a cellular neoplasm composed of a haphazard and/or fascicular arrangement of highly pleomorphic and spindle-shaped cells. Multinucleated giant cells with monomorphic or pleomorphic nuclei are frequently present. The cytoplasm is as a rule easily discernible, eosinophilic, or amphophilic, and may occasionally contain lipid droplets; variable amounts of clear cell change and granular cell change may rarely be present.[10,11] Mitotic activity, including both typical and atypical mitotic figures, is generally marked (see Fig. 7.1C). A spindle-cell (nonpleomorphic) variant of AFX characterized by a fascicular proliferation of spindle-shaped cells with pale eosinophilic cytoplasm and without an overtly pleomorphic component is recognized (see Fig. 7.1D).[4] AFX has an expansile growth pattern, frequently with a "pushing" border, and may be surrounded by a mononuclear inflammatory infiltrate. The overlying epidermis is normal, but when ulceration is present, the lesion often cannot be evaluated for the presence of epidermal dysplasia or junctional activity, important in excluding the differential diagnostic options of sarcomatoid (spindle-cell) carcinoma and melanoma. Invasion into subcutaneous fat (even minimal, or deeper) or the presence of necrosis, lymphovascular, or perineural invasion are not features of AFX and exclude AFX as a diagnostic consideration.[2–6,9]

Immunohistochemistry

In addition to nonspecific staining for vimentin, the lesions are frequently positive for CD10 and characteristically show strong, diffuse staining for p53 (see Fig. 7.1E), although, in our experience, a very small number of otherwise typical examples of AFX (<5%) do not stain for p53. Weak

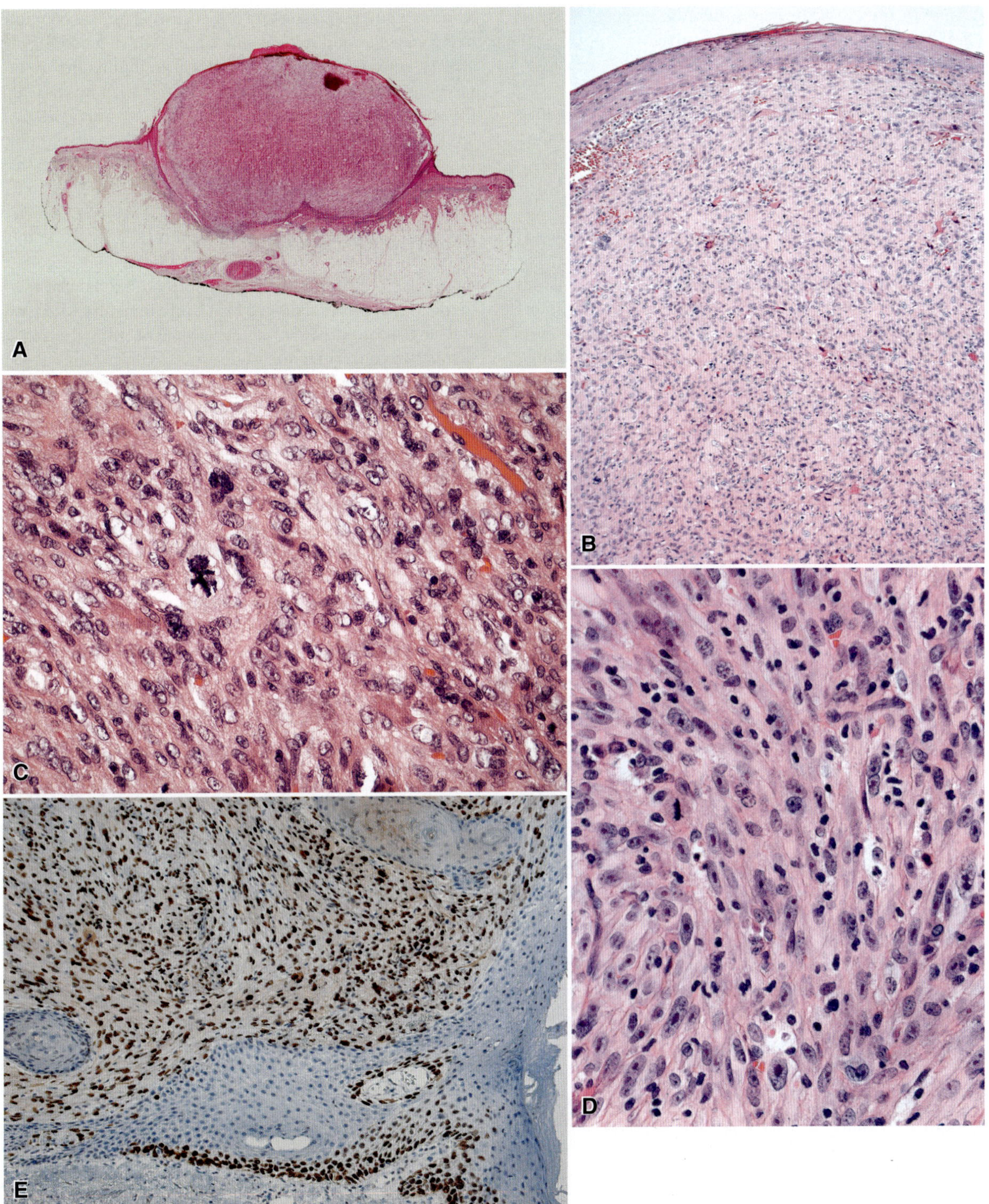

Figure 7.1 **Atypical Fibroxanthoma.** (A) Whole-mount view demonstrating the cutaneous location and sharp demarcation of the deep margin of the tumor. Note the epidermal collarette. (B) Medium-power view emphasizing the characteristic intimate approximation of the lesion to the overlying but uninvolved epidermis. (C) Pleomorphic variant of atypical fibroxanthoma. (D) Spindle cell (nonpleomorphic) variant of atypical fibroxanthoma. (E) Diffuse immunohistochemical positivity for p53 typical of this lesion.

positivity for smooth muscle actin may focally be present.[2–6,8] Most importantly, S-100 protein and keratins are negative.

Molecular Genetics

Ultraviolet light–induced *TP53* mutations, and, more recently, ultraviolet light–induced *TERT* promoter mutations, all supporting a sun exposure–induced etiology, have been identified in AFX.[6,12]

Differential Diagnosis

The differential diagnosis includes primarily spindle-cell (sarcomatoid) carcinoma, melanoma, atypical intradermal smooth muscle tumor, and cutaneous involvement by (metastatic) leiomyosarcoma, which may all exhibit a pleomorphic and spindle-cell appearance. Diligent clinical correlation (to exclude metastatic disease from a known or unknown primary lesion elsewhere), together with an appropriate immunohistochemical panel, including several keratins, melanoma markers, smooth muscle actin, and desmin, is generally sufficient to reach the correct diagnosis. Lesions otherwise typical of AFX but characterized by infiltration into subcutaneous fat, necrosis, lymphovascular, or perineural invasion, all predictive of aggressive behavior including (distant) metastases, are best classified as pleomorphic dermal sarcoma, not otherwise specified.[9] Therefore the diagnosis of AFX cannot be rendered based on superficial (shave) biopsies, where the base of the lesion cannot be visualized. In such samples, the interim designation *atypical intradermal spindle-cell/pleomorphic neoplasm*, with a comment recommending complete excision prior to definite diagnosis, is appropriate.

Prognosis and Treatment

Surgical excision with free margins is curative. Although there is some debate as to whether AFX is benign, if the previously mentioned criteria are strictly applied, AFX behaves in a benign manner with a risk of local recurrence if incompletely excised. There are rare reports of AFX with metastases, but such cases are often incompletely illustrated for optimal evaluation of the minimal diagnostic criteria for AFX (discussed earlier), or stem from the pre- and early immunohistochemistry era (without or with inadequate immunohistochemical workup).[13–15] Consequently, these lesions may not represent typical AFX and possibly include malignant nonmesenchymal tumors such as poorly differentiated and sarcomatoid carcinoma and amelanotic melanoma. A very recent and more convincing study of putative AFX with (distant) metastases has been published; nevertheless, the conclusions need to be interpreted with caution, and further studies are required to support the validity of these findings.[16]

PRACTICE POINTS: Atypical Fibroxanthoma

- Atypical fibroxanthoma (AFX) is a tumor of older adults, arising in actinically damaged skin, almost exclusively in the head and neck area.
- AFX is usually a pleomorphic tumor, although a spindle cell variant is also recognized.
- AFX does not infiltrate the subcutaneous fat and does not exhibit necrosis, vascular invasion, or perineural invasion.
- AFX is a diagnosis of exclusion; sarcomatoid carcinoma, melanoma, and leiomyosarcoma must be excluded.
- AFX is regarded as benign and does not metastasize.

Undifferentiated Pleomorphic Sarcoma

Undifferentiated pleomorphic sarcoma, previously termed *MFH*, is defined as a high-grade pleomorphic neoplasm with no identifiable line(s) of differentiation using currently available diagnostic techniques.[1] In the 1960s, Stout and colleagues first introduced MFH as a diagnostic label for a group of malignant mesenchymal tumors composed primarily of pleomorphic and spindle-shaped cells with a predominantly storiform growth pattern, which did not appear to fit into any of the recognized sarcoma categories.[17,18] The genesis of this term was based partly on (1) the fibroblast-like appearance of the neoplastic cells at a light microscopic level, and (2) the observation that tumor cells in tissue culture appeared to acquire ameboid and phagocytic properties—hence they presumed the cells to be of "fibrohistiocytic" origin.[17,18]

Following these original studies, MFH soon gained widespread acceptance as a clinicopathologic entity, and by the end of the 1980s, storiform/pleomorphic MFH was the single largest category of sarcomas.[19–22] During this period, four additional variants were added to the MFH family: giant cell MFH, inflammatory MFH, myxoid MFH, and angiomatoid MFH.[23–28] Nevertheless, with the passage of time, skepticism concerning the validity of this diagnostic concept grew, and, facilitated by the advent of electron microscopy and the development and refinement of immunohistochemical techniques, it became increasingly clear that there was no real scientific evidence for a "fibrohistiocytic" line of differentiation in this group of tumors.[29–34] In fact, in a seminal paper in 1992, Fletcher convincingly demonstrated that so-called *storiform/pleomorphic MFH* (the "flagship" MFH category) represented a heterogeneous group of tumors including not only a variety of different sarcoma types but also melanomas, carcinomas, and lymphomas, unified by a common histologic appearance (Fig. 7.2).[29] In this retrospective re-analysis of 159 tumors diagnosed as MFH, 97 cases (61%) turned out to be specific sarcomas with an identifiable line of differentiation, 20 (13%) were nonmesenchymal neoplasms (pleomorphic carcinoma, melanoma, and lymphoma), and only 42 (26%) showed no identifiable line(s) of differentiation. Of these remaining cases, 21 (13%) were of a sufficient quality to be evaluable and potentially eligible for a diagnosis of *storiform/pleomorphic MFH*, although importantly, these lesions did not share any consistent features, negating the possibility that they might form part of a homogeneous tumor category. Clearly the terms *fibrohistiocytic* and *fibrous histiocytoma* are misnomers for this group of lesions, uniting a variety of different tumor types that are probably unrelated. The category *storiform/pleomorphic MFH* therefore seems to have served primarily as a "wastebasket" for a heterogeneous group of unclassifiable neoplasms with pleomorphic morphology. A proportion of these tumors will in all likelihood prove to be of (myo)fibroblastic lineage, but, as of yet, due to the lack of reliable and reproducible diagnostic criteria by which such a line of differentiation can be consistently recognized, accurate diagnosis of high-grade myofibroblastic sarcomas remains problematic. Diagnostic criteria for malignant "true" histiocytic neoplasms have gradually been defined in the past decade, facilitating accurate recognition of this group of tumors.[35]

The remaining four MFH variants have similarly been critically re-evaluated. Giant cell MFH, once nonmesenchymal tumors such as osteoclast-rich (metastatic) carcinoma have been excluded, appears to represent a morphologic pattern shared primarily by (malignant) giant cell tumor of soft tissue, extraskeletal osteosarcoma, and leiomyosarcoma with osteoclastic giant cells (see Chapter 11).[1,36–38] Inflammatory MFH remains a poorly defined category and, once pleomorphic lymphoreticular neoplasms and inflammatory sarcomatoid carcinomas have been excluded, probably consists predominantly of dedifferentiated liposarcoma (DDLPS) with inflammatory features and inflammatory myofibroblastic tumor (see Chapter 10).[1,39,40] Myxoid MFH, a distinct entity discussed separately later, is synonymous with myxofibrosarcoma, a term that is a more accurate representation of its fibroblastic lineage and myxoid properties.[1,26,27,41] Angiomatoid MFH shares no features with the other members of the MFH family and has been renamed *angiomatoid fibrous histiocytoma* as a result of its intermediate biologic potential (rarely metastasizing), falling within the category of tumors of "uncertain

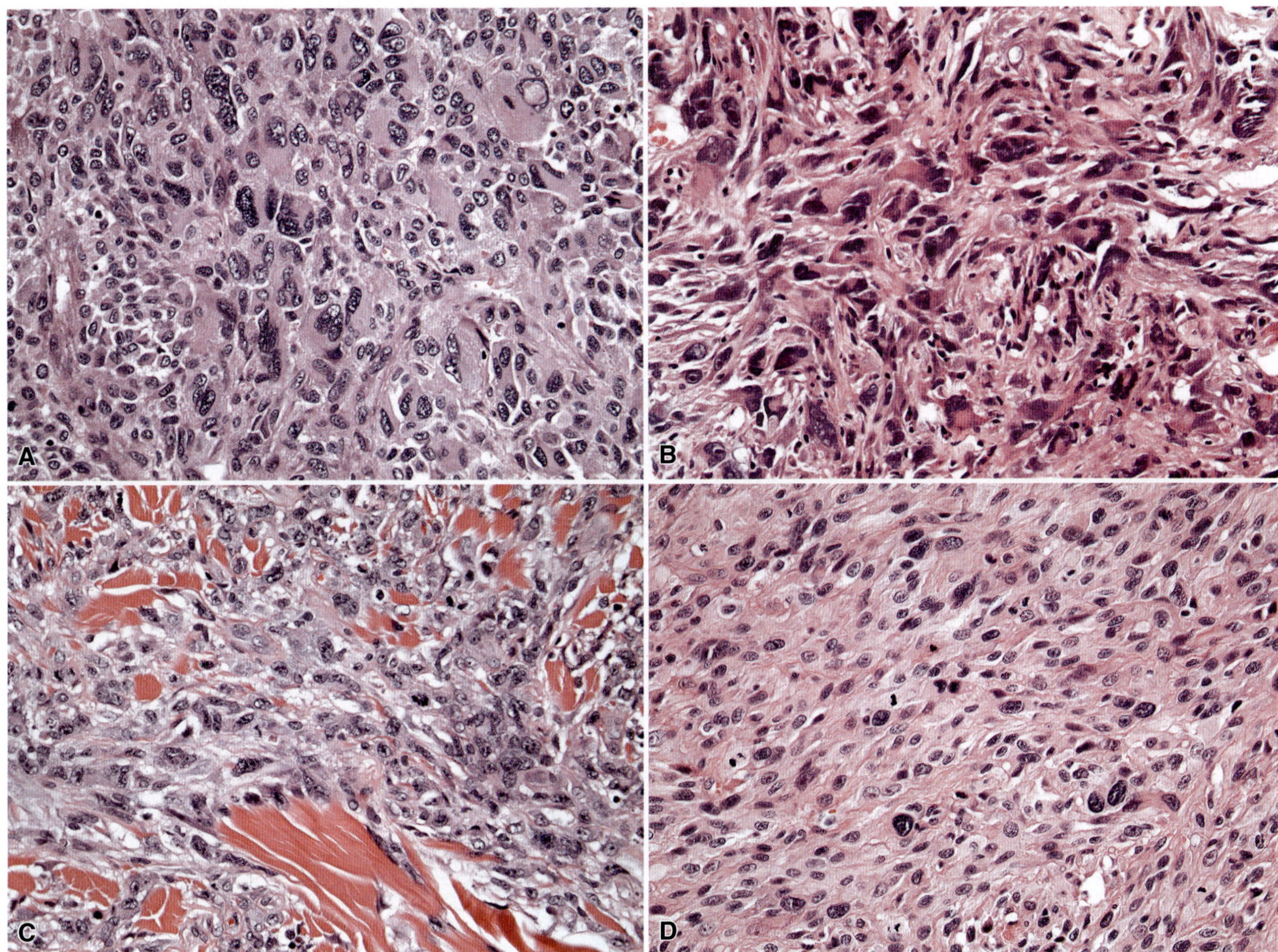

Figure 7.2 Nonmesenchymal Neoplasms Mimicking Undifferentiated Pleomorphic Sarcoma. (A) Melanoma. (B) Carcinoma. (C) Anaplastic large-cell lymphoma. (D) Undifferentiated pleomorphic sarcoma.

differentiation" (see Chapters 3 and 10).[1] Consequently the diagnostic label "undifferentiated pleomorphic sarcoma" has been gradually and informally introduced to replace "MFH" and should be regarded as a diagnosis of exclusion to be used only when all efforts to identify a specific line of differentiation have failed.

This shift in thinking is reflected in the recent WHO classifications (2002, 2013), and general consensus at last appears to have accepted that the rubric "MFH" is scientifically inaccurate, no longer of diagnostic value, and represents a collection of heterogeneous tumors with variable morphology (pleomorphic, spindle cell, epithelioid, round cell) that are not readily classifiable by current methods.[1] As such, the WHO has chosen to replace this term ("MFH") with the neutral and more accurate label of *undifferentiated (high-grade) sarcoma*, and in the most recent WHO classification (2013), this group has been further categorized to include the subcategories undifferentiated pleomorphic sarcoma, undifferentiated spindle cell sarcoma, undifferentiated round cell sarcoma, undifferentiated epithelioid sarcoma, and undifferentiated sarcoma not otherwise specified (Table 7.2).[1]

Clinical Features

Undifferentiated sarcomas as a whole probably account for 5% to 10% of sarcomas in adults older than 40 years of age.[1,29,30] These tumors generally arise in the deep (subfascial) soft tissues of older patients (in the sixth decade and older). They have a predilection for the extremities (lower limbs), followed by the trunk, and a small proportion (no more than 10%) arise in the subcutaneous tissues and retroperitoneum.[1]

Pathologic Features

Grossly, the tumors vary in size from 5 to 15 cm, are usually firm with a grayish color, are usually well circumscribed (with or without a pseudocapsule derived from adjacent compressed tissue) but may show infiltrative margins, and frequently contain visible areas of necrosis and/or hemorrhage (Fig. 7.3). Histologically, tumors are composed of a haphazard, storiform, fascicular, or nested arrangement of predominantly or variably highly pleomorphic, spindle-shaped, epithelioid or round cells, with a variable amount of eosinophilic or amphophilic cytoplasm and numerous typical and atypical mitoses. Stroma is usually collagenous with or without an inflammatory infiltrate and occasionally (osteoclastic) giant cells may be prominent (Fig. 7.4). Ancillary ultrastructural studies are, by definition, not helpful in identifying a particular line of differentiation.[29,30,33,34]

Immunohistochemistry

Usually only the nonspecific marker vimentin is convincingly positive. The degree of immunohistochemical positivity required to define a particular line of differentiation remains a controversial issue in soft tissue pathology, although generally one requires more than just rare positive cells for an immunohistochemical marker to support specific differentiation (Table 7.3).[29,30]

Molecular Genetics

Cytogenetically, karyotypes are usually highly complex and nonspecific (Table 7.4).[42]

Differential Diagnosis

The differential diagnosis includes (metastatic) sarcomatoid carcinoma, (metastatic) melanoma, anaplastic large-cell lymphoma, and other high-grade pleomorphic sarcomas (high-grade myxofibrosarcoma, pleomorphic leiomyosarcoma, pleomorphic rhabdomyosarcoma, pleomorphic liposarcoma, DDLPS, and malignant peripheral nerve sheath tumor [MPNST] without or with heterologous rhabdomyoblastic differentiation [malignant triton tumor]). The clinical context and an appropriate immunohistochemical panel usually resolve any diagnostic dilemmas in the distinction from carcinoma, melanoma, and lymphoma (see Table 7.1). Generous sampling and the judicious use of immunohistochemistry (see Table 7.3) should facilitate the identification of foci with myogenic or neurogenic features (leiomyosarcoma/rhabdomyosarcoma or MPNST), lipoblasts (pleomorphic liposarcoma), contiguous foci of atypical lipomatous tumor (ALT)/well-differentiated liposarcoma (WDLPS), or areas with myxoid stroma and curvilinear vessels (myxofibrosarcoma). Because *undifferentiated (high-grade) sarcoma* remains a diagnosis of exclusion (as detailed previously), extensive sampling is mandatory in order to maximize the chance of identifying a (histologically, immunohistochemically, or ultrastructurally) recognizable line of differentiation, facilitating accurate and clinically useful classification.

Prognosis and Treatment

Wide surgical excision with free margins and adjuvant radiotherapy is the primary therapeutic modality of choice. Prognostically, tumors are usually high grade, have distant metastases at presentation in 5% to 10% of cases, and have a 5-year survival of 50% to 60%.[1,30,43] Tumor size, tumor depth, grade, the presence of necrosis, and local recurrence appear to correlate with metastatic rate and survival, although these

Table 7.2 Old and New Terminology for Sarcomas Showing No Identifiable Lines of Differentiation Using Currently Available Diagnostic Tools

Old Terminology	New Terminology
Storiform/pleomorphic MFH	Undifferentiated sarcoma with pleomorphic, spindle cell, round cell and epithelioid subtypes
Giant cell MFH	Undifferentiated pleomorphic sarcoma with giant cells
Inflammatory MFH	Undifferentiated pleomorphic sarcoma with prominent inflammation
Myxoid MFH	Myxofibrosarcoma
Angiomatoid MFH	Angiomatoid fibrous histiocytoma

MFH, Malignant fibrous histiocytoma.

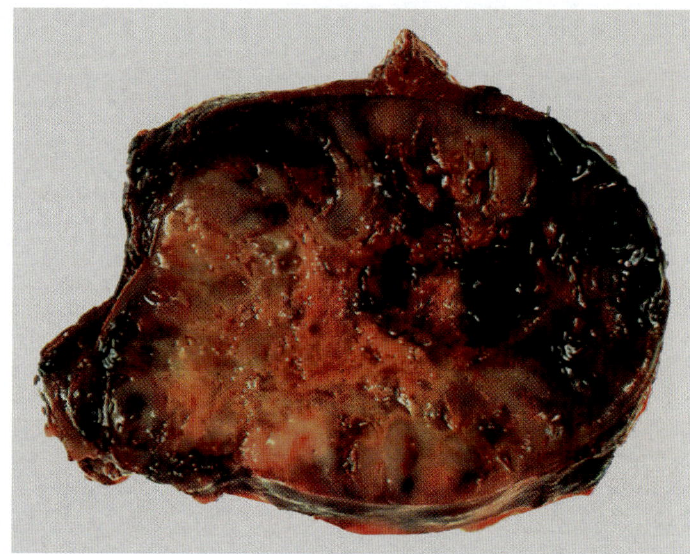

Figure 7.3 Characteristic Gross (Macroscopic) Appearance of Undifferentiated Pleomorphic Sarcoma. There are visible areas of hemorrhage and necrosis. The frequent presence of extensive necrosis in high-grade neoplasms emphasizes the need for diligent (extensive) sampling in order to identify viable tumor essential for accurate classification of the lesion.

Table 7.3 Immunohistochemical Panel for the Analysis of Pleomorphic and Spindle Cell Neoplasms

	KRT	EMA	S-100	HMB45	CD30	ALK	SMA	DES	h-CD	MYOG
Carcinoma	+	±	–	–	–	–	–	–	–	–
Melanoma	–	–	+	±	–	–	–	–	–	–
ALCL	–	–	–	–	+	±	–	–	–	–
PLMS	±	±	–	–	–	–	+	+	+	–
PRMS	–	–	–	–	–	–	±	+	–	+
PLPS	–	–	±	–	–	–	±	–	–	–
DDLPS	–	–	–	–	–	–	±	±	–	–
MPNST-R	–	±	±	–	–	–	±	+	–	+
MFS	–	–	–	–	–	–	±	–	–	–
IMT	–	–	–	–	–	±	±	±	–	–

ALCL, Anaplastic large-cell lymphoma; *DDLPS,* dedifferentiated liposarcoma; *DES,* desmin; *EMA,* epithelial membrane antigen; *h-CD,* h-caldesmon; *IMT,* inflammatory myofibroblastic tumor; *KRT,* pan-keratin; *MFS,* high-grade myxofibrosarcoma; *MPNST-R,* malignant peripheral nerve sheath tumor with heterologous rhabdomyoblastic differentiation (malignant triton tumor); *MYOG,* myogenin; *PLMS,* pleomorphic leiomyosarcoma; *PLPS,* pleomorphic liposarcoma; *PRMS,* pleomorphic rhabdomyosarcoma; *SMA,* smooth muscle actin.

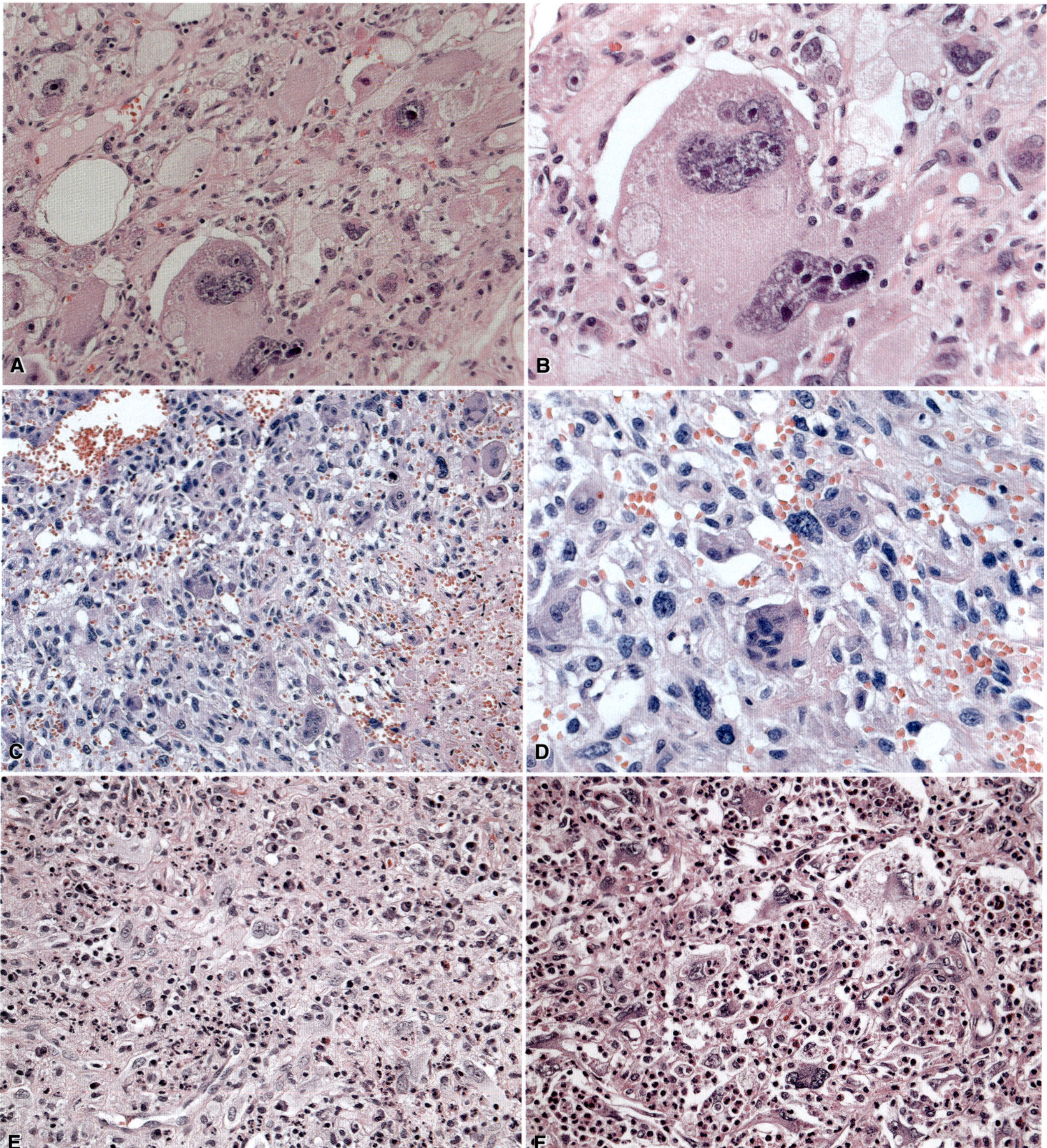

Figure 7.4 **Undifferentiated Pleomorphic Sarcoma.** Medium-power (A) and high-power (B) views of undifferentiated pleomorphic sarcoma. Medium-power (C) and high-power (D) views of undifferentiated pleomorphic sarcoma with giant cells. (E and F) Medium-power views of undifferentiated pleomorphic sarcoma with inflammatory cells.

Table 7.4 Cytogenetic Abnormalities in Pleomorphic Soft Tissue Sarcomas

Type of Sarcoma	Cytogenetic Abnormality
MFS	Nonspecific complex karyotypes
PLMS	Nonspecific complex karyotypes
PRMS	Nonspecific complex karyotypes
PLPS	Nonspecific complex karyotypes
DDLPS	Ring and giant marker chromosomes derived from amplification of 12q13–15 (variable amplification of *MDM2, SAS, CDK4, HMGA2*) Additional nonspecific complex abnormalities
EO	Nonspecific complex karyotypes
PHAT/MIFS/HFLT	t(1;10)(p22;q24) (maps to *TGFBR3* and *MGEA5*) and loss of chromosomes 3 and 13 Supernumerary ring chromosomes derived from segments of chromosome 3 and a derivative chromosome 13 der(10)t(1;10) in combination with aberrations of chromosome 3 t(2;6)(q31;p21.3)
UPS	Nonspecific complex karyotypes Extensive intratumoral heterogeneity Aneuploidy (haploid, triploid, tetraploid) Genomic imbalances, mutations in *TP53, RB1, CDKN2A*

DDLPS, Dedifferentiated liposarcoma; *EO,* extraskeletal osteosarcoma; *HFLT,* hemosiderotic fibrolipomatous tumor; *MFS,* high-grade myxofibrosarcoma; *MIFS,* myxoinflammatory fibroblastic sarcoma; *PLMS,* pleomorphic leiomyosarcoma; *PLPS,* pleomorphic liposarcoma; *PRMS,* pleomorphic rhabdomyosarcoma; *UPS,* undifferentiated pleomorphic sarcoma.

do not per se appear to be independent variables for the prediction of outcomes.[1,2,44–48]

The importance of maximizing efforts in accurate classification becomes apparent when one realizes that DDLPS has a 5-year metastatic rate of only 15% to 20%, compared with a 5-year metastatic rate of 30% to 35% for high-grade myxofibrosarcoma, and a far higher 5-year metastatic rate (>60%), together with a significantly inferior relapse-free survival rate, for pleomorphic leiomyosarcoma and rhabdomyosarcoma.[1,2,44–48]

PRACTICE POINTS: Undifferentiated Sarcoma

- MFH is a meaningless rubric, does not exhibit convincing "fibrohistiocytic" differentiation, represents a "wastebasket" for a heterogeneous collection of unclassifiable neoplasms with pleomorphic, spindle cell, epithelioid or round cell morphology, and has been designated *undifferentiated sarcoma* in the current World Health Organization classification.
- When confronted with a morphologically unclassifiable neoplasm, all efforts need to be made to exclude poorly differentiated carcinoma, melanoma, and lymphoma.
- The realization that sarcomas exhibit a wide range of biologic behavior, varying from indolent to highly aggressive, underscores the need for maximal effort in the accurate classification of sarcomas.
- Undifferentiated sarcoma is a diagnosis of exclusion and should be used only when all efforts to identify a specific line of differentiation have failed.
- Accurate classification of sarcomas allows for a better definition of their clinical behavior and facilitates participation in meaningful clinical trials.

Pleomorphic Hyalinizing Angiectatic Tumor

PHAT (of soft parts) is a recently described and enigmatic pleomorphic mesenchymal neoplasm.[1,49–52] Although (distant) metastases and tumor-related mortality have not as yet been described, PHAT is reviewed in this section because it may represent an indolent low-grade sarcoma with disease-related morbidity and mortality after longer-term follow-up.

PHAT is currently defined as an (as yet) nonmetastasizing locally aggressive tumor of uncertain lineage characterized by mitotically inert spindle-shaped and pleomorphic cells; ectatic thin-walled vessels exhibiting fibrinoid change; and a variable inflammatory infiltrate composed predominantly of eosinophils, lymphocytes, and plasma cells.[1,49–52]

Recognition of putative morphologic and (cyto)genetic overlap with hemosiderotic fibrolipomatous tumor (HFLT) and myxoinflammatory fibroblastic sarcoma (MIFS) would appear to support a morphologic continuum within a single entity (with associated implications for management and follow-up), although the exact nature of this relationship remains an active area of debate.[53–55]

Clinical Features

PHAT is a rare tumor occurring in adults (age range 10 to 80 years; median age 50 years) with an equal gender distribution. It arises primarily in the subcutaneous tissues of the lower limbs and less frequently at other sites. Patients usually present with a slowly enlarging painless swelling, which not infrequently has been present for a long period of time before medical attention is sought.

Pathologic Features

Grossly, tumors are usually poorly circumscribed with infiltrative margins and vary in size from less than 1 cm to more than 10 cm in diameter, with an average size of 3 to 4 cm. On sectioning, tumors are grayish-brown to tan in color, depending on the extent of intralesional vascularity and hemosiderin deposition. Histologically, clusters of thin-walled ectatic vessels, which may be either hyalinized or show extensive fibrinoid change involving the full thickness of the vessel wall, frequently with intraluminal thrombosis, are prominent (Fig. 7.5A and B). The stromal cells vary from being spindle-shaped to highly pleomorphic with bizarre, hyperchromatic nuclei often containing intranuclear pseudoinclusions (derived from the cytoplasm; see Fig. 7.5C and D). Mitoses are scarce, usually less than 1 per 50 high-power fields, and any increase in mitotic activity is generally regarded as not being compatible with a diagnosis of PHAT. A variable inflammatory infiltrate composed of eosinophils, lymphocytes, and plasma cells is usually present, and deposits of hemosiderin may occasionally be prominent.[1,49–51] Importantly, in a number of cases of putative PHAT, primarily in peripheral regions of the tumor, variably cellular areas composed of hemosiderin-laden spindle-shaped cells with wavy nuclei and a fascicular orientation morphologically similar to HFLT are present, infiltrating adjacent fat, while cases of putative PHAT with morphologic overlap with MIFS have also been reported, supporting grounds for a morphologic continuum within these three entities.[50,53,54]

Ancillary ultrastructural studies to date have not been of help in identifying a line of differentiation.[52]

Immunohistochemistry

The neoplastic cells do not demonstrate a specific immunohistochemical profile. Lesional cells are positive for CD34 in roughly half of cases, but they are negative for S-100 protein, important in the distinction from "ancient" schwannoma.[1,49–51]

Molecular Genetics

At a cytogenetic level, a variety of molecular alterations have been identified in PHAT, some of which (primarily a t[1;10]) appear to be shared (to a limited extent) with MIFS and HFLT, and consequently additional data are required to define the exact nature of the relationship between these three entities.[55–57]

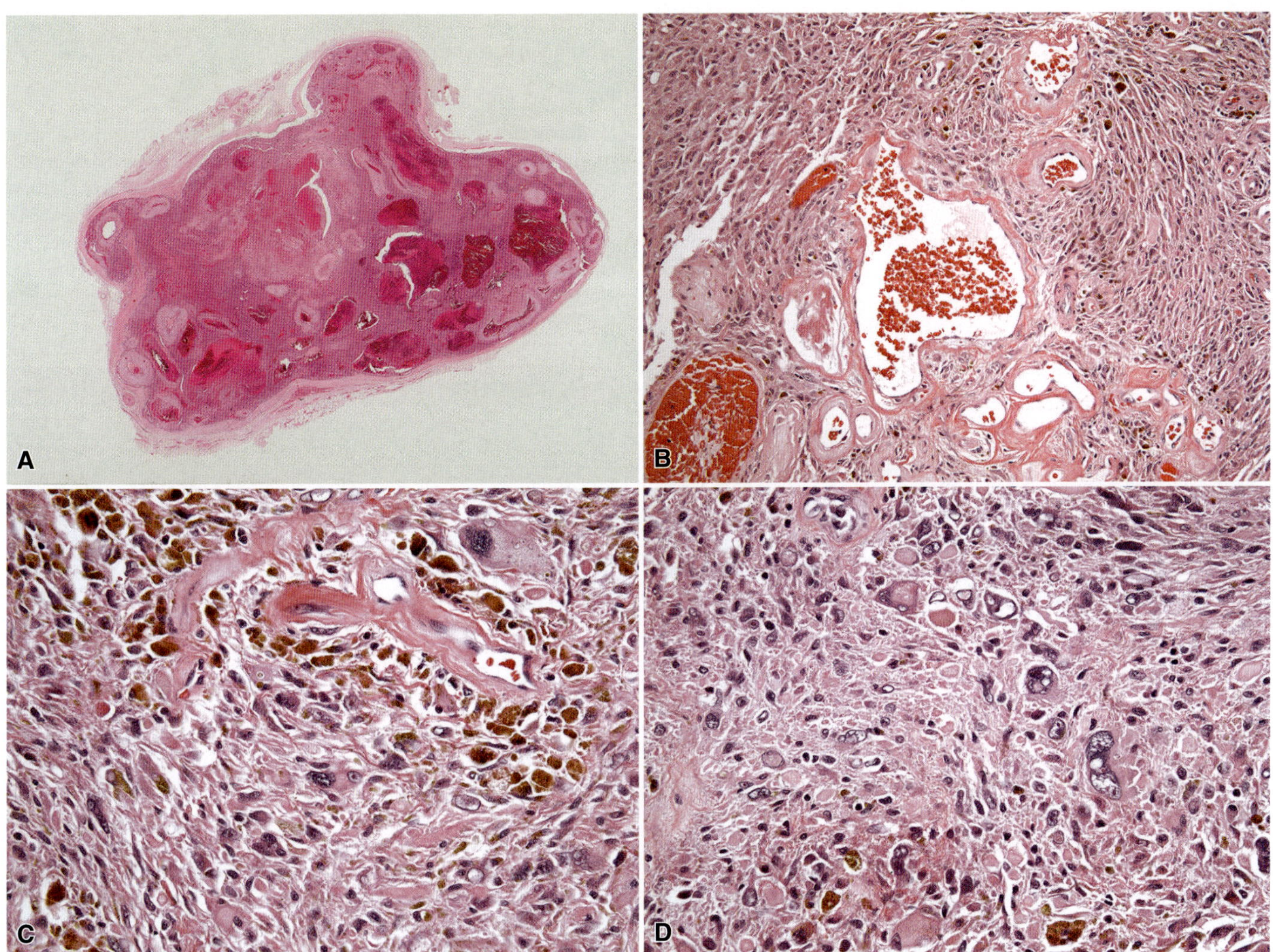

Figure 7.5 Pleomorphic Hyalinizing Angiectatic Tumor. (A) Whole-mount view illustrating the prominent lesional vascularity. Medium-power (B) and high-power (C and D) views demonstrating the cellular characteristics of the tumor.

Differential Diagnosis

The differential diagnosis primarily includes ancient schwannoma and a hemangioma with degenerative changes (symplastic hemangioma). The immunohistochemical negativity for S-100 protein excludes schwannoma, whereas the presence of a vascular component intimately associated with obviously atypical stromal cells argues against a vascular lesion.

As a result of the increasing recognition and awareness of overlapping morphologic and cytogenetic features between PHAT, HFLT, and MIFS, although still preliminary, experts are beginning to believe that PHAT, HFLT, and MIFS may fall within one morphologic spectrum.[50,53–55]

Prognosis and Treatment

Wide surgical excision with free margins is the primary therapeutic modality of choice. Typical cases of PHAT are characterized primarily by nondestructive local recurrences, although longer-term follow-up data are needed to determine more accurately the exact biologic behavior of this entity; if indeed there is a biologic continuum with MIFS (which may show high-grade progression, as discussed later) and HFLT, this will have implications for treatment and follow-up guidelines.

PRACTICE POINTS: Pleomorphic Hyalinizing Angiectatic Tumor

- PHAT may be mistaken for ancient schwannoma or hemangioma with degenerative changes (symplastic hemangioma).
- Many experts now believe that, based on unifying morphology and cytogenetics, PHAT, HFLT, and MIFS may fall within one morphologic spectrum.

Myxoinflammatory Fibroblastic Sarcoma

MIFS, also discussed in some detail in Chapters 5 and 10, has previously also been referred to as acral MIFS, inflammatory myxohyaline tumor of the distal extremities with virocyte or Reed-Sternberg–like cells, and inflammatory myxoid tumor of the soft parts with bizarre giant cells.[1,58–60] The tumor is defined as a low-grade sarcoma occurring primarily in the distal extremities. It is characterized by myxoid stroma, an inflammatory infiltrate, and distinctive virocyte- or Reed-Sternberg–like cells.[1,58–60] Recognition of putative histologic overlap with HFLT and PHAT, the identification of hybrid lesions, and the discovery of unifying cytogenetic data support a morphologic continuum within a single entity.[61–65]

Clinical Features

MIFS is a rare tumor occurring principally in adults with an equal gender distribution. Clinically, tumors present as a slowly growing swelling that has usually been present for a long period of time and may be associated with pain or discomfort and limit optimal function of the involved limb. Most lesions arise in the subcutaneous tissues of the distal extremities—more commonly in the upper limb than lower limb, with a ratio of 3:1. Infrequently, cases arising outside the extremities have been described.[1,58–60]

Pathologic Features

Grossly, tumors are usually multinodular and ill-defined with infiltrative margins, varying in size from 1 to 8 cm with an average size of 3 to 4 cm. On sectioning, tumors are generally soft with a yellow-grayish appearance and may be variably gelatinous depending on the degree of intralesional myxoid change. Histologically, tumors are characterized by distinctive pleomorphic or ganglion-like neoplastic cells with large nuclei, striking viral inclusion-like nucleoli, and eosinophilic cytoplasm. They are distributed singly or as clusters in a variably myxoid and hyaline stroma containing a prominent mixed inflammatory infiltrate (Fig. 7.6). In addition to the typical virocyte-like cells, more spindle-shaped cells, bubbly pseudolipoblasts, and hemosiderin-containing macrophages may be present.[1,58–60] Necrosis is uncommon.

Despite the variably marked cellular pleomorphism, mitotic activity is limited, usually not more than 2 mitotic figures per 50 high-power fields. Infrequently, foci consisting of low-grade hemosiderin-rich spindle cells and variably prominent thick-walled hyalinized vessels, very similar to those seen respectively in HFLT and PHAT, are identified adjacent to the more typical areas of MIFS, supporting a morphologic continuum within a single entity. Recently, high-grade sarcomatous progression within MIFS has been reported, broadening its biologic spectrum.[66]

Ultrastructurally, the tumor cells show predominantly fibroblastic features (oval clefted nuclei, a prominent endoplasmic reticulum, a well-developed Golgi system, variable numbers of lysosomes, and occasional bundles of densely packed actin filaments). However, electron microscopy has no diagnostic value for this tumor type.[58–60]

Immunohistochemistry

The neoplastic cells do not exhibit a distinctive immunohistochemical profile. However, importantly, in the differential diagnosis with Hodgkin lymphoma, the lymphoid markers CD30, CD15, and PAX5 are negative.

Molecular Genetics

The increasing availability of cytogenetic data for MIFS has identified a number of distinctive tumor-specific alterations, predominantly a balanced or unbalanced t(1;10)(p22;q24) with alterations of chromosomes 3 and 13 (see Table 7.4).[61–65] The breakpoints map to the *TGFBR3* gene in 1p22 and to, or near to, the *MGEA5* locus in 10q24; similar genetic alterations have been identified in HFLT and rarely in PHAT, providing support for a putative morphologic continuum within a single entity.[62–65]

Differential Diagnosis

Because the histologic appearance is quite distinctive, the only realistic differential diagnosis (as alluded to earlier) is with Hodgkin lymphoma, which is readily excluded with an appropriate immunohistochemical panel of lymphoid markers.

As a result of the increasing recognition and awareness of overlapping morphologies between PHAT, HFLT, and MIFS, supplemented by the increasing availability of (cyto)genetic data for these entities, many experts now believe that PHAT, HFLT, and MIFS may fall within one morphologic spectrum.

Prognosis and Treatment

Wide surgical excision with free margins is the primary therapeutic modality of choice. Prognostically, the tumor generally demonstrates an indolent clinical course, with reported rates of local recurrence varying between 20% and 70%. Nevertheless, cases with aggressive local behavior and progression to high-grade pleomorphic sarcoma have been described, and rare cases with metastases to regional lymph nodes and lung exist; worryingly, although not unexpectedly, a recent report documented the first case of a putative disease-related death.[54,66]

PRACTICE POINTS: Myxoinflammatory Fibroblastic Sarcoma

- MIFS may be mistaken for Hodgkin lymphoma.
- Based on unifying morphology and cytogenetics, many experts now believe that PHAT, HFLT, and MIFS may fall within one morphologic spectrum.

Myxofibrosarcoma

Myxofibrosarcoma, also discussed in Chapter 5, is defined as a malignant fibroblastic neoplasm with variably myxoid stroma, cellular pleomorphism, and a distinctive curvilinear vasculature.[1,26,27,41] It is a soft tissue tumor with a broad spectrum of histologic grade, which was first recognized as a specific entity in the late 1970s.[26,27] At the high-grade end of the spectrum, the terms *myxoid MFH* and *myxofibrosarcoma* have been used interchangeably in the literature for what is essentially the same entity, leading to confusion regarding this lesion. It is now apparent that the tumor cells do not demonstrate convincing histiocytic differentiation, and consequently, the more accurate designation *myxofibrosarcoma*, which emphasizes the fibroblastic nature and myxoid stroma of this neoplasm, has been accepted in the more recent WHO classifications as the preferred nomenclature.[1,41]

Clinical Features

Myxofibrosarcoma is a tumor of older adults (average age 65 to 70 years), occurring predominantly in the subcutaneous tissues of the extremities, with a roughly equal gender distribution. Deeper localization (subfascial and intramuscular) is less frequent, observed in approximately 30% of cases.[1,26,27,41] Occurrence in the retroperitoneum or abdominal cavity is rare, and such tumors usually represent DDLPS with myxofibrosarcoma-like features.[67] Most patients present with a slowly enlarging painless subcutaneous swelling.

Pathologic Features

Grossly, the lesions are of variable size, but the majority are less than 10 cm in diameter. Deeper lesions tend to be larger than their subcutaneous counterparts. The tumors are usually multinodular, with deceptively infiltrative margins. On sectioning, tumors are variably gelatinous, with the higher-grade lesions being firmer with a more grayish appearance, frequently with visible areas of hemorrhage and necrosis.

Histologically, myxofibrosarcoma exhibits a wide range of grade with a broad spectrum of cellularity, cytologic pleomorphism, and mitotic activity.[1,26,27,41,68–70] Nevertheless, all lesions share distinctive features that define this entity: a myxoid matrix consisting of hyaluronidase-sensitive acidic mucopolysaccharides containing fusiform to stellate cells with variably pleomorphic, hyperchromatic nuclei, and a characteristic delicate curvilinear vasculature with perivascular condensation of tumor cells, particularly in the myxoid areas.[1,26,27,41,68–70] Empirically, it has been accepted that in order to qualify for this diagnosis, roughly 10% of the tumor should contain myxoid areas. Tumors at the high-grade end of

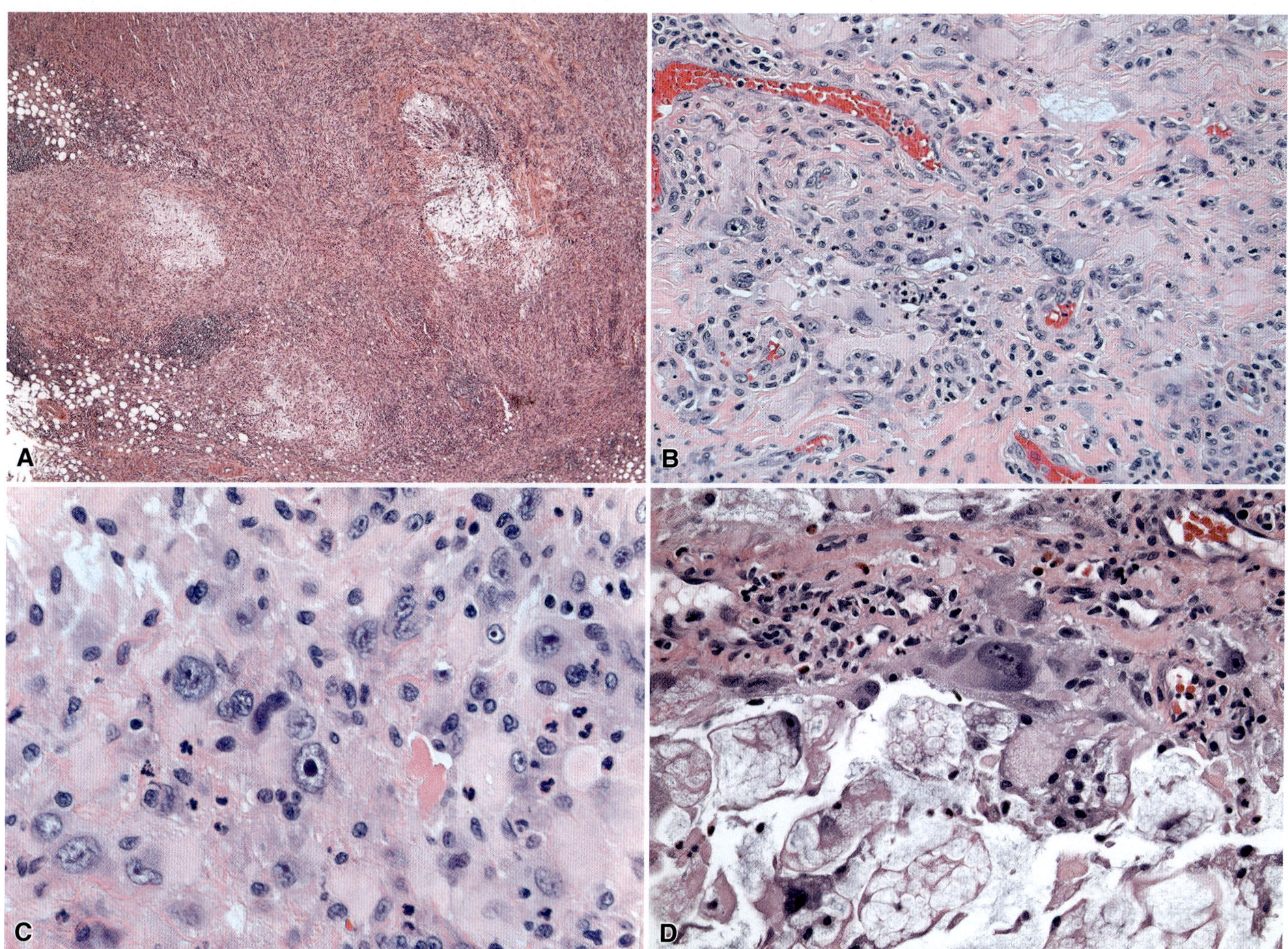

Figure 7.6 Myxoinflammatory Fibroblastic Sarcoma. Low-power (A), medium-power (B), and high-power (C and D) views of this unusual neoplasm. Note the inflammatory background, myxoid foci, and virocyte-like pleomorphic cells typical of this entity.

the spectrum are highly cellular and composed of pleomorphic cells and more spindle-shaped cells with a predominantly solid, sheet-like, storiform, and/or fascicular arrangement; the amount of cytoplasm is variable and usually amphophilic in nature (Fig. 7.7). Areas of necrosis may be present, and, in addition to the cellular pleomorphism, mitotic activity is marked. A prominent mixed inflammatory infiltrate may be seen, particularly at the periphery of the tumor. In high-grade lesions, extensive sampling is often necessary to identify the myxoid component that defines this entity. Recently, the histologic spectrum of myxofibrosarcoma has been expanded with the recognition of a variant exhibiting predominantly epithelioid morphology.[68] In this variant, the cells do not demonstrate the striking pleomorphism that is seen in typical cases of high-grade myxofibrosarcoma, but are more epithelioid ("carcinoma-like") in appearance, complicating distinction from (metastatic) carcinoma (see Fig. 7.7E). Pseudolipoblasts with mucin-containing vacuolated cytoplasm may be present (see Fig. 7.7F).

Ultrastructurally, the tumor cells are fusiform with oval clefted nuclei, a prominent and partially distended endoplasmic reticulum, a well-developed Golgi system, variable numbers of lysosomes, and occasional bundles of densely packed actin filaments, features typical of (myo) fibroblastic differentiation.[34,71,72]

Immunohistochemistry

With the exception of (nonspecific) vimentin, CD34, and focal actin-positivity (reflecting its putative fibroblastic nature), immunohistochemical markers are negative (see Table 7.3).

Molecular Genetics

Cytogenetically, karyotypes are typically complex with intratumoral heterogeneity and aneuploidy; progression in grade appears to be associated with an increase in cytogenetic abnormalities. No tumor-specific cytogenetic alterations have been described to date, although there appear to be diverse *NF1* alterations in up to 10% of myxofibrosarcomas analyzed.[73] In contrast to intramuscular myxomas, no mutations involving *GNAS* have been identified in myxofibrosarcomas (see Table 7.4).[1,42,74,75]

Differential Diagnosis

The diagnostic difficulties at the high-grade end of the spectrum are due to an increase in lesional cellularity, loss of the characteristic myxoid matrix, and absence of the typical curvilinear vasculature. The main differential diagnostic considerations include pleomorphic liposarcoma, pleomorphic myogenic sarcomas, anaplastic large-cell

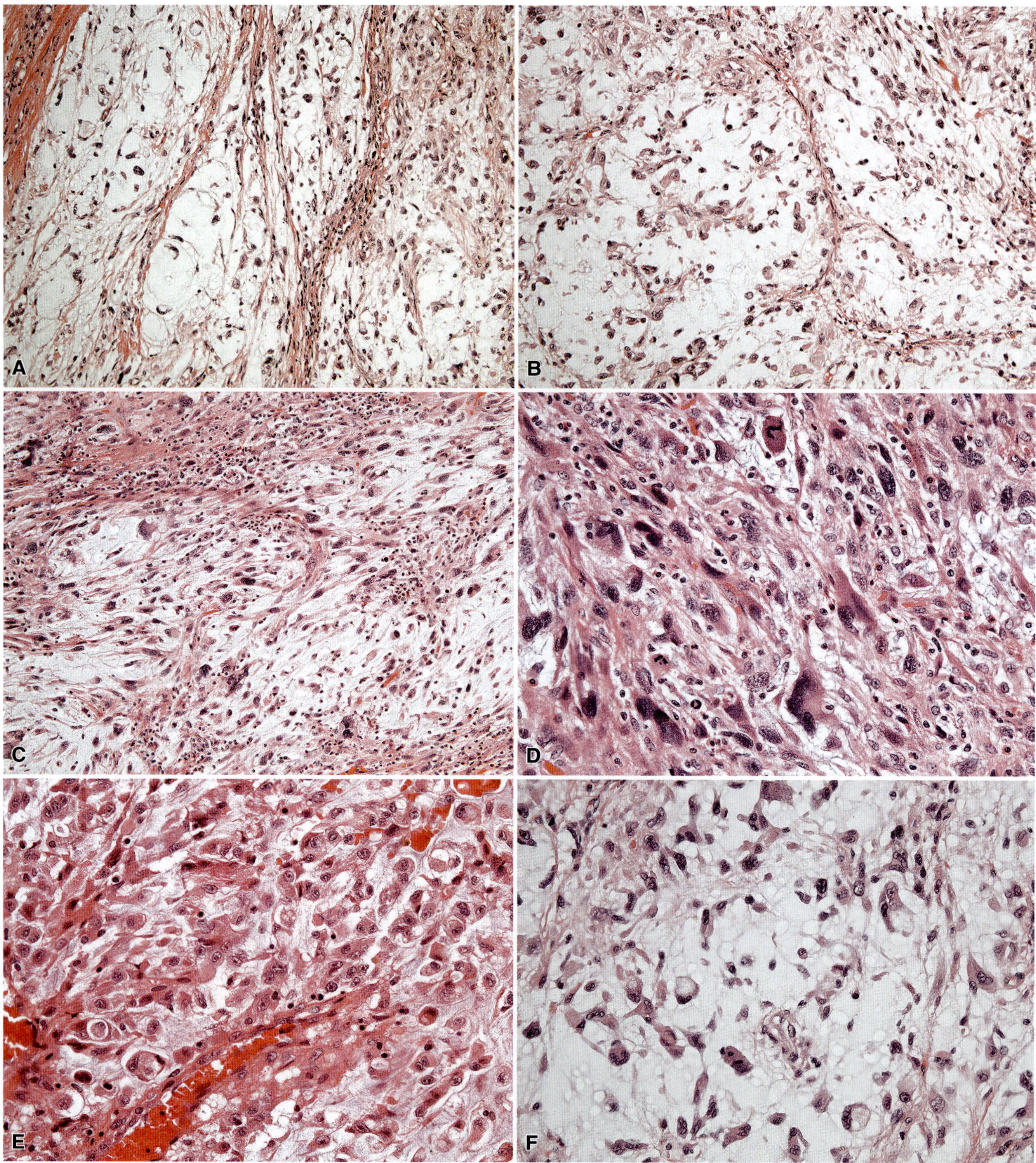

Figure 7.7 High-Grade Myxofibrosarcoma. Medium-power (A–C) and high-power (D–F) views illustrating the typical features of myxofibrosarcoma. Note the prominent cellular atypia, curvilinear vasculature, myxoid stroma, and pseudolipoblasts (F). The epithelioid variant (E) can mimic poorly differentiated carcinoma.

lymphoma, (metastatic) carcinoma, and (metastatic) melanoma. Identification of areas with myxoid stroma and the more typical features of myxofibrosarcoma are essential to establish the diagnosis, whereas an immunohistochemical panel including myogenic markers, CD45, CD30, S-100 protein and additional melanoma markers, and pankeratins generally excludes the other differential diagnostic options (see Table 7.3).

Prognosis and Treatment

Wide surgical excision with free margins and adjuvant radiotherapy is the primary therapeutic modality of choice. Given the typical strikingly infiltrative margins (usually much farther along connective tissue planes than is clinically apparent), local recurrences are common, and grade often increases with each recurrence. Prognostically, the potential for metastasis and mortality is closely associated with an increase in histologic grade and appears to be greater for deep-seated lesions. High-grade tumors are associated with a 30% to 35% risk of metastasis. Survival correlates with histologic grade, but overall 5-year survival is 50% to 70%.[1,30,41]

PRACTICE POINTS: Myxofibrosarcoma

- A variably myxoid stroma containing delicate curvilinear vessels with perivascular condensation of atypical spindle and pleomorphic cells is typical of myxofibrosarcoma.
- Generous sampling of high-grade (unclassifiable) pleomorphic sarcomas is often required to identify the myxoid foci typical of myxofibrosarcoma.
- Empirically, 10% of the tumor should consist of the typical myxoid foci to establish a diagnosis of myxofibrosarcoma.

Pleomorphic Myogenic Sarcomas

Both leiomyosarcoma and rhabdomyosarcoma, discussed in Chapters 3, 4, and 8, include a subgroup demonstrating a predominantly pleomorphic phenotype. These lesions are classified as pleomorphic leiomyosarcoma and pleomorphic rhabdomyosarcoma.[1]

Pleomorphic leiomyosarcoma is defined as a malignant tumor composed of pleomorphic and spindle-shaped cells showing features of smooth muscle differentiation.[1] Within the category of leiomyosarcoma as a whole (nonpleomorphic and pleomorphic variants), intraabdominal leiomyosarcoma (retroperitoneum, mesentery, and omentum) accounts for 40% to 45% of cases, subcutaneous and deep extremity tumors account for 30% to 35% of cases, vascular leiomyosarcoma accounts for about 5% of cases and arises primarily from the inferior vena cava and larger veins of the lower limbs, and cutaneous leiomyosarcoma and leiomyosarcoma in genital locations account for the remainder.[1,76–82] Nevertheless, although leiomyosarcoma at all sites may exhibit a pleomorphic phenotype, the vast majority of pleomorphic leiomyosarcomas arise in the extremities and retroperitoneum and only rarely in cutaneous or genital locations.[83]

Pleomorphic rhabdomyosarcoma is defined as a high-grade sarcoma occurring almost exclusively in older adults. It consists of bizarre polygonal, round, and spindle cells that display evidence of skeletal muscle differentiation and lack an identifiable embryonal or alveolar component.[1,84,85]

Clinical Features

Pleomorphic leiomyosarcoma is a tumor primarily of middle-aged and older adults, presenting most often as a mass or with pain and discomfort in the involved anatomic region. Deep-seated tumors are usually larger than their subcutaneous counterparts.[1,76–83]

Pleomorphic rhabdomyosarcoma occurs in older adults, more frequently in men than women. It arises most commonly in the deep soft tissues of the lower limbs. The two most frequent presenting symptoms are the presence of a mass and the existence of pain/discomfort.[1,84,85]

Pathologic Features

Grossly, pleomorphic leiomyosarcomas and pleomorphic rhabdomyosarcomas vary in size from 5 to 15 cm and are usually relatively well circumscribed (with or without a pseudocapsule derived from compressed adjacent tissues). They are reddish-brown in color and often have areas of visible necrosis or hemorrhage.

Histologic recognition of pleomorphic leiomyosarcoma and pleomorphic rhabdomyosarcoma may be challenging. Tumors are composed of round to spindle-shaped to highly pleomorphic cells; the focal presence of deeply eosinophilic cytoplasm should raise the suspicion of myogenic differentiation. In leiomyosarcoma, areas with a fascicular architecture may focally be present (Fig. 7.8), whereas in rhabdomyosarcoma, the architecture is less well defined, and tumor cells are loosely and more haphazardly arranged (Fig. 7.9A and B). When compared with pleomorphic leiomyosarcoma, the tumor cells of pleomorphic rhabdomyosarcoma are generally more pleomorphic, have larger nucleoli, and have more striking eosinophilia. Tadpole-shaped rhabdomyoblasts and cells with rhabdoid cytoplasmic inclusions may be encountered, but cross striations are rarely identified in pleomorphic rhabdomyosarcoma. Pleomorphic rhabdomyosarcomas that occur in children almost always contain small foci with embryonal or alveolar features, in which case they are classified as anaplastic rhabdomyosarcoma to emphasize their poorer prognosis (see Chapter 8).

Ultrastructural features of leiomyosarcoma, although not entirely tumor specific, include the presence of complete or incomplete external laminae, abundant densely packed cytoplasmic bundles of thin actin filaments (including cytoplasmic membrane attachment sites), cell junctions, pinocytotic vesicles, and abundant glycogen deposits.[34] Ultrastructural demonstration of sarcomere formation and Z-band material are highly specific features of normal striated muscle and support rhabdomyoblastic differentiation when present in (unclassifiable) pleomorphic sarcomas.[34] However, electron microscopy has largely been supplanted by immunohistochemistry and is therefore rarely used clinically in the diagnosis of pleomorphic sarcomas.

Immunohistochemistry

Immunohistochemical positivity for the myogenic markers smooth muscle actin and desmin does not reliably discriminate between leiomyosarcoma and rhabdomyosarcoma. Although h-caldesmon is reasonably specific for smooth muscle differentiation, nuclear positivity for myogenin (MYF4) or MYOD1 is required to support unequivocal rhabdomyoblastic differentiation (see Fig. 7.9C and Table 7.3).[85–87]

Molecular Genetics

Cytogenetically, karyotypes of pleomorphic leiomyosarcoma and pleomorphic rhabdomyosarcoma are complex and bewildering. They have no diagnostic or prognostic value (see Table 7.4).[1,42]

Interestingly, recent identification of a putative translocation specific for leiomyosarcoma and novel studies of gene expression profiles in leiomyosarcoma identifying a number of tumor-specific molecular subtypes may (1) facilitate the distinction between high-grade undifferentiated sarcoma and high-grade leiomyosarcoma important for possible tumor-specific therapy, (2) facilitate a prediction of clinical outcome, and (3) provide opportunities to treat leiomyosarcoma subtypes in a targeted manner.[88–90]

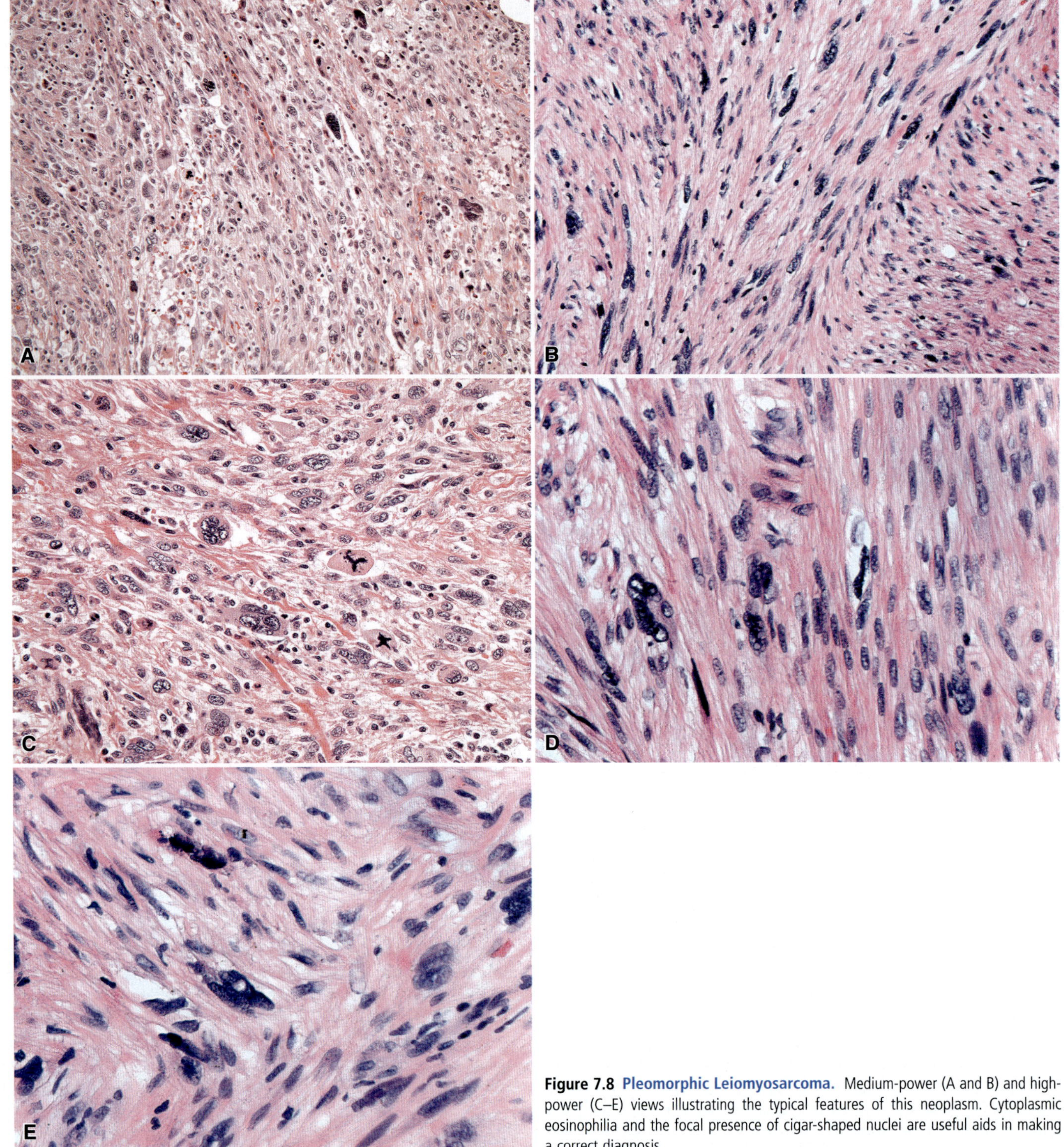

Figure 7.8 **Pleomorphic Leiomyosarcoma.** Medium-power (A and B) and high-power (C–E) views illustrating the typical features of this neoplasm. Cytoplasmic eosinophilia and the focal presence of cigar-shaped nuclei are useful aids in making a correct diagnosis.

Differential Diagnosis

The differential diagnosis for pleomorphic myogenic sarcomas is similar to that detailed previously (see the discussion of undifferentiated sarcoma): metastatic sarcomatoid carcinoma, metastatic melanoma, anaplastic large-cell lymphoma, and other high-grade pleomorphic sarcomas (high-grade myxofibrosarcoma, pleomorphic liposarcoma, DDLPS, and MPNST with or without heterologous rhabdomyoblastic differentiation [malignant triton tumor]). The clinical context, adequate tissue sampling, and an appropriate immunohistochemical panel (see Table 7.3) usually resolve any diagnostic dilemmas, although it is very important to bear in mind that immunohistochemical positivity for keratins and epithelial membrane antigen is seen in roughly 20% to 40% of leiomyosarcomas, which may be a pitfall for the unwary.[87]

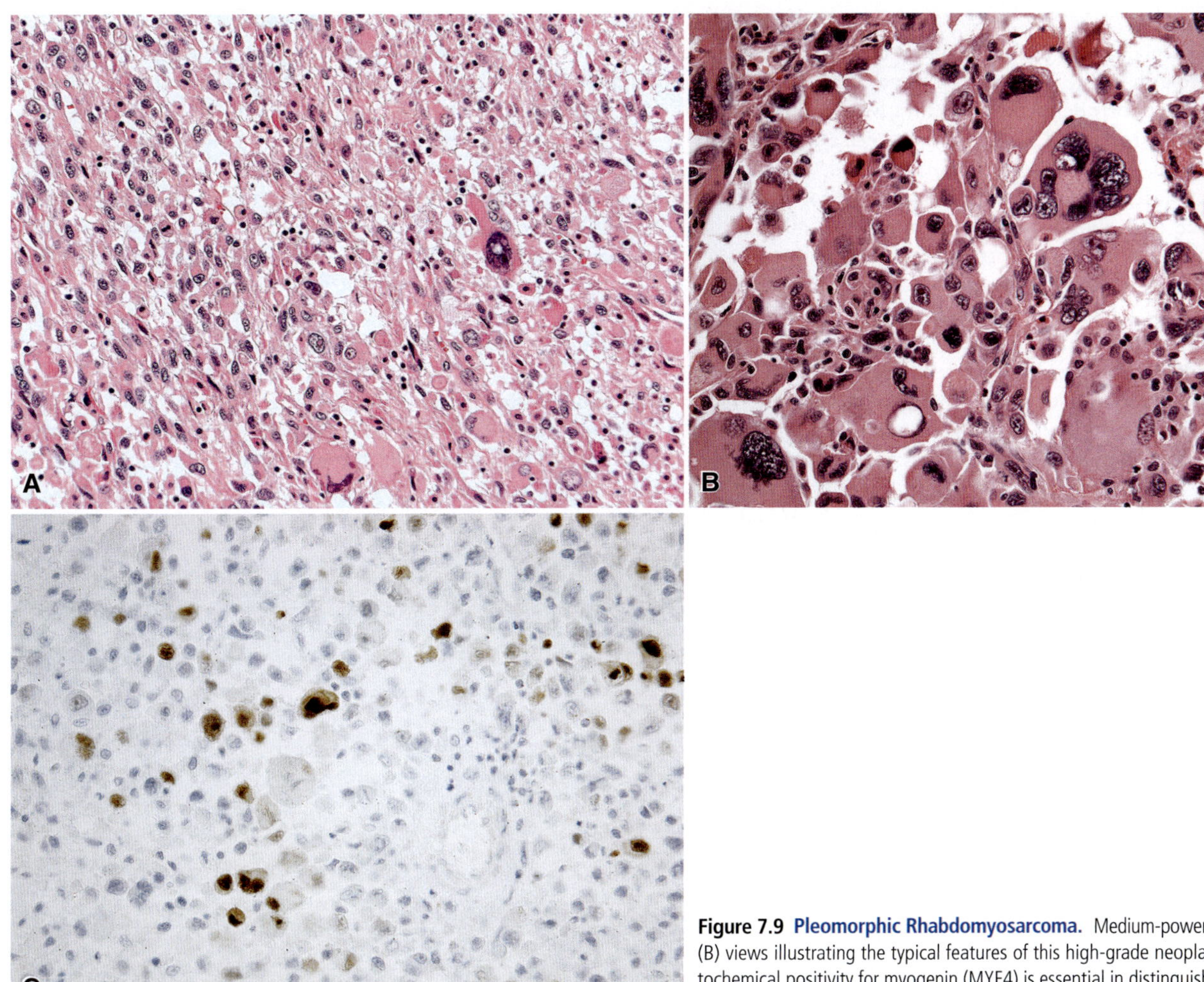

Figure 7.9 Pleomorphic Rhabdomyosarcoma. Medium-power (**A**) and high-power (B) views illustrating the typical features of this high-grade neoplasm. (C) Immunohistochemical positivity for myogenin (MYF4) is essential in distinguishing this tumor from pleomorphic leiomyosarcoma.

Prognosis and Treatment

Wide surgical excision with free margins and adjuvant radiotherapy is the primary therapeutic modality of choice. Pleomorphic leiomyosarcoma and pleomorphic rhabdomyosarcoma are extremely aggressive high-grade sarcomas, with a 5-year metastatic rate of more than 60% for leiomyosarcoma and more than 80% for rhabdomyosarcoma, which are significantly worse than for other pleomorphic sarcomas. Both lesions also have inferior relapse-free survival rates.[1,2,30]

PRACTICE POINTS: Pleomorphic Myogenic Sarcomas

- Nuclear immunohistochemical positivity for myogenin (MYF4) or MYOD1 is critical for confirming rhabdomyoblastic differentiation; smooth muscle actin and desmin do not discriminate between pleomorphic leiomyosarcoma and rhabdomyosarcoma.
- Identification of a myoid phenotype is of prognostic value: pleomorphic myogenic sarcomas have a significantly increased risk of metastasis and an inferior relapse-free survival rate compared with other pleomorphic sarcomas.

Pleomorphic Lipogenic Sarcomas

Within the group of liposarcomas, pleomorphic liposarcoma and DDLPS may both be characterized by areas of marked cellular pleomorphism, creating problems in the differential diagnosis with other pleomorphic sarcomas. These tumor types are also discussed in Chapter 12.

Pleomorphic Liposarcoma

Pleomorphic liposarcoma is defined as a pleomorphic, high-grade sarcoma containing a variable number of intralesional pleomorphic lipoblasts, without areas of ALT/WDLPS or other lines of differentiation. Pleomorphic liposarcoma is the rarest subtype of liposarcoma, accounting for roughly 5% of all liposarcomas.[1,91–99]

Clinical Features

Pleomorphic liposarcoma is essentially a tumor of adults older than 50 years of age. Although it has been described at a wide variety of sites, it shows a marked predilection for the deep soft tissues of the extremities and less frequently involves the retroperitoneum. Patients most often present with an enlarging mass frequently associated with mild discomfort or pain.[91–99]

Pathologic Features

Grossly, tumors are usually firm and, depending on the adipocytic content, yellowish to gray-white in color. The tumors are either well circumscribed or more poorly defined with infiltrative margins, often have areas of visible necrosis, and are usually between 5 and 10 cm in diameter. Histologically, the defining feature is the identification of unequivocal lipoblasts. Classical multivacuolated lipoblasts are easiest to recognize and consist of two or more optically clear cytoplasmic vacuoles that indent a centrally or eccentrically placed hyperchromatic nucleus, resulting in the typical scalloped appearance of these nuclei (Fig. 7.10). Other variants of lipoblasts include giant cells with or without multinucleation, numerous cytoplasmic vacuoles of varying size and bizarre hyperchromatic scalloped nuclei, and small univacuolated lipoblasts that resemble signet-ring cells. A frequent but nonspecific finding is the presence of cytoplasmic eosinophilic hyaline droplets that are presumed to be of lysosomal origin. Tumors are highly cellular and are composed of lipoblasts in a background of high-grade pleomorphic sarcoma. Although a number of histologic patterns have been described (pleomorphic-type, myxofibrosarcoma-like, epithelioid-type, round cell–type), lipoblasts remain the key feature for the diagnosis. The presence of lipoblasts is highly variable and may be ubiquitous, either as individual cells or in sheets, or may be extremely scarce, requiring extensive sampling of the tumor for their identification and hence a correct diagnosis.[91–99]

Ultrastructurally, lipoblasts recapitulate features as seen in the various stages of normal lipogenesis. The predominant and defining feature is the presence (in the cytoplasm) of numerous dense, non-membrane-bound lipid droplets of varying sizes with scalloping of the adjacent nucleus. In addition, the cells have incomplete external laminae, abundant mitochondria, and deposits of glycogen.[34,100] However, electron microscopy does not play a role in the diagnosis of pleomorphic liposarcoma, which is entirely morphologic.

Immunohistochemistry

Immunohistochemical stains are generally not helpful. S-100 protein staining, although positive in normal adipocytes, stains lipoblasts in less than 20% of cases.

Molecular Genetics

Cytogenetically, karyotypes are complex and are of no diagnostic or prognostic value (see Table 7.4).[42,101]

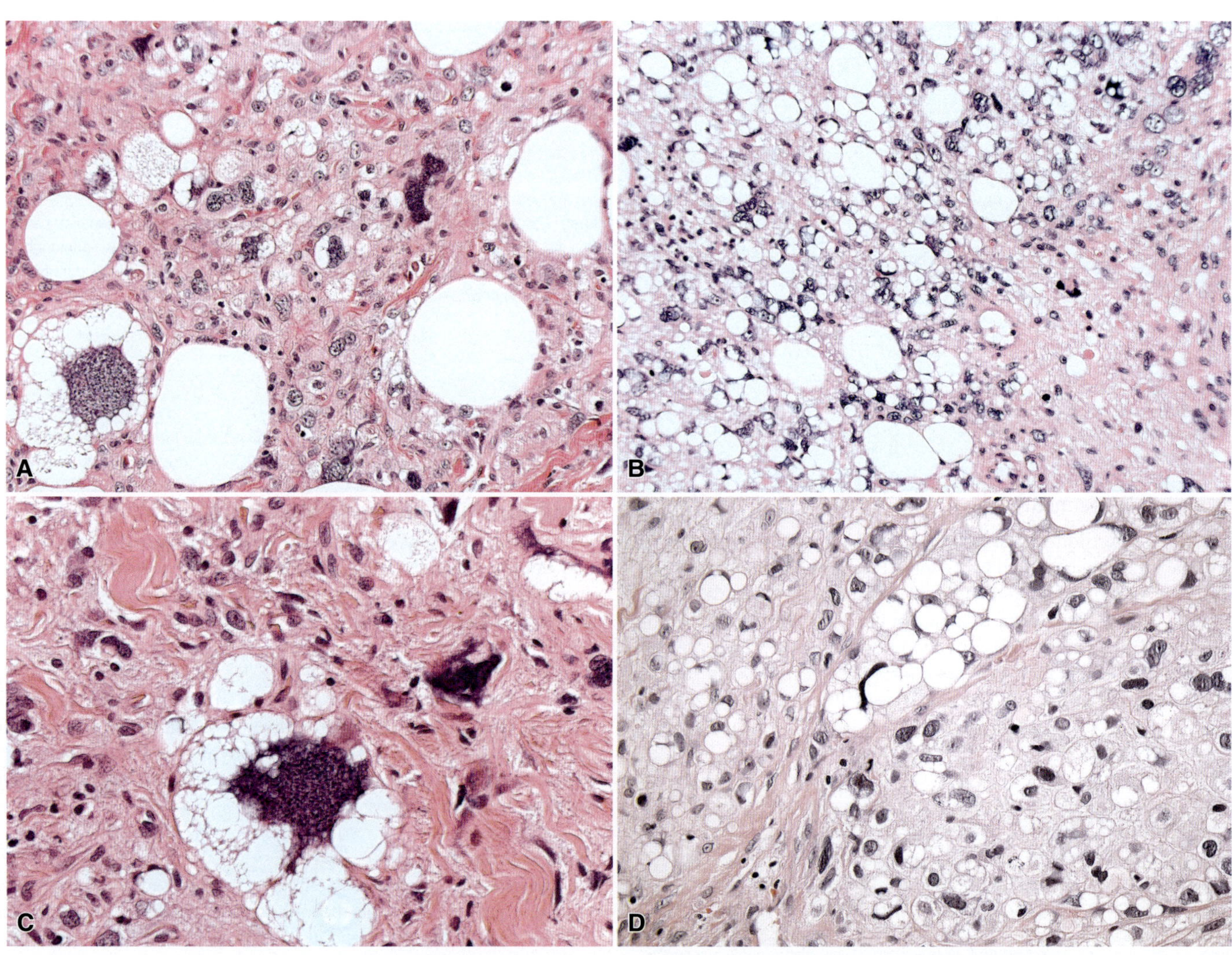

Figure 7.10 Pleomorphic Liposarcoma. Medium-power (A and B) and high-power (C and D) views illustrating the typical features of pleomorphic liposarcoma. Note the typical lipoblasts essential for making the correct diagnosis. (D) The epithelioid variant may be mistaken for metastatic clear cell carcinoma.

Differential Diagnosis

The differential diagnosis is essentially with pleomorphic nonmesenchymal tumors (poorly differentiated carcinoma, melanoma, anaplastic large-cell lymphoma) and other high-grade pleomorphic sarcomas as described earlier (see "Undifferentiated Pleomorphic Sarcoma"). Importantly, the rare epithelioid variant of pleomorphic liposarcoma may be confused with a primary or metastatic carcinoma, in particular adrenal cortical carcinoma and renal cell carcinoma, or melanoma. In all cases, the identification of lipoblasts is essential for making the correct diagnosis.

Prognosis and Treatment

Wide surgical excision with free margins and adjuvant radiotherapy is the primary therapeutic modality of choice. Pleomorphic liposarcoma is an aggressive high-grade neoplasm with a 5-year metastatic rate of around 50%, and most patients die in a short period of time; in a study from the 1960s, the 5-year survival rate was 21%.[1,2,30,93,94]

Dedifferentiated Liposarcoma

DDLPS, described in more detail in Chapter 12, is defined as a malignant adipocytic neoplasm showing transition from a well-differentiated lipomatous neoplasm (ALT/WDLPS) to a nonlipogenic sarcoma of either low or high histologic grade; DDLPS accounts for approximately 10% to 15% of all liposarcomas.[1]

Clinical Features

DDLPS arises principally in older adults, with a male predominance; the male-to-female ratio is roughly 3 : 1. The majority of tumors arise in the retroperitoneum, followed distantly by the deep soft tissues of the extremities. Fewer than 20% of tumors arise outside these two anatomic locations, with fewer than 1% occurring in the subcutaneous tissues. Approximately 90% of cases of DDLPS arise de novo, whereas only 10% arise in recurrences of previously excised ALT/WDLPS.

Clinical presentation is usually as an asymptomatic swelling or mass associated with mild discomfort. Retroperitoneal tumors are frequently discovered by chance as a consequence of imaging procedures for unrelated clinical complaints. In the limbs, the presence of a long-standing swelling that has recently begun to increase in size should be regarded with suspicion, because this frequently represents dedifferentiation in an ALT.[39,102–108]

PRACTICE POINTS: Pleomorphic Liposarcoma

- The identification of unequivocal lipoblasts within a pleomorphic sarcoma is essential for diagnosing pleomorphic liposarcoma.
- S-100 protein stains lipoblasts in fewer than 20% of cases of pleomorphic liposarcoma and is therefore not a particularly helpful diagnostic tool.

Pathologic Features

Tumors may reach a very large size (>20 cm), especially in the retroperitoneum, and may either be well or poorly circumscribed. Grossly, tumors are typically soft and yellowish-white in color (representing the well-differentiated component) with reasonably well-circumscribed nodular areas of firm grayish-white tissue representing foci of dedifferentiation. During surgery, the dedifferentiated tumor mass is generally easy to identify, whereas the well-differentiated fatty component, resembling normal adipose tissue, is not always recognized as being part of the neoplasm and may be left behind. Furthermore, the circumferential boundaries of the tumor, particularly the well-differentiated component, may be difficult to identify, complicating efforts at complete surgical removal of the tumor. This is not only a problem for the unfortunate surgeon; it is imperative for the pathologist to conscientiously sample all areas of adjacent fibro-fatty tissue to avoid missing a possible well-differentiated component.

Histologically, tumors consist of areas of ALT/WDLPS with an abrupt transition to nonlipogenic pleomorphic sarcoma, morphologically usually high-grade. Occasionally, the transition is less abrupt with comingling of the lipogenic and nonlipogenic areas; it has been proposed that a component of dedifferentiation be macroscopically visible (>1 cm) for a diagnosis of DDLPS, whereas smaller foci of dedifferentiation may be diagnosed as "incipient dedifferentiation."[1] The high-grade nonlipogenic component is composed of a cellular proliferation of pleomorphic and spindle-shaped cells very similar to undifferentiated pleomorphic sarcoma (Fig. 7.11) and usually shows no evidence of specific lines of differentiation; heterologous leiomyosarcomatous, rhabdomyosarcomatous, or osteo/chondrosarcomatous foci may be present in roughly 5% to 10% of cases. Occasional tumors also show "homologous" lipoblastic differentiation in the dedifferentiated component, mimicking pleomorphic liposarcoma.[109] Dedifferentiation may also be morphologically low-grade and characterized by a cellular proliferation of spindle-shaped cells with a variably fascicular architecture and mild cytologic atypia. An additional infrequent but morphologically distinctive pattern is the presence of nodules and whorls of spindle-shaped cells with a neural or meningioma-like appearance. Rarely, the dedifferentiated component has a prominent (mixed) inflammatory infiltrate, which probably accounts for the majority of tumors classified in the past as *inflammatory MFH*.[39] Ultrastructural analysis is generally not helpful for diagnostic purposes.

Immunohistochemistry

The majority (>90%) of ALT/WDLPS and DDLPS are characterized by immunohistochemically detectable overexpression of the MDM2 (see Fig. 7.11D) and CDK4 gene products (see later discussion), which may be diagnostically helpful in the analysis of small biopsies.[110] However, once areas of atypical adipocytic tissue have been identified in association with a nonlipogenic neoplasm, immunohistochemistry plays only a minor role in the diagnostic process and is primarily useful for identifying foci of heterologous differentiation.[39,110]

Molecular Genetics

Cytogenetically, in contrast to other nonlipogenic (high-grade) sarcomas, karyotypes of the nonlipogenic component are relatively simple and resemble the genetic background seen in ALT/WDLPS (see Table 7.4). The predominant karyotypic features are the presence of ring and giant marker chromosomes, typical of ALT/WDLPS, with some additional, and more complex, abnormalities. The ring and giant marker chromosomes arise from amplification of 12q13–15 and contain multiple copies of *MDM2, CDK4*, and *HMGA2*, among other genes.[42,101] It has been speculated that the additional presence of the more complex alterations in DDLPS is responsible (in part) for the process of dedifferentiation.[42,101,111] Interestingly, in a study of 14 cases of DDLPS, mutations in *TP53*, present in the majority of high-grade pleomorphic sarcomas, were found in only one of the 14 tumors studied. It is possible that the relatively simple karyotypic aberrations and the presence of wild-type *TP53* may play a role in the less aggressive clinical course of DDLPS, as compared with other pleomorphic sarcomas (see subsequent discussion).[112]

Differential Diagnosis

Once the combination of an ALT/WDLPS and a nonlipogenic tumor has been identified, there are no realistic differential diagnostic options. When confronted with a problematic unclassifiable pleomorphic neoplasm without a fatty component (small biopsy specimen or larger

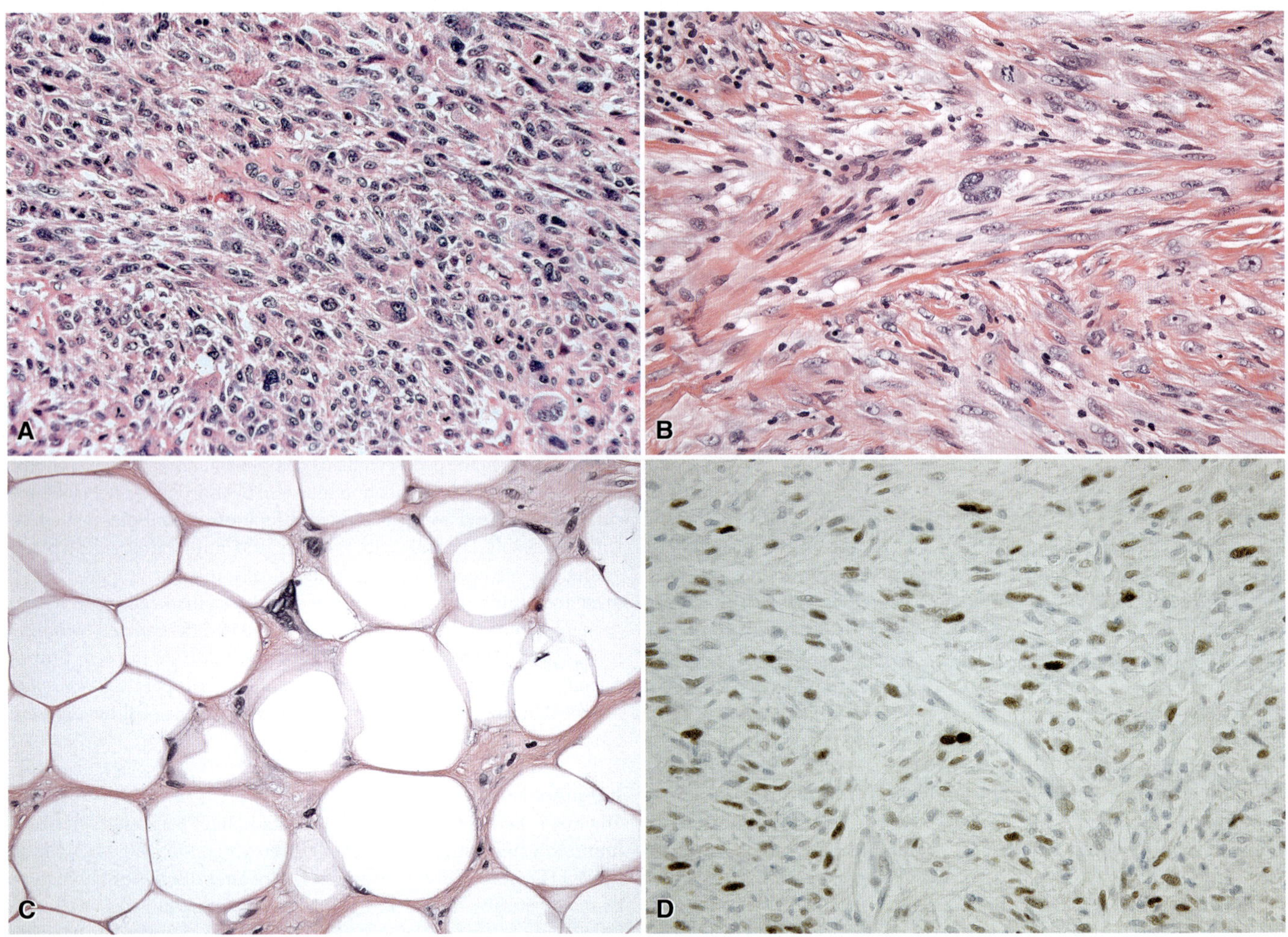

Figure 7.11 Dedifferentiated Liposarcoma. Medium-power (A) and high-power (B) views of dedifferentiated liposarcoma, indistinguishable from undifferentiated pleomorphic sarcoma unless the adjacent well-differentiated liposarcomatous component is identified (C). (D) Diffuse immunohistochemical reactivity for MDM2 is present in nearly all cases.

surgical specimen in which a fatty component is absent), in which DDLPS is a differential diagnostic possibility, immunohistochemical positivity for MDM2 and CDK4, demonstrable amplification of the chromosomal region 12q13–15 (by fluorescence in situ hybridization for *MDM2*), or cytogenetic identification of ring or giant marker chromosomes are useful in facilitating the correct diagnosis.

Prognosis and Treatment

Wide surgical excision with free margins and adjuvant radiotherapy is the primary therapeutic modality of choice. Prognostically, anatomic location has a strong influence on the clinical course. Tumors in an extraperitoneal location are characterized by a local recurrence rate of about 40% and a better clinical outcome compared with retroperitoneal tumors, which, probably because of the more limited surgical possibilities for radical excision at this site, almost always recur if patients are followed long enough; interestingly, DDLPS may recur as pure ALT/WDLPS and vice versa.[44,108] DDLPS is associated with a 5-year metastatic rate of only 15% to 20% and is significantly better than that for other pleomorphic high-grade sarcomas; overall mortality at 5-year follow-up appears to be about 30%.[2,44] Recent studies have suggested that histologic grade and the presence of a heterologous rhabdomyosarcomatous component may influence 5-year survival; further research in this area is needed to confirm these findings.[2,44,113–115]

PRACTICE POINTS: Dedifferentiated Liposarcoma

- Dedifferentiated liposarcoma (DDLPS) may be a morphologically low-grade or high-grade lesion.
- Nuclear immunohistochemical staining for MDM2 and CDK4 and amplification of *MDM2* by FISH are helpful to confirm the diagnosis of DDLPS, particularly in small biopsies.
- Recent studies suggest that histologic grade may influence prognosis.
- DDLPS has a significantly better 5-year metastatic rate and 5-year survival rate compared with other pleomorphic sarcomas.

Extraskeletal Osteosarcoma

Extraskeletal osteosarcoma, discussed in more detail in Chapter 14, is defined as a malignant mesenchymal tumor of soft tissue, not associated with underlying skeletal structures, containing neoplastic osteoid produced by a population of malignant cells recapitulating osteoblasts. A proportion of tumors also contain chondroblastic and/or fibroblastic lines of differentiation, similar to their skeletal counterparts.[1] By definition, no other lines of differentiation are present. Extraskeletal osteosarcoma accounts for approximately 5% of all osteosarcomas and 1% to 2% of all soft tissue sarcomas.[1,37,116–118]

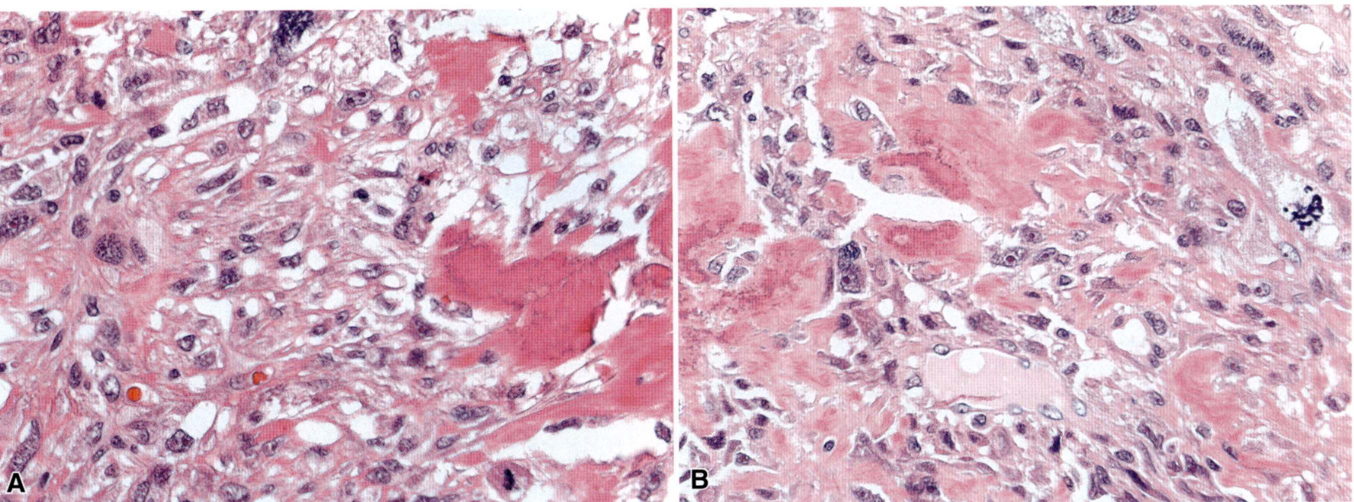

Figure 7.12 Extraskeletal Osteosarcoma. High-power views (A and B) of this neoplasm, indistinguishable from undifferentiated pleomorphic sarcoma unless the "malignant" osteoid is identified.

Clinical Features

In contrast to conventional (skeletal) osteosarcoma, which is primarily a tumor of children and adolescents, extraskeletal osteosarcoma arises in older adults, occurring more frequently in males than females (ratio, roughly 1.5–2 : 1). About half of extraskeletal osteosarcomas occur in the thigh; the shoulder and pelvic girdle, trunk, and retroperitoneum are also frequently involved. At least 90% of tumors arise in the deep soft tissues. In approximately 10% of cases, there is a previous history of trauma to or irradiation of the involved site. Clinical presentation is most commonly as a swelling that may or may not be painful. Imaging studies demonstrate a mass with variable mineralization.[1,37,116–121]

Pathologic Features

Grossly, tumors are usually well circumscribed, 5 to 10 cm in diameter, and grayish-tan in color, with visible areas of necrosis and hemorrhage and a gritty surface on sectioning. Histologically, in addition to a number of nonpleomorphic variants (osteoblastic, chondroblastic, fibroblastic, small cell, and telangiectatic), a highly pleomorphic (previously known as *MFH-like*) subtype is also recognized. The common denominator of all subtypes is the presence of osteoid produced by the neoplastic cells and deposited in a delicate lace-like or trabecular pattern (Fig. 7.12). In contrast to myositis ossificans, in which the cellular nonosseous zone is centrally situated and shows gradual transition to a less cellular peripheral zone with metaplastic bone formation, osteoid in extraskeletal osteosarcoma is most abundant in the less cellular central part of the tumor, with cellularity increasing, and osteoid production decreasing, in a centripetal fashion. The matrix-producing cells show variable cytologic atypia, are mitotically active, and may be spindle-shaped (in the fibroblastic variant), epithelioid (in the osteoblastic and chondroblastic variants), resemble tumor cells of Ewing sarcoma or non-Hodgkin lymphoma (in the small cell variant), or be highly pleomorphic (in the pleomorphic variant). The telangiectatic variant is a morphologically distinctive pleomorphic and spindle-cell neoplasm characterized by numerous pseudovascular blood-filled cavities.[1,120,121]

Ultrastructurally, the neoplastic cells essentially demonstrate fibroblastic features (prominent rough endoplasmic reticulum, well-developed Golgi apparatus, abundant extracellular collagen), but osteoid and early bone formation can be seen with the deposition of hydroxyapatite crystals and/or foci of intracytoplasmic calcification.[1,34] However, electron microscopy has little clinical diagnostic value for this tumor type.

Immunohistochemistry

The recognition of osteoid formation by the neoplastic cells defines extraskeletal osteosarcoma, and, consequently, immunohistochemistry is generally unnecessary. It is important to realize that the neoplastic component may express smooth muscle actin, desmin, epithelial membrane antigen, and keratin in a proportion of cases, occasionally complicating accurate classification when osteoid is not readily apparent.[1,116–121]

Recently SATB2, a nuclear protein that plays an important role in osteoblast lineage commitment, has been shown to be very useful in identifying osteoblastic differentiation in benign and malignant mesenchymal tumors. Although clearly not a specific marker for (extraskeletal) osteosarcoma, it may be helpful in distinguishing between sclerotic/hyalinized collagen and osteoid when the differential diagnosis with an (extraskeletal) osteosarcoma is being considered.[122]

Immunohistochemical detection of CDK4 and MDM2, typically seen in ALT/DDLPS (resulting from amplification of 12q13–15, which harbors, among others, the *MDM2* and *CDK4* genes), has also been described in a subgroup of extraskeletal osteosarcomas, potentially complicating the accurate distinction from metastatic DDLPS with heterologous osteosarcomatous differentiation.[123,124]

Molecular Genetics

Cytogenetically, karyotypes are uniformly complex and uninformative (see Table 7.4).[42]

Differential Diagnosis

Once malignant osteoid is identified, there are no realistic differential diagnostic considerations, except, particularly for tumors arising in the retroperitoneum, to exclude DDLPS with heterologous osteosarcomatous differentiation, which requires adequate sampling to exclude a well-differentiated adipocytic component. Because a subgroup of extraskeletal osteosarcomas share immunohistochemical expression of CDK4 and MDM2, distinction from metastatic DDLPS (with heterologous osteosarcomatous differentiation) may be extremely difficult, requiring careful clinical correlation to exclude a primary lesion elsewhere.[123,124] The rare variant of MPNST exhibiting heterologous osteosarcomatous differentiation may also result in diagnostic confusion, but a clinical history of type 1 neurofibromatosis and/or variable immunohistochemical positivity for S-100 protein, glial fibrillary acidic protein, or SOX10 should facilitate the correct diagnosis. Needless to say, in all cases of extraskeletal osteosarcoma, a skeletal origin needs to be excluded with adequate radiologic imaging.

Prognosis and Treatment

Neoadjuvant chemotherapy and wide surgical excision with free margins are the primary therapeutic modalities of choice. Prognostically, extraskeletal osteosarcoma is a highly aggressive tumor, with a 5-year survival rate of 15% to 25%.[1,123,124] Although the intensive chemotherapeutic regimens used for treating its skeletal counterpart also appear to be effective for extraskeletal osteosarcoma, such protocols are usually less well tolerated by the older patient group, hence reducing their therapeutic impact.[1,123–126]

PRACTICE POINT: Extraskeletal Osteosarcoma

The identification of malignant osteoid within a pleomorphic sarcoma is required for the diagnosis of extraskeletal osteosarcoma.

Nuclear immunohistochemical staining for SATB2 is helpful to distinguish extraskeletal osteosarcoma from other sarcomas with prominent hyalinized stromal collagen.

Malignant Mesenchymoma

Malignant mesenchymoma is an extremely rare and contentious entity defined as a malignant mesenchymal neoplasm demonstrating two or more distinct lines of sarcomatous differentiation.[1,127,128] Excluded from this definition are DDLPS (which may show heterologous elements); MPNST with a heterologous rhabdomyosarcomatous (malignant triton tumor), chondrosarcomatous, or osteosarcomatous component; and specific sarcomas with an undifferentiated pleomorphic (MFH-like) or hemangiopericytoma-like component. One particular (very rare) entity meeting the requirements of this definition is leiomyosarcoma, demonstrating osteosarcomatous or rhabdomyosarcomatous foci. Experience with these tumors to date indicates that malignant mesenchymoma is best regarded and treated as an aggressive sarcoma.[1,127,128]

Algorithmic Approach When Confronted With a Pleomorphic Sarcomatoid Neoplasm

The following approach should be taken:

1. Determine whether the tumor is cutaneous or more deeply situated (subcutaneous and deep soft tissue).
2. If the lesion is cutaneous:
   - Accurate clinical correlation is required to exclude the possibility of a primary malignancy elsewhere with cutaneous metastasis.
   - Sarcomatoid carcinoma, melanoma, and atypical intradermal smooth muscle neoplasm/leiomyosarcoma should be excluded with an appropriate immunohistochemical panel (pan-keratins, S-100 protein, HMB45, melan A, smooth muscle actin, desmin).
   - Important question: Are the histologic features compatible with AFX?
   - If not compatible with AFX, spindle cell and/or pleomorphic dermal sarcoma not otherwise specified is a possibility if an identifiable line of differentiation cannot be established.
3. If the lesion is more deeply situated, exclude metastatic disease (pleomorphic/anaplastic carcinoma and melanoma) and anaplastic large-cell lymphoma. This requires careful clinical correlation, together with the use of an appropriate immunohistochemical panel (see Table 7.1).
4. When the mesenchymal nature of the lesion has been established:
   - Benign mimics of sarcoma must be excluded (see Box 7.1).
   - Important question: Are there histologic features of a specific entity: PHAT, MIFS, myxofibrosarcoma?
   - Areas of atypical fat adjacent to the pleomorphic sarcomatous tissue: DDLPS
   - Unequivocal lipoblasts within the pleomorphic sarcomatous tissue: pleomorphic liposarcoma
   - Malignant osteoid: extraskeletal osteosarcoma
   - Evidence of myogenic differentiation: pleomorphic leiomyosarcoma or pleomorphic rhabdomyosarcoma (myogenin or MYOD1 diagnostic of rhabdomyosarcoma)
   - No identifiable line(s) of differentiation: undifferentiated pleomorphic sarcoma

Grading of Pleomorphic Sarcomas

Although a more extensive discussion concerning the grading of soft tissue sarcomas is provided in Chapter 2, some additional detail with respect to pleomorphic sarcomas in particular is warranted. As for sarcomas as a whole, sarcomas with a pleomorphic phenotype also represent a heterogeneous group of neoplasms with a broad spectrum of biologic behavior. At one end of the spectrum are indolent tumors with an excellent prognosis characterized primarily by local recurrence with little risk of metastasizing, whereas the other end of the spectrum is characterized by highly aggressive lesions with a poor prognosis and a high mortality rate.

Ideally, the clinicopathologic study of sarcomas with the identification of parameters predictive of tumor grade, and hence biologic behavior, should aim to be histotype-specific (as has recently been recognized for gastrointestinal stromal tumors). However, because of the relative rarity of sarcomas, studying and comparing large groups of specific tumor types remain problematic, and consequently the histologic parameters that form the mainstay of the available grading schemes have been based on studies of histologically diverse lesions. Of the various grading schemes in use, the three-tiered grading systems of the American National Cancer Institute (NCI grading system) and the French Federation of Cancer Centers Sarcoma Group (FNCLCC grading system) remain the most popular, although the French system would appear to be somewhat more reproducible for pathologists.[129–133] Nevertheless, the grading of pleomorphic sarcomas presents certain difficulties: while those sarcomas with an aggressive clinical course (pleomorphic myogenic and lipogenic sarcomas) are invariably high-grade on the basis of grading parameters, other pleomorphic mesenchymal neoplasms (e.g., PHAT and MIFS), which are essentially indolent tumors, are designated as intermediate grade (grade 2) tumors using conventional grading parameters. However, as our experience with these low-grade tumors increases, it may be that metastases occur much later in their clinical course, validating their grade 2 status. Recent developments in genomic and expression profiling would appear to offer promising improvements in attempts at grading specific sarcoma types.[134]

The Role of Imaging Studies in the Diagnosis of Pleomorphic Sarcomas

The diagnosis and management of patients with soft tissue tumors is critically dependent on a multidisciplinary approach, including accurate pre- and postoperative radiologic evaluation.[135] Radiologic assessment is essential for confirming a primary soft tissue origin. Although conventional radiography and computed tomography are historically deeply ingrained in the primary assessment of any bone tumor, magnetic resonance imaging (MRI), particularly dynamic contrast-enhanced MRI, is the preferred procedure for identifying and characterizing soft tissue lesions. This modality provides accurate information concerning the site and size of the tumor and is the most sensitive technique for defining tumor margins and relationships to adjacent anatomic structures. Early and rapid enhancement of the tumor on dynamic MRI studies favors sarcoma, and the identification of necrosis is indicative of an aggressive neoplasm, but the procedure is not particularly helpful for further delineation of possible tumor types. Nevertheless, MRI is an essential component of the diagnostic workup, providing important information for planning biopsy procedures and definitive surgery. In addition, it is the mainstay of postoperative patient follow-up for the identification of local recurrence and/or metastatic disease.[135]

References

1. Fletcher CDM, Bridge JA, Hogendoorn PCW, et al, editors: *WHO classification of tumours of soft tissue and bone*, Lyon, France, 2013, IARC Press.
2. Dei Tos AP: The classification of pleomorphic sarcomas: where are we now?, *Histopathology* 48:51–62, 2006.
3. Fretzin D, Helwig EB: Atypical fibroxanthoma of the skin. A clinicopathological study of 140 cases, *Cancer* 39:1541–1552, 1973.
4. Calonje E, Wadden C, Wilson-Jones E, et al: Spindle cell non-pleomorphic atypical fibroxanthoma: analysis of a series and delineation of a distinctive variant, *Histopathology* 22:247–254, 1993.
5. de Feraudy S, Mar N, McCalmont TH: Evaluation of CD10 and procollagen 1 expression in atypical fibroxanthoma and dermatofibroma, *Am J Surg Pathol* 32:1111–1122, 2008.
6. Dei Tos AP, Maestro R, Doglioni C, et al: Ultraviolet-induced p53 mutations in atypical fibroxanthoma, *Am J Pathol* 145:11–17, 1994.
7. Barr RJ, Wuerker RB, Graham JH: Ultrastructure of atypical fibroxanthoma, *Cancer* 40:736–743, 1977.
8. Beer TW, Drury P, Heenan PJ: Atypical fibroxanthoma: a histological and immunohistochemical review of 171 cases, *Am J Dermatopathol* 32:533–540, 2010.
9. Miller K, Goodlad JR, Brenn T: Pleomorphic dermal sarcoma: adverse histologic features predict aggressive behavior and allow distinction from atypical fibroxanthoma, *Am J Surg Pathol* 36:1317–1326, 2012.
10. Requena L, Sangueza OP, Sanchez Yus E, et al: Clear cell atypical fibroxanthoma: an uncommon histopathologic variant of atypical fibroxanthoma, *J Cutan Pathol* 24:176–182, 1997.
11. Rudisaile SN, Hurt MA, Santa Cruz DJ: Granular cell atypical fibroxanthoma, *J Cutan Pathol* 32:314–317, 2005.
12. Griewank KG, Schilling B, Murali R, et al: TERT promoter mutations are frequent in atypical fibroxanthomas and pleomorphic dermal sarcomas, *Mod Pathol* 27:502–508, 2014.
13. Jacobs DS, Edwards WD, Ye RC: Metastatic atypical fibroxanthoma of the skin, *Cancer* 35:457–463, 1975.
14. Helwig EB, May D: Atypical fibroxanthomas of the skin with metastases, *Cancer* 57:368–376, 1986.
15. Glavin FL, Cornwell ML: Atypical fibroxanthoma of the skin metastatic to lung. Report of a case, features by conventional and electron microscopy, and a review of the relevant literature, *Am J Dermatopathol* 7:57–63, 1985.
16. Wang WL, Torres-Cabala C, Curry JL, et al: Metastatic atypical fibroxanthoma: a series of 11 cases including with minimal and no subcutaneous involvement, *Am J Dermatopathol* 37:455–461, 2015.
17. Ozzello L, Stout AP, Murray MR: Culture characteristics of malignant histiocytomas and fibrous xanthomas, *Cancer* 16:331–344, 1963.
18. O'Brien JE, Stout AP: Malignant fibrous xanthomas, *Cancer* 17:1445–1455, 1964.
19. Kempson RL, Kyriakos M: Fibroxanthosarcoma of the soft tissues. A type of malignant fibrous histiocytoma, *Cancer* 29:961–976, 1972.
20. Weiss SW, Enzinger FM: Malignant fibrous histiocytoma. An analysis of 200 cases, *Cancer* 41:2250–2266, 1978.
21. Weiss SW: Malignant fibrous histiocytoma: a reaffirmation, *Am J Surg Pathol* 6:773–784, 1982.
22. Kearney MM, Soule EH, Ivins JC: Malignant fibrous histiocytoma. A retrospective study of 167 cases, *Cancer* 45:167–178, 1980.
23. Guccion JG, Enzinger FM: Malignant giant cell tumor of soft parts. An analysis of 32 cases, *Cancer* 29:1518–1529, 1972.
24. Kyriakos M, Kempson RL: Inflammatory fibrous histiocytoma. An aggressive and lethal lesion, *Cancer* 37:1584–1606, 1976.
25. Khalidi HS, Singleton TP, Weiss SW: Inflammatory malignant fibrous histiocytoma: a distinction from Hodgkin's disease and non-Hodgkin's lymphoma by a panel of leukocyte markers, *Mod Pathol* 10:438–442, 1997.
26. Angervall L, Kindblom L-G, Merck C: Myxofibrosarcoma. A study of 30 cases, *Acta Pathol Microbiol Scand [A]* 85:127–140, 1977.
27. Weiss SW, Enzinger FM: Myxoid variant of malignant fibrous histiocytoma, *Cancer* 39:1672–1685, 1977.
28. Enzinger FM: Angiomatoid malignant fibrous histiocytoma. A distinct fibrohistiocytic tumor of children and young adults simulating a vascular neoplasm, *Cancer* 44:2147–2157, 1979.
29. Fletcher CD: Pleomorphic malignant fibrous histiocytoma: fact or fiction? A critical reappraisal of 159 tumors diagnosed as pleomorphic sarcomas, *Am J Surg Pathol* 16:213–228, 1992.
30. Fletcher CD, Gustafson P, Rydholm A, et al: Clinicopathologic re-evaluation of 100 malignant fibrous histiocytomas: prognostic relevance of subclassification, *J Clin Oncol* 19:3045–3050, 2001.
31. Akerman M: Malignant fibrous histiocytoma—the commonest soft tissue sarcoma or a nonexistent entity?, *Acta Orthop Scand* 68(Suppl 273):41–46, 1997.
32. Hollowood K, Fletcher CD: Malignant fibrous histiocytoma: morphologic pattern or pathologic entity, *Semin Diagn Pathol* 12:210–220, 1995.
33. Erlandson RA, Antonescu CR: The rise and fall of malignant fibrous histiocytoma, *Ultrastruct Pathol* 28:283–289, 2004.
34. Kindblom LG, Widéhn S, Meis-Kindblom JM: The role of electron microscopy in the diagnosis of pleomorphic sarcomas of soft tissue, *Semin Diagn Pathol* 20:72–81, 2003.
35. Hornick JL, Jaffe ES, Fletcher CD: Extranodal histiocytic sarcoma: clinicopathologic analysis of 14 cases of a rare epithelioid malignancy, *Am J Surg Pathol* 28:1133–1144, 2004.
36. Folpe AL, Morris RJ, Weiss SW: Soft tissue giant cell tumor of low malignant potential: a proposal for the reclassification of malignant giant cell tumor of soft parts, *Mod Pathol* 12:894–902, 1999.
37. Lee JS, Fetsch JF, Wasdahl DA, et al: A review of 40 patients with extraskeletal osteosarcoma, *Cancer* 76:2253–2259, 1995.
38. Mentzel T, Calonje E, Fletcher CDM: Leiomyosarcoma with prominent osteoclast-like giant cells: analysis of eight cases closely mimicking the so-called giant cell variant of 'MFH, *Am J Surg Pathol* 18:258–265, 1994.
39. Coindre JM, Hostein I, Maire G, et al: Inflammatory fibrous histiocytoma and dedifferentiated liposarcoma: histological review, genomic profile, and MDM2 and CDK4 status favour a single entity, *J Pathol* 203:822–830, 2004.
40. Coffin CM, Hornick JL, Fletcher CD: Inflammatory myofibroblastic tumor: comparison of clinicopathologic, histologic, and immunohistochemical features including ALK expression in atypical and aggressive cases, *Am J Surg Pathol* 31:509–520, 2007.
41. Mentzel T, Calonje E, Wadden C, et al: Myxofibrosarcoma. Clinicopathologic analysis of 75 cases with emphasis on the low-grade variant, *Am J Surg Pathol* 20:391–405, 1996.
42. Mertens F, Fletcher CD, Dal Cin P, et al: Cytogenetic analysis of 46 pleomorphic sarcomas and correlation with morphologic and clinical features: a report of the CHAMP Study Group. Chromosomes and MorPhology, *Genes Chromosomes Cancer* 22:16–25, 1998.
43. Gustafson P: Soft tissue sarcoma. Epidemiology and prognosis in 508 patients, *Acta Orthop Scand* 65(Suppl 259):1–31, 1994.
44. McCormick D, Mentzel T, Beham A, et al: Dedifferentiated liposarcoma: a clinicopathologic analysis of 32 cases suggesting a better prognostic subgroup among pleomorphic sarcomas, *Am J Surg Pathol* 18:1213–1223, 1994.
45. Miyajima K, Oda Y, Tamiya S, et al: Clinicopathological prognostic factors in soft tissue leiomyosarcoma: a multivariate analysis, *Histopathology* 40:353–359, 2002.
46. Schürch W, Bégin LR, Seemayer TA, et al: Pleomorphic soft tissue myogenic sarcomas of adulthood. A reappraisal in the mid-1990s, *Am J Surg Pathol* 20:131–147, 1996.
47. Deyrup AT, Haydon RC, Huo D, et al: Myoid differentiation and prognosis in adult pleomorphic sarcomas of the extremety: an analysis of 92 cases, *Cancer* 98:805–813, 2003.
48. Massi D, Beltrami G, Capanna R, et al: Histopathological reclassification of extremity pleomorphic soft tissue sarcoma has clinical relevance, *Eur J Surg Oncol* 30:1131–1136, 2004.
49. Smith MEF, Fisher C, Weiss SW: Pleomorphic hyalinizing angiectatic tumor of soft parts. A low grade neoplasm resembling neurilemmoma, *Am J Surg Pathol* 21:21–29, 1996.
50. Folpe AL, Weiss SW: Pleomorphic hyalinizing angiectatic tumor: analysis of 41 cases supporting evolution from a distinctive precursor lesion, *Am J Surg Pathol* 28:1417–1425, 2004.
51. Silverman JS, Dana MM: Pleomorphic hyalinizing angiectatic tumor of soft parts: immunohistochemical case study shows cellular composition by CD34+ fibroblasts and factor XIIIa+ dendrophages, *J Cutan Pathol* 24:377–383, 1997.
52. Capovilla M, Birembaut P, Cucherousset J, et al: Pleomorphic hyalinizing angiectatic tumor of soft parts: ultrastructural analysis of a case with original features, *Ultrastruct Pathol* 30:59–64, 2006.
53. Michal M, Kazakov DV: Relationship between pleomorphic hyalinizing angiectatic tumor and hemosiderotic fibrohistiocytic lipomatous lesion, *Am J Surg Pathol* 29:1256–1257, 2005.
54. Michal M, Kazakov DV, Hadravsky L, et al: Pleomorphic hyalinizing angiectatic tumor revisited: all tumors manifest typical morphologic features of myxoinflammatory fibroblastic sarcoma, further suggesting 2 morphologic variants of a single entity, *Ann Diagn Pathol* 20:40–43, 2016.
55. Carter JM, Sukov WR, Montgomery E, et al: TGFBR3 and MGEA5 rearrangements in pleomorphic hyalinizing angiectatic tumors and the spectrum of related neoplasms, *Am J Surg Pathol* 38:1182–1192, 2014.
56. Wei S, Pan Z, Siegel GP, et al: Complex analysis of a recurrent pleomorphic hyalinizing angiectatic tumor of soft parts, *Hum Pathol* 43:121–126, 2012.
57. Mohajeri A, Kindblom LG, Sumathi VP, et al: SNP array and FISH findings in two pleomorphic hyalinizing angiectatic tumors, *Cancer Genet* 205:673–676, 2012.
58. Meis-Kindblom JM, Kindlom L-G: Acral myxoinflammatory fibroblastic sarcoma. A low grade tumor of the hands and feet, *Am J Surg Pathol* 22:911–924, 1998.
59. Montgomery EA, Devaney KO, Giordano TJ, et al: Inflammatory myxohyaline tumor of distal extremities with virocyte or Reed-Sternberg-like cells: a distinctive lesion with features simulating inflammatory conditions, Hodgkin's disease and various sarcomas, *Mod Pathol* 11:384–391, 1998.

60. Michal M: Inflammatory myxoid tumor of the soft parts with bizarre giant cells, *Pathol Res Pract* 194:529–533, 1998.
61. Lambert I, Debiec-Rychter M, Guelinckz P, et al: Acral myxoinflammatory fibroblastic sarcoma with unique clonal chromosomal changes, *Virchows Arch* 438:509–512, 2001.
62. Elco CP, Mariño-Enríquez A, Abraham JA, et al: Hybrid myxoinflammatory fibroblastic sarcoma/hemosiderotic fibrolipomatous tumor: report of a case providing further evidence for a pathogenetic link, *Am J Surg Pathol* 34:1723–1727, 2010.
63. Antonescu CR, Zhang L, Nielsen GP, et al: Consistent t(1;10) with rearrangements of TGFBR3 and MGEA5 in both myxoinflammatory fibroblastic sarcoma and hemosiderotic fibrolipomatous tumor, *Genes Chromosomes Cancer* 50:757–764, 2011.
64. Hallor KH, Sciot R, Staaf J, et al: Two genetic pathways, t(1;10) and amplification of 3p11-12, in myxoinflammatory fibroblastic sarcoma, haemosiderotic fibrolipomatous tumour, and morphologically similar lesions, *J Pathol* 217:716–727, 2009.
65. Zreik RT, Carter JM, Sukov WR, et al: TGFBR3 and MGEA5 rearrangements are much more common in "hybrid" hemosiderotic fibrolipomatous tumor-myxoinflammatory fibroblastic sarcomas than in classical myxoinflammatory fibroblastic sarcomas: a morphologic and fluorescence in situ hybridization study, *Hum Pathol* 53:14–24, 2016.
66. Michal M, Kazakov DV, Hadravsky L, et al: High grade myxoinflammatory fibroblastic sarcoma: a report of 23 cases, *Ann Diagn Pathol* 19:157–163, 2015.
67. Hisaoka M, Morimitsu Y, Hashimoto H, et al: Retroperitoneal liposarcoma with combined well-differentiated and myxoid malignant fibrous histiocytoma-like myxoid areas, *Am J Surg Pathol* 23:1480–1492, 1999.
68. Nascimento AF, Bertoni F, Fletcher CD: Epithelioid variant of myxofibrosarcoma: expanding the clinicopathologic spectrum of myxofibrosarcoma in a series of 17 cases, *Am J Surg Pathol* 31:99–105, 2007.
69. Willems SM, Szuhai K, Hartgrink H, et al: Myxoid tumours of soft tissue: the so-called myxoid extracellular matrix is heterogeneous in composition, *Histopathology* 52:465–474, 2008.
70. Graadt van Roggen JF, Hogendoorn PCW, Fletcher CDM: Myxoid tumours of soft tissue, *Histopathology* 35:291–312, 1999.
71. Kindblom L-G, Merck C, Angervall L: The ultrastructure of myxofibrosarcoma. A study of 11 cases, *Virchows Arch [A]* 381:121–139, 1979.
72. Wood GS, Beckstead JH, Turner RR, et al: Malignant fibrous histiocytoma tumor cells resemble fibroblasts, *Am J Surg Pathol* 10:323–335, 1986.
73. Barretina J, Taylor BS, Banerji S, et al: Subtype-specific genomic alterations define new targets for soft-tissue sarcoma therapy, *Nat Genet* 42:715–721, 2010.
74. Willems SM, Debiec-Rychter M, Szuhai K, et al: Local recurrence of myxofibrosarcoma is associated with increase in tumour grade and cytogenetic aberrations, suggesting a multistep tumour progression model, *Mod Pathol* 19:407–416, 2006.
75. Willems SM, Mohseny AB, Balog C, et al: Cellular/intramuscular myxoma and grade I myxofibrosarcoma are characterized by distinct specific genetic alterations and specific composition of their extracellular matrix, *J Cell Mol Med* 13:1291–1301, 2009.
76. Wile AG, Evans HL, Romsdahl MM: Leiomyosarcoma of soft tissue: a clinicopathologic study, *Cancer* 48:1022–1032, 1981.
77. Gustafson P, Willén H, Baldetrop B, et al: Soft tissue leiomyosarcoma. A population-based epidemiologic and prognostic study of 48 patients, including cellular DNA content, *Cancer* 70:114–119, 1992.
78. Hashimoto H, Tsuneyoshi M, Enjoji M: Malignant smooth muscle tumors of the retroperitoneum and mesentery: a clinicopathologic analysis of 44 cases, *J Surg Oncol* 28:177–186, 1985.
79. Farshid G, Pradhan M, Goldblum J, et al: Leiomyosarcoma of somatic soft tissues: a tumor of vascular origin with multivariate analysis of outcome in 42 cases, *Am J Surg Pathol* 26:14–24, 2002.
80. Hashimoto H, Daimaru Y, Tsuneyoshi M, et al: Leiomyosarcoma of the external soft tissues. A clinicopathologic, immunohistochemical and electron microscopic study, *Cancer* 57:2077–2088, 1986.
81. Fields JP, Helwig EB: Leiomyosarcoma of the skin and subcutaneous tissue, *Cancer* 47:156–169, 1981.
82. Newman PL, Fletcher CDM: Smooth muscle tumours of the external genitalia: clinicopathologic analysis of a series, *Histopathology* 18:523–529, 1991.
83. Oda Y, Miyajima K, Kawaguchi K, et al: Pleomorphic leiomyosarcoma: a clinicopathologic and immunohistochemical study with special emphasis on its distinction from ordinary leiomyosarcoma and malignant fibrous histiocytoma, *Am J Surg Pathol* 25:1030–1038, 2001.
84. Gaffney EF, Dervan PA, Fletcher CDM: Pleomorphic rhabdomyosarcoma in adulthood: analysis of 11 cases with definition of diagnostic criteria, *Am J Surg Pathol* 17:601–609, 1993.
85. Furlong MA, Mentzel T, Fanburg-Smith JC: Pleomorphic rhabdomyosarcoma in adults: a clinicopathologic study of 38 cases with emphasis on morphologic variants and recent skeletal muscle-specific markers, *Mod Pathol* 14:595–603, 2001.
86. Kumar S, Perlman E, Harris CA, et al: Myogenin is a specific marker for rhabdomyosarcoma. An immunohistochemical study in paraffin-embedded tissues, *Mod Pathol* 13:988–993, 2000.
87. Iwata J, Fletcher CDM: Immunohistochemical detection of cytokeratin and epithelial membrane antigen in leiomyosarcoma: a systematic study of 100 cases, *Pathol Int* 50:7–14, 2000.
88. Guo X, Jo VY, Mills AM, et al: Clinically relevant molecular subtypes in leiomyosarcoma, *Clin Cancer Res* 21:3501–3511, 2015.
89. Mills AM, Beck AH, Montgomery KD, et al: Expression of subtype-specific group 1 leiomyosarcoma markers in a wide variety of sarcomas by gene expression analysis and immunohistochemistry, *Am J Surg Pathol* 35:583–589, 2011.
90. De Graaf MA, de Jong D, Briaire-de Bruin IH, et al: A translocation t(6;14) in two cases of leiomyosarcoma: molecular cytogenetic and array-based comparative genomic hybridization characterization, *Cancer Genet* 208:537–544, 2015.
91. Gebhard S, Coindre JM, Michels JJ, et al: Pleomorphic liposarcoma: clinicopathologic, immunohistochemical, and follow-up analysis of 63 cases: a study from the French Federation of Cancer Centers Sarcoma Group, *Am J Surg Pathol* 26:601–616, 2002.
92. Hornick JL, Bosenberg MW, Mentzel T, et al: Pleomorphic liposarcoma: clinicopathologic analysis of 57 cases, *Am J Surg Pathol* 28:1257–1267, 2004.
93. Enzinger FM, Winslow DJ: Liposarcoma: a study of 103 cases, *Virchows Arch [Pathol Anat]* 335:367–388, 1963.
94. Downes KA, Goldblum JR, Montgomery EA, et al: Pleomorphic liposarcoma: a clinicopathologic analysis of 19 cases, *Mod Pathol* 14:179–184, 2001.
95. Oliveira AM, Nascimento AG: Pleomorphic liposarcoma, *Semin Diagn Pathol* 18:274–285, 2001.
96. Dei Tos AP, Mentzel T, Fletcher CD: Primary liposarcoma of the skin: a rare neoplasm with unusual high grade features, *Am J Dermatopathol* 20:332–338, 1998.
97. Miettinen M, Enzinger FM: Epithelioid variant of pleomorphic liposarcoma: a study of 12 cases of a distinctive variant of high-grade liposarcoma, *Mod Pathol* 12:722–728, 1999.
98. Cai YC, McMenamin ME, Rose G, et al: Primary liposarcoma of the orbit: a clinicopathologic study of seven cases, *Ann Diagn Pathol* 5:255–266, 2001.
99. Klimstra DS, Moran CA, Perino G, et al: Liposarcoma of the anterior mediastinum and thymus. A clinicopathologic study of 28 cases, *Am J Surg Pathol* 19:782–791, 1995.
100. Weiss LM, Warhol MJ: Ultrastructural distinctions between adult pleomorphic rhabdomyosarcomas, pleomorphic liposarcomas, and pleomorphic malignant fibrous histiocytomas, *Human Pathol.* 15:1025–1033, 1984.
101. Meiss-Kindblom JM, Sjögren H, Kindblom LG, et al: Cytogenetic and molecular genetic analysis of liposarcoma and its soft tissue simulators: recognition of new variants and differential diagnosis, *Virchows Arch* 439:141–151, 2001.
102. Evans HL: Liposarcoma: a study of 55 cases with a reassessment of its classification, *Am J Surg Pathol* 3:507–523, 1979.
103. Henricks WH, Chu YC, Goldblum JR, et al: Dedifferentiated liposarcoma: a clinicopathological analysis of 155 cases with a proposal for an expanded definition of dedifferentiation, *Am J Surg Pathol* 21:271–281, 1997.
104. Elgar F, Goldblum JR: Well-differentiated liposarcoma of the retroperitoneum: a clinicopathologic analysis of 20 cases, with particular attention to the extent of low-grade differentiation, *Mod Pathol* 10:113–120, 1997.
105. Evans HL, Khurana KK, Kemp BL, et al: Heterologous elements in the dedifferentiated component of dedifferentiated liposarcoma, *Am J Surg Pathol* 18:1150–1157, 1994.
106. Tallini G, Erlandson RA, Brennan MF, et al: Divergent myosarcomatous differentiation in retroperitoneal liposarcoma, *Am J Surg Pathol* 17:546–556, 1993.
107. Nascimento AG, Kurtin PJ, Guillou L, et al: Dedifferentiated liposarcoma. A report of nine cases with a peculiar neural-like whorling pattern associated with metaplastic bone formation, *Am J Surg Pathol* 22:945–955, 1998.
108. Weiss SW, Rao VK: Well-differentiated liposarcoma (atypical lipoma) of deep soft tissue of the extremities, retroperitoneum, and miscellaneous sites. A follow-up study of 92 cases with analysis of the incidence of "dedifferentiation.", *Am J Surg Pathol* 16:1051–1058, 1992.
109. Mariño-Enríquez A, Fletcher CD, Dal Cin P, et al: Dedifferentiated liposarcoma with "homologous" lipoblastic (pleomorphic liposarcoma-like) differentiation: clinicopathologic and molecular analysis of a series suggesting revised diagnostic criteria, *Am J Surg Pathol* 34:1122–1131, 2010.
110. Binh MB, Sastre-Garau X, Guillou L, et al: MDM2 and CDK4 immunostainings are useful adjuncts in diagnosing well-differentiated and dedifferentiated liposarcoma subtypes: a comparative analysis of 559 soft tissue neoplasms with genetic data, *Am J Surg Pathol* 29:1340–1347, 2005.
111. Fletcher CD, Akerman M, Dal Cin P, et al: Correlation between clinicopathological features and karyotype in lipomatous tumors. A report of 178 cases from the Chromosomes and Morphology (CHAMP) Collaborative Study Group, *Am J Pathol* 148:623–630, 1996.
112. Dei Tos AP, Doglioni C, Piccinin S, et al: Molecular abnormalities of the p53 pathway in dedifferentiated liposarcoma, *J Pathol* 181:8–13, 1997.
113. Mussi C, Collini P, Miceli R, et al: The prognostic impact of dedifferentiation in retroperitoneal liposarcoma. A series of surgically treated patients at a single institution, *Cancer* 113:1657–1665, 2008.
114. Keung EZ, Hornick JL, Bertagnolli MM, et al: Predictors of outcomes in patients with primary retroperitoneal dedifferentiated liposarcoma undergoing surgery, *J Am Coll Surg* 218:206–217, 2014.
115. Gronchi A, Collini P, Miceli R, et al: Myogenic differentiation and histologic grading are major prognostic determinants in retroperitoneal liposarcoma, *Am J Surg Pathol* 39:383–393, 2015.
116. Allan CJ, Soule EH: Osteogenic sarcoma of the somatic soft tissues. Clinicopathologic study of 26 cases and review of the literature, *Cancer* 27:1121–1133, 1971.
117. Sordillo PP, Hajdu SI, Magill GB, et al: Extraosseous osteosarcoma. A review of 48 patients, *Cancer* 71:727–734, 1983.
118. Chung EB, Enzinger FM: Extraskeletal osteosarcoma, *Cancer* 60:1132–1142, 1987.
119. Lidang Jensen M, Schumacher B, Myhre Jensen O, et al: Extraskeletal osteosarcoma: a clinicopathologic study of 25 cases, *Am J Surg Pathol* 22:588–594, 1998.
120. Mirra JM, Fain JS, Ward WG, et al: Extraskeletal telangiectatic osteosarcoma, *Cancer* 71:3014–3019, 1993.

121. Graadt van Roggen JF, Zonderland HM, Welvaart K, et al: Local recurrence of a phyllodes tumour of the breast presenting with widespread differentiation to a telangiectatic osteosarcoma, *J Clin Pathol* 51:706–708, 1998.
122. Conner JR, Hornick JL: SATB2 is a novel marker of osteoblastic differentiation in bone and soft tissue tumours, *Histopathology* 63:36–49, 2013.
123. Von Baer A, Ehrhardt A, Baumhoer D, et al: Immunohistochemical and FISH analysis of MDM2 and CDK4 in a dedifferentiated extraskeletal osteosarcoma arising in the vastus lateralis muscle: differential diagnosis and diagnostic algorithm, *Pathol Res Pract* 210:698–703, 2014.
124. Kriazoglou AI, Vieira J, Dimitriadis E, et al: 12q amplification defines a subtype of extraskeletal osteosarcoma with good prognosis that is the soft tissue homologue of parosteal osteosarcoma, *Cancer Genet* 205:332–336, 2012.
125. Goldstein-Jackson SY, Gosheger G, Delling G, et al: Extraskeletal osteosarcoma has a favourable prognosis when treated like conventional osteosarcoma, *J Cancer Res Clin Oncol* 131:520–526, 2005.
126. Berner K, Bjerkehagen B, Bruland OS, et al: Extraskeletal osteosarcoma in Norway, between 1975 and 2009, and a brief review of the literature, *Anticancer Res* 35:2129–2140, 2015.
127. Stout AP: Mesenchymoma, the mixed tumor of mesenchymal derivatives, *Ann Surg* 127:278–290, 1948.
128. Brady MS, Perino G, Tallini G, et al: Malignant mesenchymoma, *Cancer* 77:467–473, 1996.
129. Trojani M, Contesso G, Coindre JM, et al: Soft-tissue sarcomas of adults; study of pathological prognostic variables and definition of a histopathological grading system, *Int J Cancer* 33:7–42, 1984.
130. Costa J, Wesley RA, Glatstein E, et al: The grading of soft tissue sarcomas. Results of a clinicopathologic correlation in a series of 163 cases, *Cancer* 53:530–541, 1984.
131. Coindre J-M, Terrier P, Bui NB, et al: Prognostic factors in adult patients with locally controlled soft tissue sarcoma: a study of 546 patients from the French Federation of Cancer Centers Sarcoma Group, *J Clin Oncol* 14:869–877, 1996.
132. Guillou L, Coindre J-M, Bonichon F, et al: Comparative study of the National Cancer Institute and French Federation of Cancer Centers Sarcoma Group grading systems in a population of 410 adult patients with soft tissue sarcoma, *J Clin Oncol* 15:350–362, 1997.
133. Graadt van Roggen JF: The histopathological grading of soft tissue sarcomas: current concepts, *Curr Diagn Pathol.* 7:1–7, 2001.
134. Chibon F, Lagarde P, Salas S, et al: Validated prediction of clinical outcome in sarcomas and multiple types of cancer on the basis of a gene expression signature related to genome complexity, *Nat Med* 16:781–787, 2010.
135. Graadt van Roggen JF, Bovée JVMG, van der Woude HJ, et al: An update of diagnostic strategies using molecular genetic and magnetic resonance imaging techniques for musculoskeletal tumors, *Curr Opin Rheumatol* 12:7–83, 2000.

8

Round Cell Tumors

Enrique de Alava, MD, PhD, David Marcilla, MD, and Michele Biscuola, PhD

The term *small round blue cell tumors* is used to refer to a group of generally highly aggressive malignant neoplasms, seen under the microscope as monotonous proliferations of small cells with scant cytoplasm. This category classically includes certain subtypes of sarcomas, carcinomas, lymphomas, melanoma, and neuroblastoma (Box 8.1). Many of these tumor types are more common in young patients (e.g., small cell osteosarcoma), but several entities (e.g., metastatic small cell carcinoma) are more common in older adults. Small round cell sarcomas of soft tissue include Ewing sarcoma, rhabdomyosarcoma, desmoplastic small round cell tumor (DSRCT), poorly differentiated synovial sarcoma (round cell variant), "round cell" liposarcoma, and undifferentiated round cell sarcomas, the latter including a growing number of new entities collectively termed Ewing-like sarcomas. Some of these (i.e., round cell variants of liposarcoma, synovial sarcoma) are discussed in more detail in other chapters.

Despite their low frequency, small round cell sarcomas have interested the scientific community for decades. On the one hand, the histogenesis and differential diagnosis of these entities have been intriguing problems for diagnostic pathology. Approximately 80% of soft tissue round cell sarcomas can be diagnosed with careful attention to a combination of clinical examination, imaging techniques, and conventional histopathology.[1] First electron microscopy and then in the last three decades immunohistochemistry have become widely available for routine diagnostic use; they provide valuable complementary information for differential diagnosis. On the other hand, beyond the monotonous appearance and clinical overlap of this group of tumors (they are more frequently found in children and adolescents), a huge wealth of molecular data is available; this chapter shows that this information can be useful not only for accurate diagnosis in round cell sarcomas of soft tissue but also for prognosis and clinical management. One of the current challenges for pathologists is to be able to handle, manage, and integrate molecular pathology into the routine diagnosis of round cell sarcomas when needed. There is a further reason to provide accurate diagnosis in soft tissue round cell sarcomas of childhood: the high response rate of many of them to appropriately applied specific neoadjuvant/adjuvant chemotherapeutic protocols. Finally, uncommon tumors, especially soft tissue sarcomas in children and adolescents, require a multidisciplinary approach, with collaboration between pathologists and their colleagues in pediatric and medical oncology, orthopedic oncology, surgical oncology, pediatric surgery, radiation oncology, radiology, and nuclear medicine. At cancer centers, these physicians should ideally serve on a single sarcoma tumor board.

The Role of Immunohistochemistry and Molecular Genetics

Sarcomas are generally classified according to their specific line of differentiation. However, round cell sarcomas often lack a definable differentiation program that can suggest any normal tissue type. The role of immunohistochemistry in the diagnosis of small round blue cell tumors is, first, to exclude nonsarcomatous entities and, second, to determine which line of mesenchymal differentiation (if any) the tumor cells exhibit (Fig. 8.1).[2] Therefore appropriate panels of antibodies must be applied in the workup of small round cell tumors. A suggested initial panel is shown in Table 8.1; the application of immunohistochemistry is discussed in more detail for each entity in its corresponding section.

Another notable feature of most round cell sarcomas is their relatively simple cytogenetic alterations, usually balanced translocations (see also Chapter 18). Gene fusions generated from these translocations are the initiating events of many sarcoma types. Because gene fusions and their products are nearly specific for each tumor type and they are found in essentially all cases of a large group of sarcomas, their characterization offers wide opportunities for differential diagnosis (Table 8.2).[3]

In addition, a deeper knowledge of these genetic alterations, specifically, the target molecules of the translocation-derived fusion proteins, has led to development of new antibodies for immunohistochemistry. Several current markers can detect proteins that are either overexpressed or aberrantly expressed as a result of such translocations. Examples of these antibodies in sarcomas include TFE3 (alveolar soft part sarcoma), ALK (inflammatory myofibroblastic tumor), WT1 (DSRCT), and FLI1 (Ewing sarcoma) (see Box 8.2 and Chapter 1).[2] New technologies such as massively parallel sequencing and associated computational algorithms (next-generation sequencing; see Chapter 18) will likely affect the diagnosis of small round cell tumors and result in the generation of considerable new information, some of which could be used to identify and validate targetable molecular alterations in sarcomas (reviewed in reference 3).

Box 8.1 Small Round Cell Tumors

Primarily Extraskeletal Round Cell Sarcomas
- Rhabdomyosarcomas: alveolar and embryonal
- Ewing sarcoma
- Desmoplastic small round cell tumor
- *CIC*-rearranged Ewing-like sarcomas

Sarcomas That Can Have a Round Cell Component (Discussed in Other Chapters)
- Round cell (high-grade myxoid) liposarcoma
- Poorly differentiated synovial sarcoma, small cell variant
- Mesenchymal chondrosarcoma
- Small cell osteosarcoma

Nonsarcomatous Small Round Cell Tumors (Should Always Be Ruled Out)
- Lymphoma/leukemia
- Neuroblastoma
- Small cell melanoma
- Small cell (neuroendocrine) carcinoma

How Should Small Round Cell Sarcoma Samples Be Handled?

The role of the pathologist dealing with a small round cell sarcoma specimen (Fig. 8.2) is time-honored and includes the following: to render a diagnosis; to establish the presence of key prognostic elements, such as stage and response to induction chemotherapy; and to discuss with the surgeon and the oncologist the features of the resection specimen.[4] At the same time, the pathologist should manage the sample in a timely fashion to allow for a rapid and accurate assessment of immunohistochemical and molecular markers. In particular, material should be quickly submitted to pathology; on arrival and before formalin fixation, tumor imprints (touch preps) on coated/treated slides should be taken (useful for fluorescence in situ hybridization [FISH]), and tissue/cell suspensions should be kept frozen. Another option is to establish primary cell cultures for cytogenetics. Another interesting resource is the generation of patient-derived xenografts from the primary small round cell tumor samples, as they represent a closer model to the clinical setting than regular cell line xenografts.[5] It is important to emphasize the central role that pathologists play in translational research, specifically in creating and maintaining biobanks. Biobanks are instrumental for diagnostic and translational research in the molecular pathology of cancer.[6] Informed consent for biobanking that allows for later analysis and research should be sought.

Should Molecular Techniques to Detect Translocations Always Be Performed?

When round cell sarcomas present in unusual clinicopathologic contexts (e.g., age, location), pathologic diagnosis can be difficult. To address this issue, we would like to make a distinction between essential and optional indications for the application of molecular techniques.[3,4] In the following circumstances, molecular diagnostic approaches are essential:

- Appearance of an unusual morphologic variant (e.g., a poorly differentiated synovial sarcoma that appears at a typical site in a patient of usual age, such as close to the knee joint in a 27-year-old man; a tumor morphologically similar to an adamantinoma on the anterior aspect of the tibia, but containing areas with round cells, may suggest the differential diagnosis with Ewing sarcoma).

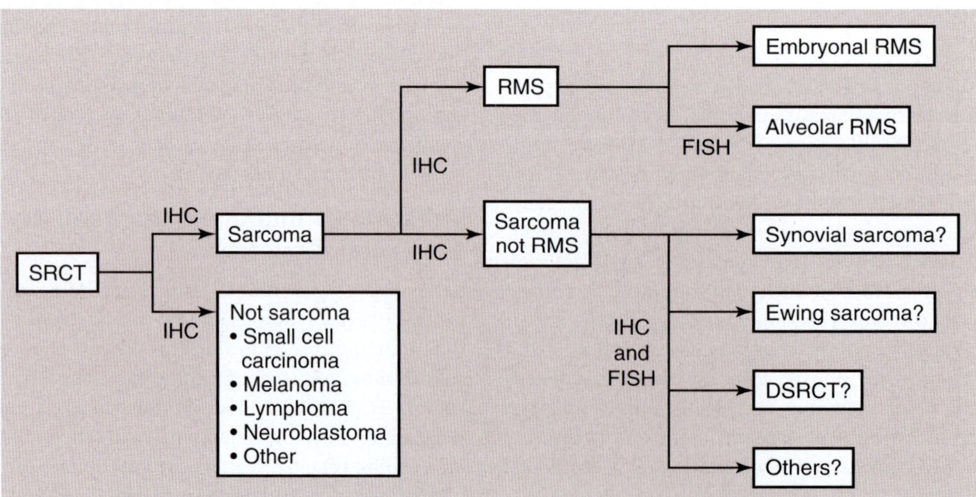

Figure 8.1 Diagnostic Algorithm for Round Cell Sarcomas. *DSRCT,* Desmoplastic small round cell tumor; *FISH,* fluorescence in situ hybridization; *IHC,* immunohistochemistry; *RMS,* rhabdomyosarcoma; *SRCT,* small round cell tumor.

Table 8.1 Expected Immunophenotype in Small Round Cell Tumors

	Epithelial Membrane Antigen/Keratins	S-100 Protein	Lymphoid Markers[a]	Desmin	Myogenin	FLI1	WT1	CD99
Ewing sarcoma	+	–	–	–	–	++	–	++
Rhabdomyosarcoma	–	–	–	++	++[b]	–	–	+
Desmoplastic small round cell tumor	++	–	–	++	–	–	++[c]	+
Poorly differentiated synovial sarcoma	++	–	–	–	–	–	–	+
CIC-rearranged Ewing-like sarcoma[d]	+	–	–	+	–	++	++	++ (patchy)
BCOR-rearranged Ewing-like sarcoma[e]	–	–	–	–	–	–	–	+ (patchy)
Lymphoma/leukemia	–	–	++	–	–	+	–	+
Mesenchymal chondrosarcoma	–	–[f]	–	–	–	–	–	++
Neuroblastoma	–	–[g]	–	–	–	–	–	–
Wilms tumor	–	–	–	–	–	–	++	–
Melanoma	–	++	–	–	–	–	–	–

[a]CD45, terminal deoxynucleotidyl transferase, CD3, CD20, CD79a (as appropriate).
[b]Stronger and more diffuse in alveolar rhabdomyosarcoma.
[c]Only carboxyl-terminal epitopes in desmoplastic small round cell tumor.
[d]Consider also ETV4 or DUX4.
[e]Consider CCNB3 or BCOR.
[f]Except in overtly cartilaginous areas.
[g]Except in schwannian stromal areas.
++, Usually or almost always positive (>50%); +, occasionally positive (10% to 50%); –, never or almost never positive (<10%).

Table 8.2 Most Prevalent Gene Fusions of Diagnostic Utility in Sarcomas With Usual or Occasional Small Round Cell Morphology

Entity	Gene Fusion
Ewing sarcoma	*EWSR1-FLI1* *EWSR1-ERG*
Alveolar rhabdomyosarcoma	*PAX3-FOXO1A* *PAX7-FOXO1A*
Embryonal rhabdomyosarcoma	None
Desmoplastic small round cell tumor	*EWSR1-WT1*
Poorly differentiated synovial sarcoma	*SS18-SSX1* *SS18-SSX2*
Round cell (high-grade myxoid) liposarcoma	*FUS-DDIT3* *EWSR1-DDIT3*
Mesenchymal chondrosarcoma	*HEY1-NCOA2*
CIC-rearranged Ewing-like sarcoma[a]	*CIC-DUX4* *CIC-FOXO4*
BCOR-rearranged Ewing-like sarcoma[a]	*BCOR-CCNB3* *BCOR-MAML3* *ZC3H7B-BCOR*

[a]Some tumors with *CIC* or *BCOR* rearrangements have unknown fusion partners.

- Appearance of a sarcoma with typical morphologic features, but at an unusual age. This applies to round cell sarcomas, which have characteristic translocations, in patients older than 40 years.
- Appearance of a sarcoma with typical morphologic features, but at an unusual location (e.g., cutaneous, renal, or bladder Ewing sarcoma, which may be mistaken for small cell/neuroendocrine carcinoma).

Box 8.2 Immunohistochemistry to Detect Translocations in Round Cell Sarcomas

- BCOR (Ewing-like sarcomas with *BCOR* rearrangements)[a]
- DUX4 (most Ewing-like sarcomas with *CIC* rearrangements)
- FLI1 or ERG (Ewing sarcoma)
- WT1 (desmoplastic small round cell tumor)[b]

[a]*BCOR* gene fusions or internal tandem duplications
[b]Using antibodies directed against the C-terminus of WT1

- Distinguishing between a sarcoma and other (nonsarcomatous) tumor types that it may mimic. The most frequent examples, in our experience, do not belong to the small round cell tumor category. One example is a spindle cell tumor in the pleura, which might suggest the differential diagnosis of synovial sarcoma, malignant mesothelioma, and a malignant solitary fibrous tumor; another example is the differential diagnosis between clear cell sarcoma of soft tissues and metastatic melanoma.

Ewing Sarcoma

The most recent World Health Organization (WHO) classification considers Ewing sarcoma a single entity that encompasses different clinical presentations and histologic appearances: bone and soft tissue sites, peripheral primitive neuroectodermal tumor (PNET), skin tumors, and other less frequent examples.[7]

Until relatively recently, however, Ewing sarcoma and PNET were considered distinct tumor types from a histogenetic point of view. Interestingly, both tumors were initially reported in New York City, in the same journal, 3 years apart.[8] In 1921 James Ewing reported an undifferentiated tumor in the diaphysis of long bones that was radiosensitive. He considered this tumor endothelial in origin.

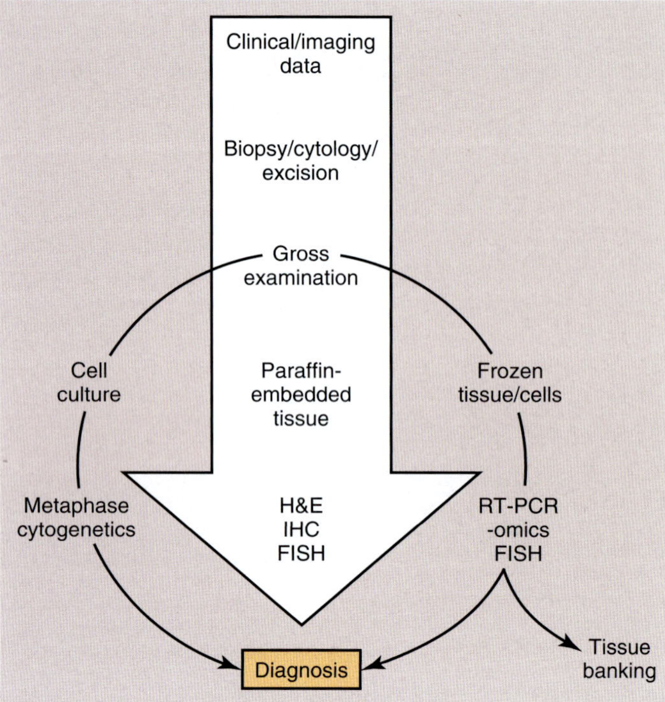

Figure 8.2 **How to Handle Samples of Small Round Cell Tumors.** *FISH,* Fluorescence in situ hybridization; *H&E,* hematoxylin and eosin; *IHC,* immunohistochemistry; *RT-PCR,* reverse transcriptase-polymerase chain reaction.

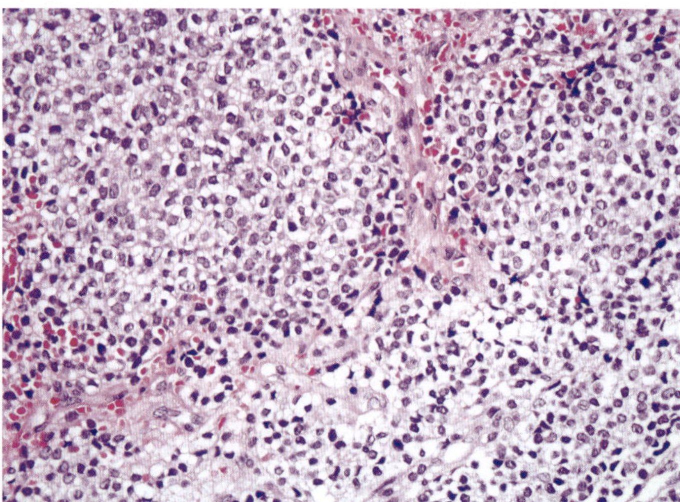

Figure 8.3 **Ewing Sarcoma.** Conventional appearance of Ewing sarcoma. Note the vaguely lobulated pattern and clear cytoplasm secondary to abundant glycogen.

In 1918 Arthur Purdy Stout described a "tumor of the ulnar nerve" with the gross features of a sarcoma, but microscopically composed of small round cells forming rosettes. He later called this tumor *neuroepithelioma*, which was later known as PNET. Whatever the clinicopathologic presentation, the cells of Ewing sarcoma show high levels of expression of CD99 (MIC2 or p30/32 glycoprotein; O13) on the cell membrane, and cytogenetic techniques reported similar consistent balanced translocations in Ewing sarcoma of bone and PNET in 1983 and 1984, respectively. These translocations generate specific molecular markers, gene fusions between the *EWSR1* gene and one of the members of the ETS family of transcription factors (*FLI1* and *ERG* being the most frequent).[7]

Clinical Features

Ewing sarcoma is the second most common bone/soft tissue sarcoma in the pediatric age group. It usually affects male patients 10 to 25 years of age, although well-documented cases with molecular confirmation have been reported in patients older than 40 years. Extraskeletal Ewing sarcoma usually arises (in descending order of frequency) in the thigh, pelvis, paraspinal area, and foot.[9] Approximately 25% of patients have clinically detectable metastases at the time of diagnosis, although it is likely that nearly all patients have micrometastases at diagnosis because the cure rate using only local treatment (resection and radiation therapy) is less than 20%.[10]

Pathologic Features

Gross examination of untreated Ewing sarcoma specimens is now uncommon because of the standard use of neoadjuvant chemotherapy. The cut surface is gray-white and soft, frequently with areas of hemorrhage and necrosis. Extraskeletal Ewing sarcoma can be large; in fact, the volume of a Ewing sarcoma is one important prognostic factor. Resection specimens of treated tumors show reparative features, such as marked sclerosis and hemorrhage, often with no visible residual foci of viable tumor.

Histologically, *conventional* Ewing sarcoma is composed of sheets of closely packed cells with relatively small, round nuclei, displaying a monomorphous pattern under low-power examination (Fig. 8.3). The chromatin is finely granular, and nucleoli are inconspicuous. A small number of darker cells are seen among more common lighter cells; electron microscopy suggests that dark cells are probably undergoing apoptosis.[11] There are usually extensive deposits of glycogen in the cytoplasm; periodic acid–Schiff stain is positive in more than half of tumors, especially in well-fixed specimens. Nevertheless, many other round cell sarcomas can show variable proportions of cells that are positive by periodic acid–Schiff staining. This feature is therefore not useful for differential diagnosis. Reticulin stains show a lack of matrix among tumor cells. A *large cell*, or *atypical*, variant has been reported,[12] which shows a low-magnification appearance similar to that of conventional Ewing sarcoma. The main differences are the larger size and the more irregular contours of the nuclei; conspicuous nucleoli can be seen, and periodic acid–Schiff stain is frequently negative (Fig. 8.4). The immunophenotypic and molecular features are similar to those of conventional Ewing sarcoma, and no consistent prognostic importance has been assigned to this variant. The availability of molecular diagnostics, and growing awareness by soft tissue pathologists, has helped categorize some of these cases into *CIC-DUX4* Ewing-like sarcomas, whereas bona fide atypical Ewing sarcoma has *EWSR1-ETS* fusions.

Ewing sarcomas showing a higher degree of neural differentiation (formerly called PNET) contain Homer-Wright rosettes, with a central fibrillary core lacking vascular lumina, similar to those seen in neuroblastoma. More frequently, tumors with a rosette-like configuration are seen in ill-defined groups of up to 10 cells oriented toward a central space (Fig. 8.5). They show higher expression of neuron-specific enolase and other (nonspecific) neuroectodermal markers, such as CD57 (Leu-7), than conventional (undifferentiated) Ewing sarcoma. No consistent prognostic differences have been found between these two groups.

Tumor cells show a variable degree of necrosis after induction chemotherapy; they are replaced by loose connective tissue. Histopathologic assessment of tumor necrosis after therapy correlates with overall survival. Several different grading systems have been reported. Similar to osteosarcoma, the prognostically relevant cutoff in most systems is 10% residual viable tumor cells.[10]

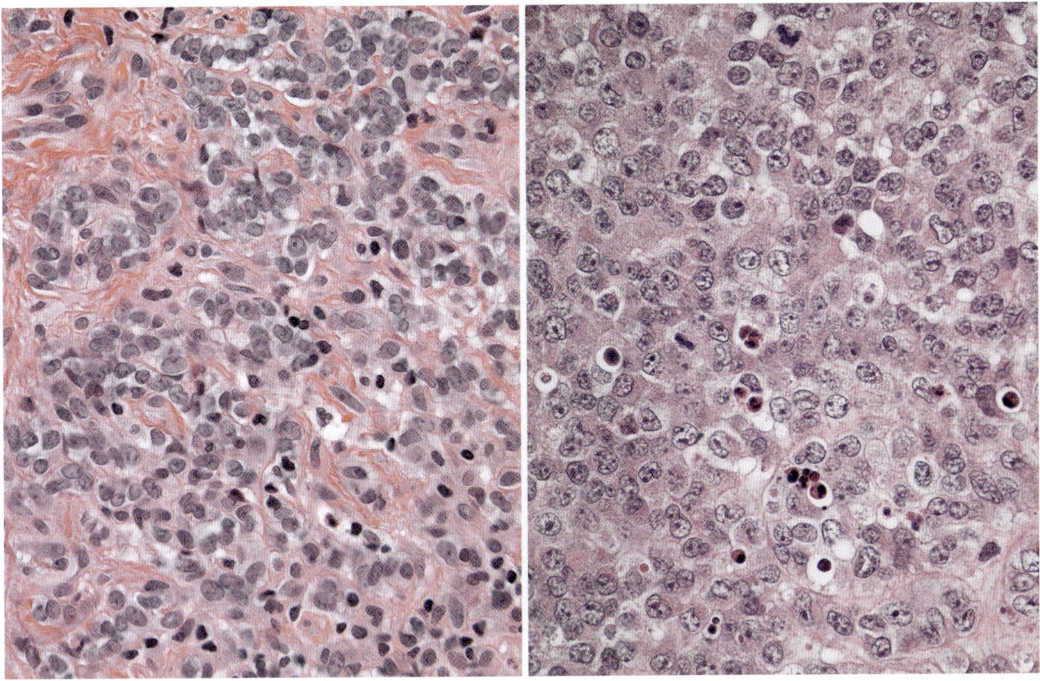

Figure 8.4 **Ewing Sarcoma.** Large cell variant of Ewing sarcoma *(right)*, compared with conventional Ewing sarcoma *(left)* in terms of nuclear size, nuclear irregularity, and prominent nucleoli.

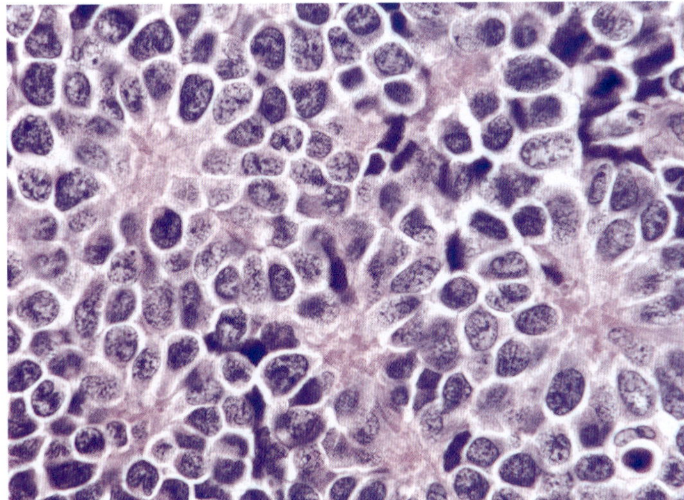

Figure 8.5 **Ewing Sarcoma.** Well-formed pseudorosettes in a Ewing sarcoma with extensive neural differentiation (formerly known as peripheral primitive neuroectodermal tumor). Note the absence of nucleoli and the finely granular chromatin.

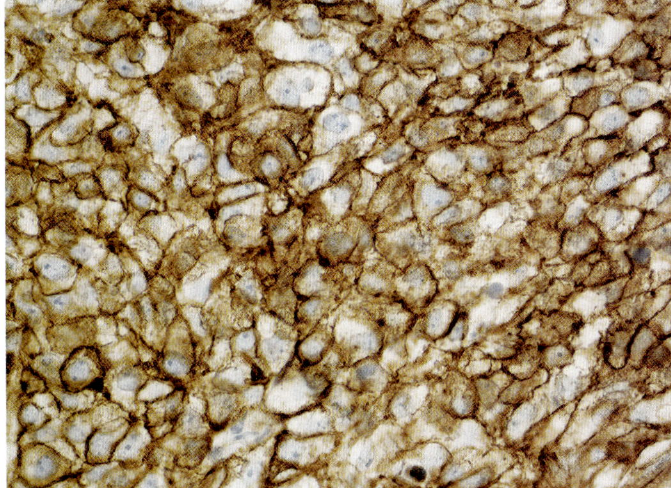

Figure 8.6 **CD99 in Ewing Sarcoma.** Diffuse membranous immunoreactivity for CD99 is characteristic of Ewing sarcoma.

Immunohistochemistry

CD99 is a cell surface glycoprotein (also known as MIC2) that is recognized by the monoclonal antibody O13. Strong, diffuse membranous expression of CD99 is seen in nearly all Ewing sarcomas (Fig. 8.6).[7] CD99 expression is unrelated to the gene products of the specific translocations found in Ewing sarcomas. CD99 is not specific for Ewing sarcoma and has been reported in a large group of normal tissues and tumor types, including other round cell sarcomas. For example, between 71% and 93% of lymphoblastic lymphomas and leukemias express CD99,[13] as did all cases of small cell osteosarcoma (albeit with weak cytoplasmic staining in few neoplastic cells) in a recent series[14]; almost all mesenchymal chondrosarcomas,[15] the large majority of *CIC-DUX4* sarcomas, between 10% and 25% of rhabdomyosarcomas, and approximately 20% of DSRCTs are also positive for CD99.[16] In DSRCTs and rhabdomyosarcomas, CD99 usually shows a cytoplasmic staining pattern, in contrast to the membranous pattern typical of Ewing sarcoma. Importantly, neuroblastomas lack CD99 immunoreactivity in all locations and age groups.[17] Therefore CD99 is a sensitive but not specific marker for Ewing sarcoma.

Immunohistochemical detection of FLI1 (as a consequence of the *EWSR1-FLI1* fusion) is somewhat more specific for Ewing sarcoma than CD99, although specificity of FLI1 is limited by its expression in lymphoblastic leukemias/lymphomas, non-Hodgkin lymphomas, endothelial cells and derived neoplasms, and a subset of a wide range of other mesenchymal tumor types. Although the sensitivity of FLI1 for Ewing sarcoma is high, occasional cases show low levels of

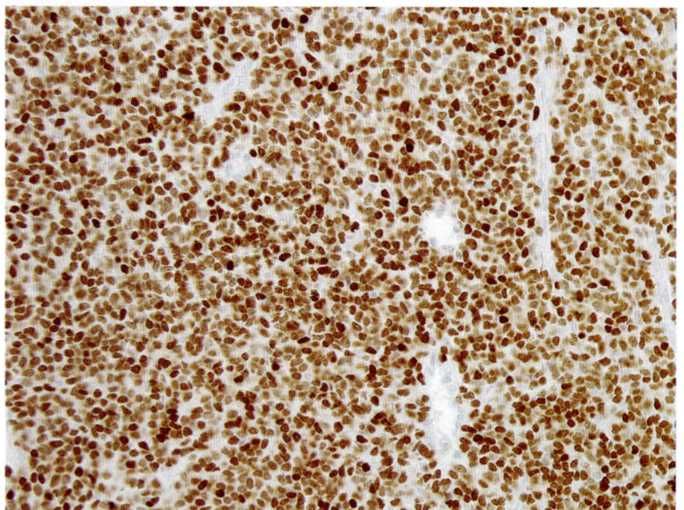

Figure 8.7 NKX2-2 in Ewing Sarcoma. Diffuse nuclear immunoreactivity for NKX2-2 is characteristic of Ewing sarcoma.

expression, and tumors with variant translocations that do not involve the *FLI1* gene are typically negative.[2]

The transcription factor NKX2-2 is a downstream target of EWSR1-FLI1 signaling identified by gene expression profiling.[18] NKX2-2 is a highly sensitive and relatively specific immunohistochemical marker for Ewing sarcoma (Fig. 8.7); mesenchymal chondrosarcomas are also often positive.[19-21] The combination of CD99 and NKX2-2 is highly specific for Ewing sarcoma.[20]

Molecular Genetics

Approximately 85% of Ewing sarcomas have *EWSR1-FLI1* fusions; *EWSR1-ERG* fusions are identified in 10% of cases, whereas in 3% of cases, fusions between *EWSR1* and other members of the ETS family of transcription factors are detected (see Chapter 18).[7] Ewing sarcomas may rarely harbor fusions between *EWSR1* and non-ETS family members (*PATZ1, SP3, NFATc2, SMARCA5*); these tumors sometimes show atypical morphology (scattered larger cells, more prominent nucleoli) or present at older ages, but they show significant histologic overlap with conventional Ewing sarcoma with ETS-containing fusions. Finally, a small group of Ewing sarcomas shows *FUS* gene rearrangements instead of *EWSR1*, with an *ERG* or *FEV* fusion partner; *FUS*-positive tumors appear to be morphologically and immunohistochemically similar to *EWSR1*-positive Ewing sarcomas.[22] *FUS* gene rearrangements should be evaluated in small round cell sarcomas with morphology consistent with Ewing sarcoma and strong membranous CD99 expression but lacking *EWSR1* rearrangements.[23]

All these rearrangements are characteristic of Ewing sarcoma; reverse transcriptase-polymerase chain reaction (RT-PCR) and FISH studies of other small round cell tumors that enter into the differential diagnosis—such as neuroblastoma, rhabdomyosarcomas, adamantinoma, and giant cell tumor of bone—are negative for these particular fusion genes. A reference laboratory for sarcoma diagnosis may have either FISH or RT-PCR (or both) methods available. The introduction of next-generation sequencing will likely change the diagnostic approach for round cell sarcoma in the near future. The choice of technique depends on the specific experience of the laboratory,[24] although RT-PCR is suitable when frozen tissue is available, whereas FISH is a good choice when only formalin-fixed, paraffin-embedded tissue is available. There are several commercial sources for *EWSR1* break-apart probes; however, it is important to note that assays using *EWSR1* break-apart probes do not detect *EWSR1-FLI1* fusions per se but only *EWSR1* gene rearrangements (see also Chapter 18), which should not be a problem in most cases. Next-generation sequencing applications for Ewing sarcoma have demonstrated the potential pitfall of relying only on FISH-based assays to detect *EWSR1*-containing fusions.[23] For a list of tumors showing *EWSR1* gene rearrangements, see Table 8.2.

Differential Diagnosis

A basic immunohistochemical panel for small round cell tumors, such as the one shown in Table 8.1, should, in the appropriate clinical and histologic context, be sufficient to reach a confident diagnosis of Ewing sarcoma and, in particular, to exclude nonsarcomatous entities. Moreover, FISH or RT-PCR analysis is helpful to confirm the diagnosis in difficult cases, as discussed earlier.

In our experience, the two major differential diagnostic considerations for extraskeletal Ewing sarcoma within the round cell sarcoma category are poorly differentiated synovial sarcoma and alveolar rhabdomyosarcoma. Useful hints for this differential diagnosis are shown in Table 8.3. The differential diagnosis with round cell sarcomas with *CIC* and *BCOR* gene rearrangements is discussed in the last section of this chapter.

Ewing sarcoma can have an infiltrative pattern (sometimes referred to in the literature as a "filigree" pattern), with irregular strands of tumor cells in a fibrous stroma. If such a tumor arises in the abdomen and imaging techniques do not show an organ-specific location, the differential diagnosis of DSRCT is likely to arise. Attention should be paid to subtle morphologic features: fibrosis should not be mistaken for true desmoplasia, and a capillary vascular proliferation is characteristic of DSRCT. Both entities can share keratin and CD99 expression, although desmin (not myogenin) is usually expressed only in DSRCT and NKX2-2 only in Ewing sarcoma. *EWSR1-WT1* fusions characteristic of DSRCT lead to overexpression of the carboxyl-terminal portion of the WT1 protein, which can be detected by immunohistochemistry, although available antibodies show somewhat inconsistent results. FISH analysis with commercial *EWSR1* break-apart probes is useless for this differential diagnosis because both entities share gene fusions with *EWSR1* rearrangements. RT-PCR, if frozen tissue is available, is the technique of choice.

Soft tissue involvement by small cell osteosarcoma (Fig. 8.8) can pose particular diagnostic problems in core biopsy specimens, when osteoid may be scarce or absent. However, even if osteoid deposition is limited, tumor cell nuclei usually have mild variability in size and shape, an uncommon finding in Ewing sarcoma. Expression of SATB2, a nuclear protein important for osteoblast differentiation, may be helpful to differentiate osteoid from hyalinized collagen[25]; however, SATB2 expression in round cell sarcomas should be interpreted with caution, as this marker is usually positive in *BCOR-CCNB3* Ewing-like sarcomas of bone as well. A somewhat similar problem can arise in mesenchymal chondrosarcoma, because the cartilaginous component may be missed in small biopsy specimens. Moreover, membranous CD99 expression is often detected in the undifferentiated round cell component of mesenchymal chondrosarcomas, and NKX2-2 is often positive as well.[15,21] Molecular analysis can solve the problem in both situations by confirming the presence of *EWSR1* gene rearrangement and the diagnosis of Ewing sarcoma.

Ewing sarcoma shares a variable degree of neural differentiation with neuroblastoma. There is a subgroup of schwannian stroma-poor neuroblastomas, designated *undifferentiated neuroblastomas,* which can have small round cell morphologic features overlapping with those of Ewing sarcoma. Age is helpful in this situation, because this subset of neuroblastomas typically presents in patients younger than 18 months of age, which would be exceptional for Ewing sarcoma.

Table 8.3 Differential Diagnosis for Ewing Sarcoma, Alveolar Rhabdomyosarcoma, and Poorly Differentiated Synovial Sarcoma, Small Cell Variant

	Useful?	Ewing Sarcoma	Alveolar Rhabdomyosarcoma	Poorly Differentiated Synovial Sarcoma
Age	No	10–25 years	10–25 years	10–30 years
Location	Not much	Extremities and trunk	Extremities and pelvis	Extremities
Morphologic features	Yes	Monotonous appearance; usually indistinct nucleoli	Look for nascent alveolar pattern and giant cells	Look for primitive epithelial structures
CD99 expression	No	>95%	25%	65%
Focal keratin or epithelial membrane antigen expression	Not much	30%	50%	90%
Myogenin expression	Yes	—	>95%	—
FLI1 expression	Rather useful	90%	—	—
Fluorescence in situ hybridization analysis	Yes	*EWSR1* break-apart probes	*FOXO1A* break-apart probes	*SS18* break-apart probes
Reverse transcriptase-polymerase chain reaction	Yes	*EWSR1-FLI1/ERG*	*PAX3/PAX7-FOXO1A*	*SS18-SSX1/2*

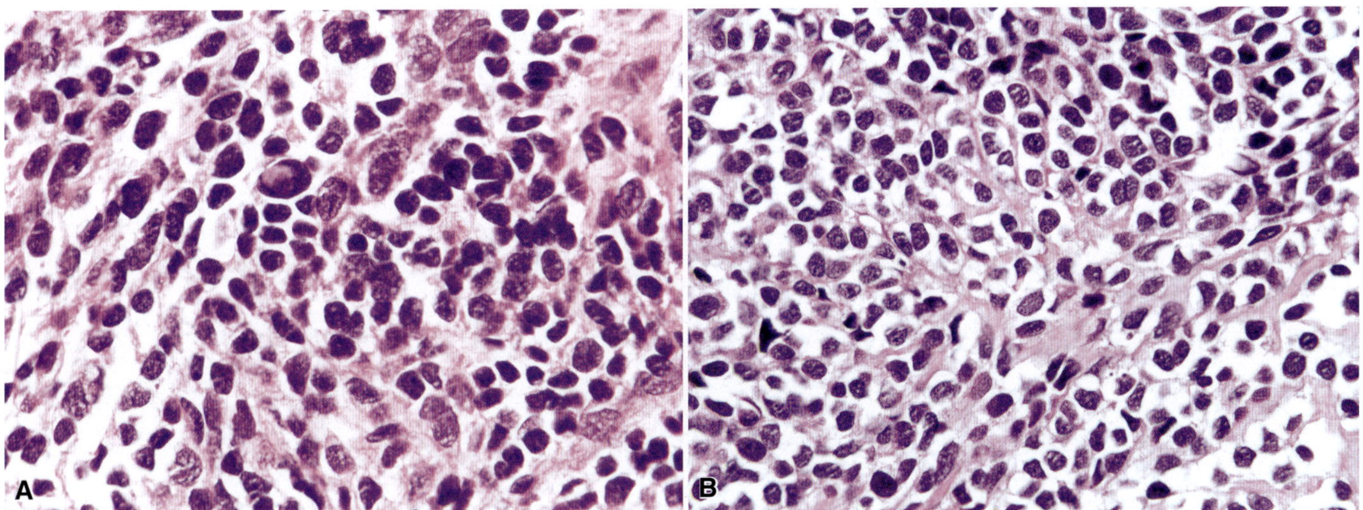

Figure 8.8 **Small Cell Osteosarcoma.** (A) Soft tissue invasion by a small round cell tumor located in the femur of a 13-year-old boy. Mild pleomorphism and nuclear hyperchromasia suggest the diagnosis of small cell osteosarcoma; compare the chromatin quality with that seen in Fig. 8.5. (B) Osteoid produced by tumor cells was found after thorough sampling of the specimen, confirming the diagnosis of small cell osteosarcoma.

Neuroblastoma typically lacks CD99 expression and translocations involving the *EWSR1* gene, whereas the nuclear transcription factor PHOX2B is specific for neuroblastoma in this differential diagnosis.[26]

Ewing sarcoma can arise in the kidney. At this site, monophasic blastemal Wilms tumors can enter the differential diagnosis. Again, age is of help, because 90% of Wilms tumors arise before 6 years of age, which would be very uncommon for Ewing sarcoma. In addition, Wilms tumors lack rearrangements involving the *EWSR1* gene and are typically negative for NKX2-2.

Prognosis and Treatment

Prognostic factors in Ewing sarcoma include stage, tumor location and volume, age, and response to induction chemotherapy.[10]

Multimodal approaches within clinical trials, employing combination chemotherapy and surgery or radiation therapy, have improved 5-year survival rates from less than 10% to close to 80%. Current standard trials employ 3 to 6 cycles of initial chemotherapy after biopsy, followed by local therapy and another 6 to 10 cycles of chemotherapy. Local control is attempted by surgery or radiation therapy (if complete surgical resection is impossible) or if histologic response in the surgical specimen was poor (i.e., >10% viable tumor cells).[4] Patients with extraskeletal Ewing sarcoma have a better prognosis than those with osseous Ewing sarcoma independent of age, ethnic group, or primary site.[9]

Alveolar Rhabdomyosarcoma

Rhabdomyosarcoma is the most common soft tissue sarcoma in children and adolescents. On the basis of histologic criteria, rhabdomyosarcomas in this age group are classified into two major subgroups, the more common embryonal rhabdomyosarcoma (60%) and the rarer alveolar rhabdomyosarcoma (20%). Embryonal rhabdomyosarcoma is associated with a more favorable prognosis.[27] Alveolar rhabdomyosarcoma is a prototypical round cell sarcoma and is discussed first.

Clinical Features

Alveolar rhabdomyosarcoma usually arises in the extremities (typically, the forearm) or in the head and neck, trunk, or pelvic area of adolescents and young adults, with a peak between 10 and 25 years of age.

Pathologic Features

Alveolar rhabdomyosarcoma is composed of small round cells that are attached to connective tissue septa. Formalin fixation induces an artifact in the form of partial cell detachment from these septa, giving the tumor its classic microcystic or alveolar appearance. Depending on the amount of intervening stroma, cells grow in nests or cords/trabeculae with either nascent (microalveolar) or frank central cystic change (Fig. 8.9A). Sometimes this artifact is not observed, in which case alveolar rhabdomyosarcoma has a paradoxically solid appearance ("solid" alveolar rhabdomyosarcoma). This variant is particularly difficult to diagnose because it can be mistaken for many other tumor types in this age group (see Fig. 8.9B).[27] The tumor cells are monomorphic and large, with characteristic nuclear features, either nuclei with coarse chromatin and prominent nucleoli or evenly distributed chromatin (see Fig. 8.9C). Prominent wreath-like tumor giant cells are seen in a subset of cases of alveolar rhabdomyosarcoma. Rare cases show marked clear cell change (Fig. 8.10).

The 2013 WHO classification of skeletal muscle neoplasms includes a type of rhabdomyosarcoma, the sclerosing variant, which is not strictly a small round cell tumor.[28,29] Sclerosing rhabdomyosarcoma is characterized by rounded cells with a microalveolar or cord-like pattern embedded in a hyalinized, matrix-rich stroma (Fig. 8.11). This variant is closely related to spindle cell rhabdomyosarcoma, showing overlapping clinical and pathological features; in addition, both variants share *MYOD1* point mutations.[30] The 2013 WHO classification considers them as a single entity, different from embryonal and alveolar rhabdomyosarcomas. However, spindle cell/sclerosing rhabdomyosarcoma is a heterogeneous genetic group of tumors among different age groups.[31]

Immunohistochemistry

Immunohistochemistry is a very helpful technique to diagnose this particular tumor type because of the specificity of several available antibodies, namely, myogenin (Myf4) and MyoD1. MyoD1 and myogenin are nuclear transcription factors; their expression is specific for skeletal muscle differentiation.[32] Therefore only nuclear staining should be considered a positive result. Stronger and more uniform myogenin expression is seen in alveolar rhabdomyosarcoma compared with embryonal rhabdomyosarcoma (Fig. 8.12). Diffuse myogenin expression by immunohistochemistry is an unfavorable prognostic factor in rhabdomyosarcoma, independent of histologic features and the presence of fusion genes (discussed later).[33] In addition, alveolar rhabdomyosarcoma usually shows strong, diffuse reactivity for desmin and muscle-specific actin. A subset of cases express keratins or neuroendocrine markers (especially synaptophysin), which can lead to their misdiagnosis as neuroendocrine carcinoma, particularly when tumors arise in the

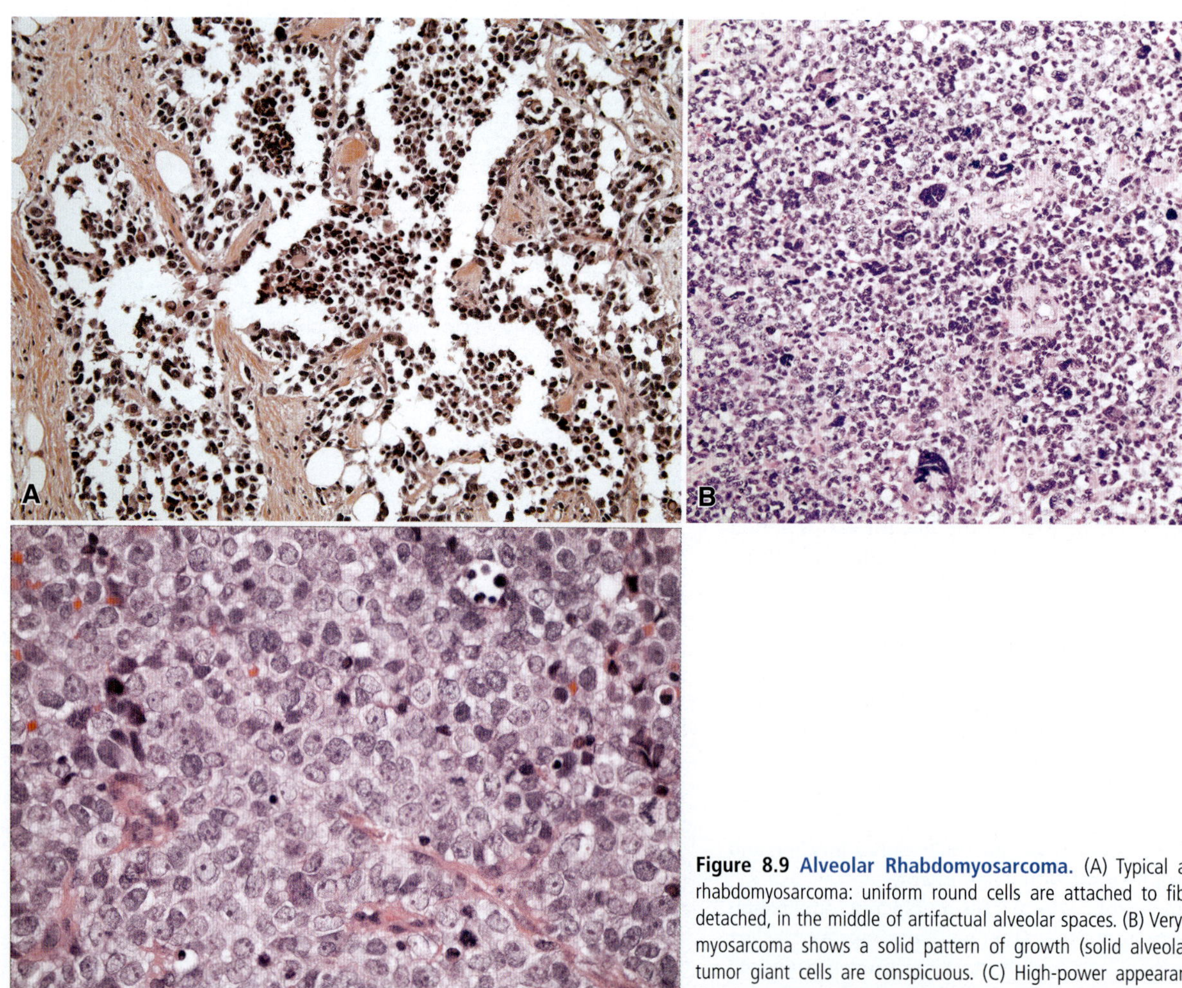

Figure 8.9 Alveolar Rhabdomyosarcoma. (A) Typical appearance of alveolar rhabdomyosarcoma: uniform round cells are attached to fibrous septa, or appear detached, in the middle of artifactual alveolar spaces. (B) Very often alveolar rhabdomyosarcoma shows a solid pattern of growth (solid alveolar rhabdomyosarcoma); tumor giant cells are conspicuous. (C) High-power appearance of a solid alveolar rhabdomyosarcoma composed of uniform large cells with even chromatin and prominent nucleoli. Note the resemblance to Ewing sarcoma.

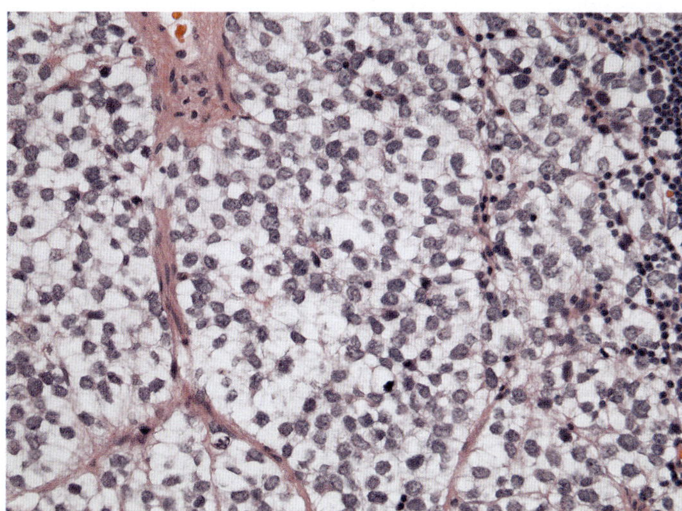

Figure 8.10 Alveolar Rhabdomyosarcoma. Rare cases of alveolar rhabdomyosarcoma show striking clear cell change.

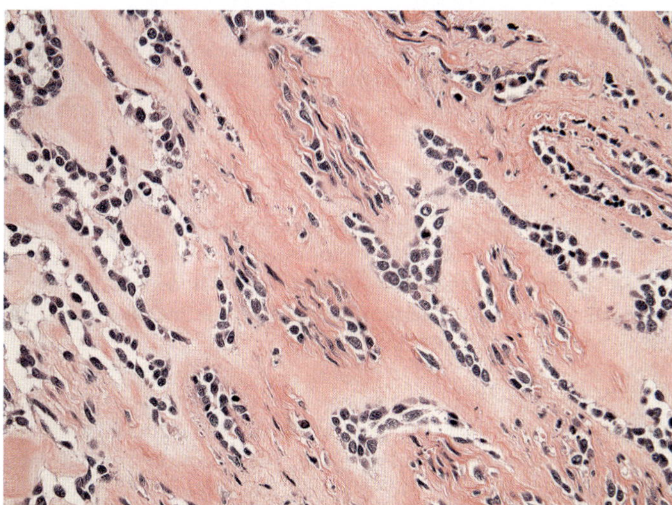

Figure 8.11 Sclerosing Rhabdomyosarcoma. Rhabdomyoblastic tumor cells embedded in a densely sclerotic stroma, showing a pseudovascular growth pattern much smaller than the usual alveolar spaces of alveolar rhabdomyosarcoma. This tumor was negative for *FOXO1A* gene rearrangements.

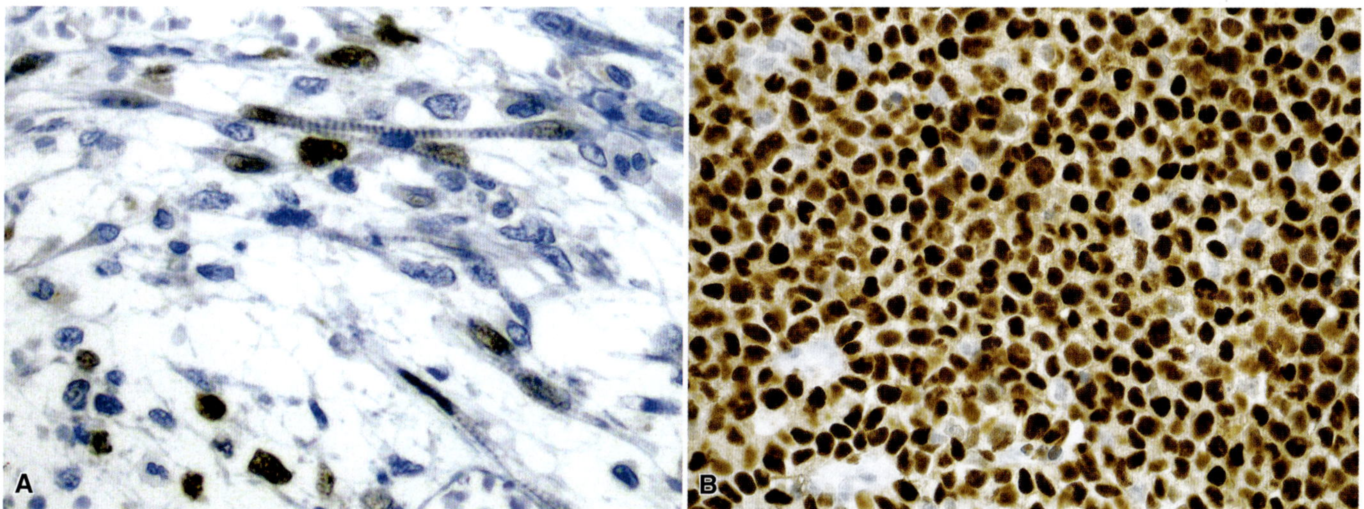

Figure 8.12 Myogenin in Rhabdomyosarcoma. (A) All rhabdomyosarcomas show nuclear expression of myogenin; in this embryonal rhabdomyosarcoma, expression of myogenin is more intense in undifferentiated cells than in those showing well-developed cross striations. (B) Expression of myogenin is more extensive in alveolar rhabdomyosarcoma than in embryonal rhabdomyosarcoma.

sinonasal region in adults.[34] PAX7 has been reported as a potential immunohistochemical marker of skeletal muscle differentiation, with the only exception being Ewing sarcoma; PAX7 was negative in 99.7% of a large series of small round cell tumors other than rhabdomyosarcoma.[35]

Molecular Genetics

Approximately 80% of alveolar rhabdomyosarcomas are associated with recurrent chromosomal translocations, including t(2;13) (60%) and less commonly, t(1;13) (20%), which result in fusion of the *PAX3* and *PAX7* genes, respectively, to the *FOXO1A* gene located at 13q14 (previously designated *FKHR*, or forkhead in rhabdomyosarcoma). Fusions can be detected routinely by FISH or RT-PCR.[36] Fusion gene amplification has been detected in some tumors with *PAX7-FOXO1A* fusions, suggesting that translocation and amplification might be not only sequential but also complementary mechanisms in the genesis of this neoplasm. *PAX7-FOXO1A* tumors tend to arise in younger patients and are usually associated with lower metastatic rates and better survival compared with those with *PAX3-FOXO1A* fusions despite having similar morphologic features.[37]

The remaining 20% of alveolar rhabdomyosarcomas lack the usual translocations ("fusion-negative" alveolar rhabdomyosarcoma) and form a more heterogeneous, unexplored group. Distinguishing between this group and embryonal rhabdomyosarcoma based on histologic features is challenging because of the lack of discriminatory immunohistochemical or molecular markers. Gene expression studies have been of help to further explore this subgroup of tumors.[38] This group includes (1) those with cryptic *PAX3* or *PAX7* fusions or low expression levels of "normal" fusions that cannot be identified by classic PCR-based diagnostics; (2) those with alternative rare fusions, such as *PAX3-NCOA1* or *PAX3-AFX*; and (3) truly fusion-negative tumors. The only morphologic factors that may be associated with the absence of a translocation in alveolar rhabdomyosarcoma are the presence of extensive solid foci and "mixed" alveolar and embryonal patterns.[39] Most but not all sclerosing rhabdomyosarcomas are also fusion-negative (and instead harbor *MYOD1* mutations, as mentioned earlier).[40] Clinical outcomes of this translocation-negative subtype are as favorable as those of embryonal rhabdomyosarcoma.[41] Analyses of gene expression microarray data have helped distinguish fusion status in rhabdomyosarcoma by the use of surrogate immunohistochemical markers. These include myogenin, AP2β, NOS-1, and HMGA2.[42]

Differential Diagnosis

Morphologic clues to alveolar rhabdomyosarcoma include wreath-like giant cells and mildly eccentric nuclei. Distinction between alveolar rhabdomyosarcoma and other round cell sarcomas is shown in Table 8.3. However, the distinction from embryonal rhabdomyosarcoma can be difficult, especially with either the solid variant of alveolar rhabdomyosarcoma or a translocation-negative alveolar rhabdomyosarcoma. Histologically, embryonal rhabdomyosarcoma usually shows some degree of intratumoral heterogeneity, including small undifferentiated round cells and spindle cells, in contrast to the uniform appearance and larger cells of alveolar rhabdomyosarcoma. As already mentioned, the extent of staining for myogenin can be helpful in distinguishing between these tumor types because myogenin typically shows uniform, strong expression in alveolar rhabdomyosarcoma, whereas heterogeneous staining in a subset of cells is typical of embryonal rhabdomyosarcoma (see Fig. 8.12). Gene expression studies, followed by immunohistochemical confirmation of tumor samples, have suggested that the combined expression of AP2β and P-cadherin may be specific for fusion-positive alveolar rhabdomyosarcoma, whereas the combined expression of epidermal growth factor receptor and fibrillin-2 may be specific for embryonal rhabdomyosarcoma.[42] These findings require confirmation in additional studies.

Prognosis and Treatment

The prognosis of alveolar rhabdomyosarcoma is much worse than that of embryonal rhabdomyosarcoma, even with the currently available treatment modalities. Spindle cell/sclerosing pediatric or adult rhabdomyosarcomas with *MYOD1* mutations (with or without *PIK3CA* mutations) have a very aggressive behavior. In contrast, infantile/congenital spindle cell rhabdomyosarcomas with *VGLL2* or *NCOA2* rearrangements carry an excellent prognosis.[31] The most frequent metastatic sites include the lung and lymph nodes. Treatment includes initial first-line chemotherapy, followed by alternate second-line chemotherapy in the event of a poor response to initial treatment. Most groups also include radiation therapy for alveolar rhabdomyosarcoma.

Embryonal Rhabdomyosarcoma

Clinical Features

Embryonal rhabdomyosarcoma appears to arise from the undifferentiated mesoderm, most commonly in the head and neck region (orbit, nasopharynx, oral cavity, and ear), genitourinary tract, retroperitoneum, and biliary tract. This tumor type is uncommon in the somatic soft tissues of the extremities and in the skin. The typical age at presentation is 3 to 12 years.

Pathologic Features

Grossly, an ill-defined, whitish, friable tumor is seen. When growing beneath a mucosal surface, such as in the bladder, vagina, or upper respiratory tract, it often shows a polypoid, grape-like ("botryoid") appearance. Classically named *botryoid sarcoma*, this form of rhabdomyosarcoma is currently considered a clinicopathologic variant of embryonal rhabdomyosarcoma; it has an excellent prognosis.

Histologically, the tumor cells are small and variably rounded or spindle-shaped (Fig. 8.13), a small subset of which usually shows dense, eosinophilic cytoplasm. In some better-differentiated cases, cross-striations may be seen (Fig. 8.14), but this finding is not always present and other histologic features should be considered. A helpful diagnostic clue is a tendency toward perivascular cellular condensation, in contrast to other hypocellular myxoid areas. A classic and useful finding, specific to the botryoid subtype, is the densely cellular "cambium layer" immediately beneath the mucosa. Less commonly, embryonal rhabdomyosarcoma may contain scattered large and irregular cells, leading to a more anaplastic appearance (Fig. 8.15).

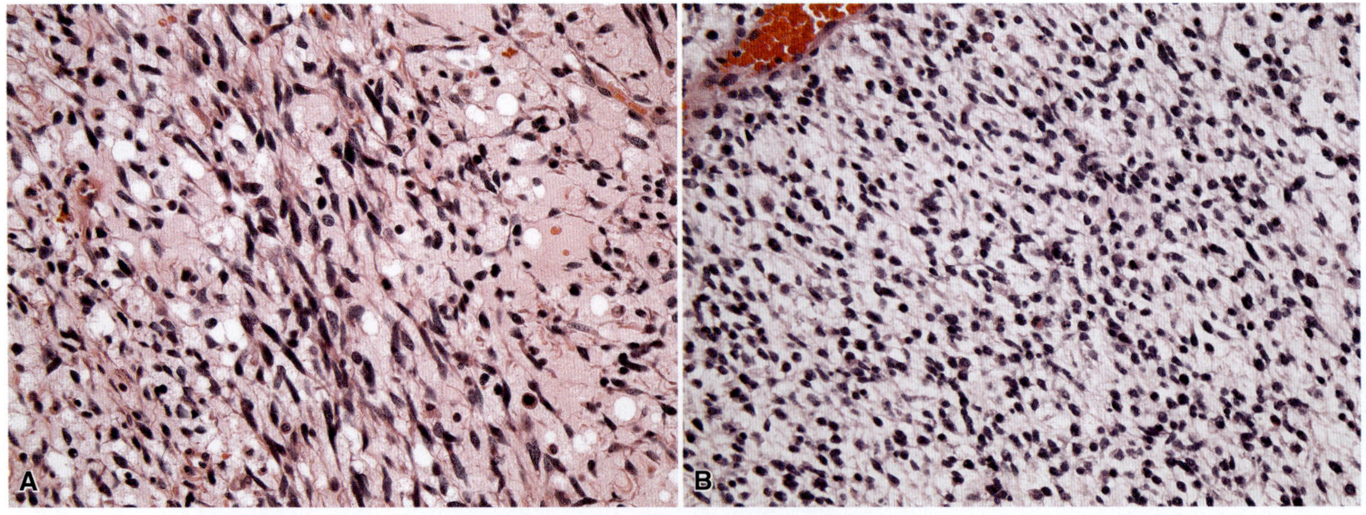

Figure 8.13 Embryonal Rhabdomyosarcoma. (A) The classic appearance of embryonal rhabdomyosarcoma is that of a round to spindle cell sarcoma with abundant loose myxoid stroma. (B) This example shows a more undifferentiated appearance.

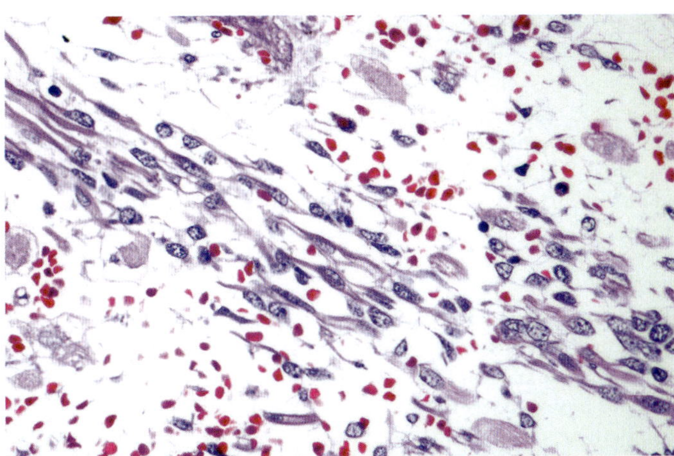

Figure 8.14 Embryonal Rhabdomyosarcoma. The cytoplasm of occasional tumor cells has a fibrillary quality, and cross striations are sometimes seen.

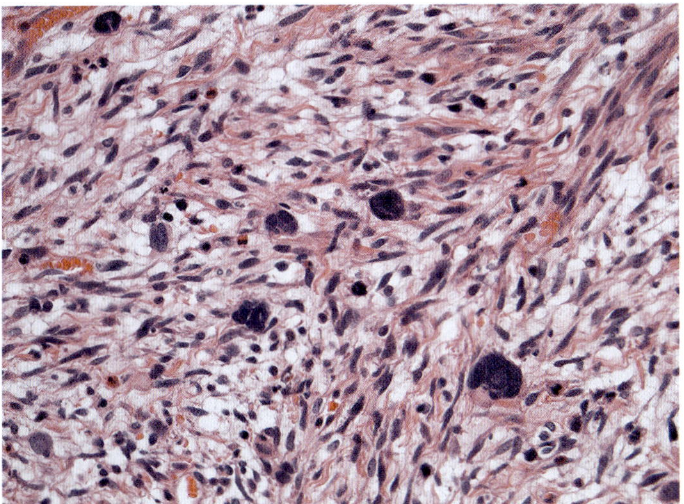

Figure 8.15 Embryonal Rhabdomyosarcoma. Scattered large pleomorphic ("anaplastic") cells in an embryonal rhabdomyosarcoma.

Immunohistochemistry

See the earlier discussion of alveolar rhabdomyosarcoma.

Molecular Genetics

No specific molecular genetic features of diagnostic utility have been identified in embryonal rhabdomyosarcoma. The absence of a transloca-tion in a rhabdomyosarcoma, however, is not synonymous with the embryonal subtype, because at least 20% of alveolar rhabdomyosarcomas are translocation-negative (discussed earlier in the molecular genetics section of alveolar rhabdomyosarcoma).

Differential Diagnosis

See the earlier discussion of alveolar rhabdomyosarcoma.

Prognosis and Treatment

The prognosis of embryonal rhabdomyosarcoma is very favorable when no metastatic disease is present. The most common sites of metastasis are the lung, soft tissues, serosal surfaces, and lymph nodes. Lymph nodes are the most common site of metastasis for pelvic and extremity tumors. Besides the botryoid subtype, another subtype associated with an excellent prognosis in the pediatric group is spindle cell rhabdo-myosarcoma, which usually arises in the paratesticular region and in which spindle-shaped tumor cells are arranged in long fascicles (see Chapter 4).[31,41]

Treatment includes first-line chemotherapy followed by alternate second-line chemotherapy in the event of a poor response to initial treatment. There is some debate among different groups regarding the timing and intensity of local therapy. Surgical resection is the preferred local therapy, with radiation therapy used only after incomplete surgical resection, documented nodal involvement, or poor clinical response to combination chemotherapy.

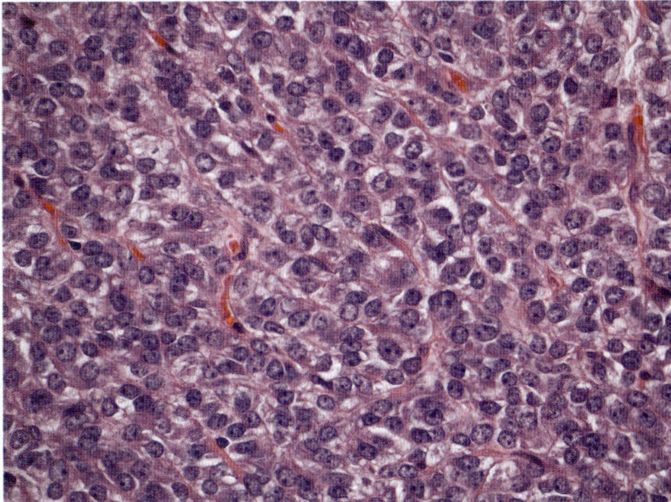

Figure 8.16 Round Cell Liposarcoma. Hypercellular/round cell areas are commonly observed in myxoid liposarcoma, but relatively pure round cell tumors, such as the one depicted, are seldom seen. The plexiform ("crow's feet") vascular pattern is a helpful clue to the correct diagnosis.

"Round Cell" Liposarcoma

Pure "round cell" liposarcoma is a rare variant of myxoid liposarcoma in which hypercellularity or round cell morphologic features account for the majority of the tumor tissue (Fig. 8.16). Most frequently, early foci of hypercellularity begin to form in a perivascular distribution; a 5% cutoff has been proposed as a helpful marker of poor prognosis. Because transition to hypercellular/round cell areas is commonly observed in typical myxoid liposarcoma and myxoid and round cell liposarcoma share the same characteristic chromosome translocations, this distinction was abandoned in the 2002 World Health Organization classification of soft tissue tumors; round cell liposarcoma is now referred to as high-grade myxoid liposarcoma in the 2013 classification.[1] This topic is discussed in detail in Chapter 12.

Desmoplastic Small Round Cell Tumor

DSRCT is a rare, poorly understood, aggressive neoplasm with distinctive clinical, histologic, immunophenotypic, and cytogenetic features.[43] It affects mainly children and adolescent males, usually in the form of widespread intraabdominal growth unrelated to any organ system.

Clinical Features

There is a striking male predominance (>85%), with age at presentation ranging from 6 to 79 years (mean 22 years). Presenting symptoms and signs are usually related to the primary site of tumor involvement and include pain, distention, palpable mass, acute abdomen, ascites, and obstruction of organs, such as the esophagus, bowel, ureter, or bile duct.[44] Some patients (~5%) present with tumor outside the abdominal cavity. The most prevalent sites outside the abdomen include the thoracic cavity, lung, kidney, lymph node, hand, and posterior cranial fossa.[44]

Pathologic Features

Histologically, DSRCT is typically characterized by angulated nests of small round cells within an abundant desmoplastic stroma (Fig. 8.17). The stroma contains a prominent component of spindle-shaped fibroblasts and myofibroblasts embedded in a matrix of loose or myxoid extracellular material and collagen. Prominent stromal vascularity is also present, suggesting a hyperplastic response induced by the tumor.[43] However, there are considerable variations in the histologic appearance.[44] The degree of cellularity can vary significantly from tiny clusters to large sheet-like expanses. Central necrosis and cystic degeneration are common. In some cases, a more infiltrative pattern is present, particularly in association with areas of necrosis and after antineoplastic therapy. Occasional tumors exhibit a definite epithelial architecture focally, with a glandular, rosette-like, or trabecular arrangement, but this is rarely a prominent feature.

Immunohistochemistry

The tumor cells show polyphenotypic differentiation, expressing epithelial, muscle, and neural markers. The majority of cases are immunoreactive with antibodies to keratin, epithelial membrane antigen (EMA), vimentin, desmin, and neuron-specific enolase. Other muscle-specific antigens, including muscle-specific actin and myogenin, are not detected in DSRCT. CD99, when present, usually shows a cytoplasmic pattern of expression instead of the typical membranous staining pattern of Ewing sarcoma.[44] Because the *EWSR1-WT1* fusion gene (discussed later) leads to overexpression of a fusion protein that includes a truncated WT1 protein, immunohistochemistry using antibodies directed against the C-terminus of WT1 may be helpful,[45] although the available antibodies show somewhat inconsistent results.

Molecular Genetics

In DSRCT, the *EWSR1* gene is fused to the *WT1* gene. *WT1* was initially described as a tumor suppressor gene in Wilms tumor. In fact, *EWSR1-WT1* is the first example of a constant rearrangement involving a tumor suppressor gene. The *EWSR1-WT1* chimeric transcript has been found in 97% of studied cases, which makes this a very useful diagnostic marker.[46] It also suggests that the chimeric protein is important for tumor development. As in many other sarcoma types, this chimeric protein acts as an aberrant transcription factor, which modulates the expression of genes that coincide, at least partially, with *WT1* gene targets.

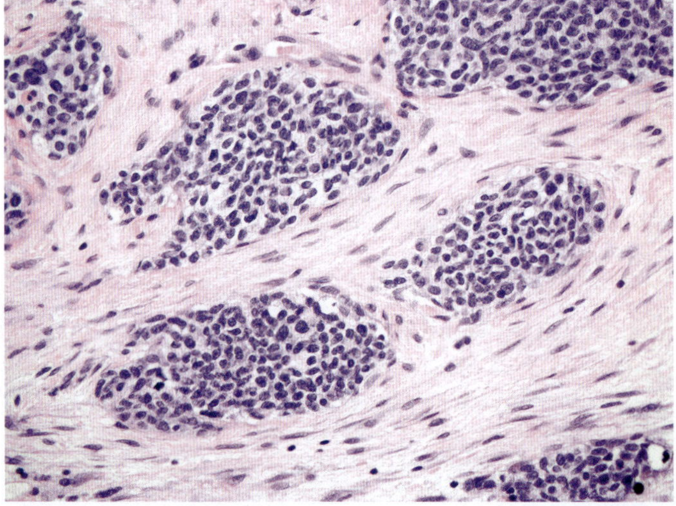

Figure 8.17 Desmoplastic Small Round Cell Tumor. Classic appearance, with sharply demarcated nests of small round cells within a desmoplastic stroma containing spindle-shaped myofibroblasts embedded in a matrix of loose or myxoid extracellular material and collagen.

Differential Diagnosis

The differential diagnosis for DSRCT includes other round cell sarcomas, especially Ewing sarcoma and alveolar rhabdomyosarcoma.[47] Although both Ewing sarcoma and DSRCT can express keratins and CD99, Ewing sarcoma rarely shows diffuse staining for keratins, and the distinct membranous pattern of CD99 expression typical of Ewing sarcoma is very rarely seen in DSRCT; nuclear staining for NKX2-2 favors Ewing sarcoma.[19,21] Immunoreactivity for desmin and EMA supports the diagnosis of DSRCT. When attempting to differentiate between Ewing sarcoma and DSRCT by molecular diagnostic approaches, it is important to identify the partner gene to *EWSR1* by RT-PCR. FISH with *EWSR1* break-apart probes is not useful for this purpose, because gene fusions in both tumor types share *EWSR1* as a fusion partner. Alveolar rhabdomyosarcoma rarely arises in the abdomen and pelvis, where DSRCT is most common. Although both tumor types show extensive expression of desmin, only alveolar rhabdomyosarcoma is positive for myogenin. DSRCT rarely affects older adults; metastatic neuroendocrine carcinoma (which is much more common in this age group) could also be considered, especially because both tumor types express epithelial markers. Reactivity for chromogranin favors a neuroendocrine carcinoma, whereas desmin expression is not observed in this tumor type.

Prognosis and Treatment

Experience indicates that aggressive multimodal therapy—including surgical debulking, multiagent chemotherapy, and whole abdominopelvic intensity-modulated radiation therapy (IMRT)—improves tumor control. Overall survival remains poor.[47]

Poorly Differentiated Synovial Sarcoma, Round Cell Variant

Clinical Features

The round cell variant of poorly differentiated synovial sarcoma usually arises in deep soft tissues of the limbs, more frequently in male patients averaging 30 to 35 years of age.[48]

Pathologic Features

The classic patterns of monophasic and biphasic synovial sarcomas are described in Chapters 3 and 9, respectively. Poorly differentiated synovial sarcoma has three morphologic subvariants: the most common round cell variant, a large cell epithelioid variant, and a high-grade spindle cell variant. The round cell variant of poorly differentiated synovial sarcoma, compared with other synovial sarcoma variants, more frequently shows necrosis, a high mitotic rate (>10 mitoses per 10 high-power fields), vascular invasion, and a hemangiopericytoma-like pattern of growth (Fig. 8.18).[49]

Immunohistochemistry

The immunohistochemical profile of poorly differentiated synovial sarcoma, round cell variant, is similar to that of more conventional subtypes; patchy expression of EMA and keratin in scattered cells is typical. TLE1 is a highly sensitive and moderately specific marker of synovial sarcoma; greater than 90% of poorly differentiated synovial

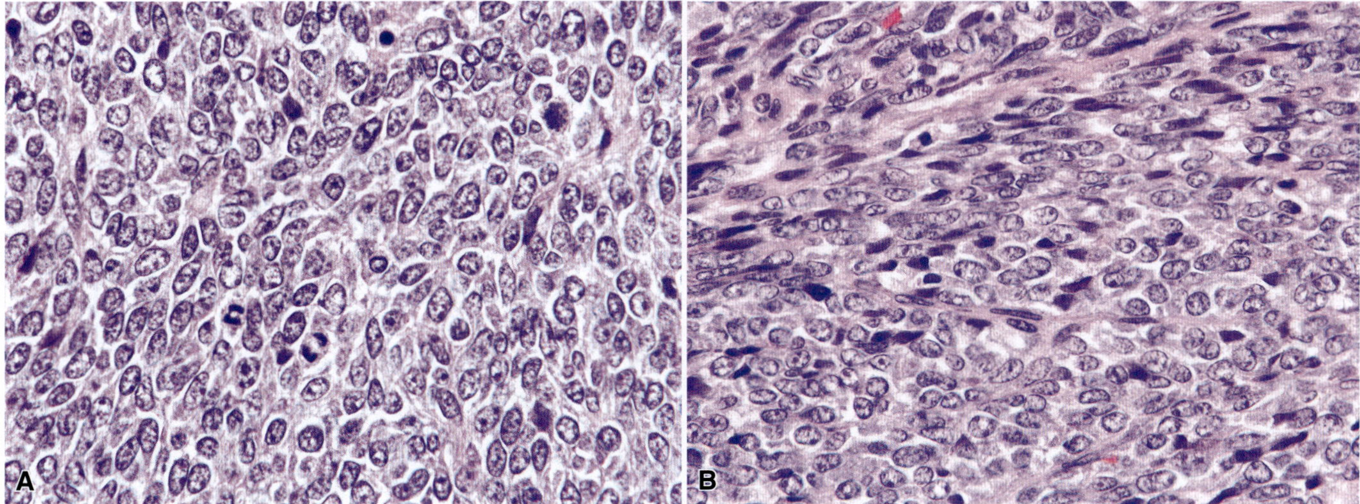

Figure 8.18 Poorly Differentiated Synovial Sarcoma. (A) This neoplasm is composed of small round cells. Subtle spindling is often at least focally present. (B) Transition to an overt spindle cell pattern is sometimes present, especially when extensive sampling is performed.

sarcomas show strong nuclear staining.[2,50,51] CD99 expression can become a source of diagnostic confusion because it is also expressed in Ewing sarcoma. Molecular studies can resolve this dilemma.[52]

Molecular Genetics

Synovial sarcoma has a characteristic chromosomal translocation, t(X;18), which results in fusion of the *SS18* (*SYT*) gene at chromosome 18 to *SSX* genes; these have two different copies, *SSX1* and *SSX2*, located in two subregions of chromosome Xp11 (23 and 21, respectively). Some rarer fusions also exist. Transcripts are detected in almost all synovial sarcomas with RT-PCR. Synovial sarcoma provides a clear example of the correlation that can exist between the fusion transcript type and tumor phenotype. Interestingly, *SS18-SSX1* fusions are associated with biphasic synovial sarcoma (in both epithelioid and spindle cell elements), whereas the monophasic variant usually contains *SS18-SSX2* fusions. No significant correlations exist between the round cell variant of poorly differentiated synovial sarcoma and a specific transcript subtype.[53]

Differential Diagnosis

The most important differential diagnosis for the round cell variant of poorly differentiated synovial sarcoma is Ewing sarcoma, as previously discussed, especially because of the lack of a specific immunohistochemical profile, other than TLE1, which is relatively specific for synovial sarcoma in this differential diagnosis. EMA and keratin expression in poorly differentiated synovial sarcoma can be limited, and these markers may be completely negative in small biopsy specimens. As discussed earlier, a subset of Ewing sarcomas are positive for keratin. NKX2-2 is consistently positive in Ewing sarcoma but rarely positive in poorly differentiated synovial sarcoma. Although the diffuse membranous pattern of CD99 staining is characteristic of Ewing sarcoma, synovial sarcoma can also be positive, albeit usually with a more cytoplasmic pattern. Again, in small samples (e.g., needle biopsy specimens), the pattern of CD99 staining may be equivocal. In this context, molecular testing is crucial, not only for proper diagnosis but also for treatment strategies or protocol inclusion (especially for Ewing sarcoma).

Prognosis and Treatment

Poorly differentiated synovial sarcoma has an especially poor prognosis, with an even higher metastatic rate than conventional forms of synovial sarcoma.[53]

Undifferentiated Round Cell Sarcomas

Occasional round cell tumors encountered in soft tissue lack any identifiable clues as to their lineage, and, even after extensive immunohistochemical and molecular genetic investigations, these tumors have been classified as *undifferentiated*. These are rare tumors, as attested by the fact that only 8% of pediatric sarcomas in the Intergroup Rhabdomyosarcoma Study III and Intergroup Rhabdomyosarcoma Study IV pilot series were classified as undifferentiated soft tissue sarcomas with the use of immunohistochemistry and without molecular pathology.[22] This category also includes some sarcomas with spindle cell morphology, similar to infantile fibrosarcoma. The incidence of undifferentiated (round cell or spindle cell) sarcomas in adults is unknown. The increasing use of next-generation sequencing techniques has defined a growing number of new gene fusions in these categories. This is especially true in the area of small round cell sarcomas negative for *EWSR1* or *FUS* rearrangements, with morphologic features that do not fit perfectly with Ewing sarcoma (reviewed in references 22 and 54). These tumors are collectively referred to as Ewing-like sarcomas in the current WHO classification[7]; they are the main subject of this section.

CIC-Rearranged Sarcomas

About two thirds of Ewing-like sarcomas harbor *CIC* gene rearrangements, either *CIC-DUX4* (by far the most common) or *CIC-FOXO4* fusions; some tumors have *CIC* rearrangements with unknown fusion partners. Tumors with *CIC* rearrangements show similar clinical presentations and histologic findings. A recent review summarizes the current experience with this neoplasm.[54] Most affected patients are between 20 and 40 years of age; these tumors arise almost exclusively at extraskeletal locations, although visceral and bone cases have also been reported.[55-57] Histologically, clues suggesting a possible diagnosis of *CIC*-rearranged sarcoma (as opposed to Ewing sarcoma) include increased heterogeneity in nuclear shape and size, more prominent nuclei, more abundant cytoplasm, and focal spindle cell or epithelioid morphology, with areas of myxoid or fibrous stroma (Fig. 8.19A). No rosette formation is seen.[55,56] However, the differential diagnosis with atypical Ewing sarcoma with *EWSR1* rearrangements relies heavily on immunohistochemistry and molecular genetics. CD99 expression is observed in most cases, ranging from strong and diffuse membranous staining similar to Ewing sarcoma to patchy cytoplasmic staining. Three potentially useful

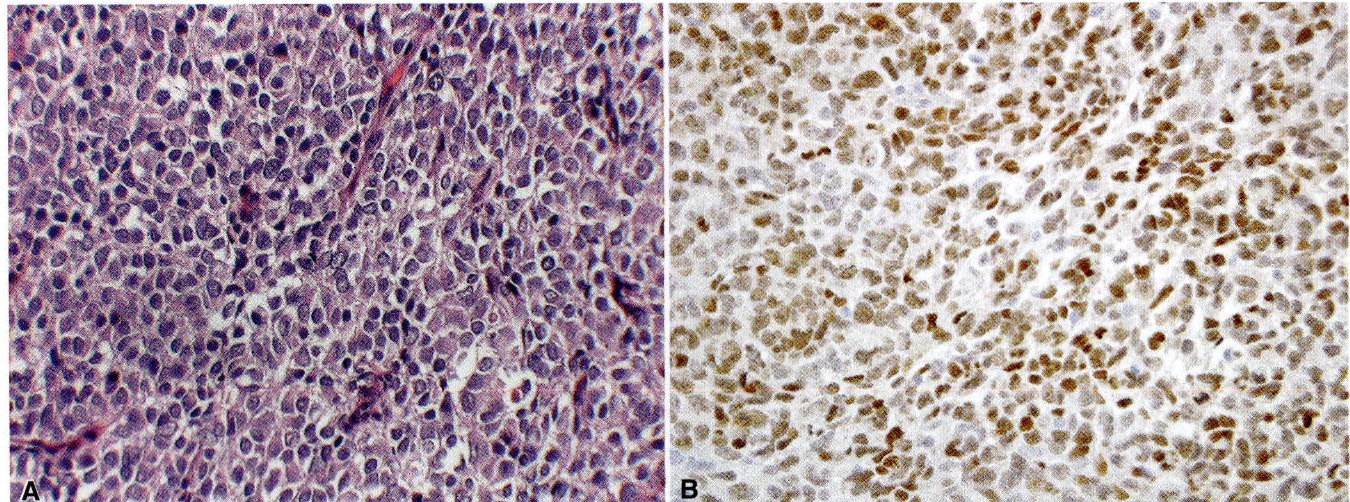

Figure 8.19 ***CIC*-Rearranged Sarcoma.** (A) Small round cell sarcoma of soft tissue with increased heterogeneity in nuclear shape and size and relatively abundant cytoplasm. (B) Nuclear expression of ETV4 is characteristic of *CIC*-rearranged sarcomas.

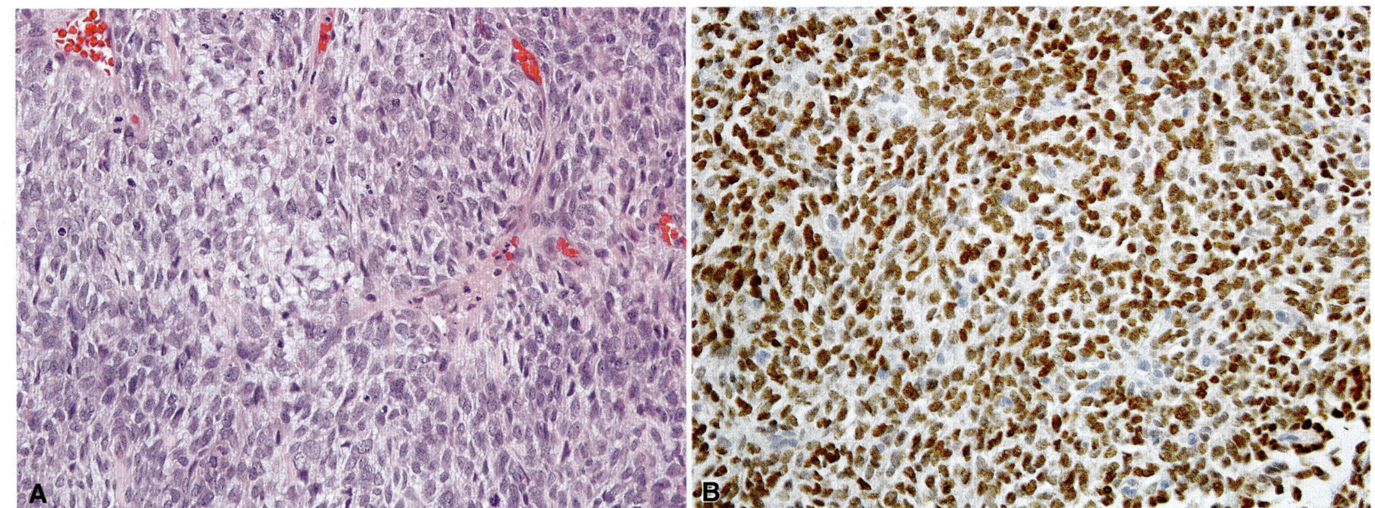

Figure 8.20 ***BCOR*-Rearranged Sarcoma** (A) This tumor is composed of an admixture of round cells and short spindle cells with fine chromatin in a scant myxoid stroma. (B) Nuclear immunoreactivity for CCNB3 is observed in tumors with *BCOR-CCNB3* fusion.

immunohistochemical markers for *CIC*-rearranged sarcoma are WT1, ETV4 (see Fig. 8.19B), and DUX4 (all nuclear).[22,57-59] Therefore a diagnosis of *CIC*-rearranged sarcoma should be suspected in a young adult with an extraskeletal small round cell sarcoma negative for *EWSR1* or *FUS* rearrangements with extensive ETV4 and WT1 expression and patchy CD99 expression. FISH analysis or sequencing (conventional or next-generation) can be used to confirm the diagnosis. The prognosis of *CIC*-rearranged sarcoma is significantly worse than that of Ewing sarcoma.[60] The aggressive nature of these neoplasms suggests that affected patients should be treated according to Ewing sarcoma protocols instead of conventional adult soft tissue sarcoma treatment protocols until better therapeutic strategies are developed.

BCOR-Rearranged Sarcomas

These tumors (first reported with *BCOR-CCNB3* fusion)[61] account for around 5% of all *EWSR1* and *FUS* rearrangement negative Ewing-like sarcomas; the initial clinical experience with small series of cases suggested that such neoplasms share similarities with Ewing sarcoma, such as their occurrence in the long bones or pelvises of teenagers (rare cases presenting in soft tissue have also been reported). Nevertheless, clear differences from Ewing sarcoma are also evident, such as a strong male predilection and a less aggressive clinical course for *BCOR-CCNB3* sarcomas as well as a distinct gene expression profile without a *EWSR1-ETS* expression signature. Other *BCOR* gene fusion partners in addition to *CCNB3*, such as *MAML3* and *ZC3H7B*, have also been described.[62] Sarcomas with *BCOR* rearrangements with unknown partners have also been reported, hence the collective term *BCOR-rearranged sarcomas* could be used.[54] Histologically, clues to the diagnosis of *BCOR*-rearranged sarcomas include a bone neoplasm with a uniform small round to ovoid tumor cell proliferation intermixed with a spindle cell component (Fig. 8.20A). CD99 expression is usually strong but can be patchy. Nuclear CCNB3 expression by immunohistochemistry is seen in *BCOR-CCNB3* cases (see Fig. 8.20B)[61]; nuclear BCOR expression is observed in *BCOR*-rearranged sarcomas irrespective of the fusion partner (in addition to the rare sarcomas with *BCOR* internal tandem duplication and those with *YWHAE-NUTM2B* fusions, including primitive myxoid mesenchymal tumor of infancy and clear cell sarcoma of the kidney).[63] Therefore a diagnosis of *BCOR*-rearranged sarcoma should be suspected in a teenager with a bone sarcoma with morphology similar to that of Ewing sarcoma but with focal spindle cell morphology, negative for *EWSR1* and *FUS* rearrangements, with CCNB3 and/or BCOR expression, and patchy staining for CD99. The clinical and histologic overlap of poorly differentiated synovial sarcoma with soft tissue *BCOR*-rearranged sarcoma is a potential pitfall.[64] Molecular analysis should be used to confirm the diagnosis. The limited number of reported cases seems to show a more favorable prognosis than that of Ewing sarcoma.

Despite thorough immunohistochemical and molecular studies of undifferentiated/unclassified sarcomas, some tumors still remain in this WHO category.[1,22] Next-generation sequencing technologies as well as new FISH-based assays will likely identify additional novel gene fusions and help better subclassify undifferentiated sarcomas with round cell morphology.

References

1. Fletcher CDM, Bridge JA, Hogendoorn PCW, et al, editors: *WHO classification of tumours of soft tissue and bone*, Lyon, France, 2013, IARC Press.
2. Hornick JL: Novel uses of immunohistochemistry in the diagnosis and classification of soft tissue tumors, *Mod Pathol* 27:S47–S63, 2014.
3. Marino-Enriquez A: Advances in the molecular analysis of soft tissue tumors and clinical implications, *Surg Pathol Clin* 8:525–537, 2015.
4. ESMO/European Sarcoma Network Working Group: Bone sarcomas: ESMO Clinical Practice Guidelines for diagnosis, treatment and follow-up, *Ann Oncol* 25(Suppl 3):iii113–iii123, 2014.
5. Ordóñez JL, Amaral AT, Carcaboso AM, et al: The PARP inhibitor olaparib enhances the sensitivity of Ewing sarcoma to trabectedin, *Oncotarget* 6:18875–18890, 2015.
6. Morente MM, Fernández PL, de Alava E: Biobanking: old activity or young discipline?, *Semin Diagn Pathol* 25:317–322, 2008.
7. de Alava E, Lessnick SL, Sorensen PH: Ewing sarcoma. In Fletcher CDM, Bridge JA, Hogendoorn PCW, et al, editors: *WHO classification of tumours of soft tissue and bone*, Lyon, France, 2013, IARC Press.
8. Dehner L: Primitive neuroectodermal tumour and Ewing's sarcoma, *Am J Surg Pathol* 17:1–13, 1993.
9. Cash T, McIlvaine E, Krailo MD, et al: Comparison of clinical features and outcomes in patients with extraskeletal versus skeletal localized Ewing sarcoma: a report from the Children's Oncology Group, *Pediatr Blood Cancer* 63:1771–1779, 2016.
10. Gaspar N, Hawkins DS, Dirksen U, et al: Ewing sarcoma: current management and future approaches through collaboration, *J Clin Oncol* 33:3036–3046, 2015.
11. de Alava E, Pardo J: Ewing tumor. Tumor biology and clinical applications, *Int J Surg Pathol* 9:7–18, 2001.
12. Nascimento AG, Unni KK, Pritchard DJ, et al: A clinicopathologic study of 20 cases of large-cell (atypical) Ewing's sarcoma of bone, *Am J Surg Pathol* 4:29–36, 1980.
13. Kang LC, Dunphy CH: Immunoreactivity of MIC2 (CD99) and terminal deoxynucleotidyl transferase in bone marrow clot and core specimens of acute myeloid leukemias and myelodysplastic syndromes, *Arch Pathol Lab Med* 130:153–157, 2006.
14. Righi A, Gambarotti M, Longo S, et al: Small cell osteosarcoma: clinicopathologic, immunohistochemical, and molecular analysis of 36 cases, *Am J Surg Pathol* 39:691–699, 2015.
15. Granter SR, Renshaw AA, Fletcher CD, et al: CD99 reactivity in mesenchymal chondrosarcoma, *Hum Pathol* 27:1273–1276, 1996.
16. Gerald WL, Ladanyi M, de Alava E, et al: Clinical, pathologic, and molecular spectrum of tumours associated with t(11;22)(p13;q12): desmoplastic small round-cell tumor and its variants, *J Clin Oncol* 16:3028–3036, 1998.
17. Hasegawa T, Hirose T, Ayala AG, et al: Adult neuroblastoma of the retroperitoneum and abdomen: clinicopathologic distinction from primitive neuroectodermal tumour, *Am J Surg Pathol* 25:918–924, 2001.
18. Smith R, Owen LA, Trem DJ, et al: Expression profiling of EWS/FLI identifies NKX2.2 as a critical target gene in Ewing's sarcoma, *Cancer Cell* 9:405–416, 2006.
19. Yoshida A, Sekine S, Tsuta K, et al: NKX2.2 is a useful immunohistochemical marker for Ewing sarcoma, *Am J Surg Pathol* 36:993–999, 2012.
20. Shibuya R, Matsuyama A, Nakamoto M, et al: The combination of CD99 and NKX2.2, a transcriptional target of EWSR1-FLI1, is highly specific for the diagnosis of Ewing sarcoma, *Virchows Arch* 465:599–605, 2014.
21. Hung YP, Fletcher CD, Hornick JL: Evaluation of NKX2-2 expression in round cell sarcomas and other tumors with EWSR1 rearrangement: imperfect specificity for Ewing sarcoma, *Mod Pathol* 29:370–380, 2016.
22. Antonescu C: Round cell sarcomas beyond Ewing: emerging entities, *Histopathology* 64:26–37, 2014.
23. Chen S, Deniz K, Sung YS, et al: Ewing sarcoma with ERG gene rearrangements: a molecular study focusing on the prevalence of FUS-ERG and common pitfalls in detecting EWSR1-ERG fusions by FISH, *Genes Chromosomes Cancer* 55:340–349, 2016.
24. Machado I, Noguera R, Pellin A, et al: Molecular diagnosis of Ewing sarcoma family of tumors: a comparative analysis of 560 cases with FISH and RT-PCR, *Diagn Mol Pathol* 18:189–199, 2009.
25. Conner JR, Hornick JL: SATB2 is a novel marker of osteoblastic differentiation in bone and soft tissue tumours, *Histopathology* 63:36–49, 2013.
26. Bielle F, Fréneaux P, Jeanne-Pasquier C, et al: PHOX2B immunolabeling: a novel tool for the diagnosis of undifferentiated neuroblastomas among childhood small round blue-cell tumors, *Am J Surg Pathol* 36:1141–1149, 2012.
27. Rudzinski ER, Anderson JR, Hawkins DS, et al: The World Health Organization classification of skeletal muscle tumors in pediatric rhabdomyosarcoma: a report from the Children's Oncology Group, *Arch Pathol Lab Med* 139:1281–1287, 2015.
28. Chiles MC, Parham DM, Qualman SJ, et al: Sclerosing rhabdomyosarcomas in children and adolescents: a clinicopathologic review of 13 cases from the Intergroup Rhabdomyosarcoma Study Group and Children's Oncology Group, *Pediatr Dev Pathol* 7:583–594, 2004.
29. Kuhnen C, Herter P, Leuschner I, et al: Sclerosing pseudovascular rhabdomyosarcoma: immunohistochemical, ultrastructural, and genetic findings indicating a distinct subtype of rhabdomyosarcoma, *Virchows Arch* 449:572–578, 2006.
30. Agaram NP, Chen CL, Zhang L, et al: Recurrent MYOD1 mutations in pediatric and adult sclerosing and spindle cell rhabdomyosarcomas: evidence for a common pathogenesis, *Genes Chromosomes Cancer* 53:779–787, 2014.
31. Alaggio R, Zhang L, Sung YS, et al: A molecular study of pediatric spindle and sclerosing rhabdomyosarcoma: identification of novel and recurrent VGLL2-related fusions in infantile cases, *Am J Surg Pathol* 40:224–235, 2016.
32. Cessna MH, Zhou H, Perkins SL, et al: Are myogenin and myoD1 expression specific for rhabdomyosarcoma? A study of 150 cases, with emphasis on spindle cell mimics, *Am J Surg Pathol* 25:1150–1157, 2001.
33. Heerema-McKenney A, Wijnaendts LC, Pulliam JF, et al: Diffuse myogenin expression by immunohistochemistry is an independent marker of poor survival in pediatric rhabdomyosarcoma: a tissue microarray study of 71 primary tumors including correlation with molecular phenotype, *Am J Surg Pathol* 32:1513–1522, 2008.
34. Bahrami A, Gown AM, Baird GS, et al: Aberrant expression of epithelial and neuroendocrine markers in alveolar rhabdomyosarcoma: a potentially serious diagnostic pitfall, *Mod Pathol* 21:795–806, 2008.
35. Charville GW, Varma S, Forgó E, et al: PAX7 expression in rhabdomyosarcoma, related soft tissue tumors, and small round blue cell neoplasms, *Am J Surg Pathol* 40:1305–1315, 2016.
36. Nishio J, Althof PA, Bailey JM, et al: Use of a novel FISH assay on paraffin-embedded tissues as an adjunct to diagnosis of alveolar rhabdomyosarcoma, *Lab Invest* 86:547–556, 2006.
37. Sorensen PH, Lynch JC, Qualman SJ, et al: PAX3/FKHR and PAX7/FKHR gene fusions are prognostic indicators in alveolar rhabdomyosarcoma: a report from the Children's Oncology Group, *J Clin Oncol* 20:2672–2679, 2002.
38. Wachtel M, Runge T, Leuschner I, et al: Subtype and prognostic classification of rhabdomyosarcoma by immunohistochemistry, *J Clin Oncol* 24:816–822, 2006.
39. Parham DM, Qualman SJ, Teot L, et al: Correlation between histology and PAX/FKHR fusion status in alveolar rhabdomyosarcoma: a report from the Children's Oncology Group, *Am J Surg Pathol* 31:895–901, 2007.
40. Matsumura T, Yamaguchi T, Seki K, et al: Advantage of FISH analysis using FKHR probes for an adjunct to diagnosis of rhabdomyosarcomas, *Virchows Arch* 452:251–258, 2008.
41. Hiniker SM, Donaldson SS: Recent advances in understanding and managing rhabdomyosarcoma, *F1000Prime Rep* 7:59, 2015.
42. Rudzinski ER, Anderson JR, Lyden ER, et al: Myogenin, AP2β, NOS-1, and HMGA2 are surrogate markers of fusion status in rhabdomyosarcoma: a report from the soft tissue sarcoma committee of the children's oncology group, *Am J Surg Pathol* 38:654–659, 2014.
43. Gerald WL, Miller HK, Battifora H, et al: Intra-abdominal desmoplastic small round-cell tumor. Report of 19 cases of a distinctive type of high-grade polyphenotypic malignancy affecting young individuals, *Am J Surg Pathol* 15:499–513, 1991.
44. Gerald WL, Ladanyi M, de Alava E, et al: Clinical, pathologic, and molecular spectrum of tumors associated with t(11;22)(p13;q12): desmoplastic small round-cell tumor and its variants, *J Clin Oncol* 16:3028–3036, 1998.
45. Arnold MA, Schoenfield L, Limketkai BN, et al: Diagnostic pitfalls of differentiating desmoplastic small round cell tumor (DSRCT) from Wilms tumor (WT): overlapping morphologic and immunohistochemical features, *Am J Surg Pathol* 38:1220–1226, 2014.
46. de Alava E, Ladanyi M, Rosai J, et al: Detection of chimeric transcripts in desmoplastic small round cell tumor and related developmental tumors by RT-PCR. A specific diagnostic assay, *Am J Pathol* 147:1584–1591, 1995.
47. de Alava E, Marcilla D: Birth and evolution of the desmoplastic small round-cell tumor, *Semin Diagn Pathol* 33:254–261, 2016.
48. van de Rijn M, Barr FG, Xiong QB, et al: Poorly differentiated synovial sarcoma: an analysis of clinical, pathologic, and molecular genetic features, *Am J Surg Pathol* 23:106–112, 1999.

49. de Silva MV, McMahon AD, Paterson L, et al: Identification of poorly differentiated synovial sarcoma: a comparison of clinicopathological and cytogenetic features with those of typical synovial sarcoma, *Histopathology* 43:220–230, 2003.
50. Terry J, Saito T, Subramanian S, et al: TLE1 as a diagnostic immunohistochemical marker for synovial sarcoma emerging from gene expression profiling studies, *Am J Surg Pathol* 31:240–246, 2007.
51. Foo WC, Cruise MW, Wick MR, et al: Immunohistochemical staining for TLE1 distinguishes synovial sarcoma from histologic mimics, *Am J Clin Pathol* 135:839–844, 2011.
52. Coindre JM, Pelmus M, Hostein I, et al: Should molecular testing be required for diagnosing synovial sarcoma? A prospective study of 204 cases, *Cancer* 98:2700–2707, 2003.
53. Guillou L, Benhattar J, Bonichon F, et al: Histologic grade, but not SYT-SSX fusion type, is an important prognostic factor in patients with synovial sarcoma: a multicenter, retrospective analysis, *J Clin Oncol* 22:4040–4050, 2004.
54. Machado I, Navarro S, Llombart-Bosch A: Ewing sarcoma and the new emerging Ewing-like sarcomas: (CIC and BCOR-rearranged-sarcomas). A systematic review, *Histol Histopathol* 31:1169–1181, 2016.
55. Italiano A, Sung YS, Zhang L, et al: High prevalence of CIC fusion with double-homeobox (DUX4) transcription factors in EWSR1-negative undifferentiated small blue round cell sarcomas, *Genes Chromosomes Cancer* 51:207–218, 2012.
56. Gambarotti M, Benini S, Gamberi G, et al: CIC-DUX4 fusion-positive round-cell sarcomas of soft tissue and bone: a single-institution morphological and molecular analysis of seven cases, *Histopathology* 69:624–634, 2016.
57. Hung YP, Fletcher CD, Hornick JL: Evaluation of ETV4 and WT1 expression in CIC-rearranged sarcomas and histologic mimics, *Mod Pathol* 29:1324–1334, 2016.
58. Le Guellec S, Velasco V, Pérot G, et al: ETV4 is a useful marker for the diagnosis of CIC-rearranged undifferentiated round-cell sarcomas: a study of 127 cases including mimicking lesions, *Mod Pathol* 29:1523–1531, 2016.
59. Siegele B, Roberts J, Black JO, et al: DUX4 immunohistochemistry is a highly sensitive and specific marker for CIC-DUX4 fusion-positive round cell tumor, *Am J Surg Pathol* 41:423–429, 2017.
60. Antonescu CR, Owosho AA, Zhang L, et al: Sarcomas with CIC-rearrangements are a distinct pathologic entity with aggressive outcome: a clinicopathologic and molecular study of 115 cases, *Am J Surg Pathol* 41:941–949, 2017.
61. Pierron G, Tirode F, Lucchesi C, et al: A new subtype of bone sarcoma defined by BCOR-CCNB3 gene fusion, *Nat Genet* 44:461–466, 2012.
62. Specht K, Zhang L, Sung YS, et al: Novel BCOR-MAML3 and ZC3H7B-BCOR gene fusions in undifferentiated small blue round cell sarcomas, *Am J Surg Pathol* 40:433–442, 2016.
63. Kao YC, Sung YS, Zhang L, et al: BCOR overexpression is a highly sensitive marker in round cell sarcomas with BCOR genetic abnormalities, *Am J Surg Pathol* 40:1670–1678, 2016.
64. Kao YC, Sung YS, Zhang L, et al: BCOR upregulation in a poorly differentiated synovial sarcoma with SS18L1-SSX1 fusion-A pathologic and molecular pitfall, *Genes Chromosomes Cancer* 56:296–302, 2017.

9

Biphasic Tumors and Tumors With Mixed Patterns

Jason L. Hornick, MD, PhD

Soft tissue tumors with biphasic histology are uncommon. The "biphasic" designation is often applied to tumors with mixed spindle cell and overtly epithelial (often glandular) components but can also be applied to tumors with mixed spindle cell and epithelioid morphology without epithelial differentiation. The classic example of a soft tissue tumor with such a pattern is biphasic synovial sarcoma, which, when arising at typical anatomic sites, is sufficiently histologically distinctive to allow for straightforward recognition in most cases. However, a small group of other soft tissue tumors may include similar combinations of morphologic cell types and may therefore be confused with biphasic synovial sarcoma (Box 9.1).

In addition, some soft tissue tumors characteristically show marked intratumoral heterogeneity in terms of both cell types and growth patterns (see Box 9.1). Awareness of the tumors that most often show such mixed patterns can facilitate proper diagnosis. A relatively common example is dedifferentiated liposarcoma (DDLPS), which, in addition to the obvious combination of well-differentiated liposarcoma (WDLPS) and a nonlipogenic component (see Chapters 7 and 12), often shows striking heterogeneity when sampled thoroughly. Such heterogeneity in a retroperitoneal or intraabdominal tumor, for example, can be a helpful clue to the diagnosis.

Finally, some soft tissue sarcomas contain heterologous elements (especially bone, cartilage, and skeletal muscle) in a subset of cases; when such a tumor is encountered, with an appropriately high index of suspicion, additional sampling and judicious application of immunohistochemistry and molecular genetic techniques can lead to the correct diagnosis. The soft tissue sarcomas that sometimes show heterologous osseous or cartilaginous differentiation are also discussed in Chapter 14. Occasionally, other (nonmesenchymal) tumor types may also be biphasic or may show mixed histologic patterns (Box 9.2). Depending on the clinical presentation (especially the anatomic site), such tumors may be mistaken for soft tissue sarcomas with mixed patterns.

Biphasic Synovial Sarcoma

Although biphasic synovial sarcoma was the first variant recognized, the monophasic variant is more common (see Chapter 3). It is now clear that "synovial" sarcoma has no relationship to the synovial lining of joints, although this nomenclature has been retained. Synovial sarcoma is generally classified with soft tissue tumors of uncertain lineage, although epithelial differentiation is observed not only in the glandular elements but also to a more limited extent in the spindle cell component. Synovial sarcoma is also discussed in detail in Chapter 3 (monophasic synovial sarcoma) and Chapter 8 (poorly differentiated synovial sarcoma).

Clinical Features

Synovial sarcoma is most common in adolescents and young adults, with a median age of 35 years, although the age range is broad. Males are slightly more often affected than females.

Characteristically, patients seek medical attention because of a deep-seated mass, with or without pain, present for a variable interval. The most common sites of involvement are the extremities, especially in proximity to the large joints of the lower limbs, with thighs and knees being the most common locations.[1-5] However, synovial sarcoma may arise in a wide range of anatomic sites, including the lung and pleura,[6,7] mediastinum,[8] kidney,[9] retroperitoneum and pelvis,[10] stomach,[11] and head and neck,[12] among others.

Synovial sarcoma is usually associated with fascia or tendinous tissue. Only rarely are tumors located within joint spaces. Radiologically, synovial sarcoma usually presents as an extraarticular soft tissue mass, often showing calcification (which can be a helpful diagnostic clue) and no involvement of underlying bone.

Pathologic Features

Grossly, the tumor is usually well circumscribed and sometimes shows a fibrous pseudocapsule. The cut surface is usually soft, tan, and

Box 9.1 Biphasic Tumors and Tumors With Mixed Patterns

Biphasic synovial sarcoma
Myoepithelial tumors of soft tissue (including mixed tumor)
Malignant peripheral nerve sheath tumor (MPNST) with heterologous differentiation (including glandular MPNST)
Gastrointestinal stromal tumor, mixed type
Dedifferentiated liposarcoma
Melanotic neuroectodermal tumor of infancy

Box 9.2 Nonmesenchymal Tumors With Biphasic and Mixed Patterns

Ectopic hamartomatous thymoma
Sarcomatoid carcinoma
Biphasic malignant mesothelioma
Germ cell tumors
Carcinosarcoma (malignant mixed müllerian tumor)

homogeneous and may show foci of cystic degeneration. Calcifications are usually too small to be identified grossly.

Histologically, two major subtypes of synovial sarcoma are recognized, namely, monophasic and biphasic. The former is characterized by a monotonous, fascicular spindle cell proliferation and is discussed in Chapter 3.

Biphasic synovial sarcoma shows an intimate juxtaposition of a spindle cell component and clusters of epithelial cells, forming nests or glandular structures (Fig. 9.1). Other than the shape, the nuclear features of the epithelial component are usually similar to those of the spindle cells (Fig. 9.2). These epithelial cells are often cuboidal, with round vesicular nuclei, small nucleoli, and pale eosinophilic cytoplasm (Fig. 9.3). Most commonly, the spindle cell component is the predominant histologic pattern, and recognition of the epithelial component may require extensive sampling. On occasion, there is an extensive glandular component, and rarely, the epithelial component may predominate. In such cases the spindle cell component may be subtle; the diagnosis requires a high index of suspicion and identification of the spindle cell component.

Stromal collagen is often prominent (see Fig. 9.3), and foci of dystrophic calcifications may be seen. Frequent mast cells are common, and the vasculature is characterized by thin-walled, branching "hemangiopericytoma-like" vessels. Extensive cystic change in synovial sarcoma may make recognition of the tumor more difficult. Again, a high index of suspicion is needed to identify a spindle cell component within the septa of the cystic cavity. Rarely, synovial sarcomas may show stromal myxoid change. Likewise, diagnosis requires recognition of an area with typical histology.

Poorly differentiated synovial sarcoma is usually dominated by round cells and may be confused with other round cell sarcomas (see Chapter 8).

Immunohistochemistry

Although recognition of biphasic synovial sarcoma is usually straightforward, immunohistochemistry can be helpful to confirm the diagnosis. The glandular component shows strong and diffuse staining for keratins (Fig. 9.4) and epithelial membrane antigen (EMA). In most tumors the spindle cell component is also positive for keratins (AE1/AE3 is among the most sensitive) and EMA, although staining is variable and often focal (see Fig. 9.4). Even limited expression of epithelial markers in the spindle cell component can be helpful.

In addition, approximately 30% of synovial sarcomas are positive for S-100 protein. Bcl-2, cytoplasmic CD99, and α-smooth muscle actin

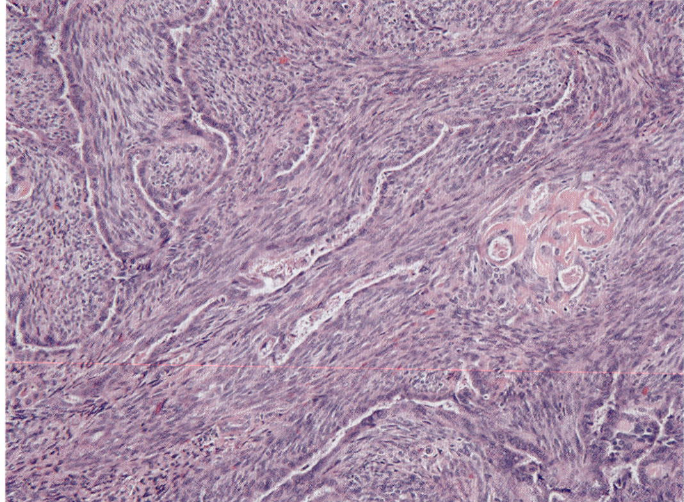

Figure 9.1 Biphasic Synovial Sarcoma. This tumor is composed of glands and cleftlike epithelial-lined structures admixed with fascicles of hyperchromatic spindle cells.

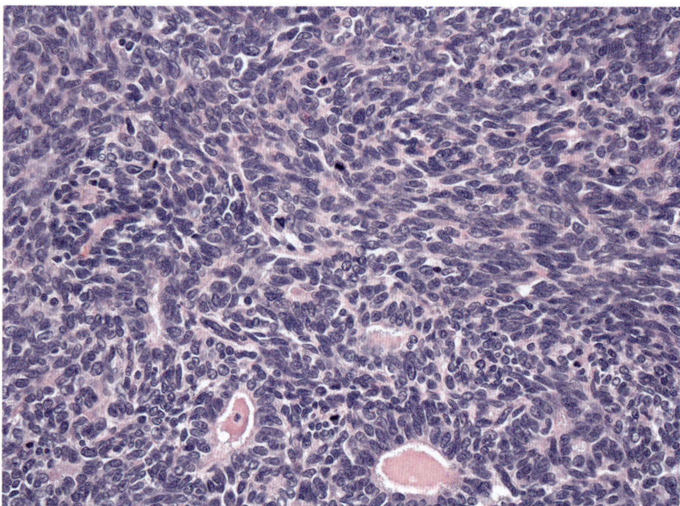

Figure 9.2 Biphasic Synovial Sarcoma. In this example, the glandular elements merge imperceptibly with the spindle cell component. The nuclei in both components show similar features.

(SMA) may also be detected but are not specific.[13] Rarely, neoplastic cells may express CD34.

TLE1, a member of a family of transcriptional corepressors that inhibit Wnt and other cell fate determination signals, is overexpressed in synovial sarcoma.[14] Although this marker may occasionally be expressed in other soft tissue tumors that mimic synovial sarcoma, such as a subset of malignant peripheral nerve sheath tumors (MPNSTs) and solitary fibrous tumors, TLE1 is highly sensitive and moderately specific for synovial sarcoma, being positive in more than 90% of cases, usually with moderate or strong nuclear staining (Fig. 9.5).[14-18] Synovial sarcomas usually show markedly reduced (but not complete loss of) nuclear staining for SMARCB1 (INI1).[19]

Molecular Genetics

Synovial sarcoma is characterized in virtually 100% of cases by a recurrent balanced translocation, namely t(X;18)(p11;q11), in which the *SS18* gene on chromosome 18 is juxtaposed to an *SSX* gene on chromosome X. To date, at least six *SSX* genes have been identified on Xp11, three

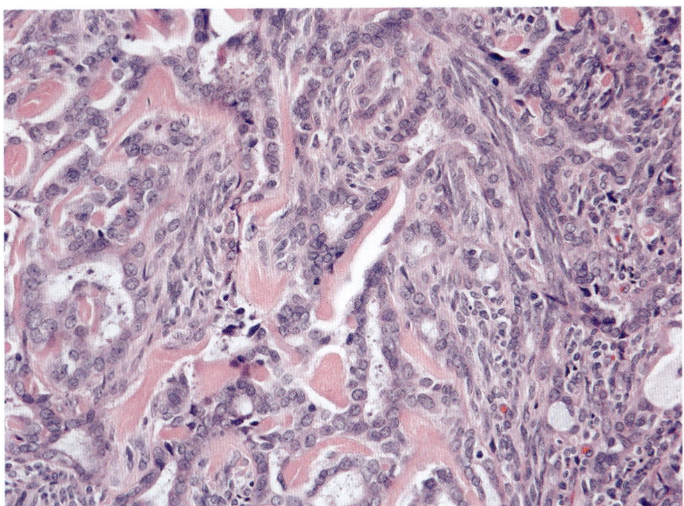

Figure 9.3 **Biphasic Synovial Sarcoma.** The glands are lined by cuboidal epithelial cells. In this case, the spindle cell component is relatively inconspicuous. Note the prominent stromal collagen.

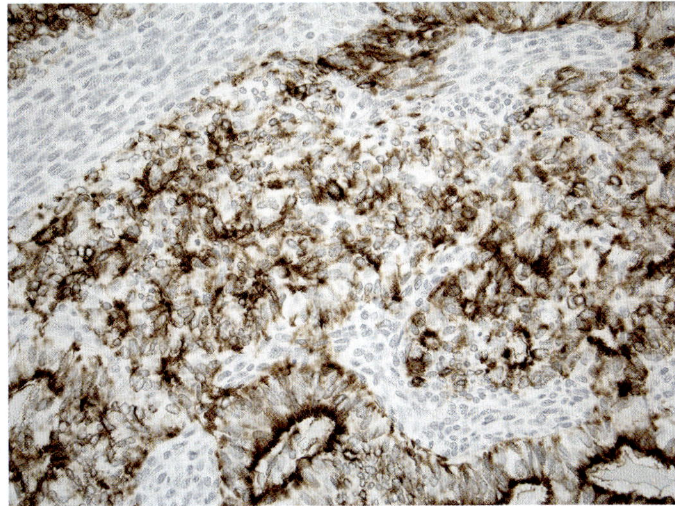

Figure 9.4 **Biphasic Synovial Sarcoma.** Keratin is diffusely positive in the glandular component but is usually only focally expressed by the spindle cells.

of which may be rearranged with *SS18*, giving rise to three fusion proteins, SS18-SSX1, SS18-SSX2, and SS18-SSX4. The first two are the most common (see Chapter 18).[20]

These fusion transcripts are mutually exclusive and are believed by some authors to correlate with morphologic subtypes of synovial sarcoma.[21] Kawai and colleagues found that monophasic tumors harbor translocations involving either the *SSX1* or *SSX2* gene, whereas biphasic tumors only had translocations involving *SSX1*.[21] However, since then, biphasic tumors harboring the *SS18-SSX2* fusion transcript have also been reported. The extent of glandular elements in synovial sarcoma may be limited; tumors initially believed to be monophasic may be biphasic if sampled more extensively. This may account for the differences in fusion partners detected.

Differential Diagnosis

The differential diagnosis of synovial sarcoma depends on the histologic subtype. Immunohistochemistry is helpful to support the diagnosis; however, in difficult cases, identification of t(X;18) by fluorescence in situ hybridization (FISH) or reverse transcriptase polymerase chain reaction (RT-PCR) can be used for confirmation.

Monophasic synovial sarcoma should be distinguished from other spindle cell sarcomas, such as MPNST, as well as solitary fibrous tumor (see Chapter 3).

The differential diagnosis for biphasic synovial sarcoma is shown in Table 9.1 and includes other spindle cell neoplasms containing admixed glandular elements, such as biphasic malignant mesothelioma, sarcomatoid carcinoma, glandular MPNST, mixed tumor (myoepithelioma), and müllerian carcinosarcoma (malignant mixed müllerian tumor [MMMT]).

Biphasic malignant mesothelioma usually involves the pleura or peritoneum. In contrast to synovial sarcoma, the sarcomatoid component of malignant mesothelioma usually shows considerable nuclear atypia, and the epithelioid component often shows a tubulopapillary growth pattern with uniform, cuboidal cells. Similar to synovial sarcoma, malignant mesothelioma is positive for keratins and EMA, but it also shows expression of calretinin and nuclear WT1. Immunoreactivity for TLE1 is observed in the majority of mesotheliomas[22]; therefore TLE1 cannot be used to make this distinction. Loss of BAP1 expression is observed in a significant subset of biphasic mesotheliomas, although somewhat less often than epithelioid mesotheliomas.[23,24]

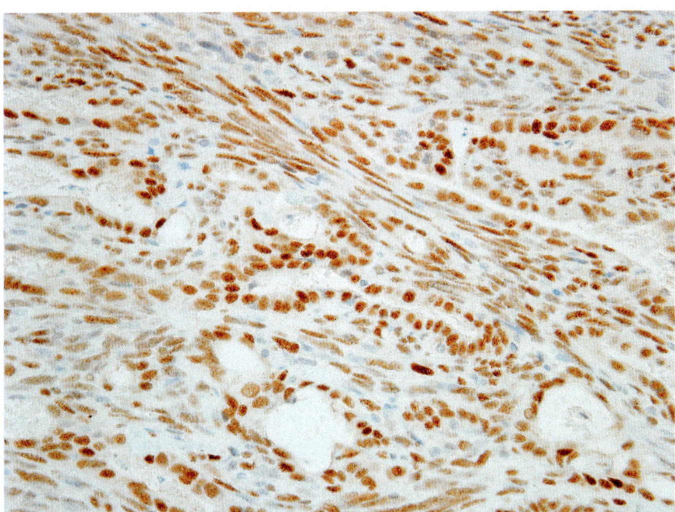

Figure 9.5 **Biphasic Synovial Sarcoma.** TLE1 shows strong nuclear staining in almost all cases of synovial sarcoma.

Sarcomatoid carcinoma often arises in the lung, breast, or kidney and may contain a minor conventional component in addition to the spindle cell or pleomorphic component. Focal expression of keratin and EMA is also seen in sarcomatoid carcinomas. However, sarcomatoid carcinomas usually show significant pleomorphism and marked nuclear atypia, which are not observed in synovial sarcoma.

Rarely, MPNST contains a glandular component admixed with the fascicles of spindle cells. This variant usually arises in patients with neurofibromatosis type 1 (NF1) and carries a particularly poor prognosis.[25] Diagnostic clues to MPNST include varying cellularity, perivascular accentuation, and tapering nuclei. Unlike biphasic synovial sarcoma, in MPNSTs the glands are sharply demarcated from the spindle cell component and are often bland and intestinal-like in appearance, including columnar cells, goblet cells, and cells with neuroendocrine differentiation. Similar to synovial sarcoma, the epithelial component is positive for keratins and EMA, but unlike synovial sarcoma, the glandular elements often express CK20 and carcinoembryonic antigen (CEA) as well. The conventional spindle cell component in MPNSTs shows focal staining for S-100 protein, glial fibrillary acidic protein

Table 9.1 Differential Diagnosis for Biphasic Synovial Sarcoma

	Keratin	Epithelial Membrane Antigen	S-100 Protein	Glial Fibrillary Acidic Protein	SOX10	Nuclear WT1	Calretinin
Biphasic synovial sarcoma	+	+	30%	–	–	–	–
Biphasic malignant mesothelioma	+	±	–	–	–	+	+
Sarcomatoid carcinoma	+	±	–	–	–	–	–
Glandular malignant peripheral nerve sheath tumor	+ (glands)	+ (glands)	±	±	±	–	–
Carcinosarcoma (malignant mixed müllerian tumor)	+ (carcinoma)	+ (carcinoma)	–	–	–	+ (carcinoma)	–

(GFAP), and/or SOX10, each in 30% to 50% of cases. S-100 protein may also be positive in synovial sarcoma (in ~30% of cases), although GFAP and SOX10 expression is not observed. TLE1 is positive in a small subset of MPNSTs. Loss of histone H3 with lysine 27 trimethylation (H3K27me3) is highly specific for MPNST in this differential diagnosis.[26,27]

Only 10% to 15% of myoepitheliomas of soft tissue show ductal differentiation (mixed tumors). Most cases are dominated by epithelioid cells with eosinophilic to clear cytoplasm, growing in nests and cords in a variably myxoid stroma, although a spindle cell component may also be present. The combination of keratin, EMA, S-100 protein, and GFAP is the typical phenotype for myoepithelioma; expression of epithelial markers is usually extensive, unlike in the spindle cell component of synovial sarcoma. Many mixed tumors of soft tissue show nuclear staining for PLAG1 (reflecting the presence of *PLAG1* gene rearrangements).[28,29]

Usually arising in the endometrium, ovary, or fallopian tube, müllerian carcinosarcoma secondarily spreads to the peritoneum and omentum, all extremely rare sites for synovial sarcoma. In contrast to synovial sarcoma, carcinosarcoma usually shows considerable heterogeneity, including epithelioid and round cell morphology, as well as marked nuclear atypia and pleomorphism. Carcinosarcoma often contains a high-grade serous carcinomatous component, in contrast to the relatively bland and uniform cytology of the glandular component in synovial sarcoma. Nuclear WT1 or PAX8 expression supports a müllerian tumor over synovial sarcoma.

The differential diagnosis for the myxoid and poorly differentiated variants of synovial sarcoma includes other myxoid neoplasms and other round cell sarcomas, respectively (see Chapters 5 and 8 for further discussion).

Prognosis and Treatment

The prognosis and treatment of synovial sarcoma are discussed in Chapter 3.

PRACTICE POINTS: Biphasic Synovial Sarcoma

- Spindle cell sarcoma with scattered glands and nests of epithelial cells
- Highly variable extent of the glandular component
- Consistently positive for epithelial membrane antigen, keratins, and TLE1
- Characterized by t(X;18)(p11;q11) translocation
- Prognosis similar to that of monophasic synovial sarcoma

Mixed Tumor/Myoepithelioma/ Myoepithelial Carcinoma

Mixed tumors and myoepitheliomas of soft tissue lie on a morphologic continuum and are composed of variable cell types. Myoepithelial tumors of soft tissue are also discussed in Chapters 5 and 6.

Clinical Features

Myoepithelial neoplasms occur in both children and adults, with males and females equally affected. These tumors most often arise in the limbs and limb girdles, with approximately 50% of cases occurring in subcutaneous tissue.[30] Myoepithelial carcinomas appear to be more frequent in children.[31,30]

Pathologic Features

Myoepithelial tumors are a morphologically heterogeneous group of tumors composed of epithelioid or spindled cells arranged in sheets, cords, nests, or clusters, within a variably abundant myxoid or chondromyxoid matrix (Fig. 9.6). Neoplastic cells are most often epithelioid or ovoid, with vesicular chromatin and small or inconspicuous nucleoli and eosinophilic cytoplasm (Fig. 9.7). In occasional examples, neoplastic cells show eccentrically placed nuclei and hyaline cytoplasmic inclusions ("plasmacytoid" cells) (Fig. 9.8A). When epithelial (ductal) differentiation is present, the designation *mixed tumor* may be applied (Fig. 9.9). This finding is uncommon, as is the presence of mesenchymal elements, such as metaplastic cartilage, bone, and adipose tissue, which are seen in at most 10% of cases.

Myoepithelial carcinoma is usually characterized by high-grade cytology with prominent nucleoli or coarse chromatin. Infiltrative margins, necrosis, and a high mitotic rate are less reliable predictors of malignant behavior.[30]

Immunohistochemistry

Myoepithelial tumors of soft tissue are characteristically positive for keratins, EMA, and S-100 protein, often with extensive staining.[31,30] Approximately half of cases also express GFAP; a subset of tumors are positive for SMA and p63.[31,30] The majority of myoepithelial tumors of soft tissue show nuclear staining for SOX10; myoepithelial carcinomas are less often positive.[32] Some myoepithelial carcinomas show loss of SMARCB1 (INI1) protein expression, most often in pediatric cases.[31,33] Myoepithelial neoplasms with *PLAG1* rearrangements show nuclear staining for PLAG1 (see Fig. 9.8B).[28,29]

Molecular Genetics

Myoepithelial tumors of soft tissue (both benign and malignant examples) are characterized by translocations involving the *EWSR1* gene in approximately half of cases.[34,35] Multiple fusion partners have been identified, including *PBX1*, *POU5F1*, *ZNF444*, *KLF17*, *ATF1*, and *PBX3*, but these partners are only found in less than 50% of cases with *EWSR1* rearrangement.[34-40] The *EWSR1* fusion partners in other cases have yet to be identified. Of note, *EWSR1* rearrangements are uncommon in myoepithelial tumors with ductal differentiation (mixed tumors) and a chondroid or osseous matrix.[35] In contrast, similar to their salivary gland counterparts, mixed tumors of skin and soft tissue often harbor *PLAG1* rearrangements; occasional myoepitheliomas without ductal differentiation also have such gene fusions.[28,29] *EWSR1* and *PLAG1* rearrangements are mutually exclusive.

Differential Diagnosis

The chief differential diagnostic considerations for myoepithelioma (extraskeletal myxoid chondrosarcoma, ossifying fibromyxoid tumor, and epithelioid schwannoma) and myoepithelial carcinoma (metastatic carcinoma, metastatic melanoma, and proximal-type epithelioid sarcoma) are discussed in Chapters 5 and 6.

Myoepitheliomas showing ductal differentiation (mixed tumors) should be distinguished in particular from biphasic synovial sarcoma and glandular MPNST. The spindle cell component of biphasic synovial sarcoma is remarkably uniform, composed of intersecting fascicles of spindle cells with scant cytoplasm, in contrast to the intratumoral heterogeneity and plump cells with eosinophilic cytoplasm seen in myoepithelial tumors. Mixed tumors generally show more extensive immunoreactivity for keratins, EMA, and S-100 protein, whereas the spindle cell component of synovial sarcoma usually shows at most limited staining for these markers. Strong TLE1 expression is typical of synovial sarcoma, whereas SOX10 expression is limited to myoepithelial neoplasms in this differential diagnosis.[32] The majority of mixed tumors show nuclear staining for PLAG1.

Glandular MPNST is a rare variant that usually arises in deep soft tissues or central body sites of patients with NF1. Unlike the ducts in mixed tumors, the glandular component in MPNST often shows enteric features (with columnar cells, goblet cells, and neuroendocrine cells), along with immunoreactivity for CK20. In contrast to myoepithelial tumors, the spindle cells in MPNST usually contain slender, tapering nuclei and inconspicuous cytoplasm. Other characteristic features of MPNST include perivascular hypercellularity and alternating cellular and myxoid areas. Diffuse expression of keratins and EMA is not seen

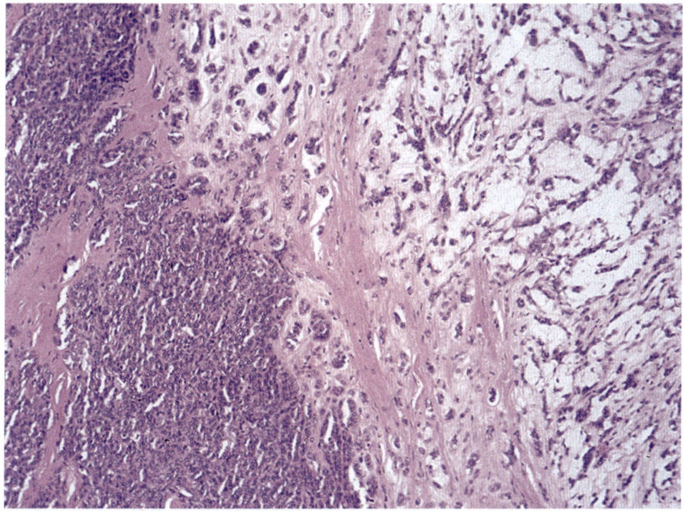

Figure 9.6 Soft Tissue Myoepithelioma. Myoepithelial tumors of soft tissue typically show intratumoral heterogeneity, ranging from a sheetlike growth pattern *(left)* to reticular architecture *(right)*. Note the abundant myxoid stroma.

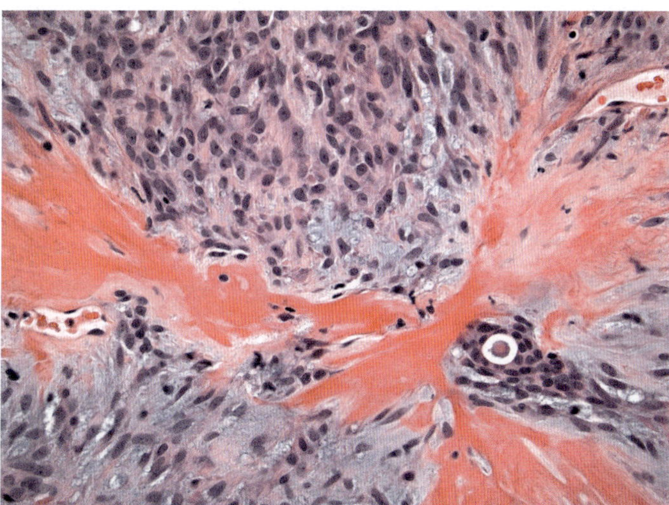

Figure 9.7 Soft Tissue Myoepithelioma. Myoepithelioma composed of uniform, bland spindle cells with palely eosinophilic cytoplasm and scant myxoid stroma. Note the areas of hyalinized stroma and rare ducts.

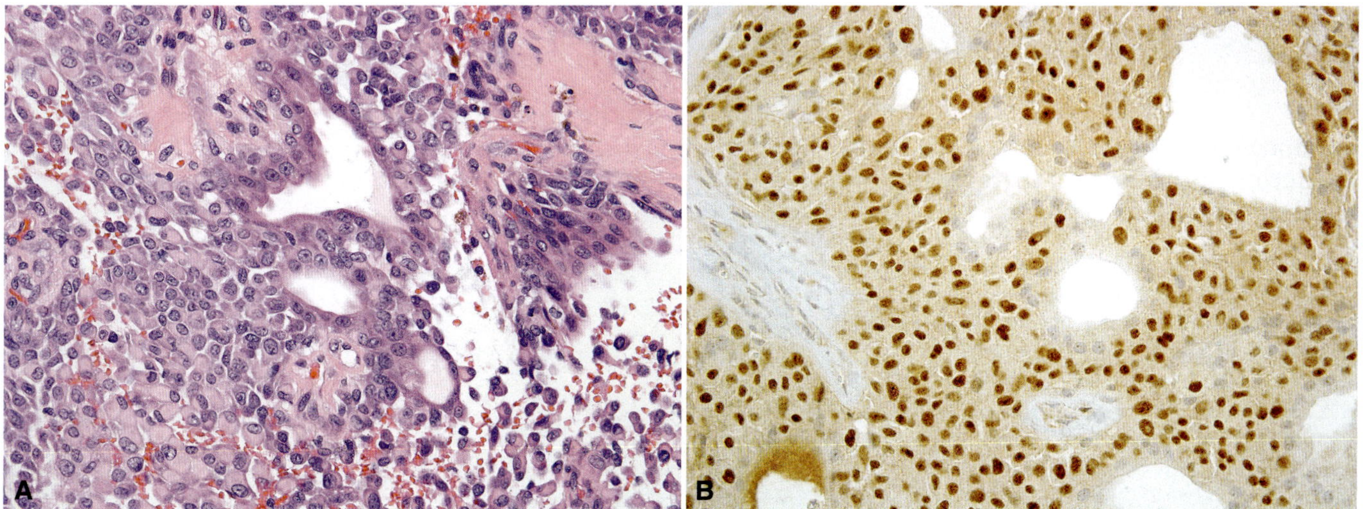

Figure 9.8 Soft Tissue Myoepithelioma. (A) Myoepitheliomas of soft tissue sometimes contain prominent hyaline cells (epithelioid cells with eccentric nuclei and eosinophilic cytoplasmic inclusions). This tumor also contained rare ducts *(center of field)*. (B) PLAG1 shows strong nuclear staining; this finding correlates with *PLAG1* gene rearrangement, a common finding in mixed tumors (but rare in myoepitheliomas without ductal differentiation).

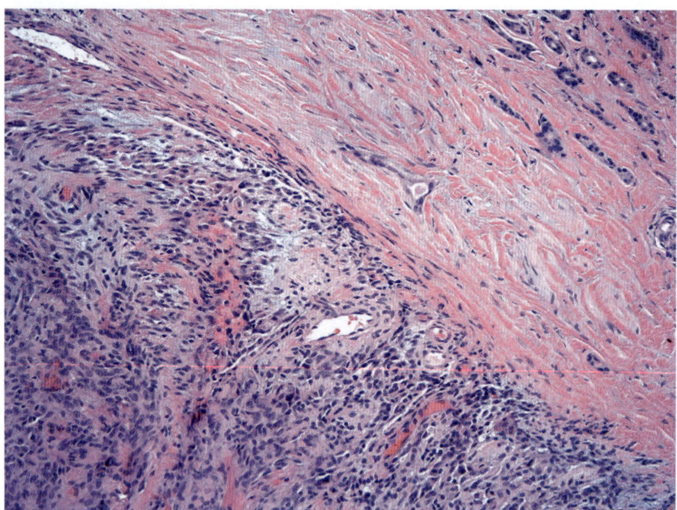

Figure 9.9 Mixed Tumor of Soft Tissue. A soft tissue myoepithelioma showing ductal differentiation *(upper right field)*; in such cases the term *mixed tumor* may be applied. The predominant myoepithelial component is composed of bland spindle cells with eosinophilic cytoplasm.

in MPNST. Most high-grade MPNSTs show loss of expression of H3K27me3.[26,27]

Prognosis and Treatment

The prognosis and treatment of myoepithelial tumors is discussed in Chapters 5 and 6.

PRACTICE POINTS: Mixed Tumor/Myoepithelial Tumors of Soft Tissue

- Typically show heterogeneous architecture (solid, reticular, nested), stroma (myxoid, hyalinized), and cell types (epithelioid, spindle cell, clear cell, plasmacytoid)
- Similar to salivary gland tumors, "mixed tumor" may be applied to myoepitheliomas with ductal differentiation
- Myoepithelial carcinoma is characterized by high-grade cytology, with cells showing prominent nucleoli or coarse chromatin
- Myoepithelial carcinoma is overrepresented in the pediatric population
- Usually express keratins, epithelial membrane antigen, and S-100 protein; often SOX10; 50% glial fibrillary acidic protein
- *EWSR1* gene rearrangement in 50% of myoepitheliomas
- *PLAG1* rearrangement is characteristic of mixed tumor

Malignant Peripheral Nerve Sheath Tumor With Divergent (Heterologous) Differentiation (Including Glandular Type)

MPNST occurs in three distinct settings, namely, sporadically, in patients with NF1, and following radiation therapy. In patients with NF1 the incidence is 4000 to 5000 times higher than in the general population.[41,42] MPNST is discussed in Chapter 3.

Heterologous mesenchymal elements are relatively common in MPNST and occur in up to 20% of tumors, with the majority seen in patients with NF1.[41,42] In contrast, glandular elements are rare but are also more often seen in the setting of NF1.[25,43]

Clinical Features

Patients with MPNST usually present with a large, deep-seated mass, arising most commonly on the trunk (especially paraspinal) or lower extremities, followed by the upper extremities, head and neck, and retroperitoneum. Glandular MPNST also has a wide anatomic distribution but seems particularly common in the retroperitoneum.[25]

Men and women are equally affected, with a peak incidence in the fourth and fifth decades.[41,42] Overall, MPNST arises in patients with NF1 approximately a decade earlier than in patients with sporadic tumors.[41,42] Patients may present with neurologic symptoms related to the involved nerve, or more frequently, a mass effect with impingement on adjacent structures or organs.

Pathologic Features

Grossly, tumors are usually large and may be associated with nerves. The cut surface is typically firm and heterogeneous, with areas of hemorrhage and necrosis.

Histologically, conventional MPNST is a spindle cell neoplasm with a fascicular growth pattern, characteristically with alternating hypocellular and hypercellular areas (Fig. 9.10). Tumor cells tend to aggregate around blood vessels. The presence of necrosis and mitotic activity is highly variable; a recent study has suggested that histologic grading of MPNST predicts metastasis and survival.[44] In a subset of cases (depending in part on the extent of sampling), a neurofibromatous precursor can be identified.

Glandular MPNST is characterized by the presence of scattered glands arranged singly or in small clusters within the spindle cell neoplasm (see Fig. 9.10). The glands are usually well defined, appear to be of low grade, and are lined by cuboidal to columnar cells, often with an intestinal-like appearance (Figs. 9.11 and 9.12), sometimes including goblet cells and neuroendocrine cells. Squamous metaplasia, clear cell change, and stromal mucin pools are rare findings.

More common in patients with NF1, MPNST with other forms of heterologous differentiation account for approximately 20% of cases.[41,42] These tumors are characterized by the presence of malignant mesenchymal elements, most often rhabdomyosarcoma (malignant Triton tumor; Figs. 9.13 and 9.14A), chondrosarcoma, and osteosarcoma, and more rarely angiosarcoma. The rhabdomyosarcomatous component is usually composed of relatively well-differentiated rhabdomyoblasts with brightly eosinophilic cytoplasm. The presence of heterologous elements is variable in extent, although these elements are usually only focal.

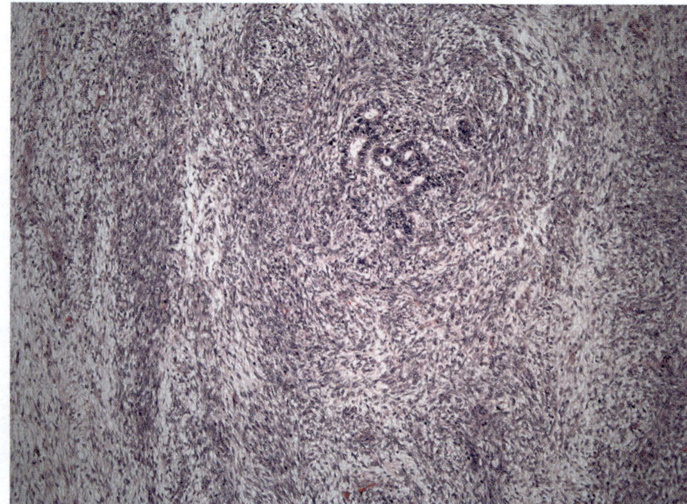

Figure 9.10 Malignant Peripheral Nerve Sheath Tumor. A characteristic feature is the presence of alternating hypocellular areas with myxoid stroma and hypercellular, fascicular areas.

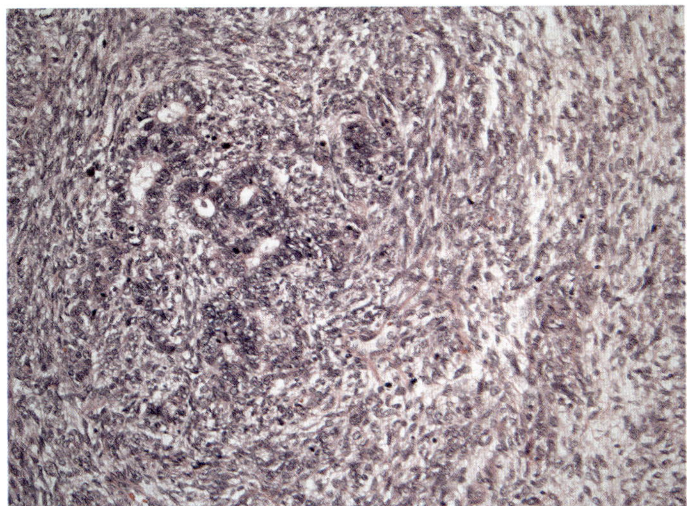

Figure 9.11 Glandular Malignant Peripheral Nerve Sheath Tumor. Malignant peripheral nerve sheath tumor characterized by a highly cellular spindle cell proliferation containing a cluster of glands with an intestinal-like appearance.

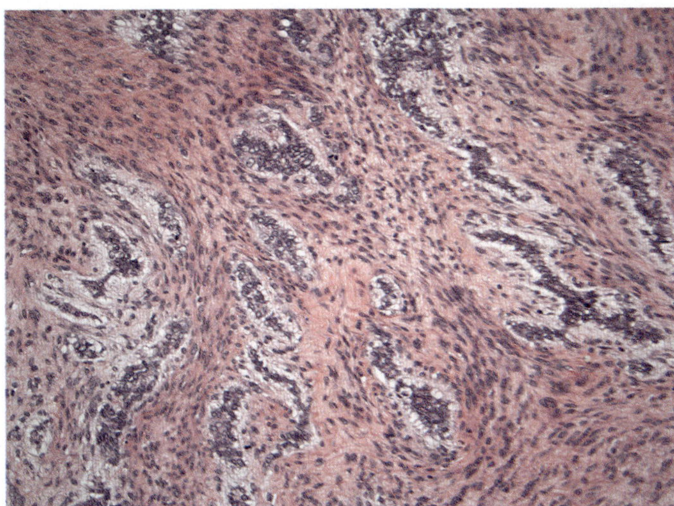

Figure 9.12 Glandular Malignant Peripheral Nerve Sheath Tumor. Malignant peripheral nerve sheath tumor composed of elongated spindle cells with tapering nuclei. Note the scattered glandular structures lined by cuboidal cells with bland nuclei.

Immunohistochemistry

Until recently, immunohistochemistry was of limited utility in confirming the diagnosis of MPNST because these tumors show variable and focal positivity for S-100 protein, GFAP, and/or SOX10, each in only 30% to 50% of cases. Expression of these markers is inversely related to histologic grade. Low-grade tumors show more extensive positivity, whereas high-grade MPNST is more often negative. Recent studies have shown that loss of expression of H3K27me3 (see Chapter 3) is a highly specific marker for MPNST; however, the sensitivity of this finding depends upon histologic grade: although more than 90% of high-grade MPNSTs show loss of H3K27me3, only 40% and 67% of low-grade and intermediate-grade tumors (respectively) show loss of this marker (see Fig. 9.14B).[26,27] CD34 is commonly positive in MPNST; expression of EMA and keratins may occasionally be focally detected. TLE1 is usually negative, but approximately 20% of tumors show nuclear staining, sometimes extensively.

The glandular component is positive for keratins and EMA, and it usually shows an intestinal phenotype, with expression of CEA and CK20 and variable positivity for neuroendocrine markers in a subset of cells.[41,45] The heterologous mesenchymal elements are positive for appropriate lineage markers, such as desmin and myogenin in rhabdomyosarcoma and CD31 or CD34 in angiosarcoma.

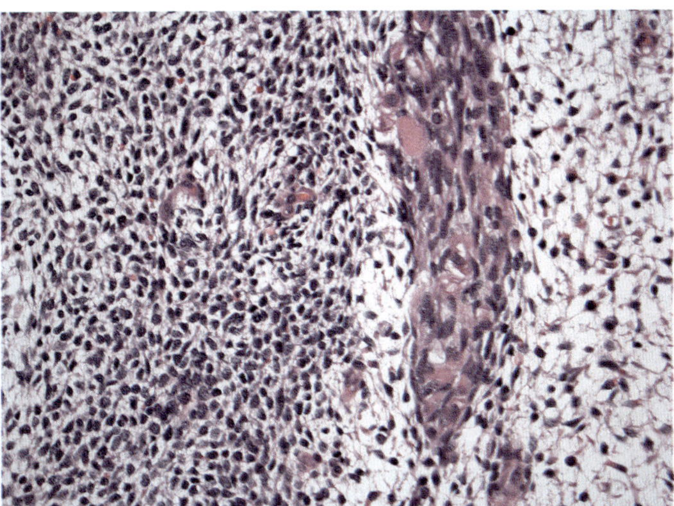

Figure 9.13 Malignant Peripheral Nerve Sheath Tumor With Heterologous Rhabdomyoblastic Differentiation. High-grade malignant peripheral nerve sheath tumor composed of spindle cells in a myxoid stroma with focal rhabdomyoblastic differentiation (malignant Triton tumor). Note the bundle of rhabdomyoblasts with brightly eosinophilic cytoplasm. Heterologous elements are more common in patients with neurofibromatosis type 1.

Molecular Genetics

The molecular genetics of MPNST is discussed in Chapters 3 and 18.

Differential Diagnosis

The differential diagnosis of glandular MPNST mainly includes müllerian carcinosarcoma and biphasic synovial sarcoma (see Table 9.1). Clinically, patients with carcinosarcoma are usually older women with large tumor masses arising in the uterus or pelvis. In contrast to MPNST, the glandular component in carcinosarcoma is histologically malignant (high-grade serous or other adenocarcinoma), with hyperchromatic nuclei and frequent mitoses, and it is positive for CK7 and often for WT1 and PAX8. The glands in MPNST usually appear benign or low-grade malignant, with an intestinal phenotype, including goblet cells, and immunoreactivity for CK20. The spindle cell component in MPNST shows focal staining for S-100 protein, GFAP, and/or SOX10 in 30% to 50% of cases; these markers are usually negative in müllerian carcinosarcoma. Heterologous mesenchymal elements (e.g., rhabdomyosarcoma and chondrosarcoma) may be seen in both tumor types.

Biphasic synovial sarcoma shows a variable extent of glandular structures, which are intimately admixed with the spindle cell component. In contrast to MPNST, the nuclear characteristics in the epithelial component of synovial sarcoma are similar to those in the spindle cells. Unlike in synovial sarcoma, the glands in MPNST often contain goblet cells and are usually positive for CK20. The spindle cell component of synovial sarcoma is usually remarkably homogeneous, in contrast to the varying cellularity, areas of myxoid stroma, and perivascular accentuation seen in MPNST. EMA and keratin expression in the spindle cell component favors synovial sarcoma. S-100 protein is not specific because it may be focally positive in approximately 30% of synovial sarcomas,

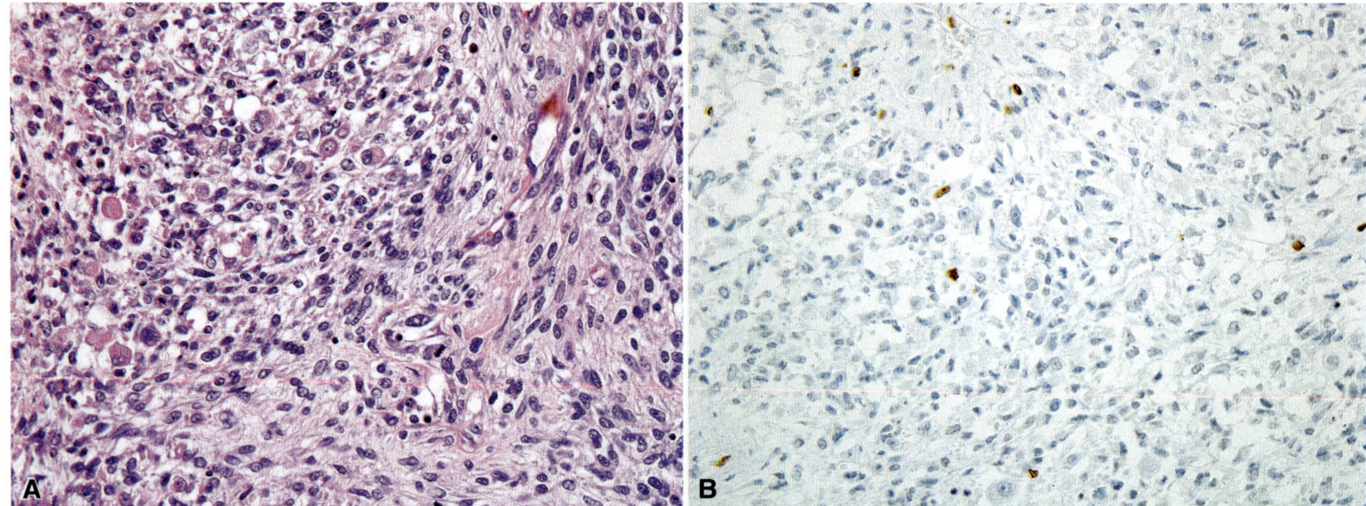

Figure 9.14 Malignant Peripheral Nerve Sheath Tumor With Heterologous Rhabdomyoblastic Differentiation. (A) In some cases the rhabdomyoblasts are very limited in number. Note the scattered polygonal rhabdomyoblasts. (B) Loss of nuclear H3K27me3 (histone H3 with trimethylated lysine 27) is highly specific for malignant peripheral nerve sheath tumor. Note the positive staining in occasional stromal cells and lymphocytes, which serve as internal controls.

although GFAP and SOX10 are not expressed. Strong nuclear staining with TLE1 is usually seen in synovial sarcoma; TLE1 is typically (but not always) negative in MPNST. Loss of H3K27me3 is specific for MPNST in this differential diagnosis. In equivocal cases the t(X;18) translocation that characterizes synovial sarcoma can be demonstrated by FISH or RT-PCR.

Cases of MPNST with heterologous mesenchymal differentiation should mainly be differentiated from DDLPS. DDLPS usually affects older patients and has a predilection for the retroperitoneum. Histologically, the diagnosis of DDLPS relies on identification of a well-differentiated adipocytic component; therefore gross recognition of a fatty component and proper sampling are critical. In the absence of an adipocytic component and in small biopsy specimens, immunohistochemistry and FISH can be helpful to support the diagnosis. DDLPS is uniformly positive for MDM2 and CDK4 in more than 95% of cases; however, MPNST also commonly expresses MDM2 (in approximately 60% of cases) but only rarely expresses CDK4.[46] Therefore these markers should be interpreted with caution with this differential diagnosis. FISH showing *MDM2* amplification is a more specific finding.

Prognosis and Treatment

Complete surgical resection combined with postoperative radiation therapy for close margins is the cornerstone of treatment of MPNST. MPNST has a high local recurrence rate (~45%), a metastatic rate of up to 40%, and a mortality rate of approximately 70%.[41,42] Histologic grading appears to predict metastasis.[44] The most common sites of metastasis are the lung, soft tissue, abdominal cavity, and retroperitoneum.[41,42] MPNST with heterologous rhabdomyoblastic differentiation (malignant Triton tumor) pursues a particularly aggressive clinical course.[47] Similarly, glandular MPNST has a very poor prognosis, with a mean survival of 2 years and a mortality rate of approximately 80%.

PRACTICE POINTS: Malignant Peripheral Nerve Sheath Tumor With Heterologous Differentiation (Including Glandular Type)

- Heterologous differentiation is seen in 20% of cases
- Most common heterologous elements are cartilage, bone, and skeletal muscle
- Glandular MPNST is characterized by low-grade appearance of glands, often with intestinal features, arranged singly or in clusters
- Occurs much more commonly in patients with neurofibromatosis type 1
- MPNST is difficult to confirm by conventional immunohistochemistry because S-100 protein, GFAP, and/or SOX10 are positive in <50% of cases
- Loss of H3K27me3 is highly specific for MPNST, with highest sensitivity in high-grade tumors
- MPNST with heterologous elements is very aggressive, with a high metastatic rate

Ectopic Hamartomatous Thymoma

Ectopic hamartomatous thymoma was first described by Smith and McClure, who reported an unusual subcutaneous tumor in the left supraclavicular fossa of a 55-year-old woman. The tumor was composed of a mixture of benign squamous epithelium, "fibroblasts," and mature adipose tissue.[48] Soon afterward, a series of similar lesions was published by Rosai and colleagues, who coined the term *ectopic hamartomatous thymoma*.[49] This tumor is believed to be of branchial origin.[49,50] Based on a comprehensive immunohistochemical analysis, it has been suggested that this tumor type is not in fact thymic in origin but instead contains a myoepithelial component and should be classified as a form of mixed tumor.[50]

Clinical Features

Ectopic hamartomatous thymoma affects adults, with a median age of 40 years and a striking predilection for men (male-to-female ratio, 10:1).[49,51] Most lesions are long-standing and painless. The tumors nearly always involve the supraclavicular, suprasternal, and neck regions.[49,50] The lesion may be either subcutaneous or subfascial.

Pathologic Features

Ectopic hamartomatous thymoma is a well-circumscribed but unencapsulated, lobulated mass averaging 5 cm.[48–50] The cut surface is tan or gray, with scattered foci of yellow adipose tissue. Foci of cystic degeneration are common.

Histologically, the tumor is composed of an admixture of plump spindle cells, smaller fibroblast-like spindle cells, mature adipose tissue, and islands and nests of epithelial cells (Figs. 9.15 and 9.16), including cysts.[49,50] The plump spindle cells contain ovoid nuclei with blunt ends, vesicular chromatin, inconspicuous nucleoli, and palely eosinophilic cytoplasm with indistinct cell borders, arranged in a fascicular or storiform pattern. The smaller fibroblast-like cells contain small slender nuclei and less cytoplasm. Mitotic activity is low, and necrosis is not observed. The proportion of adipose tissue is highly variable, ranging from less than 5% to 50%.[50] The epithelial component consists predominantly of nests and islands of squamous epithelium (Fig. 9.15), occasionally showing clear cell change or keratinization. Squamous epithelium also lines the cysts. A minor glandular component is often present, usually composed of small ducts with cuboidal epithelium (Fig. 9.17). A patchy lymphoid or lymphoplasmacytic infiltrate may be observed. Rarely, skeletal muscle (myoid) cells may be present.[51]

Immunohistochemistry

Both the epithelial and spindle cell components are positive for high- and low-molecular-weight keratins; diffuse keratin staining is usually observed in the plump spindle cells, and SMA may also be positive.[50] The fibroblast-like small spindle cells are typically positive for CD34.[50] EMA, S-100 protein, and desmin are negative in the spindle cell component. PAX8 is negative in all elements.[52]

Differential Diagnosis

After the characteristic anatomic site and distinctive histologic features are recognized, diagnosing ectopic hamartomatous thymoma is usually straightforward. However, the differential diagnosis might include mixed tumor of salivary glands (pleomorphic adenoma), biphasic synovial sarcoma, teratoma, and sarcomatoid carcinoma. Pleomorphic adenoma is usually dominated by myoepithelial cells showing variably spindled, epithelioid, or plasmacytoid (hyaline) morphology and contains scattered ducts. Unlike in ectopic hamartomatous thymoma, chondromyxoid stroma and foci of cartilaginous differentiation are common in mixed tumors of salivary glands. Origin in the salivary gland (especially parotid) is usually obvious. Both tumor types are extensively positive for keratins, but unlike mixed tumors of salivary glands, the spindle cell component in ectopic hamartomatous thymoma is usually negative for EMA, S-100 protein, and GFAP. PLAG1 is positive in most pleomorphic adenomas; CD34 is not expressed in myoepithelial tumors.

Ectopic hamartomatous thymoma with a prominent glandular component might be confused with biphasic synovial sarcoma. The spindle cells in synovial sarcoma contain hyperchromatic nuclei and scant cytoplasm, whereas the spindle cells in ectopic hamartomatous thymoma contain more abundant eosinophilic cytoplasm. Diffuse keratin expression is characteristic of ectopic hamartomatous thymoma, in contrast to the limited staining for keratin in the spindle cell component of synovial sarcoma, and CD34 is rarely positive in synovial sarcoma. The presence of squamous islands and an adipocytic component favor ectopic hamartomatous thymoma.

Teratoma is a germ cell tumor containing mature elements derived from ectoderm, mesoderm, and endoderm. In contrast to ectopic hamartomatous thymoma, teratoma arises in the mediastinum (not subcutaneous tissue), and the types of tissues encountered in teratoma are much more variable and include bone, cartilage, neural tissue, and diverse epithelia.

Both the spindle cells and the epithelial component in sarcomatoid carcinoma usually show frankly malignant cytology, and radiologic evaluation usually reveals a visceral primary site.

Prognosis and Treatment

Simple surgical excision is adequate therapy for ectopic hamartomatous thymoma. A small subset of tumors recur in a nondestructive fashion,

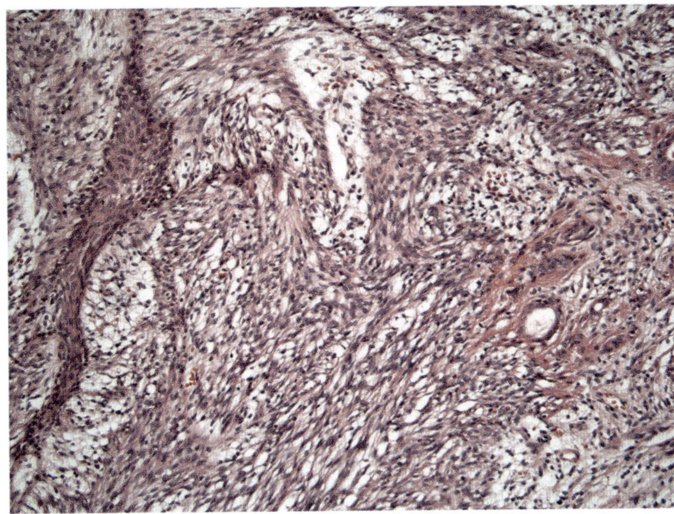

Figure 9.15 Ectopic Hamartomatous Thymoma. This distinctive tumor is composed of loose fascicles of plump spindle cells with eosinophilic cytoplasm and islands of epithelial cells, often with a squamoid appearance.

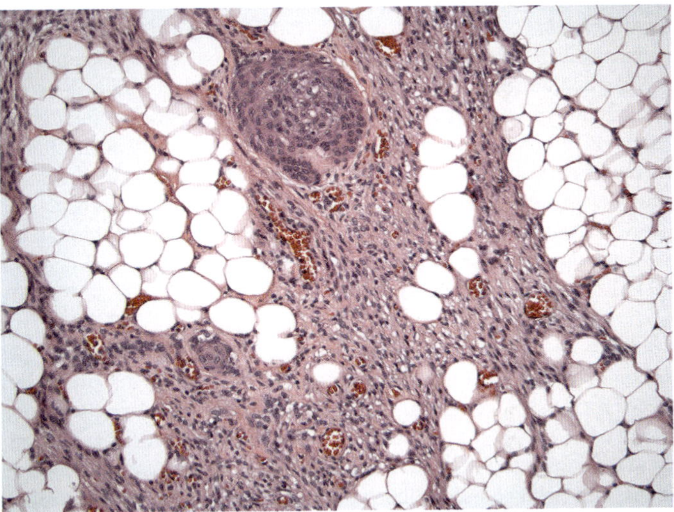

Figure 9.16 Ectopic Hamartomatous Thymoma. This tumor is an admixture of sheets of bland spindle cells, mature adipose tissue, and nests of squamoid epithelial cells.

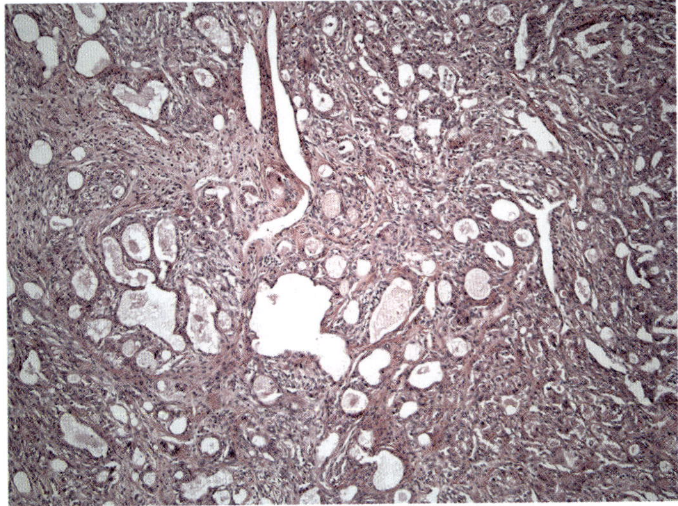

Figure 9.17 Ectopic Hamartomatous Thymoma. When a glandular component is prominent, ectopic hamartomatous thymoma may mimic biphasic synovial sarcoma.

generally after incomplete excision.[49,50] Rarely, carcinoma may arise in this lesion.[53]

PRACTICE POINTS: Ectopic Hamartomatous Thymoma

- Affects young to middle-aged adults, with a striking male predominance
- Arises in the supraclavicular, suprasternal, and neck regions
- Composed of plump spindle cells with eosinophilic cytoplasm, small fibroblast-like spindle cells, mature adipose tissue, and islands and nests of usually squamoid epithelial cells
- Spindle cell component is diffusely positive for keratins; fibroblast-like cells are positive for CD34
- Benign and rarely recurs after simple excision

Gastrointestinal Stromal Tumor, Mixed Type

Gastrointestinal stromal tumor (GIST) is the most common clinically significant mesenchymal neoplasm of the gastrointestinal tract. Most GISTs contain activating mutations of either *KIT* or *PDGFRA* tyrosine kinase receptor genes.[54] GIST is discussed in detail in Chapter 16.

Clinical Features

Men and women are equally affected. Most patients are older than 50 years. The majority of GISTs arise in the stomach (60%) or small intestine (30%); the duodenum, colon, and rectum are less commonly affected. Rarely, GIST arises primarily in the esophagus, mesentery, or omentum.[55] Occasionally, children and young adults may be affected. Such tumors are nearly exclusive to the stomach.[56,57] Some gastric GISTs are associated with Carney triad (GIST, paraganglioma, pulmonary chondroma) or Carney-Stratakis syndrome (GIST, paraganglioma); such tumors (and similar sporadic tumors; see later) are known as succinate dehydrogenase (SDH)-deficient GISTs (see Chapter 16).[54]

Pathologic Features

The majority of GISTs show spindle cell morphology, being composed of cells with slender nuclei, vesicular chromatin, small nucleoli, and fibrillary, eosinophilic cytoplasm with indistinct cell borders. Less often, GISTs show epithelioid morphology, with cells containing rounded nuclei and palely eosinophilic cytoplasm with a syncytial appearance or clear cytoplasm with more sharply defined cell borders.

In 10% to 20% of cases, GISTs show mixed spindle cell and epithelioid morphology.[58] Such tumors may show a distinctly biphasic appearance, with discrete spindle cell and epithelioid areas (Fig. 9.18), or may contain an intimate admixture of cell types that merge imperceptibly (Fig. 9.19).[54] SDH-deficient GISTs are nearly always of epithelioid or mixed epithelioid and spindle cell type; such tumors show a distinctive multinodular architecture and can therefore usually be recognized histologically.[54] With rare exceptions, GISTs are composed of remarkably uniform, bland cells without pleomorphism.

Immunohistochemistry

Nearly all GISTs (95%) are positive for KIT, which is highly specific for GIST among intraabdominal mesenchymal tumors.[59] KIT usually shows strong cytoplasmic staining, although epithelioid and mixed-type tumors may sometimes show a dotlike staining pattern. Epithelioid GISTs are more likely to show weak and focal staining for KIT or to be completely negative for this marker; such tumors often harbor *PDGFRA* mutations.[60–62] DOG1 (ANO1) is also positive in the vast majority of GISTs, including some KIT-negative tumors.[63–66]

Other markers that are commonly positive in GISTs include CD34 and h-caldesmon, although they are less specific. Expression of SMA is observed in a subset of cases, and S-100 protein and desmin are rarely expressed. Epithelioid gastric tumors are more likely to show reactivity for desmin.

SDH-deficient GISTs (Carney triad and Carney-Stratakis syndrome–associated GISTs and up to 10% of gastric GISTs overall) show loss of staining for SDHB.[67,68]

Molecular Genetics

Genetically, GISTs can be subdivided into three main categories: those containing mutations in the *KIT* gene (~80%); those with mutations in the *PDGFRA* gene (5% to 10%); and those lacking mutations in either gene ("wild-type" GISTs).[54] Although mutations in *KIT* may be seen in all histologic subtypes, *PDGFRA* mutations are more common in epithelioid and mixed-type tumors.[62,69–71] SDH-deficient GISTs (a large subset of "wild-type" GISTs) are driven by mutations in *SDHA*, *SDHB*, *SDHC*, or *SDHD*, or *SDHC* promoter hypermethylation; SDH-deficient GISTs are nearly always of epithelioid or mixed type.[67,68,72,73] The molecular findings in GISTs are discussed in more detail in Chapters 16 and 18.

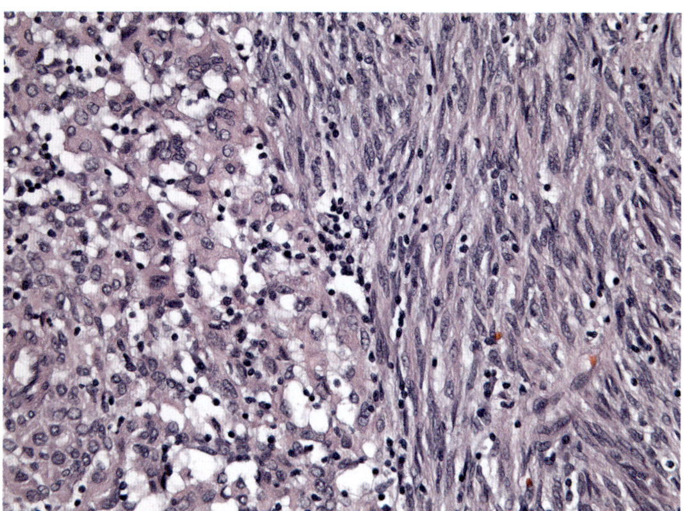

Figure 9.18 Gastrointestinal Stromal Tumor, Mixed Type. This tumor is composed of sharply demarcated spindle cell and epithelioid components. Note the uniform, bland nuclei and fibrillary cytoplasm.

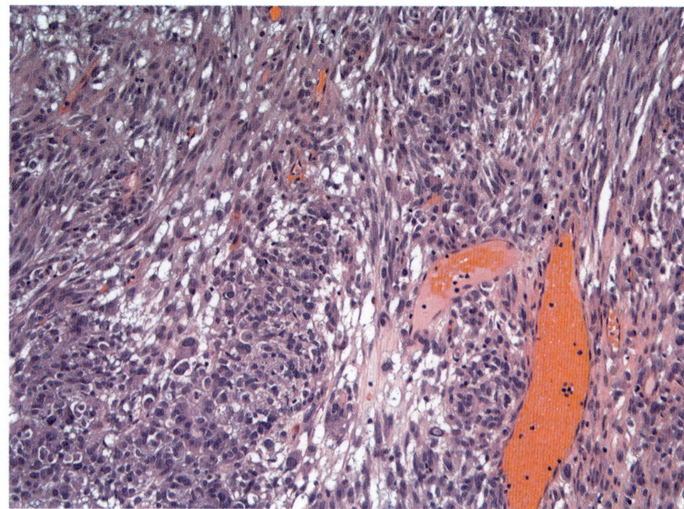

Figure 9.19 Gastrointestinal Stromal Tumor, Mixed Type. Some tumors contain an intimate admixture of epithelioid and spindle cells.

Differential Diagnosis

Because of its anatomic location and uniform morphology, the diagnosis of GIST is usually straightforward with application of a limited immunohistochemical panel. The differential diagnosis of mixed-type GIST may include carcinomas with a spindle cell (sarcomatoid) component, smooth muscle neoplasms, and malignant mesothelioma, although the distinction among these neoplasms can easily be made with the use of immunohistochemistry (Table 9.2).

Sarcomatoid carcinoma may contain both epithelioid and spindle cell components. In contrast to the uniform, bland cytology of GIST, carcinomas usually show marked nuclear atypia and pleomorphism. KIT is rarely positive in carcinomas, although DOG1 is positive in 25% to 30% of gastric adenocarcinomas, which represents a potential diagnostic pitfall.[65] Conversely, keratins are rarely positive in GIST (at most, in 1% of cases).

Both leiomyomas and leiomyosarcomas of the gastrointestinal tract are nearly always composed of spindle cells. Smooth muscle tumors with epithelioid morphology are rare and are usually malignant. Typical histologic features include brightly eosinophilic cytoplasm and well-defined cell borders. The most helpful discriminatory markers are KIT (only positive in GIST) and desmin (usually strongly positive in smooth muscle tumors; rarely positive in GIST).

Primary peritoneal malignant mesothelioma is rare and mostly affects men with a history of asbestos exposure. Most cases show purely epithelioid morphology, with tubular or tubulopapillary architecture, whereas a smaller subset of tumors are sarcomatoid or biphasic. Although mesotheliomas show relatively uniform cytology compared with carcinomas, they usually show more nuclear atypia than GISTs. In contrast to GIST, mesothelioma is usually strongly positive for keratins, EMA, and calretinin, and most tumors show nuclear staining for WT1. D2-40 (podoplanin) is not specific for mesothelioma in this context; a subset of GISTs is also positive.

Table 9.2 Differential Diagnosis for Mixed-Type Gastrointestinal Stromal Tumor

	KIT	DOG1	Desmin	Keratin	Nuclear WT1
Gastrointestinal stromal tumor	+	+	Rare	–	–
Sarcomatoid carcinoma	–	–	–	+	–
Leiomyosarcoma	–	Rare	+	±	–
Biphasic malignant mesothelioma	–	–	+	+	+

Prognosis and Treatment

The main prognostic factors in assessing the risk of malignant behavior of GISTs are anatomic location, mitotic rate, and tumor size. However, these features do not predict outcome for SDH-deficient GISTs.[74] The treatment and prognosis of GIST are discussed in Chapter 16. Overall, GISTs of the small intestine with epithelioid or mixed morphology may behave more aggressively,[75–77] although histologic subtype is not a significant prognostic factor compared with the factors listed previously.

Dedifferentiated Liposarcoma

DDLPS is defined as a nonlipogenic sarcoma arising in association with WDLPS. DDLPS usually presents as a primary tumor but may also appear as a recurrence of WDLPS. DDLPS is discussed in Chapters 7 and 12.

Clinical Features

Affecting predominantly adults, DDLPS is slightly more common in male patients. It most often arises in retroperitoneal, intraabdominal, pelvic, or mediastinal locations[78] and is rarely seen in the extremities.[78,79]

Pathologic Features

Usually, DDLPS is large and has a tan-gray and firm or fleshy cut surface. In some cases, discrete dedifferentiated and fatty areas are easily identified. Other cases are dominated by the nonlipogenic component and grossly resemble other high-grade sarcomas. DDLPS is generally well circumscribed, sometimes with a thin fibrous pseudocapsule. Areas of hemorrhage and necrosis may be seen. Sampling of the surrounding adipose tissue to identify WDLPS is critical in cases in which a fatty component is not obvious.

Histologically, DDLPS often shows considerable intratumoral heterogeneity, with mixed histologic patterns (Fig. 9.20), which is a helpful diagnostic clue. However, this characteristic makes proper diagnosis of core biopsy specimens challenging. Most tumors are characterized by a nondistinctive spindle cell proliferation, with varying cellularity and pleomorphism and fascicular, storiform, or mixed growth patterns.[78–81] DDLPS shows a range of morphology from relatively uniform, bland cytology ("low-grade dedifferentiation") to striking pleomorphism (see Fig. 9.20B). It may also contain epithelioid (Fig. 9.20C) and round cell components and hemangiopericytoma-like blood vessels (see Fig. 9.20D). Other histologic features include an inflammatory malignant fibrous histiocytoma–like pattern (Fig. 9.21), a neural (or meningioma)-like whorling architecture, and a myxofibrosarcoma-like pattern.[82–85] Again, a heterogeneous histologic appearance suggests DDLPS.

Heterologous elements are seen in a subset of DDLPS (approximately 10%), most often osteosarcoma, chondrosarcoma, rhabdomyosarcoma (Fig. 9.22), and leiomyosarcoma. Occasional cases may also show areas of "homologous" lipoblastic differentiation in the higher-grade component, mimicking pleomorphic LPS (Fig. 9.23).[86]

Immunohistochemistry

In more than 95% of cases, DDLPS expresses both MDM2 and CDK4 (see Fig. 9.21B).[46] Although these markers are sensitive for DDLPS, they are not entirely specific because they also stain a subset of other sarcomas that are included in the differential diagnosis.[46] However, in the context of a retroperitoneal, intraabdominal, or pelvic tumor with nondistinctive spindle cell morphology, detecting MDM2 and CDK4 can be very helpful in supporting the diagnosis. Other markers that may be positive in DDLPS include desmin, SMA, and CD34. Heterologous rhabdomyoblastic elements are positive for the skeletal muscle markers desmin and myogenin.

Molecular Genetics

The molecular findings of DDLPS are discussed in Chapters 12 and 18. DDLPS is characterized by the presence of ring and giant marker chromosomes derived from amplified material from chromosomal region 12q13-15, leading to overexpression of *MDM2*, *CDK4*, and *HMGA2*.[46,87] Conventional karyotyping and FISH are useful in showing these abnormalities.

Differential Diagnosis

The differential diagnosis of DDLPS depends on the dominant histologic findings and may include myxoid LPS, myxofibrosarcoma, MPNST, leiomyosarcoma, undifferentiated pleomorphic sarcoma, and sarcomatoid carcinoma.

Myxoid LPS and myxofibrosarcoma virtually never arise in central body sites (retroperitoneum, abdomen) as primary lesions. The former

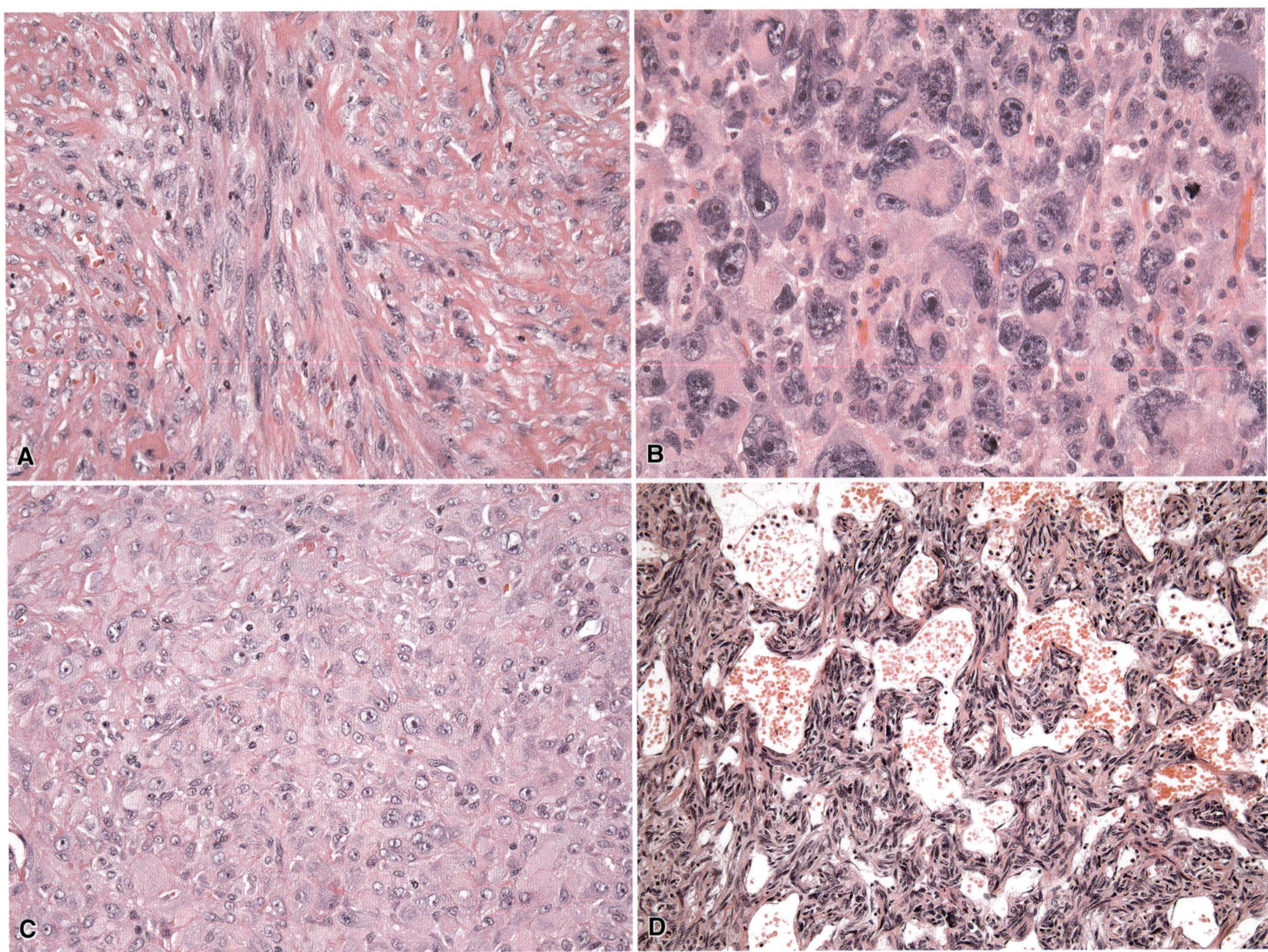

Figure 9.20 Dedifferentiated Liposarcoma. Dedifferentiated liposarcoma often shows striking intratumoral heterogeneity, ranging from fascicles of relatively uniform spindle cells (A) to sheets of highly pleomorphic cells with striking nuclear atypia (B). Some cases show areas with epithelioid morphology (C) and branching hemangiopericytoma-like blood vessels (D).

is characteristically seen in the limbs and limb girdles of young adults, whereas the latter is usually diagnosed in the extremities of elderly patients. Therefore primary lesions in retroperitoneal, mediastinal, or pelvic locations with histologic features resembling either of these tumor types most likely represent DDLPS.[88] Although DDLPS may contain prominent myxoid stroma and delicate plexiform blood vessels, the degree of nuclear atypia and pleomorphism in such areas is generally greater than that observed in myxoid LPS. Finding a well-differentiated liposarcomatous component confirms the diagnosis. Although expression of MDM2 and CDK4 favors DDLPS, these markers are not completely specific and may also be seen in a subset of myxoid LPSs and myxofibrosarcomas. However, in the appropriate clinical context (e.g., a large retroperitoneal mass), staining for MDM2 and CDK4 strongly favors DDLPS. Similarly, finding ring chromosomes by cytogenetics or *MDM2* amplification by FISH is helpful in confirming the diagnosis of DDLPS; FISH is more specific than immunohistochemistry and is used as the preferred diagnostic modality for DDLPS in many institutions.

Often arising in the same anatomic locations as DDLPS, MPNST may also contain heterologous elements. However, MPNST generally lacks the marked intratumoral heterogeneity of DDLPS, contains relatively uniform spindle cells with tapering nuclei, and characteristically shows perivascular hypercellularity. In addition, a neurofibromatous precursor may be seen in MPNST. MDM2 overexpression is commonly observed in both tumor types; however, because CDK4 is rarely positive in MPNST, the combination of these two markers is diagnostically helpful. MPNST shows cytogenetic findings distinct from those of DDLPS (i.e., complex nondistinctive karyotypes), and amplification of *MDM2* is not seen in MPNST. Loss of H3K27me3 is specific for MPNST in this differential diagnosis.

Leiomyosarcoma is usually characterized by a relatively uniform fascicular proliferation of spindle cells containing broad, blunt-ended nuclei and brightly eosinophilic cytoplasm, in contrast to the striking heterogeneity of DDLPS. DDLPS may show heterologous smooth muscle differentiation, but this finding is usually only focal. Leiomyosarcoma expresses SMA, desmin, and h-caldesmon. The former two markers may also be positive in DDLPS but generally not in a strong and diffuse fashion. MDM2 and CDK4 are rarely positive in leiomyosarcoma; amplification of *MDM2* detected by FISH is not observed in leiomyosarcoma.

Undifferentiated pleomorphic sarcoma is a diagnosis of exclusion; the overwhelming majority of sarcomas with such an appearance in the retroperitoneum represent DDLPS. This distinction is clinically important because DDLPS has a low metastatic rate. Therefore a

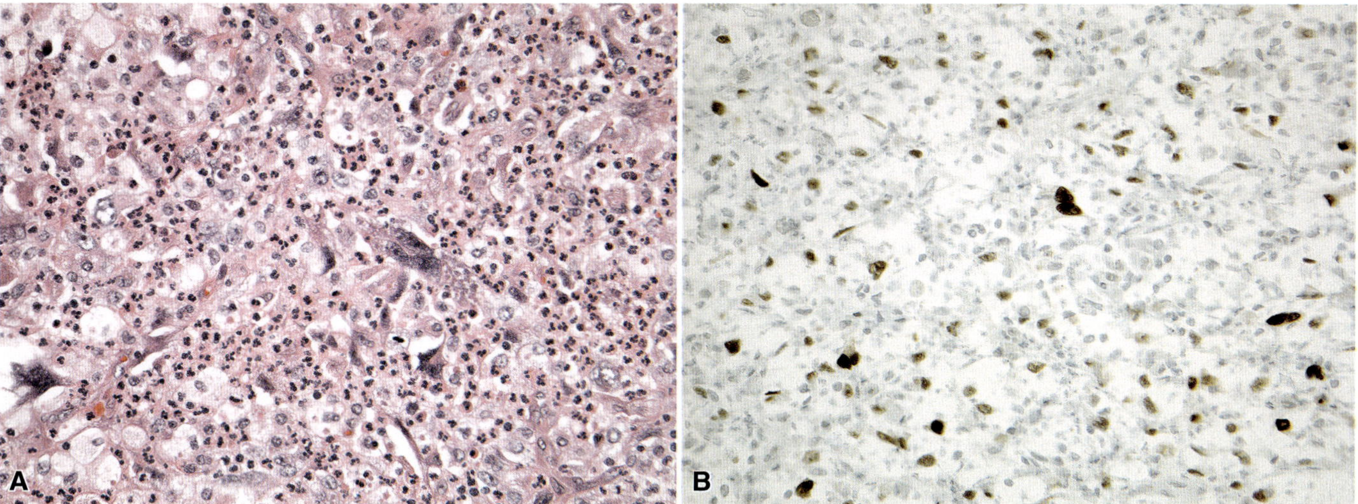

Figure 9.21 Dedifferentiated Liposarcoma. (A) Nearly all cases of inflammatory malignant fibrous histiocytoma are dedifferentiated liposarcomas with prominent inflammation. Note the abundant neutrophils and foamy histiocytes. (B) Nuclear reactivity for MDM2 is helpful to confirm the diagnosis.

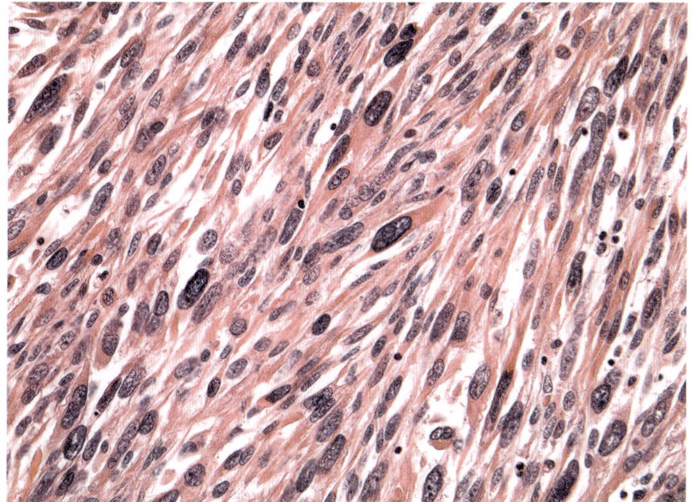

Figure 9.22 Dedifferentiated Liposarcoma. The brightly eosinophilic cytoplasm is a diagnostic clue to heterologous rhabdomyoblastic differentiation. A biopsy specimen showing this appearance from a retroperitoneal or intraabdominal tumor in an adult should suggest dedifferentiated liposarcoma.

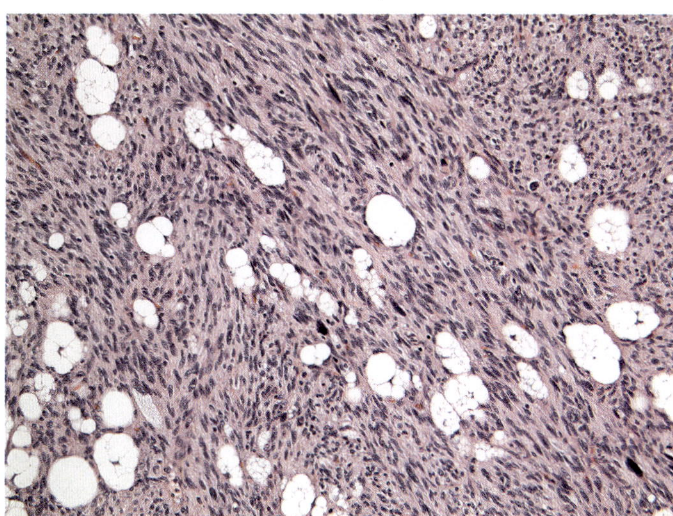

Figure 9.23 Dedifferentiated Liposarcoma. Lipoblastic differentiation may occasionally be found in the otherwise nonlipogenic component of dedifferentiated liposarcoma, mimicking pleomorphic liposarcoma.

careful search for a well-differentiated liposarcomatous appearance and immunohistochemistry for MDM2 and CDK4 (or FISH for *MDM2*) are mandatory before undifferentiated pleomorphic sarcoma can be diagnosed in the retroperitoneum. DDLPS usually shows considerable heterogeneity, including morphologically lower-grade spindle cell areas.

A visceral origin is usually obvious for sarcomatoid carcinomas. The most common primary sites are the kidney and lung. Proper sampling may show a conventional epithelial component. Detection of keratin expression helps support the diagnosis of sarcomatoid carcinoma, but several broad-spectrum keratin antibodies may be required and staining may be limited. In general, sarcomatoid carcinomas usually lack more specific lineage markers, although sarcomatoid renal cell carcinoma may be positive for PAX8. MDM2 and CDK4 may also be positive in carcinomas. Amplification of *MDM2* by FISH favors DDLPS.

Prognosis and Treatment

The prognosis of DDLPS is discussed in Chapter 12.

PRACTICE POINTS: Dedifferentiated Liposarcoma

- Defined as a nonlipogenic sarcoma associated with well-differentiated liposarcoma (atypical lipomatous tumor)
- May occur de novo or as a recurrence of well-differentiated liposarcoma
- Affects middle-aged and elderly adults
- Most common in intraabdominal, retroperitoneal, pelvic, or mediastinal locations
- Typically shows considerable morphologic heterogeneity; 10% contain heterologous elements
- Positive for MDM2 and CDK4 in >95% of cases; FISH for *MDM2* is helpful to confirm the diagnosis
- Tendency for local recurrence and 15%–20% rate of distant metastasis

Melanotic Neuroectodermal Tumor of Infancy

Melanotic neuroectodermal tumor of infancy (MNTI) is a rare tumor of young children that has previously been referred to as *congenital melanoma, melanotic adamantinoma, retinal anlage tumor, melanotic progonoma,* and *pigmented epulis of infancy.*[89] Although MNTI usually behaves in a benign fashion, a small subset of cases pursue a malignant clinical course. This tumor type is believed to be of neuroectodermal origin, with some cells showing neuroblastic differentiation and others producing melanin pigment.[90]

Clinical Features

Mainly affecting young infants with a median age of 5 to 6 months, MNTI has no apparent sex predilection.[89–92] Patients usually present with a rapidly growing mass. The most common sites include the head and neck (especially the maxilla and mandible), skull, epididymis, testis, and brain.[89–92] Rarely, urinary excretion of vanillylmandelic acid is found, further supporting a neural crest origin.[93] Imaging studies usually show a cystic radiolucent lesion with destruction of bone.[92]

Pathologic Features

Grossly, MNTI is usually well-circumscribed and lobulated, with an average size of 4 cm. The cut surface is often firm and gray to black, depending on the amount of melanin pigment.

Histologically, MNTI is a biphasic neoplasm consisting of cellular nests separated by a fibrous stroma (Fig. 9.24A). The nests may resemble alveolar structures. Two distinct populations of cells are observed. Larger epithelioid cells with eosinophilic cytoplasm containing variably prominent melanin pigment (Fig. 9.25) sometimes line the alveolar structures, and small cells that resemble neuroblasts with round nuclei, fine chromatin, inconspicuous nucleoli, and scant cytoplasm (see Fig. 9.24A) are usually located toward the center of the nests. These cells may be embedded within a neurofibrillary matrix, similar to glial tissue. Although atypia may be present, mitotic figures are rare.

Immunohistochemistry

The large, pigment-producing epithelioid cells are consistently positive for keratin (see Fig. 9.24B), HMB-45, and neuron-specific enolase (NSE), and variably positive for EMA.[90,92,94,95] The small cell (neuroblastic) component is also positive for NSE, as well as synaptophysin, but negative for keratin.[90,92,95] Both cell types are negative for S-100 protein, chromogranin, neurofilament protein, desmin, and CEA.

Differential Diagnosis

After the distinctive admixture of cell types is recognized, there is no realistic differential diagnosis for MNTI. The small cell component of MNTI should be differentiated from other small round cell tumors of childhood, namely, alveolar rhabdomyosarcoma, desmoplastic small round cell tumor (DSRCT), and metastatic neuroblastoma, whereas the larger cell component might be mistaken for melanoma. These lesions can be distinguished with the use of immunohistochemistry and molecular genetic studies.

Alveolar rhabdomyosarcoma consistently expresses desmin and myogenin and is usually negative for keratins. Similar to the small cell component of MNTI, alveolar rhabdomyosarcoma may also be positive for synaptophysin.

In contrast to MNTI, DSRCT is usually associated with markedly desmoplastic stroma. DSRCT shows a polyphenotypic staining pattern, with reactivity for NSE, desmin, keratin, and EMA. The small cell component of MNTI is generally positive only for NSE. DSRCT harbors a t(11;22)(p13;q12) translocation, juxtaposing the *EWSR1* gene on chromosome 22 with the *WT1* gene on chromosome 11. RT-PCR or FISH can be used to detect this rearrangement.

Similar to MNTI, neuroblastoma is characterized by a proliferation of small round cells with neuronal differentiation, evidenced by the expression of NSE and synaptophysin and occasional Homer Wright rosettes. Recognition of the pigment-producing larger epithelioid cell component facilitates the diagnosis of MNTI.

In contrast to the epithelioid cells in MNTI, melanocytic neoplasms are consistently positive for S-100 protein and negative for keratins, although HMB-45 is positive in both tumor types.

Prognosis and Treatment

The treatment for MNTI is complete surgical excision, if possible. Most tumors behave in a benign fashion, with a 20% risk of local recurrence. Metastases are rare (<5%); histologic features cannot predict which tumors will behave aggressively.[90,92]

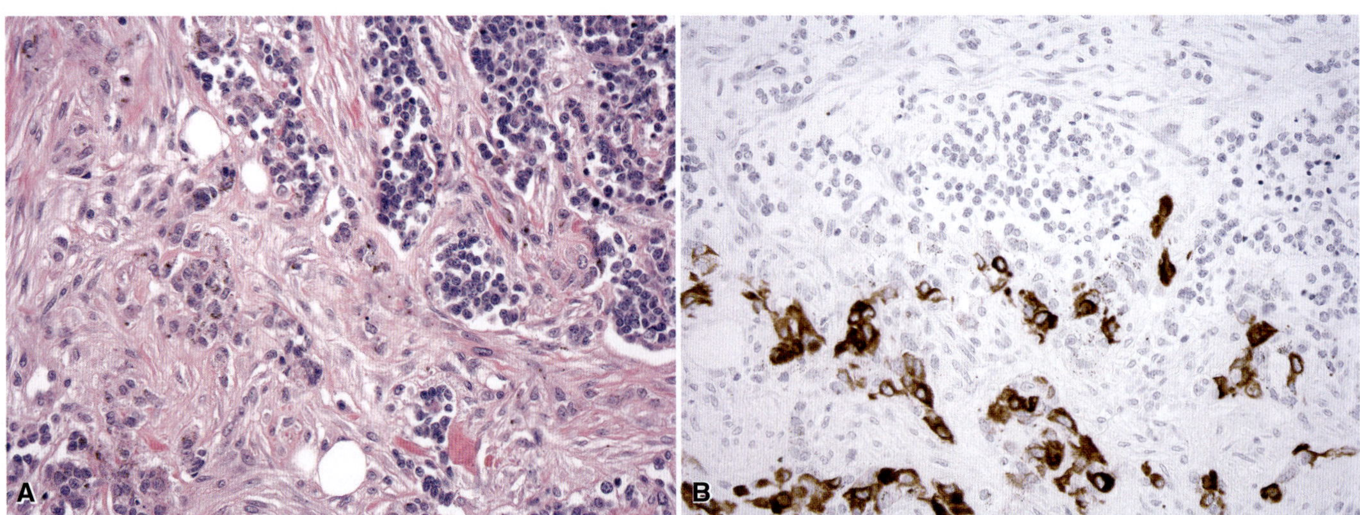

Figure 9.24 Melanotic Neuroectodermal Tumor of Infancy. (A) This tumor is composed of nests of small round cells separated by fibrous stroma *(right)*, in addition to larger epithelioid cells *(left)*. (B) The epithelioid cells are consistently positive for keratin.

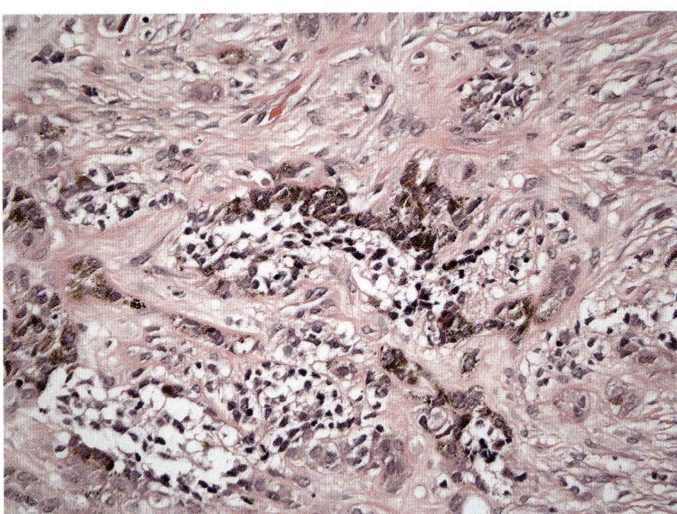

Figure 9.25 **Melanotic Neuroectodermal Tumor of Infancy.** The epithelioid cells contain melanin pigment and often line alveolar structures. Note the small round cells in the center of the nests.

PRACTICE POINTS: Melanotic Neuroectodermal Tumor of Infancy

- Affects mainly infants
- Presents as a rapidly growing mass
- Arises most often in head and neck, skull, epididymis, testis, and brain
- Characterized by biphasic nests of cells separated by fibrous tissue
- Small cell component resembles neuroblasts, whereas the larger epithelioid component contains melanin pigment
- Most cases are benign, with a recurrence rate of 20%
- Rarely metastasize; histologic features cannot predict malignant behavior

Nonmesenchymal Tumors With Biphasic and Mixed Patterns

A small group of nonmesenchymal tumors characteristically show biphasic or mixed histologic patterns, which may also include heterologous elements. These tumor types merit brief discussion because they can be considered in the differential diagnosis of mesenchymal tumors. Such tumors include sarcomatoid carcinoma, malignant mesothelioma, germ cell tumor, and müllerian carcinosarcoma (MMMT).

Clinical Features

Sarcomatoid carcinomas are uncommon, aggressive histologic variants. Although they may rarely arise in almost any organ, the lung and kidney are the most common primary sites. These tumors affect the same population as their nonsarcomatoid counterparts.

Malignant mesothelioma is an uncommon neoplasm that arises in the pleura, or less commonly, the peritoneum. It is linked to occupational exposure to asbestos, which is more strongly associated with pleural disease and less clearly identified as a risk factor in peritoneal cases.[96] Men in the seventh and eighth decades are most commonly affected.

Germ cell tumors affect primarily young men, ranging from 20 to 40 years, and most commonly arise in the testis but can more rarely arise at extragonadal sites, including the retroperitoneum and mediastinum. Symptoms are related to anatomic location, and laboratory findings often include elevated tumor markers, such as α-fetoprotein and β-human chorionic gonadotrophin.

A gynecologic tumor that usually arises in the uterus, müllerian carcinosarcoma may occasionally involve the ovary or peritoneum.[97,98] Affected patients are predominantly older postmenopausal women, with a median age of 65 years, who usually present with a large pelvic mass, mainly involving the uterus.[99-103]

Pathologic Features

Sarcomatoid carcinoma is typically a spindle cell neoplasm with marked nuclear atypia. The degree of pleomorphism is variable, and occasionally lesions may be deceptively bland. Areas of conventional carcinoma may be identified with thorough sampling of the tumor.

Biphasic malignant mesothelioma contains an admixture of epithelioid and sarcomatoid components (Fig. 9.26A). Within the epithelioid areas, several distinct growth patterns (tubular, nested, papillary) can be identified, whereas the sarcomatoid component shows variable morphology, ranging from a fascicular growth pattern with elongated spindle cells with mild atypia to more compact spindle cells or occasionally cells with more prominent pleomorphism.

Germ cell tumors may be composed of a highly variable mixture of seminomatous and nonseminomatous elements, including embryonal carcinoma, yolk sac tumor, choriocarcinoma, and teratoma (see Fig. 9.26B). Occasionally, a somatic malignancy may develop from the teratomatous component, including sarcoma (e.g., rhabdomyosarcoma [see Fig. 9.26C] and angiosarcoma).

Characterized by variable amounts of carcinoma and malignant mesenchymal (sarcomatous) components (see Fig. 9.26D), müllerian carcinosarcoma usually has an epithelial component that is of high grade and often shows features of endometrioid or serous carcinoma. The sarcomatous component shows a mixture of nondistinctive spindle cell and undifferentiated round cell sarcoma and may also contain differentiated elements, such as rhabdomyosarcoma, leiomyosarcoma, chondrosarcoma, and osteosarcoma.

Immunohistochemistry

The typical immunohistochemical findings are summarized in Table 9.3. Sarcomatoid carcinomas are usually at least focally positive for one or more broad-spectrum keratins; however, specific lineage markers, such as TTF-1, are usually negative. Epithelioid malignant mesothelioma is consistently positive for keratins, calretinin, WT1 (nuclear), and D2-40 (podoplanin), whereas the latter three markers are less consistently expressed in sarcomatoid areas. Loss of BAP1 expression is more common in epithelioid malignant mesotheliomas than sarcomatoid mesotheliomas.[23,24] Most components of germ cell tumors are positive for keratins, placental-like alkaline phosphatase, and SALL4; α-fetoprotein and glypican-3 are usually positive in yolk sac tumors, and β-human chorionic gonadotrophin is positive in choriocarcinoma. Embryonal carcinoma is positive for CD30 and shows nuclear staining for the embryonic stem cell transcription factors OCT4 and SOX2.[104,105] In contrast to other components, seminomas are most often positive for KIT and podoplanin (D2-40)[106,107]; OCT4 is also positive in seminoma.[104,105] In müllerian carcinosarcoma the epithelial component expresses keratins, whereas in a subset of cases the sarcomatous component is also variably positive for keratins. WT1 and PAX8 are usually also positive in the carcinomatous component. Other markers, such as desmin, SMA, and S-100 protein, are variably expressed, depending on the differentiated mesenchymal elements present.

Molecular Genetics

One tumor type in this group for which molecular genetics can occasionally play a role in the differential diagnosis is germ cell tumors. Up to 80% of germ cell tumors are characterized by isochromosome 12p, whereas other cases contain excess genetic material from 12p in derivative

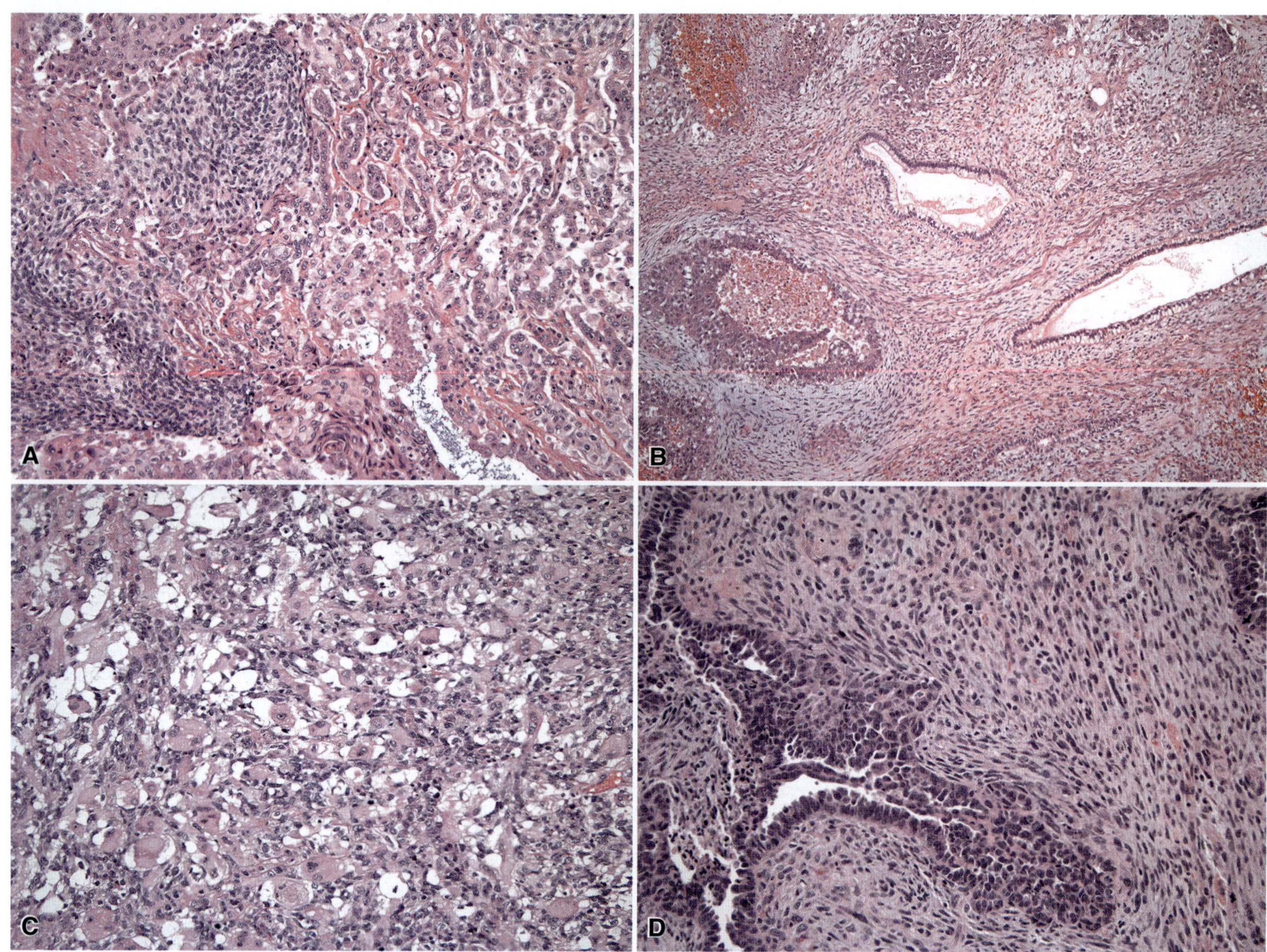

Figure 9.26 Nonmesenchymal Tumors With Biphasic and Mixed Patterns. (A) Biphasic malignant mesothelioma characterized by a spindle cell component admixed with an epithelioid component with tubulopapillary architecture. Note the uniform cytology. (B) Nonseminomatous malignant germ cell tumor composed of teratoma (with epithelial and mesenchymal elements) and islands of embryonal carcinoma. (C) Rarely, the teratomatous component of a germ cell tumor may give rise to a sarcomatous somatic malignancy such as rhabdomyosarcoma. Without a high index of suspicion, such tumors may be misdiagnosed as sarcomas. (D) Carcinosarcoma (malignant mixed müllerian tumor) showing an admixture of high-grade serous carcinoma and a nondescript spindle cell sarcoma.

chromosomes.[108-110] FISH can be used to assess for the presence of isochromosome 12p in difficult cases of a poorly differentiated malignant neoplasm where a germ cell tumor is suspected but the immunohistochemical findings are equivocal.

Differential Diagnosis

Sarcomatoid carcinoma and biphasic malignant mesothelioma should be differentiated from each other, as well as from biphasic synovial sarcoma. In contrast to synovial sarcoma, the sarcomatoid components of both malignant mesothelioma and sarcomatoid carcinoma usually show considerable nuclear atypia; pleomorphism is common in sarcomatoid carcinoma, whereas the spindle cells in mesothelioma and synovial sarcoma are relatively uniform. Similar to synovial sarcoma, both sarcomatoid mesothelioma and sarcomatoid carcinoma are focally positive for keratins, but EMA is rarely expressed in the sarcomatoid components of these tumors (with the exception of sarcomatoid renal cell carcinoma). Expression of calretinin and WT1 in the epithelioid component of mesothelioma is helpful in distinguishing between these tumor types. Loss of BAP1 expression is specific for mesothelioma in this differential diagnosis. TLE1 is positive in both synovial sarcomas and mesotheliomas; therefore this marker cannot be used in the differential diagnosis. In difficult cases, cytogenetics or molecular studies showing t(X;18) can confirm the diagnosis of synovial sarcoma.

The differential diagnosis of germ cell tumors depends on the components present within the neoplasm; however, recognition of the characteristic elements and the use of appropriate immunohistochemistry usually make the diagnosis relatively straightforward. In small core biopsy specimens, various sarcomas (e.g., MPNST and DDLPS with heterologous differentiation when mesenchymal teratomatous elements are encountered), poorly differentiated carcinoma, metastatic melanoma, and even large cell lymphoma may be considered. Because OCT4 is expressed in embryonal carcinoma and seminoma, nuclear staining for this marker in a poorly differentiated epithelioid malignant neoplasm is most helpful to confirm the diagnosis of germ cell tumor.

Tumors that might be considered in the differential diagnosis with müllerian carcinosarcoma include DDLPS and MPNST with heterologous

Table 9.3 Differential Diagnosis for Nonmesenchymal Tumors With Biphasic and Mixed Patterns

	Keratin	Calretinin	Nuclear WT1	OCT4	Placental-Like Alkaline Phosphatase
Sarcomatoid carcinoma	+	–	–	–	–
Biphasic malignant mesothelioma	+	+	+	–	–
Germ cell tumors	+	–	–	+	+
Carcinosarcoma (malignant mixed müllerian tumor)	+ (carcinoma)	–	+ (carcinoma)	–	–

elements. DDLPS characteristically shows marked intratumoral heterogeneity similar to that of carcinosarcoma, but it lacks a true epithelial component; a well-differentiated adipocytic component should be sought to confirm the diagnosis. Keratins are not expressed in DDLPS. In the rare cases of MPNST with glandular differentiation, the glands usually appear benign or low-grade malignant, in contrast to the high-grade carcinomatous component of carcinosarcoma. The spindle cell component in MPNST characteristically shows varying cellularity with myxoid areas and perivascular accentuation.

References

1. Ladanyi M, Antonescu CR, Leung DH, et al: Impact of SYT-SSX fusion type on the clinical behavior of synovial sarcoma: a multi-institutional retrospective study of 243 patients, *Cancer Res* 62:135–140, 2002.
2. Lewis JJ, Antonescu CR, Leung DH, et al: Synovial sarcoma: a multivariate analysis of prognostic factors in 112 patients with primary localized tumors of the extremities, *J Clin Oncol* 18:2087–2094, 2000.
3. Miettinen M, Limon J, Niezabitowski A, et al: Pattern of keratin polypeptides in 110 biphasic, monophasic, and poorly differentiated synovial sarcoma, *Virchows Arch* 437:275–283, 2000.
4. Trassard M, Le Doussal V, Hacène K, et al: Prognostic factors in localized primary synovial sarcoma: a multicentric study on 128 adult patients, *J Clin Oncol* 19:525–534, 2001.
5. Coindre JM, Pelmus M, Hostein I, et al: Should molecular testing be required for diagnosing synovial sarcoma?, *Cancer* 98:2700–2707, 2003.
6. Gaertner E, Zeren HE, Fleming MV, et al: Biphasic synovial sarcoma arising in the pleural cavity: a clinicopathologic study of 5 cases, *Am J Surg Pathol* 20:36–45, 1996.
7. Bégueret H, Galateau-Salle F, Guillou L, et al: Primary intrathoracic synovial sarcoma. A clinicopathologic study of 40 t(X;18)-positive cases from the French Sarcoma Group and the Mesopath Group, *Am J Surg Pathol* 29:339–346, 2005.
8. Suster S, Moran CA: Primary synovial sarcomas of the mediastinum. A clinicopathologic, immunohistochemical, and ultrastructural study of 15 cases, *Am J Surg Pathol* 29:569–578, 2005.
9. Argani P, Faria PA, Epstein JI, et al: Primary renal synovial sarcoma: molecular and morphologic delineation of an entity previously included among embryonal sarcomas of the kidney, *Am J Surg Pathol* 24:1087–1096, 2000.
10. Fisher C, Folpe AL, Hashimoto H, et al: Intra-abdominal synovial sarcoma: a clinicopathologic study, *Histopathology* 45:245–253, 2004.
11. Makhlouf HR, Ahrens W, Agarwal B, et al: Synovial sarcoma of the stomach. A clinicopathologic, immunohistochemical, and molecular genetic study of 10 cases, *Am J Surg Pathol* 32:275–281, 2008.
12. Harb WJ, Luna MA, Patel SR, et al: Survival in patients with synovial sarcoma of the head and neck: association with tumor location, size, and extension, *Head Neck* 29:731–740, 2007.
13. Pelmus M, Guillou L, Hostein I, et al: Monophasic fibrous and poorly differentiated synovial sarcoma: immunohistochemical reassessment of 60 t(X;18)(SYT-SSX)-positive cases, *Am J Surg Pathol* 26:1434–1440, 2002.
14. Terry J, Saito T, Subramanian S, et al: TLE1 as a diagnostic immunohistochemical marker for synovial sarcoma emerging from gene expression profiling studies, *Am J Surg Pathol* 31:240–246, 2007.
15. Kosemehmetoglu K, Vrana JA, Folpe AL: TLE1 expression is not specific for synovial sarcoma: a whole section study of 163 soft tissue and bone neoplasms, *Mod Pathol* 22:872–878, 2009.
16. Jagdis A, Rubin BP, Tubbs RR, et al: Prospective evaluation of TLE1 as a diagnostic immunohistochemical marker in synovial sarcoma, *Am J Surg Pathol* 33:1743–1751, 2009.
17. Knösel T, Heretsch S, Altendorf-Hofmann A, et al: TLE1 is a robust diagnostic biomarker for synovial sarcomas and correlates with t(X;18): analysis of 319 cases, *Eur J Cancer* 46:1170–1176, 2010.
18. Foo WC, Cruise MW, Wick MR, et al: Immunohistochemical staining for TLE1 distinguishes synovial sarcoma from histologic mimics, *Am J Clin Pathol* 135:839–844, 2011.
19. Kohashi K, Oda Y, Yamamoto H, et al: Reduced expression of SMARCB1/INI1 protein in synovial sarcoma, *Mod Pathol* 23:981–990, 2010.
20. Ladanyi M: Fusions of the SYT and SSX genes in synovial sarcoma, *Oncogene* 20:5755–5762, 2001.
21. Kawai A, Woodruff JM, Healey JH, et al: SYT-SSX gene fusion as a determinant of morphology and prognosis in synovial sarcoma, *N Engl J Med* 338:153–160, 1998.
22. Matsuyama A, Hisaoka M, Iwasaki M, et al: TLE1 expression in malignant mesothelioma, *Virchows Arch* 457:577–583, 2010.
23. Wu D, Hiroshima K, Yusa T, et al: Usefulness of p16/CDKN2A fluorescence in situ hybridization and BAP1 immunohistochemistry for the diagnosis of biphasic mesothelioma, *Ann Diagn Pathol* 26:31–37, 2017.
24. Cigognetti M, Lonardi S, Fisogni S, et al: BAP1 (BRCA1-associated protein 1) is a highly specific marker for differentiating mesothelioma from reactive mesothelial proliferations, *Mod Pathol* 28:1043–1057, 2015.
25. Woodruff JM, Christensen WN: Glandular peripheral nerve sheath tumors, *Cancer* 15:3618–3628, 1993.
26. Schaefer IM, Fletcher CD, Hornick JL: Loss of H3K27 trimethylation distinguishes malignant peripheral nerve sheath tumors from histologic mimics, *Mod Pathol* 29:4–13, 2016.
27. Prieto-Granada CN, Wiesner T, Messina JL, et al: Loss of H3K27me3 expression is a highly sensitive marker for sporadic and radiation-induced MPNST, *Am J Surg Pathol* 40:479–489, 2016.
28. Bahrami A, Dalton JD, Krane JF, et al: A subset of cutaneous and soft tissue mixed tumors are genetically linked to their salivary gland counterpart, *Genes Chromosomes Cancer* 51:140–148, 2012.
29. Antonescu CR, Zhang L, Shao SY, et al: Frequent PLAG1 gene rearrangements in skin and soft tissue myoepithelioma with ductal differentiation, *Genes Chromosomes Cancer* 52:675–682, 2013.
30. Hornick JL, Fletcher CDM: Myoepithelial tumors of soft tissue: a clinicopathologic and immunohistochemical study of 101 cases with evaluation of prognostic parameters, *Am J Surg Pathol* 27:1183–1196, 2003.
31. Gleason BC, Fletcher CDM: Myoepithelial carcinoma of soft tissue in children: an aggressive neoplasm analyzed in a series of 29 cases, *Am J Surg Pathol* 31:1813–1824, 2007.
32. Miettinen M, McCue PA, Sarlomo-Rikala M, et al: Sox10–a marker for not only schwannian and melanocytic neoplasms but also myoepithelial cell tumors of soft tissue: a systematic analysis of 5134 tumors, *Am J Surg Pathol* 39:826–835, 2015.
33. Hornick JL, Dal Cin P, Fletcher CD: Loss of INI1 expression is characteristic of both conventional and proximal-type epithelioid sarcoma, *Am J Surg Pathol* 33:542–550, 2009.
34. Antonescu CR, Zhang L, Chang NE, et al: EWSR1-POU5F1 fusion in soft tissue myoepithelial tumors. A molecular analysis of sixty-six cases, including soft tissue, bone, and visceral lesions, showing common involvement of the EWSR1 gene, *Genes Chromosomes Cancer* 49:1114–1124, 2010.
35. Flucke U, Palmedo G, Blankenhorn N, et al: EWSR1 gene rearrangement occurs in a subset of cutaneous myoepithelial tumors: a study of 18 cases, *Mod Pathol* 24:1444–1450, 2011.
36. Brandal P, Panagopoulos I, Bjerkehagen B, et al: Detection of a t(1;22)(q23;q12) translocation leading to an EWSR1-PBX1 fusion gene in a myoepithelioma, *Genes Chromosomes Cancer* 47:558–564, 2008.
37. Brandal P, Panagopoulos I, Bjerkehagen B, et al: t(19;22)(q13;q12) translocation leading to the novel fusion gene EWSR1-ZNF444 in soft tissue myoepithelial carcinoma, *Genes Chromosomes Cancer* 48:1051–1056, 2009.
38. Flucke U, Mentzel T, Verdijk MA, et al: EWSR1-ATF1 chimeric transcript in a myoepithelial tumor of soft tissue: a case report, *Hum Pathol* 43:764–768, 2012.
39. Agaram NP, Chen HW, Zhang L, et al: EWSR1-PBX3: a novel gene fusion in myoepithelial tumors, *Genes Chromosomes Cancer* 54:63–71, 2015.
40. Huang SC, Chen HW, Zhang L, et al: Novel FUS-KLF17 and EWSR1-KLF17 fusions in myoepithelial tumors, *Genes Chromosomes Cancer* 54:267–275, 2015.
41. Ducatman BS, Scheithauer BW, Piepgras DG, et al: Malignant peripheral nerve sheath tumors. A clinicopathologic study of 120 cases, *Cancer* 57:2006–2021, 1986.
42. Hruban RH, Shiu MH, Senie RT, et al: Malignant peripheral nerve sheath tumors of the buttock and lower extremity. A study of 43 cases, *Cancer* 66:1253–1265, 1990.
43. Woodruff JM: Peripheral nerve tumors showing glandular differentiation (glandular schwannomas), *Cancer* 37:2399–2413, 1976.
44. Le Guellec S, Decouvelaere AV, Filleron T, et al: Malignant peripheral nerve sheath tumor is a challenging diagnosis: a systematic pathology review, immunohistochemistry, and molecular analysis in 160 patients from the French Sarcoma Group database, *Am J Surg Pathol* 40:896–908, 2016.

45. Daimaru Y, Hashimoto H, Enjoji M: Malignant peripheral nerve-sheath tumors (malignant schwannomas). An immunohistochemical study of 29 cases, *Am J Surg Pathol* 9:434–444, 1985.
46. Binh MB, Sastre-Garau X, Guillou L, et al: MDM2 and CDK4 immunostainings are useful adjuncts in diagnosing well-differentiated and dedifferentiated liposarcoma subtypes. A comparative analysis of 559 soft tissue neoplasms with genetic data, *Am J Surg Pathol* 29:1340–1347, 2005.
47. Kamran SC, Howard SA, Shinagare AB, et al: Malignant peripheral nerve sheath tumors: prognostic impact of rhabdomyoblastic differentiation (malignant triton tumors), neurofibromatosis 1 status and location, *Eur J Surg Oncol* 39:46–52, 2013.
48. Smith PS, McClure J: Unusual subcutaneous mixed tumour exhibiting adipose, fibroblastic, and epithelial components, *J Clin Pathol* 35:1074–1077, 1982.
49. Rosai J, Limas C, Husband EM: Ectopic hamartomatous thymoma. A distinctive benign lesion of lower neck, *Am J Surg Pathol* 8:501–513, 1984.
50. Fetsch JF, Laskin WB, Michal M, et al: Ectopic hamartomatous thymoma. A clinicopathologic and immunohistochemical analysis of 21 cases with data supporting reclassification as a branchial anlage mixed tumor, *Am J Surg Pathol* 28:1360–1370, 2004.
51. Saeed IT, Fletcher CD: Ectopic hamartomatous thymoma containing myoid cells, *Histopathology* 17:572–574, 1990.
52. Weissferdt A, Kalhor N, Petersson F, et al: Ectopic hamartomatous thymoma-new insights into a challenging entity: a clinicopathologic and immunohistochemical study of 9 cases, *Am J Surg Pathol* 40:1571–1576, 2016.
53. Michal M, Neubauer L, Fakan F: Carcinoma arising in ectopic hamartomatous thymoma. An ultrastructural study, *Pathol Res Pract* 192:610–618, 1996.
54. Doyle LA, Hornick JL: Gastrointestinal stromal tumours: from KIT to succinate dehydrogenase, *Histopathology* 64:53–67, 2014.
55. Miettinen M, Sobin LH, Lasota J: Gastrointestinal stromal tumors presenting as omental masses—a clinicopathologic analysis of 95 cases, *Am J Surg Pathol* 33:1267–1275, 2009.
56. Miettinen M, Lasota J, Sobin LH: Gastrointestinal stromal tumors of the stomach in children and young adults. A clinicopathologic, immunohistochemical, and molecular genetic study of 44 cases with long-term follow-up and review of the literature, *Am J Surg Pathol* 29:1373–1381, 2005.
57. Rege TA, Wagner AJ, Corless CL, et al: "Pediatric-type" gastrointestinal stromal tumors in adults: distinctive histology predicts genotype and clinical behavior, *Am J Surg Pathol* 35:495–504, 2011.
58. Miettinen M, Lasota J: Gastrointestinal stromal tumors: review on morphology, molecular pathology, prognosis, and differential diagnosis, *Arch Pathol Lab Med* 130:1466–1478, 2006.
59. Hornick JL, Fletcher CD: Immunohistochemical staining for KIT (CD117) in soft tissue sarcomas is very limited in distribution, *Am J Clin Pathol* 117:188–193, 2002.
60. Medeiros F, Corless CL, Duensing A, et al: KIT-negative gastrointestinal stromal tumors. Proof of concept and therapeutic implications, *Am J Surg Pathol* 28:889–894, 2004.
61. Debiec-Rychter M, Wasag B, Stul M, et al: Gastrointestinal stromal tumours (GISTs) negative for KIT (CD117 antigen) immunoreactivity, *J Pathol* 202:430–438, 2004.
62. Wong NA: Mangwana S. KIT and PDGFRα mutational analyses of mixed cell-type gastrointestinal stromal tumours, *Histopathology* 51:758–762, 2007.
63. Espinosa I, Lee CH, Kim MK, et al: A novel monoclonal antibody against DOG1 is a sensitive and specific marker for gastrointestinal stromal tumors, *Am J Surg Pathol* 32:210–218, 2008.
64. Liegl B, Hornick JL, Corless CL, et al: Monoclonal antibody DOG1.1 shows higher sensitivity than KIT in the diagnosis of gastrointestinal stromal tumors, including usual subtypes, *Am J Surg Pathol* 33:437–446, 2009.
65. Miettinen M, Wang ZF, Lasota J: DOG1 antibody in the differential diagnosis of gastrointestinal stromal tumors: a study of 1840 cases, *Am J Surg Pathol* 33:1401–1408, 2009.
66. Novelli M, Rossi S, Rodriguez-Justo M, et al: DOG1 and CD117 are the antibodies of choice in the diagnosis of gastrointestinal stromal tumours, *Histopathology* 57:259–270, 2010.
67. Miettinen M, Wang ZF, Sarlomo-Rikala M, et al: Succinate dehydrogenase-deficient GISTs: a clinicopathologic, immunohistochemical, and molecular genetic study of 66 gastric GISTs with predilection to young age, *Am J Surg Pathol* 35:1712–1721, 2011.
68. Doyle LA, Nelson D, Heinrich MC, et al: Loss of succinate dehydrogenase subunit B (SDHB) expression is limited to a distinctive subset of gastric wild-type gastrointestinal stromal tumours: a comprehensive genotype-phenotype correlation study, *Histopathology* 61:801–809, 2012.
69. Wasag B, Debiec-Rychter M, Pauwels P, et al: Differential expression of KIT/PDGFRA mutant isoforms in epithelioid and mixed variants of gastrointestinal stromal tumors depends predominantly on the tumor site, *Mod Pathol* 17:889–894, 2004.
70. Penzel R, Aulmann S, Moock M, et al: The location of KIT and PDGFRA gene mutations in gastrointestinal stromal tumours is site and phenotype associated, *J Clin Pathol* 58:634–639, 2005.
71. Wardelmann E, Hrychyk A, Merkelbach-Bruse S, et al: Association of platelet-derived growth factor α mutations with gastric primary site and epithelioid or mixed cell morphology in gastrointestinal stromal tumors, *J Mol Diagn* 6:197–204, 2004.
72. Killian JK, Miettinen M, Walker RL, et al: Recurrent epimutation of SDHC in gastrointestinal stromal tumors, *Sci Transl Med* 6:268ra177, 2014.
73. Boikos SA, Pappo AS, Killian JK, et al: Molecular subtypes of KIT/PDGFRA wild-type gastrointestinal stromal tumors: a report from the National Institutes of Health gastrointestinal stromal tumor clinic, *JAMA Oncol* 2:922–928, 2016.
74. Mason EF, Hornick JL: Conventional risk stratification fails to predict progression of succinate dehydrogenase-deficient gastrointestinal stromal tumors: a clinicopathologic study of 76 cases, *Am J Surg Pathol* 40:1616–1621, 2016.
75. Reith JD, Goldblum JR, Lyles RH, et al: Extragastrointestinal (soft tissue) stromal tumors: an analysis of 48 cases with emphasis on histologic predictors of outcome, *Mod Pathol* 13:577–585, 2000.
76. Singer S, Rubin BP, Lux ML, et al: Prognostic value of *KIT* mutation type, mitotic activity, and histologic subtype in gastrointestinal stromal tumors, *J Clin Oncol* 20:3898–3905, 2002.
77. Trupiano JK, Stewart RE, Misick C, et al: Gastric stromal tumors. A clinicopathologic study of 77 cases with correlation of features with nonaggressive and aggressive clinical behaviors, *Am J Surg Pathol* 26:705–714, 2002.
78. Henricks WH, Chu YC, Goldblum JR, et al: Dedifferentiated liposarcoma: a clinicopathological analysis of 155 cases with a proposal for an expanded definition of dedifferentiation, *Am J Surg Pathol* 21:271–281, 1997.
79. Le Guellec S, Chibon F, Ouali M, et al: Are peripheral purely undifferentiated pleomorphic sarcomas with MDM2 amplification dedifferentiated liposarcomas?, *Am J Surg Pathol* 38:293–304, 2014.
80. Coindre JM, Mariani O, Chibon F, et al: Most malignant fibrous histiocytomas developed in the retroperitoneum are dedifferentiated liposarcomas: a review of 25 cases initially diagnosed as malignant fibrous histiocytoma, *Mod Pathol* 16:256–262, 2003.
81. Fabre-Guillevin E, Coindre JM, Somerhausen Nde S, et al: Retroperitoneal liposarcomas: follow-up analysis of dedifferentiation after clinicopathologic reexamination of 86 liposarcomas and malignant fibrous histiocytomas, *Cancer* 106:2725–2733, 2006.
82. Coindre JM, Hostein I, Maire G, et al: Inflammatory malignant fibrous histiocytomas and dedifferentiated liposarcomas: histological review, genomic profile, and MDM2 and CDK4 status favour a single entity, *J Pathol* 203:822–830, 2004.
83. Nascimento AG, Kurtin PJ, Guillou L, et al: Dedifferentiated liposarcoma: a report of nine cases with a peculiar neurallike whorling pattern associated with metaplastic bone formation, *Am J Surg Pathol* 22:945–955, 1998.
84. Fanburg-Smith JC, Miettinen M: Liposarcoma with meningothelial-like whorls: a study of 17 cases of a distinctive histological pattern associated with dedifferentiated liposarcoma, *Histopathology* 33:414–424, 1998.
85. Huang HY, Brennan MF, Singer S, et al: Distant metastasis in retroperitoneal dedifferentiated liposarcoma is rare and rapidly fatal: a clinicopathological study with emphasis on the low-grade myxofibrosarcoma-like pattern as an early sign of dedifferentiation, *Mod Pathol* 18:976–984, 2005.
86. Mariño-Enríquez A, Fletcher CD, Dal Cin P, et al: Dedifferentiated liposarcoma with "homologous" lipoblastic (pleomorphic liposarcoma-like) differentiation: clinicopathologic and molecular analysis of a series suggesting revised diagnostic criteria, *Am J Surg Pathol* 34:1122–1131, 2010.
87. Fletcher CDM, Akerman M, Dal Cin P, et al: Correlation between clinicopathological features and karyotype in lipomatous tumors. A report of 178 cases from the Chromosome and Morphology (CHAMP) Collaborative Study Group, *Am J Pathol* 148:623–630, 1996.
88. Sioletic S, Dal Cin P, Fletcher CD, et al: Well-differentiated and dedifferentiated liposarcomas with prominent myxoid stroma: analysis of 56 cases, *Histopathology* 62:287–293, 2013.
89. Allen MS, Jr, Harrison W, Jahrsdoerfer RA: "Retinal anlage" tumors. Melanotic progonoma, melanotic adamantinoma, pigmented epulis, melanotic neuroectodermal tumor of infancy, benign melanotic tumor of infancy, *Am J Clin Pathol* 51:309–314, 1969.
90. Pettinato G, Manivel JC, d'Amore ES, et al: Melanotic neuroectodermal tumor of infancy. A reexamination of a histogenetic problem based on immunohistochemical, flow cytometric, and ultrastructural study of 10 cases, *Am J Surg Pathol* 15:233–245, 1991.
91. Johnson RE, Scheithauer BW, Dahlin DC: Melanotic neuroectodermal tumor of infancy. A review of seven cases, *Cancer* 52:661–666, 1983.
92. Kapadia SB, Frisman DM, Hitchcock CL, et al: Melanotic neuroectodermal tumor of infancy. Clinicopathological, immunohistochemical, and flow cytometric study, *Am J Surg Pathol* 17:566–573, 1993.
93. Borello ED, Gorlin RJ: Melanotic neuroectodermal tumor of infancy—a neoplasm of neural crest origin. Report of a case associated with high urinary excretion of vanilmandelic acid, *Cancer* 19:196–206, 1966.
94. Cutler LS, Chaudhry AP, Topazian R: Melanotic neuroectodermal tumor of infancy: an ultrastructural study, literature review, and reevaluation, *Cancer* 48:257–270, 1981.
95. Stirling RW, Powell G, Fletcher CD: Pigmented neuroectodermal tumour of infancy: an immunohistochemical study, *Histopathology* 12:425–435, 1988.
96. Zellos L, Christiani DC: Epidemiology, biologic behavior, and natural history of mesothelioma, *Thorac Surg Clin* 14:469–477, 2004.
97. Bitterman P, Chun B, Kurman RJ: The significance of epithelial differentiation in mixed mesodermal tumors of the uterus, *Am J Surg Pathol* 14:317–328, 1990.
98. McCluggage WG: Uterine carcinosarcoma (malignant mixed Müllerian tumors) are metaplastic carcinoma, *Int J Gynecol Cancer* 12:687–690, 2002.
99. Garamvoelgyi E, Guillou L, Gebhard S, et al: Primary malignant mixed Müllerian tumor (metaplastic carcinoma) of the female peritoneum. A clinical, pathologic, and immunohistochemical study of three cases and a review of the literature, *Cancer* 74:854–863, 1994.
100. Shen DH, Khoo US, Xue WC, et al: Primary peritoneal malignant mixed Müllerian tumors. A clinicopathologic, immunohistochemical, and genetic study, *Cancer* 91:1052–1060, 2001.
101. Barwick KW, LiVolsi VA: Malignant mixed Müllerian tumors of the uterus. A clinicopathologic assessment of 34 cases, *Am J Surg Pathol* 3:125–135, 1979.

102. De Brito PA, Silverberg SG, Orenstein JM: Carcinosarcoma (malignant mixed Müllerian [mesodermal] tumor) of the female genital tract: immunohistochemical and ultrastructural analysis of 28 cases, *Hum Pathol* 24:132–142, 1993.
103. King ME, Kramer EE: Malignant Müllerian mixed tumors of the uterus. A study of 21 cases, *Cancer* 45:188–190, 1980.
104. Jones TD, Ulbright TM, Eble JN, et al: OCT4 staining in testicular tumors: a sensitive and specific marker for seminoma and embryonal carcinoma, *Am J Surg Pathol* 28:935–940, 2004.
105. Santagata S, Ligon KL, Hornick JL: Embryonic stem cell transcription factor signatures in the diagnosis of primary and metastatic germ cell tumors, *Am J Surg Pathol* 31:836–845, 2007.
106. Leroy X, Augusto D, Leteurtre E, et al: CD30 and CD117 (c-kit) used in combination are useful for distinguishing embryonal carcinoma from seminoma, *J Histochem Cytochem* 50:283–285, 2002.
107. Yu H, Pinkus GS, Hornick JL: Diffuse membranous immunoreactivity for podoplanin (D2-40) distinguishes primary and metastatic seminomas from other germ cell tumors and metastatic neoplasms, *Am J Clin Pathol* 128:767–775, 2007.
108. Bosl GJ, Ilson DH, Rodriguez E, et al: Clinical relevance of the i(12p) marker chromosome in germ cell tumors, *J Natl Cancer Inst* 86:349–355, 1994.
109. Rodriguez E, Houldsworth J, Reuter VE, et al: Molecular cytogenetic analysis of i(12p)-negative human male germ cell tumors, *Genes Chromosomes Cancer* 8:230–236, 1993.
110. Sung MT, Maclennan GT, Lopez-Beltran A, et al: Primary mediastinal seminoma: a comprehensive assessment integrated with histology, immunohistochemistry, and fluorescence in situ hybridization for chromosome 12p abnormalities in 23 cases, *Am J Surg Pathol* 32:146–155, 2008.

10

Soft Tissue Tumors With Prominent Inflammatory Cells

Jason L. Hornick, MD, PhD

Although a sparse lymphocytic infiltrate is relatively common in mesenchymal neoplasms, few histologic types of soft tissue tumors characteristically contain prominent inflammatory cells. In some such cases, the presence of an inflammatory infiltrate can be a diagnostic clue, whereas in other cases the infiltrate may obscure the neoplastic component and potentially lead to an erroneous diagnosis of either a reactive process or even a lymphoma. The types of inflammatory cells that can be prominent in soft tissue tumors are diverse, and they include lymphocytes, plasma cells, neutrophils, eosinophils, histiocytes, and mast cells. In many cases, the specific inflammatory cell types may help generate a differential diagnosis (Boxes 10.1–10.3). In contrast, histiocytes are usually not diagnostically useful in isolation (with rare exceptions), but may be seen in combination with other inflammatory cell types. An infiltrate of eosinophils is characteristic of only a small number of neoplasms, most of which are either hematopoietic (notably, Langerhans cell histiocytosis [LCH] and cutaneous and systemic mastocytosis) or vascular in nature (especially epithelioid endothelial lesions such as epithelioid hemangioma). A prominent eosinophilic infiltrate may occasionally be seen in isolated examples of soft tissue tumors apparently as an idiosyncratic phenomenon (which may be more distracting than helpful). Finally, mast cells are often prominent in myxoid soft tissue tumors and in select other mesenchymal neoplasms (e.g., synovial sarcoma and desmoid fibromatosis) and are mentioned when appropriate in other chapters, but they will not be discussed further in this chapter.

The prototypical examples of soft tissue tumors with prominent inflammatory cells are inflammatory myofibroblastic tumor (IMT) and so-called inflammatory malignant fibrous histiocytoma (MFH). Most examples of IMT contain a prominent lymphoplasmacytic infiltrate, interspersed between the myofibroblastic spindle cells, although some cases may be notable for eosinophils and occasionally neutrophils (see also Chapters 4 and 16). In contrast, inflammatory MFH classically contains a prominent infiltrate of neutrophils and foamy histiocytes; this infiltrate is usually much more abundant than the neoplastic cellular component. Most examples of inflammatory MFH represent an unusual histologic variant of dedifferentiated liposarcoma (see also Chapters 7 and 12). These tumor types will be covered only briefly in this chapter.

Histiocytic and dendritic cell tumors often contain frequent inflammatory cells, which can be a helpful clue to their diagnosis. Such tumors arise not only in lymph nodes but may also present at extranodal sites such as skin, soft tissue, and the gastrointestinal tract. This group of rare tumors will be discussed in detail in this chapter.

There is also a group of mass-forming idiopathic fibroinflammatory lesions that are not uncommonly confused with mesenchymal neoplasms (e.g., sclerosing mesenteritis and idiopathic retroperitoneal fibrosis). A select subset of these lesions will be discussed briefly at the end of the chapter, with an emphasis on differential diagnosis.

Inflammatory Myofibroblastic Tumor

Clinical Features

IMT usually affects children and young adults and is especially rare in adults older than 50 years of age (see Chapters 4 and 16).[1-4] Although the most common anatomic sites are the lung, abdominal cavity, and retroperitoneum, nearly any site may be involved. Up to one third of patients (predominantly children) present with a systemic syndrome of fever, weight loss, anemia, hypergammaglobulinemia, and an elevated erythrocyte sedimentation rate, which usually remits following surgical excision of the tumor.[2]

Box 10.1 Tumors Often Associated With Prominent Lymphocytes and/or Plasma Cells

Inflammatory myofibroblastic tumor
Inflammatory leiomyosarcoma
Follicular dendritic cell sarcoma
Fibroblastic reticular cell sarcoma
Interdigitating dendritic cell sarcoma
Indeterminate cell histiocytosis
Rosai-Dorfman disease
Histiocytic sarcoma
Well-differentiated inflammatory liposarcoma
Angiomatoid fibrous histiocytoma
Myxoinflammatory fibroblastic sarcoma
Thymoma

Box 10.2 Tumors Often Associated With Prominent Neutrophils

Dedifferentiated liposarcoma (inflammatory malignant fibrous histiocytoma)
Undifferentiated pleomorphic sarcoma with prominent inflammation
Rosai-Dorfman disease
Histiocytic sarcoma
Epithelioid inflammatory myofibroblastic sarcoma
Pseudomyogenic hemangioendothelioma
Myxoinflammatory fibroblastic sarcoma
Undifferentiated carcinoma
Anaplastic large-cell lymphoma

Box 10.3 Tumors Often Associated With Prominent Eosinophils

Langerhans cell histiocytosis/Langerhans cell sarcoma
Systemic mastocytosis/mastocytoma/mast cell sarcoma
Epithelioid hemangioma (and other epithelioid endothelial neoplasms)
Hodgkin lymphoma

Pathologic Features

Histologically, IMT is composed of variably cellular fascicles of uniform plump spindle cells with elongated, tapering nuclei, vesicular chromatin, small nucleoli, and palely eosinophilic cytoplasm with ill-defined cell borders (Fig. 10.1).[1,5] The presence of more than mild nuclear atypia or pleomorphism should suggest an alternative diagnosis (i.e., a sarcoma).[2] Areas of myxoid stroma with prominent vessels or hyalinized collagenous stroma are often seen. About 50% of tumors contain a population of polygonal ganglion-like myofibroblasts with eccentric nuclei and eosinophilic to amphophilic cytoplasm (see Fig. 10.1D). Most IMTs contain a prominent infiltrate of plasma cells and lymphocytes (Fig. 10.2), which is a helpful clue to the diagnosis; eosinophils and neutrophils are less often encountered. A distinctive variant of IMT with a predilection for the mesentery and omentum is dominated by epithelioid cells with vesicular nuclei and large nucleoli, in a prominent myxoid stroma (epithelioid inflammatory myofibroblastic sarcoma).[6] This variant characteristically contains a prominent infiltrate of neutrophils (Fig. 10.3).

Immunohistochemistry

By immunohistochemistry, IMTs show a similar phenotype as other myofibroblastic tumors. Smooth muscle actin (SMA) is positive in 80% of IMTs, desmin in 60% of tumors, and keratins in about one third of cases.[2,3] About 50% of IMTs show reactivity for anaplastic lymphoma kinase (ALK), which reflects the presence of *ALK* gene rearrangements.[7-9] The pattern of ALK staining is determined by the fusion partner; most tumors show diffuse cytoplasmic staining (Fig. 10.4A), whereas epithelioid inflammatory myofibroblastic sarcoma usually shows a nuclear membrane pattern (see Fig. 10.4B), less often a cytoplasmic pattern with perinuclear accentuation.[6,10] Around 5% to 10% of IMTs are positive for ROS1 (Fig. 10.5), which correlates with the presence of *ROS1* gene rearrangements.[11]

Molecular Genetics

About 50% of IMTs contain translocations involving the *ALK* gene, with diverse fusion partners (see Chapter 18 for more details).[12-14] Epithelioid inflammatory myofibroblastic sarcomas usually harbor an *RANBP2-ALK* fusion (correlating with a nuclear membrane pattern of ALK staining); a small subset harbors an *RRBP1-ALK* fusion.[6,10] Of the IMTs that lack *ALK* gene rearrangements, 5% to 10% harbor *ROS1* gene fusions.[15-17] Rare IMTs harbor *ETV6* rearrangements (including *ETV6-NTRK3*)[17,18]; individual cases with *PDGFRB* or *RET* fusions have also been reported.[15,16]

Differential Diagnosis

The differential diagnosis of IMT may include various spindle cell sarcomas (especially leiomyosarcoma and low-grade myofibroblastic sarcoma), dedifferentiated liposarcoma, desmoid fibromatosis, gastrointestinal stromal tumor (GIST), and dendritic cell sarcomas. When IMT is positive for ALK or ROS1, the diagnosis is relatively straightforward; ALK and ROS1-negative IMTs pose particular diagnostic problems. Even low-grade spindle cell sarcomas show a greater degree of nuclear atypia and variability than IMT; this is one of the most important features to help exclude the diagnosis of IMT. In contrast, prominent plasma cells favor IMT over various sarcoma types.

Leiomyosarcomas generally contain cells with broader nuclei and more brightly eosinophilic cytoplasm than IMT. Inflammatory leiomyosarcoma is a rare variant that may easily be confused with IMT. The presence of prominent foamy histiocytes and areas of the tumor with typical histologic features of leiomyosarcoma (i.e., tight fascicles, broad and blunt-ended nuclei, brightly eosinophilic cytoplasm) are helpful diagnostic clues. SMA, desmin, and keratin expression are shared by IMT and leiomyosarcoma; caldesmon expression (when present) favors leiomyosarcoma, and reactivity for ALK or ROS1 supports IMT. Unlike IMT, low-grade myofibroblastic sarcoma typically arises in somatic soft tissues, rarely contains a prominent inflammatory infiltrate, and shows more notable nuclear atypia and infiltrative margins. Morphologically low-grade areas of dedifferentiated liposarcoma may closely mimic IMT.[19] However, dedifferentiated liposarcoma affects older individuals and characteristically shows intratumoral heterogeneity, including pleomorphic areas, which is not a feature of IMT. Dedifferentiated liposarcoma may express SMA and desmin but is negative for ALK and ROS1. Identification of the well-differentiated adipocytic component confirms the diagnosis of dedifferentiated liposarcoma.

IMT with stromal hyalinization may be confused with desmoid fibromatosis, particularly cases that arise in the mesentery. However, desmoid tumors characteristically contain longer fascicles than IMT, and although a lymphocytic infiltrate may be present, plasma cells are usually absent. Aberrant nuclear staining for β-catenin can help confirm the diagnosis of desmoid fibromatosis. IMT may mimic spindle cell GIST, given its propensity to arise in the abdomen. In contrast to IMT, GIST has a syncytial appearance with fibrillary cytoplasm and lacks the plump myofibroblastic nuclei of IMT. Some GISTs contain prominent stromal lymphocytes, but the presence of plasma cells favors IMT. This differential diagnosis may easily be resolved with immunohistochemistry, because spindle cell GISTs are nearly always positive for KIT and DOG1, whereas ALK and ROS1 are negative.

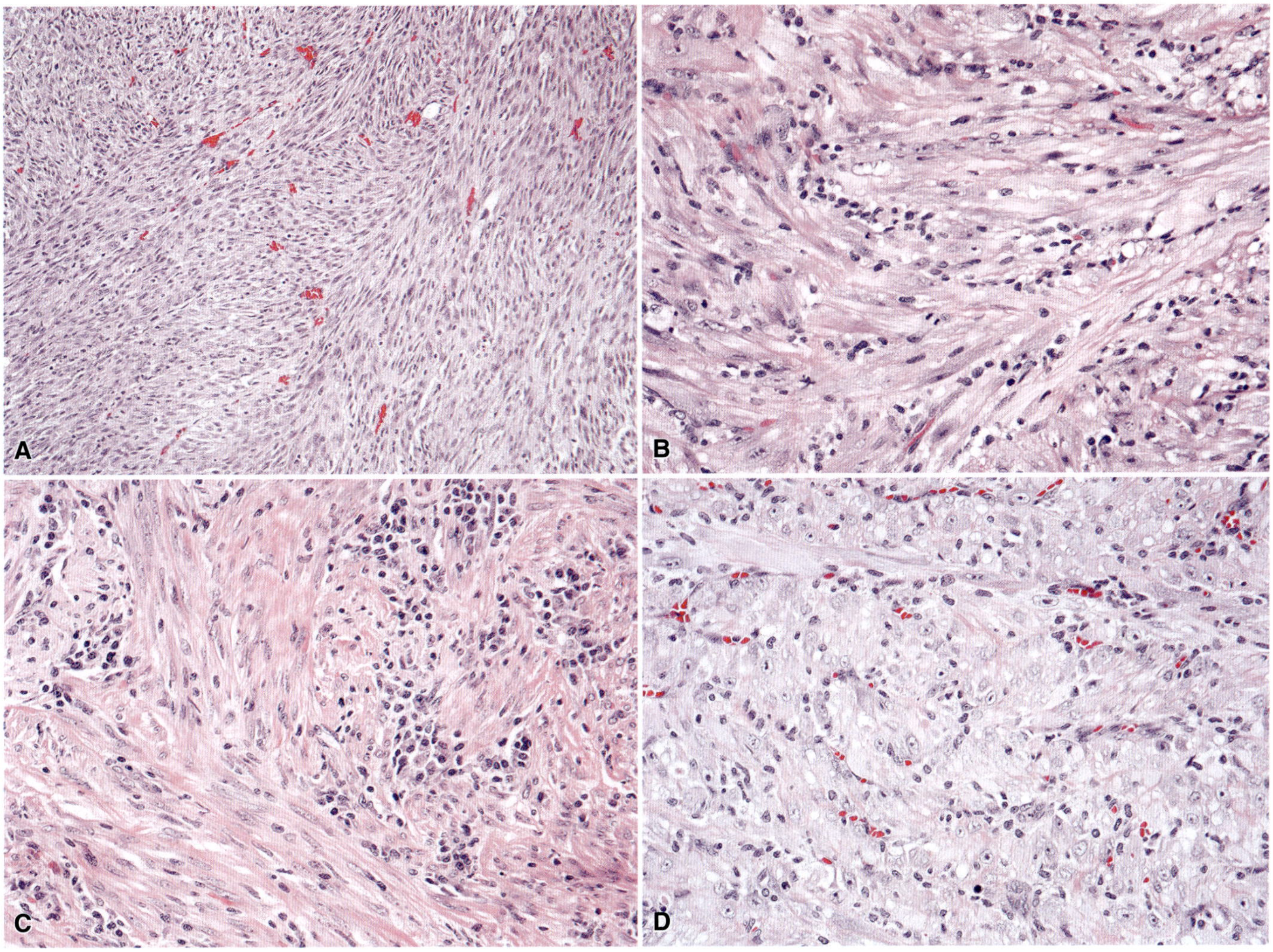

Figure 10.1 Inflammatory Myofibroblastic Tumor. (A) The tumor is composed of fascicles of uniform spindle cells with palely eosinophilic cytoplasm. (B) The tumor cells contain vesicular nuclei with small nucleoli and are admixed with lymphocytes. (C) Some tumors contain areas with collagenous stroma. Note the prominent plasma cells. (D) Polygonal tumor cells with prominent nucleoli. Note the scattered lymphocytes.

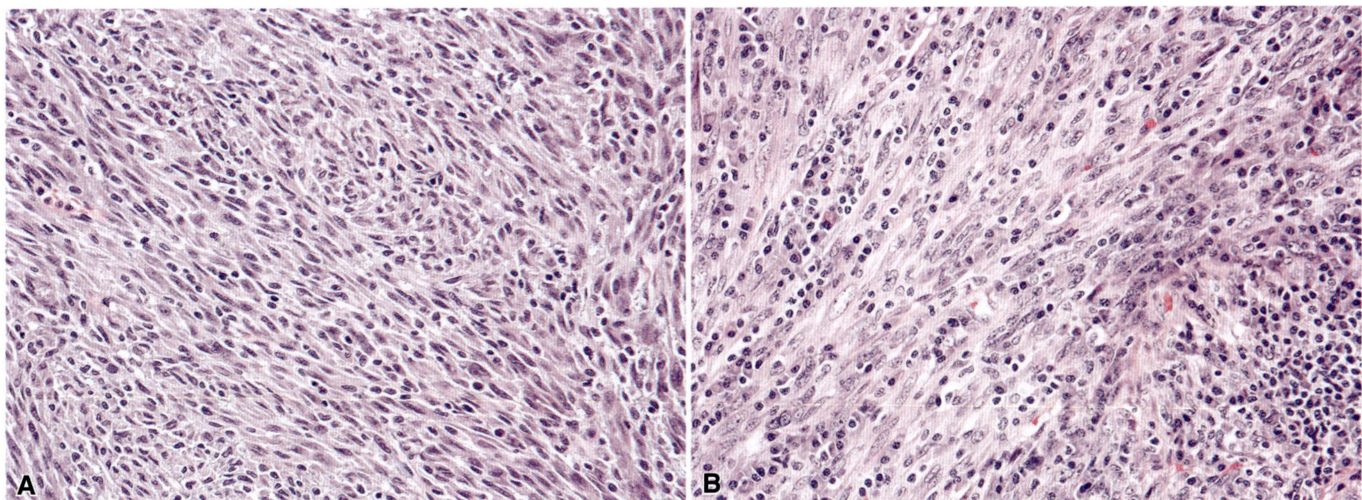

Figure 10.2 Inflammatory Myofibroblastic Tumor. Prominent small lymphocytes (A) and plasma cells (B) are a characteristic feature. Note the uniform cytology of the spindle cells.

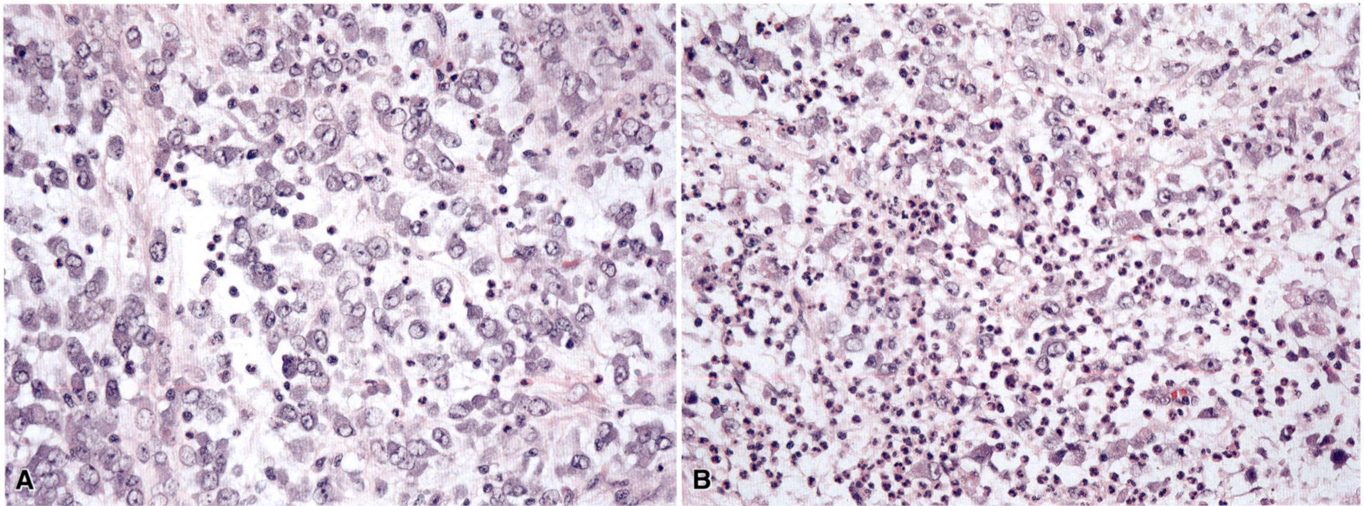

Figure 10.3 **Epithelioid Inflammatory Myofibroblastic Sarcoma.** (A) This distinctive aggressive variant of inflammatory myofibroblastic tumor is composed of epithelioid cells with amphophilic cytoplasm and prominent nucleoli. (B) Myxoid stroma and prominent stromal neutrophils are characteristic findings.

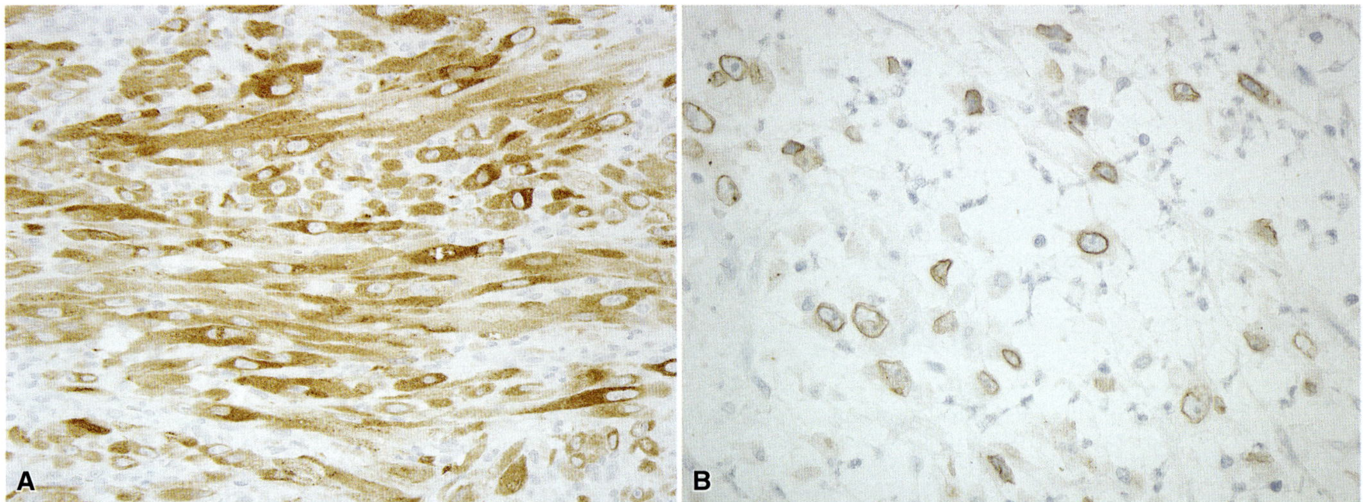

Figure 10.4 **ALK Expression in Inflammatory Myofibroblastic Tumor.** (A) About 50% of inflammatory myofibroblastic tumors are positive for ALK, usually with a diffuse cytoplasmic staining pattern. (B) Epithelioid inflammatory myofibroblastic sarcoma with a *RANBP2-ALK* fusion shows a nuclear membrane pattern of ALK staining.

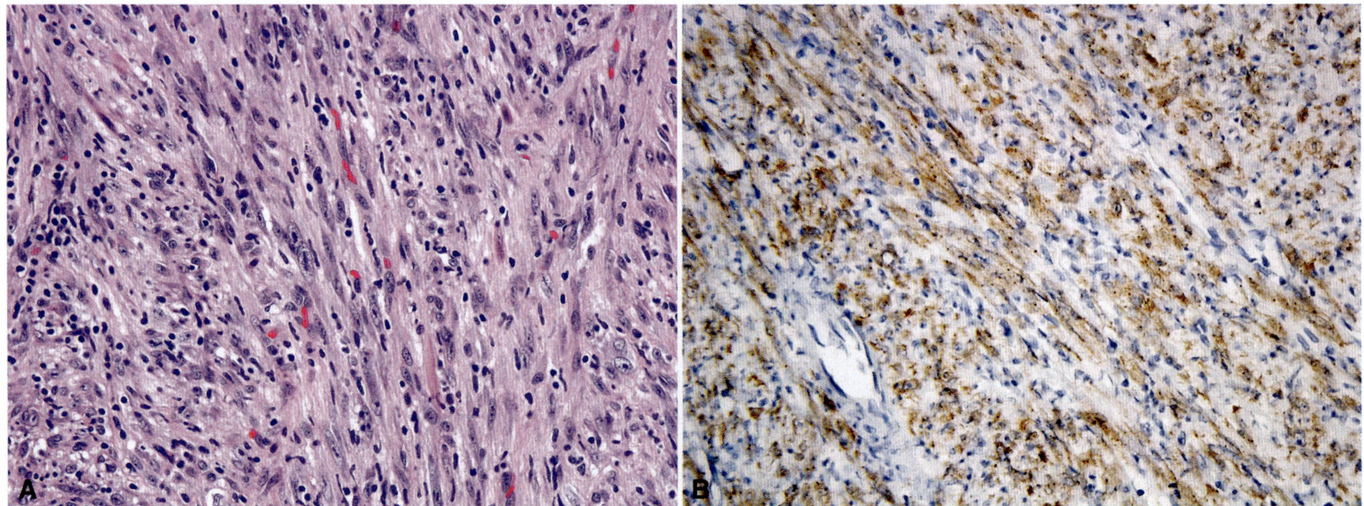

Figure 10.5 **Inflammatory Myofibroblastic Tumor With *ROS1* Rearrangement.** (A) The tumor is composed of fascicles of plump spindle cells with vesicular nuclei and eosinophilic cytoplasm. Note the prominent stromal lymphocytes. (B) The tumor cells are positive for ROS1, with a diffuse and dot-like cytoplasmic staining pattern.

Several dendritic cell neoplasms are also composed of spindle cells with a prominent chronic inflammatory infiltrate. Follicular dendritic cell sarcoma typically shows a more storiform or whorled growth pattern and a more syncytial appearance than IMT. Expression of CD21, CD35, and podoplanin (D2-40) confirms the diagnosis of follicular dendritic cell sarcoma in this differential diagnosis. Interdigitating dendritic cell sarcoma is exceedingly rare and usually arises in lymph nodes. This tumor type is diffusely positive for S-100 protein, whereas SMA, desmin, and ALK are negative.

Prognosis and Treatment

IMT belongs to the group of mesenchymal neoplasms of intermediate biologic potential, because of the significant risk of local recurrence and low rate of metastasis (<5%).[2] Intraabdominal and retroperitoneal tumors are particularly prone to recur locally (at least 25% risk), whereas the chance of recurrence of pulmonary IMT is much lower (about 5%).[1-3,5] Complete surgical excision without adjuvant therapy is appropriate treatment. Histologic features do not correlate with clinical behavior, with rare exceptions.[1] The distinctive intraabdominal variant of IMT with epithelioid morphology (epithelioid inflammatory myofibroblastic sarcoma) pursues an aggressive clinical course.[6] Patients with aggressive, recurrent or metastatic IMTs (including epithelioid inflammatory myofibroblastic sarcoma) with *ALK* or *ROS1* rearrangements may be effectively treated with targeted kinase inhibitor therapies.[15,20]

PRACTICE POINTS: Inflammatory Myofibroblastic Tumor

- Usually affects children and young adults
- Lung, abdominal cavity, and retroperitoneum most common sites
- Fascicles of uniform plump spindle cells with vesicular chromatin and palely eosinophilic cytoplasm
- Pleomorphism is not a feature
- Prominent infiltrate of lymphocytes and plasma cells is typical
- Fifty percent positive for ALK and harbors *ALK* gene rearrangement
- Five percent to 10% positive for ROS1 and harbors *ROS1* gene rearrangement
- Intermediate biologic potential: significant risk of local recurrence (lung: 5%; intraabdominal: at least 25%), but low metastatic rate (<5%)

Inflammatory Leiomyosarcoma

Inflammatory leiomyosarcoma is a rare leiomyosarcoma variant with a prominent inflammatory infiltrate, which may obscure the neoplastic cell population and may easily be mistaken for other tumor types.[21] This lesion was originally buried within the inflammatory MFH category. This variant has a peak incidence in young adults, and it may also affect children, with no gender predilection. Inflammatory leiomyosarcoma has a predilection for somatic soft tissue, particularly the extremities and trunk.[21,22]

Histologically, the tumor is composed of spindle cells with a variably fascicular or storiform architecture, in large areas masked by prominent inflammation (Fig. 10.6). The inflammatory component is often dominated by histiocytes, including aggregates of foam cells (see Fig. 10.6B); lymphocytes are also prominent (see Fig. 10.6C). Occasional cases may contain a neutrophilic infiltrate. In areas with less prominent inflammation, the typical cytoarchitectural features of leiomyosarcoma can be identified.

By immunohistochemistry, most cases of inflammatory leiomyosarcoma are positive for SMA and desmin (see Fig. 10.6D), and they may also express caldesmon. By cytogenetics, hyperhaploidy (karyotype with 24–34 chromosomes), a rare finding in tumors, has been identified in nearly all cases studied[23,24]; the gene expression signature of inflammatory leiomyosarcoma is distinct from conventional leiomyosarcoma.[24]

The differential diagnosis of inflammatory leiomyosarcoma includes IMT, dendritic cell tumors, and so-called inflammatory MFH (i.e., dedifferentiated liposarcoma). In contrast to inflammatory leiomyosarcoma, the inflammatory infiltrate in IMT often includes prominent plasma cells, and the degree of nuclear atypia is usually greater in inflammatory leiomyosarcoma. There is significant immunophenotypic overlap between these tumor types, although strong, diffuse staining for desmin and caldesmon expression favor leiomyosarcoma, whereas ALK or ROS1 expression confirms the diagnosis of IMT. Follicular dendritic cell sarcoma rarely contains prominent foamy histiocytes and is positive for CD21 and CD35. Interdigitating dendritic cell sarcoma is strongly positive for S-100 protein and lacks smooth muscle marker expression. Dedifferentiated liposarcoma has a predilection for the retroperitoneum and abdominal cavity of older adults and rarely arises in somatic soft tissue. When dedifferentiated liposarcoma shows the inflammatory MFH pattern, neutrophils usually predominate, and the tumor cells are scattered pleomorphic cells within the dense inflammatory background; the cellular, fascicular spindle cell component of inflammatory leiomyosarcoma is absent. Thorough sampling usually reveals heterogeneous histologic patterns in the dedifferentiated component, as well as areas of well-differentiated liposarcoma. Dedifferentiated liposarcoma often also expresses SMA and desmin; detection of MDM2 and CDK4 overexpression by immunohistochemistry or *MDM2* amplification by FISH is helpful to confirm the diagnosis.

Although experience is limited, inflammatory leiomyosarcoma appears to pursue a less aggressive clinical course than conventional leiomyosarcoma.[21,22] The metastatic rate seems to be relatively low.

Histiocytic and Dendritic Cell Tumors

Tumors composed of histiocytes (phagocytic cells) and dendritic cells (antigen-presenting cells) are rare. Such tumors typically arise at lymphoid tissue–rich anatomic sites (e.g., lymph nodes, tonsils, and spleen), but many of them can also occur in the abdominal cavity, soft tissues, and skin, among other locations.[25]

In a broad sense, dendritic cell tumors can be separated into those that are hematopoietic in origin (bone marrow derived from the myeloid/monocytic lineage, such as histiocytic sarcoma) and those that are mesenchymal (stromal) in origin (Box 10.4). The former category also includes the relatively common LCH, its exceedingly rare malignant counterpart Langerhans cell sarcoma, indeterminate cell histiocytosis, and interdigitating dendritic cell sarcoma. The plasticity of myeloid-derived histiocytic and dendritic cell tumors is illustrated by the occasional occurrence of clonally related metachronous (or synchronous) lymphoid neoplasms (such as T-lymphoblastic lymphoma and LCH

Box 10.4 Histiocytic and Dendritic Cell Tumors

Hematopoietic Origin (Myeloid/Monocyte Lineage)

- Langerhans cell histiocytosis
- Langerhans cell sarcoma
- Interdigitating dendritic cell sarcoma
- Indeterminate cell histiocytosis
- Histiocytic sarcoma
- Rosai-Dorfman disease

Mesenchymal Origin

- Follicular dendritic cell sarcoma
- Fibroblastic reticular cell sarcoma

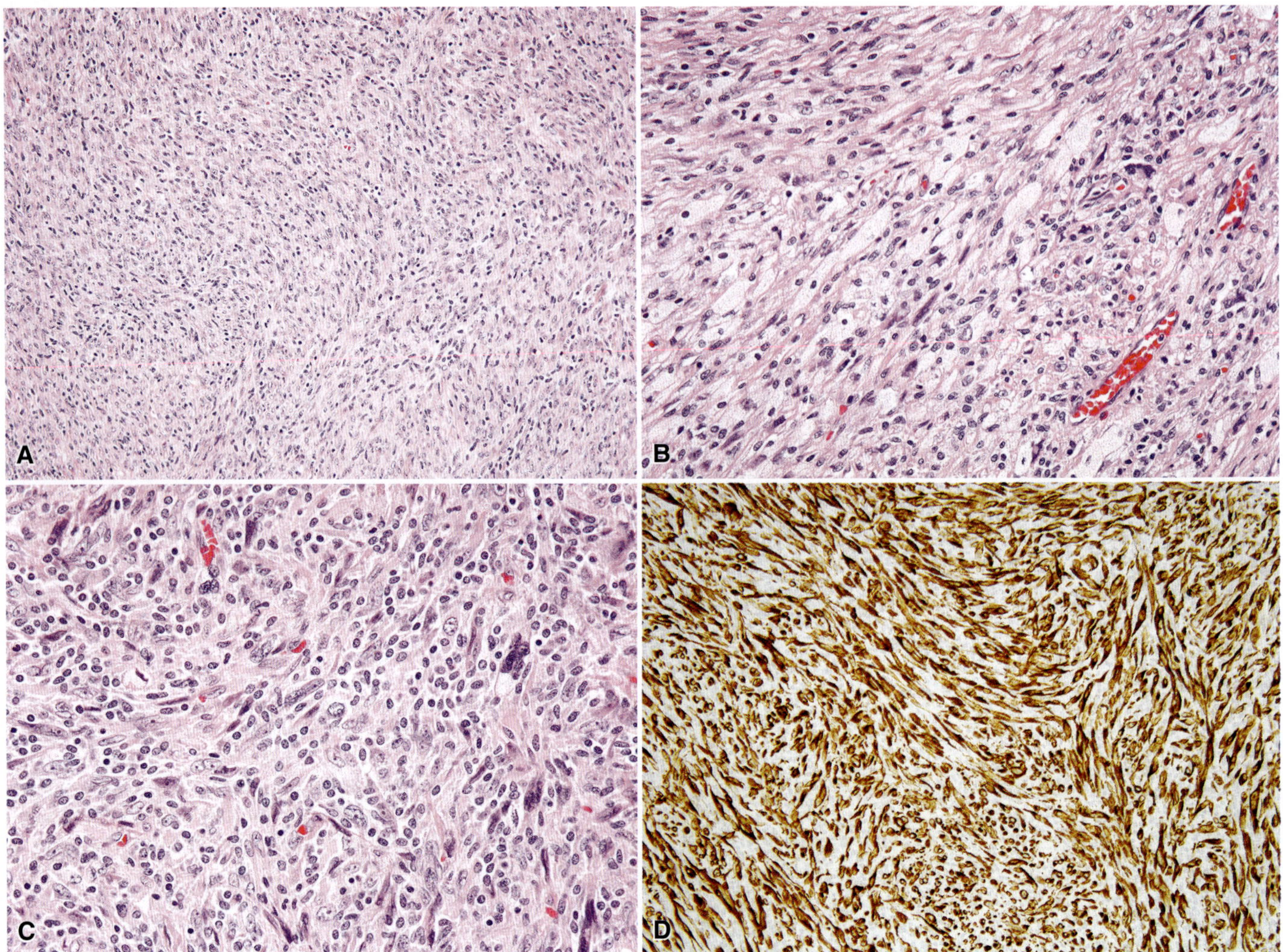

Figure 10.6 **Inflammatory Leiomyosarcoma.** (A) The tumor shows a uniform fascicular architecture with scattered lymphocytes. (B) Prominent foam cells are a characteristic finding. (C) The tumor cells are admixed with numerous lymphocytes. Note the mild nuclear atypia. (D) Strong and diffuse staining for desmin is typical.

harboring identical T-cell receptor gene rearrangements, and follicular lymphoma or chronic lymphocytic leukemia and histiocytic or interdigitating dendritic cell sarcomas harboring identical immunoglobulin gene rearrangements and/or translocations).[26-29] Stromal-derived dendritic cell tumors include follicular dendritic cell sarcoma and the poorly characterized and exceptionally rare fibroblastic reticular cell sarcoma.

The most common dendritic cell tumor in this group overall is LCH, which is familiar to and well recognized by surgical pathologists. LCH presenting as a solitary lesion is usually clinically benign. The most common malignant dendritic cell tumor is follicular dendritic cell sarcoma. This rare tumor type may mimic other more common mesenchymal (and nonmesenchymal) neoplasms histologically, arise at anatomic sites where other tumor types would be clinically much more likely (e.g., gastrointestinal tract, retroperitoneum, and mediastinum), and metastasize to the liver and lungs. Thus, follicular dendritic cell sarcoma continues to be underrecognized by pathologists and is not uncommonly misdiagnosed. Because histiocytic and dendritic cell tumors often contain a prominent inflammatory infiltrate (which is a helpful diagnostic clue), they will be discussed in this chapter.

Follicular Dendritic Cell Sarcoma

Follicular dendritic cells normally reside in (and provide architectural support for) lymphoid follicles and present antigens to B lymphocytes. As such, follicular dendritic cell sarcomas typically arise at lymphoid tissue–rich anatomic sites.[30-34] Among dendritic cell tumors, follicular dendritic cell sarcoma is most likely to be confused with other soft tissue tumors.

Clinical Features

Follicular dendritic cell sarcoma affects adults over a wide age range, with a peak in young to middle-aged adults, with no gender predilection.[35,36] Although it may develop primarily in lymph nodes (most commonly in the abdomen, axilla, mediastinum, and neck), it more often arises at extranodal sites, such as the gastrointestinal tract, mediastinum, and tonsils.[30,33-37] Follicular dendritic cell sarcoma arises in a background of hyaline-vascular Castleman disease in 5% to 10% of cases.[36] There are reports of follicular dendritic cell sarcoma associated with myasthenia gravis and other autoimmune disorders in rare cases.[38,39]

The very rare inflammatory pseudotumor-like variant of follicular dendritic cell sarcoma shows a female predominance and occurs almost exclusively in the liver and spleen.[40-42]

Pathologic Features

Grossly, most follicular dendritic cell sarcomas are between 3 and 12 cm in greatest dimension, with a mean size of 5 to 7 cm.[30,35,36] The cut surface is fleshy in appearance.

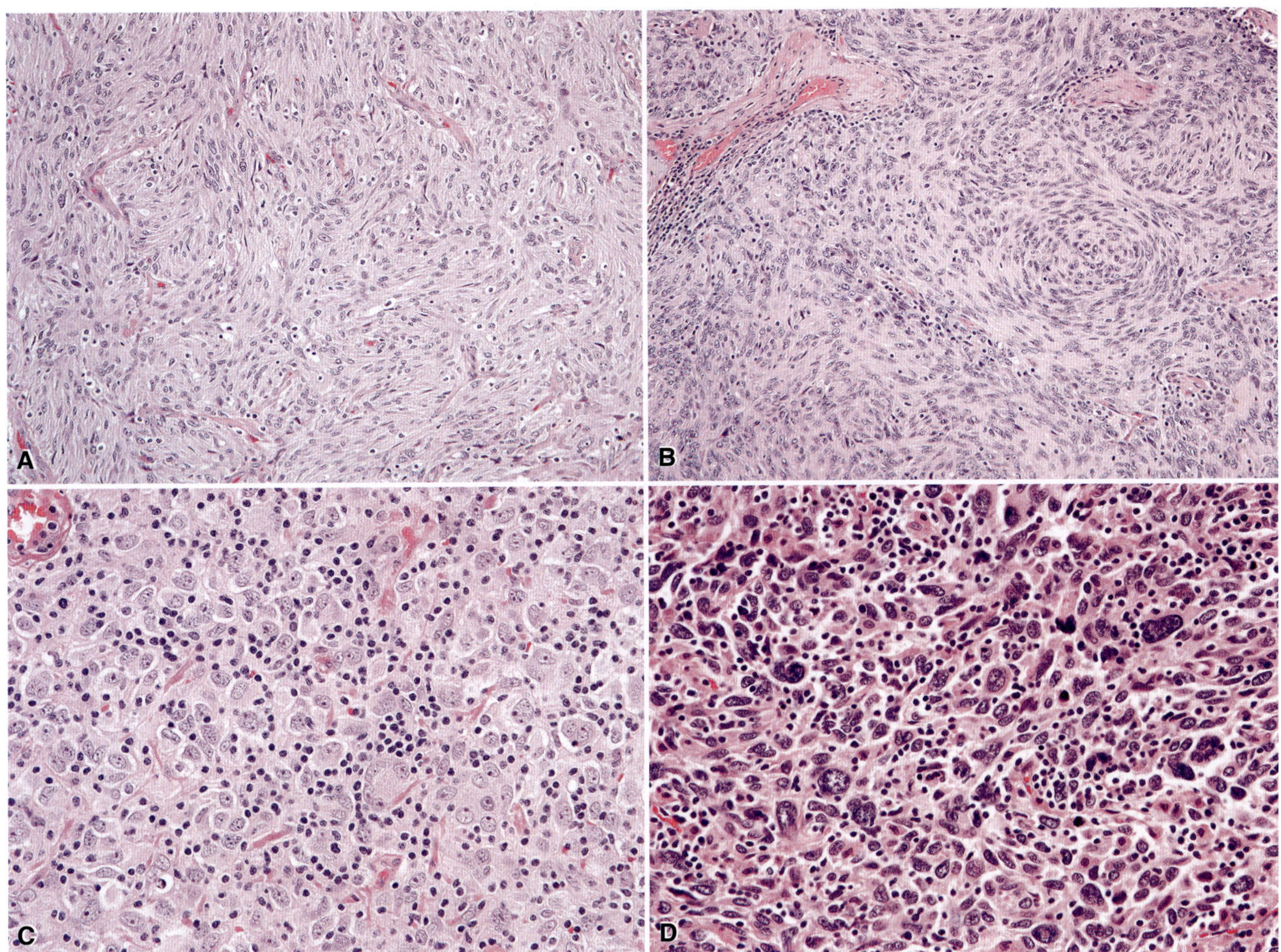

Figure 10.7 Follicular Dendritic Cell Sarcoma. This tumor type usually shows a storiform (A) or whorled architecture (B). Note the pale cytoplasm, ill-defined cell borders, and scattered lymphocytes. Some tumors are composed of epithelioid cells (C). Note the syncytial appearance and prominent lymphocytes. Focal areas of notable nuclear pleomorphism may be observed (D).

Histologically, follicular dendritic cell sarcoma is composed of ovoid to spindled cells with vesicular chromatin, small nucleoli, and moderate amounts of palely eosinophilic cytoplasm with ill-defined cell borders, arranged in a storiform, whorled (meningioma-like), or fascicular growth pattern (Fig. 10.7). Some tumors show epithelioid cytomorphology (see Fig. 10.7C). Scattered multinucleated cells are common. Prominent admixed lymphocytes and occasional plasma cells are typically seen. Although most cases show relatively bland, uniform cytomorphology, occasional examples show notable nuclear atypia and may contain pleomorphic cells (see Fig. 10.7D).

The inflammatory pseudotumor-cell variant of follicular dendritic cell sarcoma shows a loose fascicular and sheet-like growth pattern of spindle cells with more variable cytomorphology. These cells are admixed with a prominent chronic inflammatory infiltrate, which may occasionally obscure the neoplastic cells (Fig. 10.8).[40]

Immunohistochemistry

Follicular dendritic cell sarcoma is usually positive for the normal follicular dendritic cell markers CD21, CD23, and/or CD35 (Fig. 10.9).[30,36] Clusterin, podoplanin (D2-40), and CXCL13 are also highly expressed in follicular dendritic cell sarcoma.[43-45] Epithelial membrane antigen (EMA) is at least focally positive in about 50% of cases (see Fig. 10.9B), and S-100 protein is weakly expressed in about 10% of cases.[30,36] The interspersed lymphocytes may be either CD20-positive B cells or CD3-positive T cells. The rare cases associated with myasthenia gravis contain immature (TdT-positive) T cells.[38,39] Approximately 50% of follicular dendritic cell sarcomas show strong and diffuse expression of PD-L1.[46] In contrast to conventional follicular dendritic cell sarcoma, Epstein-Barr virus–encoded RNA (EBER) is positive in the inflammatory pseudotumor-like variant (see Fig. 10.8B).[40-42]

Molecular Genetics

Few studies have investigated the genetics of follicular dendritic cell sarcoma. Preliminary data include recurrent mutations in NF-κB regulatory genes (*NFKBIA*, *CYLD*, and *TNFAIP3*), *BRAF* V600E mutations, loss of tumor suppressor genes (*CDKN2A* and *RB1*), and copy number gain at chromosome 9p24, including the *PDCD1LG1* (PD-L1) and *PDCD1LG2* (PD-L2) loci in a subset of cases.[47,48] However, a unifying pathogenetic basis for this neoplasm has not yet been identified.

Differential Diagnosis

The differential diagnosis of follicular dendritic cell sarcoma includes thymoma, interdigitating dendritic cell sarcoma, metastatic undifferentiated (e.g., nasopharyngeal) carcinoma, and GIST.

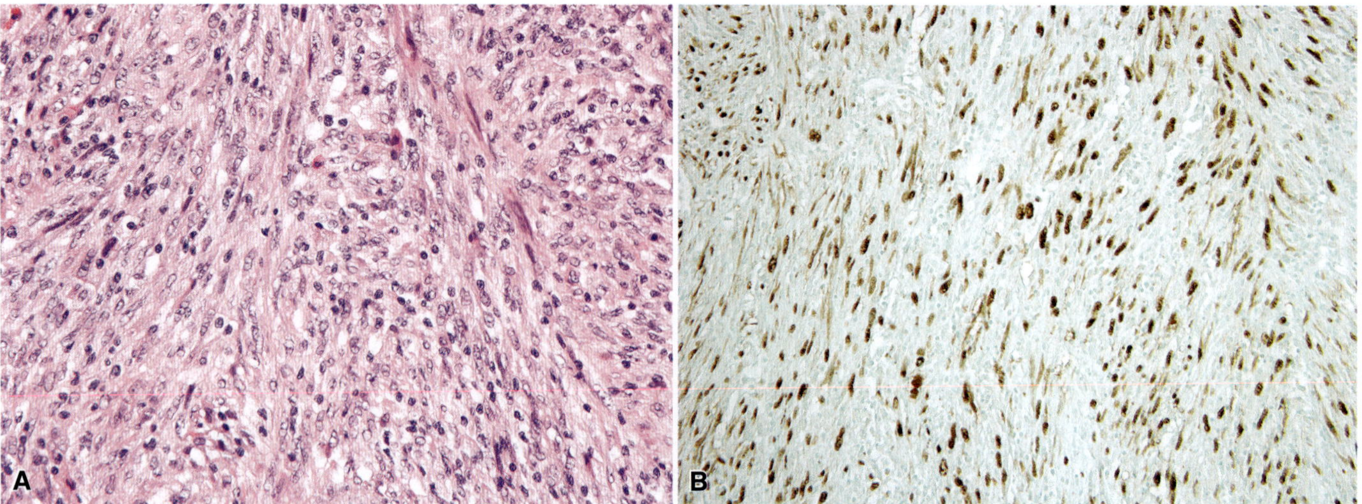

Figure 10.8 **Inflammatory Pseudotumor-Like Follicular Dendritic Cell Sarcoma.** (A) The tumor may closely resemble inflammatory myofibroblastic tumor. Note the fascicular architecture, eosinophilic cytoplasm, and scattered lymphocytes. (B) In situ hybridization for Epstein-Barr virus–encoded RNA is (EBER) positive.

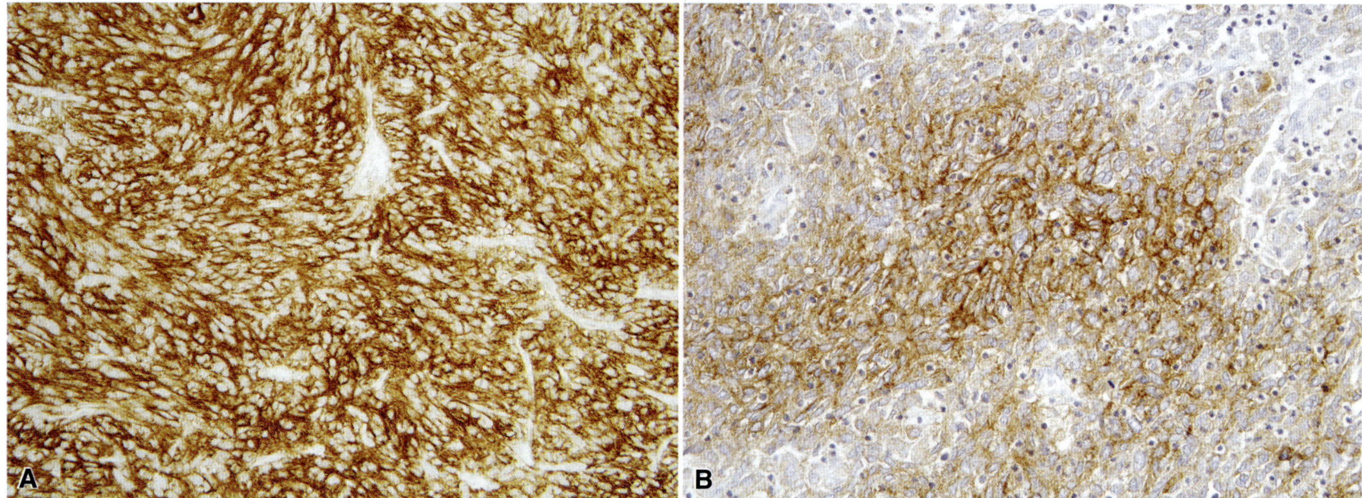

Figure 10.9 **Follicular Dendritic Cell Sarcoma.** (A) CD21 is usually strongly positive. (B) Focal staining for epithelial membrane antigen is a potential diagnostic pitfall.

When follicular dendritic cell sarcoma arises in the mediastinum, it may easily be confused with thymoma because of its whorled growth pattern, spindle cell morphology, and admixed lymphocytes. However, keratins and p63 are diffusely positive in thymomas, whereas follicular dendritic cell markers (CD21, CD35) are consistently negative. When follicular dendritic cell sarcoma arises in lymph nodes or the spleen, interdigitating dendritic cell sarcoma is a diagnostic consideration (Table 10.1). Interdigitating dendritic cell sarcoma shows a paracortical distribution in lymph nodes and lacks the storiform and whorled growth pattern of follicular dendritic cell sarcoma. Unlike follicular dendritic cell sarcoma, interdigitating dendritic cell sarcoma is diffusely positive for S-100 protein, usually also expresses CD45RO, and is negative for CD21, CD35, and other follicular dendritic cell markers.

EMA-positive follicular dendritic cell sarcomas involving lymph nodes (particularly in the neck) may be mistaken for metastatic undifferentiated or sarcomatoid carcinomas, especially because follicular dendritic cell markers are not usually included in typical immunohistochemical panels. However, keratins are nearly always negative in follicular dendritic cell sarcoma. Metastatic nasopharyngeal undifferentiated carcinoma is also positive for p63 and EBER; Epstein-Barr virus markers are only positive in the inflammatory pseudotumor-like variant of follicular dendritic cell sarcoma of the spleen and liver. Given its pale cytoplasm, indistinct cell borders, and propensity to metastasize to the liver, follicular dendritic cell sarcomas that arise in the gastrointestinal tract may be mistaken for KIT-negative GISTs. However, a dense lymphocytic infiltrate is uncommon in GIST. CD21 and CD35 are also negative in GIST, whereas DOG1 and CD34 are consistently negative in follicular dendritic cell sarcoma.

The inflammatory pseudotumor-like variant of follicular dendritic cell sarcoma may closely mimic IMT. The anatomic site (spleen or liver) is a helpful clue to the diagnosis. In addition, unlike follicular dendritic cell sarcoma, IMT is usually positive for SMA. Many tumors also express desmin, whereas 50% of tumors are positive for ALK (and harbor *ALK* gene rearrangements). CD21 and CD35 are negative in IMT.

Table 10.1 Immunohistochemistry in the Differential Diagnosis of Histiocytic and Dendritic Cell Tumors

	LCA	CD45RO	CD68	CD163	S-100	CD1a	CD21/CD35	Other
Histiocytic sarcoma	±	+	+	+	±	–	–	PU.1 (SPI1), lysozyme, CD4, CD31 positive
Rosai-Dorfman disease	+	+	±	±	+	–	–	—
Langerhans cell histiocytosis/Langerhans cell sarcoma	±	±	±	–	+	+	–	Langerin positive
Follicular dendritic cell sarcoma	–	–	–	–	~10%	–	+	D2-40, clusterin, CXCL13 positive; ~50% focal EMA positive
Inflammatory pseudotumor-like follicular dendritic cell sarcoma	–	–	–	–	–	–	+	EBER+
Interdigitating dendritic cell sarcoma	±	+	±	–	+	–	–	—
Indeterminate cell histiocytosis	±	±	±	–	+	+	–	Langerin negative
Fibroblastic reticular cell sarcoma	–	–	–	–	–	–	–	Keratin, desmin, SMA variably positive

EBER, Epstein-Barr virus–encoded RNA; *EMA*, epithelial membrane antigen; *LCA*, leukocyte common antigen; *SMA*, smooth muscle actin.

Prognosis and Treatment

Follicular dendritic cell sarcoma has a variable clinical course. Tumors arising in lymph nodes are often clinically indolent, with a small risk of metastasis (about 10%).[31,34,36] In contrast, extranodal tumors (especially intraabdominal examples) have significant metastatic potential (>50%).[30,35] The most common metastatic sites include the liver, lung, lymph nodes, and bones. Large tumor size, a high mitotic rate, marked pleomorphism, and extensive necrosis may be adverse prognostic features.[30,35] Complete surgical excision should be attempted. The role of radiation therapy and chemotherapy has not been well established.

PRACTICE POINTS: Follicular Dendritic Cell Sarcoma

- Arise in lymph nodes or at extranodal sites (e.g., gastrointestinal tract, mediastinum, tonsil)
- Ovoid, spindled, or epithelioid cells with vesicular chromatin and pale, syncytial cytoplasm
- Storiform and whorled growth pattern
- Prominent infiltrate of lymphocytes is typical
- Positive for CD21, CD23, CD35, podoplanin (D2-40), clusterin, and CXCL13
- Variable expression of epithelial membrane antigen (EMA) and S-100 is a diagnostic pitfall
- Extranodal tumors have significant metastatic potential
- Inflammatory pseudotumor-like variant arises in liver and spleen, resembles inflammatory myofibroblastic tumor, and is positive for Epstein-Barr virus–encoded RNA (EBER)

Fibroblastic Reticular Cell Sarcoma

The fibroblastic reticular cell is another type of lymphoid tissue–associated dendritic cell that is believed to be mesenchymal in origin. This cell type is found in lymph nodes, spleen, and tonsils, among other sites. The keratin-positive cells with dendritic morphology that are often encountered in small numbers in lymph nodes belong to this group of specialized mesenchymal cells. Fibroblastic reticular cell sarcomas are exceedingly rare; only very few cases have been reported.[31,49,50] Consequently, formal diagnostic criteria have not been established. Like other dendritic cell sarcomas, fibroblastic reticular cell sarcomas affect adults and have been described in lymph nodes, spleen, and soft tissues.[31,49,50]

Histologically, fibroblastic reticular cell sarcomas show some morphologic overlap with interdigitating dendritic cell sarcoma (see later discussion) but seem to have more cytologic heterogeneity.[49,50] The tumors are composed of sheets of spindled to polygonal cells with irregular nuclei and palely eosinophilic cytoplasm, admixed with small lymphocytes, which are a helpful clue to the possible diagnosis (Fig. 10.10). Some tumors show significant pleomorphism (see Fig. 10.10C). By immunohistochemistry, like their normal cellular counterparts, fibroblastic reticular cell sarcomas show variable expression of desmin, keratin, and SMA but are negative for S-100 protein and follicular dendritic cell markers (CD21 and CD35) (see Table 10.1).[49,50] Desmin and keratin stains highlight characteristic dendritic cytoplasmic processes (Fig. 10.11).

Given this nonspecific immunophenotype, this tumor type can be very difficult to diagnose. For example, myofibroblastic tumors show overlapping features. Keratin-positive fibroblastic reticular cell sarcomas of lymph nodes can easily be mistaken for metastatic sarcomatoid carcinoma, the distinction from which may be extremely difficult.

Fibroblastic reticular cell sarcomas have a variable clinical course, ranging from indolent to highly aggressive behavior with disseminated metastasis.[31,49,50]

Interdigitating Dendritic Cell Sarcoma

Interdigitating dendritic cells reside in the paracortex of lymph nodes and other lymphoid organs. Such dendritic cells are related to Langerhans cells and are involved in antigen presentation to T lymphocytes. Interdigitating dendritic cell sarcomas are exceedingly rare and may easily be mistaken for other tumor types, especially metastatic melanoma.

Clinical Features

Interdigitating dendritic cell sarcoma occurs over a wide age range. This tumor chiefly affects adults and has a male predominance[25,31,51,52]; children are rarely affected.[53] Most tumors present as painless masses. The majority of interdigitating dendritic cell sarcomas arise primarily in lymph nodes; other sites include the soft tissues, gastrointestinal tract, skin, and spleen.[31,51,52] As previously mentioned, some cases of interdigitating dendritic cell sarcoma arise in patients with a prior low-grade B-cell lymphoma as a form of clonal evolution ("transdifferentiation").[26,27]

Pathologic Features

Grossly, interdigitating dendritic cell sarcoma usually ranges from 2 to 10 cm in greatest dimension, with either a fibrous or fleshy cut surface.[52]

Histologically, interdigitating dendritic cell sarcoma usually shows a predominantly fascicular growth pattern, in areas with a more storiform

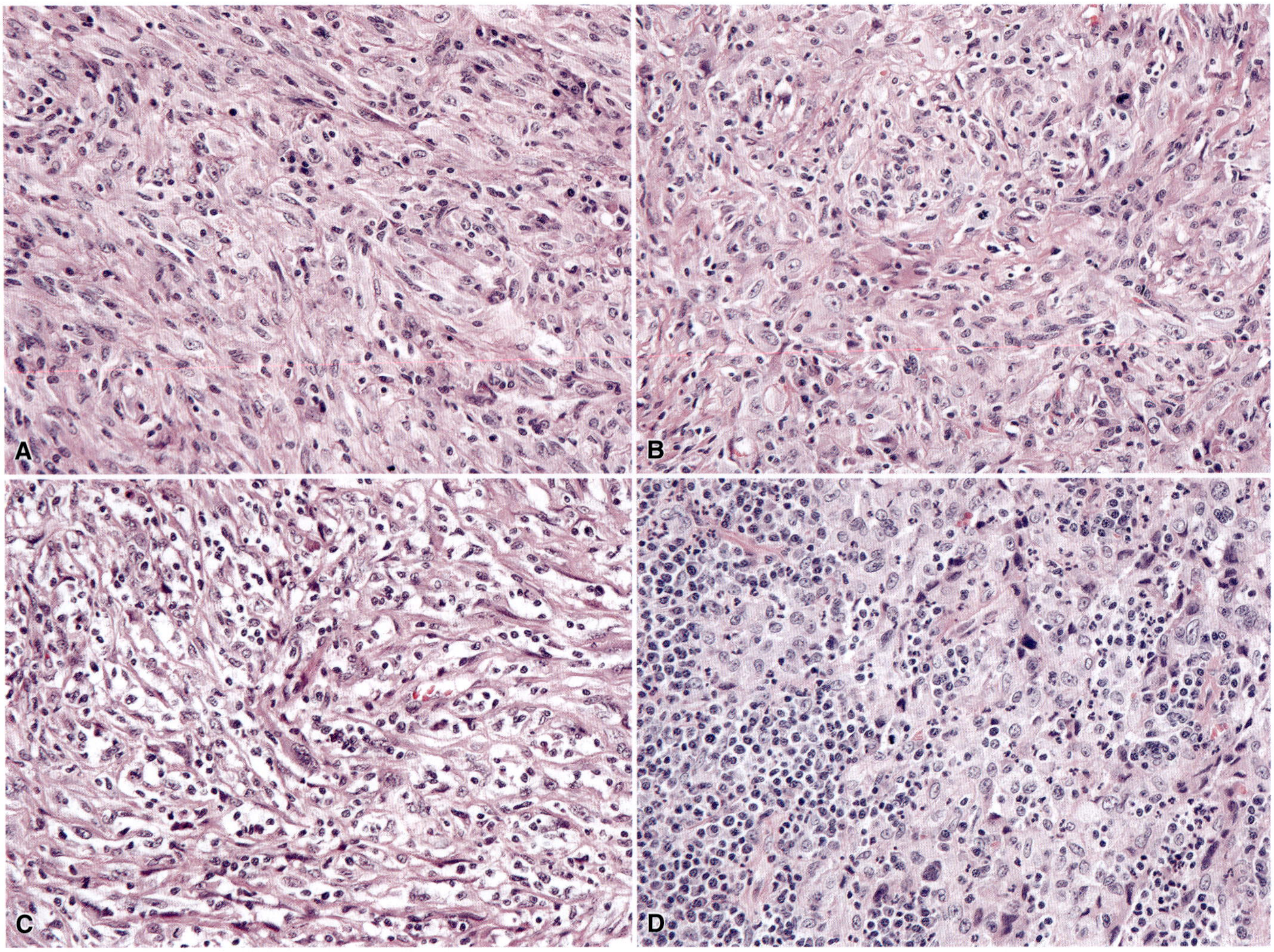

Figure 10.10 **Fibroblastic Reticular Cell Sarcoma.** (A) The tumor is composed of spindled to polygonal cells with collagenous stroma and prominent lymphocytes. (B) Some examples contain focal areas with epithelioid cytomorphology. Note the mild nuclear atypia and inflammatory infiltrate. (C) This tumor shows notable pleomorphism. Note the numerous lymphocytes. (D) An area with epithelioid cytomorphology, pale cytoplasm, and a mixed inflammatory infiltrate with lymphocytes, plasma cells, and occasional neutrophils.

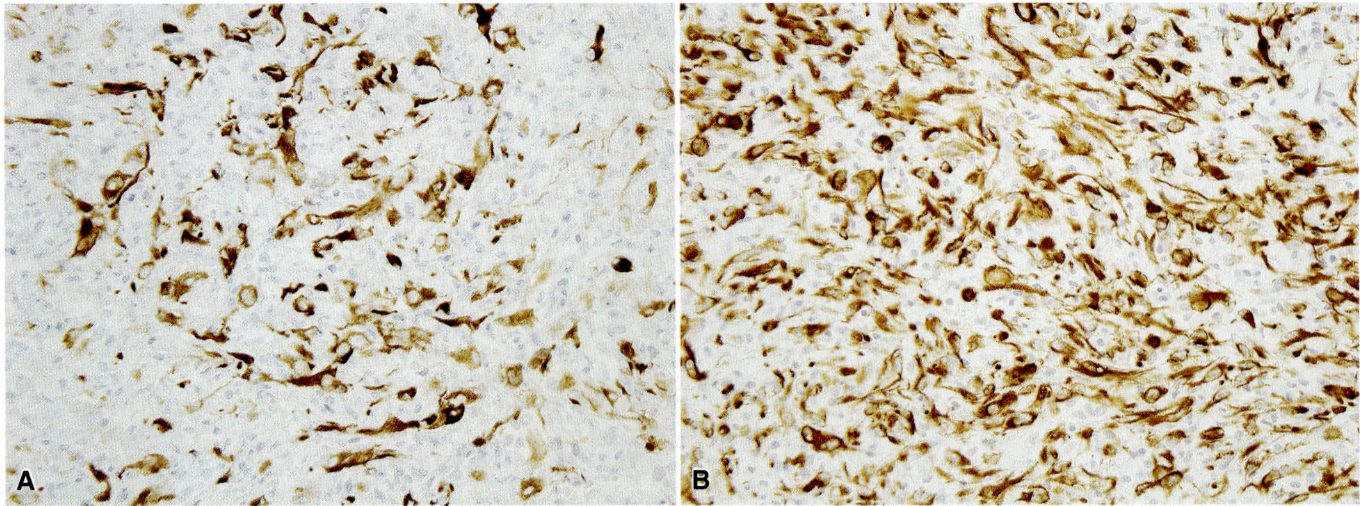

Figure 10.11 **Fibroblastic Reticular Cell Sarcoma.** These tumors show variable expression of desmin (A) and broad-spectrum keratins (B). Note the dendritic cytoplasmic processes.

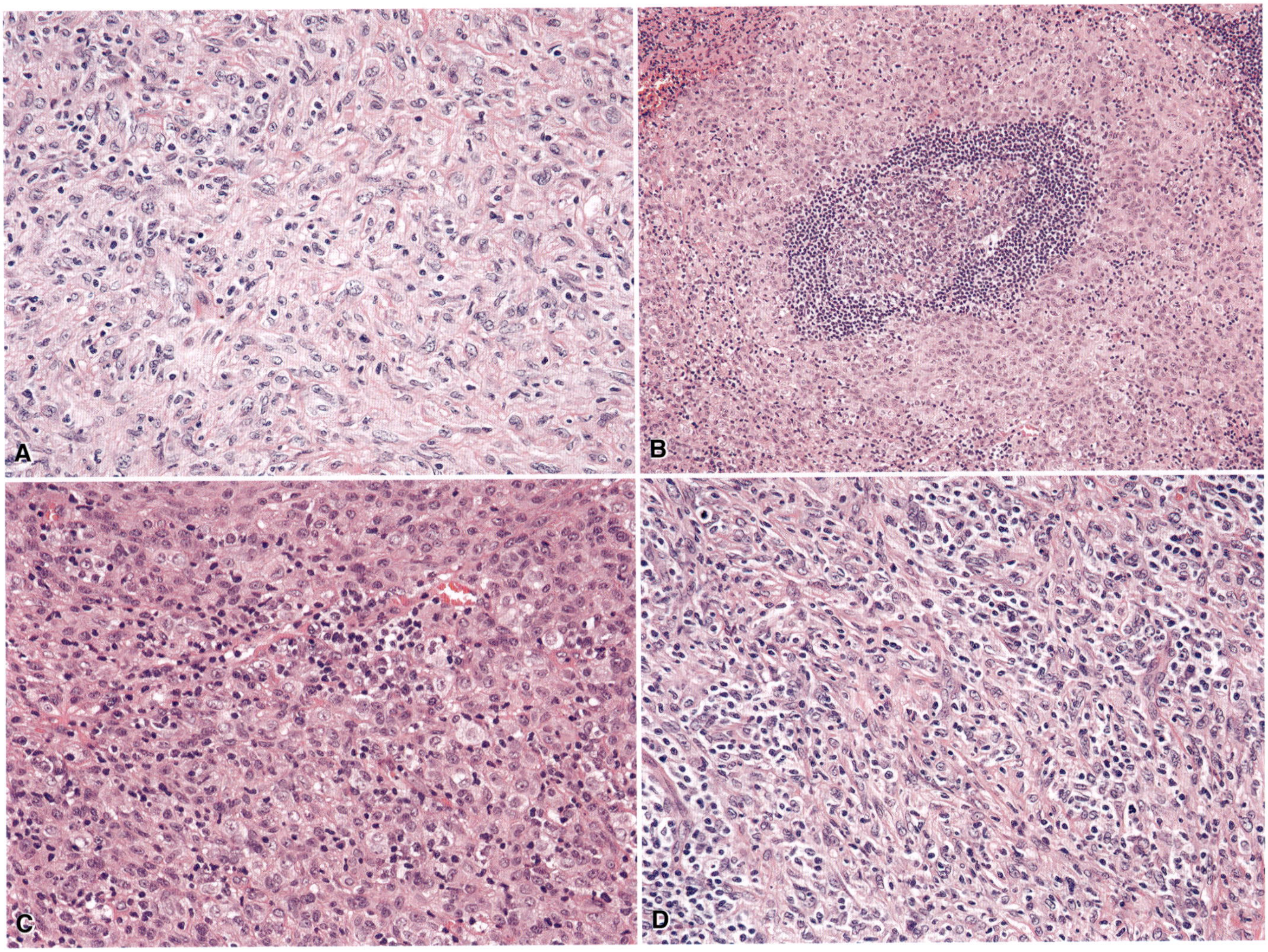

Figure 10.12 **Interdigitating Dendritic Cell Sarcoma.** (A) The tumor is composed of relatively uniform spindle cells with mild nuclear atypia and admixed lymphocytes. (B) Tumors involving lymph nodes show a paracortical distribution with sparing of follicles. (C) Some tumors show more epithelioid cytomorphology. Note the scattered lymphocytes. (D) A tumor composed of spindle cells in a collagenous stroma with numerous lymphocytes.

architecture (Fig. 10.12). In lymph nodes, interdigitating dendritic cell sarcoma characteristically involves the paracortex with sparing of lymphoid follicles (see Fig. 10.12B). The tumors are composed of ovoid to spindled cells with vesicular chromatin, small nucleoli, and abundant palely eosinophilic cytoplasm with ill-defined cell borders. There is a wide range in nuclear atypia, although most tumors are relatively uniform. Occasional tumors show notable pleomorphism. A subset of interdigitating dendritic cell sarcomas shows focal areas with epithelioid cytomorphology, mimicking histiocytic sarcoma (see Fig. 10.12C).[52] Scattered small lymphocytes are often prominent (see Fig. 10.12D); less often, admixed plasma cells may be seen.

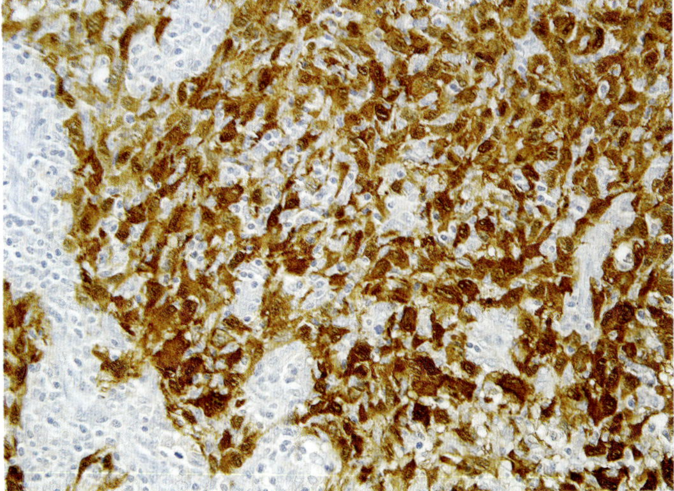

Figure 10.13 **Interdigitating Dendritic Cell Sarcoma.** The tumor cells are strongly positive for S-100 protein, which highlights dendritic cytoplasmic processes.

Immunohistochemistry

Interdigitating dendritic cell sarcoma is strongly and diffusely positive for S-100 protein, and nearly all cases also express CD45RO or LCA (the latter less consistently).[25,52] S-100 protein highlights dendritic processes (Fig. 10.13). About 20% of cases show focal expression of CD163, CD68, and lysozyme, typically in epithelioid areas resembling histiocytic sarcoma.[52] Follicular dendritic cell markers (CD21, CD35, podoplanin), CD1a, HMB-45, melan A, EMA, and keratins are consistently negative. The prominent admixed lymphocytes are CD3-positive T cells.

Differential Diagnosis

Chief differential diagnostic considerations are histiocytic sarcoma, follicular dendritic cell sarcoma, and metastatic melanoma.

In contrast to interdigitating dendritic cell sarcoma, histiocytic sarcoma is dominated by large epithelioid cells with abundant cytoplasm and shows extensive staining for CD163 and relatively limited (if any) expression of S-100 protein. Occasional tumors (particularly those with significant nuclear atypia) may be very difficult to classify; the dominant cytology (spindle cell vs. epithelioid) seems to be the most reliable distinguishing feature. Follicular dendritic cell sarcoma shows a more consistently whorled architecture. It is positive for CD21, CD35, and podoplanin and lacks diffuse expression of S-100 protein (see Table 10.1).

Both interdigitating dendritic cell sarcoma and metastatic melanoma often involve lymph nodes and are strongly positive for S-100 protein; thus, these tumor types may be confused with one another. This is particularly difficult for spindle cell melanomas, because such tumors are usually negative for second-line melanocytic markers such as melan A and HMB-45. In this context, obtaining clinical history (i.e., that of a prior skin lesion) is critical. Bland, uniform cytology and paracortical lymph node distribution favor interdigitating dendritic cell sarcoma. SOX10 is consistently positive in metastatic melanoma but is not expressed by interdigitating dendritic cell sarcoma; CD45RO is not expressed in melanoma.

Prognosis and Treatment

Interdigitating dendritic cell sarcoma shows a variable clinical course, with some tumors behaving in an aggressive fashion with disseminated metastases to the lungs, liver, and lymph nodes, whereas others are clinically indolent, particularly localized nodal tumors.[25,51-53] Large tumor size, a high mitotic rate, and the presence of a histiocytic sarcoma-like component may be adverse prognostic features.[52] Because of the rarity of this tumor type, the efficacy of chemotherapy (and the optimal combination of specific agents) has not been established.

Langerhans Cell Histiocytosis and Langerhans Cell Sarcoma

Langerhans cells are specialized dendritic cells that reside in the skin and at mucosal sites, where they are involved in presenting antigens to T lymphocytes and then migrate to lymph nodes. LCH is the most common dendritic cell neoplasm, whereas Langerhans cell sarcoma is exceptionally rare. The differential diagnosis of LCH of the skin is discussed in Chapter 15 in the section on juvenile xanthogranuloma.

Clinical Features

LCH most often affects children and young adults, with a male predominance. It often occurs as a solitary lytic tumor in the bone (so-called eosinophilic granuloma), usually several centimeters in size.[54-56] Other sites of involvement include the skin and lymph nodes.[54] LCH may also occur in older adult smokers as small, sometimes multifocal lung nodules.[54,57] Involvement of the gastrointestinal tract as small mucosal polyps is rare.[58] The presence of multifocal bony lesions has previously been referred to as Hand-Schüller-Christian disease, whereas disseminated multiorgan disease was known as Letterer-Siwe disease.[56] The latter disorder is nearly exclusive to young infants. The exceedingly rare Langerhans cell sarcoma presents in adults as a cutaneous, soft tissue, or gastrointestinal mass.[25,59,60]

Pathologic Features

Histologically, LCH is composed of sheets of relatively uniform ovoid cells with folded or grooved nuclei, fine chromatin, inconspicuous nucleoli, and moderate amounts of palely eosinophilic cytoplasm (Fig. 10.14). Prominent admixed eosinophils are usually present and may be striking with the formation of eosinophilic microabscesses. Smaller numbers of other inflammatory cell types may also be seen.

Langerhans cell sarcoma closely resembles histiocytic sarcoma (see subsequent discussion) and other pleomorphic epithelioid malignant neoplasms with eosinophilic cytoplasm (Fig. 10.15), although the tumor cells often contain less copious cytoplasm than in histiocytic sarcoma.[25] Nuclear grooves (when present) are a diagnostic clue, but some tumors are cytologically relatively nondistinctive; prominent eosinophils are another helpful feature (see Fig. 10.15B).

Immunohistochemistry

LCH is strongly positive for S-100 protein, CD1a, and langerin (CD207; Fig. 10.16),[25,57,61,62] the latter localized to Birbeck granules, which are the distinctive ultrastructural feature specific to Langerhans cells. In the past, Birbeck granules were sought to confirm the diagnosis. However, with the availability of CD1a and langerin, electron microscopy is no longer used routinely for diagnostic purposes. LCH shows variable expression of CD68 but is typically negative for CD163.

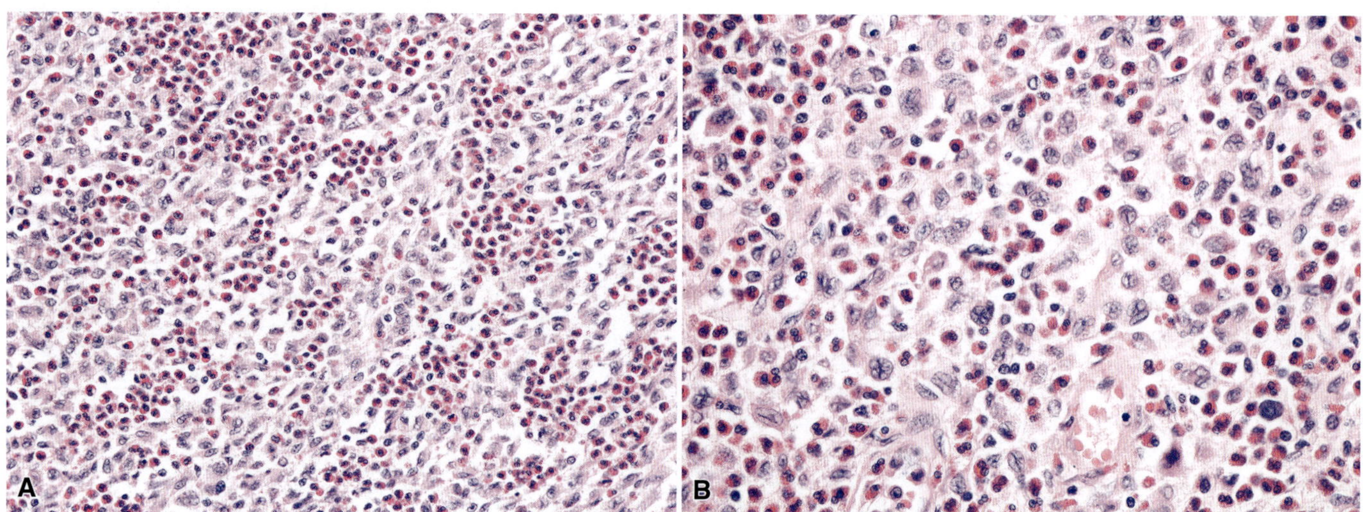

Figure 10.14 Langerhans Cell Histiocytosis. (A) The tumor is composed of sheets of mononuclear cells with pale cytoplasm admixed with numerous eosinophils. (B) The tumor cells contain irregular nuclei with nuclear grooves.

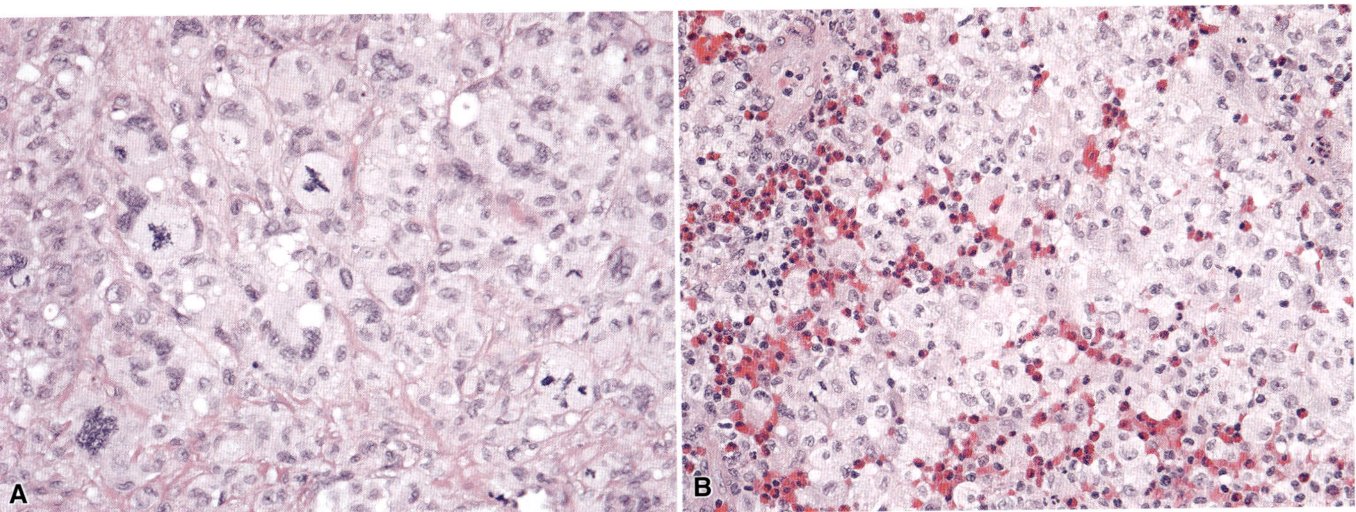

Figure 10.15 Langerhans Cell Sarcoma. (A) The tumor is composed of large histiocytoid cells with abundant pale cytoplasm. Note the pleomorphism and frequent mitotic figures. (B) Some areas show more uniform cytology. Note the prominent eosinophils, which are a helpful diagnostic clue, when present.

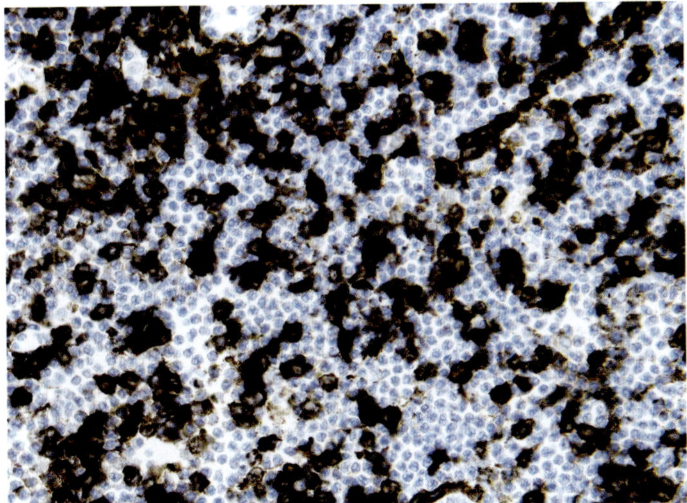

Figure 10.16 Langerhans Cell Histiocytosis. The tumor cells show strong staining for langerin (CD207).

Langerhans cell sarcoma is also positive for S-100 protein, CD1a, and langerin. However, the extent of staining for specialized Langerhans cell markers is often more limited than in LCH.[25,60]

Molecular Genetics

BRAF V600E mutations are common in LCH, found in 50% to 60% of cases.[63-66] The aggressive variants of this disorder are associated with the presence of *BRAF* mutations in hematopoietic precursor cells, whereas in localized disease, the mutation is only found in the differentiated dendritic cell compartment.[64] LCH lacking such mutations often harbors *MAP2K1* mutations.[65,66] These findings have implications for targeted therapy for patients with aggressive systemic disease.

Differential Diagnosis

Once the diagnosis of LCH is considered, the diagnosis is relatively straightforward using immunohistochemistry. The differential diagnosis might include systemic mastocytosis because of the prominent eosinophils. However, mast cells in systemic mastocytosis are round or spindled in shape. They are positive for KIT, tryptase, and CD25 and negative for Langerhans cell markers.

The differential diagnosis for Langerhans cell sarcoma includes other epithelioid malignant neoplasms, including histiocytic sarcoma, melanoma, anaplastic large-cell lymphoma, undifferentiated carcinoma, and mast cell sarcoma. The presence of focal nuclear grooves and an eosinophilic inflammatory infiltrate should at least raise the possibility of Langerhans cell sarcoma when histiocytic sarcoma is being considered. Histiocytic sarcoma is typically positive for CD163, whereas CD1a and langerin are usually negative (see Table 10.1). Although both melanoma and Langerhans cell sarcoma are positive for S-100 protein, only Langerhans cell sarcoma expresses CD1a and langerin, whereas melanocytic markers (e.g., HMB-45 and melan A) are limited to melanoma in this differential diagnosis. Anaplastic large-cell lymphoma and Langerhans cell sarcoma show considerable morphologic overlap. However, anaplastic large-cell lymphoma is strongly positive for CD30 (and a subset for ALK) and negative for S-100 protein, CD1a, and langerin. Undifferentiated carcinoma should be positive for keratins and is negative for Langerhans cell markers. Clinical history or radiologic evidence of a visceral primary is also helpful to suggest the diagnosis of metastatic carcinoma. Mast cell sarcoma is an exceedingly rare tumor composed of mast cells that may arise in skin, bone, or visceral organs. Although some affected patients have an established history of urticaria pigmentosa (maculopapular cutaneous mastocytosis) or systemic mastocytosis, other patients have no prior mast cell disorder. Mast cell sarcoma is composed of atypical epithelioid cells with clear cytoplasm and sharply defined cell borders (Fig. 10.17).[67,68] In contrast to Langerhans cell sarcoma, KIT and tryptase are positive (see Fig. 10.17B), whereas S-100, CD1a, and langerin are negative.

Prognosis and Treatment

Solitary LCH of bone and other sites is usually clinically benign, whereas infants with multiorgan involvement have a high mortality rate.[54,55]

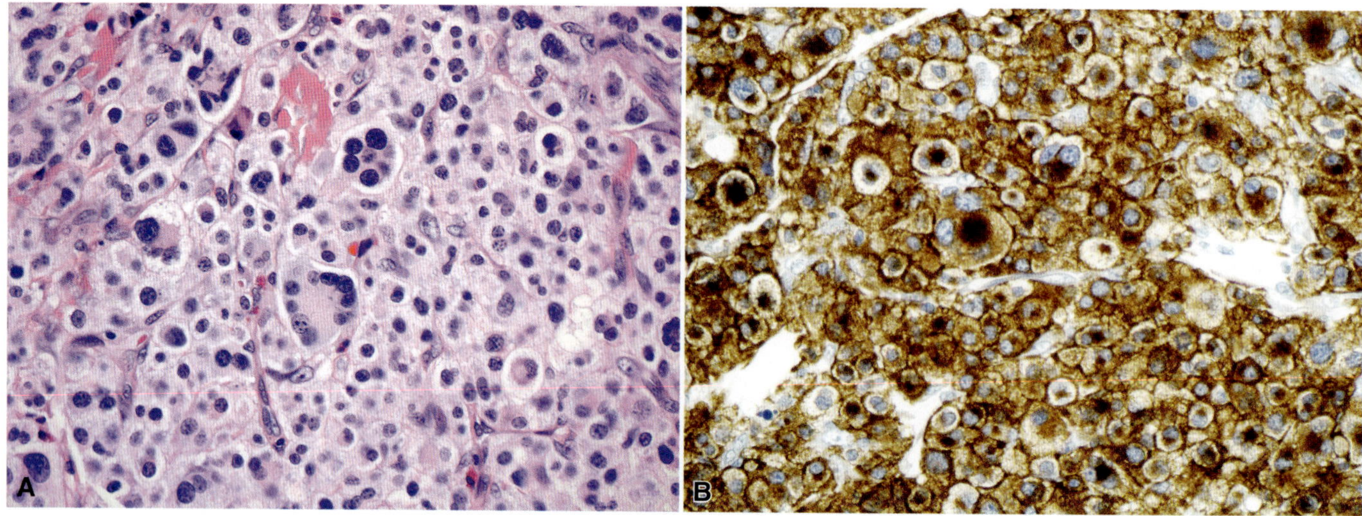

Figure 10.17 Mast Cell Sarcoma. This rare tumor type may be confused with histiocytic sarcoma, Langerhans cell sarcoma, and other epithelioid malignant neoplasms. (A) The tumor is composed of epithelioid cells with abundant pale cytoplasm and sharply defined cell borders. Note the pleomorphic and multinucleated cells. (B) The tumor cells show strong staining for KIT and tryptase (the latter not shown).

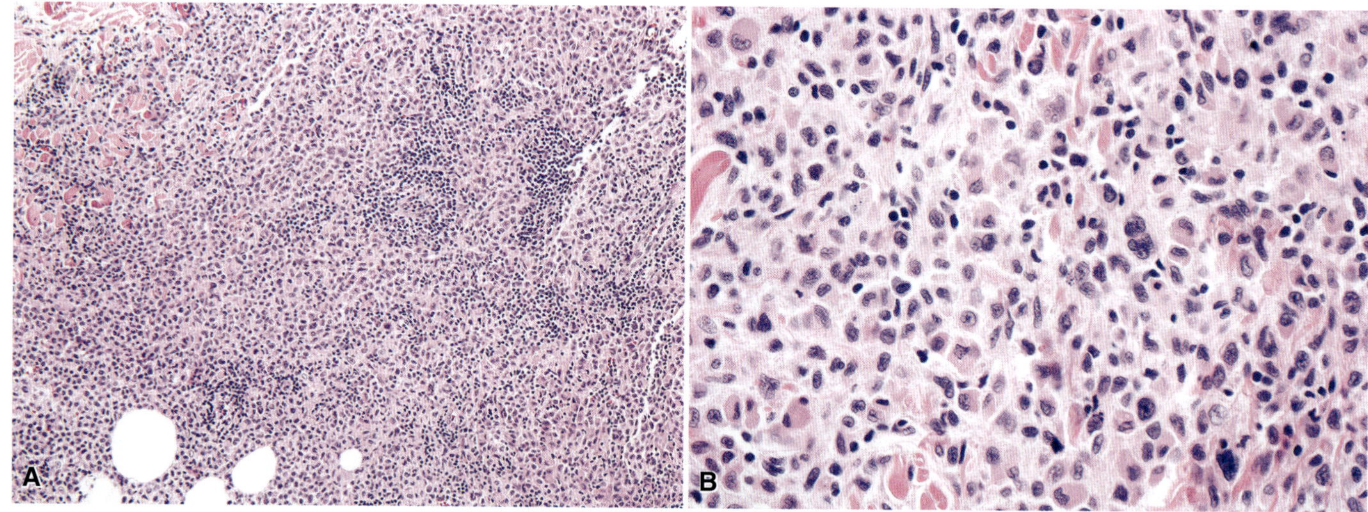

Figure 10.18 Indeterminate Cell Histiocytosis. (A) The tumor is composed of sheets of histiocytoid cells with pale cytoplasm infiltrating dermal collagen and subcutaneous tissue. Note the prominent lymphocytes. (B) The tumor cells contain irregular nuclei and include occasional pleomorphic forms.

Langerhans cell sarcoma often has an aggressive clinical course; disseminated disease is relatively common at presentation.[59,60]

PRACTICE POINTS: Langerhans Cell Histiocytosis/Langerhans Cell Sarcoma

- Langerhans cell histiocytosis usually affects children and young adults
- Solitary lytic bone lesion most common ("eosinophilic granuloma"), usually clinically benign
- Skin and lymph nodes more rarely involved
- Multiorgan disease nearly exclusive to young infants, high mortality
- Sheets of uniform ovoid cells with folded or grooved nuclei and pale cytoplasm
- Dense infiltrate of eosinophils is typical
- Positive for S-100, CD1a, and langerin
- *BRAF* V600E and *MAP2K1* mutations are common
- Exceedingly rare Langerhans cell sarcoma resembles histiocytic sarcoma; difficult to recognize; more limited staining for Langerhans cell markers

Indeterminate Cell Histiocytosis

Indeterminate cell histiocytosis (also referred to as indeterminate cell tumor) is a rare dendritic cell neoplasm with a predilection for the skin.[69,70] So-called "indeterminate cells" are thought to be the precursors to Langerhans cells. Most patients with indeterminate cell histiocytosis are adults who present with a single nodule or multiple painless cutaneous nodules.[69,70] Splenic involvement has also been documented.[71]

Histologically, indeterminate cell histiocytosis somewhat resembles LCH in terms of irregular nuclei with nuclear grooves but with more abundant pale cytoplasm, more nuclear variability, including occasional pleomorphic cells, and a lack of interspersed eosinophils (Fig. 10.18).[70] Instead, admixed small lymphocytes are commonly observed. Similar to LCH, indeterminate cell histiocytosis is positive for S-100 protein and CD1a (Fig. 10.19), but by definition, langerin is negative (and Birbeck granules are not detected by electron microscopy).[70,71] Several cases of indeterminate cell histiocytosis with *ETV3-NCOA2* gene fusions have been reported.[72]

In some patients with indeterminate cell histiocytosis, the lesions may regress spontaneously, whereas others pursue an aggressive clinical course with widespread disseminated disease.[70] Pathologic parameters to predict behavior have not been established.

Extranodal Rosai-Dorfman Disease

Rosai-Dorfman disease, originally described as sinus histiocytosis with massive lymphadenopathy, is an idiopathic histiocytic proliferative disorder that may present either as lymphadenopathy or as a mass lesion.[73,74] Rosai-Dorfman disease may arise at almost any anatomic site; among the most common extranodal sites are skin, bone, upper respiratory tract, and soft tissues.[75-77] The disorder usually occurs in children and young adults with a male predominance and a predilection for black patients.[74,75] Purely cutaneous Rosai-Dorfman disease shows distinct clinical features with a female predominance and a different racial distribution (see Chapter 15).[78,79]

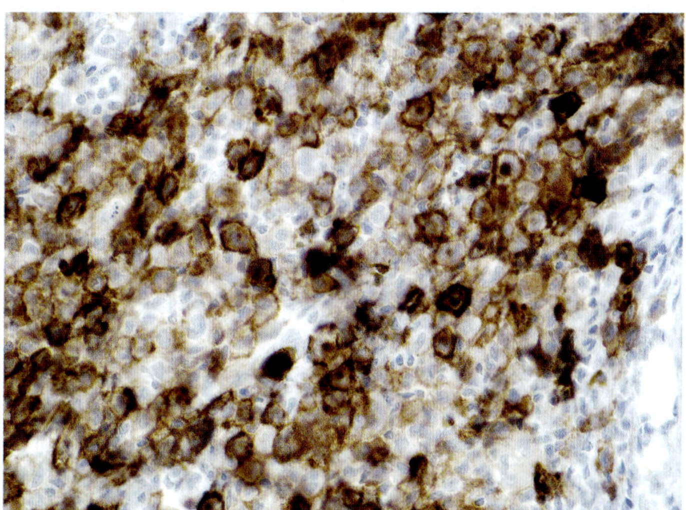

Figure 10.19 Indeterminate Cell Histiocytosis. The tumor cells are strongly positive for CD1a, but langerin is negative.

Histologically, extranodal Rosai-Dorfman disease is composed of large, distinctive histiocytes with round central nuclei, fine chromatin, small nucleoli, and voluminous pale cytoplasm with indistinct cell borders, buried within a dense mixed inflammatory infiltrate of neutrophils, lymphocytes, and plasma cells (Fig. 10.20). Associated stromal fibrosis is variable in extent. The diagnostic cells may be obscured by the background inflammation and are sometimes difficult to appreciate without immunohistochemistry. A characteristic diagnostic finding is the presence of emperipolesis (i.e., intact inflammatory cells within the cytoplasm of the large histiocytes; see Fig. 10.20B).

By immunohistochemistry, the distinctive histiocytes are strongly positive for S-100 protein, which stains the cytoplasm and often highlights emperipolesis (Fig. 10.21).[80] CD68 and CD163 are also often positive,[81] whereas CD1a and langerin are negative.

Once the characteristic histiocytes are identified, the diagnosis is relatively straightforward. The chief differential diagnostic considerations include a nonspecific inflammatory process and a lymphoproliferative disorder. When the large histiocytes are numerous, other histiocytic disorders may be considered, especially juvenile xanthogranuloma and reticulohistiocytoma (see Chapter 15) and occasionally histiocytic sarcoma. In histiocytic sarcoma, in contrast to Rosai-Dorfman disease, tumor cells show nuclear atypia and variability, S-100 protein usually shows only weak or focal staining, and emperipolesis is generally absent.

Very rarely, systemic Rosai-Dorfman disease may be aggressive, although most of the rare associated deaths are caused by infectious complications.[82] Extranodal Rosai-Dorfman disease usually pursues a benign clinical course. Spontaneous regression may occur, and most of the remaining cases are cured by simple surgical excision, when feasible.[75,82] For patients with extensive involvement, radiation and systemic therapies have been used, with variable results.[83]

Histiocytic Sarcoma

Prior to the development and widespread availability of antibodies for diagnostic immunohistochemistry, many aggressive lymphomas with abundant cytoplasm were mistakenly classified as histiocytic sarcoma (previously also referred to as true histiocytic lymphoma), including anaplastic large-cell lymphoma, diffuse large B-cell lymphoma, and enteropathy-associated T-cell lymphoma.[25,84] Bona fide histiocytic sarcoma

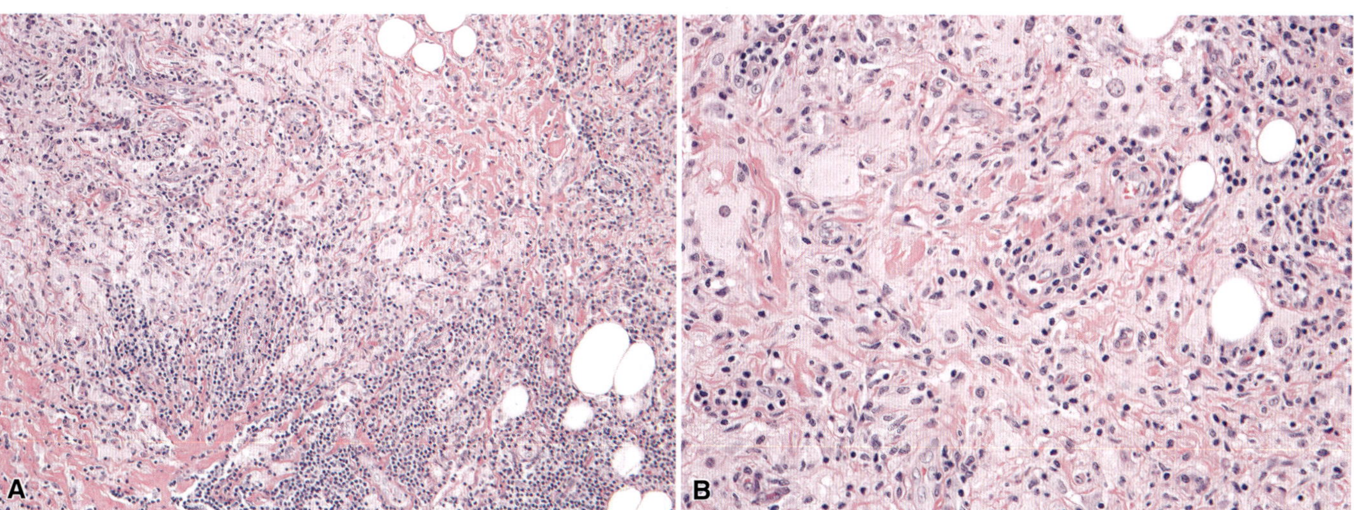

Figure 10.20 Extranodal Rosai-Dorfman Disease. (A) The lesion shows a dense inflammatory infiltrate, stromal hyalinization, and distinctive large histiocytes with abundant cytoplasm. (B) The histiocytes contain rounded nuclei with small nucleoli and voluminous pale cytoplasm. Note the prominent inflammatory cells.

(a mass-forming malignant neoplasm showing histiocytic differentiation) is very rare.

Clinical Features

Histiocytic sarcoma most commonly arises at extranodal sites, such as the soft tissue, gastrointestinal tract, and skin; however, lymph nodes, spleen, bone, central nervous system, and other visceral sites may also be affected.[84-86] Tumors occur in patients over a wide age range, mostly in adulthood. A solitary mass is the most common clinical presentation. Some patients present with systemic symptoms. As previously mentioned (similar to interdigitating dendritic cell sarcoma), histiocytic sarcoma may occur in patients with a prior history of follicular lymphoma, mantle cell lymphoma, or chronic lymphocytic leukemia as a form of clonal evolution.[26,29] This sort of "transdifferentiation" is perhaps not surprising, because the ETS family transcription factor PU.1 (SPI1) plays an important role in regulating gene expression of both the myeloid/monocytic and B-lymphoid lineages during hematopoiesis.[87]

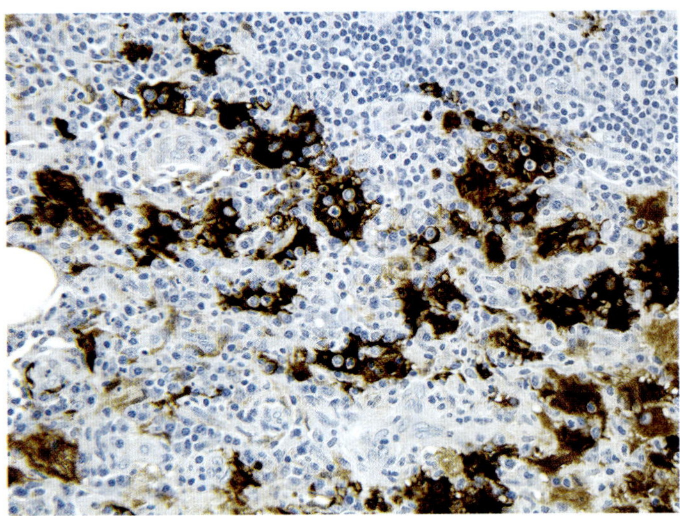

Figure 10.21 **Extranodal Rosai-Dorfman Disease.** S-100 protein is strongly positive and highlights emperipolesis.

Pathologic Features

Grossly, most histiocytic sarcomas are 5 to 10 cm in greatest dimension. They have a fleshy cut surface, often with areas of hemorrhage and necrosis.[84]

Histologically, histiocytic sarcoma is typically composed of diffuse sheets of large epithelioid cells with ovoid or irregular nuclei with vesicular chromatin, prominent nucleoli, and abundant palely eosinophilic or foamy cytoplasm (Fig. 10.22). Marked nuclear atypia, binucleated forms, and scattered pleomorphic cells are often present (see Fig. 10.22B). The tumor cells are usually admixed with variable numbers of small lymphocytes. Neutrophils, plasma cells, eosinophils, and reactive histiocytes may also be observed. Some cases contain a minor spindle cell component. A small subset of histiocytic sarcomas is morphologically low grade, with uniform nuclear features and only mild atypia.[84]

Immunohistochemistry

Histiocytic sarcoma is nearly always positive for CD68, CD163, lysozyme, CD4, CD45RO, and PU.1 (SPI1); CD163 is the most specific diagnostic marker (Fig. 10.23).[25,81,84,86] Leukocyte common antigen (LCA) and S-100 protein are also often expressed, although the latter is typically only focal in distribution. CD31 is also often positive.[84] CD1a and langerin are typically negative, as are CD21, CD35, keratins, EMA, and CD30.

Molecular Genetics

A subset of histiocytic sarcomas harbor *BRAF* V600E mutations; other *BRAF* mutations have also been reported.[47,88] Histiocytic sarcomas that arise through "transdifferentiation" harbor the same IgH gene rearrangements and translocations as the precursor B-cell lymphomas.[26,27]

Differential Diagnosis

The differential diagnosis of histiocytic sarcoma can be quite broad, including not only large-cell lymphomas (especially anaplastic large-cell lymphoma and diffuse large B-cell lymphoma) but also undifferentiated carcinomas, melanoma, and pleomorphic sarcomas. Judicious application of a sufficiently broad immunohistochemical panel is essential to exclude these other much more common possibilities. The combination of CD163 and PU.1 (SPI1) is highly specific for histiocytic sarcoma. Histiocytic sarcoma is negative for CD30, as well as B-cell, T-cell, epithelial, and melanocytic markers. Intraabdominal or retroperitoneal histiocytic

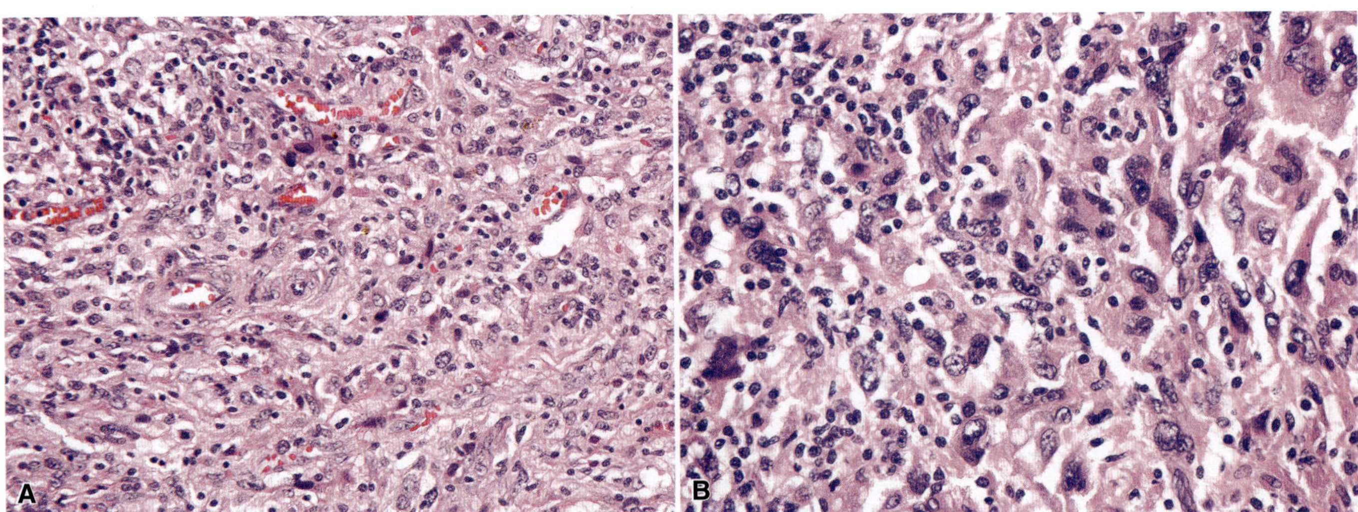

Figure 10.22 **Histiocytic Sarcoma.** (A) The tumor is composed of large epithelioid cells with foamy cytoplasm and scattered inflammatory cells. (B) The tumors often contain multinucleated cells and show nuclear pleomorphism. Note the scattered lymphocytes.

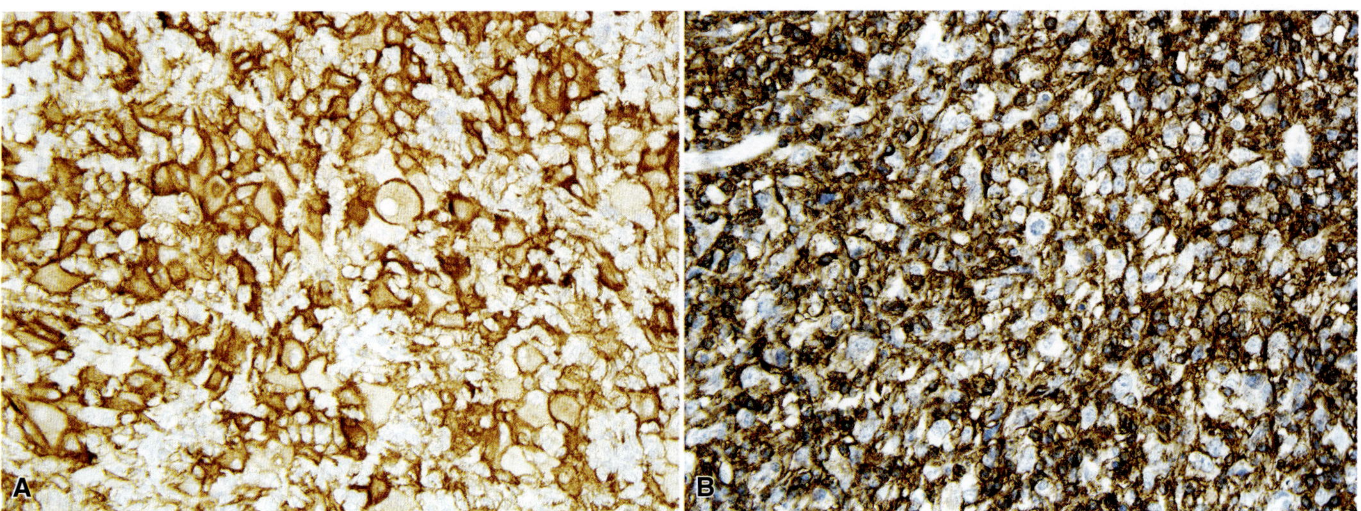

Figure 10.23 **Histiocytic Sarcoma.** (A) CD163 is the most specific histiocytic marker. (B) CD45RO is also usually positive.

sarcomas with prominent neutrophilic inflammation may be mistaken for inflammatory MFH (i.e., dedifferentiated liposarcoma). Detection of overexpression of MDM2 and CDK4 by immunohistochemistry (or *MDM2* gene amplification by FISH) can be used to confirm the diagnosis of dedifferentiated liposarcoma.

Prognosis and Treatment

Histiocytic sarcoma usually pursues an aggressive clinical course.[84,85] Typical sites of metastasis include lymph nodes, lung, and bone. Combination chemotherapy generally shows limited efficacy; protocols similar to those used for large-cell lymphoma are often attempted. Morphologically low-grade tumors and small, completely excised tumors arising on the extremities may be clinically more indolent.[84]

PRACTICE POINTS: Histiocytic Sarcoma

- Wide anatomic distribution (especially gastrointestinal tract, soft tissues, skin, lymph nodes, spleen)
- May occur in patients with history of follicular lymphoma, chronic lymphocytic leukemia, and rarely other B-cell lymphomas ("transdifferentiation")
- Sheets of large epithelioid cells with abundant palely eosinophilic cytoplasm
- Marked nuclear atypia and pleomorphism are common
- Infiltrate of lymphocytes is common; variable neutrophils, eosinophils, and reactive histiocytes
- Positive for CD68, CD163, CD45RO, and PU.1 (SPI1); variable leukocyte common antigen (LCA) and S-100
- Usually pursues aggressive clinical course

Angiomatoid Fibrous Histiocytoma

Angiomatoid fibrous histiocytoma (formerly angiomatoid MFH) is a distinctive translocation-associated mesenchymal neoplasm of uncertain lineage and intermediate biologic potential, which has no relationship with either cutaneous fibrous histiocytoma (see Chapter 15) or sarcomas formerly included in the MFH category (see Chapter 7).[89-91] This tumor type is discussed in detail in Chapter 3 and will be covered only briefly in this chapter.

Clinical Features

Angiomatoid fibrous histiocytoma usually affects children and young adults and typically arises in superficial soft tissues.[89-91] The extremities are most commonly involved, especially the antecubital fossa and popliteal fossa, followed by the head and neck. Systemic symptoms, including fever, anemia, and weight loss, may accompany the appearance of a usually painless mass.[90,91]

Pathologic Features

Grossly, angiomatoid fibrous histiocytoma is typically between 2 and 4 cm in greatest dimension. It has a firm cut surface, often showing areas of hemorrhage.

Histologically, angiomatoid fibrous histiocytoma often superficially resembles a lymph node, being well circumscribed with a peripheral fibrous pseudocapsule containing a prominent lymphoplasmacytic inflammatory infiltrate, including germinal centers (Fig. 10.24). Dilated blood-filled pseudovascular spaces are typical but may be absent ("solid" variant). The tumor is composed of nodules of cytologically uniform ovoid to histiocytoid cells with abundant palely eosinophilic cytoplasm and ill-defined cell borders, imparting a syncytial appearance (see Fig. 10.24B). Interspersed small lymphocytes may be seen. Occasional cases contain myxoid stroma or pleomorphic cells, which is of no clinical consequence.[89,92,93]

Immunohistochemistry

About 50% of angiomatoid fibrous histiocytomas are positive for EMA and desmin.[91,94] This unusual combination is diagnostically helpful. CD68, muscle-specific actin, and CD99 are also often positive.[91,95] Keratins, S-100 protein, CD21, and CD35 are negative.

Molecular Genetics

The predominant translocation in angiomatoid fibrous histiocytoma is t(2;22), resulting in an *EWSR1-CREB1* fusion gene (see Chapter 18).[96,97] Variant translocations include t(12;22) with an *EWSR1-ATF1* fusion and t(12;16) with an *FUS-ATF1* fusion.[96-101]

Differential Diagnosis

The differential diagnosis for typical angiomatoid fibrous histiocytoma is discussed in Chapter 3. For cases with prominent intratumoral lymphocytes, a histiocytic or dendritic cell tumor (e.g., follicular dendritic cell sarcoma) may be considered. Although CD68 may be positive, in contrast to histiocytic neoplasms, CD163 is negative. CD21 and CD35 are also consistently negative, unlike in follicular dendritic cell sarcoma.

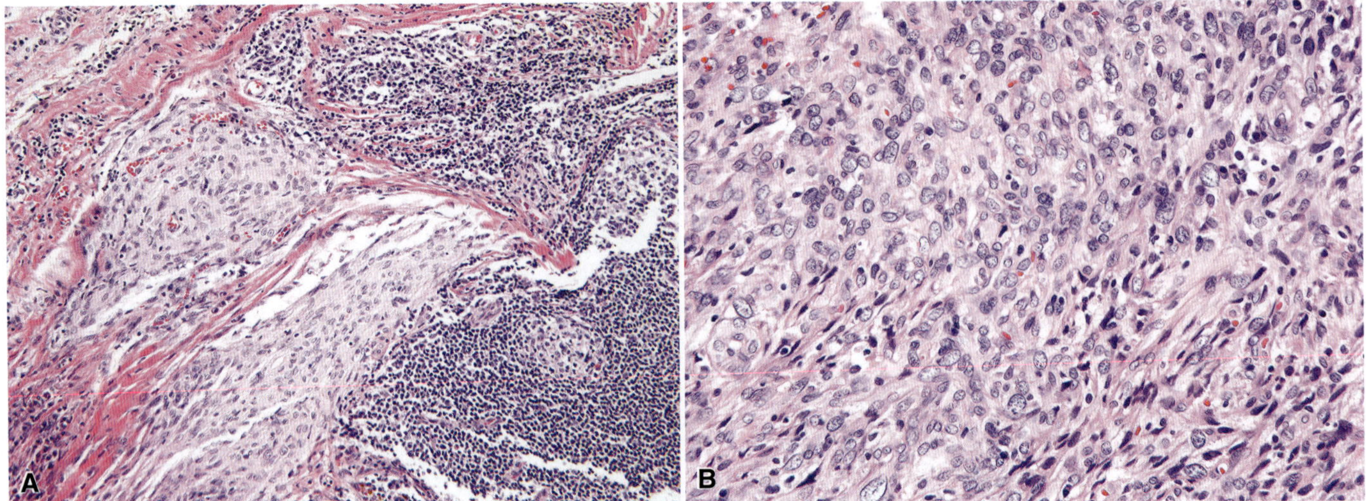

Figure 10.24 Angiomatoid Fibrous Histiocytoma. (A) The tumor is composed of nodules of pale histiocytoid cells with an adjacent lymphoplasmacytic infiltrate including germinal centers and hyalinized fibrosis. (B) The tumor cells are uniform with ovoid nuclei and fine chromatin. Note the scattered lymphocytes.

Demonstration of *EWSR1* rearrangement by FISH is helpful to confirm the diagnosis.[102,103]

Prognosis and Treatment

Angiomatoid fibrous histiocytoma belongs to the group of mesenchymal tumors of intermediate biologic potential, with a 10% to 15% risk of local recurrence and rare metastasis (about 1%) to lymph nodes or lung.[89-91] Complete surgical excision is adequate therapy.

Myxoinflammatory Fibroblastic Sarcoma

Myxoinflammatory fibroblastic sarcoma (MIFS) is a distinctive mesenchymal neoplasm of intermediate biologic potential that is likely closely related to hemosiderotic fibrolipomatous tumor.[104-107] This tumor type is discussed in more detail in Chapters 5 and 7. MIFS affects middle-aged to elderly adults with an equal gender distribution.[106,107] Most tumors arise in the subcutaneous tissues of the distal upper extremities (especially wrists and hands), followed by distal lower extremities.[106-108] Nonacral sites are rarely affected.

MIFS is grossly ill defined with infiltrative margins. Histologically, as the name implies, the tumor has a heterogeneous appearance, with both myxoid areas (often with prominent pseudolipoblasts) and cellular, inflammatory areas containing lymphocytes and neutrophils, with bland fibroblastic spindle cells and variable stromal fibrosis (Fig. 10.25). The neoplastic cells include occasional pleomorphic cells with large, viral inclusion-like nucleoli and eosinophilic or amphophilic cytoplasm (see Fig. 10.25D). Occasional tumor cells can be binucleated and closely resemble Reed-Sternberg cells. The relative contribution by myxoid areas and cellular, fibroinflammatory areas is variable; some tumors are dominated by one component. Occasional tumors show hybrid features of MIFS and hemosiderotic fibrolipomatous tumor (see Chapters 5, 7, and 12).[104]

MIFS is often focally positive for CD34 and sometimes for SMA; desmin, S-100 protein, EMA, and keratins are rarely positive.[106,109] MIFS typically harbors a t(1;10) translocation (resulting in *TGFBR3* and *MGEA5* rearrangement), in addition to alterations of chromosome 3.[104,105] Similar findings have been documented in hemosiderotic fibrolipomatous tumor and hybrid lesions.[104,105] Some studies have identified this gene fusion in only a small subset of MIFS cases.[110] A recent study identified BRAF gene rearrangements in some cases lacking TGFBR3-MGEA5 fusions.[111]

When dominated by myxoid stroma, MIFS may be confused with myxofibrosarcoma; however, MIFS lacks the characteristic curvilinear blood vessels of myxofibrosarcoma, and the latter tumor type lacks the fibroinflammatory areas of MIFS. When dominated by inflammation, MIFS may be particularly difficult to recognize, being easily mistaken for an inflammatory process or occasionally Hodgkin lymphoma. The presence of the bizarre pleomorphic cells are a clue to the correct diagnosis. Hodgkin lymphoma essentially never occurs in somatic soft tissues, and MIFS is negative for CD30 and PAX5.

MIFS has a significant potential for local recurrence, and it may recur repeatedly, sometimes resulting in amputation.[106,107,109] As such, complete surgical excision with wide margins is advisable. Radiation therapy may be helpful to prevent local recurrence.[108] Lymph node and pulmonary metastases have been reported but are rare.[106,109]

Well-Differentiated Inflammatory Liposarcoma

Well-differentiated liposarcoma (atypical lipomatous tumor) includes adipocytic (lipoma-like), sclerosing, spindle cell, and inflammatory variants (see Chapter 12). The uncommon inflammatory variant has a predilection for the retroperitoneum, but may also involve the mediastinum and paratesticular area.[112] This variant is rarely encountered in the extremities. Like other more common variants, well-differentiated inflammatory liposarcoma typically affects middle-aged to elderly adults.[112]

Histologically, well-differentiated inflammatory liposarcoma is dominated by a dense chronic inflammatory infiltrate, composed predominantly of lymphocytes (Fig. 10.26), including germinal centers, but plasma cells may also be notable. The diagnostic clue is the presence of scattered atypical stromal cells with hyperchromatic nuclei (see Fig. 10.26B), and multinucleated forms may also be identified. Although the inflammatory pattern is sometimes seen in isolation, it is often accompanied by other patterns of well-differentiated liposarcoma (especially adipocytic), which is helpful for recognizing this variant. By immunohistochemistry, well-differentiated liposarcoma shows overexpression of MDM2 and CDK4 (Fig. 10.27), reflecting amplification of 12q13–15 in the form of ring and giant marker chromosomes (see Chapters 12 and 18), which can also be demonstrated by FISH for *MDM2*.[113]

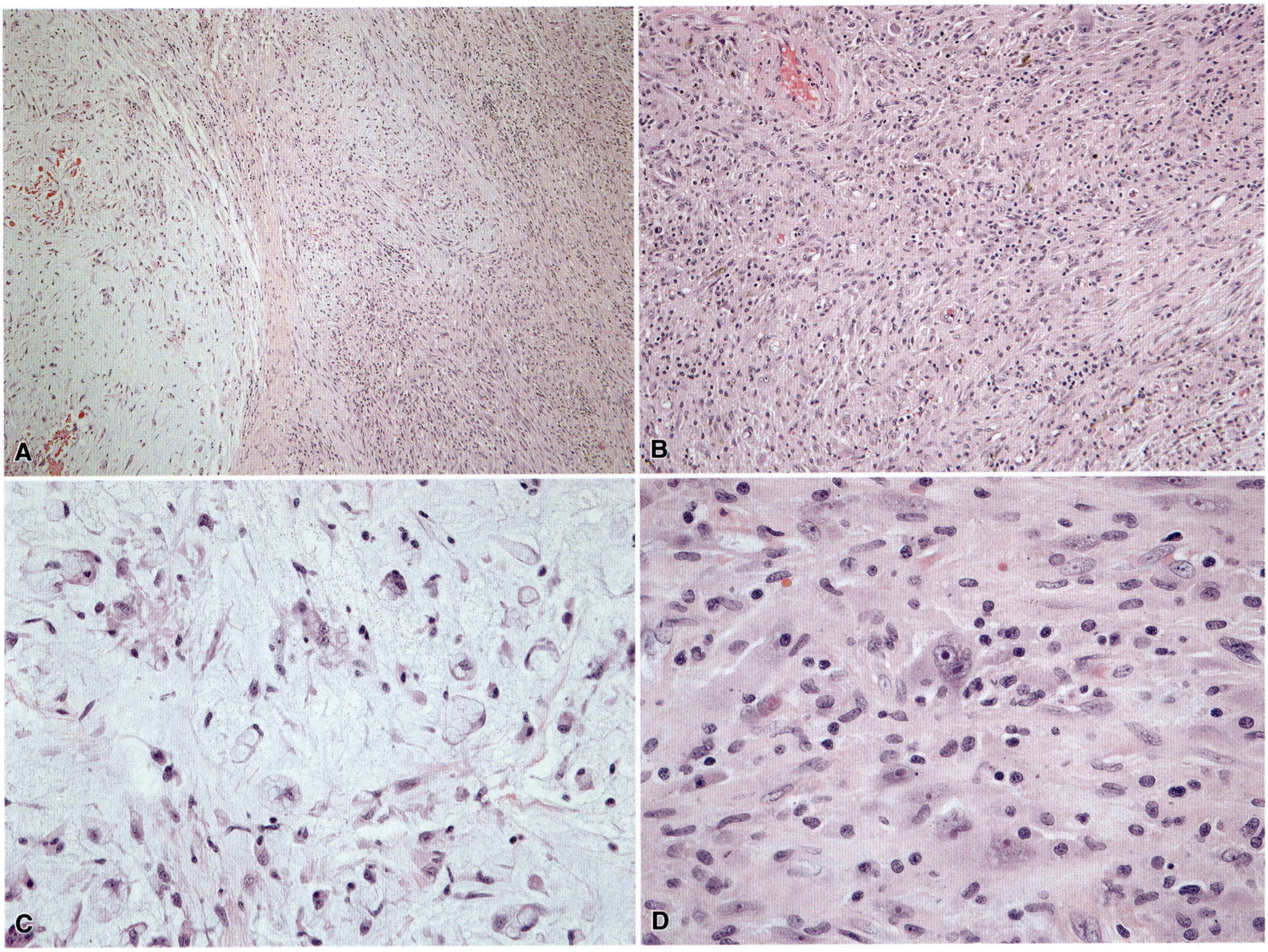

Figure 10.25 **Myxoinflammatory Fibroblastic Sarcoma.** (A) The tumor shows a heterogeneous appearance with cellular, fibroinflammatory areas and foci with abundant myxoid stroma. (B) Many tumors are composed in large part of sheets of bland spindle cells with prominent admixed lymphocytes. (C) In the myxoid areas, pseudolipoblasts may be prominent. (D) Occasional cells with large, inclusion-like nucleoli (resembling Reed-Sternberg cells) are a characteristic finding.

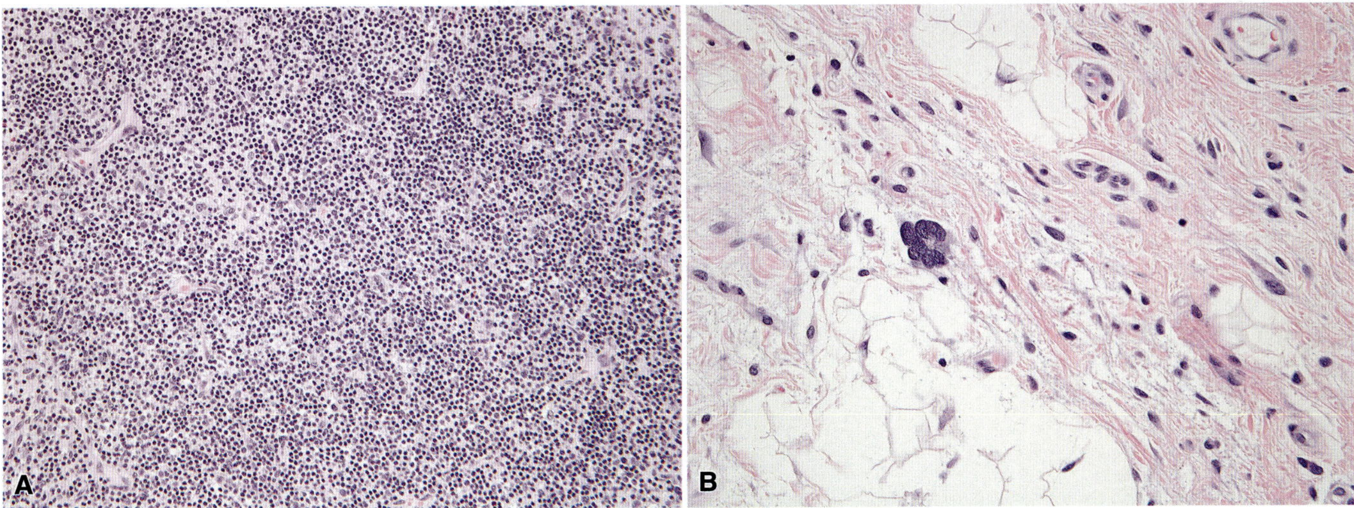

Figure 10.26 **Well-Differentiated Inflammatory Liposarcoma.** (A) The tumor shows a dense lymphocytic infiltrate, obscuring its neoplastic nature. (B) The presence of occasional atypical stromal cells is a clue to the diagnosis.

Well-differentiated inflammatory liposarcoma may easily be mistaken for an inflammatory process or a lymphoma, especially on core needle biopsy; the index of suspicion for this diagnosis must be high when evaluating a biopsy of a large retroperitoneal mass. The differential diagnosis also includes an idiopathic fibroinflammatory lesion (such as retroperitoneal fibrosis) and IMT. Idiopathic retroperitoneal fibrosis is usually bilateral, with characteristic impingement on both ureters and consequent hydronephrosis. In contrast to well-differentiated inflammatory liposarcoma, idiopathic retroperitoneal fibrosis is usually dominated by collagenous fibrosis with a minor chronic inflammatory component, and atypical stromal cells are not a feature. Immunohistochemistry for MDM2 and CDK4, or FISH for *MDM2*, can usually help resolve this differential diagnosis on limited material. IMT typically shows a fascicular spindle cell appearance, which is not seen in well-differentiated inflammatory liposarcoma. MDM2 can be positive in both tumor types, but ALK or ROS1 expression is limited to IMT.

Like other variants of well-differentiated liposarcoma, the inflammatory variant pursues a protracted clinical course with a significant potential for local recurrence, often repeatedly, with a high mortality rate over decades.[112] Dedifferentiated liposarcoma may appear as a recurrence of well-differentiated liposarcoma, at which point there is a small risk of distant metastasis, especially to the lungs.

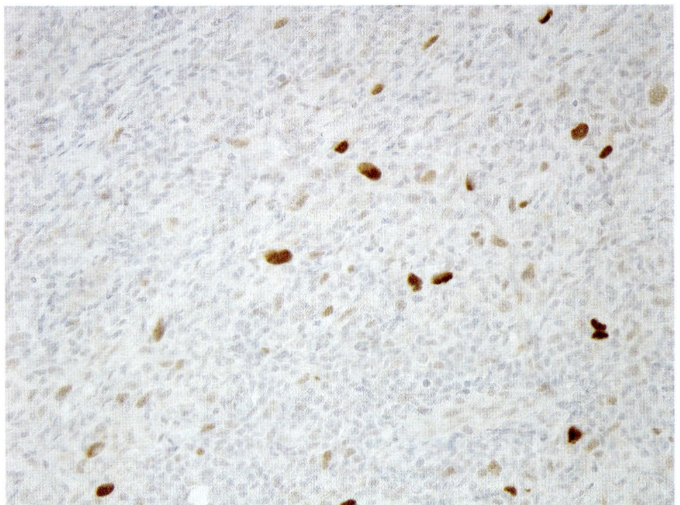

Figure 10.27 Well-Differentiated Inflammatory Liposarcoma. Occasional large cells show nuclear staining for MDM2.

Inflammatory Malignant Fibrous Histiocytoma

Inflammatory MFH was originally believed to represent a discrete pleomorphic sarcoma variant (i.e., a variant of MFH) with prominent inflammation. As discussed in Chapters 7 and 12, this histologic pattern does not in fact reflect a distinct tumor type. Rather, it is a pattern that is most often seen in dedifferentiated liposarcoma[114] but may also be observed in undifferentiated sarcomas and occasionally in nonmesenchymal neoplasms. This section will focus on dedifferentiated liposarcoma with prominent inflammation, with a brief discussion of the differential diagnosis.

Like other cases of dedifferentiated liposarcoma, tumors showing features of inflammatory MFH most often arise in the retroperitoneum of older adults as very large masses. Occasional affected patients present with fever and leukocytosis.[115]

Histologically, the tumors are composed of scattered atypical histiocytoid to pleomorphic cells within a marked inflammatory background, composed predominantly of neutrophils and foam cells (Fig. 10.28) with smaller numbers of lymphocytes and eosinophils.[114] Other histologic patterns of dedifferentiated liposarcoma (e.g., pleomorphic, spindle cell), as well as a well-differentiated liposarcomatous component, may also be identified.

The tumors show typical immunophenotypic and cytogenetic features of dedifferentiated liposarcoma. By immunohistochemistry, the tumor cells are strongly positive for MDM2 and CDK4 (Fig. 10.29).[113,114] Cytogenetic analysis usually reveals ring and giant marker chromosomes and an otherwise relatively simple karyotype. Amplification of *MDM2* is a consistent feature, which can be demonstrated by FISH, among other techniques.[114]

The chief differential diagnostic considerations include Hodgkin lymphoma, anaplastic large-cell lymphoma, histiocytic sarcoma, undifferentiated carcinoma, and other undifferentiated sarcomas. Although Hodgkin lymphoma typically shows a mixed inflammatory background, eosinophils and lymphocytes usually predominate. Binucleated or polylobated Reed-Sternberg cells with large nucleoli can usually be

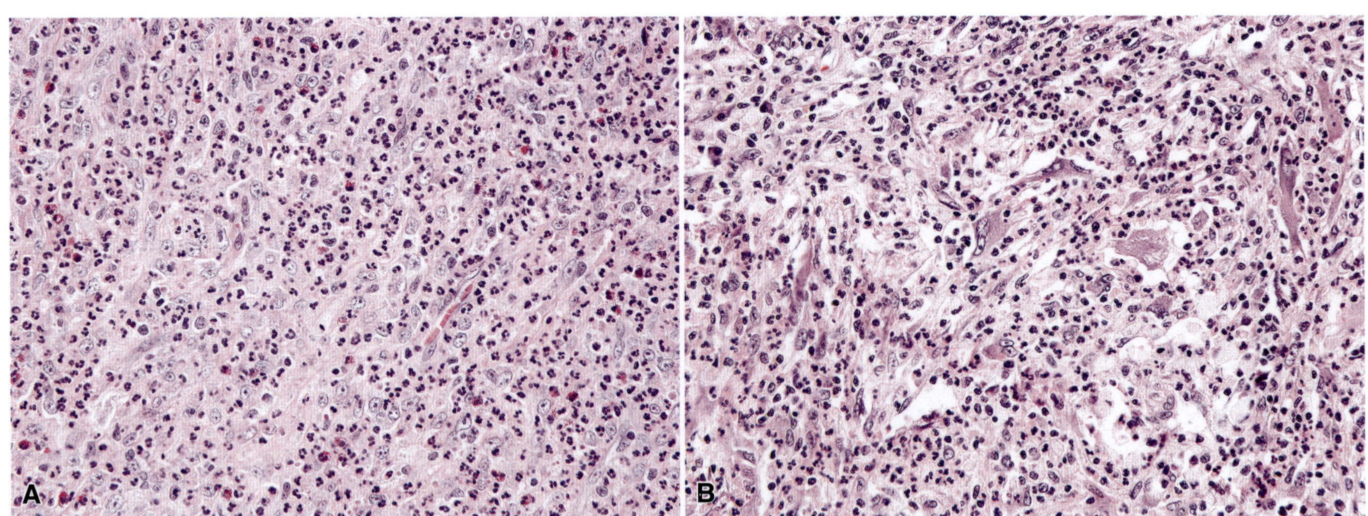

Figure 10.28 Inflammatory Malignant Fibrous Histiocytoma (Dedifferentiated Liposarcoma). (A) The tumor is composed of sheets of atypical histiocytoid cells admixed with numerous neutrophils. (B) Some tumors contain scattered bizarre, pleomorphic cells. Note the prominent stromal neutrophils and foam cells.

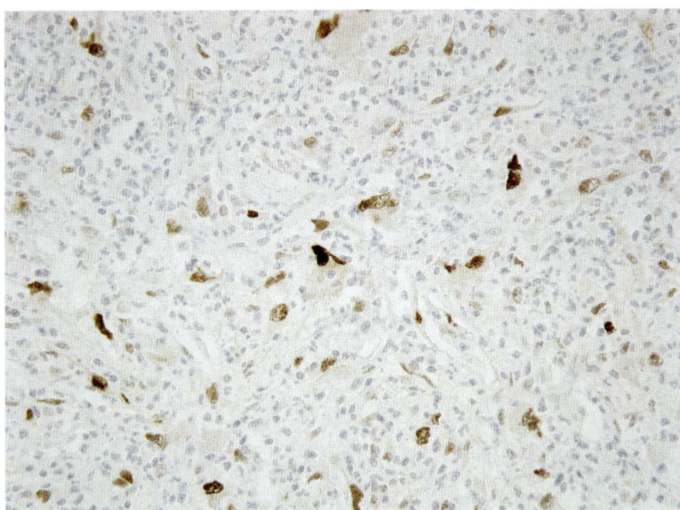

Figure 10.29 Inflammatory Malignant Fibrous Histiocytoma (Dedifferentiated Liposarcoma). MDM2 is positive in tumor cells, confirming the diagnosis of dedifferentiated liposarcoma.

seen. Hodgkin cells are positive for CD30 and PAX5. Anaplastic large-cell lymphoma is sometimes accompanied by a marked neutrophilic inflammatory infiltrate. Like Hodgkin lymphoma, anaplastic large-cell lymphoma is strongly positive for CD30. Histiocytic sarcoma is typically dominated by large epithelioid neoplastic cells with a minor inflammatory component. Unlike dedifferentiated liposarcoma, histiocytic sarcoma expresses CD163, PU.1 (SPI1), and CD45RO. However, the presence of numerous foam cells (which express histiocytic markers) is a potential diagnostic pitfall. Undifferentiated carcinomas are at least focally positive for keratins; in most cases, a visceral primary site can be identified by radiologic studies. Although most sarcomas showing features of inflammatory MFH are dedifferentiated liposarcomas, a small subset of such tumors cannot be subclassified using currently available techniques and are therefore designated "undifferentiated pleomorphic sarcoma with prominent inflammation" (see Chapter 7). Of note, sarcomas with an inflammatory MFH pattern arising in somatic soft tissue (e.g., the extremities) are less likely to be dedifferentiated liposarcoma.

Like conventional dedifferentiated liposarcoma, tumors with prominent inflammation have a high risk of local recurrence but a low metastatic rate (10% to 15%). Most affected patients succumb to uncontrolled local recurrence, often following repeated surgical debulking of recurrent disease.

PRACTICE POINTS: Inflammatory Malignant Fibrous Histiocytoma

- Histologic pattern most often seen in dedifferentiated liposarcoma
- Predilection for retroperitoneum of older adults
- Scattered atypical histiocytoid to pleomorphic cells in a background of inflammatory cells, chiefly neutrophils and foam cells
- Dedifferentiated liposarcoma positive for MDM2 and CDK4 (amplification of 12q13–15)
- Inflammatory malignant fibrous histiocytoma pattern occasionally seen in undifferentiated pleomorphic sarcomas

Mass-Forming Idiopathic Fibroinflammatory Disorders

Sclerosing Mesenteritis

Sclerosing mesenteritis (previously also known as retractile mesenteritis, mesenteric lipodystrophy, and mesenteric panniculitis, depending on the predominant histologic feature) is the most common of the idiopathic fibroinflammatory tumefactive lesions.[116,117] Sclerosing mesenteritis usually presents with abdominal pain, bowel obstruction, or a painless mass.[117] Sclerosing mesenteritis may also be discovered incidentally on abdominal computed tomography or positron emission tomography (PET) scan (the lesions are often PET–avid). The lesions occur in adults over a wide age range, with a peak incidence in middle age, and there is no gender predilection. Most patients present with a single mass lesion, ranging from several centimeters to over 20 cm in greatest dimension (mean size, 10 cm). However, a small subset presents with multiple intraabdominal masses or diffuse mesenteric thickening.[117] Sclerosing mesenteritis may be clinically mistaken for lymphoma, among other neoplasms.

Histologically, sclerosing mesenteritis typically shows a combination of fibrosis, chronic inflammation, and fat necrosis (Fig. 10.30); fibrosis usually predominates.[117] The chronic inflammatory infiltrate consists mainly of lymphocytes and histiocytes, and occasional germinal centers may be present. In the past, lesions dominated by fat necrosis and chronic inflammation were designated "mesenteric lipodystrophy" and "mesenteric panniculitis," respectively; most pathologists prefer to use the term *sclerosing mesenteritis* irrespective of the relative contribution of the histologic features.[117] A subset of cases of sclerosing mesenteritis (especially those presenting with visceral organ involvement) may fall within the spectrum of immunoglobulin G4 (IgG4)–related disease (see later discussion).[118]

The differential diagnosis may include lymphoma (especially in a small biopsy), well-differentiated liposarcoma, IMT, and a secondary reactive process (associated with either carcinoma or bowel perforation). Well-differentiated liposarcoma may contain prominent (obscuring) chronic inflammation; a careful search usually reveals scattered atypical stromal cells. Immunohistochemistry for MDM2 and CDK4 or FISH for *MDM2* amplification can help confirm the diagnosis of well-differentiated liposarcoma.[119] Of note, histiocytes may show nuclear staining for MDM2 (but not CDK4), especially in association with fat necrosis. IMT usually shows a cellular, fascicular appearance with plump myofibroblasts containing vesicular nuclei, in contrast to the hypocellular appearance, small indistinct fibroblasts, and more prominent stromal collagen typical of sclerosing mesenteritis. Plasma cells are often a notable finding in IMT, whereas they are usually absent or scarce in sclerosing mesenteritis. Metastatic carcinoma often provokes a desmoplastic stromal response that may be mistaken for sclerosing mesenteritis; a careful search for carcinoma is warranted. Organizing serositis/mesenteritis secondary to bowel perforation usually contains foci of acute inflammation and fibrin deposition, as well as fibrosis.

Sclerosing mesenteritis is usually self-limited. Simple surgical excision is curative in most cases; some lesions remain stable following biopsy alone.[117]

Idiopathic Retroperitoneal Fibrosis

Idiopathic retroperitoneal fibrosis is a usually bilateral fibroinflammatory process that often surrounds the abdominal aorta and ureters.[116,120] A subset of cases appears to be a manifestation of IgG4-related disease.[121,122] The most common presenting symptoms are back and abdominal pain.[120] The condition affects middle-aged to elderly adults, with a marked male predominance. Radiologic imaging is usually diagnostic; bilateral impingement on ureters, sometimes associated with hydronephrosis, is the typical finding, with a variably prominent soft tissue component in the retroperitoneum (Fig. 10.31). Acute renal failure is a common associated finding secondary to ureteral obstruction.[120] Patients often have elevated erythrocyte sedimentation rates or C-reactive protein levels.[120] Retroperitoneal fibrosis may also arise secondary to radiation therapy and various tumor types, especially lymphoma.

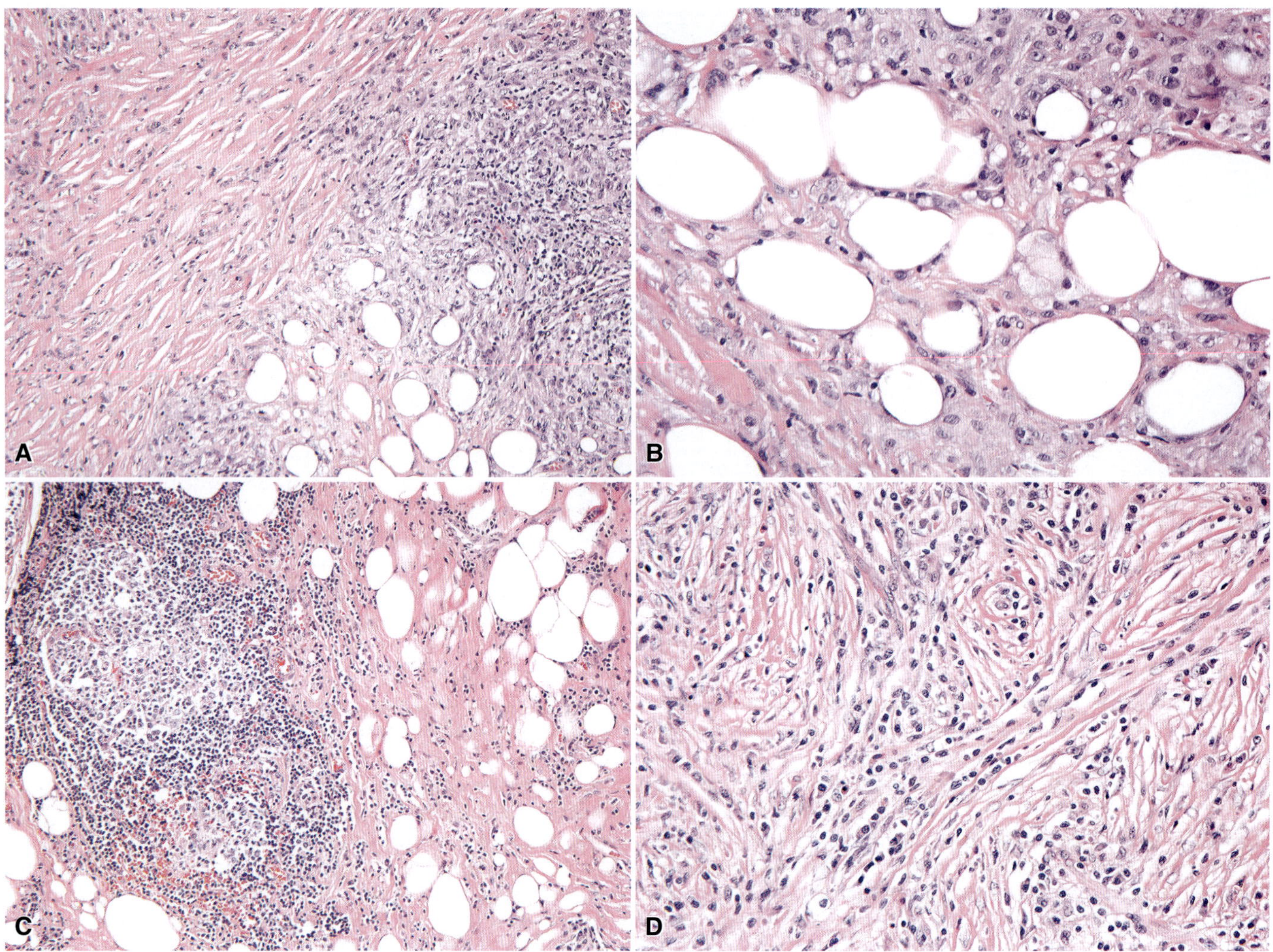

Figure 10.30 Sclerosing Mesenteritis. (A) The lesion shows a combination of fibrosis, fat necrosis, and chronic inflammation. (B) In areas of fat necrosis, histiocytic inflammation may be prominent. (C) Occasional germinal centers are often present. Note the fibrosis. (D) Many lesions are dominated by dense fibrosis. Note the scattered lymphocytes and occasional plasma cells.

The diagnosis is usually clear based on radiologic findings; thus, the primary role of biopsy is to exclude lymphoma. Histologically, idiopathic retroperitoneal fibrosis is characterized by dense fibrosis and variably prominent chronic inflammation, composed predominantly of small lymphocytes (Fig. 10.32). A high IgG4/IgG plasma cell ratio (generally >40%) helps define IgG4-related retroperitoneal fibrosis.[123]

The main differential diagnostic consideration is lymphoma. Lymphoma in the retroperitoneum (especially follicular lymphoma) is not uncommonly associated with marked stromal sclerosis and can therefore easily be mistaken for a reactive process in small biopsy samples. The diagnosis is usually relatively straightforward by immunohistochemistry, because the lymphocytic infiltrate is dominated by CD20 and PAX5-positive B lymphocytes (which in the case of follicular lymphoma are also positive for CD10), in contrast to the mixed lymphocytic infiltrate and predominance of CD3-positive T cells observed in idiopathic retroperitoneal fibrosis. In cases where a tumor is suspected, the differential diagnosis may also include liposarcoma, especially sclerosing well-differentiated liposarcoma. Similar to idiopathic retroperitoneal fibrosis, sclerosing liposarcoma is hypocellular with a paucity of inflammatory cells, but the presence of occasional atypical, pleomorphic stromal cells distinguishes well-differentiated liposarcoma from idiopathic retroperitoneal fibrosis. MDM2 and CDK4 expression by immunohistochemistry, or demonstration of *MDM2* amplification by FISH, can be used to confirm the diagnosis.

Idiopathic retroperitoneal fibrosis usually responds well to corticosteroid therapy, although some patients require ureteral stenting to relieve renal failure. Idiopathic retroperitoneal fibrosis often recurs following cessation of therapy (especially the IgG4-related subset), necessitating long-term treatment with corticosteroids.[120,124]

Immunoglobulin G4–Related Disease

IgG4-related disease is a systemic disorder characterized by predominantly visceral mass lesions, sometimes associated with organ dysfunction and variably elevated serum IgG4.[118,125,126] The prototype for (and earliest recognized manifestation of) this disease is autoimmune pancreatitis (also known as lymphoplasmacytic sclerosing pancreatitis), which usually presents as a pancreatic mass with a clinical suspicion for cancer.[118] The other most commonly affected anatomic sites are the liver and biliary tree, orbit, and salivary gland, although a wide range of other sites have also been described (including nearly every visceral organ, the skin, central nervous system, aorta, and retroperitoneum).[118] Lymph nodes may also be involved, either draining nodes of an affected visceral organ, or occasionally as isolated lymphadenopathy. The disorder usually presents with symptoms attributable to a mass lesion, or with vague abdominal symptoms, after which a mass is detected on radiologic studies. There is a male predominance, with a peak incidence in middle-aged to elderly adults. Fever and constitutional symptoms are uncommon. Elevated serum IgG4 titers are often detected, although the disorder is frequently unsuspected until after the mass is surgically resected, at which point IgG4 levels may be normal.[118,125,126]

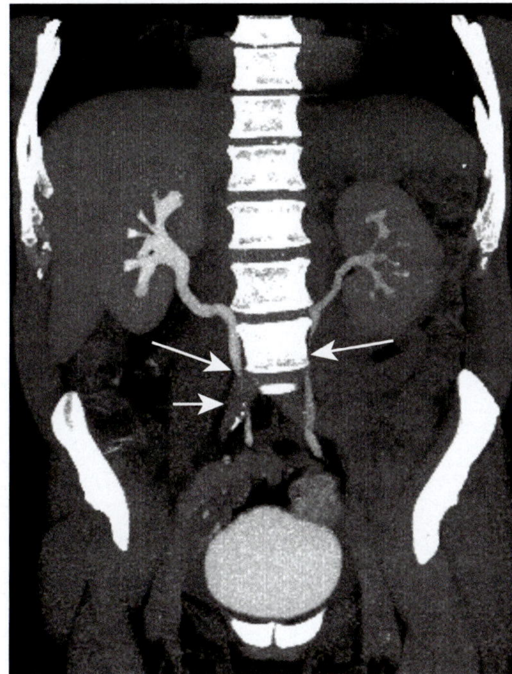

Figure 10.31 **Idiopathic Retroperitoneal Fibrosis.** A coronal image from the excretory phase of a computed tomography urogram shows narrowing of both ureters (*long arrows*) at the level of abnormal retroperitoneal soft tissue (only partially visualized; *short arrow*). Note the mild hydronephrosis on the right side. (Courtesy Dr. Atul Shinagare.)

Histologically, the characteristic features of autoimmune pancreatitis are similar to those of IgG4-related sclerosing disease of other visceral sites, and include a dense lymphoplasmacytic chronic inflammatory infiltrate (often with germinal centers), storiform fibrosis, acinar atrophy, and obliterative phlebitis (Fig. 10.33). The extent of fibrosis is variable, likely related to the time course of the disease (i.e., at what point the biopsy or resection is performed). Fibrosis usually extends into the adjacent adipose tissue beyond the parenchyma of the organ involved.

In all affected sites, immunohistochemistry for IgG4 typically reveals large numbers of IgG4-positive plasma cells (Fig. 10.34). Optimal diagnostic cutoffs appear to vary somewhat depending on anatomic site.[118,123,125] The distribution of such plasma cells within an affected organ is highly variable; the highest density area on immunohistochemistry should be sought for quantitation. The ratio of IgG4-positive to IgG-positive plasma cells appears to be a more powerful predictor of the disorder; 40% is a widely used cut-off.[118,123] However, for biopsies that are paucicellular (i.e., with few plasma cells), the ratio per se is of limited diagnostic value; moreover, tissue IgG4-positive plasma cells are insufficient to confirm the diagnosis: correlation with histologic and clinical features is essential.[123]

The differential diagnosis for IgG4-related disease is broad and varies depending on the anatomic site. As mentioned previously, recent studies have suggested that a subset of cases of sclerosing mesenteritis and retroperitoneal fibrosis may fall within the spectrum of IgG4-related disease (especially those presenting with multivisceral involvement). In patients who present with more than one site of disease, assessing for the presence of prominent IgG4-positive plasma cells (and the IgG4/IgG ratio) in a biopsy specimen (and a comment suggesting the possibility of IgG4-related systemic disorder) is reasonable. For patients who present with an isolated mesenteric mass, with the typical combination of fibrosis, fat necrosis, and chronic inflammation, the predictive value of immunohistochemistry for IgG4 is uncertain. Idiopathic retroperitoneal fibrosis (in the absence of other clinical evidence of IgG4-related disease) shows a typical clinical presentation with renal failure and impingement on bilateral ureters (sometimes with hydronephrosis); fibrosis predominates histologically, whereas plasma cells are usually scarce or absent.

The differential diagnosis may also include IMT. However, IMT usually shows a more cellular appearance, being composed of fascicles of

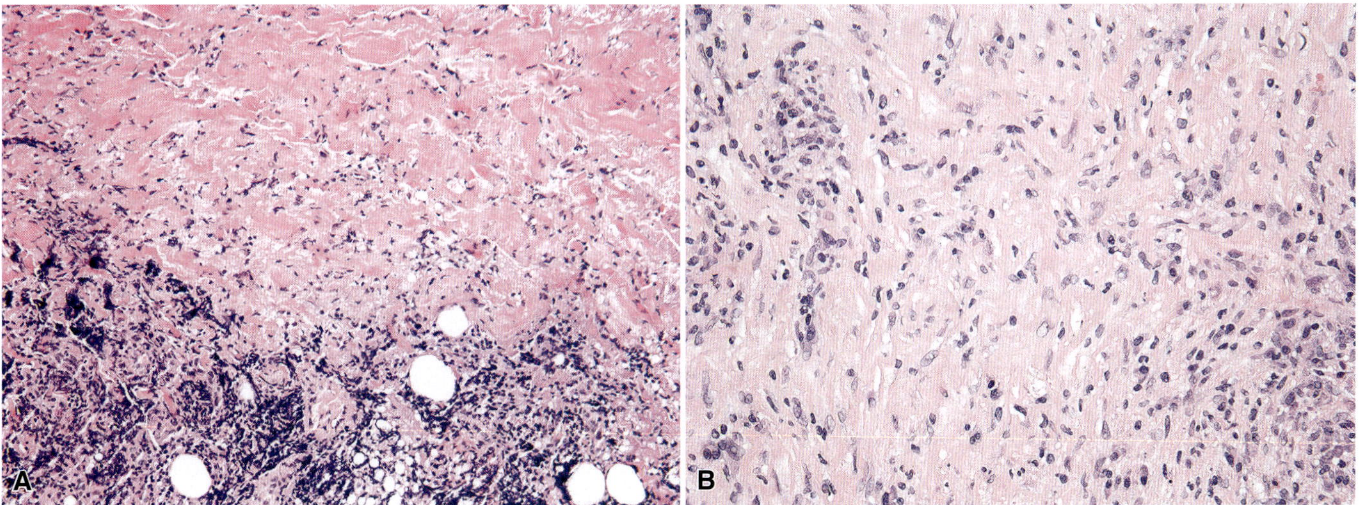

Figure 10.32 **Idiopathic Retroperitoneal Fibrosis.** (A) A biopsy shows fibrosis and a focal area of chronic inflammation. Crush artifact on a core biopsy may heighten concern for lymphoma. (B) The biopsy is dominated by dense fibrosis. Note the sparse chronic inflammatory infiltrate.

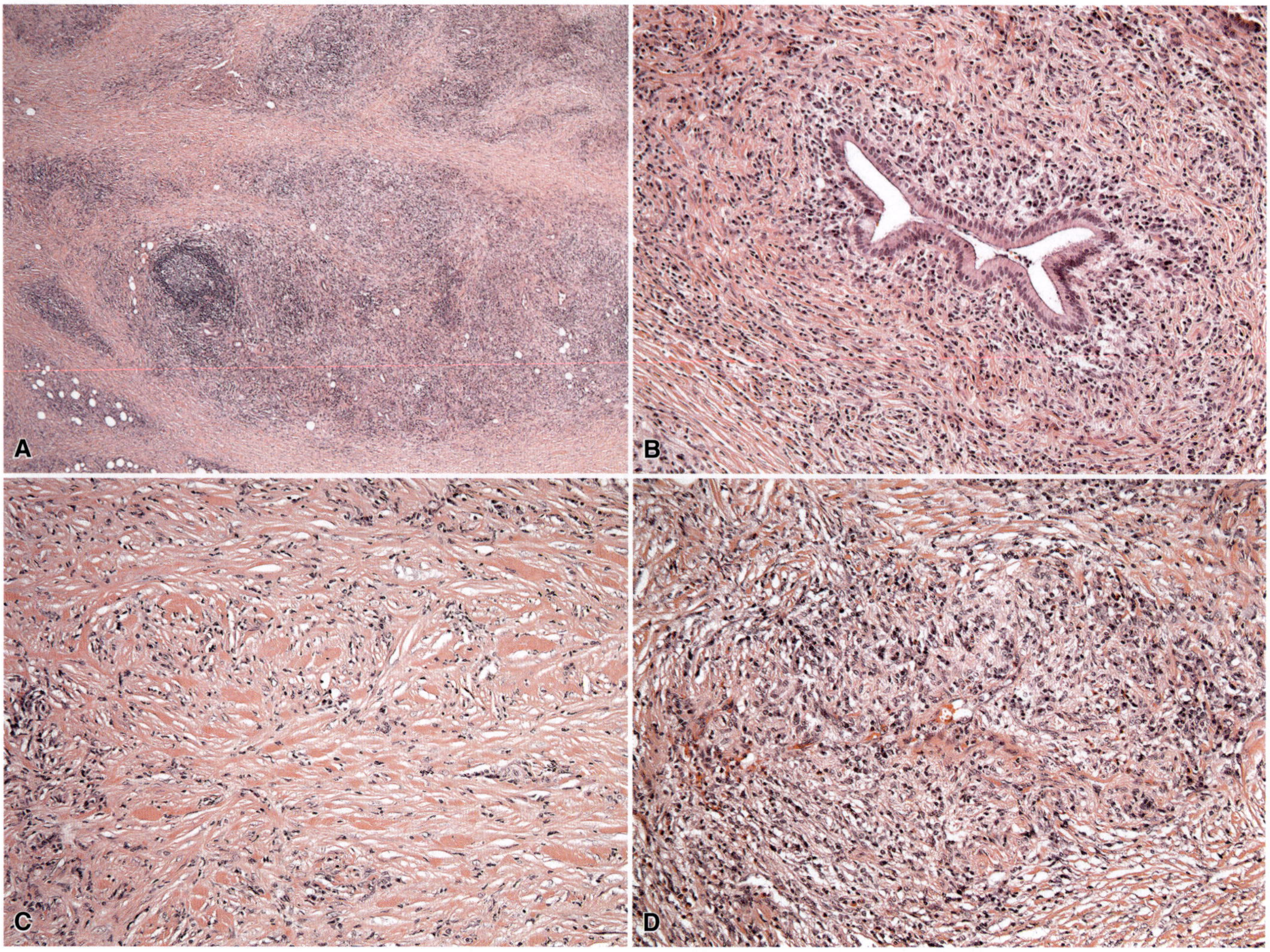

Figure 10.33 **Immunoglobulin G4–Related Sclerosing (Autoimmune) Pancreatitis.** (A) The mass consists of fibrosis and chronic inflammation, associated with acinar atrophy. (B) There is periductal fibrosis and plasma cell–rich chronic inflammation. (C) Large areas of storiform fibrosis extend into peripancreatic soft tissue. (D) Obliterative phlebitis is a characteristic feature. The remnant of a vein is infiltrated by numerous plasma cells.

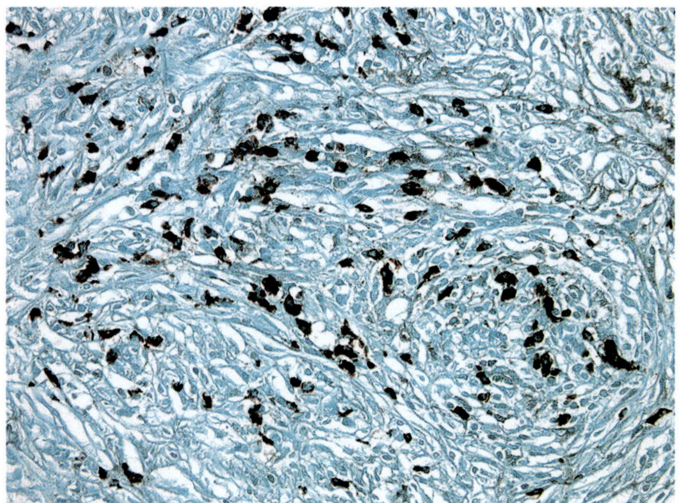

Figure 10.34 **Immunoglobulin G4 (IgG4)–Related Sclerosing (Autoimmune) Pancreatitis.** An immunostain for IgG4 highlights numerous plasma cells.

plump spindled myofibroblasts with a more limited lymphoplasmacytic infiltrate, in contrast to the paucicellular, sclerotic appearance and numerous plasma cells typical of IgG4-related disease. ALK expression (detected in 50% of cases) confirms the diagnosis of IMT. Several studies have examined the utility of immunohistochemistry for IgG4 in this distinction.[127,128] Although the density of IgG4-positive plasma cells and the IgG4/IgG ratio are significantly lower in IMT than in IgG4-related sclerosing disease, occasional IMTs contain more than 30 IgG4-positive plasma cells per high-power field, and the IgG4-to-IgG ratio in IMT is often greater than 0.10. As long as a sufficiently high cutoff is used, IgG4 may be a useful adjunct in this differential diagnosis.

Most patients with IgG4-related disease experience a dramatic clinical response to corticosteroid therapy, with a resolution in visceral mass lesions, along with a reduction in serum IgG4 titer.[118,125,126] Following discontinuation of therapy, recurrences are common. Therapeutic approaches directed against B-cell depletion (such as rituximab) appear to be effective in some corticosteroid-refractory patients.[129] Affected patients often develop other sites of involvement, sometimes years or even decades after initial presentation.

References

1. Coffin CM, Hornick JL, Fletcher CD: Inflammatory myofibroblastic tumor: comparison of clinicopathologic, histologic, and immunohistochemical features including ALK expression in atypical and aggressive cases, *Am J Surg Pathol* 31:509–520, 2007.
2. Gleason BC, Hornick JL: Inflammatory myofibroblastic tumours: where are we now?, *J Clin Pathol* 61:428–437, 2008.
3. Coffin CM, Watterson J, Priest JR, et al: Extrapulmonary inflammatory myofibroblastic tumor (inflammatory pseudotumor). A clinicopathologic and immunohistochemical study of 84 cases, *Am J Surg Pathol* 19:859–872, 1995.
4. Pettinato G, Manivel JC, De Rosa N, et al: Inflammatory myofibroblastic tumor (plasma cell granuloma). Clinicopathologic study of 20 cases with immunohistochemical and ultrastructural observations, *Am J Clin Pathol* 94:538–546, 1990.
5. Meis JM, Enzinger FM: Inflammatory fibrosarcoma of the mesentery and retroperitoneum. A tumor closely simulating inflammatory pseudotumor, *Am J Surg Pathol* 15:1146–1156, 1991.
6. Marino-Enriquez A, Wang WL, Roy A, et al: Epithelioid inflammatory myofibroblastic sarcoma: an aggressive intra-abdominal variant of inflammatory myofibroblastic tumor with nuclear membrane or perinuclear ALK, *Am J Surg Pathol* 35:135–144, 2011.
7. Cessna MH, Zhou H, Sanger WG, et al: Expression of ALK1 and p80 in inflammatory myofibroblastic tumor and its mesenchymal mimics: a study of 135 cases, *Mod Pathol* 15:931–938, 2002.
8. Chan JK, Cheuk W, Shimizu M: Anaplastic lymphoma kinase expression in inflammatory pseudotumors, *Am J Surg Pathol* 25:761–768, 2001.
9. Coffin CM, Patel A, Perkins S, et al: ALK1 and p80 expression and chromosomal rearrangements involving 2p23 in inflammatory myofibroblastic tumor, *Mod Pathol* 14:569–576, 2001.
10. Lee JC, Li CF, Huang HY, et al: ALK oncoproteins in atypical inflammatory myofibroblastic tumours: novel RRBP1-ALK fusions in epithelioid inflammatory myofibroblastic sarcoma, *J Pathol* 241:316–323, 2017.
11. Hornick JL, Sholl LM, Dal Cin P, et al: Expression of ROS1 predicts ROS1 gene rearrangement in inflammatory myofibroblastic tumors, *Mod Pathol* 28:732–739, 2015.
12. Bridge JA, Kanamori M, Ma Z, et al: Fusion of the ALK gene to the clathrin heavy chain gene, CLTC, in inflammatory myofibroblastic tumor, *Am J Pathol* 159:411–415, 2001.
13. Lawrence B, Perez-Atayde A, Hibbard MK, et al: TPM3-ALK and TPM4-ALK oncogenes in inflammatory myofibroblastic tumors, *Am J Pathol* 157:377–384, 2000.
14. Ma Z, Hill DA, Collins MH, et al: Fusion of ALK to the Ran-binding protein 2 (RANBP2) gene in inflammatory myofibroblastic tumor, *Genes Chromosomes Cancer* 37:98–105, 2003.
15. Lovly CM, Gupta A, Lipson D, et al: Inflammatory myofibroblastic tumors harbor multiple potentially actionable kinase fusions, *Cancer Discov* 4:889–895, 2014.
16. Antonescu CR, Suurmeijer AJ, Zhang L, et al: Molecular characterization of inflammatory myofibroblastic tumors with frequent ALK and ROS1 gene fusions and rare novel RET rearrangement, *Am J Surg Pathol* 3:957–967, 2015.
17. Yamamoto H, Yoshida A, Taguchi K, et al: ALK, ROS1 and NTRK3 gene rearrangements in inflammatory myofibroblastic tumours, *Histopathology* 69:72–83, 2016.
18. Alassiri AH, Ali RH, Shen Y, et al: ETV6-NTRK3 is expressed in a subset of ALK-negative inflammatory myofibroblastic tumors, *Am J Surg Pathol* 40:1051–1061, 2016.
19. Lucas DR, Shukla A, Thomas DG, et al: Dedifferentiated liposarcoma with inflammatory myofibroblastic tumor-like features, *Am J Surg Pathol* 34:844–851, 2010.
20. Butrynski JE, D'Adamo DR, Hornick JL, et al: Crizotinib in ALK-rearranged inflammatory myofibroblastic tumor, *N Engl J Med* 363:1727–1733, 2010.
21. Merchant W, Calonje E, Fletcher CD: Inflammatory leiomyosarcoma: a morphological subgroup within the heterogeneous family of so-called inflammatory malignant fibrous histiocytoma, *Histopathology* 27:525–532, 1995.
22. Chang A, Schuetze SM, Conrad EU, III, et al: So-called "inflammatory leiomyosarcoma": a series of 3 cases providing additional insights into a rare entity, *Int J Surg Pathol* 13:185–195, 2005.
23. Dal Cin P, Sciot R, Fletcher CD, et al: Inflammatory leiomyosarcoma may be characterized by specific near-haploid chromosome changes, *J Pathol* 185:112–115, 1998.
24. Nord KH, Paulsson K, Veerla S, et al: Retained heterodisomy is associated with high gene expression in hyperhaploid inflammatory leiomyosarcoma, *Neoplasia* 14:807–812, 2012.
25. Pileri SA, Grogan TM, Harris NL, et al: Tumours of histiocytes and accessory dendritic cells: an immunohistochemical approach to classification from the International Lymphoma Study Group based on 61 cases, *Histopathology* 41:1–29, 2002.
26. Feldman AL, Arber DA, Pittaluga S, et al: Clonally related follicular lymphomas and histiocytic/dendritic cell sarcomas: evidence for transdifferentiation of the follicular lymphoma clone, *Blood* 111:5433–5439, 2008.
27. Fraser CR, Wang W, Gomez M, et al: Transformation of chronic lymphocytic leukemia/small lymphocytic lymphoma to interdigitating dendritic cell sarcoma: evidence for transdifferentiation of the lymphoma clone, *Am J Clin Pathol* 132:928–939, 2009.
28. Kumar R, Khan SP, Joshi DD, et al: Pediatric histiocytic sarcoma clonally related to precursor B-cell acute lymphoblastic leukemia with homozygous deletion of CDKN2A encoding p16INK4A, *Pediatr Blood Cancer* 56:307–310, 2011.
29. Shao H, Xi L, Raffeld M, et al: Clonally related histiocytic/dendritic cell sarcoma and chronic lymphocytic leukemia/small lymphocytic lymphoma: a study of seven cases, *Mod Pathol* 24:1421–1432, 2011.
30. Chan JK, Fletcher CD, Nayler SJ, et al: Follicular dendritic cell sarcoma. Clinicopathologic analysis of 17 cases suggesting a malignant potential higher than currently recognized, *Cancer* 79:294–313, 1997.
31. Andriko JW, Kaldjian EP, Tsokos M, et al: Reticulum cell neoplasms of lymph nodes: a clinicopathologic study of 11 cases with recognition of a new subtype derived from fibroblastic reticular cells, *Am J Surg Pathol* 22:1048–1058, 1998.
32. Hollowood K, Pease C, Mackay AM, et al: Sarcomatoid tumours of lymph nodes showing follicular dendritic cell differentiation, *J Pathol* 163:205–216, 1991.
33. Hollowood K, Stamp G, Zouvani I, et al: Extranodal follicular dendritic cell sarcoma of the gastrointestinal tract. Morphologic, immunohistochemical and ultrastructural analysis of two cases, *Am J Clin Pathol* 103:90–97, 1995.
34. Perez-Ordonez B, Erlandson RA, Rosai J: Follicular dendritic cell tumor: report of 13 additional cases of a distinctive entity, *Am J Surg Pathol* 20:944–955, 1996.
35. Shia J, Chen W, Tang LH, et al: Extranodal follicular dendritic cell sarcoma: clinical, pathologic, and histogenetic characteristics of an underrecognized disease entity, *Virchows Arch* 449:148–158, 2006.
36. Facchetti F, Lorenzi L: Follicular dendritic cells and related sarcoma, *Semin Diagn Pathol* 33:262–276, 2016.
37. Viola P, Vroobel KM, Devaraj A, et al: Follicular dendritic cell tumour/sarcoma: a commonly misdiagnosed tumour in the thorax, *Histopathology* 69:752–761, 2016.
38. Hartert M, Strobel P, Dahm M, et al: A follicular dendritic cell sarcoma of the mediastinum with immature T cells and association with myasthenia gravis, *Am J Surg Pathol* 34:742–745, 2010.
39. Kim WY, Kim H, Jeon YK, et al: Follicular dendritic cell sarcoma with immature T-cell proliferation, *Hum Pathol* 41:129–133, 2010.
40. Cheuk W, Chan JK, Shek TW, et al: Inflammatory pseudotumor-like follicular dendritic cell tumor: a distinctive low-grade malignant intra-abdominal neoplasm with consistent Epstein-Barr virus association, *Am J Surg Pathol* 25:721–731, 2001.
41. Selves J, Meggetto F, Brousset P, et al: Inflammatory pseudotumor of the liver. Evidence for follicular dendritic reticulum cell proliferation associated with clonal Epstein-Barr virus, *Am J Surg Pathol* 20:747–753, 1996.
42. Shek TW, Ho FC, Ng IO, et al: Follicular dendritic cell tumor of the liver. Evidence for an Epstein-Barr virus-related clonal proliferation of follicular dendritic cells, *Am J Surg Pathol* 20:313–324, 1996.
43. Grogg KL, Lae ME, Kurtin PJ, et al: Clusterin expression distinguishes follicular dendritic cell tumors from other dendritic cell neoplasms: report of a novel follicular dendritic cell marker and clinicopathologic data on 12 additional follicular dendritic cell tumors and 6 additional interdigitating dendritic cell tumors, *Am J Surg Pathol* 28:988–998, 2004.
44. Yu H, Gibson JA, Pinkus GS, et al: Podoplanin (D2-40) is a novel marker for follicular dendritic cell tumors, *Am J Clin Pathol* 128:776–782, 2007.
45. Vermi W, Lonardi S, Bosisio D, et al: Identification of CXCL13 as a new marker for follicular dendritic cell sarcoma, *J Pathol* 216:356–364, 2008.
46. Xu J, Sun HH, Fletcher CD, et al: Expression of programmed cell death 1 ligands (PD-L1 and PD-L2) in histiocytic and dendritic cell disorders, *Am J Surg Pathol* 40:443–453, 2016.
47. Go H, Jeon YK, Huh J, et al: Frequent detection of BRAF(V600E) mutations in histiocytic and dendritic cell neoplasms, *Histopathology* 65:261–272, 2014.
48. Griffin GK, Sholl LM, Lindeman NI, et al: Targeted genomic sequencing of follicular dendritic cell sarcoma reveals recurrent alterations in NF-κB regulatory genes, *Mod Pathol* 29:67–74, 2016.
49. Chan AC, Serrano-Olmo J, Erlandson RA, et al: Cytokeratin-positive malignant tumors with reticulum cell morphology: a subtype of fibroblastic reticulum cell neoplasm?, *Am J Surg Pathol* 24:107–116, 2000.
50. Schuerfeld K, Lazzi S, De Santi MM, et al: Cytokeratin-positive interstitial cell neoplasm: a case report and classification issues, *Histopathology* 43:491–494, 2003.
51. Gaertner EM, Tsokos M, Derringer GA, et al: Interdigitating dendritic cell sarcoma. A report of four cases and review of the literature, *Am J Clin Pathol* 115:589–597, 2001.
52. Hornick JL, Kraus M, Banner B, et al: Interdigitating dendritic cell sarcoma: further clinicopathologic characterization in a study of 12 cases, *Mod Pathol* 21(Suppl 1s):257A, 2008.
53. Pillay K, Solomon R, Daubenton JD, et al: Interdigitating dendritic cell sarcoma: a report of four paediatric cases and review of the literature, *Histopathology* 44:283–291, 2004.
54. Howarth DM, Gilchrist GS, Mullan BP, et al: Langerhans cell histiocytosis: diagnosis, natural history, management, and outcome, *Cancer* 85:2278–2290, 1999.
55. Kilpatrick SE, Wenger DE, Gilchrist GS, et al: Langerhans' cell histiocytosis (histiocytosis X) of bone. A clinicopathologic analysis of 263 pediatric and adult cases, *Cancer* 76:2471–2484, 1995.
56. Lieberman PH, Jones CR, Steinman RM, et al: Langerhans cell (eosinophilic) granulomatosis. A clinicopathologic study encompassing 50 years, *Am J Surg Pathol* 20:519–552, 1996.
57. Sholl LM, Hornick JL, Pinkus JL, et al: Immunohistochemical analysis of langerin in langerhans cell histiocytosis and pulmonary inflammatory and infectious diseases, *Am J Surg Pathol* 31:947–952, 2007.
58. Singhi AD, Montgomery EA: Gastrointestinal tract langerhans cell histiocytosis: a clinicopathologic study of 12 patients, *Am J Surg Pathol* 35:305–310, 2011.
59. Bohn OL, Ruiz-Arguelles G, Navarro L, et al: Cutaneous Langerhans cell sarcoma: a case report and review of the literature, *Int J Hematol* 85:116–120, 2007.
60. Zhao G, Luo M, Wu ZY, et al: Langerhans cell sarcoma involving gallbladder and peritoneal lymph nodes: a case report, *Int J Surg Pathol* 17:347–353, 2009.

61. Chikwava K, Jaffe R: Langerin (CD207) staining in normal pediatric tissues, reactive lymph nodes, and childhood histiocytic disorders, *Pediatr Dev Pathol* 7:607–614, 2004.
62. Lau SK, Chu PG, Weiss LM: Immunohistochemical expression of Langerin in Langerhans cell histiocytosis and non-Langerhans cell histiocytic disorders, *Am J Surg Pathol* 32:615–619, 2008.
63. Badalian-Very G, Vergilio JA, Degar BA, et al: Recurrent BRAF mutations in Langerhans cell histiocytosis, *Blood* 116:1919–1923, 2010.
64. Berres ML, Lim KP, Peters T, et al: BRAF-V600E expression in precursor versus differentiated dendritic cells defines clinically distinct LCH risk groups, *J Exp Med* 211:669–683, 2014.
65. Chakraborty R, Hampton OA, Shen X, et al: Mutually exclusive recurrent somatic mutations in MAP2K1 and BRAF support a central role for ERK activation in LCH pathogenesis, *Blood* 124:3007–3015, 2014.
66. Diamond EL, Durham BH, Haroche J, et al: Diverse and targetable kinase alterations drive histiocytic neoplasms, *Cancer Discov* 6:154–165, 2016.
67. Ryan RJ, Akin C, Castells M, et al: Mast cell sarcoma: a rare and potentially under-recognized diagnostic entity with specific therapeutic implications, *Mod Pathol* 26:533–543, 2013.
68. Monnier J, Georgin-Lavialle S, Canioni D, et al: Mast cell sarcoma: new cases and literature review, *Oncotarget* 7:66299–66309, 2016.
69. Ratzinger G, Burgdorf WH, Metze D, et al: Indeterminate cell histiocytosis: fact or fiction?, *J Cutan Pathol* 32:552–560, 2005.
70. Rezk SA, Spagnolo DV, Brynes RK, et al: Indeterminate cell tumor: a rare dendritic neoplasm, *Am J Surg Pathol* 32:1868–1876, 2008.
71. Chen M, Agrawal R, Nasseri-Nik N, et al: Indeterminate cell tumor of the spleen, *Hum Pathol* 43:307–311, 2012.
72. Brown RA, Kwong BY, McCalmont TH, et al: ETV3-NCOA2 in indeterminate cell histiocytosis: clonal translocation supports sui generis, *Blood* 126:2344–2345, 2015.
73. Rosai J, Dorfman RF: Sinus histiocytosis with massive lymphadenopathy. A newly recognized benign clinicopathological entity, *Arch Pathol* 87:63–70, 1969.
74. Rosai J, Dorfman RF: Sinus histiocytosis with massive lymphadenopathy: a pseudolymphomatous benign disorder. Analysis of 34 cases, *Cancer* 30:1174–1188, 1972.
75. Foucar E, Rosai J, Dorfman R: Sinus histiocytosis with massive lymphadenopathy (Rosai-Dorfman disease): review of the entity, *Semin Diagn Pathol* 7:19–73, 1990.
76. Wenig BM, Abbondanzo SL, Childers EL, et al: Extranodal sinus histiocytosis with massive lymphadenopathy (Rosai-Dorfman disease) of the head and neck, *Hum Pathol* 24:483–492, 1993.
77. Walker PD, Rosai J, Dorfman RF: The osseous manifestations of sinus histiocytosis with massive lymphadenopathy, *Am J Clin Pathol* 75:131–139, 1981.
78. Brenn T, Calonje E, Granter SR, et al: Cutaneous Rosai-Dorfman disease is a distinct clinical entity, *Am J Dermatopathol* 24:385–391, 2002.
79. Kong YY, Kong JC, Shi DR, et al: Cutaneous Rosai-Dorfman disease: a clinical and histopathologic study of 25 cases in China, *Am J Surg Pathol* 31:341–350, 2007.
80. Eisen RN, Buckley PJ, Rosai J: Immunophenotypic characterization of sinus histiocytosis with massive lymphadenopathy (Rosai-Dorfman disease), *Semin Diagn Pathol* 7:74–82, 1990.
81. Nguyen TT, Schwartz EJ, West RB, et al: Expression of CD163 (hemoglobin scavenger receptor) in normal tissues, lymphomas, carcinomas, and sarcomas is largely restricted to the monocyte/macrophage lineage, *Am J Surg Pathol* 29:617–624, 2005.
82. Foucar E, Rosai J, Dorfman RF: Sinus histiocytosis with massive lymphadenopathy. An analysis of 14 deaths occurring in a patient registry, *Cancer* 54:1834–1840, 1984.
83. Saboo SS, Jagannathan JP, Krajewski KM, et al: Symptomatic extranodal Rosai-Dorfman disease treated with steroids, radiation, and surgery, *J Clin Oncol* 29:e772–e775, 2011.
84. Hornick JL, Jaffe ES, Fletcher CD: Extranodal histiocytic sarcoma: clinicopathologic analysis of 14 cases of a rare epithelioid malignancy, *Am J Surg Pathol* 28:1133–1144, 2004.
85. Lauritzen AF, Delsol G, Hansen NE, et al: Histiocytic sarcomas and monoblastic leukemias. A clinical, histologic, and immunophenotypical study, *Am J Clin Pathol* 102:45–54, 1994.
86. Vos JA, Abbondanzo SL, Barekman CL, et al: Histiocytic sarcoma: a study of five cases including the histiocyte marker CD163, *Mod Pathol* 18:693–704, 2005.
87. Ruzinova MB, Hornick JL: Expression of PU.1 in histiocytic and dendritic cell neoplasms and histologic mimics, *Mod Pathol* 23(Suppl 1s):320A, 2010.
88. Liu Q, Tomaszewicz K, Hutchinson L, et al: Somatic mutations in histiocytic sarcoma identified by next generation sequencing, *Virchows Arch* 469:233–241, 2016.
89. Costa MJ, Weiss SW: Angiomatoid malignant fibrous histiocytoma. A follow-up study of 108 cases with evaluation of possible histologic predictors of outcome, *Am J Surg Pathol* 14:1126–1132, 1990.
90. Enzinger FM: Angiomatoid malignant fibrous histiocytoma: a distinct fibrohistiocytic tumor of children and young adults simulating a vascular neoplasm, *Cancer* 44:2147–2157, 1979.
91. Fanburg-Smith JC, Miettinen M: Angiomatoid "malignant" fibrous histiocytoma: a clinicopathologic study of 158 cases and further exploration of the myoid phenotype, *Hum Pathol* 30:1336–1343, 1999.
92. Weinreb I, Rubin BP, Goldblum JR: Pleomorphic angiomatoid fibrous histiocytoma: a case confirmed by fluorescence in situ hybridization analysis for EWSR1 rearrangement, *J Cutan Pathol* 35:855–860, 2008.
93. Schaefer IM, Fletcher CD: Myxoid variant of so-called angiomatoid "malignant fibrous histiocytoma": clinicopathologic characterization in a series of 21 cases, *Am J Surg Pathol* 38:816–823, 2014.
94. Fletcher CD: Angiomatoid "malignant fibrous histiocytoma": an immunohistochemical study indicative of myoid differentiation, *Hum Pathol* 22:563–568, 1991.
95. Smith ME, Costa MJ, Weiss SW: Evaluation of CD68 and other histiocytic antigens in angiomatoid malignant fibrous histiocytoma, *Am J Surg Pathol* 15:757–763, 1991.
96. Antonescu CR, Dal Cin P, Nafa K, et al: EWSR1-CREB1 is the predominant gene fusion in angiomatoid fibrous histiocytoma, *Genes Chromosomes Cancer* 46:1051–1060, 2007.
97. Rossi S, Szuhai K, Ijszenga M, et al: EWSR1-CREB1 and EWSR1-ATF1 fusion genes in angiomatoid fibrous histiocytoma, *Clin Cancer Res* 13:7322–7328, 2007.
98. Hallor KH, Mertens F, Jin Y, et al: Fusion of the EWSR1 and ATF1 genes without expression of the MITF-M transcript in angiomatoid fibrous histiocytoma, *Genes Chromosomes Cancer* 44:97–102, 2005.
99. Hallor KH, Micci F, Meis-Kindblom JM, et al: Fusion genes in angiomatoid fibrous histiocytoma, *Cancer Lett* 251:158–163, 2007.
100. Raddaoui E, Donner LR, Panagopoulos I: Fusion of the FUS and ATF1 genes in a large, deep-seated angiomatoid fibrous histiocytoma, *Diagn Mol Pathol* 11:157–162, 2002.
101. Waters BL, Panagopoulos I, Allen EF: Genetic characterization of angiomatoid fibrous histiocytoma identifies fusion of the FUS and ATF-1 genes induced by a chromosomal translocation involving bands 12q13 and 16p11, *Cancer Genet Cytogenet* 121:109–116, 2000.
102. Tanas MR, Rubin BP, Montgomery EA, et al: Utility of FISH in the diagnosis of angiomatoid fibrous histiocytoma: a series of 18 cases, *Mod Pathol* 23:93–97, 2010.
103. Thway K, Gonzalez D, Wren D, et al: Angiomatoid fibrous histiocytoma: comparison of fluorescence in situ hybridization and reverse transcription polymerase chain reaction as adjunct diagnostic modalities, *Ann Diagn Pathol* 19:137–142, 2015.
104. Antonescu CR, Zhang L, Nielsen GP, et al: Consistent t(1;10) with rearrangements of TGFBR3 and MGEA5 in both myxoinflammatory fibroblastic sarcoma and hemosiderotic fibrolipomatous tumor, *Genes Chromosomes Cancer* 50:757–764, 2011.
105. Hallor KH, Sciot R, Staaf J, et al: Two genetic pathways, t(1;10) and amplification of 3p11–12, in myxoinflammatory fibroblastic sarcoma, haemosiderotic fibrolipomatous tumour, and morphologically similar lesions, *J Pathol* 217:716–727, 2009.
106. Meis-Kindblom JM, Kindblom LG: Acral myxoinflammatory fibroblastic sarcoma: a low-grade tumor of the hands and feet, *Am J Surg Pathol* 22:911–924, 1998.
107. Montgomery EA, Devaney KO, Giordano TJ, et al: Inflammatory myxohyaline tumor of distal extremities with virocyte or Reed-Sternberg-like cells: a distinctive lesion with features simulating inflammatory conditions, Hodgkin's disease, and various sarcomas, *Mod Pathol* 11:384–391, 1998.
108. Tejwani A, Kobayashi W, Chen YL, et al: Management of acral myxoinflammatory fibroblastic sarcoma, *Cancer* 116:5733–5739, 2010.
109. Laskin WB, Fetsch JF, Miettinen M: Myxoinflammatory fibroblastic sarcoma: a clinicopathologic analysis of 104 cases, with emphasis on predictors of outcome, *Am J Surg Pathol* 38:1–12, 2014.
110. Zreik RT, Carter JM, Sukov WR, et al: TGFBR3 and MGEA5 rearrangements are much more common in "hybrid" hemosiderotic fibrolipomatous tumor-myxoinflammatory fibroblastic sarcomas than in classical myxoinflammatory fibroblastic sarcomas: a morphological and fluorescence in situ hybridization study, *Hum Pathol* 53:14–24, 2016.
111. Kao YC, Ranucci V, Zhang L, et al: Recurrent BRAF gene rearrangements in myxoinflammatory fibroblastic sarcomas, but not hemosiderotic fibrolipomatous tumors, *Am J Surg Pathol* 2017 [epub ahead of print].
112. Kraus MD, Guillou L, Fletcher CD: Well-differentiated inflammatory liposarcoma: an uncommon and easily overlooked variant of a common sarcoma, *Am J Surg Pathol* 21:518–527, 1997.
113. Binh MB, Sastre-Garau X, Guillou L, et al: MDM2 and CDK4 immunostainings are useful adjuncts in diagnosing well-differentiated and dedifferentiated liposarcoma subtypes: a comparative analysis of 559 soft tissue neoplasms with genetic data, *Am J Surg Pathol* 29:1340–1347, 2005.
114. Coindre JM, Hostein I, Maire G, et al: Inflammatory malignant fibrous histiocytomas and dedifferentiated liposarcomas: histological review, genomic profile, and MDM2 and CDK4 status favour a single entity, *J Pathol* 203:822–830, 2004.
115. Hisaoka M, Tsuji S, Hashimoto H, et al: Dedifferentiated liposarcoma with an inflammatory malignant fibrous histiocytoma-like component presenting a leukemoid reaction, *Pathol Int* 47:642–646, 1997.
116. Dehner LP, Coffin CM: Idiopathic fibrosclerotic disorders and other inflammatory pseudotumors, *Semin Diagn Pathol* 15:161–173, 1998.
117. Emory TS, Monihan JM, Carr NJ, et al: Sclerosing mesenteritis, mesenteric panniculitis and mesenteric lipodystrophy: a single entity?, *Am J Surg Pathol* 21:392–398, 1997.
118. Cheuk W, Chan JK: IgG4-related sclerosing disease: a critical appraisal of an evolving clinicopathologic entity, *Adv Anat Pathol* 17:303–332, 2010.
119. Weaver J, Goldblum JR, Turner S, et al: Detection of MDM2 gene amplification or protein expression distinguishes sclerosing mesenteritis and retroperitoneal fibrosis from inflammatory well-differentiated liposarcoma, *Mod Pathol* 22:66–70, 2009.
120. Corradi D, Maestri R, Palmisano A, et al: Idiopathic retroperitoneal fibrosis: clinicopathologic features and differential diagnosis, *Kidney Int* 72:742–753, 2007.
121. Zen Y, Onodera M, Inoue D, et al: Retroperitoneal fibrosis: a clinicopathologic study with respect to immunoglobulin G4, *Am J Surg Pathol* 33:1833–1839, 2009.
122. Khosroshahi A, Carruthers MN, Stone JH, et al: Rethinking Ormond's disease: "idiopathic" retroperitoneal fibrosis in the era of IgG4-related disease, *Medicine (Baltimore)* 92:82–91, 2013.

123. Deshpande V, Zen Y, Chan JK, et al: Consensus statement on the pathology of IgG4-related disease, *Mod Pathol* 25:1181–1192, 2012.
124. Vaglio A, Palmisano A, Alberici F, et al: Prednisone versus tamoxifen in patients with idiopathic retroperitoneal fibrosis: an open-label randomised controlled trial, *Lancet* 378:338–346, 2011.
125. Stone JH, Zen Y, Deshpande V: IgG4-related disease, *N Engl J Med* 366:539–551, 2012.
126. Zen Y, Nakanuma Y: IgG4-related disease: a cross-sectional study of 114 cases, *Am J Surg Pathol* 34:1812–1819, 2010.
127. Saab ST, Hornick JL, Fletcher CD, et al: IgG4 plasma cells in inflammatory myofibroblastic tumor: inflammatory marker or pathogenic link?, *Mod Pathol* 24:606–612, 2011.
128. Yamamoto H, Yamaguchi H, Aishima S, et al: Inflammatory myofibroblastic tumor versus IgG4-related sclerosing disease and inflammatory pseudotumor: a comparative clinicopathologic study, *Am J Surg Pathol* 33:1330–1340, 2009.
129. Brito-Zerón P, Kostov B, Bosch X, et al: Therapeutic approach to IgG4-related disease: a systematic review, *Medicine (Baltimore)* 95:e4002, 2016.

11

Giant Cell–Rich Tumors

Bernadette Liegl-Atzwanger, MD, and Jason L. Hornick, MD, PhD

Multinucleated giant cells are seen in small numbers in a diverse range of soft tissue tumors. Similarly, soft tissue tumors with prominent giant cells compose a heterogeneous group of benign, intermediate, and malignant neoplasms. Recognition of the various types of morphologically distinct giant cells may provide clues to the diagnosis. In some cases, the giant cells instead distract the pathologist from paying careful attention to architectural patterns and other constituent cell types that are more helpful in arriving at the correct diagnosis of these tumors.

The multinucleated giant cells in many soft tissue tumors are derived from the monocyte-macrophage lineage.[1] These non-neoplastic giant cells contain cytologically uniform nuclei that lack atypia. In contrast, other soft tissue tumors contain small numbers of distinctive forms of tumor-derived giant cells. Finally, highly atypical, pleomorphic (non-distinctive) tumor giant cells are essentially limited to pleomorphic sarcomas, anaplastic carcinomas, lymphomas (especially anaplastic large cell lymphoma), and occasional malignant melanomas. The group of non-neoplastic giant cells and distinctive tumor giant cells includes Touton giant cells, floret-type giant cells, wreath-like giant cells, multinucleated tumor cells with glassy cytoplasm, and osteoclast-like giant cells. Each of these types of giant cells is described briefly in the following paragraphs (Table 11.1 and Fig. 11.1).

Touton giant cells, which are histiocytic in nature, contain eosinophilic cytoplasm encircled by a ring of nuclei, which are in turn surrounded by a lipid-laden rim of foamy cytoplasm. Occasionally, hemosiderin may also be seen in the cytoplasm. These giant cells are characteristically found in a few cutaneous lesions, including (juvenile) xanthogranuloma and benign fibrous histiocytoma (see Chapter 15 for details).

Floret-type giant cells are composed of hyperchromatic nuclei arranged in a semicircle surrounding deeply eosinophilic cytoplasm. This type of giant cell is typically found in pleomorphic lipoma, a benign adipocytic tumor of the neck, upper back, and shoulder region (see Chapter 12). In addition, this form of giant cell can be found in the pediatric, superficial neoplasm known as *giant cell fibroblastoma* (discussed in Chapter 15) and the solitary fibrous tumor variant previously known as *giant cell angiofibroma* (see Chapter 3), which has a predilection for the soft tissues of the orbit.[2-4] Neurofibromas may also contain floret-type giant cells in a small subset of cases.[5]

Wreath-like giant cells contain hyperchromatic, peripherally located nuclei surrounding eosinophilic cytoplasm. Typically, this type of giant cell is found in alveolar rhabdomyosarcoma (discussed in Chapter 8), clear cell sarcoma (discussed in Chapter 3), and cellular blue nevus.

Multinucleated tumor cells with glassy cytoplasm are characteristic of the rare cutaneous lesion reticulohistiocytoma (discussed in Chapter 15).

Osteoclast-like giant cells are composed of irregularly distributed, small ovoid nuclei (that resemble those found in histiocytes) within eosinophilic or amphophilic cytoplasm. In most tumors, these giant cells contain 5 to 10 nuclei; however, 20 or more nuclei may occasionally be seen, particularly in giant cell tumor of soft tissue (see later discussion). Osteoclast-like giant cells can sometimes be found in a wide range of soft tissue tumors. For example, prominent osteoclast-like giant cells are seen in about 10% of cases of nodular fasciitis (Fig. 11.2) (see Chapters 3 and 4). A relatively small group of soft tissue tumors characteristically contain osteoclast-like giant cells. These latter tumors are the focus of this chapter.

Soft tissue tumors that typically contain osteoclast-like giant cells can be divided into three main groups (Box 11.1):

1. Tumors associated with joints or arising in the soft tissues adjacent to joints (the tenosynovial giant cell tumors)
2. Tumors of superficial soft tissue (dermis and subcutis) that usually contain nodules of giant cells admixed with mononuclear cells
3. Giant cell–rich sarcomas

Attention to the anatomic site, tumor depth (superficial or deep soft tissues), architecture (plexiform, nodular, diffuse), and constituent cells other than the giant cells is helpful in the evaluation of soft tissue tumors containing prominent giant cells. For the tumors in these first two groups in particular, immunohistochemistry is of limited value in

Table 11.1 Types of Multinucleated Giant Cells Seen in Soft Tissue Tumors

Type of Giant Cell	Characteristic Tumor Types	Chapters Where Discussed
Touton giant cell	Xanthogranuloma	15
	Benign fibrous histiocytoma	15
Floret-type giant cell	Pleomorphic lipoma	12
	Giant cell fibroblastoma	15
	Giant cell angiofibroma	3
	Neurofibroma (rare)	3
Wreath-like giant cell	Alveolar rhabdomyosarcoma	8
	Clear cell sarcoma	3
	Cellular blue nevus	NA
Multinucleated giant cell with glassy cytoplasm	Reticulohistiocytoma	15
Osteoclast-like giant cell	Nodular fasciitis	3 and 4
	Giant cell tumor of tendon sheath	11
	Diffuse-type giant cell tumor	11
	Plexiform fibrohistiocytic tumor	11
	Giant cell tumor of soft tissue	11
	Leiomyosarcoma	3 and 11
	Extraskeletal osteosarcoma	7, 11, and 14
	Undifferentiated pleomorphic sarcoma	7 and 11
	Undifferentiated carcinoma	NA
Pleomorphic tumor giant cell	Undifferentiated pleomorphic sarcoma	7
	Anaplastic carcinomas	NA
	Anaplastic large cell lymphoma	NA
	Histiocytic sarcoma	10

NA, Not applicable.

Box 11.1 Soft Tissue Tumors With Prominent Osteoclast-Like Giant Cells

Tenosynovial Giant Cell Tumors

Giant cell tumor of tendon sheath
Diffuse-type giant cell tumor
Malignant diffuse-type giant cell tumor (sarcoma ex–diffuse-type giant cell tumor)

Tumors of Superficial Soft Tissues

Plexiform fibrohistiocytic tumor
Giant cell tumor of soft tissue

Giant Cell–Rich Sarcomas

Leiomyosarcoma
Extraskeletal osteosarcoma
Undifferentiated pleomorphic sarcoma

differential diagnosis. In contrast, because other malignant neoplasms (especially undifferentiated carcinoma and large cell lymphomas) may easily be confused with giant cell–rich sarcomas, immunohistochemistry is critical to exclude nonmesenchymal neoplasms before an undifferentiated sarcoma is diagnosed (see Chapter 7).

Tenosynovial Giant Cell Tumors

Tenosynovial giant cell tumors arise from tendon sheaths, joints, bursae, or adjacent soft tissues. Depending on their location, they can be subclassified clinically into intraarticular and extraarticular subtypes. Based on growth pattern, tenosynovial giant cell tumors can be separated histologically into localized and diffuse subtypes. These variants have significant differences in clinical presentation and prognosis. Rarely, tenosynovial giant cell tumors may be histologically and clinically malignant.

Giant Cell Tumor of Tendon Sheath (Localized-Type Tenosynovial Giant Cell Tumor)

Localized-type tenosynovial giant cell tumor is widely known as *giant cell tumor of tendon sheath*. In the past, this lesion was referred to as *nodular tenosynovitis* or *benign synovioma*. Giant cell tumor of tendon sheath is one of the more common types of soft tissue tumor.

Clinical Features

Most giant cell tumors of tendon sheath arise on the fingers (about 85%). Less commonly affected sites include the wrists, feet, ankles, and knees. Very rarely, this tumor type occurs in the elbow or hip. The tumor can occur in people of any age but preferentially affects young to middle-aged adults between 30 and 50 years of age. A female predominance of 2:1 has been noted.[6] The tumors are painless, slowly growing nodules, usually in the soft tissue, in close proximity to tendons or interphalangeal joints. Occasionally, these tumors erode nearby bone or involve the overlying skin.[7] Rarely, patients present with multiple discrete tumors, usually along a single tendon sheath, but exceptionally involving separate digits. A history of local trauma has been reported in a subset of cases.[6,8]

Pathologic Features

Giant cell tumors of tendon sheath are usually small nodules between 0.5 and 3 cm in size. The uncommon localized intraarticular examples within the ankle, elbow, or hip may be larger. On gross examination, giant cell tumor of tendon sheath is a well-circumscribed, lobulated mass with a white, fibrous cut surface. The presence of yellow and brown areas is variable and depends on the number of xanthoma cells and the extent of hemosiderin deposition.

Histologically, giant cell tumor of tendon sheath is surrounded by a fibrous pseudocapsule, and thin bands of fibrous tissue often separate the tumor into nodules. The nodules are usually dominated by small, mononuclear histiocytoid cells with reniform or clefted nuclei, small nucleoli, and pale cytoplasm, which are admixed with larger epithelioid cells with eosinophilic, sometimes glassy cytoplasm and eccentric nuclei, multinucleated osteoclast-like giant cells, foamy macrophages, siderophages, and chronic inflammatory cells (Figs. 11.3 and 11.4A). The larger epithelioid cells may contain fine cytoplasmic hemosiderin pigment (see Fig. 11.4B). In some cases, the histiocytoid cells have a more spindled appearance. The collagenous stroma can be variably hyalinized, and cholesterol clefts may be found. In tumors with prominent stromal hyalinization, the larger epithelioid cells can be more prominent, and only sparse osteoclast-like giant cells may be seen (Fig. 11.5). Cleft-like spaces, which are typically seen in diffuse-type tenosynovial giant cell tumor (see subsequent discussion), are generally absent. Mitotic activity is highly variable and can occasionally be brisk (>5 per 10 high-power fields). In rare cases, focal necrosis and metaplastic bone may be apparent.

Immunohistochemistry

In practice, immunohistochemistry plays no real role in the diagnosis of giant cell tumor of tendon sheath. The multinucleated osteoclast-like giant cells and many of the small mononuclear cells usually express CD68 and CD163, reflecting the histiocytic nature of these cells. The larger epithelioid cells may be positive for desmin (which often highlights dendritic cytoplasmic processes), in up to 50% of cases; the number of desmin-positive cells is highly variable but is usually less than 10%.[9,10] The larger epithelioid cells are often positive for clusterin and podoplanin (D2-40) as well.[10]

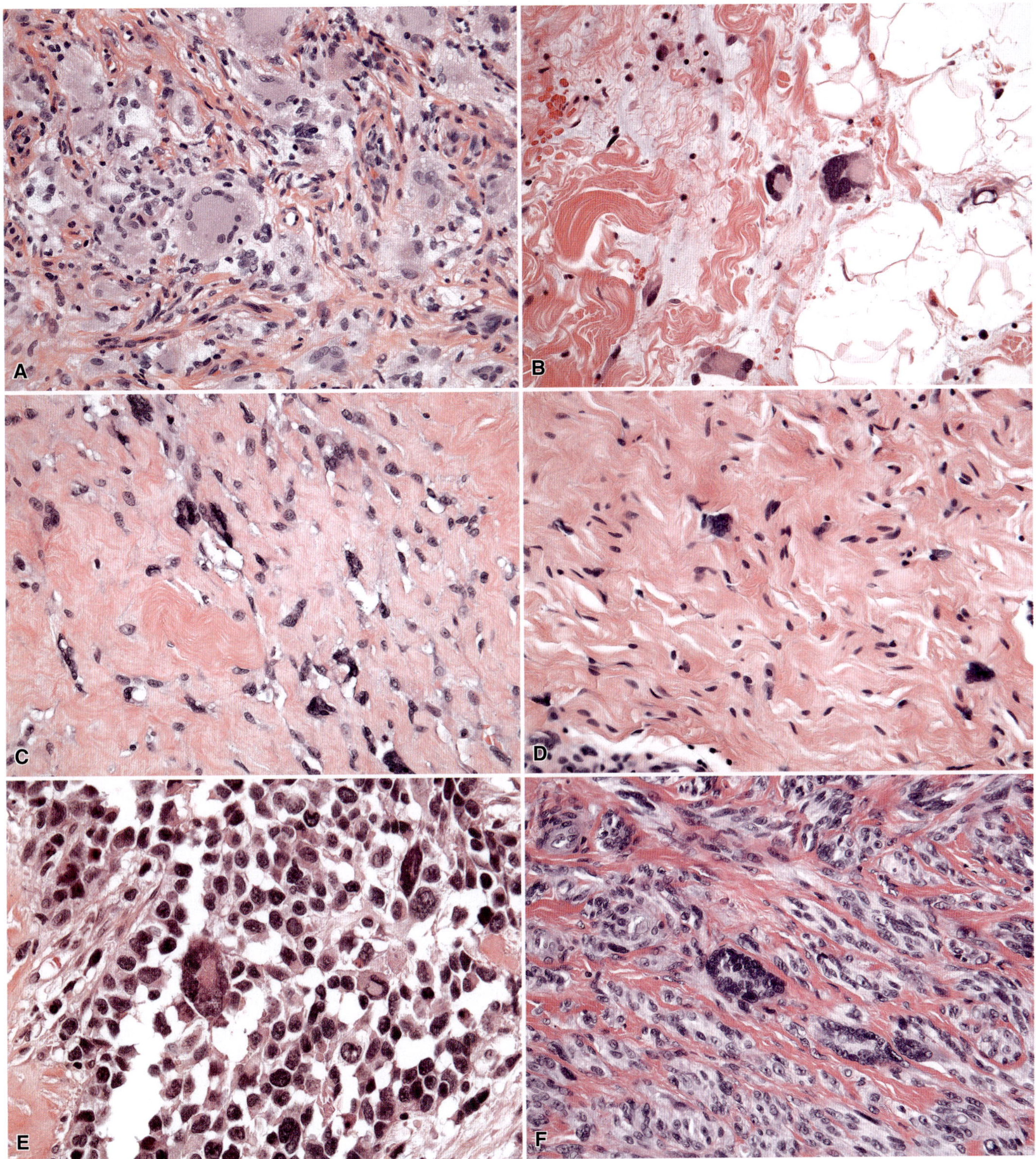

Figure 11.1 **Various Types of Giant Cells in Soft Tissue Tumors.** Touton giant cells in juvenile xanthogranuloma (A); floret-type giant cells in pleomorphic lipoma (B), giant cell fibroblastoma (C), and neurofibroma (D); wreath-like giant cells in alveolar rhabdomyosarcoma (E), clear cell sarcoma (F), *Continued*

Molecular Genetics

Clonal cytogenetic aberrations in giant cell tumor of tendon sheath commonly involve the short arm of chromosome 1 (1p13),[11-13] with rearrangement of the *CSF1* gene in the majority of cases,[14,15] indicating the neoplastic nature of this tumor type. In a subset of tumors, the fusion partner is *COL6A3*, located at 2q37, whereas in a significant number of cases the fusion partner has not yet been identified.[14,15] Recently, several cases with a novel CSF1 transcript were identified by RNA sequencing, including one with *CSF1-S100A10* fusion.[15] However, the *CSF1* translocation is only present in a minority of cells within the

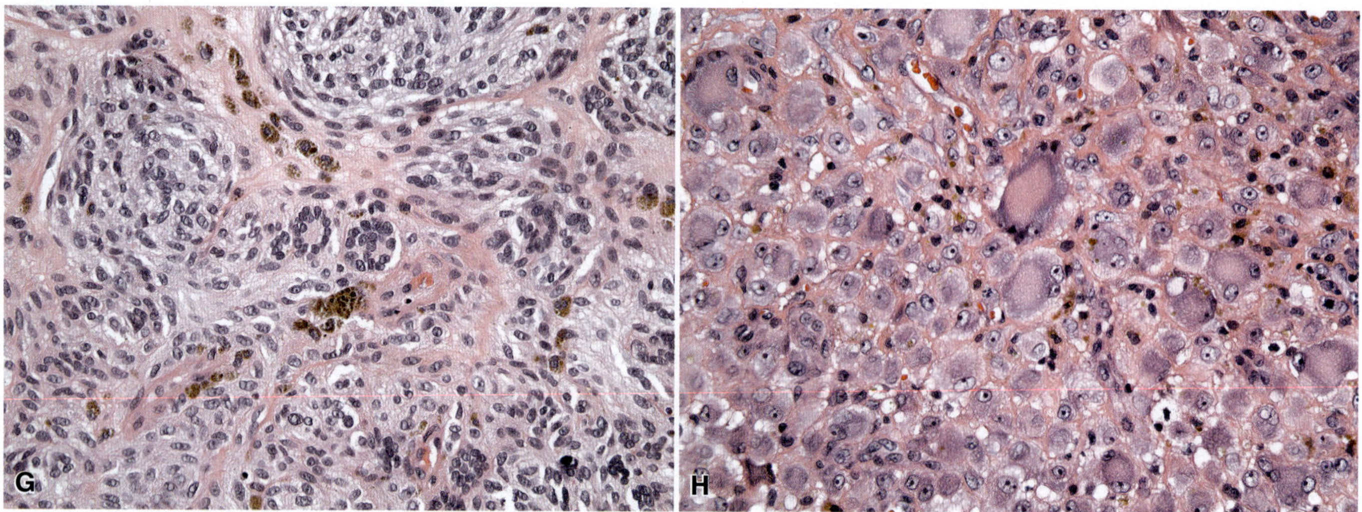

Figure 11.1, cont'd and cellular blue nevus (G); multinucleated tumor cells with glassy cytoplasm in reticulohistiocytoma (H).

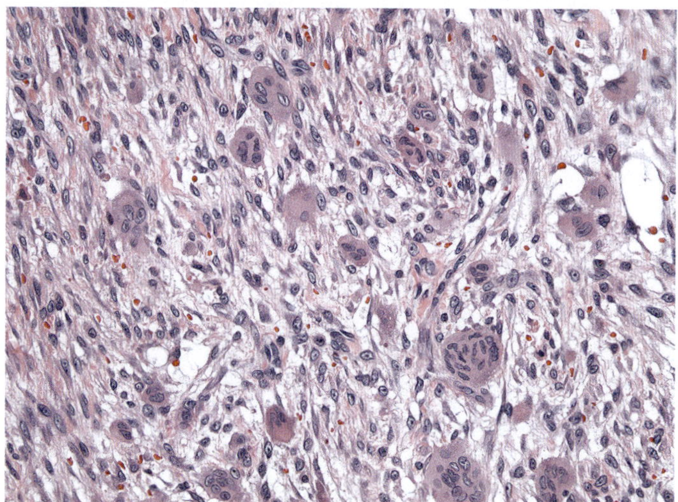

Figure 11.2 Nodular Fasciitis. Around 10% of cases contain prominent osteoclast-like giant cells.

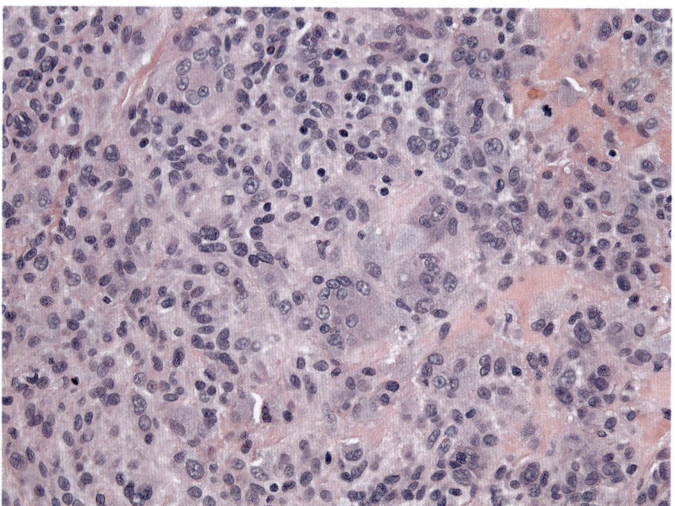

Figure 11.3 Giant Cell Tumor of Tendon Sheath. The tumor is composed of an admixture of small mononuclear histiocytoid cells with reniform nuclei, larger mononuclear cells, and osteoclast-like giant cells.

tumor (i.e., the larger epithelioid cells). These CSF1-producing neoplastic cells are believed to recruit and induce the proliferation of non-neoplastic CSF1 receptor–expressing cells of the monocyte-macrophage lineage. This "landscaping effect" is thought to account for the formation of a tumor mass with the heterogeneous cellular composition of predominantly non-neoplastic cells.[14]

Differential Diagnosis

The diagnosis of giant cell tumor of tendon sheath is generally straightforward. The most important differential diagnostic consideration is diffuse-type tenosynovial giant cell tumor (given the much higher risk of local recurrence). Diffuse-type giant cell tumor is distinguished from giant cell tumor of tendon sheath by its lack of sharp circumscription; nodules or sheets of tumor cells infiltrate into surrounding soft tissues. This tumor type most often arises within joints (preferentially the knee and the hip) but can also occur in extraarticular soft tissue. There is considerable histologic overlap between giant cell tumor of tendon sheath and diffuse-type giant cell tumor, although the latter often shows a villous appearance and contains prominent cleft-like spaces and fewer giant cells. Fibroma of tendon sheath occurs at locations similar to those of giant cell tumor of tendon sheath but is histologically quite different, being composed of fascicles of uniform small spindle cells in a collagenous stroma with slit-like blood vessels at the periphery of the tumor. Giant cells may occasionally be seen, but the mononuclear histiocytoid cells and epithelioid cells are absent. When the epithelioid cells in giant cell tumor of tendon sheath are prominent, epithelioid sarcoma may be considered. This differential diagnosis can easily be resolved with immunohistochemistry; epithelial membrane antigen (EMA) and keratins are consistently positive in epithelioid sarcoma but are negative in giant cell tumor of tendon sheath. In addition, loss of SMARCB1 (INI1) is specific for epithelioid sarcoma in this differential diagnosis. The presence of desmin expression in the epithelioid cells may raise the possibility of a myogenic tumor (such as rhabdomyosarcoma). However, giant cell tumor of tendon sheath is negative for other muscle markers such as smooth muscle actin (SMA), caldesmon, and myogenin. Awareness of this occurrence can help avoid diagnostic confusion.

Prognosis and Treatment

Giant cell tumor of tendon sheath is benign, with a low risk of nondestructive local recurrence (5% to 20%). Conservative local excision is adequate treatment.

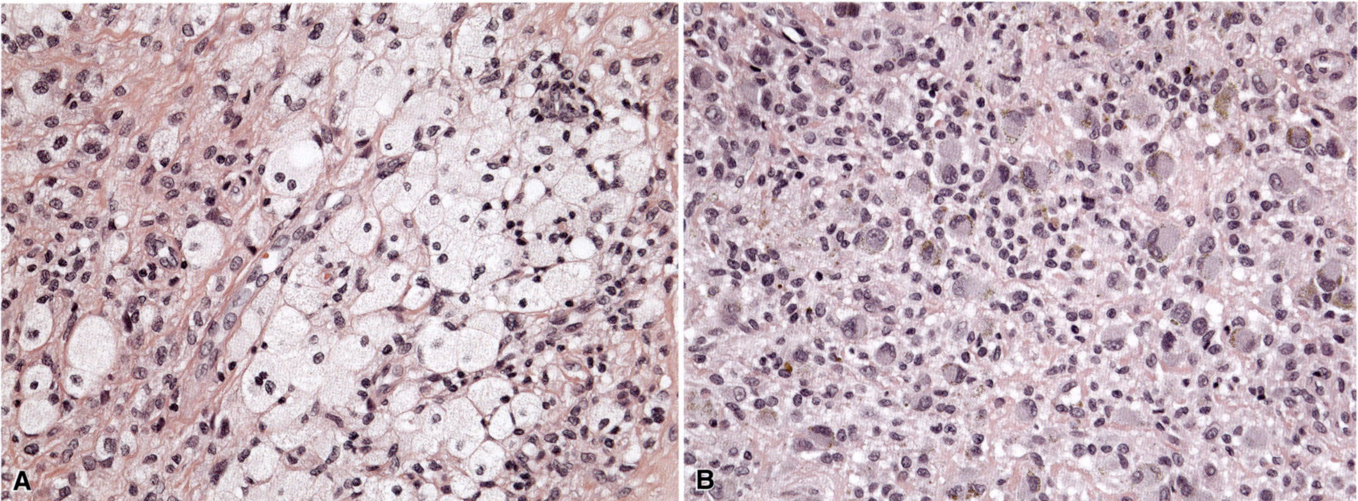

Figure 11.4 **Giant Cell Tumor of Tendon Sheath.** Focal areas in the tumor may contain prominent foamy macrophages and chronic inflammatory cells (A). The larger mononuclear cells have eccentric nuclei, and their cytoplasm often contains fine hemosiderin pigment (B).

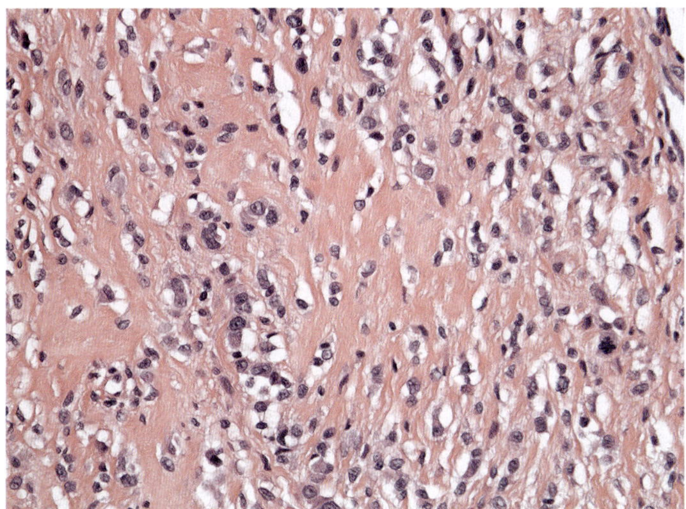

Figure 11.5 **Giant Cell Tumor of Tendon Sheath.** Tumors with prominent stromal hyalinization may contain few or no osteoclast-like giant cells.

Diffuse-Type (Tenosynovial) Giant Cell Tumor

Diffuse-type tenosynovial giant cell tumor is also widely known clinically as *pigmented villonodular (teno)synovitis* (PVNS). However, diffuse-type giant cell tumor is a clonal neoplasm with a significant potential for destructive local recurrence, as well as a small risk of metastasis (not an inflammatory process). Therefore, the misleading designation PVNS should be discouraged.

Clinical Features

According to location, diffuse-type (tenosynovial) giant cell tumors can be divided into intraarticular tumors (which often extend into adjacent soft tissue) and entirely extraarticular examples. The most common site of intraarticular diffuse-type giant cell tumor is the knee (about 70% of cases), followed by the hip (10%). Rarely, the temporomandibular joint or the spinal facet joints are involved.[16-18] Extraarticular diffuse-type giant cell tumors most commonly arise in the periarticular soft tissues around the knee, hip, or foot. The fingers, toes, wrists, and elbows are rarely affected. Entirely intramuscular tumors and subcutaneous examples are rarely observed.[19] Diffuse-type giant cell tumor preferentially occurs in patients younger than 40 years of age with a slight female predominance.[19-21] Patients often present with a long duration of symptoms, including pain, swelling, tenderness, and limitation of motion of the affected joint. The presence of hemarthrosis and joint effusion is not unusual. Radiographically, the tumor appears as an ill-defined mass, which may be associated with degenerative alterations of the affected joint. On magnetic resonance imaging, the tumor shows decreased signal intensity in T1- and T2-weighted images.[22]

Pathologic Features

Diffuse-type giant cell tumor ranges from 3 to 13 cm in size (median, 4.3 cm).[21] On gross examination, the tumors are firm and sponge-like. If located within a joint, a villous surface is typically observed. Similar to giant cell tumor of tendon sheath, the cut surface is usually white with variably prominent brown areas depending on the extent of hemosiderin deposition.

Histologically, diffuse-type giant cell tumor shows an infiltrative growth pattern with diffuse and expansile sheets of tumor cells (Fig. 11.6). At low power, these tumors demonstrate variable cellularity with alternating dense, cellular areas and loose, hypocellular, often collagenized areas. In the majority of cases, cleft-like, pseudoglandular, alveolar, or cystic spaces can be appreciated (Fig. 11.7). Cleft-like spaces are observed in about 80% of cases and are thought to represent a form of "cracking" artifact.[21] The cystic and pseudoglandular spaces are lined by mononuclear cells reminiscent of normal synovial lining. Compared with giant cell tumor of tendon sheath, prominent stromal hyalinization is less commonly seen. At higher power, the tumor has a polymorphous appearance, being composed of a variable admixture of mononuclear cells, osteoclast-like giant cells, foamy histiocytes, hemosiderophages, and chronic inflammatory cells (Fig. 11.8). The mononuclear cells consist of two different cell types: small histiocyte-like cells, which represent the main cellular component, and larger cells (two to four times larger than the small histiocytes) scattered among the small histiocytes or arranged in small clusters.[21] The small histiocytes are ovoid to spindle-shaped with irregular nuclei containing longitudinal grooves and pale cytoplasm. The larger cells have an epithelioid appearance with eosinophilic cytoplasm and eccentric nuclei (Fig. 11.9A). A peripheral rim of fine

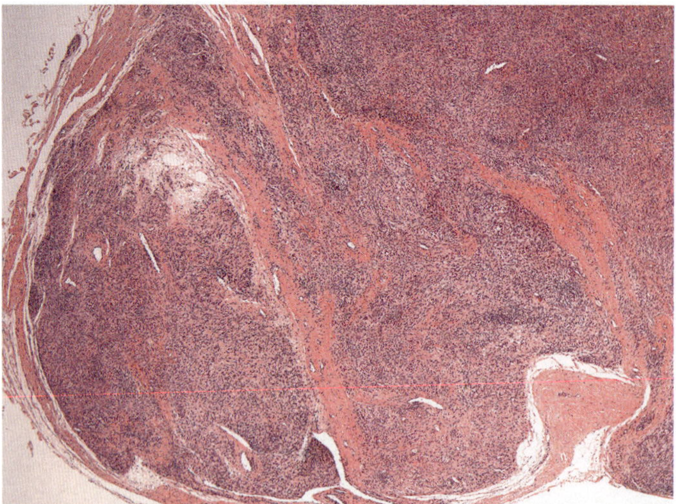

Figure 11.6 Diffuse-Type Giant Cell Tumor. The tumor often shows a nodular growth pattern. Note the irregular tumor margins.

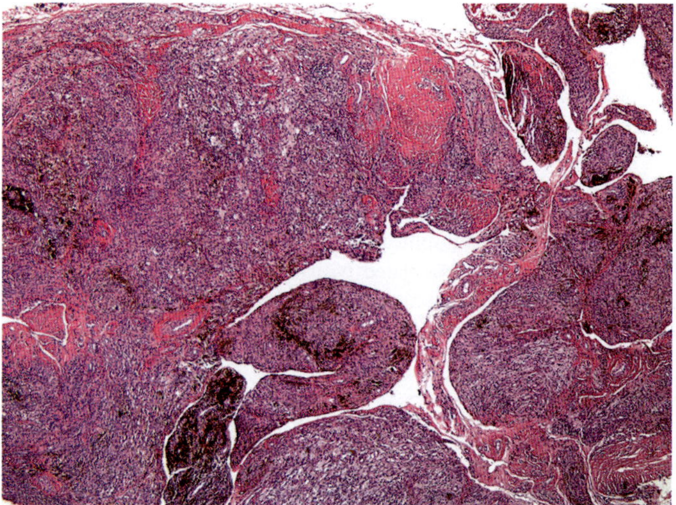

Figure 11.7 Diffuse-Type Giant Cell Tumor. Cleft-like spaces are a typical feature.

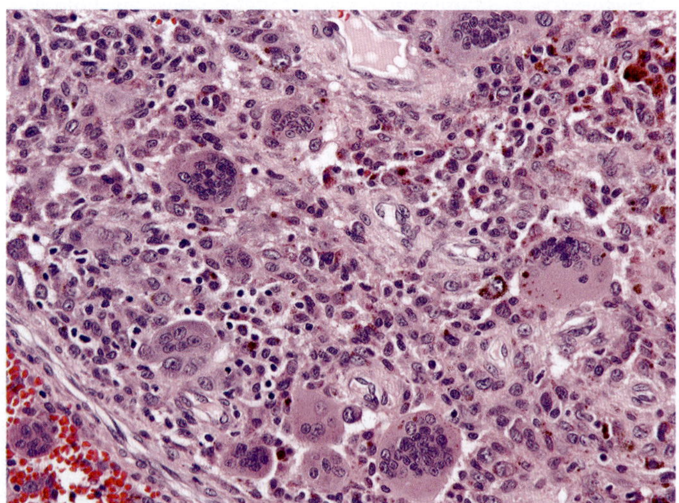

Figure 11.8 Diffuse-Type Giant Cell Tumor. The tumor consists of the same polymorphous cell population as giant cell tumor of tendon sheath. Note the osteoclast-like giant cells and hemosiderin deposition.

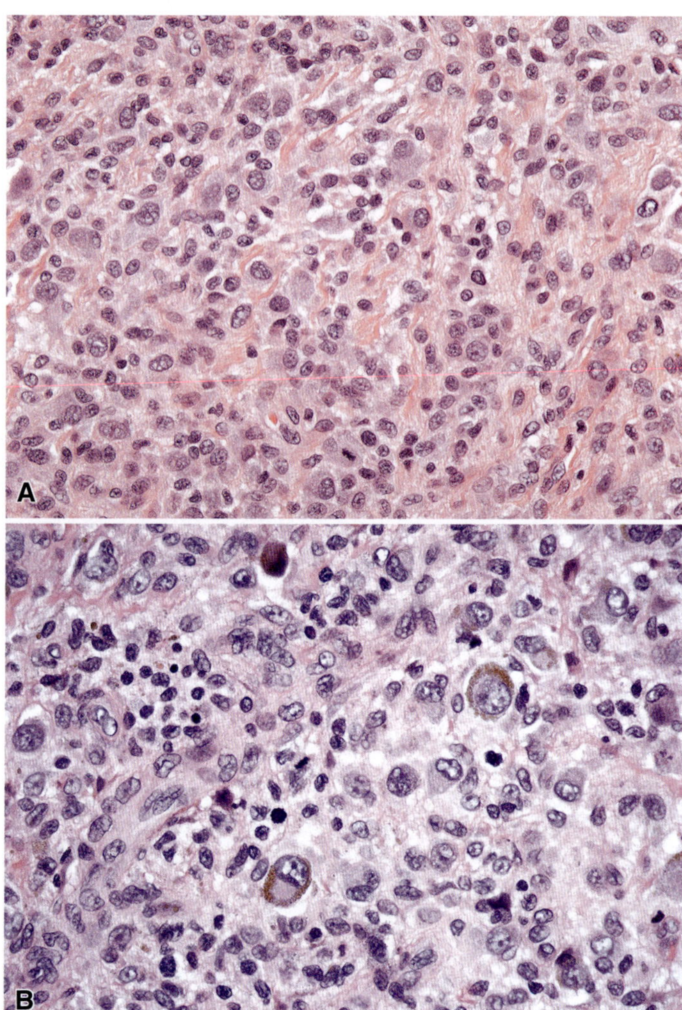

Figure 11.9 Diffuse-Type Giant Cell Tumor. The tumor contains two types of mononuclear cells: small cells with ovoid nuclei and pale cytoplasm and larger cells with eccentric nuclei and abundant eosinophilic to amphophilic cytoplasm (A). When the larger cells predominate, this tumor type may be difficult to recognize. A subset of epithelioid cells contains a rim of fine hemosiderin granules (B).

hemosiderin granules is often present in the cytoplasm of a subset of these epithelioid cells (see Fig. 11.9B) ("ladybird cells"). The nuclei are rounded or reniform, with vesicular chromatin and eosinophilic nucleoli. Paranuclear eosinophilic filamentous inclusions may be seen. The inflammatory infiltrate is composed mainly of small lymphocytes. Foci of metaplastic ossification are occasionally seen, and chondroid metaplasia is rare.[23,24] Chondroid metaplasia is predominantly seen in temporomandibular locations and is distributed in a geographic pattern. The extent of chondroid metaplasia varies widely (30% to 90%).[23,24] Mitotic activity is variable (often >5 per 10 high-power fields).

Immunohistochemistry

The immunophenotypic findings are identical to those in giant cell tumor of tendon sheath. The multinucleated osteoclast-like giant cells and a subset of the mononuclear cells and foamy histiocytes express CD68 and CD163. The large epithelioid mononuclear cells are negative for CD68 but express desmin in up to 50% of cases.[9,10,21] Desmin also highlights dendritic cytoplasmic processes in these cells. In the epithelioid cells, clusterin and podoplanin (D2-40) are also often positive.[10]

Molecular Genetics

The neoplastic nature of these tumors is supported by aneuploid DNA content[25] and clonal karyotypic abnormalities,[13,26] including recurrent trisomy 5 and 7.[26] The cytogenetic findings are the same as those in giant cell tumor of tendon sheath, including 1p13 rearrangements, sometimes in a t(1;2)(p13;q37) translocation. These rearrangements involve the *CSF1* gene,[14,15] expression of which is believed to cause proliferation of neoplastic cells in an autocrine fashion, as well as the recruitment of non-neoplastic cells of the monocyte-macrophage lineage, resulting in the heterogeneous cellular composition of this tumor type.[14] Recently, several cases with a novel *CSF1-S100A10* fusion gene and CSF1 transcript were identified by RNA sequencing, as well as a case with a t(1;17) translocation in addition to trisomy 5.[27,28]

Differential Diagnosis

As mentioned previously, diffuse-type giant cell tumor is distinguished from giant cell tumor of tendon sheath by its infiltrative borders. In addition, giant cell tumor of tendon sheath usually arises on the fingers, only very rarely in the vicinity of large joints, and usually lacks the cleft-like spaces typical of diffuse-type giant cell tumor. Immunohistochemical staining for desmin and the presence of alveolar spaces in diffuse-type giant cell tumor may raise the possibility of alveolar rhabdomyosarcoma. However, alveolar rhabdomyosarcoma lacks the heterogeneous cellular composition of diffuse-type giant cell tumor and shows strong nuclear expression of myogenin. Undifferentiated pleomorphic sarcomas with prominent inflammation might also enter the differential diagnosis. However, such tumors show marked nuclear pleomorphism and a high mitotic rate, including atypical mitoses, and the inflammatory infiltrate consists mainly of neutrophils and eosinophils, in contrast to the small lymphocytes seen in diffuse-type giant cell tumor. In cases where alveolar spaces and the chronic inflammatory component are prominent, angiomatoid fibrous histiocytoma could be considered. However, angiomatoid fibrous histiocytoma contains nodules or sheets of syncytial histiocytoid cells with ill-defined cell borders, in contrast to the single tumor cells with well-defined cell borders in diffuse-type giant cell tumor. In addition, the alveolar spaces in diffuse-type giant cell tumor are not filled with blood, and osteoclast-like giant cells are rarely seen in angiomatoid fibrous histiocytoma. Desmin positivity can be seen in both tumor types, but only angiomatoid fibrous histiocytoma shows EMA expression (about 50% of cases). Angiomatoid fibrous histiocytoma harbors *EWSR1* gene rearrangements in most cases. Diffuse-type giant cell tumors dominated by epithelioid mononuclear cells may be mistaken for histiocytic sarcoma, but the latter tumor type is usually composed of larger cells with abundant pale cytoplasm and marked nuclear atypia. It is positive for CD163, CD45RO, and often for S-100 protein, and it is consistently negative for desmin. Tumors with chondroid metaplasia in temporomandibular locations may mimic synovial chondroma, synovial chondromatosis, chondrosarcoma, or chondroblastoma. In the benign cartilage-forming lesions, chondrocytes are present in well-formed lacunae, and polymorphous inflammatory infiltrates and hemosiderin deposition are lacking. In chondrosarcomas, nuclear atypia is seen throughout the lesion in combination with bone invasion defined by entrapment of trabecular bone or invasion of cortical bone. In contrast, chondroid diffuse-type giant cell tumors only demonstrate osteoclastic resorption of the adjacent bone with a clear tumor-to-bone interface. Of note, chondroblastomas are composed of sheets of a uniform population of tumor cells with well-defined borders and eccentric grooved nuclei, in contrast to the admixture of variable cell types in diffuse-type giant cell tumors.[24]

Prognosis and Treatment

Local recurrences are common in both intraarticular (20% to 50%) and extraarticular (30% to 60%) examples of diffuse-type giant cell tumor,[18,19,21] may be multiple, and they can lead to severe limitation of joint function and joint replacement. The risk of recurrence correlates with positive excision margins. Therefore, a total synovectomy is the best treatment for intraarticular tumors,[29] and wide excision with negative margins is indicated for extraarticular cases. CSF1 receptor inhibitors are under investigation for patients with uncontrolled local recurrences or unresectable disease.[30] A retrospective study reported clinical responses to imatinib mesylate in a subset of patients.[31] Conventional diffuse-type giant cell tumor only very rarely metastasizes to lymph nodes or distant sites.

Malignant Diffuse-Type (Tenosynovial) Giant Cell Tumor

Malignant transformation in diffuse-type giant cell tumor is exceedingly rare. Only small numbers of convincing examples have been published.[21,32-34] The designation "malignant" diffuse-type giant cell tumor is used when (1) tumors contain a component of conventional diffuse-type giant cell tumor and a cytologically malignant or sarcomatous component, or (2) tumors initially diagnosed as (conventional) diffuse-type giant cell tumor recur as a sarcoma. Histologically typical cases of diffuse-type giant cell tumor very rarely metastasize, but this occurrence cannot be predicted based on histologic features. Although a very high mitotic rate (>20 per 10 high-power fields), necrosis, nuclear enlargement with prominent nucleoli, and prominent spindling of the large mononuclear cells are worrisome findings (in which cases the designation "atypical" diffuse-type giant cell tumor is reasonable), none of these features alone is sufficient for the diagnosis of malignancy, which requires overtly malignant cytology. The malignant component often consists of sheets of large histiocytoid cells somewhat reminiscent of the epithelioid mononuclear cells in conventional examples, but with marked nuclear atypia (Fig. 11.10). Some cases contain areas indistinguishable from an undifferentiated pleomorphic sarcoma, fascicles of spindle cells, focally myxoid stroma, or giant cell–rich nodules.[34] In such cases, without recognizing areas of conventional diffuse-type giant cell tumor, a specific diagnosis cannot be rendered. Malignant diffuse-type giant cell tumors have a high rate of destructive local recurrence, as well as the potential to metastasize to lymph nodes, lung, and bone.[21,34]

Molecular Genetics

Recently, aberrations of cyclin A and P53, as well as deletions on chromosome 15q, have been implicated as possible mechanisms for sarcomatous transformation of diffuse-type giant cell tumor.[35] Although expression of CSF1 has been documented, *COL6A3-CSF1* gene fusion has only been detected in a small subset of cases.[35]

PRACTICE POINTS: Tenosynovial Giant Cell Tumors

- Giant cell tumor of tendon sheath usually arises on the fingers
- Diffuse-type giant cell tumor is most common around the knees and hips
- Infiltrative borders distinguish diffuse-type giant cell tumor from localized-type
- Tenosynovial giant cell tumors are composed of sheets of small mononuclear histiocytoid cells, larger epithelioid cells with eccentric nuclei, and scattered osteoclast-like giant cells
- Rare diffuse-type giant cell tumors show progression to sarcoma
- Desmin is positive in epithelioid cells in 50% of cases
- *CSF1* gene rearrangements are typical

Tumors of Superficial Soft Tissues

Plexiform Fibrohistiocytic Tumor

Plexiform fibrohistiocytic tumor is a rare, distinctive mesenchymal neoplasm of intermediate biologic potential (rarely metastasizing) that typically has an unusual biphasic appearance.

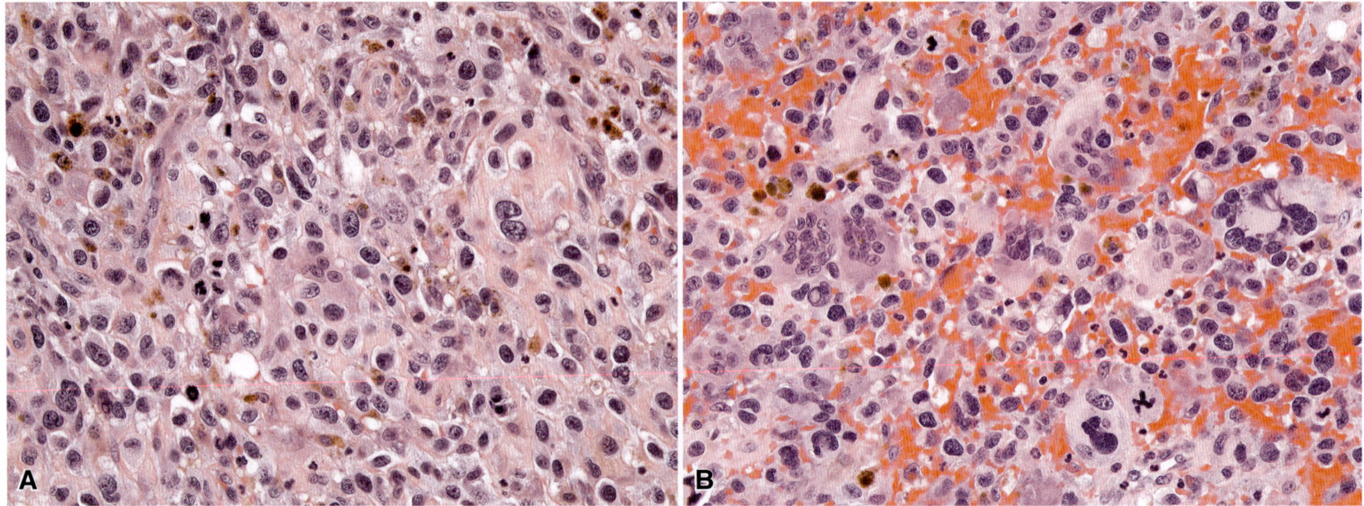

Figure 11.10 Malignant Diffuse-Type Giant Cell Tumor. The tumor is composed of sheets of histiocytoid cells with marked nuclear atypia and a high mitotic rate (A). This tumor contains both osteoclast-like giant cells and pleomorphic tumor giant cells (B).

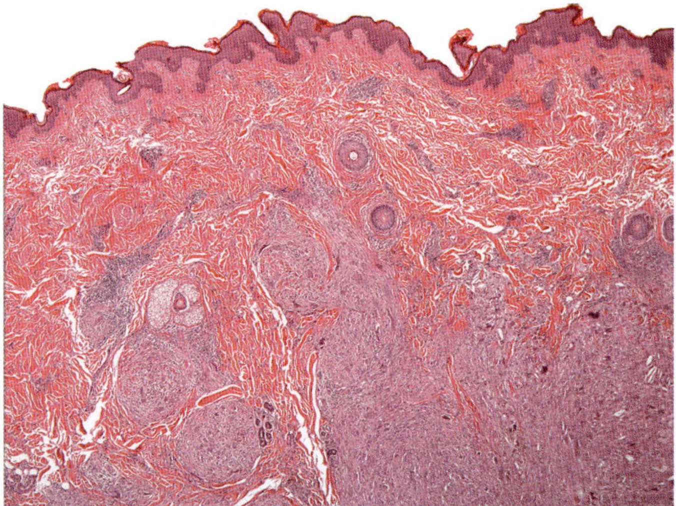

Figure 11.11 Plexiform Fibrohistiocytic Tumor. This superficial tumor shows a characteristic multinodular, infiltrative growth pattern.

Figure 11.12 Plexiform Fibrohistiocytic Tumor. The tumor often involves subcutaneous tissue. Note the plexiform architecture.

Clinical Features

Plexiform fibrohistiocytic tumor has a predilection for children and young adults. Patients typically present with a painless, slowly growing nodule located at the interface between the dermis and subcutaneous tissue.[36-38] Approximately two-thirds of cases involve the upper extremity, most commonly the hand or the wrist. Most other cases arise on the lower extremity; very rarely they involve the head and neck region.[36-38]

Pathologic Features

Most tumors are between 1 and 3 cm in size. On gross examination, the tumor is poorly circumscribed and usually has a multinodular appearance. Histologically, as its name implies, plexiform fibrohistiocytic tumor has a plexiform, multinodular architecture (Figs. 11.11 and 11.12); it is composed of discontiguous nodules or clusters of mononuclear histiocytoid or epithelioid cells with fine chromatin, small nucleoli, and palely eosinophilic cytoplasm and scattered osteoclast-like giant cells (Figs. 11.13 and 11.14), connected by fascicles of bland myofibroblastic spindle cells mimicking desmoid fibromatosis (Fig. 11.15). In addition to the classical mixed pattern (in which the elements are present in approximately equal proportions), two other histologic subtypes have been recognized: a fibrohistiocytic variant composed mainly of nodules of histiocytoid/epithelioid cells and giant cells and a fibroblastic variant composed of fascicles of spindle cells with only rare clusters of histiocytoid cells and/or giant cells. In cases lacking the nodules of mononuclear cells, sometimes they can be identified in deeper levels. Nuclear atypia and pleomorphism are not features of plexiform fibrohistiocytic tumor. Mitoses are rare, and atypical mitoses and necrosis are absent. Vascular invasion can be seen in 10% to 20% of cases. Although the tumor is usually located primarily in the dermis or subcutaneous tissue, infiltration into underlying skeletal muscle can occasionally occur.

Immunohistochemistry

In classic cases of plexiform fibrohistiocytic tumor, immunohistochemistry is not required for diagnosis. The spindle cell component is usually at least focally positive for SMA (Fig. 11.16A), the histiocytoid cells are variably positive for CD68, and the osteoclast-like giant cells show strong staining for CD68 and CD163 (see Fig. 11.16B). The tumor cells are negative for desmin, S-100 protein, and CD34.[39] In cases dominated

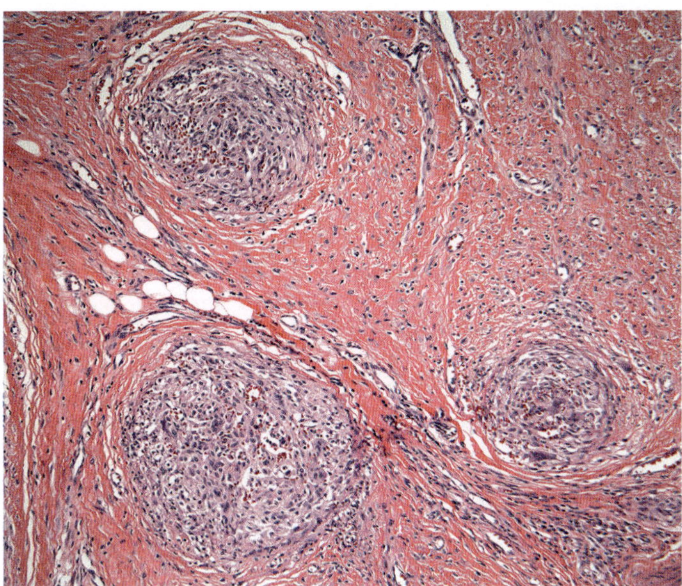

Figure 11.13 Plexiform Fibrohistiocytic Tumor. The discontiguous nodules are sharply demarcated.

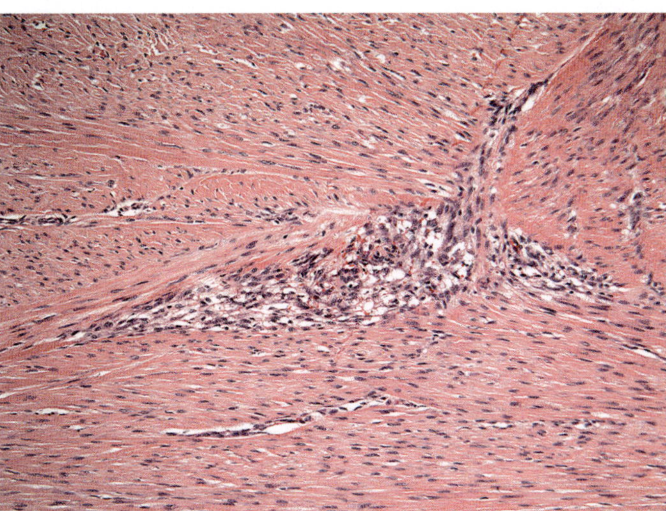

Figure 11.15 Plexiform Fibrohistiocytic Tumor. The fascicular spindle cell component resembles fibromatosis. Note the small focus of mononuclear cells in the center of the field.

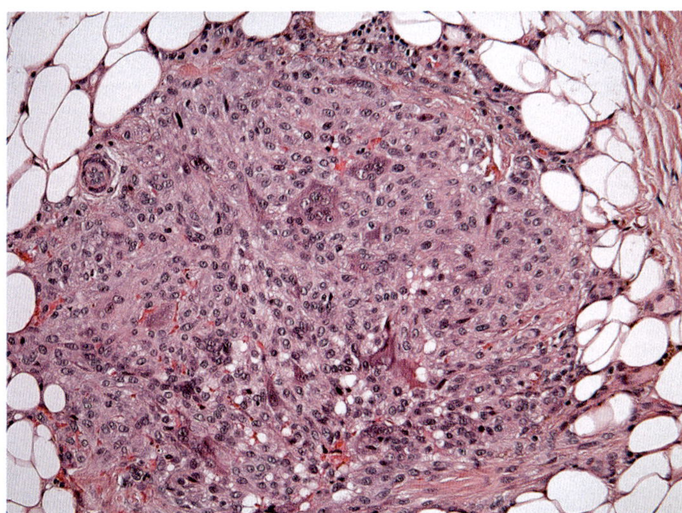

Figure 11.14 Plexiform Fibrohistiocytic Tumor. The nodules contain small mononuclear cells with abundant palely eosinophilic cytoplasm and scattered osteoclast-like giant cells.

by fascicles of spindle cells (the fibroblastic variant), CD68 or CD163 can sometimes aid in identifying nodules of mononuclear cells.

Differential Diagnosis

Once the distinctive combination of histologic features is recognized, the diagnosis of plexiform fibrohistiocytic tumor is relatively straightforward. However, particularly in cases dominated by one of the two components, differential diagnostic considerations might include giant cell tumor of soft tissue, deep fibrous histiocytoma, desmoid or palmar fibromatosis, fibrous hamartoma of infancy, and cellular neurothekeoma. Similar to plexiform fibrohistiocytic tumor, giant cell tumor of soft tissue contains cellular nodules of osteoclast-like giant cells and mononuclear cells, although the nodules are usually larger and giant cells are typically more numerous in giant cell tumor. Moreover, giant cell tumor of soft tissue often contains fibrous tissue with hemosiderin deposition between the nodules but lacks the fibromatosis-like spindle cell fascicles

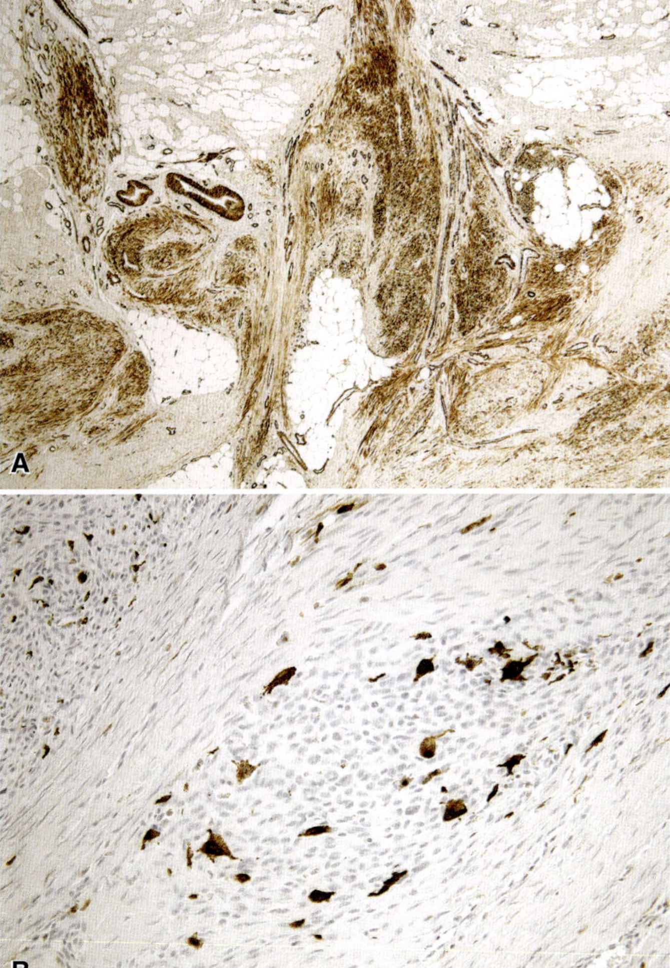

Figure 11.16 Plexiform Fibrohistiocytic Tumor. The myofibroblastic fascicles are usually positive for smooth muscle actin. Note the plexiform growth pattern through subcutaneous tissue (A). The osteoclast-like giant cells can be highlighted by staining for CD68 or CD163 (B).

characteristic of plexiform fibrohistiocytic tumor. Deep fibrous histiocytoma may contain scattered osteoclast-like giant cells, but instead of a plexiform growth pattern and discrete small nodules of mononuclear cells, deep fibrous histiocytoma contains a diffuse proliferation of short spindle cells in a variably storiform to fascicular growth pattern. The individual myofibroblastic fascicles of plexiform fibrohistiocytic tumor are histologically very similar to desmoid fibromatosis; however, desmoid tumors do not primarily involve the dermis, contain longer and wider fascicles, and do not have a plexiform growth pattern. In addition, more than 70% of desmoid tumors demonstrate nuclear β-catenin staining. Although the cellular phase of palmar fibromatosis often has a nodular appearance, it typically involves the fascia, and, unlike plexiform fibrohistiocytic tumor, the nodules are composed solely of myofibroblastic spindle cells, without a mononuclear cell component. Fibrous hamartoma of infancy usually lacks osteoclast-like giant cells and contains a primitive myxoid cellular component, in addition to a fascicular fibroblastic component and mature adipose tissue. Cellular neurothekeoma only very rarely shows histologic overlap with plexiform fibrohistiocytic tumor, when osteoclast-like giant cells and a somewhat plexiform architecture are present (see Chapter 15). However, cellular neurothekeoma typically involves the head and neck, shoulder, or upper arm, has a uniform, micronodular growth pattern, and is composed of nests of epithelioid cells with abundant palely eosinophilic cytoplasm, in contrast to the small histiocytoid cells and myofibroblastic fascicles of plexiform fibrohistiocytic tumor. Microphthalmia transcription factor (MITF) may be helpful to distinguish cellular neurothekeoma from plexiform fibrohistiocytic tumor in some cases.[40]

Prognosis and Treatment

Plexiform fibrohistiocytic tumor has a significant potential for local recurrences (35% to 40%); therefore, complete surgical excision with wide margins is indicated.[36,38,39] This tumor type rarely metastasizes to the lungs or lymph nodes.[36,38]

PRACTICE POINTS: Plexiform Fibrohistiocytic Tumor

- Most common in dermis and subcutaneous tissue of upper extremities
- Biphasic appearance: nodules of mononuclear histiocytoid cells and scattered osteoclast-like giant cells connected by fibromatosis-like spindle cell fascicles
- One component may predominate ("fibrohistiocytic variant" or "fibroblastic variant")
- Significant potential for local recurrence
- Metastases rare

Giant Cell Tumor of Soft Tissue

Giant cell tumor of soft tissue has the same histologic features as giant cell tumor of bone. Although giant cell tumor of soft tissue usually has a benign clinical course, distant metastases may rarely develop.

Clinical Features

Giant cell tumor of soft tissue affects people of a wide age range but usually occurs in adults, with a peak in the fifth decade. It has an equal gender distribution. The superficial soft tissues of the extremities are most commonly involved (70%), followed by the trunk (20%) and the head and neck region.[41-43] Giant cell tumor of soft tissue usually arises in the dermis and subcutaneous tissue, and it develops less frequently in the deep soft tissues. Patients typically present with a painless mass, with an average symptom duration of 6 months.[43] On imaging studies, peripheral bone formation may be apparent.

Pathologic Features

Giant cell tumor of soft tissue is most often between 2 and 4 cm in size, although tumors located in deep soft tissues may be larger than 5 cm.[41-43]

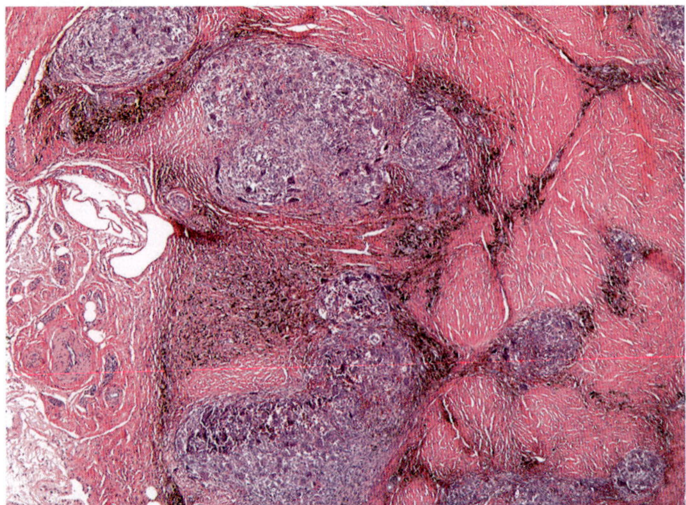

Figure 11.17 Giant Cell Tumor of Soft Tissue. The tumor shows a multinodular growth pattern. Note the prominent hemosiderin deposition.

On gross examination, giant cell tumor of soft tissue is a circumscribed, nodular mass with a red-brown or gray cut surface. Foci of bone may be observed at the periphery of the tumor.

Histologically, giant cell tumor of soft tissue shows a multinodular architecture (Fig. 11.17). The nodules vary in size and are composed of multinucleated osteoclast-like giant cells distributed evenly among mononuclear cells within a vascular stroma (Fig. 11.18). The nuclear features of the mononuclear cells are similar to those in the giant cells, namely round to oval with vesicular chromatin and small nucleoli (Fig. 11.19). The mononuclear cells are usually histiocytoid, but a spindle-cell component may also be present.[42] The nodules are surrounded by dense fibrous tissue containing prominent small blood vessels, hemosiderin deposition, and hemosiderin-laden macrophages (Fig. 11.20). In about 50% of cases, an incomplete peripheral shell of woven bone surrounds the tumor. Blood-filled cystic spaces, similar to aneurysmal bone cyst, stromal hemorrhage, and clusters of foamy histiocytes may be present. Atypia and pleomorphism are not features of giant cell tumor of soft tissue. Mitotic figures can be numerous (>10 per 10 high-power fields), but atypical mitoses are not observed. Vascular invasion is seen in about 30% of tumors.[43]

Immunohistochemistry

The multinucleated osteoclast-like giant cells express CD68 and CD163, whereas the mononuclear cells show only focal and variable staining. SMA is expressed in a subset of mononuclear cells but not in the multinucleated giant cells. The tumor cells are negative for desmin and S-100 protein. Very rarely, tumor cells show limited staining for keratin.[43]

Molecular Genetics

Giant cell tumor of soft tissue lacks the *H3F3A* mutations characteristic of giant cell tumor of bone suggesting that despite the histologic resemblance, these tumor types are not in fact related.[44] The molecular pathogenetic basis for giant cell tumor of soft tissue has not yet been elucidated.

Differential Diagnosis

The differential diagnosis includes other tumors rich in osteoclast-like giant cells. It is critical to separate giant cell tumor of soft tissue from giant cell–rich sarcomas, including undifferentiated pleomorphic sarcoma with giant cells, giant cell–rich extraskeletal osteosarcoma, and leiomyosarcoma (see Chapter 7). Giant cell–rich sarcomas generally lack

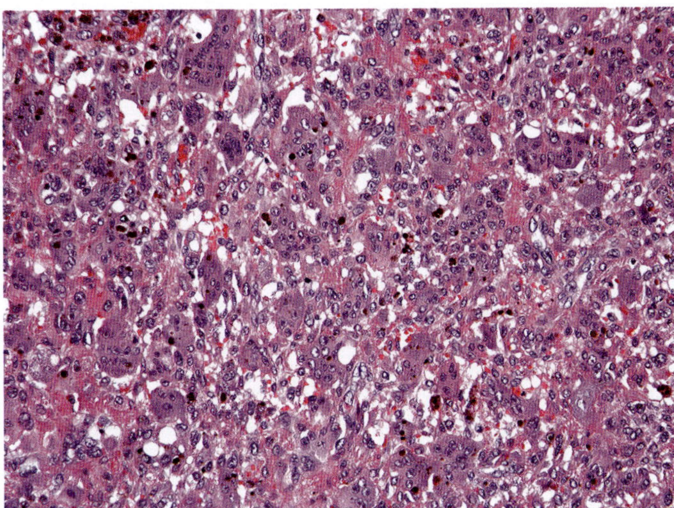

Figure 11.18 **Giant Cell Tumor of Soft Tissue.** The tumor is composed of numerous osteoclast-like giant cells evenly distributed among mononuclear cells.

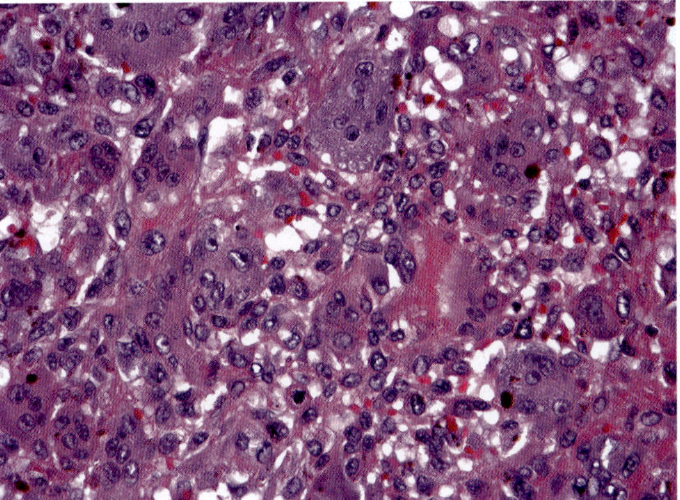

Figure 11.19 **Giant Cell Tumor of Soft Tissue.** The mononuclear cells contain round to ovoid nuclei with vesicular chromatin and small nucleoli.

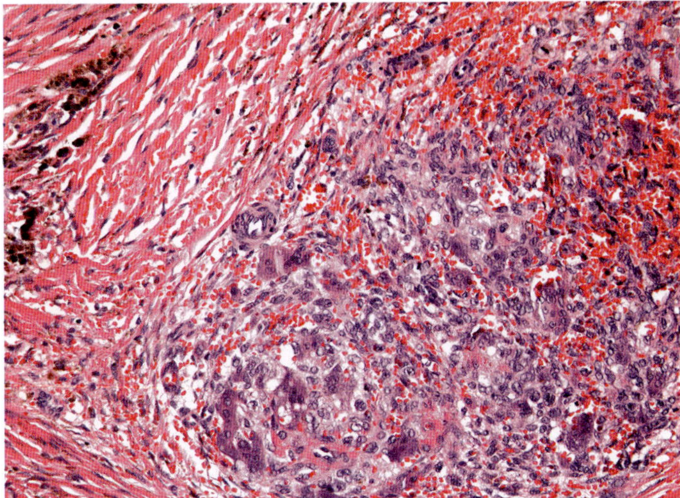

Figure 11.20 **Giant Cell Tumor of Soft Tissue.** The stroma adjacent to the nodules usually shows fibrosis and contains prominent hemosiderin deposition.

the well-defined multinodular growth pattern typical of giant cell tumor of soft tissue. Unlike giant cell tumor of soft tissue, these sarcomas contain polygonal or spindle cells with marked nuclear atypia and pleomorphic cells, admixed with osteoclast-like giant cells. Extraskeletal osteosarcoma by definition shows variably prominent "malignant osteoid" associated with cytologically malignant cells. This osteoid must be distinguished from the reactive bone commonly seen at the periphery of giant cell tumor of soft tissue: "malignant" osteoid typically surrounds individual tumor cells in a lace-like pattern, whereas the bone in giant cell tumor of soft tissue consists of woven bone with prominent osteoblastic rimming. Osteoblastic differentiation can be confirmed by nuclear SATB2 expression, although this marker does not distinguish osteosarcoma from benign mesenchymal neoplasms that produce bone.[45] Leiomyosarcoma usually has at least focal areas with typical cytoarchitectural features, including fascicles of spindle cells with brightly eosinophilic cytoplasm and broad (cigar-shaped) nuclei. Moreover, in leiomyosarcoma, SMA, desmin, and caldesmon are positive. Plexiform fibrohistiocytic tumor has a predilection for the hands and wrists and typically affects younger patients. Although the individual nodules of mononuclear cells and osteoclast-like giant cells in plexiform fibrohistiocytic tumor may mimic those in giant cell tumor of soft tissue, fibromatosis-like fascicles of myofibroblasts are observed between the nodules in plexiform fibrohistiocytic tumor, in contrast to the hemosiderin-containing dense fibrous tissue in giant cell tumor.

Prognosis and Treatment

Giant cell tumor of soft tissue has a local recurrence rate of 10% to 15%. Therefore, complete surgical excision is advisable. Lung metastases are rare and cannot be predicted based on histologic or clinical features.[43] Patients who present with large tumors showing high mitotic activity and vascular invasion should be followed carefully, and a baseline lung radiograph should be considered.

PRACTICE POINTS: Giant Cell Tumor of Soft Tissue

- Most common in dermis and subcutaneous tissue of extremities
- Histologically similar to giant cell tumor of bone
- Multinodular with nodules surrounded by dense fibrous tissue with hemosiderin deposition
- Nodules contain osteoclast-like giant cells distributed evenly among mononuclear cells with similar nuclear features as giant cells
- Surrounded by incomplete shell of bone in 50% of cases
- Vascular invasion common
- Low rate of local recurrence; rare metastasis to lung

Giant Cell–Rich Sarcomas and Histologic Mimics

The last group of tumors that are briefly discussed in this chapter include the malignant tumors rich in osteoclast-like giant cells (Box 11.2). Some of these tumors also contain highly atypical neoplastic tumor giant cells. The main tumor types in this category are undifferentiated pleomorphic sarcoma, extraskeletal osteosarcoma, leiomyosarcoma,

Box 11.2 Malignant Tumors With Prominent Osteoclast-Like Giant Cells

- Undifferentiated pleomorphic sarcoma
- Extraskeletal osteosarcoma
- Leiomyosarcoma
- Anaplastic carcinoma
- Anaplastic large cell lymphoma

anaplastic carcinoma, and large cell lymphomas (especially anaplastic large cell lymphoma). Pleomorphic sarcomas are discussed in more detail in Chapter 7. In general, these tumors affect older adults (with the exception of anaplastic large cell lymphoma, which has a predilection for children and young adults). Careful microscopic examination is essential to identify (1) better differentiated areas within an otherwise highly pleomorphic (nondistinctive) background, and (2) other (sometimes subtle) histologic clues to the proper diagnosis. Immunohistochemistry plays a critical role in the diagnosis of most of these tumor types. Giant cell–rich undifferentiated pleomorphic sarcoma (formerly known as *giant cell malignant fibrous histiocytoma*, or MFH) is a diagnosis of exclusion. This diagnosis should not be made until other pleomorphic sarcomas (and nonmesenchymal neoplasms) are excluded by both immunohistochemistry and extensive sampling (e.g., to identify foci of "malignant" osteoid).

Clinical Features

Exact clinical data for giant cell–rich sarcomas are difficult to obtain, given the diverse tumor types formerly included in this group. However, the majority of tumors in this general category occur in the deep soft tissues of the limbs and trunk of older adults with no gender predilection. Most such tumors present as large, painless masses. Tumors showing essentially indistinguishable morphology but arising in visceral organs, including the lung, thyroid gland, pancreas, breast, and kidney represent (in large part) giant cell–rich anaplastic carcinomas.

Pathologic Features

Histologically, giant cell–rich sarcomas are composed of osteoclast-like giant cells admixed with ovoid to spindle-shaped or epithelioid tumor cells showing nuclear hyperchromasia; vesicular nuclei with prominent nucleoli; pleomorphism; and mitotic activity, including atypical forms. The (non-neoplastic) osteoclast-like giant cells lack cytologic features of malignancy. Therefore, careful examination of the tumor cells admixed with the osteoclast-like giant cells is essential to determine whether a lesion is benign or malignant.

Neoplastic tumor giant cells (with unequivocal cytologic features of malignancy) may also be seen in undifferentiated pleomorphic sarcomas, giant cell–rich carcinomas, and anaplastic large cell lymphoma. In fact, nearly any high-grade sarcoma may occasionally contain pleomorphic tumor giant cells.

As mentioned, to classify tumors with such overlapping morphologic features accurately, pathologists must carefully search for better differentiated areas. Furthermore, careful sampling of these tumors is mandatory. The following paragraphs focus on the main tumor types showing this morphologic pattern, which should be considered before diagnosing a giant cell–rich undifferentiated sarcoma.

Giant Cell–Rich Extraskeletal Osteosarcoma. Before the diagnosis of a primary osteosarcoma of soft tissue is rendered, involvement of an underlying bone should be excluded by imaging studies. The hallmark of extraskeletal osteosarcoma is the production of "malignant" osteoid laid down by tumor cells, most typically in a lace-like pattern (Fig. 11.21).

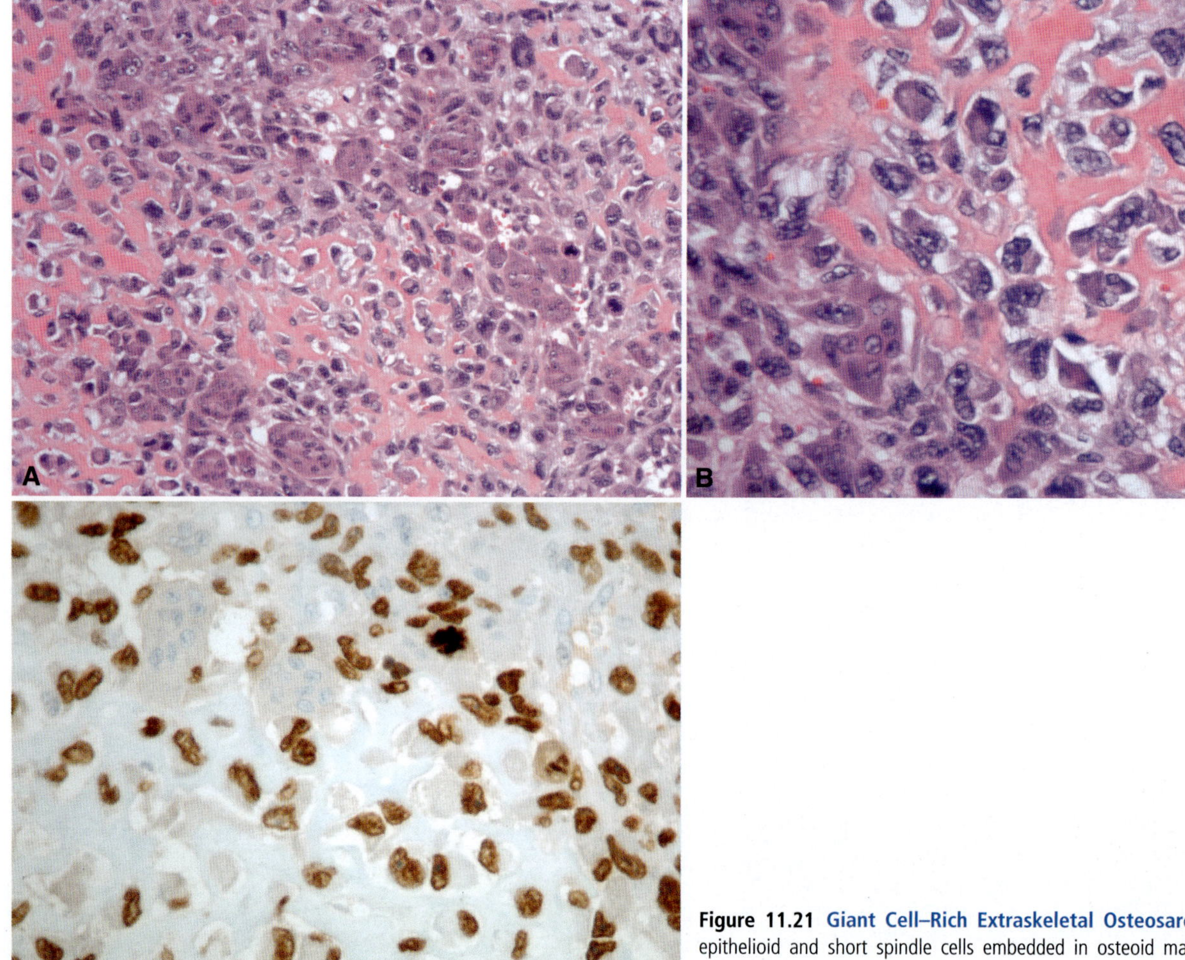

Figure 11.21 **Giant Cell–Rich Extraskeletal Osteosarcoma.** Highly atypical epithelioid and short spindle cells embedded in osteoid matrix are admixed with clusters of osteoclast-like giant cells (A). Osteoid surrounds tumor cells in a lace-like pattern (B). SATB2 shows strong nuclear staining in tumor cells (C).

Interestingly, osteoid production is often most abundant in the less cellular, central portion of the tumor. Toward the periphery of the tumor, cellularity often increases and osteoid production is scarce or absent. Extraskeletal osteosarcoma is a histologic diagnosis, and immunohistochemistry plays a limited role. Recently, nuclear SATB2 expression has been shown to be useful to demonstrate osteoblastic differentiation in soft tissue and bone tumors, particularly when the distinction between hyalinized collagen and osteoid is challenging.[45] It is important to mention that the neoplastic cells in osteosarcoma may focally express keratins, EMA, SMA, and desmin in a subset of cases, complicating accurate classification if osteoid is not readily apparent (see Chapter 14).

Leiomyosarcoma With Prominent Osteoclast-Like Giant Cells. Giant cell–rich leiomyosarcoma can be recognized by the fascicular growth pattern and the tumor cells with broad, blunt-ended (cigar-shaped) nuclei and brightly eosinophilic cytoplasm (Fig. 11.22). In addition, immunohistochemical staining for SMA, desmin, and caldesmon can help support smooth muscle differentiation (see Chapter 3).

Giant Cell–Rich Anaplastic Carcinomas. Undifferentiated carcinomas with prominent osteoclast-like giant cells presenting as soft tissue metastases should be differentiated from giant cell–rich sarcomas (Fig. 11.23A). Carcinomas with this morphologic pattern are rare and are mainly found in the pancreas, thyroid gland, lung, and breast. Clinical history of a visceral malignancy and radiologic studies can provide helpful diagnostic clues. Immunohistochemical staining for keratin is essential to render this diagnosis. It should be mentioned that the use of more than one broad-spectrum keratin (e.g., AE1/AE3, CAM5.2, and MNF116) is often required to demonstrate keratin expression, which may be limited in extent (see Fig. 11.23B).

Large Cell Lymphomas. Rarely, diffuse large B-cell lymphoma and anaplastic large cell lymphoma may contain prominent osteoclast-like giant cells and thereby mimic a giant cell–rich sarcoma. The neoplastic cells in such cases are usually dyshesive with a rounded or polygonal appearance. Immunohistochemical stains, including pan–B-cell markers (CD20, CD79a, PAX5), CD30, and anaplastic lymphoma kinase (ALK), should be performed when considering these possibilities.

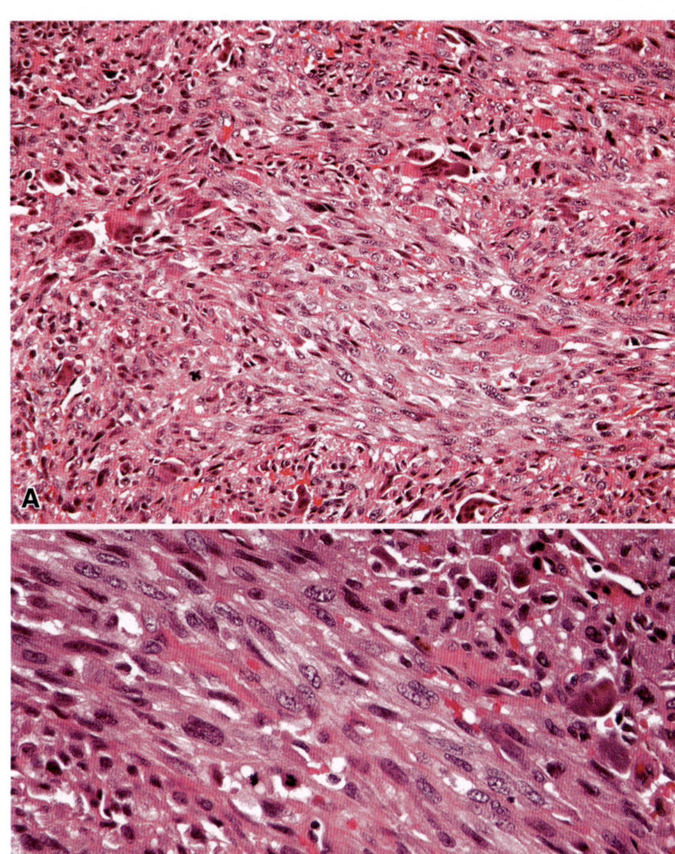

Figure 11.22 High-Grade Leiomyosarcoma With Osteoclast-Like Giant Cells. The fascicular growth pattern, brightly eosinophilic cytoplasm (A), and blunt-ended nuclei are helpful diagnostic clues (B).

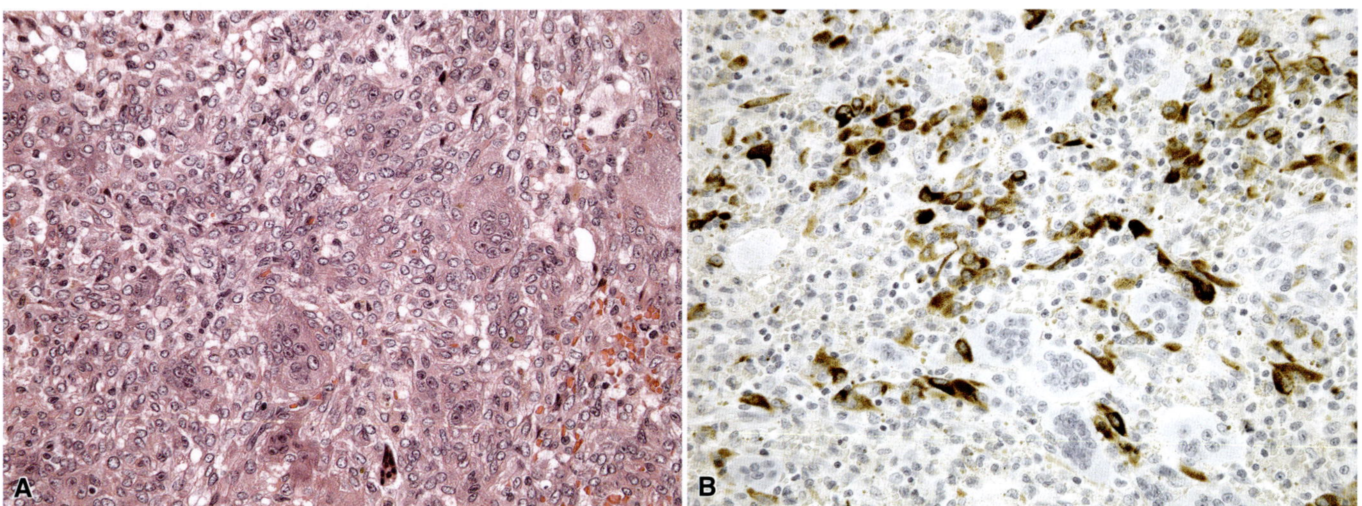

Figure 11.23 Undifferentiated Carcinoma With Osteoclast-Like Giant Cells. The tumor is composed of sheets of mononuclear cells admixed with osteoclast-like giant cells (A) Keratin expression may be relatively limited in such carcinomas (B).

References

1. Anderson JM: Multinucleated giant cells, *Curr Opin Hematol* 7:40–47, 2000.
2. Furusato E, Valenzuela IA, Fanburg-Smith JC, et al: Orbital solitary fibrous tumor: encompassing terminology for hemangiopericytoma, giant cell angiofibroma, and fibrous histiocytoma of the orbit: reappraisal of 41 cases, *Hum Pathol* 42:120–128, 2011.
3. Guillou L, Gebhard S, Coindre JM: Orbital and extraorbital giant cell angiofibroma: a giant cell-rich variant of solitary fibrous tumor? Clinicopathologic and immunohistochemical analysis of a series in favor of a unifying concept, *Am J Surg Pathol* 24:971–979, 2000.
4. Dei Tos AP, Seregard S, Calonje E, et al: Giant cell angiofibroma. A distinctive orbital tumor in adults, *Am J Surg Pathol* 19:1286–1293, 1995.
5. Magro G, Amico P, Vecchio GM, et al: Multinucleated floret-like giant cells in sporadic and NF1-associated neurofibromas: a clinicopathologic study of 94 cases, *Virchows Arch* 456:71–76, 2010.
6. Ushijima M, Hashimoto H, Tsuneyoshi M, et al: Giant cell tumor of the tendon sheath (nodular tenosynovitis). A study of 207 cases to compare the large joint group with the common digit group, *Cancer* 57:875–884, 1986.
7. Uriburu IJ, Levy VD: Intraosseous growth of giant cell tumors of the tendon sheath (localized nodular tenosynovitis) of the digits: report of 15 cases, *J Hand Surg Am* 23:732–736, 1998.
8. Monaghan H, Salter DM, Al-Nafussi A: Giant cell tumour of tendon sheath (localised nodular tenosynovitis): clinicopathological features of 71 cases, *J Clin Pathol* 54:404–407, 2001.
9. Folpe AL, Weiss SW, Fletcher CD, et al: Tenosynovial giant cell tumors: evidence for a desmin-positive dendritic cell subpopulation, *Mod Pathol* 11:939–944, 1998.
10. Boland JM, Folpe AL, Hornick JL, et al: Clusterin is expressed in normal synoviocytes and in tenosynovial giant cell tumors of localized and diffuse types: diagnostic and histogenetic implications, *Am J Surg Pathol* 33:1225–1229, 2009.
11. Dal Cin P, Sciot R, De Smet L, et al: A new cytogenetic subgroup in tenosynovial giant cell tumors (nodular tenosynovitis) is characterized by involvement of 16q24, *Cancer Genet Cytogenet* 87:85–87, 1996.
12. Dal Cin P, Sciot R, Samson I, et al: Cytogenetic characterization of tenosynovial giant cell tumors (nodular tenosynovitis), *Cancer Res* 54:3986–3987, 1994.
13. Sciot R, Rosai J, Dal Cin P, et al: Analysis of 35 cases of localized and diffuse tenosynovial giant cell tumor: a report from the Chromosomes and Morphology (CHAMP) study group, *Mod Pathol* 12:576–579, 1999.
14. West RB, Rubin BP, Miller MA, et al: A landscape effect in tenosynovial giant-cell tumor from activation of CSF1 expression by a translocation in a minority of tumor cells, *Proc Natl Acad Sci USA* 103:690–695, 2006.
15. Cupp JS, Miller MA, Montgomery KD, et al: Translocation and expression of CSF1 in pigmented villonodular synovitis, tenosynovial giant cell tumor, rheumatoid arthritis and other reactive synovitides, *Am J Surg Pathol* 31:970–976, 2007.
16. Furlong MA, Motamedi K, Laskin WB, et al: Synovial-type giant cell tumors of the vertebral column: a clinicopathologic study of 15 cases, with a review of the literature and discussion of the differential diagnosis, *Hum Pathol* 34:670–679, 2003.
17. Giannini C, Scheithauer BW, Wenger DE, et al: Pigmented villonodular synovitis of the spine: a clinical, radiological, and morphological study of 12 cases, *J Neurosurg* 84:592–597, 1996.
18. Schwartz HS, Unni KK, Pritchard DJ: Pigmented villonodular synovitis. A retrospective review of affected large joints, *Clin Orthop Relat Res* 243–255, 1989.
19. Ushijima M, Hashimoto H, Tsuneyoshi M, et al: Pigmented villonodular synovitis. A clinicopathologic study of 52 cases, *Acta Pathol Jpn* 36:317–326, 1986.
20. Myers B, Masi A: Pigmented villonodular synovitis and tenosynovitis: a clinical epidemiologic study of 166 cases and review of the literature, *Medicine (Baltimore)* 59:223–238, 1980.
21. Somerhausen NS, Fletcher CD: Diffuse-type giant cell tumor: clinicopathologic and immunohistochemical analysis of 50 cases with extraarticular disease, *Am J Surg Pathol* 24:479–492, 2000.
22. Shabat S, Kollender Y, Merimsky O, et al: The use of surgery and yttrium 90 in the management of extensive and diffuse pigmented villonodular synovitis of large joints, *Rheumatology (Oxford)* 41:1113–1118, 2002.
23. Oda Y, Izumi T, Harimaya K, et al: Pigmented villonodular synovitis with chondroid metaplasia, resembling chondroblastoma of the bone: a report of three cases, *Mod Pathol* 20:545–551, 2007.
24. Hoch L, Garcia RA, Smalberger GJ: Chondroid tenosynovial giant cell tumor: a clinicopathological and immunohistochemical analysis of 5 new cases, *Int J Surg Pathol* 19:180–187, 2011.
25. Abdul-Karim FW, el-Naggar AK, Joyce MJ, et al: Diffuse and localized tenosynovial giant cell tumor and pigmented villonodular synovitis: a clinicopathologic and flow cytometric DNA analysis, *Hum Pathol* 23:729–735, 1992.
26. Fletcher JA, Henkle C, Atkins L, et al: Trisomy 5 and trisomy 7 are nonrandom aberrations in pigmented villonodular synovitis: confirmation of trisomy 7 in uncultured cells, *Genes Chromosomes Cancer* 4:264–266, 1992.
27. Panagopoulos I, Brandal P, Gorunova L, et al: Novel CSF1-S100A10 fusion gene and CSF1 transcript identified by RNA sequencing in tenosynovial giant cell tumors, *Int J Oncol* 44:1425–1432, 2014.
28. Nishio J, Kamachi Y, Iwasaki H, et al: Diffuse-type giant cell tumor with t(1;17)(p13;p13) and trisomy 5, *In Vivo* 28:949–952, 2014.
29. Chin KR, Barr SJ, Winalski C, et al: Treatment of advanced primary and recurrent diffuse pigmented villonodular synovitis of the knee, *J Bone Joint Surg Am* 84-A:2192–2202, 2002.
30. Staals EL, Ferrari S, Donati DM, et al: Diffuse-type tenosynovial giant cell tumour: current treatment concepts and future perspectives, *Eur J Cancer* 63:34–40, 2016.
31. Cassier PA, Gelderblom H, Stacchiotti S, et al: Efficacy of imatinib mesylate for the treatment of locally advanced and/or metastatic tenosynovial giant cell tumor/pigmented villonodular synovitis, *Cancer* 118:1649–1655, 2012.
32. Bertoni F, Unni KK, Beabout JW, et al: Malignant giant cell tumor of the tendon sheaths and joints (malignant pigmented villonodular synovitis), *Am J Surg Pathol* 21:153–163, 1997.
33. Ushijima M, Hashimoto H, Tsuneyoshi M, et al: Malignant giant cell tumor of tendon sheath. Report of a case, *Acta Pathol Jpn* 35:699–709, 1985.
34. Li CF, Wang JW, Huang WW, et al: Malignant diffuse-type tenosynovial giant cell tumors: a series of 7 cases comparing with 24 benign lesions with review of the literature, *Am J Surg Pathol* 32:587–599, 2008.
35. Huang HY, West RB, Tzeng CC, et al: Immunohistochemical and biogenetic features of diffuse-type tenosynovial giant cell tumors: the potential roles of cyclin A, P53, and deletion of 15q in sarcomatous transformation, *Clin Cancer Res* 14:6023–6032, 2008.
36. Enzinger FM, Zhang RY: Plexiform fibrohistiocytic tumor presenting in children and young adults. An analysis of 65 cases, *Am J Surg Pathol* 12:818–826, 1988.
37. Hollowood K, Holley MP, Fletcher CD: Plexiform fibrohistiocytic tumour: clinicopathological, immunohistochemical and ultrastructural analysis in favour of a myofibroblastic lesion, *Histopathology* 19:503–513, 1991.
38. Remstein ED, Arndt CA, Nascimento AG: Plexiform fibrohistiocytic tumor: clinicopathologic analysis of 22 cases, *Am J Surg Pathol* 23:662–670, 1999.
39. Moosavi C, Jha P, Fanburg-Smith JC: An update on plexiform fibrohistiocytic tumor and addition of 66 new cases from the Armed Forces Institute of Pathology, in honor of Franz M. Enzinger, MD, *Ann Diagn Pathol* 11:313–319, 2007.
40. Fox MD, Billings SD, Gleason BC, et al: Expression of MiTF may be helpful in differentiating cellular neurothekeoma from plexiform fibrohistiocytic tumor (histiocytoid predominant) in a partial biopsy specimen, *Am J Dermatopathol* 34:157–160, 2012.
41. Folpe AL, Morris RJ, Weiss SW: Soft tissue giant cell tumor of low malignant potential: a proposal for the reclassification of malignant giant cell tumor of soft parts, *Mod Pathol* 12:894–902, 1999.
42. O'Connell JX, Wehrli BM, Nielsen GP, et al: Giant cell tumors of soft tissue: a clinicopathologic study of 18 benign and malignant tumors, *Am J Surg Pathol* 24:386–395, 2000.
43. Oliveira AM, Dei Tos AP, Fletcher CD, et al: Primary giant cell tumor of soft tissues: a study of 22 cases, *Am J Surg Pathol* 24:248–256, 2000.
44. Lee JC, Liang CW, Fletcher CD: Giant cell tumor of soft tissue is genetically distinct from its bone counterpart, *Mod Pathol* 30:728–733, 2017.
45. Conner JR, Hornick JL: SATB2 is a novel marker of osteoblastic differentiation in bone and soft tissue tumors, *Histopathology* 63:36–49, 2013.

12

Adipocytic Tumors

Marta Sbaraglia, MD, and Angelo Paolo Dei Tos, MD

Adipocytic tumors represent an extremely heterogeneous category of clinically and morphologically distinctive lesions, sharing variable amounts of lipomatous differentiation. Some of them (i.e., benign lipomas and well-differentiated liposarcoma [WDLPS]) are among the most commonly encountered mesenchymal neoplasms. As will be discussed in depth, diagnostic criteria have been evolving constantly, in part because of the contribution of cytogenetics and molecular genetics. These techniques have not only offered insights into the pathogenesis of many lesions but also have become valuable confirmatory diagnostic tools because the vast majority of the entities discussed in this chapter harbor specific chromosomal abnormalities.

Many adipocytic tumors present diagnostic challenges. Diagnostic difficulties are caused by the rarity of some entities (e.g., chondroid lipoma) as well as the significant morphologic overlap among these clinically and biologically distinctive lesions (e.g., benign lipoma and atypical lipomatous tumor [ALT]/WDLPS). Another potential source of diagnostic confusion has been generated by inconsistent application of terminology that has led to a significant degree of uncertainty among both pathologists and clinicians. The previous classification of mesenchymal tumors issued by the World Health Organization (WHO) in 2002 has offered semantic clarifications that are useful to enumerate.[1] First of all, it has been made clear that the terms ALT and WDLPS are synonyms because they refer to lesions that are identical morphologically and genetically. The use of one term rather than the other depends only on the anatomic location. For surgically amenable lesions, the less aggressive designation ALT is preferable, whereas the term WDLPS is used when dealing with deep-seated masses at central body sites, such as the retroperitoneum, mediastinum, and spermatic cord.

The current classification of mesenchymal tumors, issued by the WHO in 2013, has introduced minimal changes in the category of adipocytic tumors, among which are: (1) the abolition of the term "round cell liposarcoma" (in 2002 the entity had already been incorporated into the myxoid liposarcoma category), recognizing the fact that it merely represents an inaccurate description of high-grade myxoid liposarcoma; and (2) the deletion of the label "mixed type liposarcoma," as it most likely corresponds to unusual morphological patterns (most often myxofibrosarcoma-like) of dedifferentiated liposarcoma.[2]

As has already been alluded to, the interplay between morphology and genetics has greatly contributed to the field of adipocytic neoplasia, and the diagnostic workup of fatty tumors in some cases may incorporate both conventional cytogenetics and molecular genetics. However, unsophisticated techniques, such as gross sampling and microscopic examination of hematoxylin and eosin–stained slides, still represent the diagnostic mainstay in this group of tumors. The importance of proper gross sampling will be discussed in depth whenever relevant, but in general, gross examination should not be delegated to inexperienced individuals because this may hamper the diagnostic process. In addition, proper orientation of the surgical specimen (best if performed with the surgeon) and identification of the closest margins are key steps that should be performed accurately.

Last but not least, proper classification (inclusive of molecular data) may play a fundamental role in predicting the response to innovative therapeutic approaches. For example, molecular targeting of MDM2 and or CDK4-expressing neoplasms (e.g., dedifferentiated liposarcoma) and the exquisite sensitivity of myxoid liposarcoma to the relatively new compound trabectedin show the importance of correct partitioning of liposarcomas.

Lipoma

Benign solitary lipoma, a proliferation of mature white fat, is the most commonly encountered human mesenchymal neoplasm. In a small fraction of patients (~5% of all benign lipomatous tumors), lipomas present as multiple lesions. This condition is generally kept distinct from lipomatosis, an even rarer disease in which a diffuse overgrowth of fatty tissue is observed.

Clinical Features

Benign lipoma most often occurs as a subcutaneous solitary mass in adults between the fourth and sixth decades. Men are more frequently affected than women,[3,4] and obese patients tend to have lipomas with higher frequency than the normal population. Lipomas can arise at any anatomic location and can involve both superficial and deep soft tissues. Not infrequently, they can occur within or between skeletal muscles, in which case they are labeled as *intramuscular* and *intermuscular* lipomas, respectively.[5,6] The most frequently affected anatomic sites for this subgroup are the large muscles of the thigh, shoulder, and upper arm. Benign lipomas can also be encountered in the head and neck region[7] and at visceral sites in the submucosa of the small and large bowel. More rarely, lipomas can be observed in the respiratory tract.[8] Specific subsets of lipomas are represented by dermal lipoma[9] and synovial lipoma.[10] Dermal lipomas most often occur as pedunculated, skin tag–like lesions. When they are multiple and located around the lower limb girdle, the term *nevus lipomatosus superficialis* has traditionally been applied (see also Chapter 15). Synovial lipoma is also known as *lipoma arborescens*, a designation that reflects the villous-like gross appearance of this lesion arising in the joint space. Synovial lipoma occurs in adults and is almost always associated with inflammation and synovial hyperplasia. Both features support the possible reactive nature of this distinctive lipomatous proliferation. Very rarely, benign lipomas present as primary intraosseous lesions.[11] In principle, a diagnosis of benign lipoma in the abdomen or retroperitoneum should be made with extreme caution and with the support of ancillary techniques.[12] Common experience shows that most often those lesions actually represent WDLPS.

Clinically, most solitary lipomas present as a painless mass of long duration. Multicentricity is observed in approximately 5% of patients. Multiple lipomas tend to cluster in the upper half of the body. Interestingly, one third of the patients presenting with multiple lipomas appear to inherit the disorder in an autosomal dominant manner.[13]

Rarely, patients present with a diffuse overgrowth of morphologically benign adipose tissue known as *lipomatosis* that most often affects the extremities and the trunk. Clinically, lipomatosis is subclassified into symmetric, asymmetric, pelvic, and mediastino-abdominal forms.[14–18] Symmetric lipomatosis, also known as *Madelung disease* or *Launois-Bensaude syndrome*, most often affects adult patients of Mediterranean origin. Clinically, it presents as a massive, ill-defined lipomatous overgrowth localized at the neck and extending deeply into the muscular structures of the region. Asymmetric lipomatosis affects large portions of the extremities, the trunk, and rarely the viscera, and may be associated with gigantism of the involved anatomic segment. Pelvic lipomatosis is characterized by a diffuse adipose tissue overgrowth in the pelvic region associated with compression of the urinary tract, sigmoid colon, and rectum.

Pathologic Features

Grossly, solitary benign lipomas are usually well circumscribed, are surrounded by a thin capsule, and feature a yellow cut surface. Maximum size depends on the anatomic location and ranges from 1 cm to 5 cm for superficial lesions, whereas deep-seated lesions may attain larger dimensions.

The microscopic hallmark of benign lipomas is a uniform proliferation of mature adipocytes with minimal or no variation in size and shape (Fig. 12.1). Secondary changes are relatively frequent, including foci of fibrosis and microscopic fat necrosis, with foamy histiocytes and multinucleated giant cells (Fig. 12.2). Occasionally, metaplastic bone or cartilage (*osteolipoma* and *chondrolipoma*), as well as extramedullary hematopoiesis, can be observed. Lipomas can contain fibrous tissue and show myxoid change to the extent that the use of terms such as *fibrolipoma* and *myxolipoma*, respectively, can be justified. Intramuscular lipomas harbor skeletal muscle fibers showing variable degrees of atrophy (Fig. 12.3). Most intramuscular lipomas are infiltrative, whereas a minority (not exceeding 10%) of these tumors appear to be well demarcated. The same diagnostic criteria used for ordinary lipomas must be applied, and it is of particular importance to exclude nuclear atypia in both adipocytes and stromal cells, all features favoring a diagnosis of ALT/WDLPS.

Immunohistochemistry

Benign lipomas are diffusely positive for S-100 protein; however, this finding is not diagnostically relevant.

Molecular Genetics

Solitary benign lipomas feature an abnormal karyotype in approximately half of cases.[19] Three main categories are identified: (1) rearrangements of the 12q13-15 region mostly with 3q22; (2) deletion of 13q; and (3) rearrangement of 6p21-23. The target gene in 12q13-15 is *HMGA2*, which encodes a member of the high-mobility group (HMG) protein family.[20,21]

Differential Diagnosis

The diagnosis of benign lipomas (including intra- and intermuscular forms) is usually straightforward. However, the distinction from the adipocytic variant of ALT/WDLPS can occasionally be difficult. Diagnostic clues favoring a diagnosis of lipoma are the complete absence of cytologic atypia in both adipocytes and stromal cells as well as the uniform size of fat cells. The absence of lipoblasts (i.e., uni- or multivacuolated cells harboring a hyperchromatic, atypical scalloped nucleus) is not a helpful finding, because lipoblasts can be absent in ALT/WDLPS. A relatively common diagnostic pitfall is the presence of fat necrosis, a condition in which significant variation in cell size is observed as a consequence of inflammation (Fig. 12.4). Therefore, the differential diagnosis with ALT/WDLPS can be raised. The presence of foamy histiocytes as well as occasional multinucleated giant cells and the absence of nuclear atypia are the two most important diagnostic criteria. In addition, MDM2/CDK4 overexpression and amplification are never observed in benign lipomas, whereas they are usually present in ALT/WDLPS. Evaluation of MDM2 immunohistochemistry in differentiated adipocytic neoplasms is sometimes challenging; it has been suggested that in such cases fluorescence in situ hybridization (FISH) analysis may be a more valuable diagnostic tool.[22]

Not infrequently, intramuscular lipoma must be distinguished from intramuscular angioma (see Chapter 13), which, in addition to a complex vascular network, frequently features a prominent adipocytic component and fatty atrophy of muscle fibers, leading to diagnostic confusion (Fig. 12.5). The recognition of the abnormal vascular component is the most important diagnostic clue.

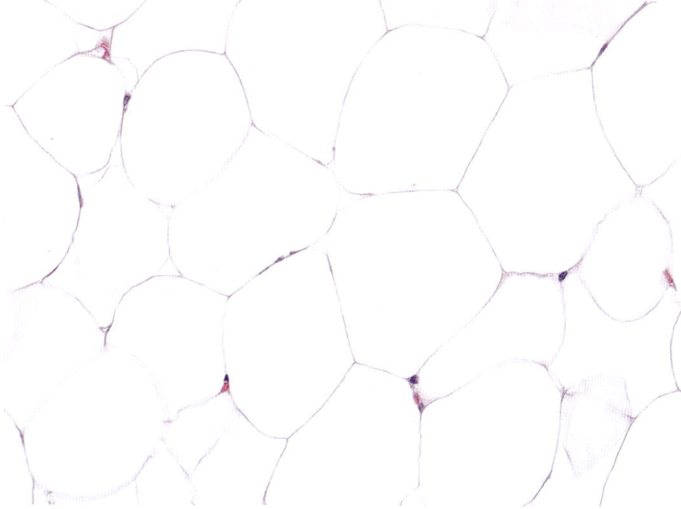

Figure 12.1 **Benign Lipoma.** Benign lipoma is characterized by uniformity of adipocytes with minimal or no variation in size and shape.

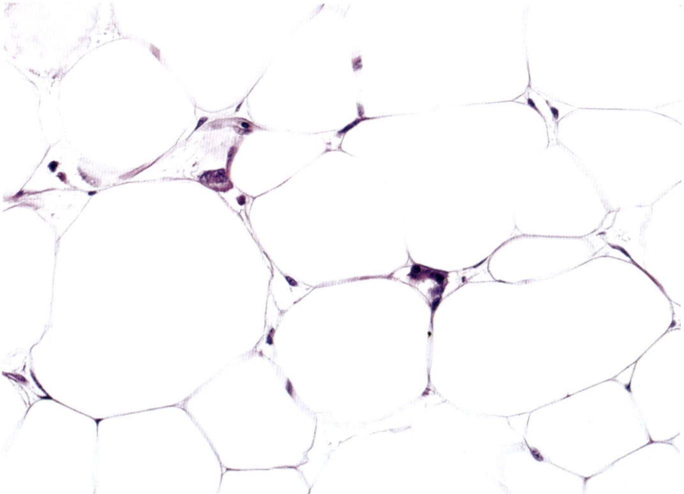

Figure 12.2 **Benign Lipoma.** Multinucleated giant cells are frequently seen with fat necrosis.

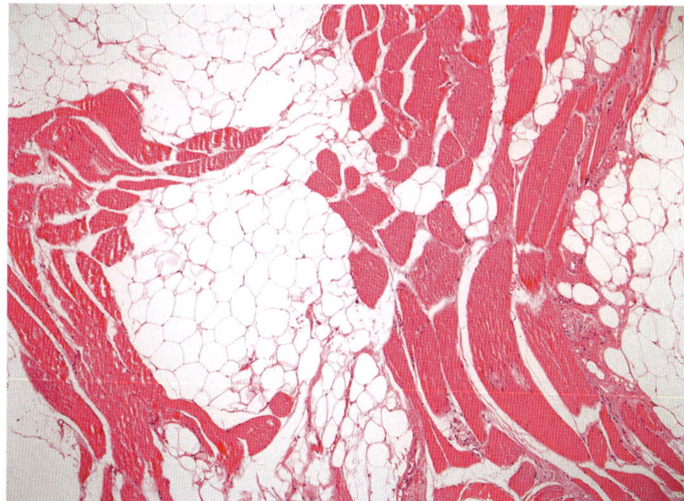

Figure 12.3 **Intramuscular Lipoma.** Striated muscle cells are separated by a mature adipocytic proliferation.

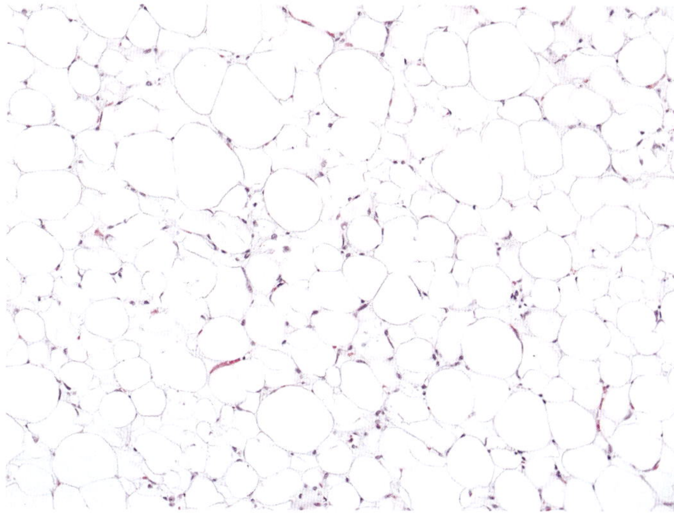

Figure 12.4 **Fat Necrosis.** Significant variation in cell size is observed with fat necrosis, representing a potential diagnostic pitfall.

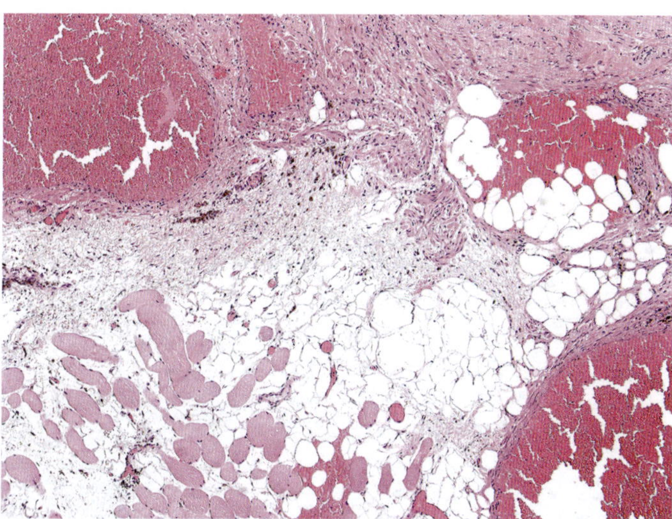

Figure 12.5 **Intramuscular Angioma.** A prominent adipocytic component and extensive fatty atrophy of muscle fibers are frequently seen in intramuscular angioma.

Prognosis and Treatment

Lipomas are benign mesenchymal lesions whose complete local excision is curative. A 5% local recurrence rate is reported. In contrast, intramuscular lipomas are characterized by a significant incidence of local recurrence (approximately 20%) that can be avoided only by complete removal of the involved muscle.

Lipofibromatosis

Lipofibromatosis is a diffuse spindle cell proliferation typically occurring in childhood that is associated with a mature adipocytic component. Lipofibromatosis should be kept separate from the clinically, morphologically, and genetically distinct entity known as *infantile (desmoid) fibromatosis* (see Chapter 4).

Clinical Features

Clinically, lipofibromatosis occurs in the pediatric population, with a peak incidence in the first decade. Not infrequently, this lesion can be detected at birth. The most common anatomic locations are the hand and upper and lower limbs, followed by the feet, trunk, and head and neck region. In the original description by Fetsch and colleagues, patient age ranged from 11 days to 12 years, with a median age of 1 year.[23] Occasionally, an association with macrodactyly has been reported.

Pathologic Features

Grossly, lipofibromatosis tends to be poorly circumscribed, with a yellow-gray, variegated cut surface. Histologically, a spindle cell fibroblastic or myofibroblastic proliferation organized in fascicles is observed (Fig. 12.6). Neoplastic cells tend to grow along fibrous septa and are associated with an abundant adipocytic component (Fig. 12.7). Cytologic atypia is generally absent.

Immunohistochemistry

Immunohistochemistry does not play a major role in the diagnosis of lipofibromatosis. Variable, focal immunoreactivity for CD99, CD34, α-smooth muscle actin, bcl-2, and less frequently, S-100 protein has been reported, whereas desmin is negative.

Molecular Genetics

A three-way t(4;9;6) translocation has been reported in a single case of lipofibromatosis.[24]

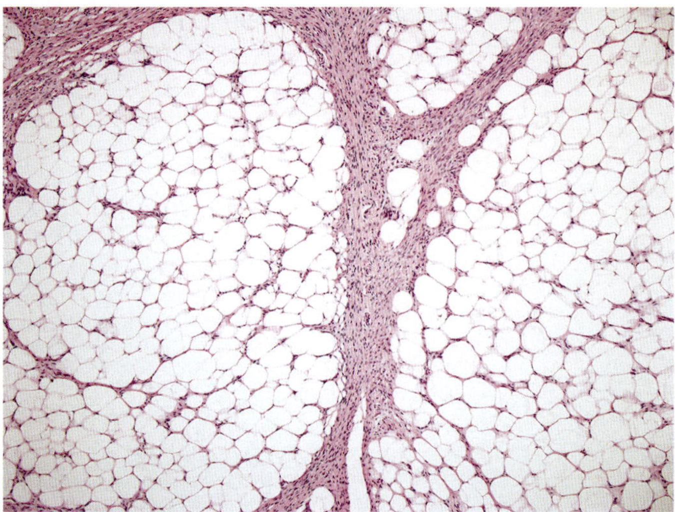

Figure 12.6 Lipofibromatosis. Fascicles of cytologically bland spindle cells are typical of lipofibromatosis.

Differential Diagnosis

The differential diagnosis includes fibrous hamartoma of infancy and desmoid fibromatosis. Lipofibromatosis lacks the distinctive organoid growth pattern, with primitive, myxoid nodules, characteristic of fibrous hamartoma. Desmoid fibromatosis lacks the adipocytic component of lipofibromatosis and is characterized by long fascicles of uniform spindle cells set in a heavily collagenous stroma. Nuclear immunopositivity for β-catenin is frequently observed in desmoid fibromatosis, which is helpful for confirming the diagnosis. Recently, a group of locally aggressive soft tissue tumors of children and young adults with distinctive lipofibromatosis-like morphology, S-100 protein immunopositivity, and *NTRK1* gene fusions has been described.[25]

Prognosis and Treatment

Persistent disease or nondestructive local recurrence is observed in more than two thirds of cases of lipofibromatosis and seems to correlate with congenital onset, distal anatomic location, incomplete excision, and possibly mitotic activity in the spindle cell component.

Lipomatosis of Nerve

Lipomatosis of nerve, also known as *fibrolipomatous hamartoma of nerve* or *neural fibrolipoma*, is a fibrolipomatous proliferation of epineurium most often occurring in the median nerve, with consequent enlargement of the affected anatomic compartment.

Clinical Features

Lipomatosis of nerve most often arises in the median nerve (followed by the ulnar, radial, peroneal, and cranial nerves) of young adults, with a peak incidence between the first and third decades; however, it can be present at birth.[26–28] Approximately one third of affected patients show macrodactyly. Expansion of the lesion is associated with compression neuropathy, causing local pain in half of affected patients.

Pathologic Features

Grossly, a soft, fusiform enlargement of the affected nerve and its branches is seen, with a yellow cut surface as a consequence of the abundant adipocytic component. Histologically, a mature adipocytic proliferation, variably associated with a fibrous component, infiltrates and expands the epineurial and perineurial compartments of the affected nerves (Figs. 12.8 and 12.9). Concentric perineurial fibrosis is invariably present,

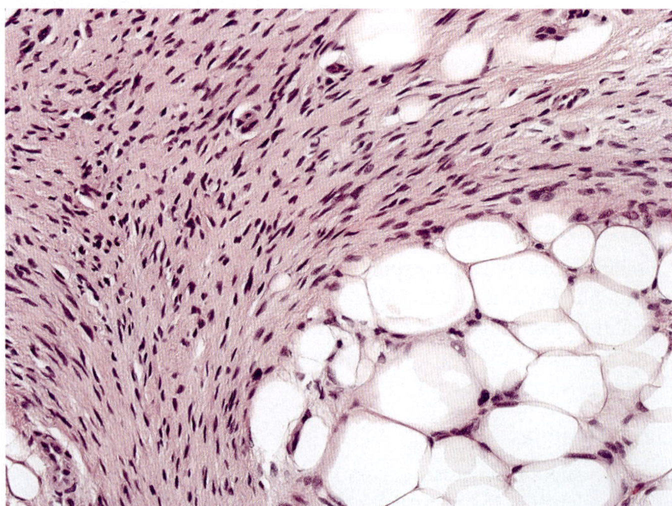

Figure 12.7 Lipofibromatosis. Spindle cells are always associated with a mature adipocytic component.

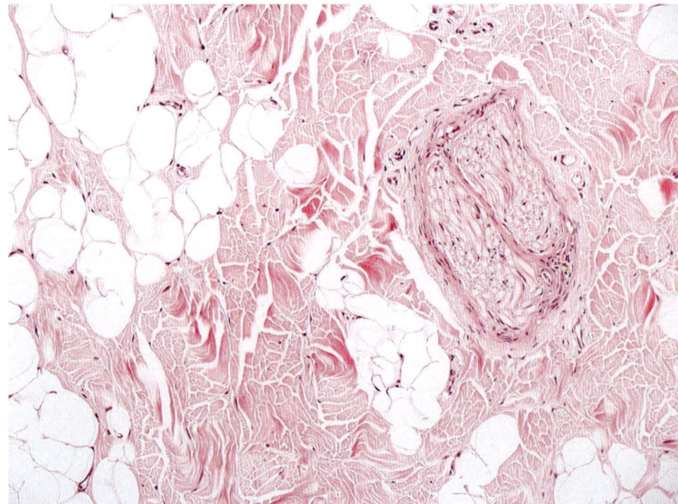

Figure 12.8 Lipomatosis of Nerve. An adipocytic proliferation expands the epi/perineurial compartment of the affected nerve.

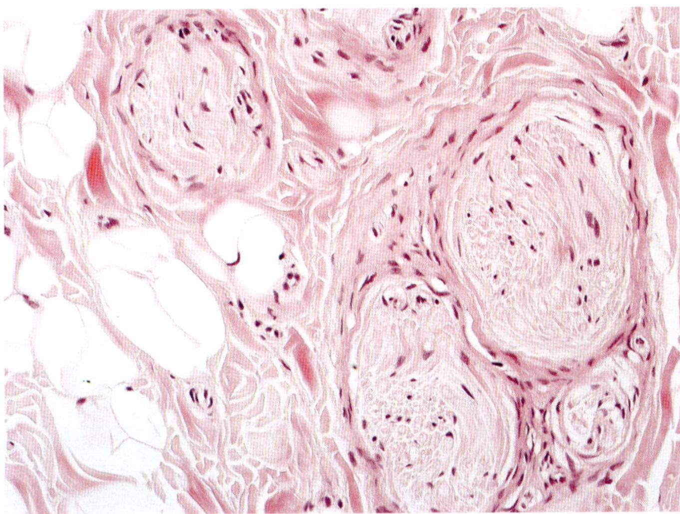

Figure 12.9 Lipomatosis of Nerve. Mature adipose tissue surrounds nerve bundles.

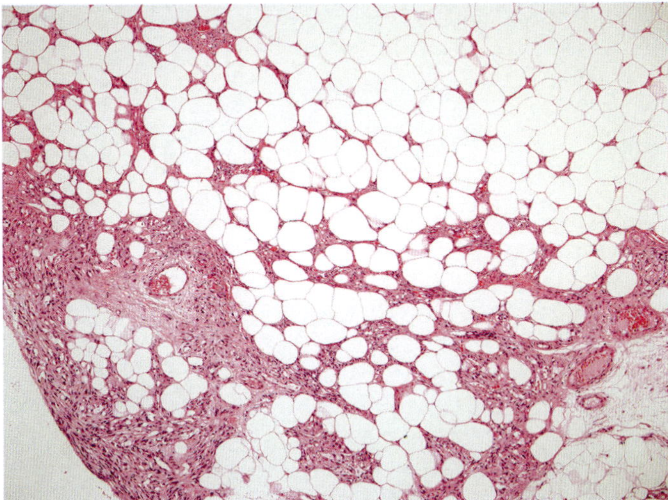

Figure 12.10 Angiolipoma. A mature adipocytic proliferation is associated with a capillary-sized vascular component.

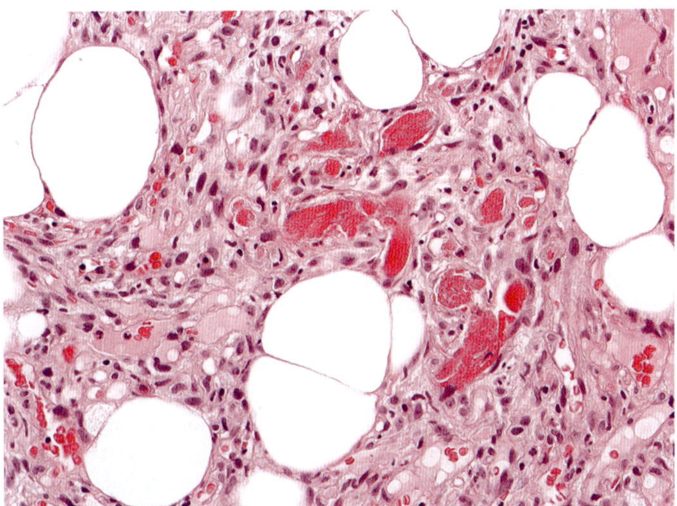

Figure 12.11 Angiolipoma. Characteristic fibrin microthrombi are seen.

whereas microfasciculation ("pseudo-onion bulb" formation, in which perineurial cells grow in concentric layers surrounding axons) is more rarely encountered.

Immunohistochemistry

Immunohistochemistry is helpful only to highlight the various components of nerve fibers and the absence of proliferation of the neural/perineurial component, which instead tends to appear atrophic.

Differential Diagnosis

Microfasciculation may occasionally raise the differential diagnosis of intraneural perineurioma, a rare, distinctive clinicopathologic entity characterized by an intraneural neoplastic proliferation of epithelial membrane antigen (EMA)–positive perineurial cells, most often arising in the upper extremities of young adults.

Prognosis and Treatment

Lipomatosis of nerve is a benign lesion whose local excision may lead to severe functional damage, sometimes greater than that generated by the disease itself. Conservative, nerve-sparing surgical approaches are therefore recommended.

Angiolipoma

Angiolipoma is a relatively common, small, benign subcutaneous adipocytic lesion with a variably prominent capillary-sized vascular network. Patients frequently present with multiple lesions that can be painful, especially on palpation.

Clinical Features

Angiolipoma usually occurs as multiple (solitary in only one third of patients), painful subcutaneous nodules, most often arising in the upper limbs (approximately two thirds are seen in the forearm), trunk, and lower limbs of young adults.[29,30] Angiolipomas most often occur sporadically, but in a minority of cases a family history can be identified.[31]

Peak incidence is between the second and third decades. They most frequently affect men. Deep-seated lesions, in the past called *infiltrating angiolipomas*, instead represent intramuscular angioma, a lesion in which an adipocytic component is frequently observed (see Chapter 13).[32]

Pathologic Features

Grossly, angiolipomas are well-circumscribed, encapsulated nodular lesions, most often smaller than 2 cm. The cut surface shows variation in color from yellow to red, depending on the relative proportions of adipocytic and vascular components. Histologically, angiolipomas have a mature adipocytic proliferation variably associated with a vascular component. The vascular network is predominantly composed of a capillary-sized proliferation that tends to be more prominent at the periphery (Fig. 12.10). Characteristically, the blood vessels contain fibrin microthrombi, an almost unique morphologic feature of angiolipoma (Fig. 12.11). The amount of capillary proliferation can vary from minimal to predominant *(cellular angiolipoma)*, and the adipocytic nature of the lesion may be overlooked (Fig. 12.12).[33]

Immunohistochemistry

S-100 protein immunopositivity is observed in the adipocytic component, whereas endothelial markers, such as CD31 and CD34, highlight the capillary network. However, immunohistochemistry generally does not play a role in the diagnosis.

Molecular Genetics

Cytogenetically, angiolipomas are almost unique among adipocytic neoplasms because they are the only entity in which the search for

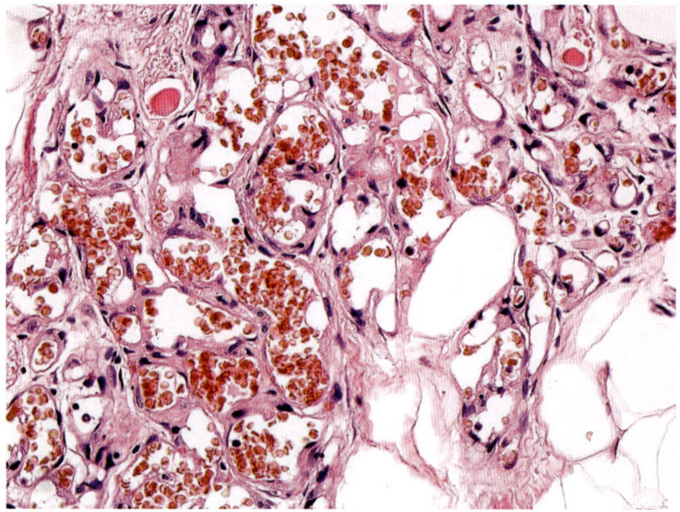

Figure 12.12 Cellular Angiolipoma. Sometimes a predominant vascular component overshadows the adipocytic nature of the lesion.

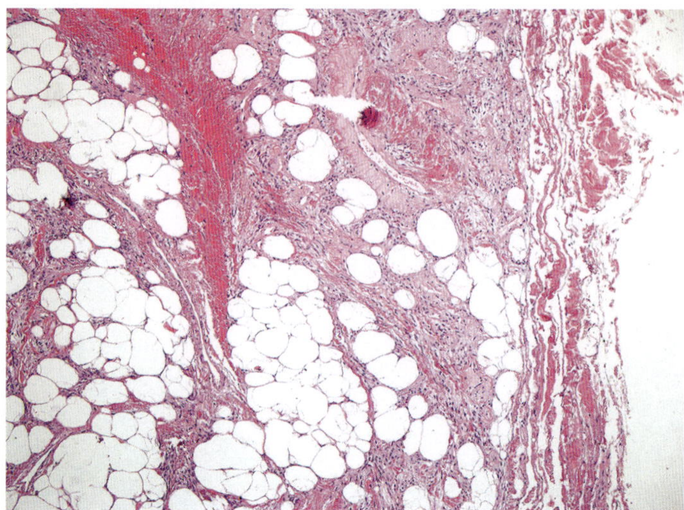

Figure 12.13 Spindle Cell Lipoma. Spindle cell lipoma is well circumscribed and is composed of bland spindle cells admixed with mature adipocytes.

karyotypic abnormalities has failed.[34] The only exception is one case in which a t(X;2) has been documented in 1 of 5 angiolipomas.[35] A recent study identified frequent *PRKD2* mutations in angiolipomas.[35a]

Differential Diagnosis

Clinically, local pain is observed not only in angiolipoma but also in other histologically unrelated subcutaneous nodular lesions, such as angioleiomyoma, eccrine spiradenoma, schwannoma, and glomus tumor ("five painful nodules of the subcutis"). Histologically, most diagnostic difficulties arise with lesions lying at the extremes of the morphologic spectrum, in which the vascular component can be minimal, and therefore overlooked, or predominant (cellular angiolipoma) to the extent that a capillary hemangioma or even Kaposi sarcoma may be considered in the differential diagnosis. Lack of immunostaining for human herpesvirus-8 (HHV8) is particularly useful in excluding Kaposi sarcoma.

Prognosis and Treatment

Angiolipomas are benign lesions. Local excision is curative, with no recurrences reported.

Spindle Cell/Pleomorphic Lipoma

Spindle cell lipoma and pleomorphic lipoma have been generally regarded as separate (but related) entities. However, the concept that spindle cell/pleomorphic lipoma actually represents a spectrum of benign adipocytic neoplasms, all sharing clinical, morphologic, immunophenotypic, and genetic features, has recently gained broad acceptance. In the past, some confusion was generated by the use of the term *atypical lipoma* as a synonym for pleomorphic lipoma. As mentioned, the terms *atypical lipoma* and ALT are alternative designations for WDLPS arising in surgically amenable soft tissue sites. ALT/WDLPS is clinically, morphologically, and genetically distinct from pleomorphic lipoma.

Clinical Features

Spindle cell/pleomorphic lipoma typically occurs as a painless subcutaneous mass, most often less than 5 cm in diameter, located on the posterior aspect of the neck or upper back of middle-aged men (men outnumbering women 10:1), with a peak incidence between the fourth and fifth decades.[36–40] The face, orbital region, and oral cavity are more rarely affected.[41,42] Uncommonly, spindle cell lipoma can be observed at a purely dermal location (see Chapter 15), which shows a more ubiquitous anatomic distribution.[43] Subcutaneous spindle cell/pleomorphic lipoma has rarely been diagnosed outside the back and head and neck regions[44]; however, caution is recommended when making such a diagnosis outside the context of the typical clinicopathologic presentation, in particular, when dealing with deeply situated masses. Common experience indicates that most (if not all) of these lesions represent ALT/WDLPS. Spindle cell lipomas can present as multiple lesions and also occur as a familial disease.[45]

Pathologic Features

Grossly, spindle cell/pleomorphic lipoma is usually well circumscribed, but less well demarcated than ordinary lipomas. The cut surface varies from yellow to white-gray, depending on the relative amount of adipocytic and spindle cell components. Focal to diffuse myxoid change can be observed.

Histologically, classic forms of spindle cell lipoma are composed of a cytologically bland spindle cell proliferation admixed with a variable amount of mature adipocytes (Fig. 12.13). Fibromyxoid stroma with brightly eosinophilic, coarse ("ropy") collagen fibers is one of the most important morphologic hallmarks of the lesion (Fig. 12.14). The amount of the spindle cell component is extremely variable, with some cases featuring rare adipocytes ("cellular spindle cell lipoma") (Fig. 12.15).[46] The degree of variation in adipocyte size is often greater than is seen in ordinary lipoma. Not infrequently, myxoid stromal change is present, which may be a source of diagnostic confusion, most often with myxofibrosarcoma and myxoid liposarcoma (Fig. 12.16). When myxoid change becomes prominent, the formation of angiectoid spaces may result in a pseudoangiomatous growth pattern.[47] Most likely, the lesion described as *dendritic fibromyxolipoma* actually corresponds to examples of spindle cell lipoma with prominent myxoid change.[48] As already mentioned, pleomorphic lipoma represents part of the spectrum of this entity, in which bizarre, hyperchromatic, and sometimes multinucleated cells are associated with the otherwise typical morphologic features of spindle cell lipoma (Fig. 12.17).[38,39] In classic cases, multinucleated giant cells show a floret-like appearance (Fig. 12.18). Interestingly, occasional lipoblasts may be seen, underscoring the idea that lipoblasts are not exclusive to liposarcoma.

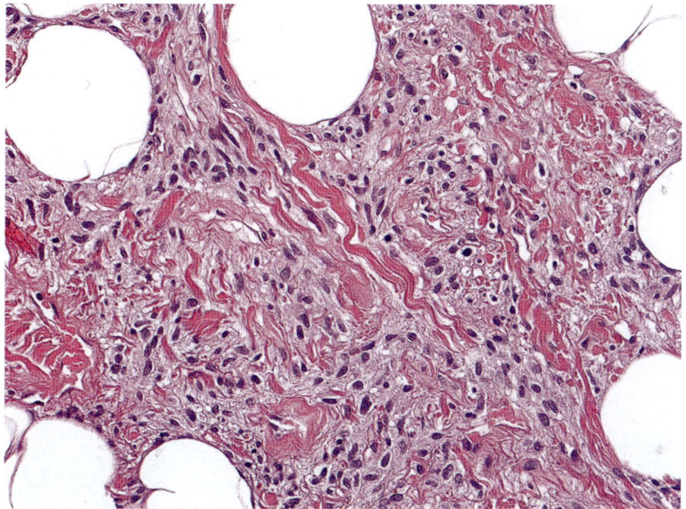

Figure 12.14 Spindle Cell Lipoma. Eosinophilic, "ropy" collagen bundles provide a useful diagnostic clue.

Immunohistochemistry

Spindle cell lipoma is characterized by diffuse positivity for CD34.[49,50] CD10 immunoreactivity has also been reported.[51] Similar to CD34, CD10 expression appears to be much more widespread than was initially believed (and is therefore of dubious diagnostic utility). Recently, loss of nuclear expression of retinoblastoma protein (Rb) has been reported in spindle cell/pleomorphic lipoma.[52]

Molecular Genetics

Cytogenetic analysis of spindle cell/pleomorphic lipoma cases has demonstrated consistent deletions of the long arm of chromosome 13, often in combination with loss of the long arm of chromosome 16.[53,54] These genetic features support distinction from both ordinary lipoma and ALT/WDLPS. Interestingly, the same alteration is seen in a morphologically similar entity know as mammary (or mammary-type) myofibroblastoma, as well as in cellular angiofibroma (see Chapters 3 and 17)[55–57]; all of these lesions show loss of Rb expression.[52]

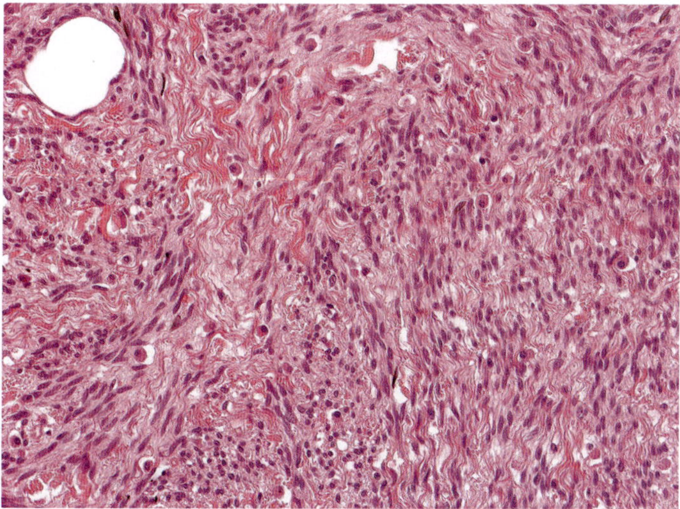

Figure 12.15 Spindle Cell Lipoma. When the adipocytic component is scarce, the term *cellular spindle cell lipoma* may be used.

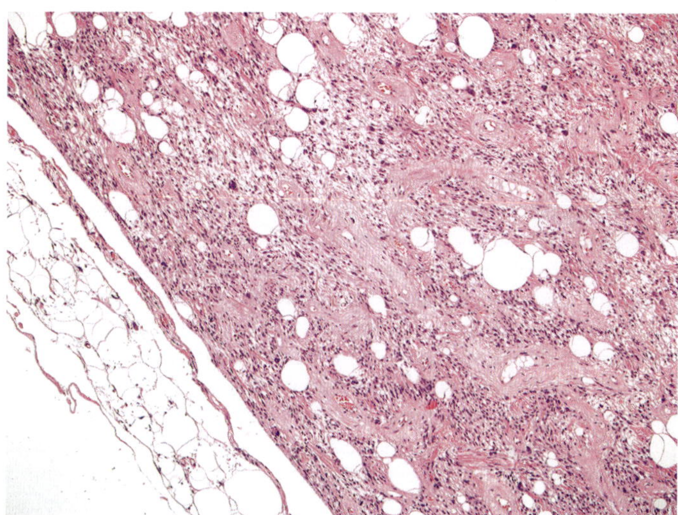

Figure 12.17 Pleomorphic Lipoma. Pleomorphic lipoma exhibits cytologic pleomorphism in association with morphologic features overlapping with those of spindle cell lipoma.

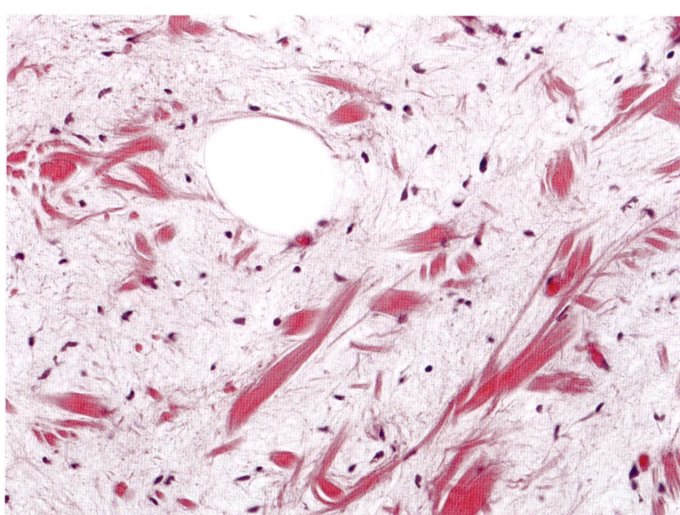

Figure 12.16 Spindle Cell Lipoma. In a minority of spindle cell lipomas, extensive myxoid stromal change is present.

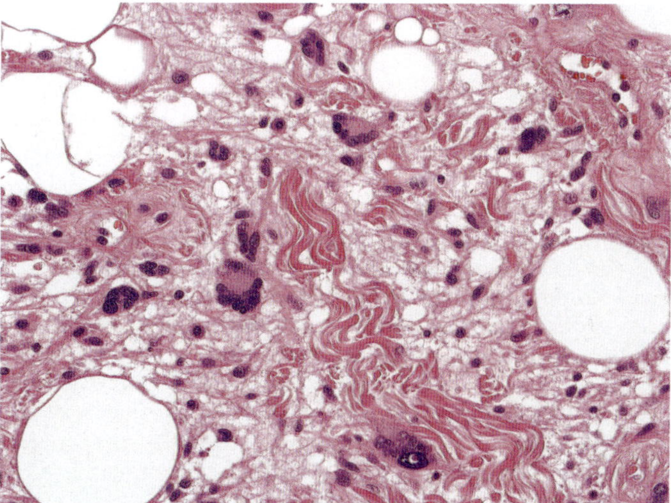

Figure 12.18 Pleomorphic Lipoma. Floret-like multinucleated giant cells are often seen.

Differential Diagnosis

The greatest morphologic overlap is with mammary-type myofibroblastoma, a benign lesion that shares the same karyotypic alterations with spindle cell lipoma. Originally reported in the breast,[58] this lesion may also arise in the soft tissues, most often in the inguinal region of middle-aged men, with a peak incidence in the fifth decade and a male predominance.[59,60] Ironically, mammary-type myofibroblastoma is far more common at extramammary sites (mammary location accounts for ~10% of cases), and in addition to the groin, it may occur in the limbs, trunk and axilla. Mammary-type myofibroblastoma is well circumscribed and composed of a cellular, cytologically bland, spindle cell proliferation in a collagenous stroma containing the same ropy collagen bundles as seen in spindle cell lipoma (Fig. 12.19). The presence of adipocytes in variable amounts makes the resemblance to spindle cell lipoma even greater. Numerous scattered mast cells are generally part of the typical morphologic picture. In contrast to spindle cell lipoma, a more fascicular architecture is generally observed in mammary-type myofibroblastoma, and strong desmin immunopositivity is usually detected (Fig. 12.20). Loss of nuclear expression of Rb is observed in approximately 90% of cases, further highlighting the genetic link with spindle cell lipoma.[52,60]

As discussed earlier, extensive myxoid change may raise the differential diagnosis of myxoid liposarcoma. However, spindle cell lipoma lacks the typical plexiform, capillary-sized (crow's feet) vascular network that is one of the diagnostic hallmarks of myxoid liposarcoma. Spindle cell lipoma also lacks the specific translocations involving the *DDIT3* gene that are characteristic of myxoid liposarcoma. Low-grade myxofibrosarcoma can also be mistaken for myxoid spindle cell lipoma; however, myxofibrosarcoma is almost always multinodular, featuring a highly distinctive curvilinear vascular pattern as well as a markedly atypical, pleomorphic neoplastic cell population. The differential diagnosis with atypical spindle cell lipomatous tumor is discussed later in the chapter; however, this distinction is based primarily on the absence of nuclear atypia.

Pleomorphic lipoma can be a diagnostic challenge, mostly because of the presence of often striking cytologic atypia. The differential diagnosis with a pleomorphic sarcoma is usually straightforward because pleomorphic lipoma is much less cellular, and in contrast to pleomorphic sarcomas, mitoses are rare. Well-differentiated sclerosing liposarcoma features bizarre neoplastic cells with hyperchromatic nuclei that may mimic those observed in pleomorphic lipoma. However, a distinctive fibrillary collagenous background (instead of the characteristic broad collagen bundles) is a useful diagnostic clue in favor of WDLPS. In addition, MDM2 immunopositivity is generally limited to WDLPS and virtually absent in spindle cell/pleomorphic lipoma (Table 12.1). Key diagnostic clues are summarized in Box 12.1.

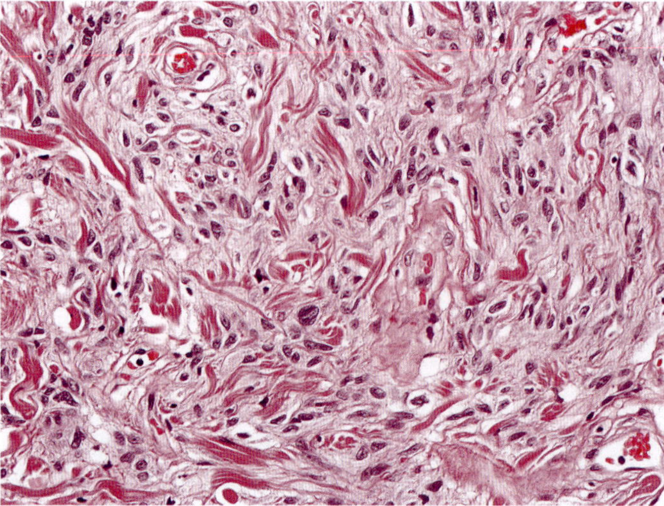

Figure 12.19 Mammary-Type Myofibroblastoma. Morphologic overlap with the spindle cell component of spindle cell lipoma is striking.

Prognosis and Treatment

Spindle cell/pleomorphic lipoma is entirely benign, and local excision is curative. Local recurrence is exceptional, even after incomplete resection.

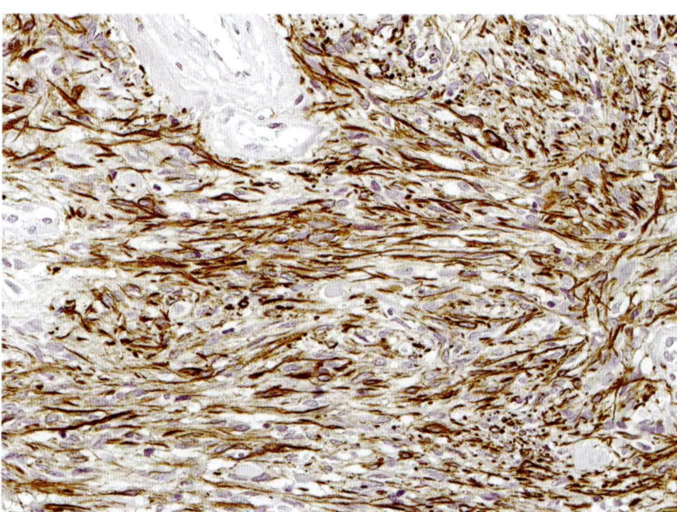

Figure 12.20 Mammary-Type Myofibroblastoma. Immunoreactivity for desmin is observed in the vast majority of cases.

Table 12.1 Differential Diagnosis Between Pleomorphic Lipoma and Well-Differentiated Sclerosing Liposarcoma

	Pleomorphic Lipoma	Well-Differentiated Sclerosing Liposarcoma
Predominant anatomic sites	Head and neck, upper back	Retroperitoneum, spermatic cord
Coarse collagen bundles	Present	Absent
Fibrillary stroma	Absent	Present
Lipoblasts	Rare	None to numerous
MDM2/CDK4 overexpression	Absent	Present
Genetics	16q and 13q deletions	12q13-15 amplification (ring chromosomes or giant markers)

Box 12.1 Spindle Cell/Pleomorphic Lipoma

Diagnose spindle cell/pleomorphic lipoma when:
- The tumor is located in the neck and shoulder region in middle-aged adults.
- The tumor is subcutaneous.
- Neoplastic cells are set in stroma rich in eosinophilic, refractile, "ropy" collagen bundles.
- Cytologic atypia is absent or degenerative.

Hemosiderotic Fibrolipomatous Tumor

Hemosiderotic fibrolipomatous tumor (HFLT) or *hemosiderotic fibrohistiocytic lipomatous lesion* (so-named in the original description)[61] is a hemosiderin-rich, fibrofatty, locally aggressive lesion that occurs predominantly in the ankle region of middle-aged adults with a female predominance.

Clinical Features

This lesion occurs most often in the ankle region of middle-aged women, with a peak incidence in the fifth decade.[61,62] Less frequent anatomic locations include the upper limbs, hands, and head and neck region. Some patients have a history of previous trauma. It has been suggested that HFLT represents a precursor to the low-grade mesenchymal lesion descriptively named *pleomorphic hyalinizing angiectatic tumor*, but this is not widely accepted.[63] In fact, recent morphologic as well as cytogenetic data support a relationship with myxoinflammatory fibroblastic sarcoma (MIFS),[64,65] which also shows a tendency to occur at acral sites (see Chapters 5, 7, and 10). The occurrence of occasional lesions showing hybrid features of HFLT and MIFS further supports this concept.

Pathologic Features

Grossly, most lesions show ill-defined borders and a yellow cut surface. Tumor size ranges from 1 cm to 20 cm, with most tumors between 2 cm and 10 cm. Histologically, a proliferation of bland, fibroblastic spindle cells is seen associated with a mature adipocytic component (Fig. 12.21). Scattered inflammatory cells and abundant iron pigment are constant findings. Iron pigment predominates in macrophages within the spindle cell component (Fig. 12.22). The spindle cells contain vesicular nuclei with indistinct nucleoli, and occasional cells show mild hyperchromasia. As already mentioned, rare cases are observed in which a morphologic transition from HFLT to MIFS is observed.

Immunohistochemistry

Immunohistochemical findings are not diagnostically useful. The spindle cell component is often positive for CD34 and negative for smooth muscle actin, desmin, and S-100 protein.

Molecular Genetics

Clonal reciprocal translocations between chromosomes 1 and 10 have recently been reported in HFLT, with a further rearrangement involving the derivative chromosome 1 and chromosome 3 in one case.[65–68] As a consequence of the t(1;10) translocation, rearrangement of the *TGFBR3* and *MGEA5* genes is observed.[65] Interestingly, the same genetic alteration also seems to be common in hybrid HFLT/MIFS.[68]

Differential Diagnosis

The differential diagnosis of HFLT includes plexiform fibrohistiocytic tumor (PFHT); giant cell tumor of soft tissue; dermatofibrosarcoma protuberans (DFSP), with which HFLT shares CD34 immunopositivity; and ALT, particularly the spindle cell variant (also known as *spindle cell liposarcoma*). PFHT is composed of fibromatosis-like fascicles of spindle cells connecting nodules of mononuclear histiocytoid cells and scattered osteoclastic giant cells, which contrasts with the uniform cytologic composition of HFLT. Although PFHT typically entraps fat, adipose tissue is not an intrinsic component of the lesion. Unlike HFLT, smooth muscle actin is positive in the spindle cells of PFHT. Giant cell tumor of soft tissue shows a multinodular proliferation of mononuclear cells and osteoclastic giant cells, separated by fibrotic tissue. Hemosiderin deposition is often seen in stromal macrophages in the fibrous septa. Fat is not a component of giant cell tumor of soft tissue. DFSP is characterized by a monotonous spindle cell proliferation organized in a storiform growth pattern and typically infiltrating the subcutaneous fat in a honeycomb fashion. DFSP is more uniformly cellular than HFLT (which is usually dominated by the adipocytic component) and lacks the prominent hemosiderin deposition. Atypical spindle cell lipomatous tumor can be excluded by the lack of variation in adipocyte size and the absence of lipoblasts and significant adipocytic or stromal atypia.

Prognosis and Treatment

Although HFLT is a benign lesion that is incapable of metastatic spread, it can recur locally in up to 50% of cases, likely as a result of incomplete excision because of the poorly demarcated borders of these lesions. Complete excision is generally curative. The rare cases exhibiting transition to MIFS tend to follow a locally aggressive but non-metastasizing clinical behavior. Personal experience indicates that morphologic progression to undifferentiated spindle cell sarcoma is possible but represents an exceptional event.

Lipoblastoma/Lipoblastomatosis

Lipoblastoma is a rare, benign adipocytic tumor of infancy composed of immature (fetal) adipose tissue that morphologically recapitulates

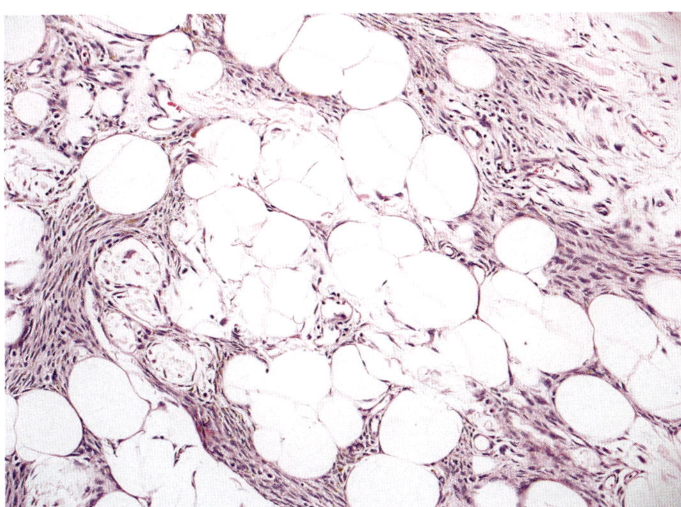

Figure 12.21 **Hemosiderotic Fibrolipomatous Tumor.** A spindle cell proliferation is associated with a mature adipocytic component.

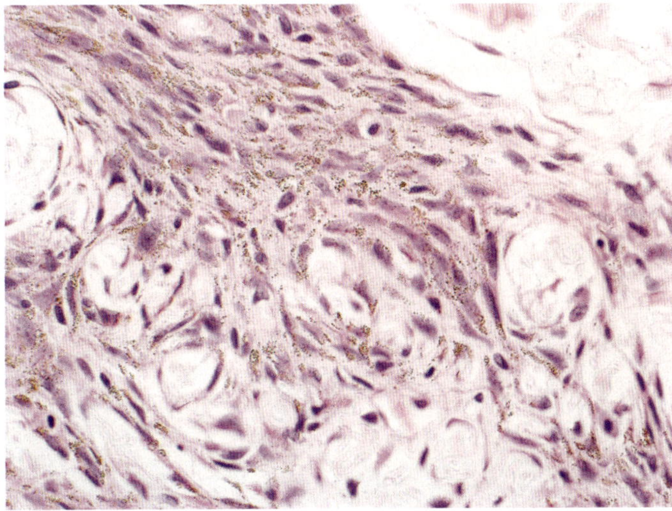

Figure 12.22 **Hemosiderotic Fibrolipomatous Tumor.** Deposition of iron pigment is one of the morphologic characteristics of these lesions.

the process of embryonic adipocytic differentiation.[69] It may occur as a localized lesion (lipoblastoma) or as a diffuse proliferation (lipoblastomatosis).

Clinical Features

Lipoblastoma occurs predominantly in boys within the first 3 years of life and most frequently affects the lower and upper extremities. Much rarer locations include the mediastinum, retroperitoneum, trunk, and head and neck region.[70–72] Lipoblastoma generally presents as a slow-growing, painless, well-demarcated nodule confined to the subcutaneous soft tissue, usually not larger than 5 cm. Lipoblastomatosis, in addition to involving the subcutis, almost invariably infiltrates the underlying muscle. The lesion known as *lipoblastoma-like tumor of the vulva* may represent a clinically distinct variant of lipoblastomatosis or (more likely) atypical spindle cell lipomatous tumor.[73]

Pathologic Features

Grossly, lipoblastoma is usually well circumscribed, with a white to yellow, lobulated cut surface. Gelatinous areas may vary from focal to predominant, according to the degree of adipocytic maturation.

Histologically, lipoblastoma is composed of lobules of adipocytes showing varying stages of differentiation (Fig. 12.23). A lobulated growth pattern is one of the distinctive features. The neoplastic cell population is composed of an admixture of immature spindle cells (preadipocytes), lipoblasts, and mature fat cells (Fig. 12.24). The number of lipoblasts is variable and most likely depends on the duration of the lesion. Long-standing lesions may exhibit almost complete maturation, making the distinction from a benign lipoma challenging. Not infrequently, the stroma can show extensive myxoid change that, when associated with a plexiform vascular network, may closely mimic myxoid liposarcoma (Fig. 12.25). In lipoblastomatosis, the lobular architecture is usually much less evident. In addition, because of the infiltrative growth pattern, residual muscle fibers are usually seen within the lesion.

Immunohistochemistry

The lesional cells exhibit immunopositivity for S-100 protein, which is of no real diagnostic utility. Most lipoblastomas show nuclear staining for PLAG1, correlating with the presence of gene fusions (see below).

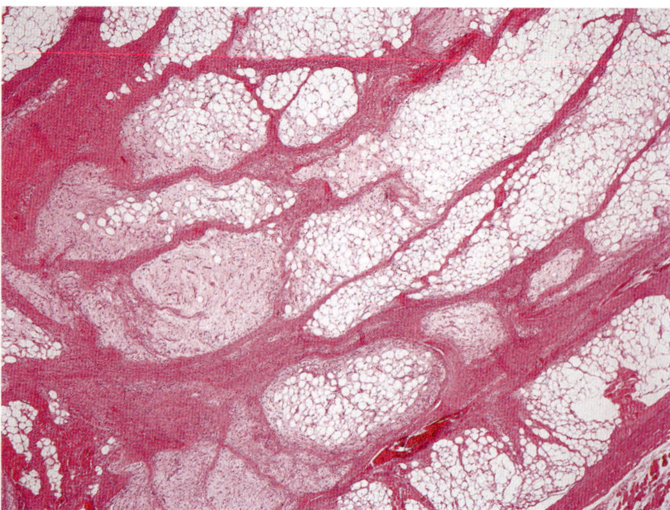

Figure 12.23 Lipoblastoma. At low power, lipoblastoma exhibits a lobular architecture.

Molecular Genetics

Lipoblastoma is characterized by *PLAG1* gene rearrangements, involving the 8q11-13 region. A range of *PLAG1* fusion partners have been reported, including *HAS2*, *COL1A2*, *COL3A1*, *RAD51L1*, and *RAB2A*. These fusion genes seem to use the promoter-swapping mechanism.[74–78]

Differential Diagnosis

Fully matured lipoblastoma can be differentiated from ordinary lipoma on the basis of its distinctive lobulation. The most important differential diagnosis, however, is with myxoid liposarcoma.[79] The young age of the patient (a diagnosis of myxoid liposarcoma should be made with great caution in a patient younger than 10 years), the lobular growth pattern, and the absence of cytologic atypia are useful clues; however, in rare cases, morphologic overlap is extreme. In such cases, genetic analysis (e.g., by FISH) to show the absence of *DDIT3* gene rearrangement is extremely useful (Table 12.2).

Prognosis and Treatment

Lipoblastoma is a benign lesion whose complete excision is curative. In contrast, as a consequence of its infiltrative growth pattern, local

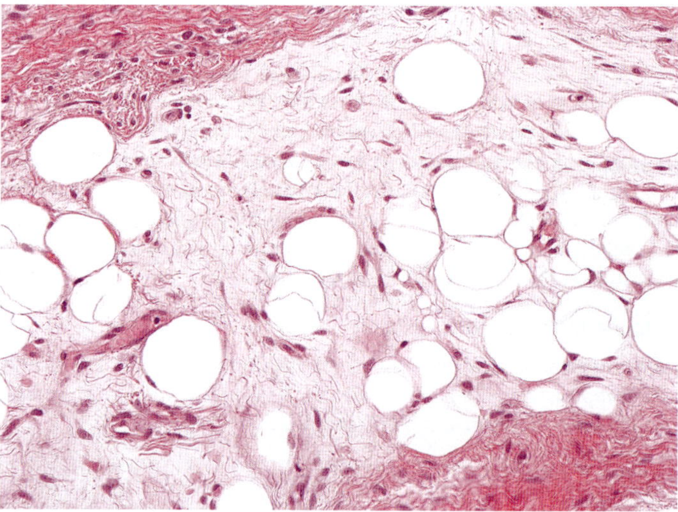

Figure 12.24 Lipoblastoma. Immature spindle cells, lipoblasts, and mature adipocytes are variably admixed.

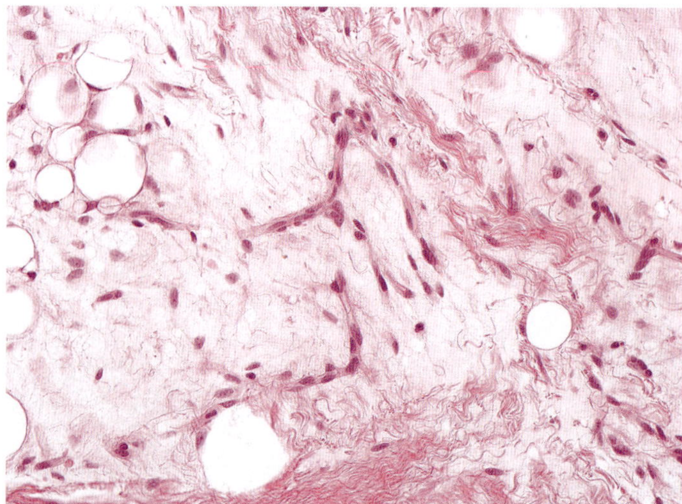

Figure 12.25 Lipoblastoma. Myxoid stromal change may lead to diagnostic confusion with myxoid liposarcoma.

Table 12.2 Differential Diagnosis Between Lipoblastoma and Myxoid Liposarcoma

	Lipoblastoma	Myxoid Liposarcoma
Typical age range	<10 years	Third to fifth decades
Lobulation	Present	Absent
Lipoblasts	Variable	Univacuolated; most often at the periphery of the lesion
Mature fat	Variable	Rare
Plexiform vascular network	Rarely present and associated with myxoid change	Present
Genetics	8q11-13 rearrangement (*PLAG1*)	12q13 rearrangement, usually t(12;16) *(DDIT3-FUS)*

recurrence is seen in up to 15% of cases of lipoblastomatosis, for which wide local excision is justified.

Hibernoma

Hibernoma is a benign adipocytic tumor of adults, the first description of which dates back to 1906,[80] before Gery introduced the term in 1914.[81] Hibernoma is composed of a predominant brown (fetal) fat cell proliferation, variably intermingled with mature white adipose tissue.

Clinical Features

Hibernoma most often presents as a long-standing, slow-growing, painless mass located in the subcutis in young adults.[82–84] Peak incidence is between the third and fourth decades; however, the age range is broad. A minority of cases (~10% to 15%) are deep-seated, located within somatic muscles. There is a slight male predominance. The most frequently affected anatomic site is the thigh, followed by the trunk, upper limbs, and head and neck. Rarely, hibernomas arise at visceral locations, such as the retroperitoneum and mediastinum.

Pathologic Features

Grossly, hibernomas are well circumscribed, ranging in size from 2 cm to 20 cm. The cut surface shows an easily recognizable lobulation, with color varying from yellow to red-brown, depending on the relative amounts of brown and white adipocytic components.

Histologically, most hibernomas are composed of a predominant population of multivacuolated brown adipocytes containing coarsely granular cytoplasm and centrally located nuclei, organized in a lobular growth pattern (Fig. 12.26). The cytoplasm of brown fat cells may vary from pale to intensely eosinophilic (Fig. 12.27). In fewer than 10% of cases, the white fat cell component is predominant and scattered or small clusters of brown fat cells are seen. A similar minority of cases feature myxoid degeneration of the stroma.[84] The brown fat component is most often admixed with a variable amount of ordinary adipose tissue. Mitotic activity is usually absent, as is cytologic atypia.

Immunohistochemistry

The diagnosis of hibernoma is relatively straightforward, and immunohistochemistry does not play a role. As in most adipocytic lesions, S-100 protein is usually positive.

Molecular Genetics

Cytogenetic analysis most often shows structural rearrangements of the 11q13-21 region and, less often, 10q22.[85] At the molecular level, deletion of the multiple endocrine neoplasia-1 (*MEN1*) gene has been reported.[86]

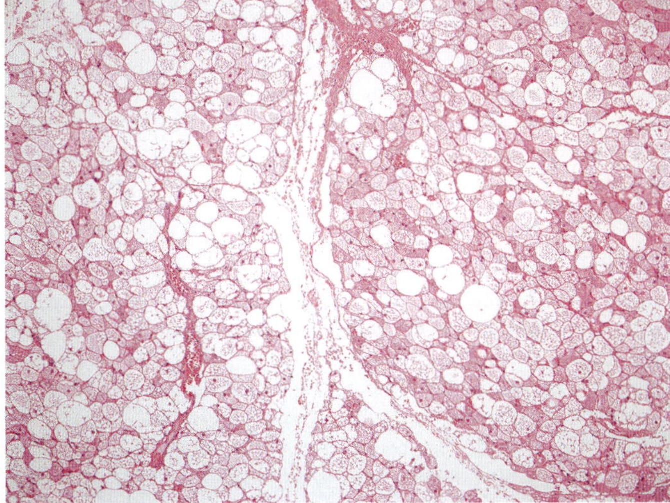

Figure 12.26 Hibernoma. Hibernoma is organized in a lobular growth pattern.

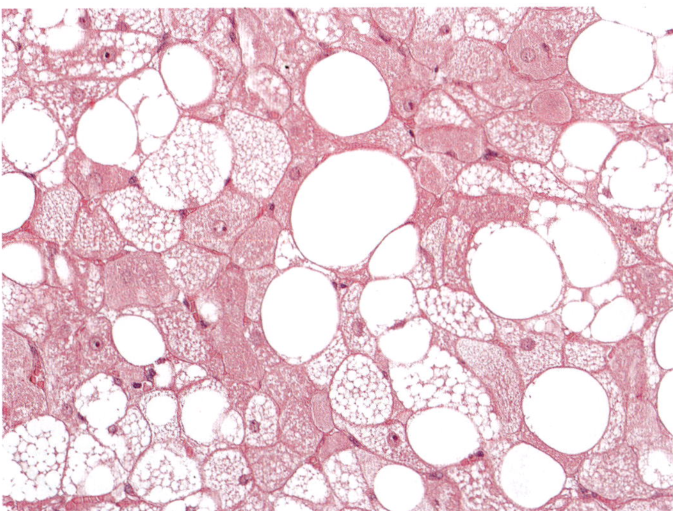

Figure 12.27 Hibernoma. Hibernoma cells are coarsely granular, with cytoplasm varying from pale to intensely eosinophilic.

Differential Diagnosis

The differential diagnosis of hibernoma is limited. Hibernoma-like features are rarely observed in ALT/WDLPS[87] as well as in myxoid liposarcoma.

Granular cell tumor may be considered, given the distinctive fine cytoplasmic granularity. Both lesions show reactivity for S-100 protein. However, granular cell tumor tends to be more superficially located, and the constituent cells show more uniformly granular (as opposed to vacuolated) cytoplasm.

Prognosis and Treatment

Hibernomas are benign neoplasms, irrespective of morphologic variation, and local excision is curative. Local recurrences are not observed, even after incomplete excision.

Myolipoma

Myolipoma, also known as *extrauterine lipoleiomyoma*, is a benign adipocytic neoplasm nearly exclusively affecting women, characterized by the coexistence of mature adipocytic and smooth muscle cell components.[88,89]

Clinical Features

Myolipoma presents as a slow growing, deep-seated, painless mass, most frequently arising in the pelvis, retroperitoneum, and abdomen of women. More rarely, it has been described in the groin and extremities. Peak incidence is between the fifth and sixth decades. Because of its deep situation, myolipoma can attain a large size, up to 15 cm to 20 cm in diameter.

Pathologic Features

Grossly, myolipoma is well circumscribed, most often appearing as a large encapsulated or partially encapsulated mass. The cut surface appears glistening, with color ranging from white to yellow. The presence of firmer areas correlates with the amount of leiomyomatous differentiation. Necrosis is absent. Histologically, myolipoma exhibits characteristic biphasic morphologic features because of the coexistence of mature adipose tissue and variable amounts of differentiated smooth muscle fibers organized in short bundles (Fig. 12.28). Notably, both the smooth muscle and adipocytic components lack cytologic atypia.

Immunohistochemistry

The distinctive biphasic adipocytic and myogenic components can be easily confirmed immunohistochemically by the finding of desmin or smooth muscle actin reactivity in the smooth muscle cells. Expression of estrogen and progesterone receptors has also been reported in both smooth muscle cells and adipocytes.[90]

Molecular Genetics

Cytogenetic alterations of the high-mobility group AT-hook 2 (*HMGA2*) gene have been reported in 2 cases of myolipoma. In one case a translocation t(9;12)(p22;q14) fusing *HMGA2* with *C9orf92* has been detected.[91,92]

Differential Diagnosis

The chief differential diagnostic consideration is leiomyoma with extensive fatty degeneration, which usually lacks the uniform distribution of adipocytes that is typically observed in myolipoma, although this distinction is of no clinical importance. ALT/WDLPS may also contain foci of smooth muscle differentiation; however, myolipoma never shows adipocytic or stromal atypia, which is the diagnostic hallmark of ALT/WDLPS.[93,94] Immunoreactivity for MDM2 and CDK4 (or amplification of *MDM2* detected by FISH) can confirm ALT/WDLPS. Angiomyolipoma is distinguished by the coexpression of myogenic and melanocytic markers, such as HMB-45 or melan A.[94]

Prognosis and Treatment

Myolipoma is a benign mesenchymal lesion whose complete surgical removal is curative. No recurrences or metastases have been reported.

Chondroid Lipoma

Chondroid lipoma is a rare, benign adipocytic neoplasm, most often arising in the limbs or limb girdles of adult women. In its first description, it was termed *extraskeletal chondroma with lipoblast-like cells*,[95] suggesting possible chondrogenic differentiation, which has subsequently been disproven. The presence of an abundant lipoblastic cell population in chondroid lipoma further underscores the fact that lipoblasts are not exclusive to malignant adipocytic neoplasms.

Clinical Features

Chondroid lipoma usually presents as a long-standing, painless, slow-growing, deep-seated lesion located in the proximal limbs and limb girdles, followed by the trunk, distal extremities, and head and neck region.[96,97] Approximately 20% of cases arise superficially. The peak incidence is in the third and fourth decades, and women outnumber men 4:1.

Pathologic Features

Chondroid lipoma is usually well circumscribed and most often (but not always) encapsulated. One third of cases appear multilobulated. The cut surface is white to yellowish, depending on the extent of the mature adipocytic component. Histologically, chondroid lipoma is composed of a variable admixture of mature adipocytes, eosinophilic chondroblast-like cells, and vacuolated cells set in a myxochondroid background, often organized in a lobular growth pattern (Fig. 12.29). One of the most striking features of this lesion is the presence of vacuolated cells that are virtually indistinguishable from ordinary lipoblasts (Fig. 12.30). In the original description, this distinctive cell type was designated as a *pseudolipoblast*; however, such terminology is misleading because it incorrectly implies that these cells are mimics of lipoblasts. Instead, these vacuolated elements exhibit all of the morphologic, histochemical, and ultrastructural features of lipoblasts and therefore

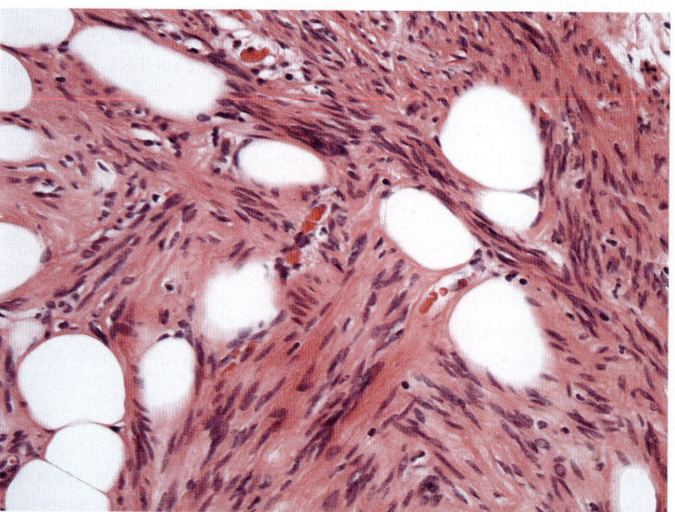

Figure 12.28 Myolipoma. Myolipoma is composed of an admixture of well-differentiated smooth muscle cells and mature adipocytes.

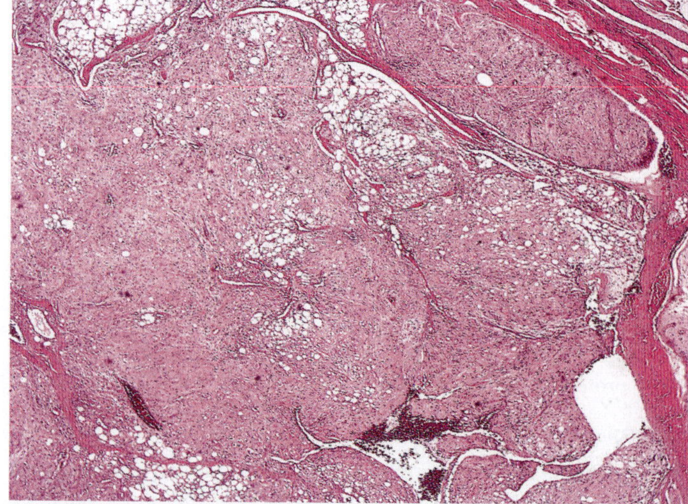

Figure 12.29 Chondroid Lipoma. At low power, a mixed population of fat cells and eosinophilic cells set in a myxochondroid background is seen.

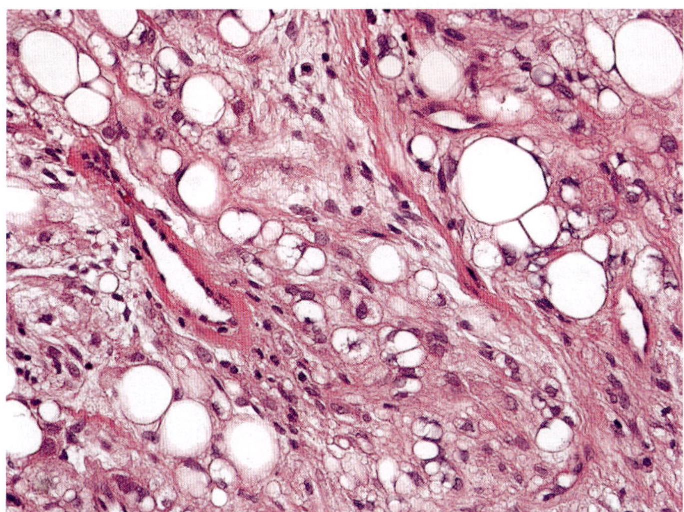

Figure 12.30 Chondroid Lipoma. A lipoblastic population is invariably seen in chondroid lipoma.

can be considered as such.[98,99] Chondroid lipoma is also characterized by a rich vascular network composed of thick-walled blood vessels alternating with large, gaping, thin-walled vascular spaces.

Immunohistochemistry

By immunohistochemistry, S-100 protein is positive in most neoplastic cells. This finding does not play a major role in the differential diagnosis.

Molecular Genetics

Chondroid lipoma is characterized by a t(11;16)(q13;p13) translocation.[100–102] This translocation results in the fusion of the *C11orf95* and *MKL2* (megakaryoblastic leukemia 2) genes.[103] One reported patient had an additional three-way translocation involving chromosomes 1, 2, and 5.[100]

Differential Diagnosis

The differential diagnosis of chondroid lipoma includes soft tissue chondroma, myxoid liposarcoma, extraskeletal myxoid chondrosarcoma, and soft tissue myoepithelioma. Soft tissue chondroma shows a predilection for the hands and feet and is composed of genuine hyaline cartilage. Myxoid liposarcoma is distinguished by its distinctive plexiform capillary-sized (crow's feet) vascular network as well as more prominent myxoid stroma. Extraskeletal myxoid chondrosarcoma shows a more pronounced lobular architecture, with abundant myxoid stroma containing a reticular arrangement of uniform, usually spindled but occasionally epithelioid cells that are positive for S-100 protein in fewer than 20% of cases. Soft tissue myoepithelioma also often contains myxoid stroma and shows a reticular architecture, but is distinguished by a distinctive immunophenotype that usually includes reactivity for S-100 protein, keratins, and EMA, as well as glial fibrillary acidic protein (GFAP) in approximately 50% of cases.

Prognosis and Treatment

Chondroid lipoma is a benign adipocytic neoplasm, and complete surgical removal is curative. No recurrences or distant metastases have been reported.

Liposarcoma

Liposarcomas are the most common malignant mesenchymal neoplasms, accounting for approximately 20% of all sarcomas. Malignant adipocytic tumors are a heterogeneous group of lesions, with both morphologically and genetically distinctive features. This biologic diversity is associated with remarkable clinical heterogeneity, ranging from neoplasms of intermediate biologic potential, incapable of systemic spread (i.e., ALT/WDLPS), to aggressive sarcomas, such as high-grade myxoid liposarcoma and pleomorphic liposarcoma, both with a significant potential for metastasis.[104–107] The 2002 WHO classification of soft tissue and bone tumors recognized five major subtypes: (1) ALT/WDLPS (which included the adipocytic, sclerosing, inflammatory, and spindle cell variants); (2) dedifferentiated liposarcoma; (3) myxoid liposarcoma (which also included "round cell liposarcoma"); (4) pleomorphic liposarcoma; and (5) the exceptionally rare "mixed type" liposarcoma, not otherwise specified.[1] In the latter group, the coexistence of two distinct liposarcoma variants (e.g., ALT/WDLPS and myxoid liposarcoma) is observed. As already mentioned, the 2013 WHO classification abolished both the term "round cell liposarcoma" and the entity "mixed-type liposarcoma."[2] Interestingly, the WHO histologic partitioning of liposarcoma is closely mirrored by cytogenetic findings, according to which three broad categories can be considered: (1) ALT/WDLPS and dedifferentiated liposarcoma, in which alterations (i.e., amplification) of the 12q13-15 region are observed; (2) myxoid liposarcoma, in which rearrangement of the *DDIT3* gene is the main genetic alteration; and (3) pleomorphic liposarcoma, in which, as in most pleomorphic sarcomas, complex (non-distinctive) karyotypic alterations are detected (Table 12.3).

Table 12.3 Classification of Liposarcomas With Associated Genetic Aberrations

	Cytogenetics	Molecular Genetics
Atypical lipomatous tumor/ well-differentiated liposarcoma	Ring chromosomes or giant markers (12q13-15 amplification)	*HMGA2/MDM2/CDK4* amplification
Atypical spindle cell lipomatous tumor	Chromosome 7 monosomy (subset)	*RB1* heterozygous deletion (subset)
Dedifferentiated liposarcoma	Ring chromosomes or giant markers (12q13-15 amplification) plus additional alterations	*HMGA2/MDM2/CDK4* amplification
Myxoid liposarcoma	t(12;16)(q13;p11) t(12;22)(q13;q22)	*DDIT3-FUS* *DDIT3-EWSR1*
Pleomorphic liposarcoma	Complex karyotypic alterations	*NF1* mutations

The clinical presentations among the main groups and even among subgroups of liposarcoma are also distinct. For example, myxoid liposarcoma arises predominantly in the limbs and is very rare in the retroperitoneum, where, in contrast, well-differentiated and dedifferentiated liposarcomas are relatively common. Furthermore, among WDLPS, the sclerosing subtype shows a striking predilection for both the retroperitoneum and spermatic cord. The main clinical features of liposarcoma variants are discussed in more detail later; however, awareness of the typical clinical presentation is critical to the diagnostic approach to lipomatous neoplasms. A second important point is management of the surgical specimen. As mentioned earlier, accurate orientation is mandatory for evaluation of the status of the surgical margins. Second, extensive sampling is strongly recommended because both diagnosis and grading of the tumor may depend on features present only focally. In general, any gross variation (even subtle ones) should be sampled and carefully analyzed microscopically. As will be discussed, these recommendations are crucial for all liposarcoma subtypes. A final general comment pertains to the diagnostic value of lipoblasts. Lipoblasts are defined as uni- or multivacuolated cells harboring hyperchromatic, indented (or scalloped) nuclei (Fig. 12.31). Lipoblasts can be variably

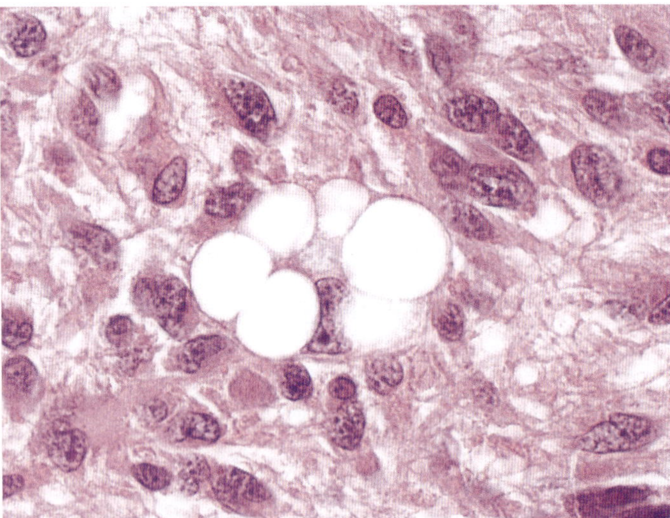

Figure 12.31 Lipoblast. Lipoblasts are defined as uni- or multivacuolated cells harboring a hyperchromatic, scalloped nucleus.

present in malignant adipocytic neoplasms, and in atypical spindle cell lipomatous tumor (in many cases a mostly nonlipogenic tumor) and pleomorphic liposarcoma, their presence is helpful for proper diagnosis. However, lipoblasts can be seen in benign lesions (e.g., lipoblastoma, spindle cell/pleomorphic lipoma, and chondroid lipoma), and in contrast, can be totally absent in WDLPS (Box 12.2). As discussed later, the histologic classification of liposarcoma is not based on a single diagnostic feature, but rather on the integration of a constellation of morphologic findings.

Box 12.2 Lipoblasts

Lipoblasts are not required for a diagnosis of liposarcoma.
Lipoblasts can be seen in benign adipocytic tumors.
Lipoblasts are mostly univacuolated in myxoid liposarcoma.
Lipoblasts are mostly multivacuolated in pleomorphic liposarcoma.

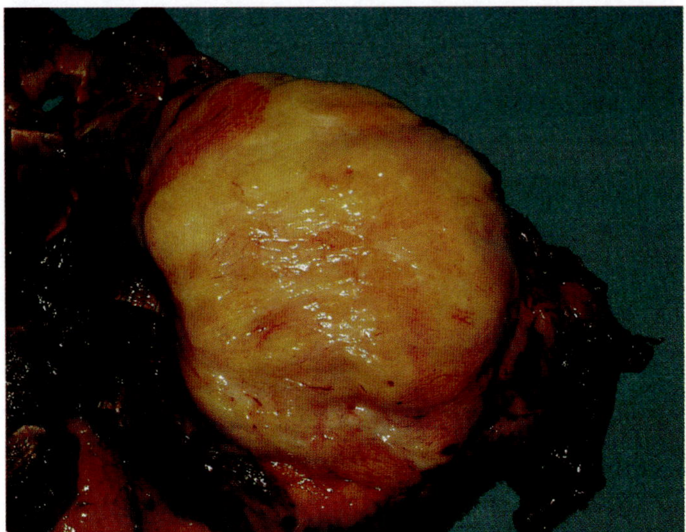

Figure 12.32 Atypical Lipomatous Tumor/Well-Differentiated Liposarcoma, Lipoma-Like Variant. The lipoma-like cut surface tends to be uniformly yellow.

Atypical Lipomatous Tumor/ Well-Differentiated Liposarcoma

WDLPS is the largest subgroup of malignant adipocytic neoplasms and accounts for approximately 40% to 45% of all liposarcomas.[108–110] Four subtypes of WDLPS were recognized in the most recent WHO classification of soft tissue tumors: (1) adipocytic (or lipoma-like), (2) sclerosing, (3) inflammatory, and (4) spindle cell.[110] As will be discussed later, atypical spindle cell lipomatous tumor (also known as spindle cell liposarcoma) deserves to be discussed separately from the MDM2-related variants of liposarcoma. As mentioned earlier, the alternative term ALT was introduced for lesions arising at surgically amenable soft tissue sites.[111–113] Although WDLPS has a tendency to recur locally, overall in approximately 30% of cases (the rate depends on the anatomic site), it is incapable of metastasizing unless it undergoes dedifferentiation. Based on this behavior, in 1979, Evans and colleagues suggested the use of alternative designations such as *atypical lipoma* or ALT.[111] Currently, there is broad consensus among experts that the choice of terminology should be based on the principle of avoiding either inadequate or excessive treatment. As a consequence, the term ALT is adequate for lesions arising at anatomic locations for which achieving compete surgical excision is relatively straightforward, whereas the term WDLPS is preferred for lesions arising in deep-seated, central body sites, such as the retroperitoneum, for which radical multivisceral surgery is considered feasible treatment.[114,115]

Clinical Features

Although WDLPS occurs equally commonly in the retroperitoneum and limbs, it is seen more rarely in the spermatic cord and mediastinum.[116,117] The head and neck region can also be involved.[118,119] In most patients, the clinical history is that of a slowly growing mass. Visceral locations are generally associated with larger size. As already mentioned, specific morphologic variants of ALT/WDLPS exhibit some degree of anatomic tropism. Although adipocytic ALT/WDLPS is observed in both the limbs and retroperitoneum, the sclerosing subtype is more often observed in the retroperitoneum and spermatic cord. Inflammatory ALT/WDLPS is also most common in the retroperitoneum, whereas the spindle cell subtype shows a predilection for the limbs and superficial soft tissues.

Pathologic Features

Grossly, ALT/WDLPS is usually well circumscribed. The appearance of the cut surface depends on the extent of the lipomatous component and tends to be uniformly yellow in the lipoma-like variant (Fig. 12.32). The variable presence of fibrous tissue correlates with white-gray areas that can predominate in the sclerosing and spindle cell subtypes (Fig. 12.33). Extensive sampling is critical because the most important diagnostic clues can be very focal and therefore easily overlooked.

The histologic hallmark of adipocytic (lipoma-like) ALT/WDLPS is the presence of a mature adipocytic proliferation, exhibiting striking variation in cell size with at least focal nuclear atypia in fat cells or stromal spindle cells (Fig. 12.34). The presence of fibrous septa is a relatively common finding, wherein hyperchromatic stromal cells are easier to find (Fig. 12.35). As emphasized earlier, the number of lipoblasts (uni- or multivacuolated fat cells containing a hyperchromatic, scalloped nucleus) in ALT/WDLPS may vary from many to none. Lipoblasts had previously long been considered the main diagnostic clue in favor of a diagnosis of liposarcoma; however, it is well established that the presence of lipoblasts does not make and is not required for a diagnosis of liposarcoma. Very rarely, foci of metaplastic bone, scattered rhabdomyoblasts, or areas of smooth muscle differentiation can be observed.[120,121]

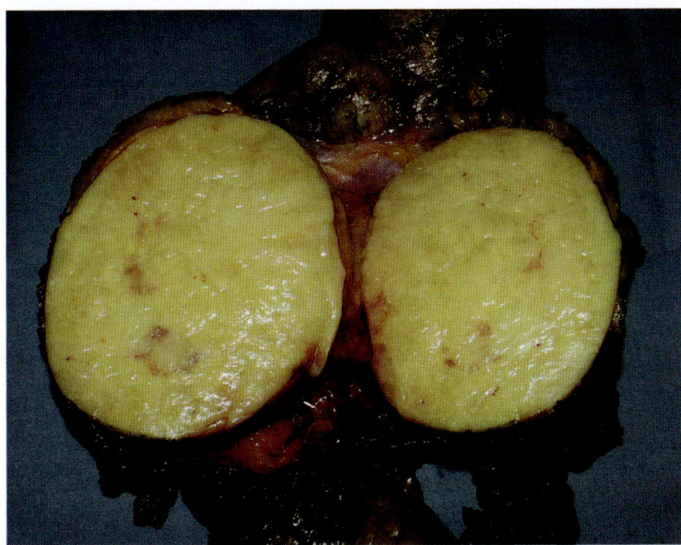

Figure 12.33 Atypical Lipomatous Tumor/Well-Differentiated Liposarcoma, Sclerosing Variant. White-gray areas reflect the amount of fibrous tissue that usually predominates in sclerosing well-differentiated liposarcoma.

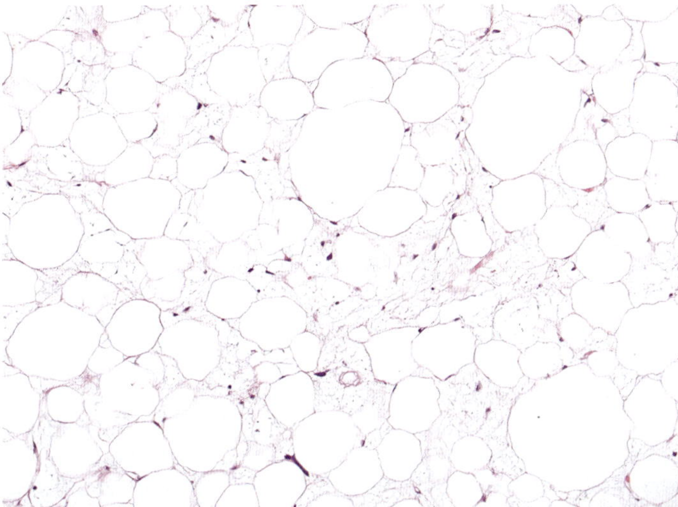

Figure 12.34 Atypical Lipomatous Tumor/Well-Differentiated Liposarcoma, Lipoma-Like Variant. Variation in cell size is a constant finding.

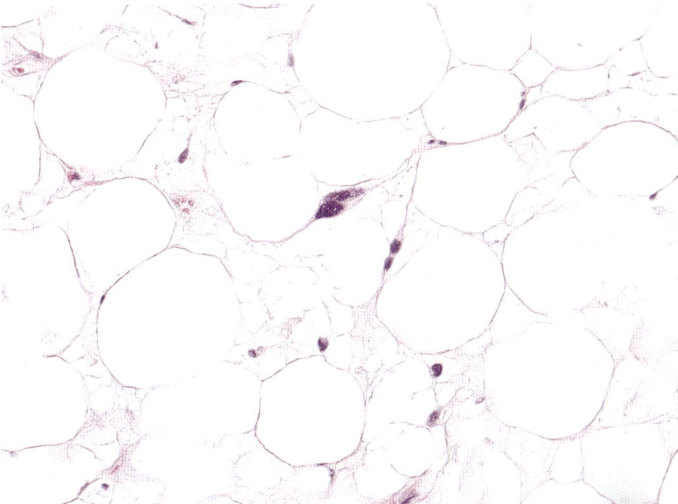

Figure 12.35 Atypical Lipomatous Tumor/Well-Differentiated Liposarcoma, Lipoma-Like Variant. Atypical hyperchromatic cells are seen.

Sclerosing ALT/WDLPS occurs most frequently in the retroperitoneum and paratesticular region. Again, the main diagnostic finding is not the presence of lipoblasts (which tend to be multivacuolated), but instead scattered bizarre, hyperchromatic stromal cells set in a fibrillary collagenous background (Fig. 12.36). Not infrequently, the fibrous component can be so extensive that lipogenic areas are overlooked, especially in small biopsy specimens (Fig. 12.37).

In rare instances, ALT/WDLPS may exhibit a dense chronic inflammatory infiltrate. The inflammation can be so prominent as to obscure the adipocytic nature of the neoplasm (Fig. 12.38). The detection of scattered atypical stromal cells is a critical diagnostic clue (Fig. 12.39). A lymphoplasmacytic infiltrate is most often seen, including lymphoid follicles, but in some cases T cells are the main inflammatory component.[122,123]

Atypical spindle cell lipomatous tumor (also known as spindle cell liposarcoma) is an adipocytic neoplasm of intermediate biologic potential (similar to ALT/WDLPS); this tumor most likely represents a rare,

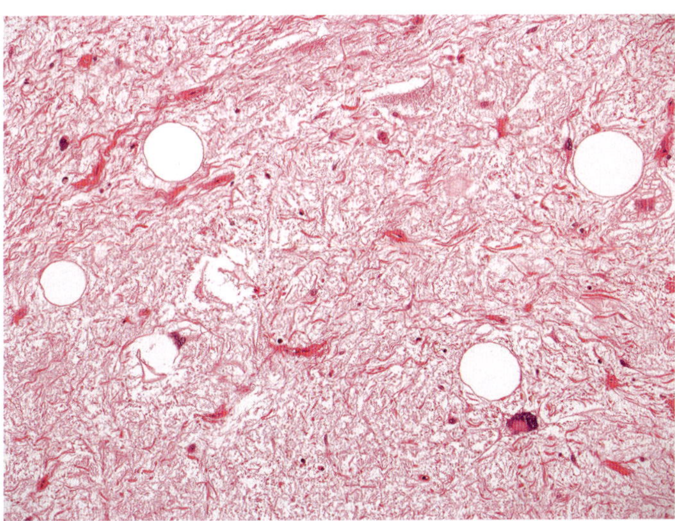

Figure 12.36 Atypical Lipomatous Tumor/Well-Differentiated Liposarcoma, Sclerosing Variant. The most important diagnostic clue is the presence of markedly atypical stromal cells.

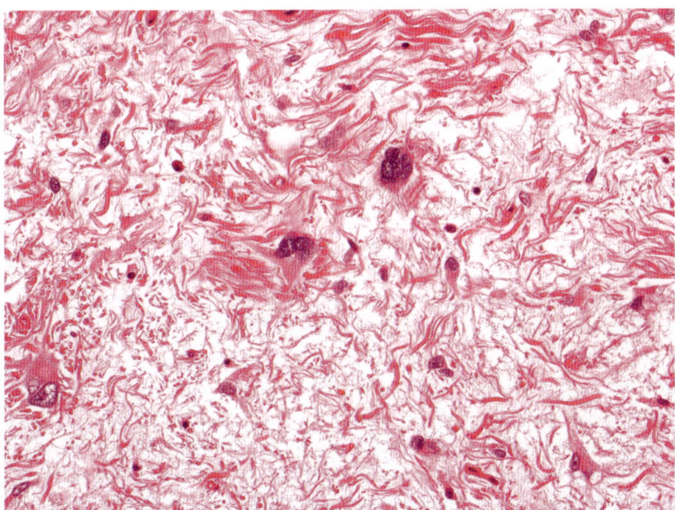

Figure 12.37 Atypical Lipomatous Tumor/Well-Differentiated Liposarcoma, Sclerosing Variant. Neoplastic cells are set in a fibrillary collagenous background that can overshadow the adipocytic component.

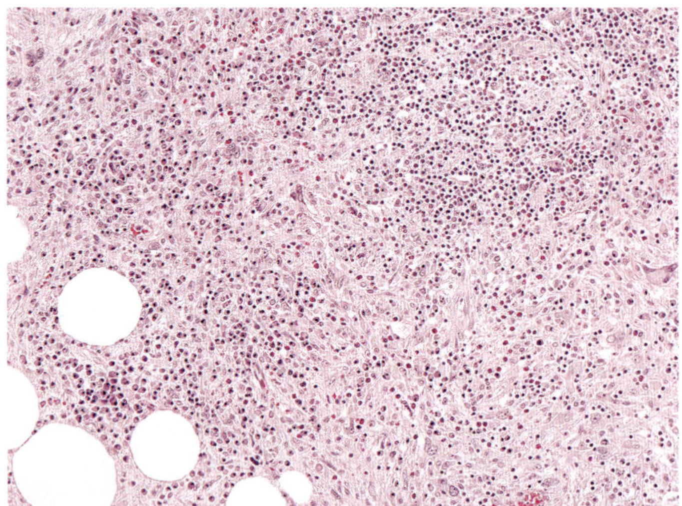

Figure 12.38 Atypical Lipomatous Tumor/Well-Differentiated Liposarcoma, Inflammatory Variant. Rarely, a marked inflammatory infiltrate obscures the adipocytic component.

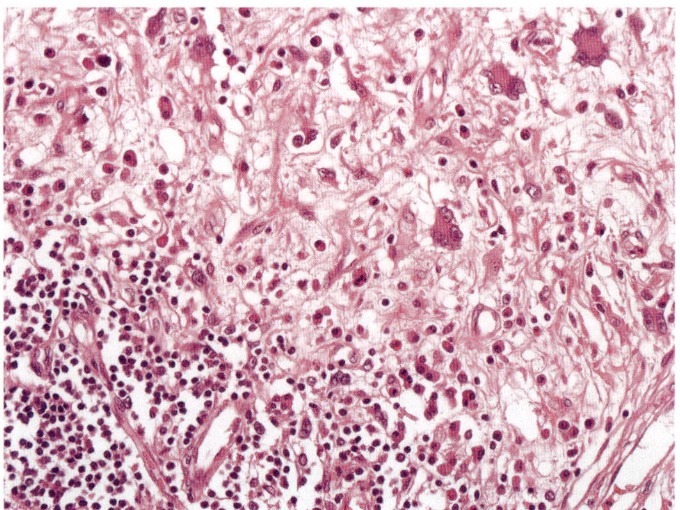

Figure 12.39 Atypical Lipomatous Tumor/Well-Differentiated Liposarcoma, Inflammatory Variant. The presence of atypical stromal elements is a key diagnostic clue.

distinct category of adipocytic neoplasm, accounting for approximately 2% of cases of ALT.[124,125] Atypical spindle cell lipomatous tumor occurs predominantly in adults and shows an anatomic distribution somewhat different than the other ALT/WDLPS subtypes. The initial impression of a tendency to be more superficial was not confirmed in a recent large study; there is an equal distribution between superficial and deep locations.[126] Approximately two thirds of cases occur in the limbs and limb girdles; this tumor type shows a predilection for the hands and feet.[126] The histologic features of atypical spindle cell lipomatous tumor are somewhat varied. More often the lesion is composed of a bland spindle cell proliferation reminiscent of a neural neoplasm set in a fibrous or myxoid background, associated with a mature or atypical lipomatous component that usually includes occasional lipoblasts. (Fig. 12.40). However, in some tumors, the cellularity is higher, the spindle cells are more atypical, and there is less extracellular matrix. Some features enabling recognition of the different ALT/WDLPS subtypes are summarized in Table 12.4.

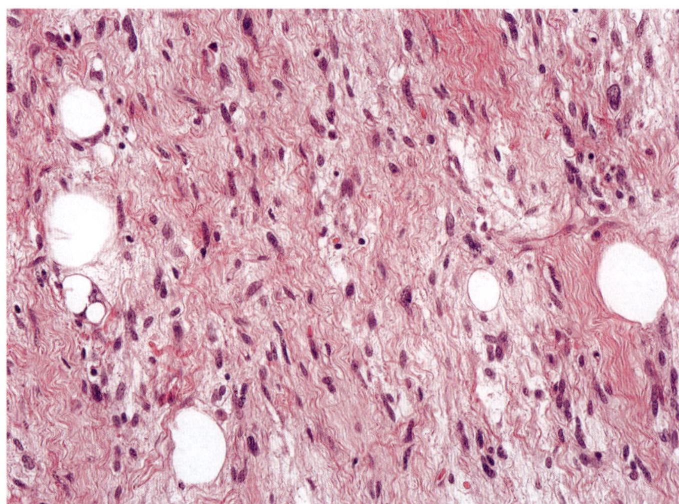

Figure 12.40 Atypical Spindle Cell Lipomatous Tumor. Atypical spindle cell lipomatous tumor is composed of a spindle cell population associated with scattered lipoblasts.

Table 12.4 Diagnostic Features of Atypical Lipomatous Tumor/Well-Differentiated Liposarcoma Subtypes

	Adipocytic	Sclerosing	Inflammatory	Spindle Cell
Size variation of adipocytes	Prominent	Focal	Focal	Focal
Nuclear atypia in stroma	Present	Marked	Present	Variable/mild
Lipoblasts	Variable	Variable	Variable	Variable
MDM2 overexpression/ amplification	Present	Present	Present	Absent

Immunohistochemistry

By immunohistochemistry, most adipocytic tumors express S-100 protein, which may play a minor role in highlighting lipoblasts. MDM2 and CDK4 are becoming increasingly popular confirmatory markers because they are essentially never overexpressed in benign lipomas (Fig. 12.41).[127–130] It is important to be aware that MDM2 can cross-react with macrophages and multinucleated giant cells, most often seen in foci of fat necrosis. However, these markers are usually negative in atypical spindle cell lipomatous tumor; therefore, they cannot be used to confirm the diagnosis of this tumor type. Variable staining for CD34, S-100 protein and desmin has been reported in atypical spindle cell lipomatous tumor; loss of nuclear expression of Rb is detected in approximately 60% of cases.[126]

Molecular Genetics

Karyotypic analysis of lipomatous lesions has provided a great amount of information (see also Chapter 18). ALT/WDLPS is characterized by distinctive ring or giant marker chromosomes containing amplified sequences derived from the 12q13-15 chromosome region, wherein map several proto-oncogenes, including *MDM2*, *CDK4*, and *HMGA2*.[131,132] Concomitant amplification of *HMGA2* and *MDM2*, as well as overexpression of the encoded proteins, is characteristic of ALT/WDLPS; immunohistochemistry and molecular genetic techniques are useful confirmatory diagnostic tools.[133–136] The cell cycle regulator *CDK4* is amplified as well in most cases, but within a distinct amplicon that may also include *DDIT3*.[137]

Interestingly, chromosome 7 monosomy was initially reported in two cases of atypical spindle cell lipomatous tumor, in the absence of

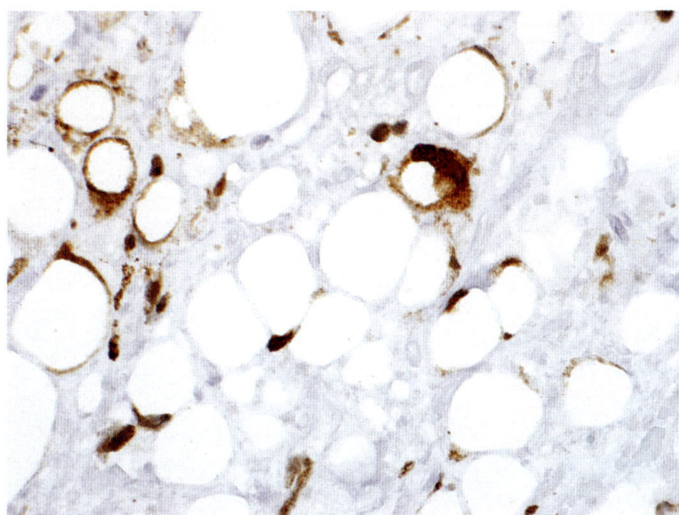

Figure 12.41 Atypical Lipomatous Tumor/Well-Differentiated Liposarcoma. As a consequence of *MDM2* gene amplification, nuclear overexpression of MDM2 is frequently observed.

12q abnormalities, suggesting a different molecular pathogenesis for this subtype.[138] Another study detected *RB1* gene deletion by FISH in six cases of spindle cell liposarcoma, suggesting a possible relationship with spindle cell lipoma.[139] These data have been confirmed in a recent series that documented loss of nuclear expression of Rb in around 60% of cases of atypical spindle cell lipomatous tumor, correlating with *RB1* heterozygous deletion.[126] The fact that MDM2 overexpression/amplification is typically absent (and loss of *RB1* is common) in atypical spindle cell lipomatous tumor supports the concept that this tumor in fact represents a distinct tumor type, likely unrelated to conventional ALT.

Because some genetic features, such as involvement of the 12q chromosome region and overexpression of HMGA2, are shared by both benign lipomas and ALT/WDLPS, it has been hypothesized that these tumor types may form a genetic and morphologic continuum.[128] Recently, eight lipomas that had unusual chromosomal features resulting in gains of 12q14-15 were reported.[140] Although three patients had simple numerical rearrangements (trisomy 12) or structural rearrangements (unbalanced translocations with 12q gains), five were particularly intriguing because of peculiar features, such as giant chromosomes, supernumerary chromosomes, or neocentromeres, which are usually the hallmarks of ALT/WDLPS. Gains of 12q14-15 sequences, including extra copies of *MDM2* and *CDK4*, were detected by FISH in all cases analyzed, but no expression of MDM2 and CDK4 was observed, suggesting that these genomic imbalances might not have functional consequence. Rearrangements of *HMGA2* in five of eight cases were also reported. These results support the view that intermediate forms between classic lipomas and classic ALT/WDLPS may exist.

Differential Diagnosis

The differential diagnosis of well-differentiated adipocytic liposarcoma is mainly with benign lipoma (Table 12.5). Variation in adipocytic size and cytologic atypia are the main diagnostic clues. As mentioned earlier, the absence of lipoblasts is meaningless because they may be difficult to find or completely absent in ALT/WDLPS. A common diagnostic pitfall is the presence of microscopic fat necrosis as well as fat atrophy. In both situations, variation in adipocytic size (associated with macrophages in fat necrosis) may lead to consideration of ALT/WDLPS. However, the absence of cytologic atypia in both fat and stromal cells is helpful to establish a benign diagnosis.

Table 12.5 Differential Diagnosis Between Benign Lipoma and Atypical Lipomatous Tumor/Lipoma-Like Well-Differentiated Liposarcoma

	Lipoma	Atypical Lipomatous Tumor
Size variation of adipocytes	Absent	Present
Nuclear atypia in adipocytes	Absent	Present
Nuclear atypia in stroma	Absent	Present
Lipoblasts	Absent	From none to several
MDM2 overexpression/ amplification	Absent	Usually present

Sclerosing liposarcoma must be distinguished from idiopathic retroperitoneal fibrosis.[141] Typical clinical presentation and radiologic findings and the absence of atypical stromal cells are helpful for diagnosing retroperitoneal fibrosis. FISH evaluation for *HMGA2* or *MDM2* gene amplification or immunohistochemistry for MDM2 and CDK4 overexpression can help confirm the diagnosis of sclerosing WDLPS.[142]

For well-differentiated inflammatory liposarcoma, the differential diagnosis includes non-adipocytic lesions, such as inflammatory myofibroblastic tumor and Castleman disease. Inflammatory myofibroblastic tumor is characterized by a proliferation of myofibroblastic spindle cells associated with an inflammatory infiltrate variably composed of plasma cells, lymphocytes, and eosinophils. Inflammatory myofibroblastic tumors variably express smooth muscle actin and desmin, and in approximately 50% of cases, they express ALK protein as a consequence of *ALK* gene rearrangements. In any case, to avoid diagnostic confusion, these lesions should be sampled extensively to prevent overlooking the adipocytic component.

The differential diagnosis of atypical spindle cell lipomatous tumor includes benign as well as malignant lesions, such as spindle cell lipoma, neurofibroma, DFSP, malignant peripheral nerve sheath tumor (MPNST), well-differentiated sclerosing liposarcoma, dedifferentiated liposarcoma, and low-grade fibromyxoid sarcoma. In this context, as spindle cell ALT is a predominantly non-lipogenic lesion, the presence of lipoblasts is a helpful diagnostic clue. However, lipoblasts can occasionally be found in spindle cell lipoma, and both spindle cell lipoma and atypical spindle cell lipomatous tumor often show loss of nuclear Rb expression; the absence of nuclear atypia and the presence of ropy collagen bundles are key discriminating features. DFSP is a CD34-positive, cytologically uniform, bland spindle cell neoplasm typically infiltrating the subcutaneous fat with a honeycomb pattern of growth. Atypical spindle cell lipomatous tumor is less cellular, with more intervening stroma, and lacks the honeycomb architecture. Benign neural lesions and low-grade MPNST arising in neurofibroma are typically extensively positive for S-100 protein (although atypical spindle cell lipomatous tumor can also express S-100 protein) and lack an adipocytic component. Conventional MPNST shows obvious cytologic atypia, and in contrast to atypical spindle cell lipomatous tumor, typically exhibits variation in cellularity from area to area, often with perivascular accentuation of cellularity. Immunohistochemistry is not particularly helpful because S-100 protein, GFAP, and SOX10 are positive in only a fraction of neoplastic cells in at most 40% of MPNSTs; S-100 protein expression is also seen in around 40% of atypical spindle cell lipomatous tumors. The differential diagnosis with dedifferentiated liposarcoma can be challenging at times, as the more cellular examples of atypical spindle cell lipomatous tumor may overlap morphologically with non-pleomorphic examples of dedifferentiated liposarcoma (DDLPS). The absence of MDM2/CDK4 expression and amplification is an important diagnostic clue in these rare cases. Low-grade fibromyxoid sarcoma shows characteristic alternating fibrous

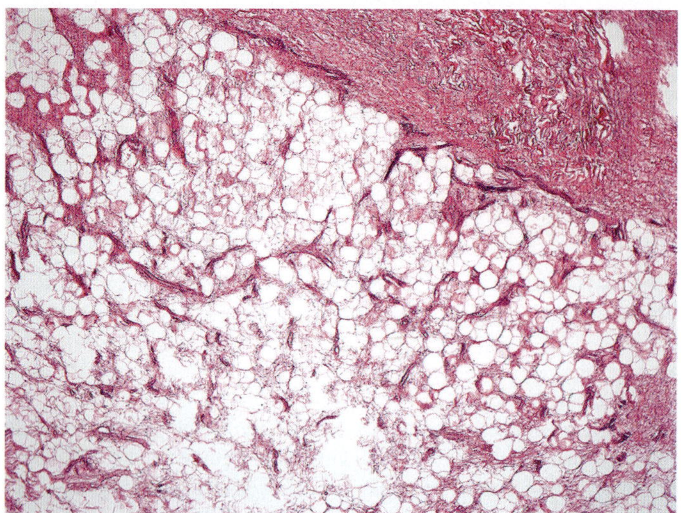

Figure 12.42 **Massive Localized Lymphedema.** Broadened fibrous septa demarcating lobules of mature fat are typically seen.

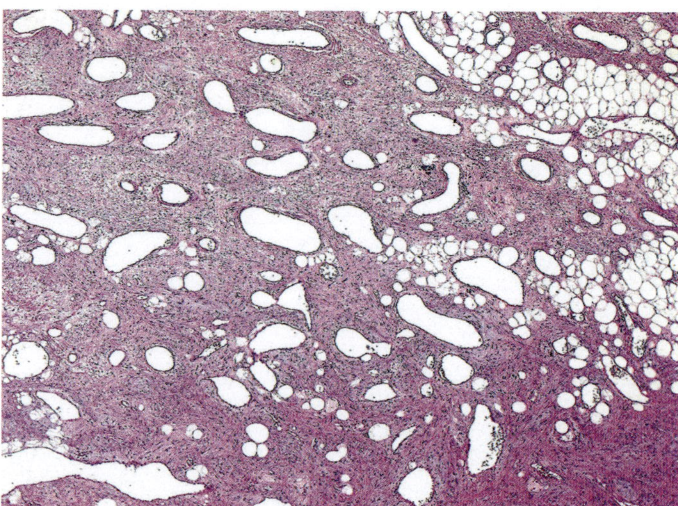

Figure 12.43 **Fat-Forming Solitary Fibrous Tumor.** The typical patternless, collagen-rich, spindle cell proliferation is intermingled with a mature adipocytic component.

and myxoid areas containing arcades of thin-walled blood vessels, lacks an adipocytic component, and is diffusely positive for MUC4. In difficult cases, detection of *FUS* gene rearrangement by FISH can confirm the diagnosis.

Another important lesion sometimes mistaken for a true adipocytic neoplasm is a condition known as *massive localized lymphedema*.[143,144] This lesion typically affects morbidly obese individuals (mostly women). Massive localized lymphedema tends to involve the proximal medial aspect of the extremities and is unilateral. Clinically, massive localized lymphedema presents as a diffuse, ill-defined mass of long duration that most often attains a very large size. Histologically, massive localized lymphedema is composed of lobules of mature fat demarcated by expanded connective tissue septa. Such widened septa simulate the fibrous bands of ALT/WDLPS; however, nuclear atypia is absent in both fat and stromal cells (Fig. 12.42). The overlying dermis usually shows lymphangiectasia and stromal edema. Massive localized lymphedema is a non-neoplastic condition.

Rarely, ALT/WDLPS undergoes extensive myxoid change to the extent that the differential diagnosis with myxoid liposarcoma can be raised.[145] The absence of a plexiform vascular pattern and the presence of significant nuclear hyperchromasia are helpful diagnostic features to support ALT. Cytogenetics or molecular genetics can be of great help because these two entities have distinctive genetic features.

Another potential diagnostic problem is the differential diagnosis with "fat-forming" solitary fibrous tumor, a lesion that in the past was first reported as *lipomatous hemangiopericytoma*, which is simply a variant of solitary fibrous tumor containing an adipocytic component (Fig. 12.43). A CD34-positive spindle cell proliferation set in a collagenous stroma and a prominent hemangiopericytoma-like vascular pattern are typical morphologic features of solitary fibrous tumor; nuclear expression of STAT6 is a helpful finding to confirm the diagnosis (see also Chapter 3).

Prognosis and Treatment

Although ALT/WDLPS is associated with a 30% to 50% overall risk of local recurrence, distant metastases are never observed unless dedifferentiation occurs (discussed later). The anatomic location is the most important prognostic factor and the main predictor of relapse. The overall mortality rate is nearly 0% for lesions arising in surgically amenable soft tissue sites (e.g., the extremities), but up to 80% for lesions occurring in the retroperitoneum or other visceral sites, wherein the risk for repeated, local (and eventually aggressive) recurrences approaches 100%.

Standard treatment for ALT/WDLPS is complete surgical removal with negative margins, if possible. Negative surgical margins are almost impossible to achieve when dealing with retroperitoneal tumors. Nonetheless, radical multivisceral surgery is currently recommended for such tumors to increase the relapse-free interval.[114,115] According to recently published data, atypical spindle cell lipomatous tumor exhibits a rate of local recurrence of approximately 12%, with no potential for systemic spread.[126]

Dedifferentiated Liposarcoma

The term *dedifferentiated liposarcoma* (DDLPS) was introduced by Evans in 1979 to define the morphologic progression from ALT/WDLPS to a non-lipogenic sarcoma.[146] Most often, the non-lipogenic component is high grade; however, there exist cases in which the dedifferentiated component is morphologically low grade.[147–149] The concept of dedifferentiation had been previously introduced by Dhalin and colleagues in the context of tumor progression in chondrosarcoma[150] and subsequently extended to other entities, such as chordoma, parosteal osteosarcoma, and ALT/WDLPS. As discussed later, DDLPS is a biologically fascinating entity, in which the morphologic features, genetics, and clinical course defy common rules of mesenchymal malignancies.

Clinical Features

Dedifferentiated liposarcoma accounts for approximately 10% of all liposarcomas, although their true incidence may be underestimated because of the previous tendency to diagnose all pleomorphic neoplasms in the retroperitoneum as "malignant fibrous histiocytoma" ("MFH"). Dedifferentiated liposarcoma occurs most frequently in the retroperitoneum in adults, followed by the deep soft tissue of the limbs, trunk, mediastinum, head and neck region, and spermatic cord.[151–153] Occurrence in the superficial soft tissues is observed in fewer than 1% of cases. Elderly men are slightly more frequently affected than women, with a peak incidence between the sixth and seventh decades. Dedifferentiation is encountered most frequently (90%) in the primary tumor (de novo DDLPS) than in recurrences of WDLPS (10%). Recently published molecular data suggest that the incidence of DDLPS arising in the limbs may be underestimated.[154]

Pathologic Features

Most cases of DDLPS present as a large, multinodular mass with a yellow cut surface, containing firm tan-gray areas (Fig. 12.44), the amount of which depends solely on the relative abundance of the dedifferentiated (non-lipogenic) component. Not infrequently, a distinct, well-demarcated firm nodule is seen in the background of the adipose tissue component. As mentioned earlier, adequate sampling is critical. The well-differentiated component may be mistakenly regarded as "normal fat" and therefore overlooked. In the past, inadequate sampling of DDLPS greatly contributed to the common misdiagnosis of retroperitoneal "MFH." Most often, histologic examination shows an abrupt transition from WDLPS to a high-grade non-lipogenic sarcoma (Fig. 12.45); however, in some cases, this transition can be more gradual, and exceptionally, low-grade and high-grade areas appear to be intermingled (Fig. 12.46). In the vast majority of cases, dedifferentiated areas exhibit complete morphologic overlap with undifferentiated pleomorphic sarcoma (formerly known as the storiform and pleomorphic variant of MFH; see Chapter 7) (Fig. 12.47). Less frequently, high-grade myxofibrosarcoma-like morphologic features are observed (Fig. 12.48). In some cases, a marked mixed inflammatory infiltrate dominated by neutrophils is present; in the past, such cases were classified as the inflammatory variant of MFH. However, morphologic, clinical, and genetic evidence show that most, if not all, cases of inflammatory MFH are actually examples of DDLPS with a prominent inflammatory component.[155] An additional fascinating aspect of DDLPS is heterologous differentiation.[156,157] This phenomenon occurs in approximately 5% to 10% of cases and is most often myogenic (rhabdomyosarcomatous or leiomyosarcomatous) (Figs. 12.49 and 12.50), but osteo/chondrosarcomatous, and more rarely, angiosarcomatous differentiation can also be seen. Occasionally, the non-lipogenic component of DDLPS may show a peculiar spindle cell proliferation organized in distinctive whorls, reminiscent of neural or meningothelial structures (Figs. 12.51 and 12.52), often associated with metaplastic bone formation, and more rarely, with a plasmacytic inflammatory infiltrate.[158,159] This peculiar variant of DDLPS exhibits the same karyotypic aberrations observed in the conventional type (discussed later).[160]

As mentioned earlier, not all cases of DDLPS exhibit "high-grade" morphologic features. Some cases contain fascicles of relatively bland

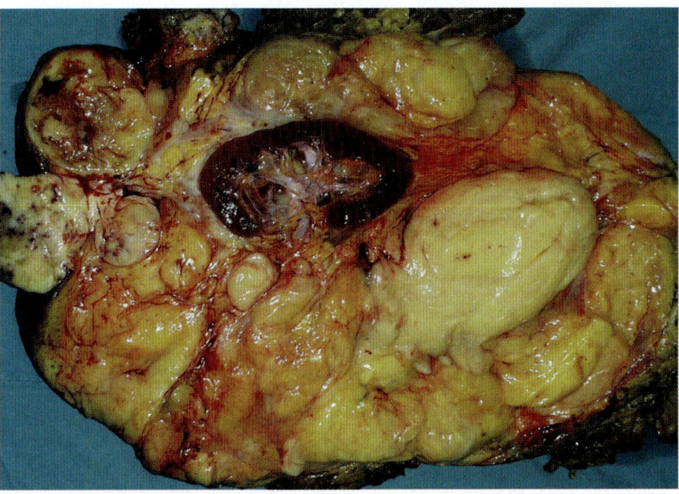

Figure 12.44 **Dedifferentiated Liposarcoma.** Grossly, dedifferentiated liposarcoma contains a variable amount of firm gray areas.

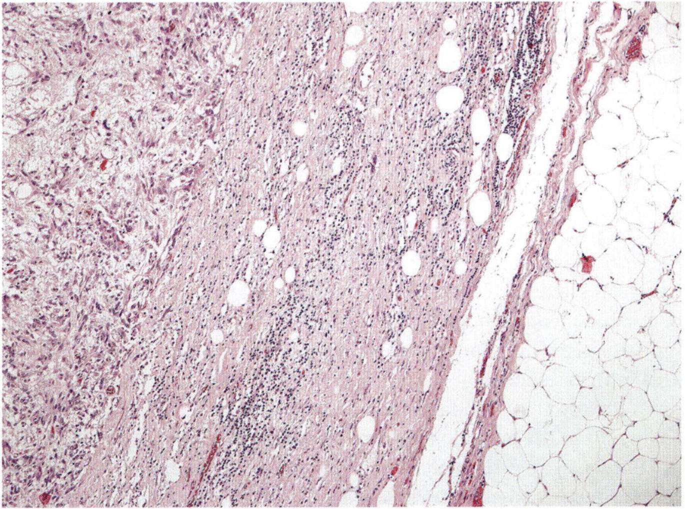

Figure 12.45 **Dedifferentiated Liposarcoma.** Abrupt transition from a well-differentiated adipocytic component to a high-grade nonlipogenic sarcoma is most often seen.

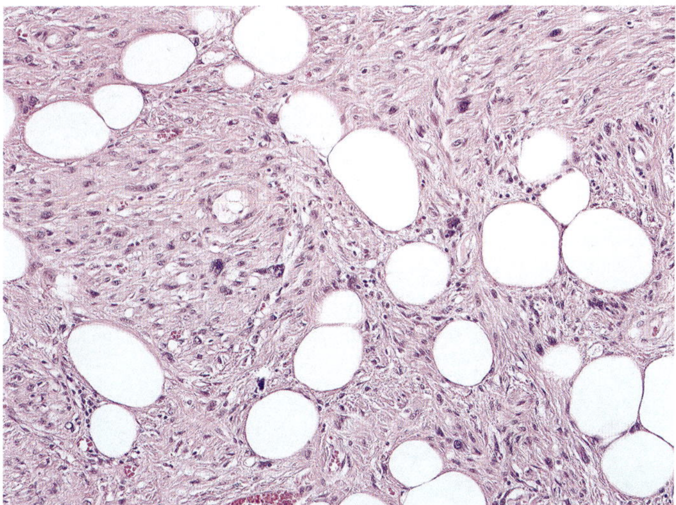

Figure 12.46 **Dedifferentiated Liposarcoma.** Rarely, well-differentiated and high-grade areas are intermingled.

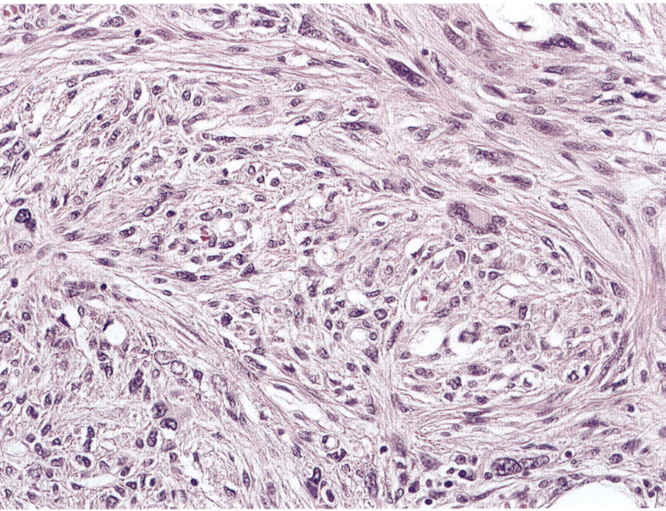

Figure 12.47 **Dedifferentiated Liposarcoma.** Most often, the high-grade component overlaps morphologically with undifferentiated pleomorphic sarcoma.

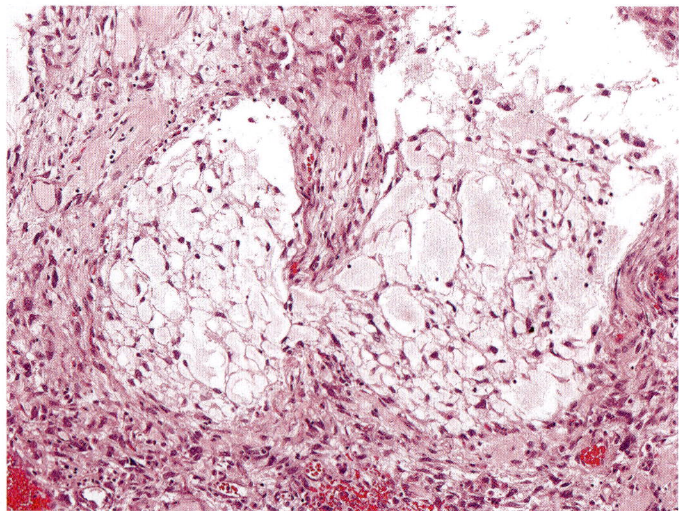

Figure 12.48 **Dedifferentiated Liposarcoma.** High-grade myxofibrosarcoma-like morphologic features are also seen.

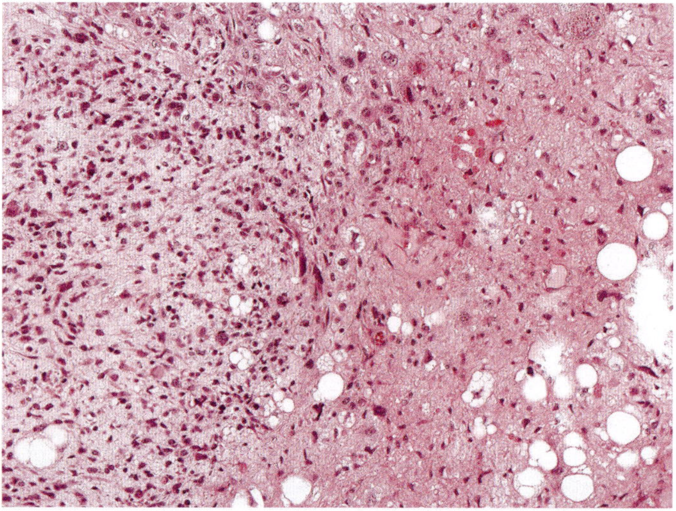

Figure 12.49 **Dedifferentiated Liposarcoma.** Heterologous differentiation (most often myogenic) is observed in a minority of cases.

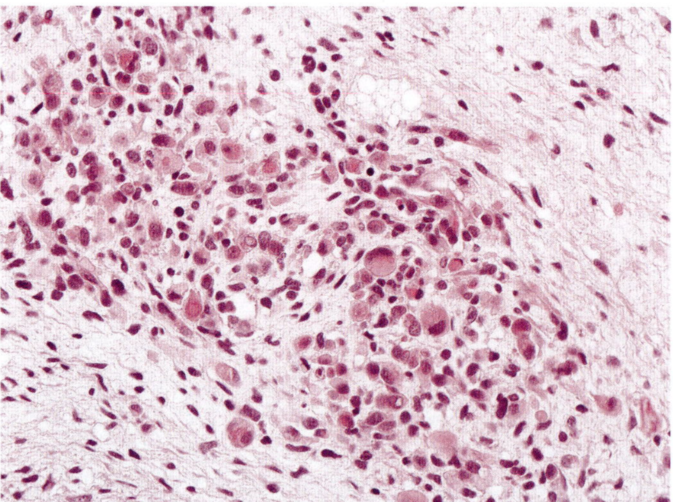

Figure 12.50 **Dedifferentiated Liposarcoma.** Neoplastic cells show focal rhabdomyoblastic differentiation.

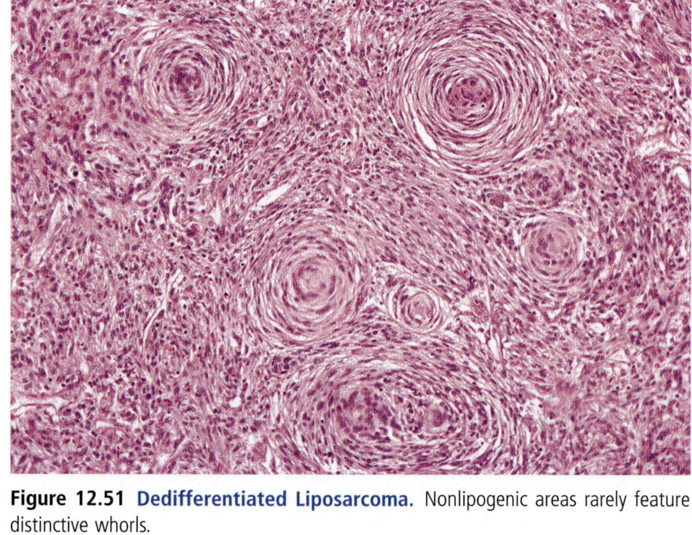

Figure 12.51 **Dedifferentiated Liposarcoma.** Nonlipogenic areas rarely feature distinctive whorls.

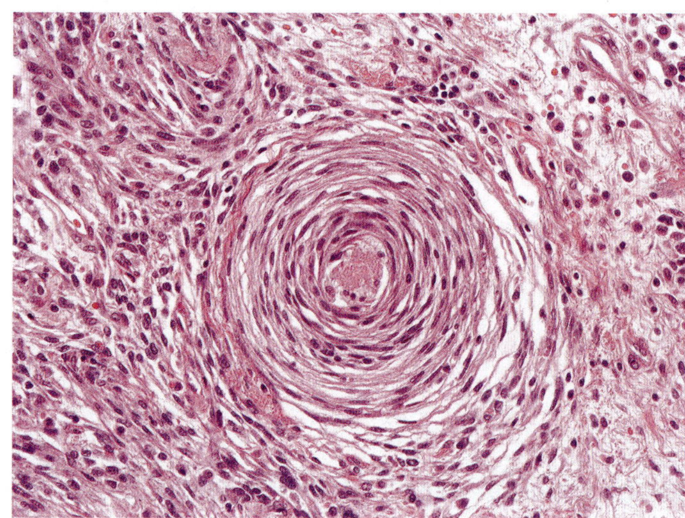

Figure 12.52 **Dedifferentiated Liposarcoma.** These peculiar structures are reminiscent of neural or meningothelial neoplasms.

spindle cells with a cellularity intermediate between that of well-differentiated sclerosing liposarcoma and usual high-grade areas of DDLPS. *Low-grade dedifferentiation* is the term proposed to describe these areas, to mark the morphologic difference with conventional "high-grade" nonlipogenic components (Fig. 12.53). It is common for DDLPS to show striking intratumoral morphologic heterogeneity, which can be a helpful diagnostic clue when the well-differentiated adipocytic component has been overlooked. Occasionally, the higher-grade component of DDLPS may show lipoblastic differentiation—either in the form of isolated lipoblasts scattered throughout the higher-grade component, or as sheets of atypical pleomorphic adipocytes—resulting in areas morphologically indistinguishable from pleomorphic LPS (see also Chapter 7).[161,162] This phenomenon has been referred to as "homologous lipoblastic differentiation" or "pleomorphic LPS-like features;" it is thought to be analogous to the heterologous differentiation observed more frequently in DDLPS. Molecular analysis has shown high-level amplification of the *MDM2* locus and expression levels of MDM2 and CDK4 comparable to conventional DDLPS, as well as a similar karyotype, supporting the classification of these lesions as DDLPS rather than pleomorphic LPS, which has a considerably worse prognosis.[161,162]

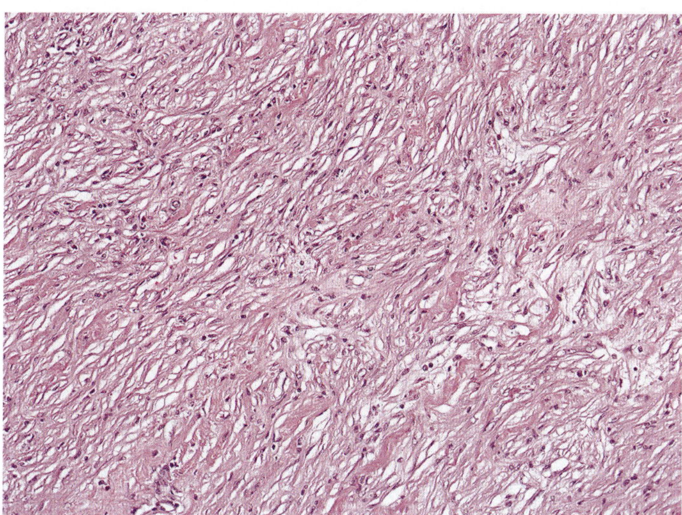

Figure 12.53 Dedifferentiated Liposarcoma. Nonlipogenic areas may exhibit low-grade spindle cell morphologic features.

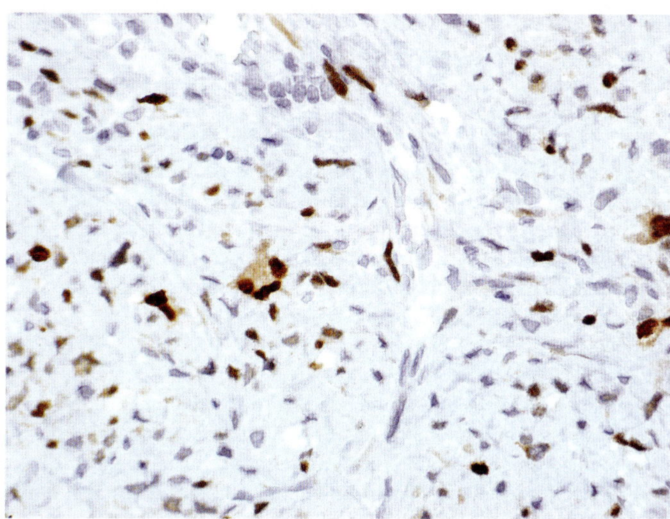

Figure 12.54 Dedifferentiated Liposarcoma. MDM2 is overexpressed in most cases of dedifferentiated liposarcoma.

Immunohistochemistry

Overexpression of MDM2 and CDK4 in both lipogenic and nonlipogenic components of DDLPS is consistently observed (Fig. 12.54); the extent of staining is much greater in the dedifferentiated component.[128–130] Recent data have suggested that immunopositivity for peroxisome proliferator-activated receptor-γ (a nuclear hormone receptor that plays a critical role in adipocyte differentiation) may also help in distinguishing DDLPS from other retroperitoneal sarcomas.[163] Pertinent differentiation markers are helpful in confirming heterologous differentiation.

Molecular Genetics

Dedifferentiated liposarcoma shows a significant genetic overlap with ALT/WDLPS, usually with ring or giant marker chromosomes, although superimposed additional aberrations have been reported (see also Chapter 18).[85,164] At the molecular level, a significant increase in both amplification and overexpression of *MDM2* in the high-grade areas has been observed, which may account for tumor progression in this subset of sarcomas.[165,166] However, at variance with other high-grade pleomorphic sarcomas, which most often harbor *TP53* mutations (significantly associated with poor clinical outcome), in DDLPS, *TP53* is almost always unaffected.[167] Similar to ALT/WDLPS, *HMGA2* tends to co-amplify with *MDM2* in DDLPS, whereas *CDK4* belongs to a distinct inconsistent amplicon that might be generated by the disruption of a fragile region 5′ of *DDIT3*. Amplification and overexpression of *YEATS4*, an oncogene that inactivates TP53, has also been reported, raising the possibility that YEATS4 might play a synergic role with MDM2 in the molecular oncogenesis of DDLPS.[137] Molecular genetics may also prove useful for developing new therapeutic strategies. Recent studies have shown that Nutlin-3a, an antagonist of MDM2, preferentially induces apoptosis and growth arrest in DDLPS cells compared with normal adipocytes, suggesting that MDM2 inhibition is a promising rationale for molecular targeted therapy in DDLPS.[168–170] CDK4, which also plays a key role in the oncogenesis of DDLPS, may also represent a promising target for molecular therapy.[171]

Differential Diagnosis

Dedifferentiated liposarcoma should be distinguished from other pleomorphic sarcomas occurring in the retroperitoneum (especially pleomorphic leiomyosarcoma),[171] as well as from other sarcomatous and nonsarcomatous lesions (Box 12.3). Pleomorphic leiomyosarcoma, once a well-differentiated liposarcomatous component has been excluded, can be recognized by the presence of better-differentiated areas containing spindle cells with the typical fibrillary eosinophilic cytoplasm and broad, cigar-shaped nuclei. Leiomyosarcoma is supported by variable expression of smooth muscle actin, desmin, and h-caldesmon. However, the immunoprofile should be interpreted with caution because DDLPS may also show reactivity for smooth muscle actin or desmin. Importantly, both MDM2 and CDK4 are only rarely detected in leiomyosarcoma. As already mentioned, most cases of inflammatory MFH are in fact DDLPS containing a dense inflammatory infiltrate.[155] When low-grade dedifferentiation is encountered, gastrointestinal stromal tumor may enter the differential diagnosis. However, immunopositivity for KIT (CD117) and DOG1, and molecular demonstration of *KIT* or *PDGFRA* mutations in KIT-negative tumors or other challenging cases, permits proper classification of most gastrointestinal stromal tumors. Sarcomatoid carcinoma can be excluded by the lack of epithelial differentiation markers, such as EMA and keratins.

Box 12.3 Dedifferentiated Liposarcoma

Dedifferentiated liposarcoma is a likely diagnosis when:
- A pleomorphic sarcoma is seen in the retroperitoneum.
- A well-differentiated liposarcomatous component is associated with a high-grade nonlipogenic sarcoma.
- MDM2 and CDK4 are overexpressed/amplified.

Prognosis and Treatment

The clinical behavior of DDLPS is as intriguing as its morphologic features. Despite having high-grade histologic appearances, DDLPS is less aggressive than other types of high-grade pleomorphic sarcoma.[152] In contrast with WDLPS, dedifferentiation is associated with a 15% to 20% metastatic rate. Mortality is more often related to uncontrolled local recurrences than to metastatic spread. Because time to relapse appears to be correlated with the extent of resection, the current recommended treatment is wide surgical resection which, for retroperitoneal lesions, should include adjacent viscera.[114,115]

The clinical and biologic peculiarities of DDLPS include local recurrences as WDLPS in which the dedifferentiated component is absent. In addition, there is no correlation between the amount of dedifferentiation and outcome. As mentioned earlier, the dedifferentiated component may exhibit a broad spectrum of histologic grade. Retrospective data have suggested that, using the French Fédération Nationale des Centres de Lutte Contre le Cancer (FNCLCC) grading system, there may be a correlation between grade and both disease-specific and local recurrence-free survival.[172] This observation has been confirmed in a larger study.[173] When dedifferentiated liposarcoma is graded according to FNCLCC system, a significantly worse prognosis is observed when comparing grade 3 versus grade 2 tumors. In addition, again at variance with previously published data, the presence of myogenic differentiation and, in particular, rhabdomyoblastic differentiation seems to correlate with more aggressive clinical behavior.[173]

Myxoid Liposarcoma

Myxoid liposarcoma is the second largest group of malignant adipocytic neoplasms, accounting for 30% to 35% of all liposarcomas.[174,175] Myxoid liposarcoma forms a morphologic continuum that includes hypercellular neoplasms composed of oval to round neoplastic cells, formerly known as *round cell liposarcoma*. As already mentioned, the 2013 WHO classification has abolished the term round cell liposarcoma, emphasizing the fact that it simply represents part of the spectrum of a single disease.[2] The presence of hypercellular areas, however, is a key prognostic determinant.[176,177] Advances in molecular genetics have greatly contributed to the acceptance of the concept of this morphologic spectrum by showing that both myxoid and round cell types of liposarcoma contain the same genetic abnormality, in most cases, a balanced translocation t(12;16)(q13;p11) that fuses the *DDIT3* gene on 12q13 with the *FUS* gene on 16p11.[178,179]

Clinical Features

The clinical presentation of myxoid liposarcoma differs significantly from that of ALT/WDLPS or DDLPS. Myxoid liposarcoma occurs predominantly in the lower limbs (especially the thigh), whereas a retroperitoneal primary site is exceptional.[180] The peak incidence is between the third and fifth decades, with an equal gender distribution. Myxoid liposarcoma, depending on the extent of hypercellularity, exhibits a significant tendency toward metastatic spread (up to 60% when a hypercellular/round cell component is present in more than 25% of the tumor mass). Interestingly, unlike most other sarcoma types, bone and soft tissue (including the retroperitoneum) are among the most common metastatic sites.[181,182] Again, because quantitative evaluation of the less differentiated areas plays a key role in grading, extensive sampling of the surgical specimen is mandatory.

Pathologic Features

Grossly, purely myxoid liposarcoma is a well-circumscribed, multinodular, gelatinous mass (Fig. 12.55). The presence of hypercellular (round cell) areas may confer a fleshy appearance that overlaps with that of other high-grade sarcomas (Fig. 12.56).

Histologically, purely myxoid liposarcoma is composed of a hypocellular bland spindle cell proliferation set in a myxoid background (Fig. 12.57), often showing pools of mucin, which have been described as imparting a "pulmonary edema–like" appearance (Fig. 12.58). Lipoblasts are most often univacuolated or bivacuolated and tend to cluster around vessels or at the periphery of the lesion (Fig. 12.59). A most helpful morphologic clue is the delicate, capillary-sized vascular network, organized in a distinctive plexiform pattern that has been variably described as *chicken wire* or *crow's feet* (Fig. 12.60).

Myxoid/round cell liposarcoma is defined by the presence of hypercellular areas (that most frequently begin to form in a perivascular distribution), featuring undifferentiated round cell morphologic features and ranging in extent from 5% to 80% (Fig. 12.61). Pure "round cell liposarcoma" is a rare neoplasm in which hypercellularity or round cell morphologic features account for more than 80% of tumor tissue

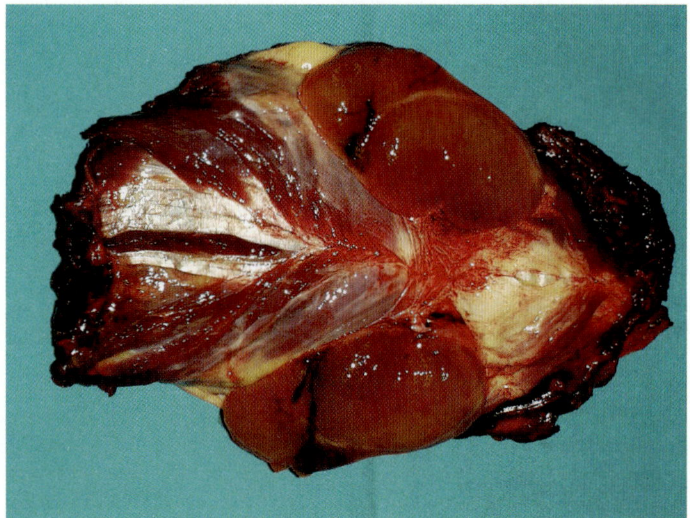

Figure 12.55 Myxoid Liposarcoma. Well-demarcated gelatinous nodules are the typical gross appearance.

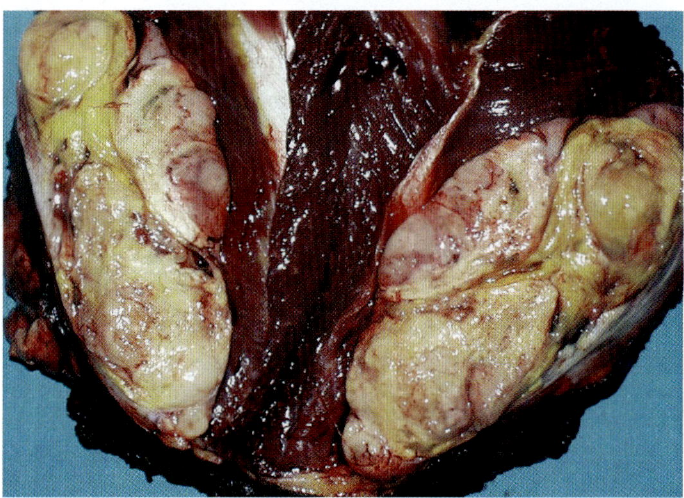

Figure 12.56 Myxoid Liposarcoma. Fleshy areas correlate with the progression to high-grade (round cell) morphologic features.

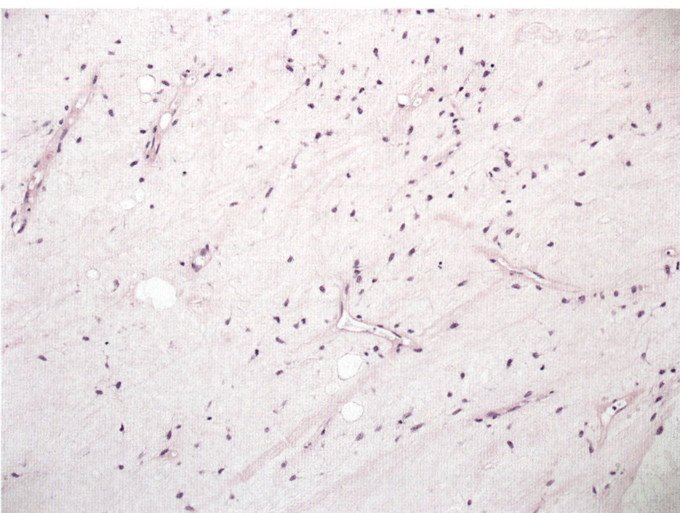

Figure 12.57 Myxoid Liposarcoma. A spindle cell proliferation set in a myxoid background is seen.

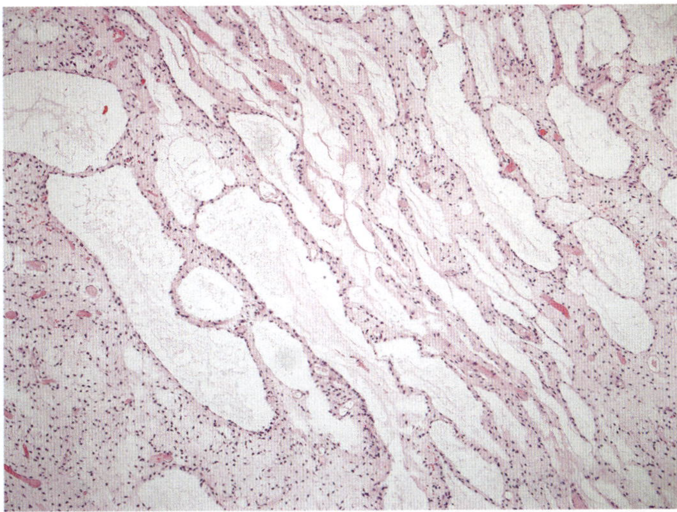

Figure 12.58 **Myxoid Liposarcoma.** Pools of mucin are frequently identified.

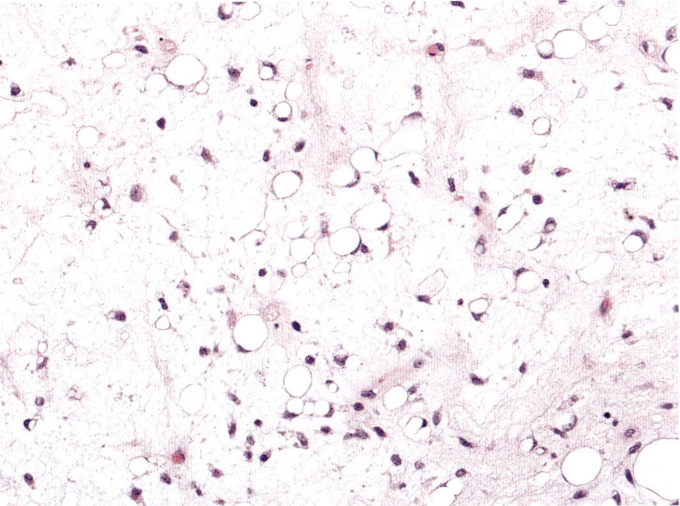

Figure 12.59 **Myxoid Liposarcoma.** Lipoblasts in myxoid liposarcoma tend to be univacuolated.

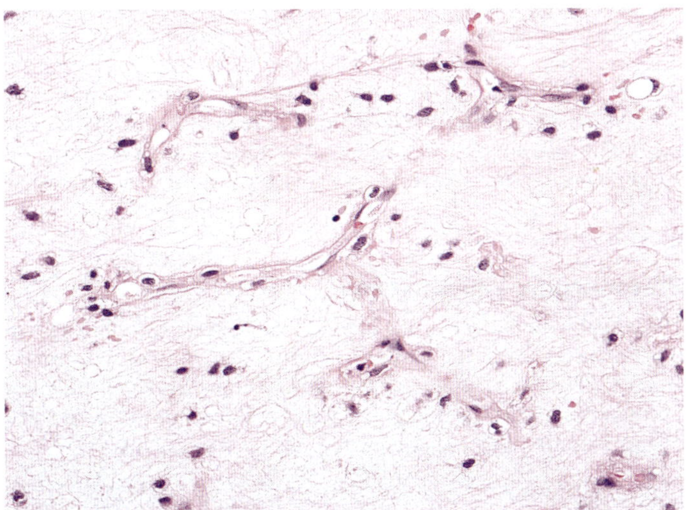

Figure 12.60 **Myxoid Liposarcoma.** One of the most important diagnostic clues is a plexiform capillary network.

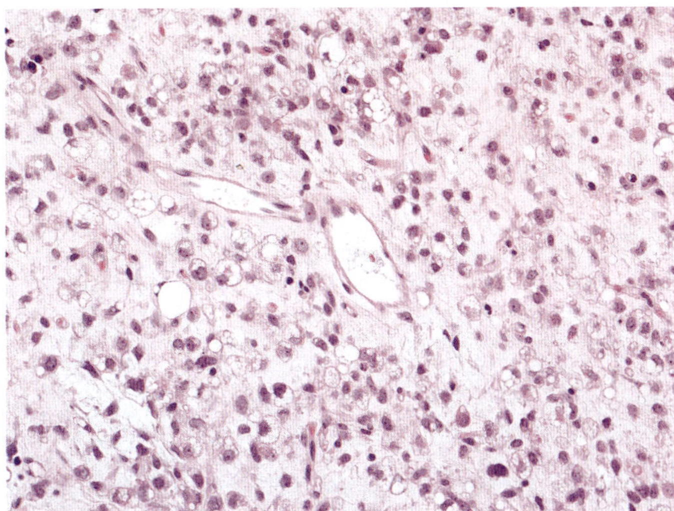

Figure 12.61 **Myxoid Liposarcoma.** Hypercellularity usually begins around blood vessels.

(Fig. 12.62). Adipocytic differentiation in pure round cell liposarcoma is often very limited or inapparent, but the presence of S-100 protein immunopositivity in the majority of cases may be diagnostically helpful.[183] High-grade myxoid liposarcoma may not have round cell morphologic features, but simply show a hypercellular appearance with the typical spindle cell morphologic features of lower-grade lesions. For this reason, the *round cell* designation has been replaced by the more accurate label "high grade myxoid liposarcoma." The transition to hypercellular/round cell areas in myxoid liposarcoma was the initial evidence supporting the concept that myxoid and round cell liposarcoma are part of a morphologic continuum. As mentioned, these morphologic observations have been validated by both cytogenetics and molecular genetics (discussed later).[178,179] In exceedingly rare cases, heterologous elements can be observed.[184]

Immunohistochemistry

Myxoid liposarcoma usually exhibits S-100 protein immunopositivity, which is often retained in the hypercellular/round cell areas. However, immunohistochemistry plays a minor role in diagnosis.

Molecular Genetics

Myxoid liposarcoma is characterized by two main karyotypic alterations (see also Chapter 18). More than 95% of cases harbor a specific t(12;16)(q13;p11) that fuses the *DDIT3* (*CHOP*) gene on 12q13 (a member of the CCAAT/enhancer binding protein family involved in adipocyte differentiation), with the *FUS* (*TLS*) gene on 16p11. A minority of cases (not exceeding 5%) carry a t(12;22)(q13;q12) that fuses *DDIT3* with *EWSR1* on 22q12. Several FUS-DDIT3 transcripts have been detected, and although they do not have any known prognostic significance, they may play a role in predicting response to the marine-derived alkaloid trabectedin.[185] The normal function of the *DDIT3* gene is to promote growth arrest and adipocytic differentiation, but as a consequence of the translocation, the anti-proliferative activity is lost, whereas the prolipogenic activity is retained.[186]

Molecular analysis of myxoid liposarcoma has shown that *TP53* gene mutations occur in approximately one third of cases, but these appear to be independent of tumor grade.[187]

Differential Diagnosis

The differential diagnosis of myxoid liposarcoma can be broad. As mentioned earlier, ALT/WDLPS can exhibit myxoid stromal change

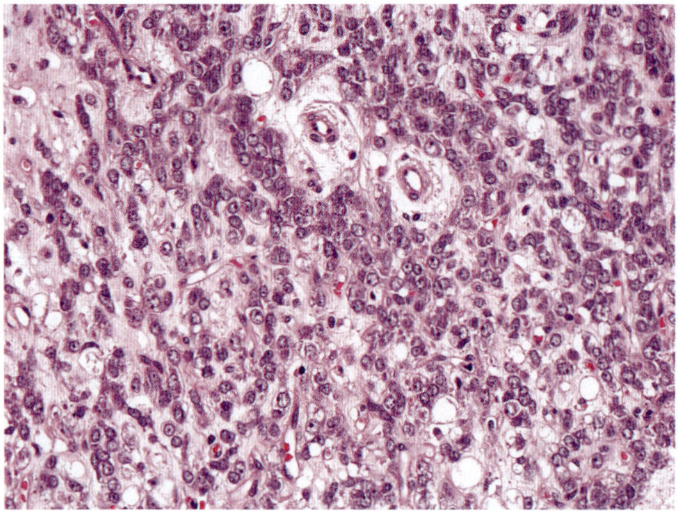

Figure 12.62 **Myxoid Liposarcoma.** In "round cell liposarcoma," hypercellular areas predominate.

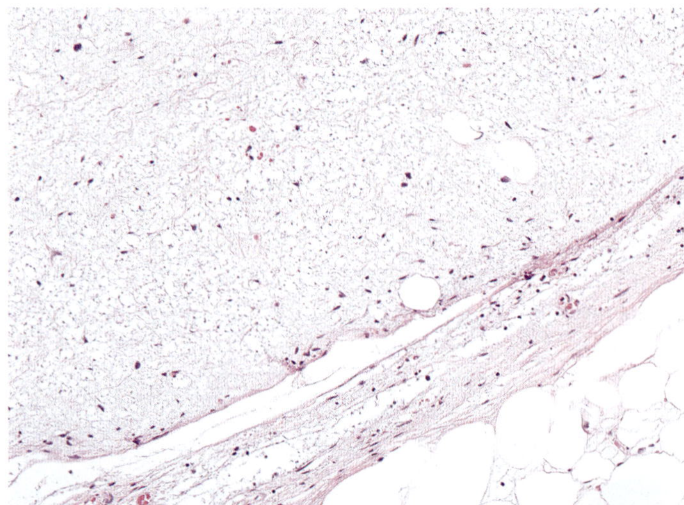

Figure 12.63 **Atypical Lipomatous Tumor/Well-Differentiated Liposarcoma With Myxoid Change.** Myxoid change can be seen. Lack of a plexiform vascular pattern and the presence of cytologic atypia are important diagnostic criteria.

and thereby closely mimic myxoid liposarcoma (Table 12.6). However, the presence of stromal atypia, the absence of a plexiform vascular pattern (Fig. 12.63), and distinct cytogenetic features (i.e., ring and giant marker chromosomes) distinguish ALT/WDLPS from myxoid liposarcoma. Purely myxoid liposarcoma must be differentiated from low-grade myxofibrosarcoma. Myxofibrosarcoma usually occurs in older patients and is more superficially located. Morphologically, it features atypical stromal cells and pseudolipoblasts (vacuolated cells containing mucin instead of lipid) set in a myxoid background, with distinctive thin-walled, elongated curvilinear blood vessels that lack the characteristic plexiform pattern of myxoid liposarcoma. Extraskeletal myxoid chondrosarcoma may also enter the differential diagnosis. Extraskeletal myxoid chondrosarcoma is a multinodular myxoid neoplasm composed of spindled or round to epithelioid cells organized in strands and cords, often clustering at the periphery of the nodules. S-100 protein immunopositivity is seen in most myxoid liposarcomas (including round cell areas), but in fewer than 20% of extraskeletal myxoid chondrosarcomas. Myxoid chondrosarcoma is characterized by a t(9;22)(q22;q12) translocation that fuses the *NR4A3* gene to *EWSR1*. However, genetic analysis may rarely lead to diagnostic errors, if FISH using split-apart probes for the *EWSR1* gene is performed, because *EWSR1* gene rearrangement can also be detected in 5% of myxoid liposarcomas. The use of FISH to detect *DDIT3* or *FUS* gene rearrangement distinguishes myxoid liposarcoma from extraskeletal myxoid chondrosarcoma in most cases. Alternatively, PCR-based techniques may be used to detect the various fusion transcripts specific to these tumor types.

Table 12.6 Differential Diagnosis Between Atypical Lipomatous Tumor/Well-Differentiated Liposarcoma With Myxoid Stromal Change and Myxoid Liposarcoma

	Atypical Lipomatous Tumor/ Well-Differentiated Liposarcoma With Myxoid Change	Myxoid Liposarcoma
Vascular network	Scarce	Prominent and plexiform
Lipoblasts	From none to numerous; often multivacuolated	Univacuolated or bivacuolated; more numerous at the periphery of the lesion
Stromal atypia	Present	Absent or minimal
Genetics	12q13-15 amplification (ring chromosomes or giant markers)	t(12;16)(q13;p11) or t(12;22)(q13;q12)

Prognosis and Treatment

As was previously emphasized, the presence of hypercellular areas (also known as *round cell differentiation* when neoplastic cells assume round cell morphologic features) is one of the most important prognostic features of myxoid liposarcoma. Different cutoff values, ranging from 5% to 25%, have been set by different studies.[176,177,188–190] A reliable assessment of the percentage of hypercellularity requires adequate sampling. Currently, it is recommended that any amount of hypercellularity should be reported, and if it exceeds 5%, the tumor should be considered high grade. In contrast with many other sarcoma types, myxoid liposarcoma tends to spread to serosal membranes, the abdominal cavity, distant soft tissues sites, and bones (notably, including the spine), even in the absence of lung metastases. Moreover, according to a recent study, it appears that spread to bone by myxoid liposarcoma has been underestimated; this may actually be among the most frequent sites of dissemination.[182] In addition, multifocality in myxoid liposarcoma represents metastatic spread to peripheral soft tissues.[191,192]

Standard treatment for myxoid liposarcoma is wide surgical resection.[190] For high-grade lesions, adjuvant therapy (radiation therapy or chemotherapy) may also be used. Recently, a marine-derived alkaloid designated trabectedin has shown efficacy in the treatment of metastatic myxoid liposarcoma.[185,193] Recently, a Phase 3 clinical trial with eribulin (a microtubule-dynamics inhibitor) has also shown significant improvement in overall survival of patients with advanced, pretreated myxoid liposarcoma.[194] The advent of new, more active as well as specific treatments, makes accurate diagnosis of myxoid liposarcoma extremely important (Box 12.4).

Pleomorphic Liposarcoma

Pleomorphic liposarcoma is a high-grade pleomorphic sarcoma that most often occurs in the limbs of elderly patients and shows variable amounts of adipocytic differentiation, ranging from very focal to extensive (see also Chapter 7). Pleomorphic liposarcoma is the rarest liposarcoma variant, accounting for approximately 5% of all cases.

Clinical Features

Pleomorphic liposarcoma is an aggressive neoplasm that most often affects older adults, with a peak incidence between the fifth and sixth

Box 12.4 Features Arguing Against Myxoid Liposarcoma

Myxoid liposarcoma is an unlikely diagnosis when:
- An adipocytic tumor with myxoid stroma occurs in the pediatric age group (most likely lipoblastoma).
- An adipocytic tumor with myxoid stroma occurs in the retroperitoneum (most likely well-differentiated liposarcoma).
- A plexiform capillary-sized vascular network is absent.
- Marked cytologic atypia is present.
- MDM2 and CDK4 are overexpressed/amplified.

decades. Men are affected slightly more often than women.[195–198] Most frequently, pleomorphic liposarcoma occurs in the lower limbs, in particular, the thigh. The trunk and retroperitoneum are much less commonly affected. Dedifferentiated liposarcoma may be misinterpreted as pleomorphic liposarcoma at these anatomic sites. Rare cases have been reported in the skin; however, as is often the case for superficially located soft tissue sarcomas, the outcome for this subset appears to be particularly favorable, and complete removal is usually curative, although some patients will eventually develop metastases.[198,199]

Pathologic Features

Pleomorphic liposarcoma exhibits similar gross features as other high-grade sarcomas. The tumor is usually well demarcated, with a fleshy cut surface featuring variable amounts of necrosis and hemorrhage (Fig. 12.64).

Histologically, pleomorphic liposarcoma is a further paradigm for the importance of careful gross sampling. In contrast to most liposarcoma subtypes, the main diagnostic feature is the presence of lipoblasts. Their identification often requires careful histologic examination because they can be very focal. Cytologic atypia is usually extreme, and lipoblasts are frequently large and contain irregular, hyperchromatic, scalloped nuclei with prominent nucleoli and multivacuolated cytoplasm (Fig. 12.65). Nuclear pseudoinclusions as well as multinucleated forms are also relatively common features of pleomorphic liposarcoma. Four main histologic patterns are seen: (1) in approximately two thirds of cases, a high-grade, MFH-like pleomorphic/spindle cell sarcoma featuring scattered lipoblasts or sheets of lipoblasts is seen (Fig. 12.66); (2) in fewer than one third of cases, a high-grade pleomorphic sarcoma with epithelioid areas and scattered lipoblasts is seen (Fig. 12.67)[200,201]; (3) rare cases overlap morphologically with intermediate to high-grade myxofibrosarcoma, except for the presence of lipoblasts (Fig. 12.68); and (4) even more rarely, pleomorphic liposarcoma is composed entirely of pleomorphic, multivacuolated lipoblasts (Fig. 12.69). Mitotic activity is usually high, and necrosis can be extensive, reflecting its clinically aggressive behavior.

Immunohistochemistry

S-100 protein immunoreactivity may help highlight the presence of multivacuolated lipoblasts in cases in which adipocytic differentiation is focal and therefore easily overlooked.

Molecular Genetics

Similar to most high-grade pleomorphic sarcomas, pleomorphic liposarcomas exhibit complex nondistinctive karyotypes. Alterations involving the *NF1* gene have been reported in approximately 10% of cases.[202]

Differential Diagnosis

The main differential diagnosis includes other subtypes of high-grade pleomorphic sarcoma and dedifferentiated liposarcoma (see Chapter 7). Recognition of even focal adipocytic differentiation in an otherwise pleomorphic sarcoma is the most important diagnostic clue and permits

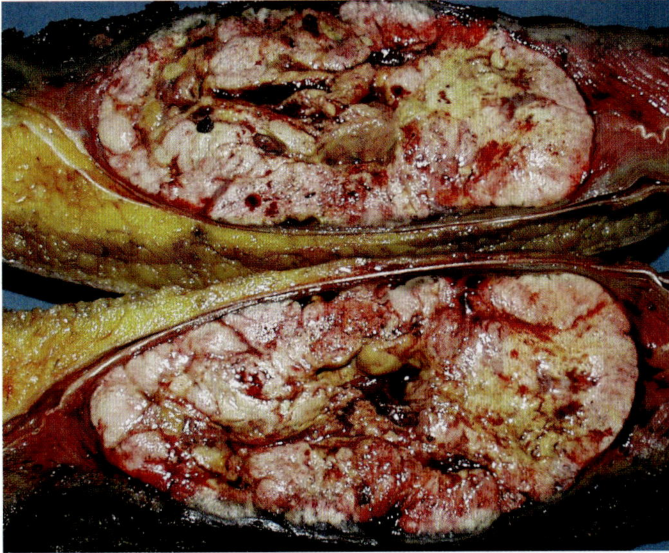

Figure 12.64 Pleomorphic Liposarcoma. A well-demarcated, fleshy cut surface is seen, with areas of necrosis and hemorrhage.

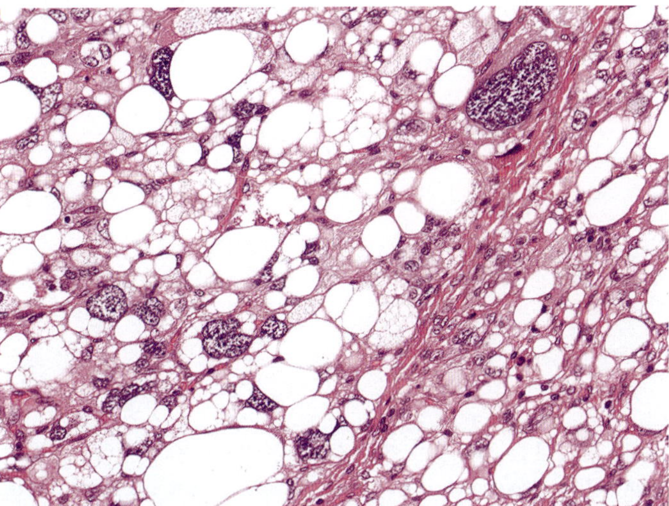

Figure 12.65 Pleomorphic Liposarcoma. Extreme cytologic atypia is frequently observed in pleomorphic liposarcoma.

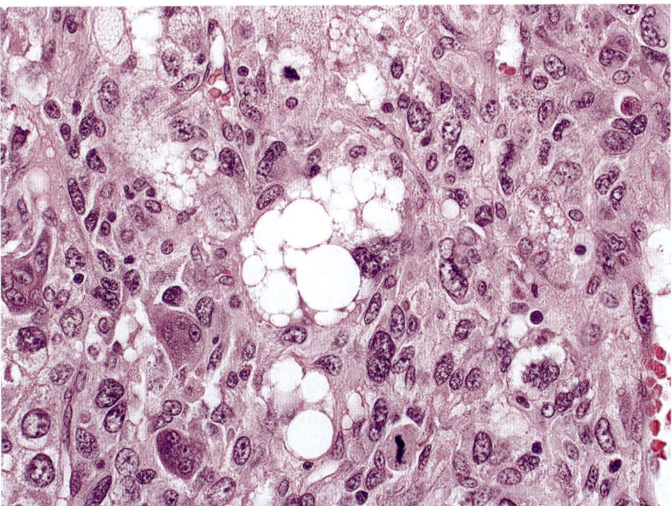

Figure 12.66 Pleomorphic Liposarcoma. Mutivacuolated lipoblasts are seen scattered among pleomorphic neoplastic cells.

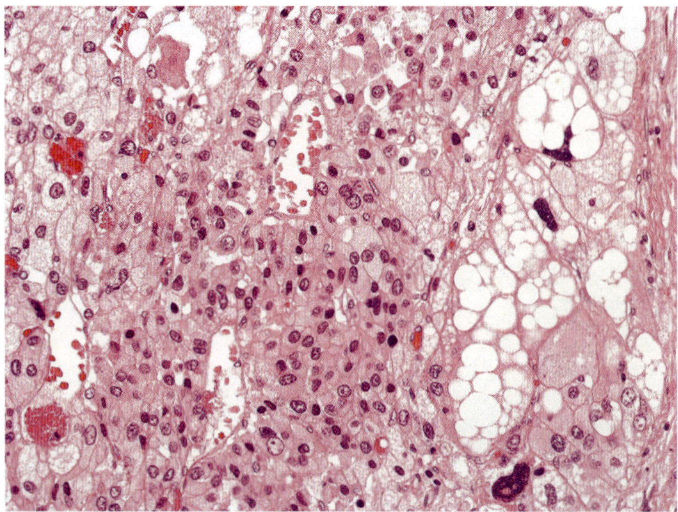

Figure 12.67 Pleomorphic Liposarcoma. Lipoblasts can be associated with an epithelioid neoplastic cell population.

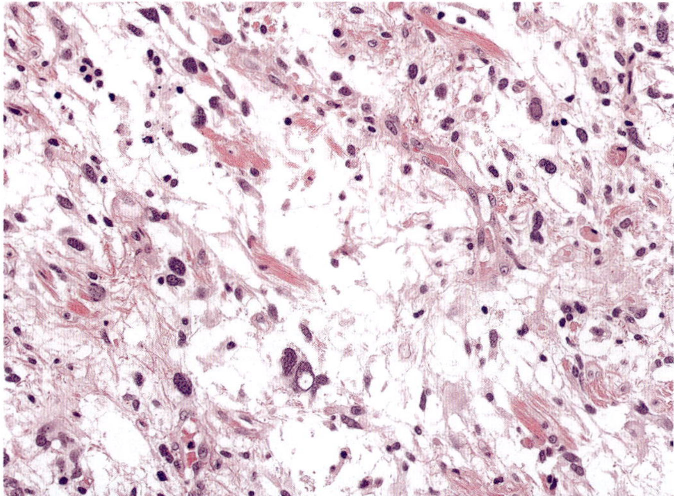

Figure 12.68 Pleomorphic Liposarcoma. Sometimes pleomorphic liposarcoma can mimic high-grade myxofibrosarcoma.

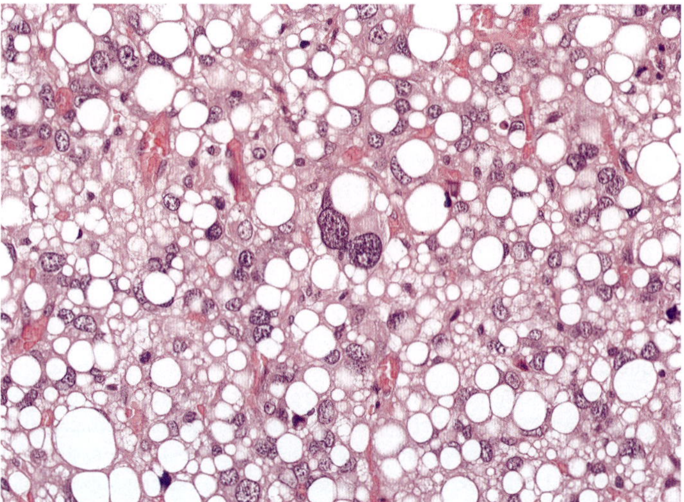

Figure 12.69 Pleomorphic Liposarcoma. Rarely, pleomorphic liposarcoma is entirely composed of uni- and multivacuolated lipoblasts.

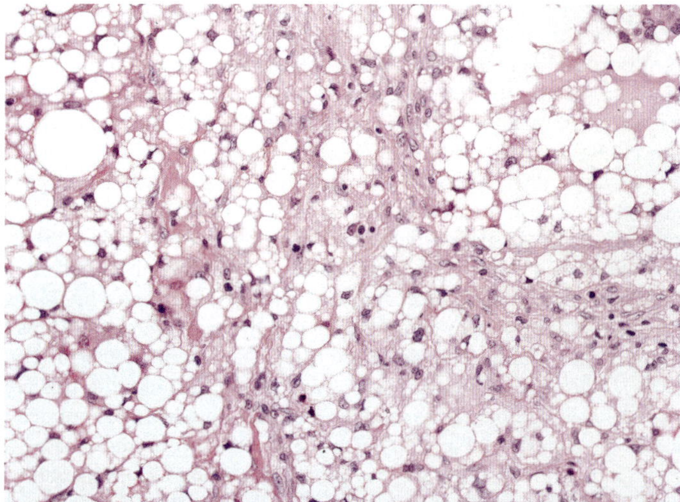

Figure 12.70 Silicone Granuloma. Foreign body reaction to silicone may mimic pleomorphic liposarcoma.

distinction from other pleomorphic sarcoma subtypes. In dedifferentiated liposarcoma, the high-grade component is usually nonlipogenic and is usually associated with a well-differentiated liposarcomatous component. The epithelioid variant of pleomorphic liposarcoma may be mistaken for carcinoma, especially adrenal cortical and renal cell carcinoma. Immunoreactivity for keratins supports a diagnosis of carcinoma. An unusual diagnostic pitfall is represented by silicone granuloma, in which the granulomatous reaction to the injected foreign material may mimic pleomorphic lipoblasts (Fig. 12.70).

Prognosis and Treatment

Pleomorphic liposarcoma is a high-grade sarcoma associated with poor survival. The metastatic rate is between 30% and 50%, and the overall mortality rate ranges from 40% to 50%. Standard treatment is wide surgical resection in addition to adjuvant therapy (radiation therapy or chemotherapy).

Acknowledgment

Gross photographs courtesy of Alessandro Gronchi, MD, National Cancer Institute, Milan, Italy.

References

1. Fletcher CD, Unni KK, Mertens F, editors: *Pathology and genetics of tumours of soft tissue and bone. World Health Organization classification of tumours*, Lyon, 2002, IARC Press.
2. Fletcher CDM, Bridge JA, Hogendoorn PCW, et al, editors: *WHO classification of tumours of soft tissue and bone*, 4th ed, Lyon, 2013, IARC Press.
3. Adair FE, Pack GT, Farrior JH: Lipoma, *Am J Cancer* 16:1104–1120, 1932.
4. Rydholm A, Berg NO: Size, site and clinical incidence of lipoma. Factors in the differential diagnosis of lipoma and sarcoma, *Acta Orthop Scand* 54:929–934, 1983.
5. Furlong MA, Fanburg-Smith JC, Childers EL: Lipoma of the oral and maxillofacial region: site and subclassification of 125 cases, *Oral Surg Oral Med Oral Pathol Oral Radiol Endod* 98:441–450, 2004.
6. Kindblom LG, Angervall L, Stener B, et al: Intermuscular and intramuscular lipomas and hibernomas. A clinical, roentgenologic, histologic, and prognostic study of 46 cases, *Cancer* 33:754–762, 1974.
7. Fletcher CD, Martin-Bates E: Intramuscular and intermuscular lipoma: neglected diagnoses, *Histopathology* 12:275–287, 1988.
8. Muraoka M, Oka T, Akamine S, et al: Endobronchial lipoma: review of 64 cases reported in Japan, *Chest* 123:293–296, 2003.
9. Jones EW, Marks R, Pongsehirun D: Naevus superficialis lipomatosus. A clinicopathological report of twenty cases, *Br J Dermatol* 93:121–133, 1975.
10. Hallel T, Lew S, Bansal M: Villous lipomatous proliferation of the synovial membrane (lipoma arborescens), *J Bone Joint Surg Am* 70:264–270, 1988.
11. Eyzaguirre E, Liqiang W, Karla GM, et al: Intraosseous lipoma. A clinical, radiologic, and pathologic study of 5 cases, *Ann Diagn Pathol* 11:320–325, 2007.

12. Macarenco RS, Erickson-Johnson M, Wang X, et al: Retroperitoneal lipomatous tumors without cytologic atypia: are they lipomas? A clinicopathologic and molecular study of 19 cases, *Am J Surg Pathol* 33:1470–1476, 2009.
13. Stoll G, Alembik Y, Truttmann M: Multiple familial lipomatosis with polyneuropathy, an inherited autosomal condition, *Ann Genet* 39:193–197, 1996.
14. Enzi G, Inelmen EM, Baritussio A, et al: Multiple symmetric lipomatosis: a defect in adrenergic-stimulated lipolysis, *J Clin Invest* 60:1221–1229, 1977.
15. Enzi G, Digito M, Marin R, et al: Mediastino-abdominal lipomatosis: deep accumulation of fat mimicking a respiratory disease and ascites. Clinical aspects and metabolic studies in vitro, *Q J Med* 53:453–463, 1984.
16. De Joanna F, Romano C: On a case of retroperitoneal sclerolipomatosis with prevailing perivesical development (simulating a neoplasm of the pelvic cavity), *Rass Int Clin Ter* 47:602–608, 1967.
17. Majewski J, Perley J, Spatz M, et al: Pelvic lipomatosis, *Urology* 2:180–182, 1973.
18. Enzi G, Busetto L, Ceschin E, et al: Multiple symmetric lipomatosis: clinical aspects and outcome in a long-term longitudinal study, *Int J Obes Relat Metab Disord* 26:253–261, 2002.
19. Willen H, Akerman M, Dal Cin P, et al: Comparison of chromosomal patterns with clinical features in 165 lipomas: a report of the CHAMP study group, *Cancer Genet Cytogenet* 102:46–49, 1998.
20. Schoenmakers EFPM, Wanchura S, Mols R, et al: Recurrent rearrangements in the high mobility group protein gene, HMGI-C, in benign mesenchymal tumours, *Nature Genet.* 10:436–444, 1995.
21. Petit MR, Mols R, Schoenmakers EFPM, et al: LPP, the preferred fusion partner gene of HMGIC in lipomas, is a novel member of the LIM protein gene family, *Genomics* 86:118–129, 1996.
22. Clay MR, Martinez AP, Weiss SW, et al: MDM2 and CDK4 immunohistochemistry: should it be used in problematic differentiated lipomatous tumors? A new perspective, *Am J Surg Pathol* 40:1647–1652, 2016.
23. Fetsch JF, Miettinen M, Laskin WB, et al: A clinicopathologic study of 45 pediatric soft tissue tumors with an admixture of adipose tissue and fibroblastic elements, and a proposal for classification as lipofibromatosis, *Am J Surg Pathol* 24:1491–1500, 2000.
24. Kenney B, Richkind KE, Friedlaender G, et al: Chromosomal rearrangements in lipofibromatosis, *Cancer Genet Cytogenet* 179:136–139, 2007.
25. Agaram NP, Zhang L, Sung YS, et al: Recurrent NTRK1 gene fusions define a novel subset of locally aggressive lipofibromatosis-like neural tumors, *Am J Surg Pathol* 40:1407–1416, 2016.
26. Silverman TA, Enzinger FM: Fibrolipomatous hamartoma of nerve. A clinicopathologic analysis of 26 cases, *Am J Surg Pathol* 9:7–14, 1985.
27. Berti E, Roncaroli F: Fibrolipomatous hamartoma of a cranial nerve, *Histopathology* 24:391–392, 1994.
28. Boren WL, Henry RE, Jr, Wintch K: MR diagnosis of fibrolipomatous hamartoma of nerve: association with nerve territory-oriented macrodactyly (macrodystrophia lipomatosa), *Skeletal Radiol* 24:296–297, 1995.
29. Howard WR, Helwig EB: Angiolipoma, *Arch Dermatol* 82:924–931, 1960.
30. Dixon AY, McGregor DH, Lee SH: Angiolipomas: an ultrastructural and clinicopathological study, *Hum Pathol* 112:739–747, 1981.
31. Hapnes SA, Boman H, Skeie SO: Familial angiolipomatosis, *Clin Genet* 17:202–208, 1980.
32. Pribyl C, Burke SW, Roberts JM, et al: Infiltrating angiolipoma or intramuscular hemangioma? A report of five cases, *J Pediatr Orthop* 6:172–176, 1986.
33. Hunt SJ, Santa Cruz DJ, Barr RJ: Cellular angiolipoma, *Am J Surg Pathol* 14:75–81, 1990.
34. Sciot R, Akerman M, Dal Cin P, et al: Cytogenetic analysis of subcutaneous angiolipoma: further evidence supporting its difference from ordinary pure lipomas: a report of the CHAMP Study Group, *Am J Surg Pathol* 21:441–444, 1997.
35. Mandahl N, Höglund M, Mertens F, et al: Cytogenetic aberrations in 188 benign and borderline adipose tissue tumors, *Genes Chromosomes Cancer* 9:207–215, 1994.
35a. Hofvander J, Arbajian E, Stenkula KG, et al: Frequent low-level mutations of protein kinase D2 in angiolipoma, *J Pathol* 241:578–582, 2017.
36. Enzinger FM, Harvey DA: Spindle cell lipoma, *Cancer* 36:1852–1859, 1975.
37. Angervall L, Dahl I, Kindblom LG, et al: Spindle cell lipoma, *Acta Pathol Microbiol Scand [A]* 84:477–487, 1976.
38. Shmookler BM, Enzinger FM: Pleomorphic lipoma: a benign tumor simulating liposarcoma. A clinicopathologic analysis of 48 cases, *Cancer* 47:126–133, 1981.
39. Azzopardi JG, Iocco J, Salm R: Pleomorphic lipoma: a tumour simulating liposarcoma, *Histopathology* 7:511–523, 1983.
40. Fletcher CDM, Martin Bates E: Spindle cell lipoma: a clinicopathologic study with some original observations, *Histopathology* 11:803–817, 1987.
41. Billings SD, Henley JD, Summerlin DJ, et al: Spindle cell lipoma of the oral cavity, *Am J Dermatopathol* 28:28–31, 2006.
42. Bartley GB, Yeatts RP, Garrity JA, et al: Spindle cell lipoma of the orbit, *Am J Ophthalmol* 100:605–609, 1985.
43. French CA, Mentzel T, Kutzner H, et al: Intradermal spindle cell/pleomorphic lipoma: a distinct subset, *Am J Dermatopathol* 22:496–502, 2000.
44. Austin CD, Tiessen JR, Gopalan A, et al: Spindle cell lipoma of the foot and the application of CD34 immunohistochemistry to atypical lipomatous tumors in unusual locations, *Appl Immunohistochem Mol Morphol* 8:222–227, 2000.
45. Fanburg-Smith JC, Devaney KO, Miettinen M, et al: Multiple spindle cell lipomas: a report of 7 familial and 11 nonfamilial cases, *Am J Surg Pathol* 22:40–48, 1998.
46. Billings SD, Folpe AL: Diagnostically challenging spindle cell lipomas: a report of 34 "low-fat" and "fat-free" variants, *Am J Dermatopathol* 29:437–442, 2007.
47. Hawley IC, Krausz T, Evans DJ, et al: Spindle cell lipoma: a pseudoangiomatous variant, *Histopathology* 24:565–569, 1994.
48. Suster S, Fisher C, Moran CA: Dendritic fibromyxolipoma: clinicopathologic study of a distinctive benign soft tissue lesion that may be mistaken for a sarcoma, *Ann Diagn Pathol* 2:111–120, 1998.
49. Templeton SF, Solomon AR, Jr: Spindle cell lipoma is strongly CD34 positive. An immunohistochemical study, *J Cutan Pathol* 23:546–550, 1996.
50. Suster S, Fisher C: Immunoreactivity for the human hematopoietic progenitor cell antigen (CD34) in lipomatous tumors, *Am J Surg Pathol* 21:195–200, 1997.
51. Magro G, Caltabiano R, Di Cataldo A, et al: CD10 is expressed by mammary myofibroblastoma and spindle cell lipoma of soft tissue: an additional evidence of their histogenetic linking, *Virchows Arch* 450:727–728, 2007.
52. Chen BJ, Mariño-Enríquez A, Fletcher CD, et al: Loss of retinoblastoma protein expression in spindle cell/pleomorphic lipomas and cytogenetically related tumors: an immunohistochemical study with diagnostic implications, *Am J Surg Pathol* 36:1119–1128, 2012.
53. Dei Tos AP, Dal Cin P: The role of cytogenetics in the classification of soft tissue tumours, *Virchows Arch* 431:83–94, 1997.
54. Dal Cin P, Sciot R, Polito P, et al: Lesions of 13q may occur independently of deletion of 16q in spindle cell/pleomorphic lipoma, *Histopathology* 31:222–225, 1997.
55. Pauwels P, Sciot R, Croiset F, et al: Myofibroblastoma of the breast: genetic link with spindle cell lipoma, *J Pathol* 191:282–285, 2000.
56. Maggiani F, Debiec-Rychter M, Vanbockrijck M, et al: Cellular angiofibroma: another mesenchymal tumour with 13q14 involvement, suggesting a link with spindle cell lipoma and (extra)-mammary myofibroblastoma, *Histopathology* 51:410–412, 2007.
57. Maggiani F, Debiec-Rychter M, Verbeeck G, et al: Extramammary myofibroblastoma is genetically related to spindle cell lipoma, *Virchows Arch* 449:244–247, 2006.
58. Wargotz EE, Weiss SW, Norris HJ: Myofibroblastoma of the breast. Sixteen cases of a distinctive benign mesenchymal tumor, *Am J Surg Pathol* 11:493–502, 1987.
59. McMenamin ME, Fletcher CD: Mammary-type myofibroblastoma of soft tissue: a tumor closely related to spindle cell lipoma, *Am J Surg Pathol* 25:1022–1029, 2001.
60. Howitt BE, Fletcher CDM: Mammary type myofibroblastoma. Clinicopathologic characterization in a series of 143 cases, *Am J Surg Pathol* 40:361–367, 2016.
61. Marshall-Taylor C, Fanburg-Smith JC: Hemosiderotic fibrohistiocytic lipomatous lesion: ten cases of a previously undescribed fatty lesion of the foot/ankle, *Mod Pathol* 13:1192–1199, 2000.
62. Browne TJ, Fletcher CD: Haemosiderotic fibrolipomatous tumour (so-called haemosiderotic fibrohistiocytic lipomatous tumour): analysis of 13 new cases in support of a distinct entity, *Histopathology* 48:453–461, 2006.
63. Folpe AL, Weiss SW: Pleomorphic hyalinizing angiectatic tumor: analysis of 41 cases supporting evolution from a distinctive precursor lesion, *Am J Surg Pathol* 28:1417–1425, 2004.
64. Elco CP, Mariño-Enríquez A, Abraham JA, et al: Hybrid myxoinflammatory fibroblastic sarcoma/hemosiderotic fibrolipomatous tumor: report of a case providing further evidence for a pathogenetic link, *Am J Surg Pathol* 34:1723–1727, 2010.
65. Antonescu CR, Zhang L, Nielsen GP, et al: Consistent t(1;10) with rearrangements of TGFBR3 and MGEA5 in both myxoinflammatory fibroblastic sarcoma and hemosiderotic fibrolipomatous tumor, *Genes Chromosomes Cancer* 50:757–764, 2011.
66. Wettach GR, Boyd LJ, Lawce HJ, et al: Cytogenetic analysis of a hemosiderotic fibrolipomatous tumor, *Cancer Genet Cytogenet* 182:140–143, 2008.
67. Hallor KH, Sciot R, Staaf J, et al: Two genetic pathways, t(1;10) and amplification of 3p11–12, in myxoinflammatory fibroblastic sarcoma, haemosiderotic fibrolipomatous tumour, and morphologically similar lesions, *J Pathol* 217:716–727, 2009.
68. Zreik RT, Carter JM, Sukov WR, et al: TGFBR3 and MGEA5 rearrangements are much more common in "hybrid" hemosiderotic fibrolipomatous tumormyxoinflammatory fibroblastic sarcomas than in classical myxoinflammatory fibroblastic sarcomas: a morphological and fluorescence in situ hybridization study, *Hum Pathol* 53:14–24, 2016.
69. Vellios F, Baez J, Shumacker HB: Lipoblastomatosis: a tumor of fetal fat different from hibernoma. Report of a case with observations on the embryogenesis of human adipose tissue, *Am J Pathol* 34:1149–1159, 1958.
70. Chung EB, Enzinger FM: Benign lipoblastomatosis. An analysis of 35 cases, *Cancer* 32:482–492, 1973.
71. Mentzel T, Calonje E, Fletcher CDM: Lipoblastoma and lipoblastomatosis: a clinicopathological study of 14 cases, *Histopathology* 23:527–533, 1993.
72. Collins MH, Chatten J: Lipoblastoma/lipoblastomatosis: a clinicopathologic study of 25 tumors, *Am J Surg Pathol* 21:1131–1137, 1997.
73. Lae ME, Pereira PF, Keeney GL, et al: Lipoblastoma-like tumour of the vulva: report of three cases of a distinctive mesenchymal neoplasm of adipocytic differentiation, *Histopathology* 40:505–509, 2002.
74. Dal Cin P, Sciot R, De Wever I, et al: New discriminative chromosomal marker in adipose tissue tumors. The chromosome 8q11-q13 region in lipoblastoma, *Cancer Genet Cytogenet* 78:232–235, 1994.
75. Hibbard MK, Kozakewich HP, Dal Cin P, et al: PLAG1 fusion gene in lipoblastoma, *Cancer Res* 60:4869–4872, 2000.

76. Gisselsson D, Hibbard MK, Dal Cin P, et al: PLAG1 alterations in lipoblastoma: involvement in varied mesenchymal cell types and evidence for alternative oncogenic mechanisms, *Am J Pathol* 159:955–962, 2001.
77. Bartuma H, Domanski HA, Von Steyern FV, et al: Cytogenetic and molecular cytogenetic findings in lipoblastoma, *Cancer Genet Cytogenet* 183:60–63, 2008.
78. de Saint Aubain Somerhausen N, Coindre JM, Debiec-Rychter M, et al: Lipoblastoma in adolescents and young adults: report of six cases with FISH analysis, *Histopathology* 52:294–298, 2008.
79. Bolen JW, Thorning D: Benign lipoblastoma and myxoid liposarcoma: a comparative light- and electron-microscopic study, *Am J Surg Pathol* 4:163–174, 1980.
80. Merkel H: On a pseudolipoma of the breast (peculiar fat tumor), *Beitr Pathol Anat* 39:152–157, 1906.
81. Gery L: Discussions, *Bull Mem Soc Anat (Paris)* 89:111–123, 1914.
82. Gaffney EF, Hargreaves HK, Semple E, et al: Hibernoma: distinctive light and electron microscopic features and relationship to brown adipose tissue, *Hum Pathol* 14:677–687, 1983.
83. Furlong MA, Fanburg-Smith JC, Miettinen M: The morphologic spectrum of hibernoma: a clinicopathologic study of 170 cases, *Am J Surg Pathol* 25:809–814, 2001.
84. Chirieac LR, Dekmezian RH, Ayala AG: Characterization of the myxoid variant of hibernoma, *Ann Diagn Pathol* 10:104–106, 2006.
85. Fletcher CDM, Akerman M, Dal Cin P, et al: Correlation between clinicopathological features and karyotype in lipomatous tumors, *Am J Pathol* 148:623–630, 1996.
86. Gisselson G, Hoglund M, Mertens F, et al: Hibernomas are characterized by homozygous deletions in the multiple endocrine neoplasia type 1 region. Metaphase fluorescence in situ hybridization reveals complex rearrangements not detected by conventional cytogenetics, *Am J Pathol* 155:61–66, 1999.
87. Hallin M, Schneider N, Thway K: Well-differentiated liposarcoma with hibernoma-like morphology, *Int J Surg Pathol* 24:620–622, 2016.
88. Meis JM, Enzinger FM: Myolipoma of soft tissue, *Am J Surg Pathol* 15:121–125, 1991.
89. Fukushima M, Schaefer IM, Fletcher CD: Myolipoma of soft tissue: clinicopathologic analysis of 34 cases, *Am J Surg Pathol* 41:153–160, 2017.
90. Fernandez-Aguilar S, Saint-Aubain N, Dargent JL, et al: Myolipoma of soft tissue: an unusual tumor with expression of estrogen and progesterone receptors. Report of two cases and review of the literature, *Acta Obstet Gynecol Scand* 81:1088–1090, 2002.
91. Hisaoka M, Sheng WQ, Tanaka A, et al: HMGIC alterations in smooth muscle tumors of soft tissues and other sites, *Cancer Genet Cytogenet* 138:50–55, 2002.
92. Panagopoulos I, Gorunova L, Agostini A, et al: Fusion of the HMGA2 and C9orf92 genes in myolipoma with t(9;12)(p22;q14), *Diagn Pathol* 11:22, 2016.
93. Evans HL: Smooth muscle in atypical lipomatous tumors. A report of three cases, *Am J Surg Pathol* 14:714–718, 1990.
94. Michal M: Retroperitoneal myolipoma. A tumour mimicking retroperitoneal angiomyolipoma and liposarcoma with myosarcomatous differentiation, *Histopathology* 25:86–88, 1994.
95. Chan JKC, Lee KC, Saw D: Extraskeletal chondroma with lipoblast-like cells, *Hum Pathol* 17:1285–1287, 1986.
96. Meis JM, Enzinger FM: Chondroid lipoma. A unique tumor simulating liposarcoma and myxoid chondrosarcoma, *Am J Surg Pathol* 17:1103–1112, 1993.
97. Kindblom LG, Meis-Kindblom JM: Chondroid lipoma: an ultrastructural and immunohistochemical analysis with further observations regarding its differentiation, *Hum Pathol* 26:706–715, 1995.
98. Nielsen GP, O'Connell JX, Dickersin GR, et al: Chondroid lipoma, a tumor of white fat cells. A brief report of two cases with ultrastructural analysis, *Am J Surg Pathol* 19:1272–1276, 1995.
99. Zamecnik M, Michal M, Fakan F: Ultrastructural study of so called chondroid lipoma, *Hum Pathol* 29:98–100, 1998.
100. Gisselsson D, Domanski HA, Hoglund M, et al: Unique cytological features and chromosome aberrations in chondroid lipoma: a case report based on fine-needle aspiration cytology, histopathology, electron microscopy, chromosome banding, and molecular cytogenetics, *Am J Surg Pathol* 23:1300–1304, 1999.
101. Thomson TA, Horsman D, Bainbridge TC: Cytogenetic and cytologic features of chondroid lipoma of soft tissue, *Mod Pathol* 12:88–91, 1999.
102. Ballaux F, Debiec-Rychter M, De Wever I, et al: Chondroid lipoma is characterized by t(11;16)(q13;p12–13), *Virchows Arch* 444:208–210, 2004.
103. Huang D, Sumegi J, Dal Cin P, et al: C11orf95-MKL2 is the resulting fusion oncogene of t(11;16)(q13;p13) in chondroid lipoma, *Genes Chromosomes Cancer* 22:810–818, 2010.
104. Stout AP: Liposarcoma: the malignant tumour of lipoblasts, *Ann Surg* 119:86–107, 1944.
105. Enzinger FM, Winslow DJ: Liposarcoma. A study of 103 cases, *Virchows Arch Path Anat* 335:367–388, 1962.
106. Azumi N, Curtis J, Kempson RL, et al: Atypical and malignant neoplasms showing lipomatous differentiation. A study of 111 cases, *Am J Surg Pathol* 11:161–183, 1987.
107. Dei Tos AP: Liposarcoma: new entities and evolving concepts, *Ann Diagn Pathol* 4:252–266, 2000.
108. Lucas DR, Nascimento AG, Sanjay BKS, et al: Well differentiated liposarcoma. The Mayo Clinic experience with 58 cases, *Am J Clin Pathol* 102:677–683, 1994.
109. Laurino L, Furlanetto A, Orvieto E, et al: Well-differentiated liposarcoma (atypical lipomatous tumors), *Semin Diagn Pathol* 18:258–262, 2001.
110. Dei Tos AP, Pedetour F: Well-differentiated liposarcoma. In Fletcher CDM, Bridge JA, Hogendoorn PCW, et al, editors: *WHO classification of tumours of soft tissue and bone*, 4th ed, Lyon, 2013, IARC Press, pp 33–36.
111. Evans HL, Soule EH, Winkelmann RK: Atypical lipoma, atypical intramuscular lipoma, and well differentiated retroperitoneal liposarcoma. A reappraisal of 30 cases formerly classified as well-differentiated liposarcoma, *Cancer* 43:574–584, 1979.
112. Kindblom LG, Angervall L, Fassina AS: Atypical lipoma, *Acta Pathol Microbiol Scand* 90:27–36, 1982.
113. Evans HL: Liposarcoma and atypical lipomatous tumors: a study of 66 cases followed for a minimum of 10 years, *Surg Pathol.* 1:41–54, 1988.
114. Gronchi A, Lo Vullo S, Fiore M, et al: Aggressive surgical policies in a retrospectively reviewed single-institution case series of retroperitoneal soft tissue sarcomas, *J Clin Oncol* 27:24–30, 2009.
115. Bonvalot S, Rivoire M, Castaing M, et al: Primary retroperitoneal sarcomas: a multivariate analysis of surgical factors associated with local control, *J Clin Oncol* 27:31–37, 2009.
116. Montgomery E, Fisher C: Paratesticular liposarcoma: a clinicopathologic study, *Am J Surg Pathol* 27:40–47, 2003.
117. Hahn HP, Fletcher CD: Primary mediastinal liposarcoma: clinicopathologic analysis of 24 cases, *Am J Surg Pathol* 31:1868–1874, 2007.
118. Nascimento AF, McMenamin ME, Fletcher CD: Liposarcomas/atypical lipomatous tumors of the oral cavity: a clinicopathologic study of 23 cases, *Ann Diagn Pathol* 6:83–93, 2002.
119. Cai YC, McMenamin ME, Rose G, et al: Primary liposarcoma of the orbit: a clinicopathologic study of seven cases, *Ann Diagn Pathol* 5:255–266, 2001.
120. Suster S, Wong TY, Moran C: Sarcomas with combined features of liposarcoma and leiomyosarcoma. Study of two cases of an unusual soft tissue tumor showing dual lineage differentiation, *Am J Surg Pathol* 17:905–911, 1993.
121. Folpe AL, Weiss SW: Lipoleiomyosarcoma (well differentiated liposarcoma with leiomyosarcomatous differentiation): a clinicopathologic study of nine cases including one with dedifferentiation, *Am J Surg Pathol* 26:742–749, 2002.
122. Kraus MD, Guillou L, Fletcher CDM: Well-differentiated inflammatory liposarcoma: an uncommon and easily overlooked variant of a common sarcoma, *Am J Surg Pathol* 21:518–527, 1997.
123. Argani P, Facchetti F, Inghirami G, et al: Lymphocyte-rich well-differentiated liposarcoma: report of nine cases, *Am J Surg Pathol* 21:884–895, 1997.
124. Dei Tos AP, Mentzel T, Newman PL, et al: Spindle cell liposarcoma: a hitherto unrecognized variant of well-differentiated liposarcoma: analysis of six cases, *Am J Surg Pathol* 18:913–921, 1994.
125. Mentzel T, Toennissen J, Rutten A, et al: Palmar atypical lipomatous tumour with spindle cell features (well-differentiated spindle cell liposarcoma): a rare neoplasm arising in an unusual anatomical location, *Virchows Arch* 446:300–304, 2005.
126. Mariño-Enriquez A, Nascimento AF, Ligon AH, et al: Atypical spindle cell lipomatous tumor: clinicopathologic characterization of 232 cases demonstrating a morphologic spectrum, *Am J Surg Pathol* 41:234–244, 2017.
127. Pilotti S, Della Torre G, Mezzelani A, et al: The expression of MDM2/CDK4 gene product in the differential diagnosis of well differentiated liposarcoma and large deep-seated lipoma, *Br J Cancer* 82:1271–1275, 2000.
128. Dei Tos AP, Doglioni C, Piccinin S, et al: Coordinated expression and amplification of the MDM2, CDK4 and HMGI-C genes in atypical lipomatous tumours, *J Pathol* 190:531–536, 2000.
129. Binh MB, Sastre-Garau X, Guillou L, et al: MDM2 and CDK4 immunostainings are useful adjuncts in diagnosing well-differentiated and dedifferentiated liposarcoma subtypes: a comparative analysis of 559 soft tissue neoplasms with genetic data, *Am J Surg Pathol* 29:1340–1347, 2005.
130. Binh MB, Garau XS, Guillou L, et al: Reproducibility of MDM2 and CDK4 staining in soft tissue tumors, *Am J Clin Pathol* 125:693–697, 2006.
131. Dal Cin P, Kools P, Sciot R, et al: Cytogenetic and fluorescence in situ hybridization investigation of ring chromosomes characterizing a specific pathologic subgroup of adipose tissue tumours, *Cancer Genet Cytogenet* 68:85–90, 1993.
132. Rosai J, Akerman M, Dal Cin P, et al: Combined morphologic and karyotypic study of 59 atypical lipomatous tumours: evaluation of their relationship and differential diagnosis with other adipose tissue tumours, *Am J Surg Pathol* 20:1182–1189, 1996.
133. Hostein I, Pelmus M, Aurias A, et al: Evaluation of MDM2 and CDK4 amplification by real-time PCR on paraffin wax-embedded material: a potential tool for the diagnosis of atypical lipomatous tumours/well-differentiated liposarcomas, *J Pathol* 202:95–102, 2004.
134. Shimada S, Ishizawa T, Ishizawa K, et al: The value of MDM2 and CDK4 amplification levels using real-time polymerase chain reaction for the differential diagnosis of liposarcomas and their histologic mimickers, *Hum Pathol* 37:1123–1129, 2006.
135. Sirvent N, Coindre JM, Maire G, et al: Detection of MDM2-CDK4 amplification by fluorescence in situ hybridization in 200 paraffin-embedded tumor samples: utility in diagnosing adipocytic lesions and comparison with immunohistochemistry and real-time PCR, *Am J Surg Pathol* 31:1476–1489, 2007.
136. Weaver J, Downs-Kelly E, Goldblum JR, et al: Fluorescence in situ hybridization for MDM2 gene amplification as a diagnostic tool in lipomatous neoplasms, *Mod Pathol* 21:943–949, 2008.
137. Italiano A, Bianchini L, Keslair F, et al: HMGA2 is the partner of MDM2 in well-differentiated and dedifferentiated liposarcomas whereas CDK4 belongs to a distinct inconsistent amplicon, *Int J Cancer* 122:2233–2241, 2008.

138. Italiano A, Chambonniere ML, Attias R, et al: Monosomy 7 and absence of 12q amplification in two cases of spindle cell liposarcomas, *Cancer Genet Cytogenet* 184:99–104, 2008.
139. Mentzel T, Palmedo G, Kuhnen C: Well-differentiated spindle cell liposarcoma ("atypical spindle cell lipomatous tumor") does not belong to the spectrum of atypical lipomatous tumor but has a close relationship to spindle cell lipoma: clinicopathologic, immunohistochemical, and molecular analysis of six cases, *Mod Pathol* 23:729–736, 2010.
140. Italiano A, Cardot N, Dupré F, et al: Gains and complex rearrangements of the 12q13–15 chromosomal region in ordinary lipomas: the "missing link" between lipomas and liposarcomas?, *Int J Cancer* 121:308–315, 2007.
141. Corradi D, Maestri R, Palmisano A, et al: Idiopathic retroperitoneal fibrosis: clinicopathologic features and differential diagnosis, *Kidney Int* 72:742–753, 2007.
142. Weaver J, Goldblum JR, Turner S, et al: Detection of MDM2 gene amplification or protein expression distinguishes sclerosing mesenteritis and retroperitoneal fibrosis from inflammatory well-differentiated liposarcoma, *Mod Pathol* 22:66–70, 2009.
143. Farshid G, Weiss SW: Massive localized lymphedema in the morbidly obese: a histologically distinct reactive lesion simulating liposarcoma, *Am J Surg Pathol* 22:1277–1783, 1998.
144. Rosenberg AE: Pseudosarcomas of soft tissue, *Arch Pathol Lab Med* 132:579–586, 2008.
145. Evans HL: Atypical lipomatous tumor, its variants, and its combined forms: a study of 61 cases, with a minimum follow-up of 10 years, *Am J Surg Pathol* 31:1–14, 2007.
146. Evans HL: Liposarcoma: a study of 55 cases with a reassessment of its classification, *Am J Surg Pathol* 3:507–523, 1979.
147. Dei Tos AP, Marino-Enriquez A, Pedetour F, et al: Dedifferentiated liposarcoma. In Fletcher CDM, Bridge JA, Hogendoorn PCW, et al, editors: *WHO classification of tumours of soft tissue and bone*, Lyon, 2013, IARC Press, pp 39–41.
148. Henricks WH, Chu YC, Goldblum JR, et al: Dedifferentiated liposarcoma: a clinicopathologic analysis of 155 cases with proposal for an expanded definition of dedifferentiation, *Am J Surg Pathol* 21:271–281, 1997.
149. Elgar F, Goldblum JR: Well-differentiated liposarcoma of the retroperitoneum: a clinicopathologic analysis of 20 cases, with particular attention to the extent of low-grade dedifferentiation, *Mod Pathol* 10:113–120, 1997.
150. Dhalin DD, Unni KK, Matsuno T: Malignant (fibrous) histiocytoma of bone: fact or fancy?, *Cancer* 39:1509–1516, 1977.
151. Weiss SW, Rao VK: Well-differentiated liposarcoma (atypical lipoma) of deep soft tissue of the extremities, retroperitoneum and miscellaneous sites. A follow-up study of 92 cases with analysis of the incidence of dedifferentiation, *Am J Surg Pathol* 16:1051–1058, 1992.
152. McCormick D, Mentzel T, Beham A, et al: Dedifferentiated liposarcoma. Clinicopathologic analysis of 32 cases suggesting a better prognostic subgroup among pleomorphic sarcomas, *Am J Surg Pathol* 18:1213–1223, 1994.
153. Nascimento AG: Dedifferentiated liposarcoma, *Sem Diagn Pathol* 18:263–266, 2001.
154. Le Guellec S, Chibon F, Ouali M, et al: Are peripheral purely undifferentiated pleomorphic sarcomas with MDM2 amplification dedifferentiated liposarcomas?, *Am J Surg Pathol* 38:293–304, 2014.
155. Coindre JM, Hostein I, Maire G, et al: Inflammatory fibrous histiocytoma and dedifferentiated liposarcoma: histological review, genomic profile, and MDM2 and CDK4 status favour a single entity, *J Pathol* 203:822–830, 2004.
156. Evans HL, Khurana KK, Kemp BL, et al: Heterologous elements in the dedifferentiated component of dedifferentiated liposarcoma, *Am J Surg Pathol* 18:1150–1157, 1994.
157. Binh MB, Guillou L, Hostein I, et al: Dedifferentiated liposarcomas with divergent myosarcomatous differentiation developed in the internal trunk: a study of 27 cases and comparison to conventional dedifferentiated liposarcomas and leiomyosarcomas, *Am J Surg Pathol* 31:1557–1566, 2007.
158. Nascimento AG, Kurtin PJ, Guillou L, et al: Dedifferentiated liposarcoma. A report of nine cases with a peculiar neurallike whorling pattern associated with metaplastic bone formation, *Am J Surg Pathol* 22:945–955, 1998.
159. Fanburg-Smith JC, Miettinen M: Liposarcoma with meningothelial-like whorls: a study of 17 cases of a distinctive histological pattern associated with dedifferentiated liposarcoma, *Histopathology* 33:414–424, 1998.
160. Macarenco RS, Erickson-Johnson M, Wang X, et al: Cytogenetic and molecular cytogenetic findings in dedifferentiated liposarcoma with neural-like whorling pattern and metaplastic bone formation, *Cancer Genet Cytogenet* 172:147–150, 2007.
161. Boland JM, Weiss SW, Oliveira AM, et al: Liposarcomas with mixed well-differentiated and pleomorphic features: a clinicopathologic study of 12 cases, *Am J Surg Pathol* 34:837–843, 2010.
162. Mariño-Enríquez A, Fletcher CD, Dal Cin P, et al: Dedifferentiated liposarcoma with "homologous" lipoblastic (pleomorphic liposarcoma-like) differentiation: clinicopathologic and molecular analysis of a series suggesting revised diagnostic criteria, *Am J Surg Pathol* 34:1122–1131, 2010.
163. Horvai AE, Schaefer JT, Nakakura EK, et al: Immunostaining for peroxisome proliferator gamma distinguishes dedifferentiated liposarcoma from other retroperitoneal sarcomas, *Mod Pathol* 21:517–524, 2008.
164. Mertens F, Fletcher CDM, Dal Cin P, et al: Cytogenetic analysis of 46 pleomorphic soft tissue sarcomas and correlation with morphologic and clinical features: a report of the CHAMP study group. CHromosomes and MorPhology, *Genes Chromosomes Cancer* 22:16–25, 1998.
165. Dei Tos AP, Doglioni C, Piccinin S, et al: Molecular abnormalities of the p53 pathway in dedifferentiated liposarcoma, *J Pathol* 181:8–13, 1997.
166. Nakayama T, Toguchida J, Wadayama B, et al: MDM2 gene amplification in bone and soft tissue tumours: association with tumour progression in differentiated adipose tissue tumours, *Int J Cancer* 64:342–346, 1995.
167. Cordon Cardo C, Latres E, Drobnjac M, et al: Molecular abnormalities of MDM2 and p53 genes in adult soft tissue sarcomas, *Cancer Res* 54:794–799, 1994.
168. Singer S, Socci ND, Ambrosini G, et al: Gene expression profiling of liposarcoma identifies distinct biological types/subtypes and potential therapeutic targets in well-differentiated and dedifferentiated liposarcoma, *Cancer Res* 67:6626–6636, 2007.
169. Muller CR, Paulsen EB, Noordhuis P, et al: Potential for treatment of liposarcomas with the MDM2 antagonist Nutlin-3A, *Int J Cancer* 121:199–205, 2007.
170. Ambrosini G, Sambol EB, Carvajal D, et al: Mouse double minute antagonist Nutlin-3a enhances chemotherapy-induced apoptosis in cancer cells with mutant p53 by activating E2F1, *Oncogene* 26:3473–3481, 2007.
171. Dickson MA, Schwartz GK, Keohan ML, et al: Progression-free survival among patients with well-differentiated or dedifferentiated liposarcoma treated with CDK4 inhibitor palbociclib: a phase 2 clinical trial, *JAMA Oncol* 2:937–940, 2016.
172. Mussi C, Collini P, Miceli R, et al: The prognostic impact of dedifferentiation in retroperitoneal liposarcoma: a series of surgically treated patients at a single institution, *Cancer* 113:1657–1665, 2008.
173. Gronchi A, Collini P, Miceli R, et al: Myogenic differentiation and histologic grading are major prognostic determinants in retroperitoneal liposarcoma, *Am J Surg Pathol* 39:383–393, 2015.
174. Orvieto E, Furlanetto A, Laurino L, et al: Myxoid and round cell liposarcoma: a spectrum of myxoid adipocytic neoplasia, *Sem Diagn Pathol* 18:267–273, 2001.
175. Antonescu C, Ladanyi M: Myxoid liposarcoma. In Fletcher CDM, Bridge JA, Hogendoorn PCW, et al, editors: *WHO classification of tumours of soft tissue and bone*, 4th ed, Lyon, 2013, IARC Press, pp 39–41.
176. Kilpatrick SE, Doyon J, Choong PFM, et al: The clinicopathologic spectrum of myxoid and round cell liposarcoma. A study of 95 cases, *Cancer* 77:1450–1458, 1996.
177. Smith TA, Easley KA, Goldblum JR: Myxoid/round cell liposarcoma of the extremities. A clinicopathologic study of 29 cases with particular attention to extent of round cell liposarcoma, *Am J Surg Pathol* 20:171–180, 1996.
178. Knight JC, Renwick PJ, Dal Cin P, et al: Translocation t(12;16)(q13:p11) in myxoid liposarcoma and round cell liposarcoma: molecular and cytogenetic analysis, *Cancer Res* 55:24–27, 1995.
179. Tallini G, Akerman M, Dal Cin P, et al: Combined morphologic and karyotypic study of 28 myxoid liposarcomas. Implications for a revised morphologic typing. A report from the CHAMP group, *Am J Surg Pathol* 20:1047–1055, 1996.
180. de Vreeze RS, de Jong D, Tielen IH, et al: Primary retroperitoneal myxoid/round cell liposarcoma is a nonexisting disease: an immunohistochemical and molecular biological analysis, *Mod Pathol* 22:223–231, 2009.
181. Estourgie SH, Nielsen GP, Ott MJ: Metastatic patterns of extremity myxoid liposarcoma and their outcome, *J Surg Oncol* 80:89–93, 2002.
182. Schwab JH, Boland PJ, Antonescu C, et al: Spinal metastases from myxoid liposarcoma warrant screening with magnetic resonance imaging, *Cancer* 110:1815–1822, 2007.
183. Dei Tos AP, Wadden C, Fletcher CDM: S-100 protein staining in liposarcoma. Its diagnostic utility in the high grade myxoid (round cell) variant, *Appl Immunohistochem.* 4:95–101, 1996.
184. Weingertner N, Neuville A, Chibon F, et al: Myxoid liposarcoma with heterologous components: dedifferentiation or metaplasia? A FISH-documented and CGH-documented case report, *Appl Immunohistochem Mol Morphol* 23:230–235, 2015.
185. Grosso F, Jones RL, Demetri GD, et al: Efficacy of trabectedin (ecteinascidin-743) in advanced pretreated myxoid liposarcomas: a retrospective study, *Lancet Oncol* 8:595–602, 2007.
186. Engstrom K, Willen H, Kabjorn-Gustafsson C, et al: The myxoid/round cell liposarcoma fusion oncogene FUS-DDIT3 and the normal DDIT3 induce a liposarcoma phenotype in transfected human fibrosarcoma cells, *Am J Pathol* 168:1642–1653, 2006.
187. Dei Tos AP, Doglioni C, Piccinin S, et al: Molecular aberrations of the G1-S cell cycle checkpoint in myxoid and round cell liposarcoma, *Am J Pathol* 151:1531–1539, 1997.
188. Fletcher CDM: Will we ever reliably predict prognosis in a patient with myxoid and round cell liposarcoma?, *Adv Anat Pathol* 2:108–113, 1997.
189. Antonescu CR, Tschernyavsky SJ, Decuseara R, et al: Prognostic impact of P53 status, TLS-CHOP fusion transcript structure, and histological grade in myxoid liposarcoma: a molecular and clinicopathologic study of 82 cases, *Clin Cancer Res* 7:3977–3987, 2001.
190. Fiore M, Grosso F, Lo Vullo S, et al: Myxoid/round cell and pleomorphic liposarcomas: prognostic factors and survival in a series of patients treated at a single institution, *Cancer* 109:2522–2531, 2007.
191. Blair SL, Lewis JJ, Leung D, et al: Multifocal extremity sarcoma: an uncommon and controversial entity, *Ann Surg Oncol* 5:37–40, 1998.
192. Antonescu CR, Elahi A, Healey JH, et al: Monoclonality of multifocal myxoid liposarcoma: confirmation by analysis of TLS-CHOP or EWS-CHOP rearrangements, *Clin Cancer Res* 6:2788–2793, 2000.
193. Demetri GD, von Mehren M, Jones RL, et al: Efficacy and safety of trabectedin or dacarbazine for metastatic liposarcoma or leiomyosarcoma after failure of conventional chemotherapy: results of a phase III randomized multicenter clinical trial, *J Clin Oncol* 34:786–793, 2016.
194. Schöffski P, Chawla S, Maki RG, et al: Eribulin versus dacarbazine in previously treated patients with advanced liposarcoma or leiomyosarcoma: a randomized open-label, multicentre, phase 3 trial, *Lancet* 387:1629–1637, 2016.

195. Oliveira AM, Nascimento AG: Pleomorphic liposarcoma, *Semin Diagn Pathol* 18:274–285, 2001.
196. Mentzel T, Pedeutour F: Pleomorphic liposarcoma. In Fletcher CDM, Mertens F, Unni KK, editors: *Pathology and genetics. WHO classification of soft tissue tumors*, Lyon, 2002, IARC Press, pp 44–45.
197. Gebhard S, Coindre JM, Michels JJ, et al: Pleomorphic liposarcoma: clinicopathologic, immunohistochemical, and follow-up analysis of 63 cases: a study from the French Federation of Cancer Centers Sarcoma Group, *Am J Surg Pathol* 26:601–616, 2002.
198. Hornick JL, Bosenberg MW, Mentzel T, et al: Pleomorphic liposarcoma: clinicopathologic analysis of 57 cases, *Am J Surg Pathol* 28:1257–1267, 2004.
199. Dei Tos AP, Mentzel T, Fletcher CD: Primary liposarcoma of the skin: a rare neoplasm with unusual high grade features, *Am J Dermatopathol* 20:332–338, 1998.
200. Miettinen M, Enzinger FM: Epithelioid variant of pleomorphic liposarcoma: a study of 12 cases of a distinctive variant of high-grade liposarcoma, *Mod Pathol* 12:722–728, 1999.
201. Huang HY, Antonescu CR: Epithelioid variant of pleomorphic liposarcoma: a comparative immunohistochemical and ultrastructural analysis of six cases with emphasis on overlapping features with epithelial malignancies, *Ultrastruct Pathol* 26:299–308, 2002.
202. Barretina J, Taylor SB, Banerji S, et al: Subtype-specific genomic alterations define new targets for soft tissue sarcoma therapy, *Nat Genet* 42:715–721, 2010.

13

Vascular Tumors

Briana C. Gleason, MD, and Jason L. Hornick, MD, PhD

The vascular system is composed of arteries and veins and their derivatives, capillaries, and lymphatic channels. Although large arteries and veins are readily distinguished histologically, their smaller counterparts can be difficult to differentiate morphologically. In general, veins have a thinner smooth muscle layer and a larger luminal diameter than arteries, and a well-defined internal elastic lamina is not seen on routine sections or with elastic stains. Lymphatic vessels tend to be compressed or elongated, with irregular contours, and may contain pale eosinophilic fluid (lymph). However, the distinction between small lymphatics and venules may be challenging, particularly because lymphatics not infrequently contain blood in histologic sections, possibly as a result of surgically induced hemorrhage or small lymphaticovenous connections in vivo. If the distinction is clinically relevant, immunohistochemistry (discussed later) can be helpful.

Immunohistochemistry

The endothelial cells of blood and lymphatic vessels show considerable immunophenotypic overlap (which is not surprising because they arise from a common embryologic precursor) (Table 13.1). Blood vessel endothelium usually expresses both CD31 and CD34, whereas lymphatic endothelium shows variable and often weak CD31 expression and is typically negative for CD34.[1,2] Several antibodies with increased sensitivity and relative specificity for lymphatic endothelial cells have recently been developed, including D2-40 (podoplanin),[3,4] vascular endothelial

Table 13.1 Antibodies Useful in the Diagnosis of Vascular Tumors[a]

Antibody (Cellular Localization)	Normal Structures in Skin/Soft Tissue	Vascular Tumors	Nonvascular Tumors
CD31 (membranous)	Endothelium (blood vessels > lymphatics), histiocytes, platelets, some plasma cells	All types	Rare carcinomas and mesotheliomas, histiocytic sarcoma, plasmacytoma/myeloma
CD34 (membranous)	Endothelium (blood vessels ≫ lymphatics), endoneurial and dermal fibroblasts	All types	Widely expressed in mesenchymal tumors, acute leukemias
FLI1 (nuclear)	Endothelium (blood vessels > lymphatics), lymphocytes	All types	Ewing sarcoma; lymphoblastic lymphoma; some DSRCT, MCC, and NHL
ERG (nuclear)	Endothelium (all types)	All types	Prostate carcinoma (45%); Ewing sarcoma (10%); AML (rare)
D2-40 (membranous)	Lymphatic endothelium, mesothelium, myoepithelium, follicular dendritic cells in lymphoid follicles, perineurium	PILA, KS, angiosarcoma (50%), EHE (subset)	Mesothelioma, skin adnexal carcinomas, follicular dendritic cell sarcoma; some germ cell tumors (especially seminoma/germinoma)
Vascular endothelial growth factor receptor 3 (cytoplasmic or membranous)	Lymphatic endothelium	KS, PILA, RHE, KHE, hemangiomas (30%–80%), EHE (30%), angiosarcoma (60%–80%)	None
LYVE-1 (membranous)	Lymphatic endothelium	KS, angiosarcoma[b]	None
Smooth muscle actin (cytoplasmic)	Pericytes	Benign: intact layer of pericytes around tumor vessels Malignant: variable positivity in tumor cells	Many mesenchymal tumors and sarcomatoid carcinomas

[a]Expressed in 90% or more of cases, if not otherwise specified.
[b]Limited data available.
AML, Acute myeloid leukemia; *DSRCT*, desmoplastic small round cell tumor; *EHE*, epithelioid hemangioendothelioma; *KHE*, kaposiform hemangioendothelioma; *KS*, Kaposi sarcoma; *MCC*, Merkel cell carcinoma; *NHL*, non-Hodgkin lymphoma; *PILA*, papillary intralymphatic angioendothelioma (Dabska tumor); *RHE*, retiform hemangioendothelioma.

growth factor receptor 3 (VEGFR-3),[5,6] LYVE-1,[7] and PROX1.[8] However, as with most immunohistochemical markers, none of these antibodies is entirely specific for lymphatic differentiation (VEGFR-3 in particular is widely expressed in benign and malignant tumors of blood vascular lineage),[9–11] and they have yet to play a significant role in the routine evaluation of vascular tumors.

Special stains (histochemical or immunohistochemical) play a relatively minor role in the diagnostic work-up of vascular neoplasms compared with other soft tissue tumors. They are particularly useful in two circumstances: (1) to highlight the architecture of a known vascular neoplasm, and (2) to confirm endothelial differentiation in a poorly differentiated tumor.

In benign tumors of blood vascular origin (i.e., excluding those of lymphatic origin), each vessel has a well-defined layer of pericytes and a basal lamina. Reticulin stains (highlighting the basal lamina) and actin immunostains (highlighting the pericytic layer) are therefore useful in delineating the architecture of vascular lesions. Solid-appearing areas composed of compressed or poorly canalized vascular channels may be seen in benign neoplasms, but true solid sheets of endothelial cells are usually indicative of malignancy, with rare exceptions (e.g., epithelioid angiomatous nodule; discussed later).

In the work-up of poorly differentiated tumors, CD31 is widely regarded as the most sensitive and specific endothelial marker. FLI1, a more recently introduced antibody, shows comparable sensitivity for vascular neoplasms and may be easier to interpret than CD31 in the setting of a crushed or poorly preserved specimen because it shows nuclear rather than cytoplasmic or membranous reactivity.[12–15] However, FLI1 is not specific; Merkel cell carcinoma, Ewing sarcoma, and lymphoblastic lymphoma, as well as a small proportion (<10%) of carcinomas, melanomas, and other non-Hodgkin lymphomas, may be positive for this marker. ERG, another Ets family transcription factor, is more specific for endothelial differentiation than FLI1 and is expressed in nearly all endothelial lesions.[16] Nuclear ERG expression is also observed in 45% of prostate carcinomas (i.e., those with *TMPRSS2-ERG* fusion) and a small subset of Ewing sarcomas and acute myeloid leukemias (which also harbor *ERG* rearrangements). The older endothelial markers *Ulex europaeus* I agglutinin and factor VIII-related antigen/von Willebrand factor are rarely used in current practice because of the lack of specificity of the former and the low sensitivity and often high background staining of the latter.[17,18]

In addition, immunohistochemistry for human herpesvirus 8 (HHV-8) can be invaluable when the differential diagnosis of a vascular neoplasm includes Kaposi sarcoma.

PRACTICE POINTS: Special Stains and Vascular Tumors

Special stains are useful to:
- Confirm endothelial differentiation (e.g., CD31, CD34, or ERG)
- Dissect vascular architecture (reticulin or actin)
- Confirm the diagnosis of Kaposi sarcoma (HHV-8)

Classification of Vascular Tumors

A general classification of vascular tumors of skin and soft tissue is shown in Box 13.1. Occasional vascular neoplasms do not fit neatly into a well-defined category, but most can be classified as benign or malignant on morphologic grounds. Features of benign vascular lesions include a lobular architecture, well-formed vessels, and a single layer of endothelial cells. Features that suggest malignancy include a dissecting growth pattern, an infiltrative margin, anastomosing vascular channels, cytologic atypia, and endothelial multilayering. Mitoses and cellularity often are not discriminatory in this regard: for example, actively growing

Box 13.1 Classification of Vascular Tumors of Skin and Soft Tissue

Vascular Ectasias
- Spider angioma
- Venous lake
- Hereditary hemorrhagic telangiectasia
- Angioma serpiginosum
- Angiokeratoma
- Port-wine stain[a]

Reactive Vascular Proliferations
- Papillary endothelial hyperplasia (Masson tumor)
- Bacillary angiomatosis
- Reactive angioendotheliomatosis
- Glomeruloid hemangioma
- Acroangiodermatitis (pseudo-Kaposi sarcoma)

Benign Vascular Tumors/Malformations[b]
- Capillary hemangiomas
- Juvenile capillary hemangioma
- Lobular capillary hemangioma (pyogenic granuloma)
- Verrucous hemangioma
- Cherry angioma
- Cavernous hemangioma/venous malformation
- Sinusoidal hemangioma
- Arteriovenous hemangioma (cirsoid aneurysm)
- Microvenular hemangioma
- Hobnail hemangioma (targetoid hemosiderotic hemangioma)
- **Spindle cell hemangioma**
- *Epithelioid hemangioma (including angiolymphoid hyperplasia with eosinophilia)*
- *Epithelioid angiomatous nodule*
- Tufted angioma
- Cavernous lymphangioma/lymphangioma circumscriptum/lymphatic malformation
- Acquired progressive lymphangioma (benign lymphangioendothelioma)
- Glomuvenous malformation
- Arteriovenous malformation
- Deep (e.g., intramuscular, synovial) vascular malformations (usually mixed vessel-type)
- Angiomatosis/lymphangiomatosis

Intermediate (Locally Aggressive or Rarely Metastasizing) Vascular Tumors
- **Kaposiform hemangioendothelioma**
- Papillary intralymphatic angioendothelioma
- Retiform hemangioendothelioma
- Composite hemangioendothelioma
- **Pseudomyogenic hemangioendothelioma** (see Chapters 3 and 15)
- **Kaposi sarcoma[c]**

Malignant Vascular Tumors
- *Epithelioid hemangioendothelioma*
- Angiosarcoma
- *Epithelioid angiosarcoma*
- **Spindle cell angiosarcoma**

[a]Considered a capillary malformation by some sources.
[b]In practice, the histologic distinction between vascular malformations and hemangiomas is difficult and often impossible.
Tumors in bold are often predominantly spindled; tumors in italics are often predominantly epithelioid; the remainder are vasoformative.

benign lesions, such as pyogenic granuloma and juvenile capillary hemangioma, often show greater cellularity and mitotic activity than low-grade angiosarcomas. A single atypical feature is generally insufficient for a diagnosis of malignancy: cytologic atypia, a dissecting growth pattern, and infiltration of normal tissues may all be found in occasional reactive and benign vascular lesions.

Tumors of "intermediate biologic potential" are a well-recognized concept in soft tissue neoplasia and are particularly common among vascular neoplasms. The term *hemangioendothelioma* has been used historically in a variety of contexts but is now applied predominantly to vascular tumors in the intermediate group. The latter category includes two groups of tumors: (1) those that may be locally aggressive but have no metastatic potential; and (2) those that have a very low and histologically unpredictable risk of metastasis. In the 2013 World Health Organization (WHO) classification, the category of intermediate vascular neoplasms included kaposiform hemangioendothelioma, papillary intralymphatic angioendothelioma (Dabska tumor), retiform hemangioendothelioma, composite hemangioendothelioma, Kaposi sarcoma, and pseudomyogenic hemangioendothelioma.[19] Kaposiform hemangioendothelioma and retiform hemangioendothelioma cause morbidity and (in the case of the former) mortality through local effects; distant metastases have not been reported in either entity. Data on the behavior of papillary intralymphatic angioendothelioma and composite hemangioendothelioma are limited because of their rarity. Kaposi sarcoma is increasingly regarded as a virus-induced hyperplasia rather than a neoplasm, but it is included with the intermediate vascular tumors in this discussion because it may lead to significant morbidity and rarely mortality. Distant metastases and death from disease have been reported in rare cases of pseudomyogenic hemangioendothelioma (despite its endothelial derivation, this tumor is morphologically nonvasoformative and therefore will be discussed in Chapters 3 and 15). Epithelioid hemangioendothelioma, formerly classified in the intermediate ("rarely metastasizing") category, is now considered to be fully malignant, based on a significant risk of distant metastasis with extended follow-up periods. Two other rare vascular neoplasms, polymorphous hemangioendothelioma and giant cell angioblastoma, were not included in the 2013 WHO classification because of a lack of sufficient data on their diagnostic criteria and biologic potential.[20]

Although there are no known risk factors for most vascular neoplasms, a small subset of kaposiform hemangioendotheliomas, papillary intralymphatic angioendotheliomas, and composite hemangioendotheliomas arise in association with an underlying vascular malformation, and in rare cases, composite hemangioendothelioma, retiform hemangioendothelioma, and angiosarcoma may develop in the setting of chronic lymphedema.

Most vascular tumors are vasoformative and are readily recognized as being vascular. Less commonly, vascular neoplasms are predominantly spindled (e.g., spindle cell hemangioma, Kaposi sarcoma, kaposiform hemangioendothelioma, pseudomyogenic hemangioendothelioma, and some angiosarcomas) or epithelioid (e.g., solid epithelioid hemangiomas, epithelioid angiomatous nodule, epithelioid hemangioendothelioma, and epithelioid angiosarcoma). Each pattern is discussed separately.

PRACTICE POINTS: Benign and Worrisome Features in Vascular Tumors

Features of benign vascular tumors:
- Well circumscribed
- Lobular architecture
- Well-formed vessels
- Single layer of endothelial cells

Worrisome features:
- Infiltrative margin
- Dissecting growth pattern
- Complex anastomosing vascular channels
- Endothelial multilayering
- Cytologic atypia

Vasoformative Pattern

Vascular tumors with a vasoformative pattern are common, particularly in the skin, where most are benign. Although numerous hemangioma variants have been described, many acquired cutaneous vascular lesions do not fit neatly into a particular diagnostic category and are best reported as *unclassified benign hemangioma* or simply *benign hemangioma*. In some cases, reactive vascular proliferations closely mimic benign vascular tumors, and it may be impossible to make the distinction histologically. The clinical history is often helpful because patients with reactive vascular lesions (e.g., bacillary angiomatosis or reactive angioendotheliomatosis) often have an underlying systemic disease and frequently have multiple lesions, in contrast to hemangiomas, which are usually solitary.

The distinction between vascular malformations and neoplasms is also challenging and may be impossible, particularly among small, superficial vascular lesions in older patients. A classification system for pediatric hemangiomas and vascular malformations based largely on clinical features[21] was adopted by the International Society for the Study of Vascular Anomalies in 1996,[22] and updated in 2015,[23] which is predominantly used in pediatric institutions. Problems arise because categorization on clinical grounds is not always straightforward. Some vascular malformations may not become clinically evident until late childhood or even adulthood, and hemangiomas are rarely fully formed at birth. Furthermore, in most cases the distinction between malformations and hemangiomas is of no clinical significance. These lesions are discussed together in this chapter.

Papillary Endothelial Hyperplasia (Masson Tumor)

Papillary endothelial hyperplasia, although initially considered a neoplasm,[24] is now generally regarded as an exuberant form of organizing thrombus that occurs in three settings: primary, secondary, and extravascular.[25-27] Primary papillary endothelial hyperplasia arises within a normal or dilated vessel (nearly always a vein) and is most common on the fingers and in the head and neck region. Secondary papillary endothelial hyperplasia occurs within a preexisting vascular lesion, such as a vascular malformation, cavernous hemangioma, venous lake, angiokeratoma, or hemorrhoid. Extravascular papillary endothelial hyperplasia arises in association with a hematoma at any site, including soft tissue, the thyroid, or the adrenal gland. More than 95% of cases are intravascular, and primary papillary endothelial hyperplasia is slightly more common than the secondary form.[28]

Clinical Features

Patients present with a slowly growing mass that is often painful or tender. Rarely, multiple discrete nodules may be present.[27,29,30] Despite a predilection for sites where minor trauma is common, most patients do not recall a specific traumatic event preceding the development of the lesion.[25,28]

Pathologic Features

Intravascular papillary endothelial hyperplasia is a small (<3 cm), well-circumscribed lesion composed of numerous thin papillary structures lined by a single layer of endothelial cells. In early lesions, the papillae have brightly eosinophilic, acellular, fibrinous cores and are often associated with an identifiable thrombus (Fig. 13.1A). Later lesions have densely hyalinized, hypocellular cores (see Fig. 13.1B), with occasional small capillaries; in some cases, granulation tissue representing a late-stage organizing thrombus may be found at the periphery of the lesion, near the vessel wall. The papillae are believed to form by progressive hyalinization and endothelialization of a preexisting thrombus.

The endothelium is usually flattened and banal appearing but may be focally prominent or hyperchromatic. Mitoses are infrequently identified. The wall of the surrounding vessel is often markedly attenuated and may not be apparent without the use of special stains (i.e., elastic stains or smooth muscle actin).

Extravascular papillary endothelial hyperplasia may form large soft tissue masses, sometimes measuring greater than 10 cm,[28] and these often raise clinical concern for malignancy. The histologic features are similar to those seen in intravascular papillary endothelial hyperplasia, although there is no surrounding vessel. The characteristic hyalinized acellular papillae and a zonation phenomenon, with granulation tissue at the periphery and a progressively less mature organizing thrombus toward the center of the lesion, are helpful in recognizing this unusual variant.

Differential Diagnosis

Papillary endothelial hyperplasia may resemble sinusoidal hemangioma because of the presence of elongated papillae lined by flattened endothelial

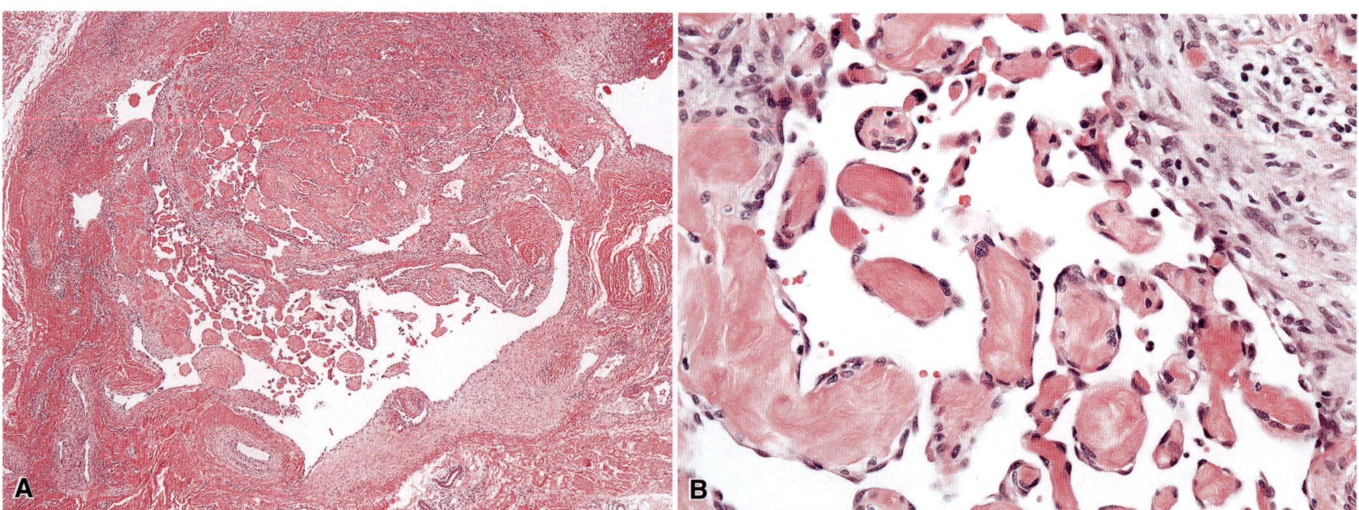

Figure 13.1 Papillary Endothelial Hyperplasia. (A) Vascular malformation containing organizing thrombus with papillary endothelial hyperplasia (Masson change). (B) Papillae with hyalinized hypocellular cores covered by flattened endothelium. Note the adjacent granulation tissue.

cells, but the latter has an orderly, sievelike appearance in contrast to the disorganized papillae of papillary endothelial hyperplasia. Although it also arises in a vein, intravascular pyogenic granuloma has well-defined lobules of tightly packed capillaries rather than complex, heterogeneous papillae.

Despite occasional marked cytologic atypia and nuclear hyperchromasia, intravascular papillary endothelial hyperplasia is readily recognized as benign because of the distinct circumscription of the lesion and the presence of a surrounding vessel wall. Extravascular papillary endothelial hyperplasia may be confused with angiosarcoma, particularly in the clinical setting of a large, deep soft tissue mass, but the absence of endothelial multilayering, numerous mitoses, necrosis, and invasion of the adjacent soft tissue argue against a malignant diagnosis.

Prognosis and Treatment

Local excision is generally curative. Rare reports of recurrence are typically caused by persistence of the underlying vascular lesion in secondary papillary endothelial hyperplasia.[25,26,31]

Chronic ("ancient") hematomas without papillary endothelial hyperplasia can also present as slowly or occasionally rapidly enlarging soft tissue masses that mimic malignancy clinically and radiologically. The masses measure from a few to more than 50 cm in greatest dimension and are most common on the lower extremities.[32,33] A history of trauma is often not given because the lesions may present a decade or more after the original injury. A central cavity filled with old or fresh hemorrhage and fibrin is surrounded by dense hypocellular fibrous tissue containing numerous granular histiocytes and amorphous eosinophilic material likely representing an old blood clot. Foreign body giant cells, dystrophic calcification, hemosiderin, cholesterol clefts, and foamy histiocytes are variably present within the fibrous pseudocapsule. These lesions should be distinguished from ancient schwannoma, which is readily achieved by the absence of S-100 protein reactivity.

PRACTICE POINTS: Papillary Endothelial Hyperplasia (Masson Tumor)

- Papillary endothelial hyperplasia (Masson tumor) typically arises in a normal vessel or preexisting vascular lesion.
- The characteristic hyalinized papillae are helpful in recognition if the surrounding vessel wall is not visible on routine sections.

Bacillary Angiomatosis

Bacillary angiomatosis is a reactive vascular proliferation induced by *Bartonella henselae* or, less often, *Bartonella quintana*. The disease was not uncommon in the United States during the acquired immunodeficiency syndrome (AIDS) epidemic of the 1980s, but it is now rarely encountered because of the routine use of prophylactic antibiotics in patients positive for human immunodeficiency virus. Although most cases of bacillary angiomatosis occur in patients with human immunodeficiency virus infection (and usually a CD4+ T-cell count <200/μL), other immunosuppressed patients may be affected, and rare cases have been reported in immunocompetent patients.[34]

Clinical Features

Patients present with solitary or, more often, multiple red papules resembling pyogenic granulomas. Subcutaneous nodules and oral, anal, conjunctival, or gastrointestinal mucosal lesions may also be present.[35] The lymph nodes, spleen, and liver may be involved in rare cases.

Pathologic Features

The cutaneous lesions are characterized by a lobular proliferation of capillaries in an edematous to myxoid stroma, often surrounded by an epidermal collarette. The endothelial cells are plump and frequently show mild to moderate atypia. Mitoses are common, and small foci of necrosis may be present in the center of the capillary lobules.[35] Stromal neutrophils and neutrophilic debris are invariably present (Fig. 13.2), even in the absence of necrosis or ulceration. Clumps of granular violaceous material representing bacteria are often visible on routine sections, but the organisms are best seen with modified silver stains (e.g., Warthin-Starry, Steiner, or Dieterle).

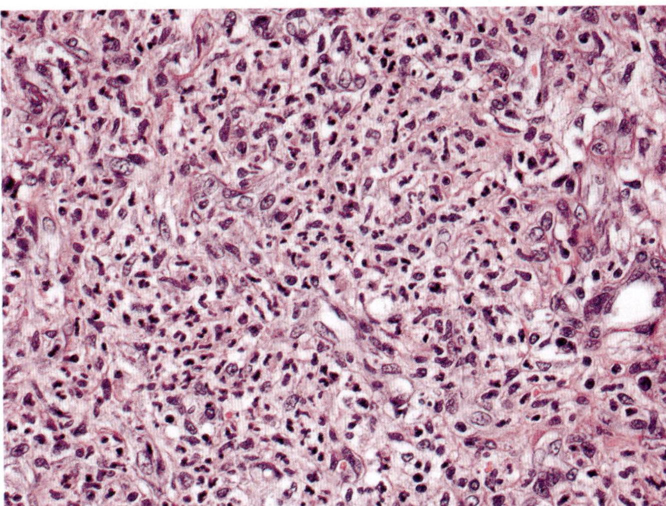

Figure 13.2 Bacillary Angiomatosis. Capillary proliferation containing plump, mildly atypical endothelial cells associated with prominent stromal neutrophils.

The subcutaneous nodules and involved lymph nodes show a vascular proliferation similar to that seen in the skin. In the liver and spleen, dilated vessels with a peliosis-like appearance are seen and clumps of bacteria may be identified.

Differential Diagnosis

Lobular capillary hemangioma has similar histologic features and, if ulcerated, can have an acute inflammatory infiltrate, but the neutrophils are predominantly localized to the superficial portion of the tumor and leukocytoclasia is absent. The characteristic granular amphophilic material is a clue to bacillary angiomatosis, and silver stain is confirmatory.

Verruga peruana is a reactive dermal or subcutaneous vascular proliferation associated with infection by *Bartonella bacilliformis*, an organism endemic to the Andes region of South America.[36] Although the infection is rare outside of endemic areas, immunocompetent travelers who have recently returned from South America may be affected.[37] The histologic features are strikingly similar to those of bacillary angiomatosis, and the clinical history is helpful in the distinction. Organisms are not visible on hematoxylin and eosin–stained sections, but Giemsa stain may highlight degraded bacteria within intracytoplasmic vacuoles (Rocha-Lima inclusions) in endothelial cells.

Prognosis and Treatment

Bacillary angiomatosis is readily cured with appropriate antibiotic therapy. However, if untreated, disseminated disease can be fatal.

PRACTICE POINTS: Bacillary Angiomatosis

- Bacillary angiomatosis shows marked clinical and histologic overlap with pyogenic granuloma but is usually multiple, occurs in immunocompromised patients, and contains bacilli.
- Organisms may be visible as amphophilic clumps on hematoxylin and eosin staining or by modified silver stains.

Reactive Angioendotheliomatosis

Reactive angioendotheliomatosis is a rare disorder defined by the development of reactive cutaneous vascular proliferations, typically in the setting of systemic disease. The original term *systemic angioendotheliomatosis* included both reactive and malignant entities, and the latter is now known to be intravascular large B-cell lymphoma.[38] Some have used the designation *diffuse dermal angiomatosis* for a variant of reactive angioendotheliomatosis in which endothelial cell proliferation is primarily extravascular rather than intravascular[39]; we prefer to use the term *reactive angioendotheliomatosis* to encompass both ends of the histologic spectrum.

Clinical Features

Reactive angioendotheliomatosis typically occurs in adults, although rare cases in infants have been reported.[40] The anatomic distribution is wide; the limbs and breast/chest wall are sites of predilection.[41] Most patients have an underlying systemic disease, including renal failure, liver failure, autoimmune diseases (including antiphospholipid antibody syndrome), lymphoproliferative disorders, cryoglobulinemia, valvular heart disease, and chronic infections.[41] Other cases have been reported in association with peripheral atherosclerotic disease or iatrogenic arteriovenous shunts,[42,43] and approximately 25% of patients are apparently otherwise healthy.[41] The pathogenesis is unknown, but systemic or localized vasoocclusion and consequent hypoxia may play a role.[44]

The clinical presentation is often dramatic. Patients have multiple purpuric patches or plaques that range from a few millimeters to several centimeters in size. These lesions may ulcerate or become necrotic; in some cases, hundreds of lesions are present. The clinical differential diagnosis often includes Kaposi sarcoma and calciphylaxis, particularly in patients with renal failure.

Pathologic Features

Reactive angioendotheliomatosis is characterized by an intravascular or extravascular proliferation of endothelial cells or pericytes in the dermis and, infrequently, the superficial subcutis. The histologic pattern varies markedly between lesions, including different lesions from the same patient, as expected for a reactive process. Commonly, a poorly circumscribed, diffuse or patchy capillary proliferation is noted in the superficial dermis and occasionally the deep dermis (Fig. 13.3A and B). Other cases have a tufted angioma-like pattern with discrete lobules of tightly packed capillaries that are widely scattered throughout the dermis.[45,46] In some lesions, endothelial proliferation is entirely intravascular, often with associated thrombosis. Less often, reactive angioendotheliomatosis has an angiosarcoma-like pattern, with slitlike, thin-walled vessels dissecting through dermal collagen (see Fig. 13.3C). Lesions in which the pericytic proliferation predominates over the endothelial proliferation, resulting in aggregates of capillaries surrounded and compressed by several layers of pericytes, have also been described.[47]

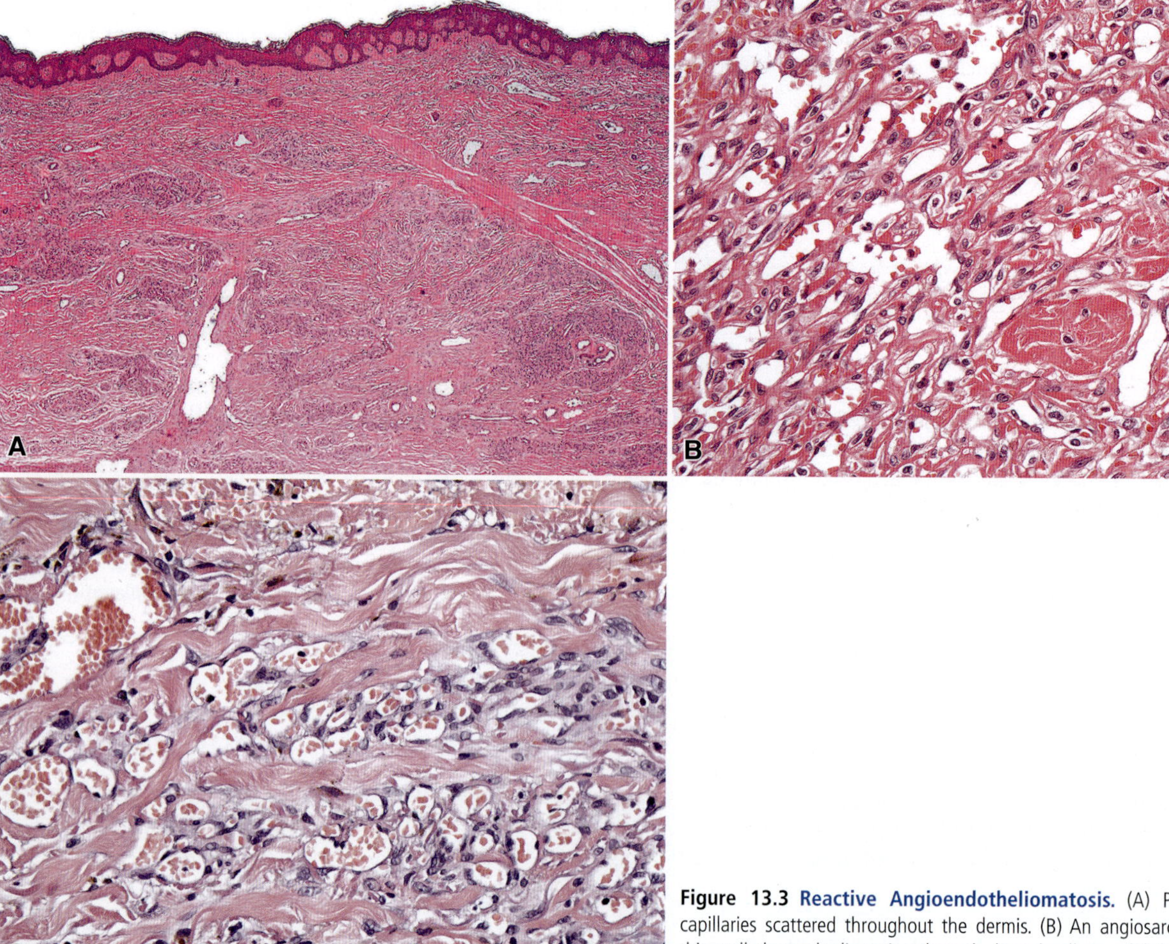

Figure 13.3 Reactive Angioendotheliomatosis. (A) Patchy proliferation of capillaries scattered throughout the dermis. (B) An angiosarcoma-like pattern with thin-walled vessels dissecting through dermal collagen. (C) Small vessels containing endothelial cells with mild cytologic atypia. Note the hemosiderin deposition.

The endothelial cells are typically flattened but may show focal cytologic atypia, particularly in association with thrombi, and infrequently, hobnail or epithelioid cytomorphologic features are seen. Occasional mitotic figures may be present. Hemosiderin deposition and a mild chronic inflammatory infiltrate are common, and a fasciitis-like myofibroblastic proliferation may be seen in association with the vascular proliferation.

Differential Diagnosis

The ill-defined margins and variable histologic features are clues to a reactive etiology. Although cytologic atypia may occur, the layer of pericytes around each vessel and the absence of endothelial multilayering argue against a diagnosis of well-differentiated angiosarcoma. The tufted angioma-like pattern of reactive angioendotheliomatosis is distinguished from tufted angioma by the clinical setting and the lack of crescentic lymphatic vessels at the periphery of the capillary tufts.

Prognosis and Treatment

The clinical course is variable.[41] Some lesions resolve spontaneously or in response to topical or systemic corticosteroids or laser therapy, whereas others are refractory to a variety of treatments. In patients with localized vasoocclusion as a result of peripheral vascular disease, the lesions usually resolve after revascularization.[39]

PRACTICE POINTS: Reactive Angioendotheliomatosis

- Reactive angioendotheliomatosis usually affects adults with an underlying systemic disease.
- Histologic patterns are widely variable, even among multiple lesions in the same patient, which is a helpful diagnostic clue.

Glomeruloid Hemangioma

Clinical Features

Glomeruloid hemangioma is a distinctive vascular proliferation that arises almost exclusively in the setting of POEMS syndrome (polyneuropathy, organomegaly, endocrinopathy, M-protein, and skin changes).[48,49] The most common cutaneous manifestations of POEMS syndrome are hyperpigmentation, hypertrichosis, hyperhidrosis, and scleroderma-like induration. Less often, patients have multiple cutaneous angiomas on the trunk, proximal extremities, and face.[50–52] Although rare cases of glomeruloid hemangioma in patients without POEMS syndrome have been reported,[53,54] based on the photographs provided, these lesions may be examples of a histologically similar entity called *papillary hemangioma* (discussed later).[55] Some authors consider glomeruloid hemangioma a distinctive pattern of reactive angioendotheliomatosis that is most often associated with POEMS syndrome, a hypothesis supported by the report of similar lesions in a patient with non-Hodgkin lymphoma and a clinical picture of reactive angioendotheliomatosis.[56]

Pathologic Features

The dermis contains widely dilated vascular spaces, with a complex intravascular capillary proliferation resembling a renal glomerulus (Fig. 13.4A and B). The endothelial lining is predominantly flattened, but occasional plump, vacuolated endothelial cells with intracytoplasmic hyaline globules are seen lining the vessels and within the stroma (see Fig. 13.4C). The inclusions are positive for periodic acid–Schiff (diastase resistant) and show polytypic reactivity for immunoglobulin.[49]

Not all cutaneous vascular lesions arising in patients with POEMS syndrome are pure glomeruloid hemangiomas. Lesions with the features of cherry angioma, tufted angioma, or reactive angioendotheliomatosis have been described, and some biopsy specimens show features of two or more patterns, including the classic glomeruloid pattern.[49,52,57]

Differential Diagnosis

Papillary hemangioma is a recently described vascular tumor that overlaps significantly with glomeruloid hemangioma histologically but presents as a solitary lesion on the head and neck of healthy patients.[55] Dilated dermal vessels show complex papillary proliferation with well-developed fibrous cores. The lesional endothelial cells are often vacuolated and contain prominent hyaline globules. The distinctly papillary architecture contrasts with the capillary tuft of glomeruloid hemangioma, and the intracytoplasmic hyaline globules are largely confined to the endothelial layer covering the papillae and are not seen in the capillaries within the fibrous cores or in stromal cells.

PRACTICE POINTS: Glomeruloid Hemangioma

- Glomeruloid hemangioma occurs in patients with POEMS syndrome.
- Key features are intravascular glomeruloid tufts and intracytoplasmic hyaline globules.
- Papillary hemangioma shows histologic overlap but occurs in healthy patients and has well-developed intravascular papillae.

Acroangiodermatitis (Pseudo-Kaposi Sarcoma)

Acroangiodermatitis is a reactive dermal capillary proliferation that occurs on the lower extremities of patients with severe chronic venous insufficiency (Mali type)[58] or congenital arteriovenous malformations (Stewart-Bluefarb syndrome).[59] A similar process has been described on the hands or fingers of patients with arteriovenous fistulas who are undergoing hemodialysis. The lesions may mimic Kaposi sarcoma both clinically and histologically, leading to the alternative designation *pseudo-Kaposi sarcoma*.[60]

Clinical Features

Patients with acroangiodermatitis of Mali present with bilateral dusky red-purple macules that progress to plaques and nodules on the distal lower extremities, particularly the dorsum of the feet and toes and the lateral malleoli. The adjacent skin shows typical changes of stasis dermatitis. Patients with Stewart-Bluefarb syndrome have violaceous macules and papules on the affected extremity during young adulthood. Varicose veins and a palpable thrill may also be noted because of the underlying arteriovenous shunt.

Pathologic Features

The histologic features are essentially those of exaggerated stasis dermatitis. The dermis contains numerous thick-walled capillaries, often in a lobular configuration, associated with extravasated erythrocytes, hemosiderin, fibrosis, and a mild chronic inflammatory infiltrate (Fig. 13.5). The endothelial cells are often plump, but nuclear atypia is absent. In acroangiodermatitis of Mali, the vascular proliferation is generally confined to the superficial dermis, whereas the entire dermis may be affected in Stewart-Bluefarb syndrome.

Differential Diagnosis

In patch- and plaque-stage Kaposi sarcoma, the vessels are thin walled, irregular, and slitlike, with a dissecting pattern through the dermis. The papillary dermis is typically uninvolved, in contrast to acroangiodermatitis. Plasma cells, hyaline globules, and a spindle cell component also favor a diagnosis of Kaposi sarcoma.[61]

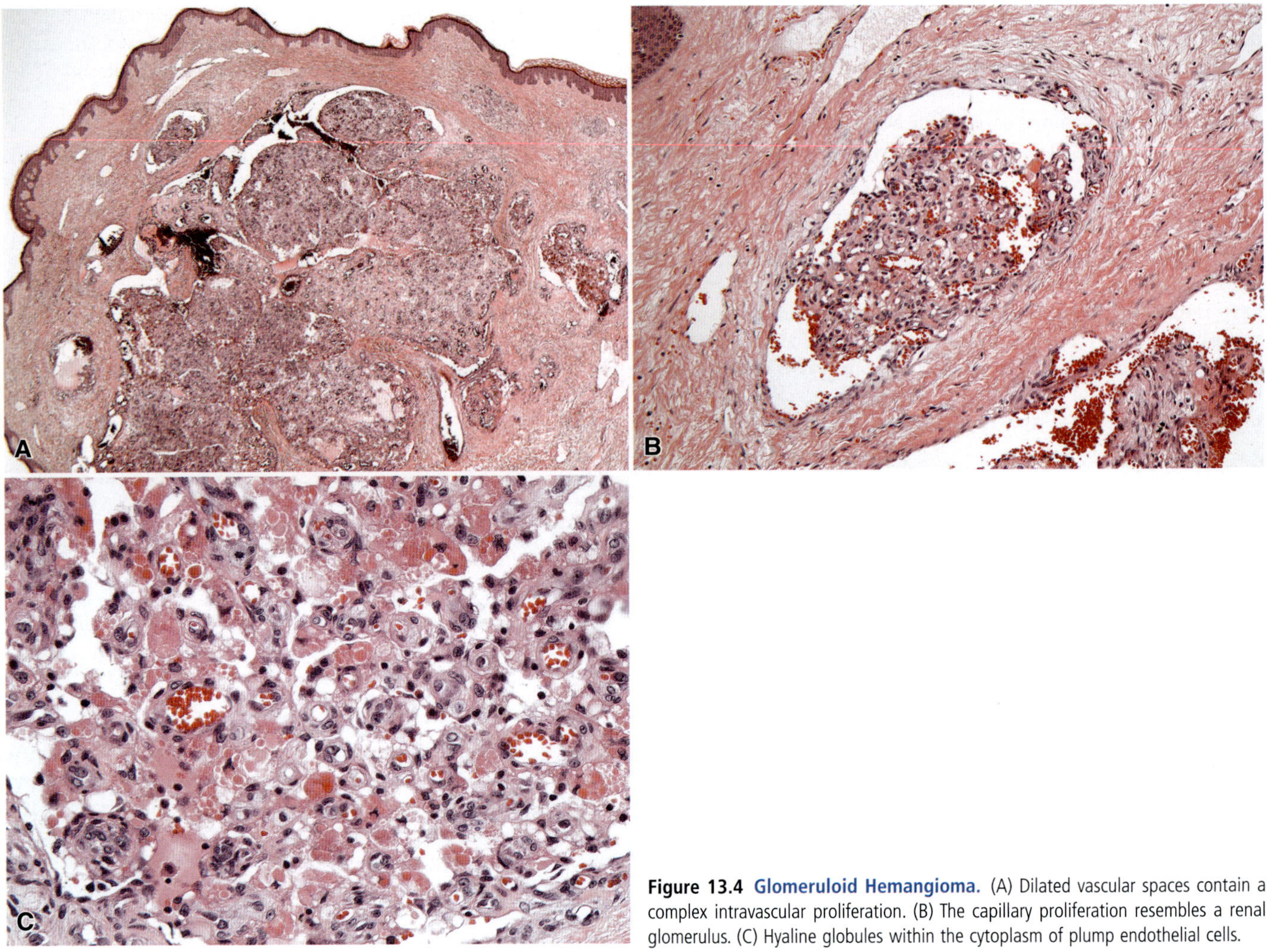

Figure 13.4 **Glomeruloid Hemangioma.** (A) Dilated vascular spaces contain a complex intravascular proliferation. (B) The capillary proliferation resembles a renal glomerulus. (C) Hyaline globules within the cytoplasm of plump endothelial cells.

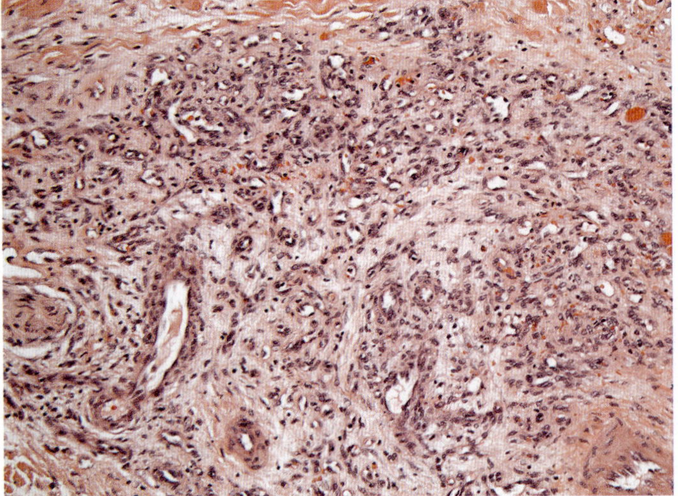

Figure 13.5 **Acroangiodermatitis.** Thick-walled capillaries associated with extravasated erythrocytes and fibrosis.

PRACTICE POINTS: Acroangiodermatitis (Pseudo-Kaposi Sarcoma)

- Acroangiodermatitis occurs on the legs of patients with severe venous stasis or arteriovenous malformations.
- There is clinical and histologic resemblance to Kaposi sarcoma.

Vascular Ectasias

Some lesions that clinically mimic vascular neoplasms are merely vascular ectasias. The most common are spider angiomas and venous lakes. A spider angioma simply represents abnormal persistence of a small artery in the dermis. The name derives from the clinical appearance of a vascular ectasia with a central red "body" and thin radiating "legs." Spider angiomas are often multiple and most commonly occur on the chest, proximal extremities, and face. They are frequently associated with liver disease, pregnancy, or estrogen use but may also arise in healthy patients, particularly children. Microscopically, the superficial dermis contains a dilated, thick-walled arteriole with numerous tiny arteriolar branches that eventually form capillary beds.[62] Venous lakes typically present as solitary or multiple 1- to 5-mm bluish macules on the ears, lips, or face of elderly patients.[63] Histologically, one or a few widely dilated venules are present in an elastotic dermis (Fig. 13.6A).

Hereditary hemorrhagic telangiectasia (Osler-Rendu-Weber syndrome) is an autosomal dominant disorder in which patients have

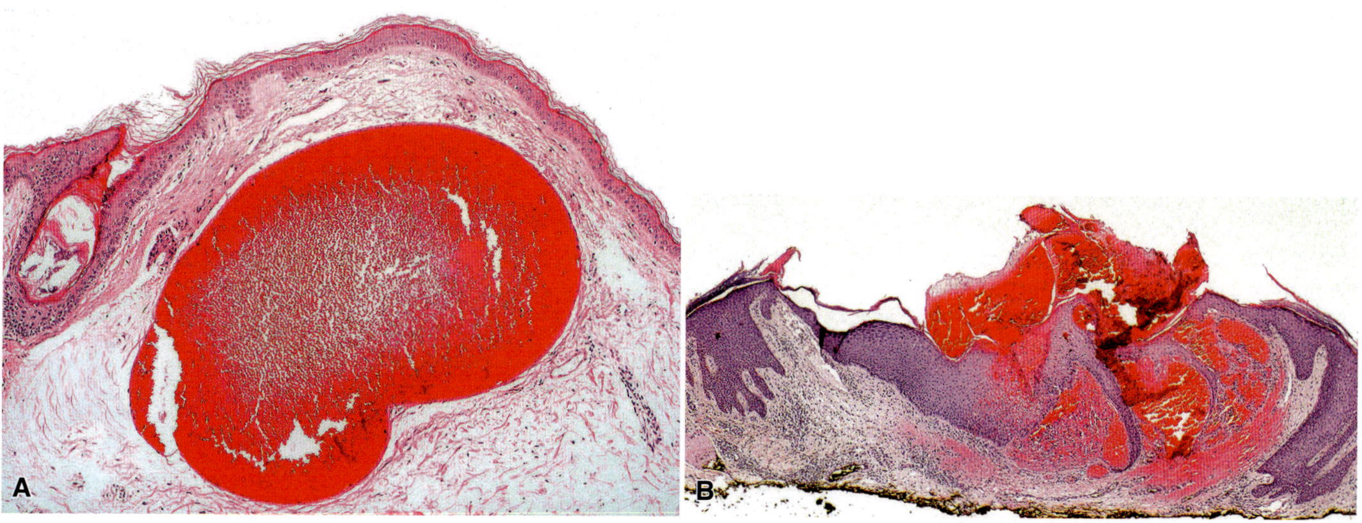

Figure 13.6 Vascular Ectasias. (A) Venous lake composed of a widely dilated venule in the dermis. (B) Angiokeratoma showing marked dilation of subepidermal vessels associated with elongated rete ridges and overlying acanthosis.

numerous mucocutaneous telangiectasias, typically presenting first on the oral and nasal mucosa and progressing to involve the face, trunk, and extremities.[64,65] Patients may have visceral involvement, including gastrointestinal telangiectasias and arteriovenous malformations of the central nervous system, lungs, liver, or gastrointestinal tract. Histologically, early lesions show only dilated postcapillary venules in the superficial dermis. In later lesions the venules and arterioles are also dilated and the venular walls are thickened.[66]

Angioma serpiginosum is a rare form of telangiectasia that most commonly arises on the extremities of girls in late childhood or adolescence.[67,68] Most cases are sporadic, but autosomal dominant inheritance has been reported.[69] The lesions consist of grouped, erythematous, pinpoint macules that form gyrate, serpiginous, or linear patterns over an area measuring several centimeters. Angioma serpiginosum typically remains stable or progresses slowly during adulthood, but complete or partial spontaneous regression has been reported. Histologically, the superficial dermal vessels are dilated and often have thick walls. In contrast to the pigmented purpuric dermatoses, which may enter the clinical differential diagnosis, extravasated erythrocytes, hemosiderin deposition, and an inflammatory infiltrate are not seen.

Angiokeratomas are telangiectasias of superficial dermal vessels that arise in four clinical settings: (1) angiokeratoma of Mibelli arises on the dorsal hands and feet of children and adolescents (girls more often than boys), often in association with pernio (chilblains); (2) angiokeratoma of Fordyce occurs as multiple 2- to 4-mm papules on the scrotum or, less often, vulva of middle-aged and elderly patients; (3) angiokeratoma corpora diffusum presents in patients with Fabry disease as symmetrical grouped lesions with a predilection for the bathing trunk region; and (4) solitary angiokeratomas arise sporadically in healthy patients, most commonly on the lower extremities.[69–72] Many, if not most, of the rare lesions reported as angiokeratoma circumscriptum likely represent verrucous hemangiomas (discussed later). Angiokeratomas initially present as soft, red papules and become blue-black and keratotic over time, ultimately resembling a melanocytic lesion or wart. Histologically, there is marked dilatation of one or more subepidermal vessels with overlying epidermal acanthosis and variably prominent hyperkeratosis (see Fig. 13.6B). Elongated rete ridges often partially or completely encase the dilated vascular channels, such that the latter may appear to be intraepidermal. Organizing thrombi are commonly found within the dilated vessels. Angiokeratoma corpora diffusum shows vacuolization of the vascular and pilar smooth muscle because of glycosphingolipid deposits.[70]

The term *nevus flammeus* encompasses two vascular lesions that present at birth: the salmon patch and the port-wine stain. Salmon patches occur in 40% of infants, most commonly on the glabella, eyelids, mid-forehead, and nape of the neck, and may be multiple.[73] Facial lesions typically fade in the first year of life, whereas nuchal salmon patches tend to persist into adulthood. Histologically, dilated capillaries are present in the papillary dermis.[74]

Port-wine stains (also known as capillary malformations) are much less common (0.3% prevalence in newborns) and are most common on the face, often in a dermatomal distribution.[73] They begin as pale pink macules and become darker and thickened over time. Between 10% and 30% of patients ultimately develop a "cobblestone" surface or discrete nodules within the lesion during adulthood.[75,76] Approximately 10% of newborns with a capillary malformation involving the distribution of the first branch of the trigeminal nerve have Sturge-Weber syndrome, a vascular malformation affecting the skin, meninges, and choroid of the eye.[77] Capillary malformations of the limbs may arise as a component of a combined vascular malformation (discussed later). Biopsy is rarely performed on port-wine stains because of their characteristic clinical presentation. Some studies have reported an increased number of vessels, whereas others have shown only telangiectasia.[78–80] A consistent finding is decreased innervation of the lesional vessels, which may be responsible for the progressive vascular dilation that occurs with age because of loss of the normal vasoconstrictive tone.[78,79,81] In children, vascular ectasia often is not evident histologically, despite a clinically visible lesion. By young adulthood, the superficial dermal vessels are widely dilated and congested, and over time, the deep dermal and superficial subcutaneous vessels also become ectatic and congested, correlating with clinical darkening of the lesion. The cobblestone appearance of some late lesions is caused by localized exaggerations of the vascular ectasia, and larger intralesional nodules are generally caused by the development of superimposed vascular proliferations.[82]

Vascular Malformations

Vascular malformations are localized or diffuse aggregates of vessels that do not have a normal organization but maintain connection to the normal vasculature. As previously mentioned, the distinction between small, superficial vascular malformations and hemangiomas is difficult on both clinical and histologic grounds, and these lesions are discussed together. Diagnosis of large, deep-seated vascular malformations is typically straightforward. Classification is based on the constituent vessel type (i.e., venous, capillary, lymphatic, or arterial) and the presence or absence of arteriovenous shunting. Mixed-type vascular malformations are common and may be associated with well-defined clinical syndromes. Combined capillary–venous and capillary–venous–lymphatic malformations are characteristic of Klippel-Trénaunay syndrome, whereas capillary–arteriovenous and capillary–arteriovenous–lymphatic malformations are seen in Parkes Weber syndrome. Both are sporadic syndromes that present at birth with a port-wine stain of the affected extremity (usually the lower extremity) and are associated with limb hypertrophy as the child grows.[22,83]

PRACTICE POINTS: Vascular Malformations

- Small, superficial vascular malformations are frequently clinically and histologically indistinguishable from hemangiomas.
- Large, deep-seated vascular malformations are classified by their constituent vessel type.
- Mixed vessel-type malformations are common.

Cavernous Hemangioma and Venous Hemangioma (Venous Malformation)

Under the International Society for the Study of Vascular Anomalies classification, most lesions formerly known as *cavernous hemangiomas* and *venous hemangiomas* are now considered venous malformations. These lesions are discussed together in this chapter because they may be histologically indistinguishable, although classic examples of each (as described later) are recognizable.

Clinical Features

These lesions most commonly present in infancy or childhood but may affect adults. Most lesions involve the skin and soft tissue; some extend into skeletal muscle. Clinically, the tumors are soft, compressible, bluish masses that may become more prominent on physical activity or in a dependent position. Large venous malformations may be associated with chronic low-grade consumptive coagulopathy as a result of stagnant blood flow within the lesion and localized activation of coagulation.[84,85] This syndrome is characterized by low fibrinogen and high D-dimer levels; in contrast to Kasabach-Merritt syndrome, the platelet count is often normal.

A small proportion of these lesions arise as part of a recognized syndrome. Multiple cutaneous and gastrointestinal venous malformations are seen in patients with blue rubber bleb nevus syndrome, a rare, typically sporadic disorder that may cause iron deficiency anemia as a result of occult (or, rarely, massive) gastrointestinal blood loss.[86,87] Patients with Maffucci syndrome have multiple superficial and deep venous malformations in addition to multiple enchondromas and spindle cell hemangiomas (discussed later). The distal extremities are the most common site for both bone and soft tissue lesions. Cerebral cavernous (venous) malformations are inherited in an autosomal dominant fashion in 10% to 50% of cases; the familial form has been linked to mutations in the *CCM1* (cerebral capillary malformation-1; *KRIT1*), *CCM2*, and *CCM3* (*PDCD10*) genes.[88]

Glomuvenous malformations (referred to in earlier literature as *infiltrating glomus tumors in children*[89]) account for approximately 5% of venous malformations.[90] Although most vascular malformations are sporadic, glomuvenous malformations are often familial. Inheritance in these cases is autosomal dominant and has been linked to a mutation in the *GLMN (glomulin)* gene on chromosome 1p.[91] In contrast to venous malformations, they usually are not compressible and may be painful on palpation.

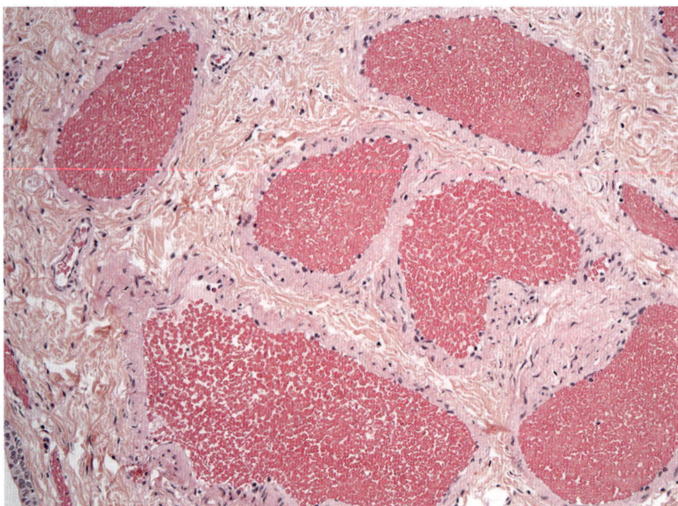

Figure 13.7 Cavernous Hemangioma. Well-circumscribed proliferation of dilated thin-walled congested vessels.

Pathologic Features

Cavernous hemangioma is a relatively circumscribed vascular proliferation composed of dilated, thin-walled, congested vessels (Fig. 13.7). In contrast, venous hemangiomas have thicker-walled, venous-type vessels that show variable dilation but also have relative circumscription and uniform histologic features. Venous malformations are classically poorly circumscribed aggregates of ectatic veins, with marked heterogeneity, including capillary- to cavernous-sized lumina and variably thickened muscular walls. Glomuvenous malformations are similar but also have one to several layers of glomus cells around the lesional vessels (Fig. 13.8). Intraluminal thrombi are common because of the slow intralesional blood flow, and intravascular papillary endothelial hyperplasia or phleboliths may be present.

Differential Diagnosis

Reported cavernous hemangiomas with a juvenile capillary hemangioma component likely represent either juvenile capillary hemangioma in the involution stage or juvenile capillary hemangioma with focally engorged vessels. Capillary proliferations are not a feature of cavernous hemangiomas. Cavernous hemangiomas with back-to-back, thin-walled channels are referred to as *sinusoidal hemangioma* (discussed later).

Sinusoidal Hemangioma

Sinusoidal hemangioma is an uncommon benign vascular tumor of adults that is notable for its propensity to arise in mammary subcutaneous tissue, where it may mimic a well-differentiated angiosarcoma.[92-94] Some authors regard sinusoidal hemangioma as a vascular malformation,[95,96] but we and others[97] consider them true acquired hemangiomas, based on their small size, overall circumscription, and histologic uniformity, as well as the acquired nature of most cases.

Clinical Features

The lesions present as solitary, bluish or flesh-colored, subcutaneous, deep dermal or, rarely, oral mucosal[98] nodules that measure up to a few centimeters. The limbs and trunk (including mammary subcutaneous tissue) are most commonly affected.[92-94,99]

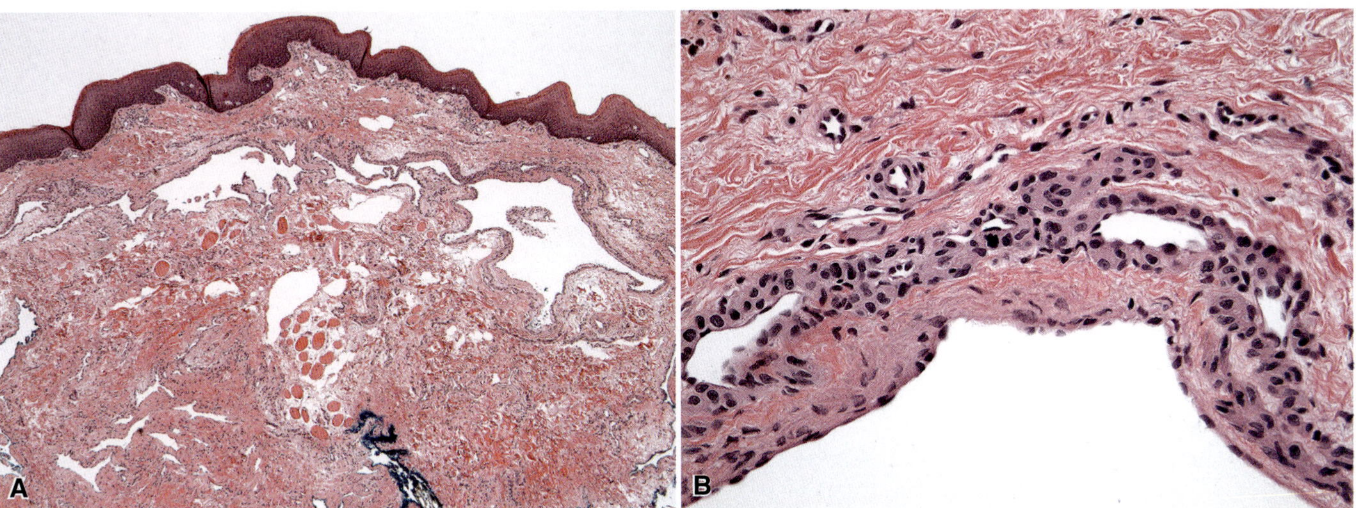

Figure 13.8 Glomuvenous Malformation. (A) The lesion shows ill-defined margins and is composed of ectatic veins of varying size and shape. (B) Some of the vessels are surrounded by a layer of rounded glomus cells.

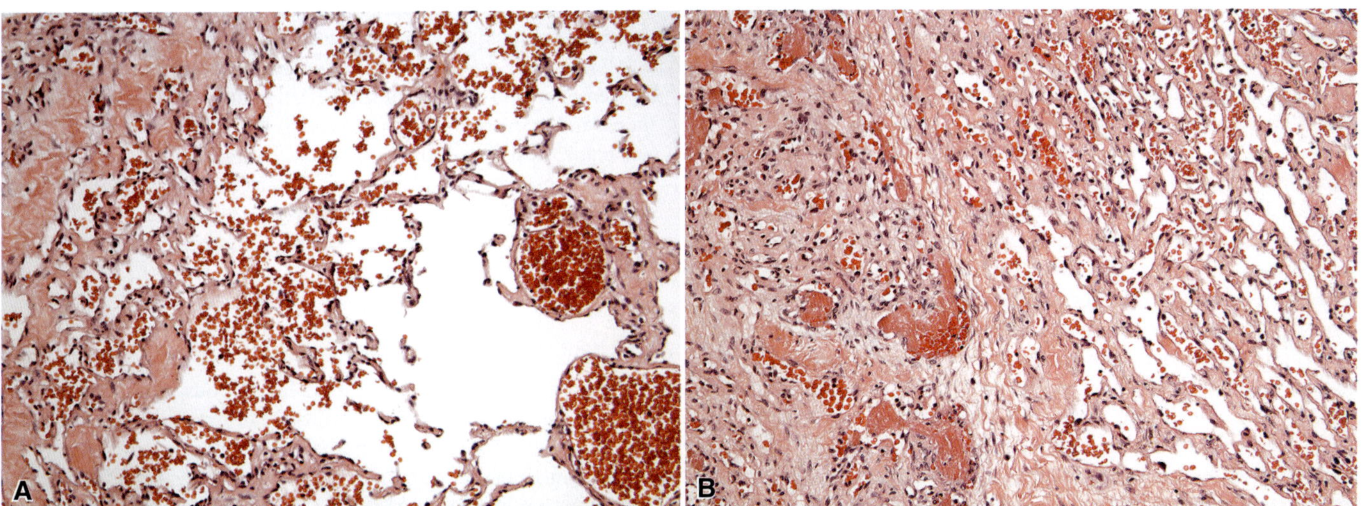

Figure 13.9 Sinusoidal Hemangioma. (A) Widely dilated thin-walled vascular channels in a back-to-back sieve-like arrangement. (B) Sinusoidal hemangioma with secondary organizing thrombus *(left)*.

Pathologic Features

The tumors are composed of widely dilated, congested vascular channels ("sinusoids") in a back-to-back arrangement, creating a sievelike appearance at low power (Fig. 13.9A). The vessels are separated by attenuated fibrous walls, and pseudopapillary structures representing thin fibrous septa cut in cross section are common. Secondary changes, including thrombi (see Fig. 13.9B), phleboliths, foamy macrophages, or cholesterol clefts, and central infarction (often as a result of previous needle localization or biopsy), may be present.[93]

In the subcutaneous tissue, the tumors characteristically completely or partially replace one or more adjacent lobules of fat. The margin is well circumscribed overall, but focally, lesional vessels may extend into adjacent soft tissue, raising concern for malignancy. The endothelial cells are typically flattened but may show focal hyperchromasia.[92] Mitoses are absent.

Differential Diagnosis

Sinusoidal hemangioma most often creates difficulties when it arises in mammary subcutaneous tissue, where the possibility of well-differentiated mammary angiosarcoma should be considered.[92–94] Although mammary angiosarcoma arises within the mammary parenchyma itself, it may extend into the overlying subcutis, and low-grade tumors are notoriously bland. Clues to low-grade angiosarcoma include focal endothelial multilayering, multifocal infiltration of adjacent soft tissue or breast parenchyma with a dissecting growth pattern, entrapment of normal lobules and ducts, diffuse mild endothelial atypia, and mitotic activity, although mitoses are rare in low-grade tumors. Even if features of malignancy are not seen, reexcision should be considered if the margins are involved, particularly if the relationship of the vascular proliferation to the mammary parenchyma cannot be evaluated.[94]

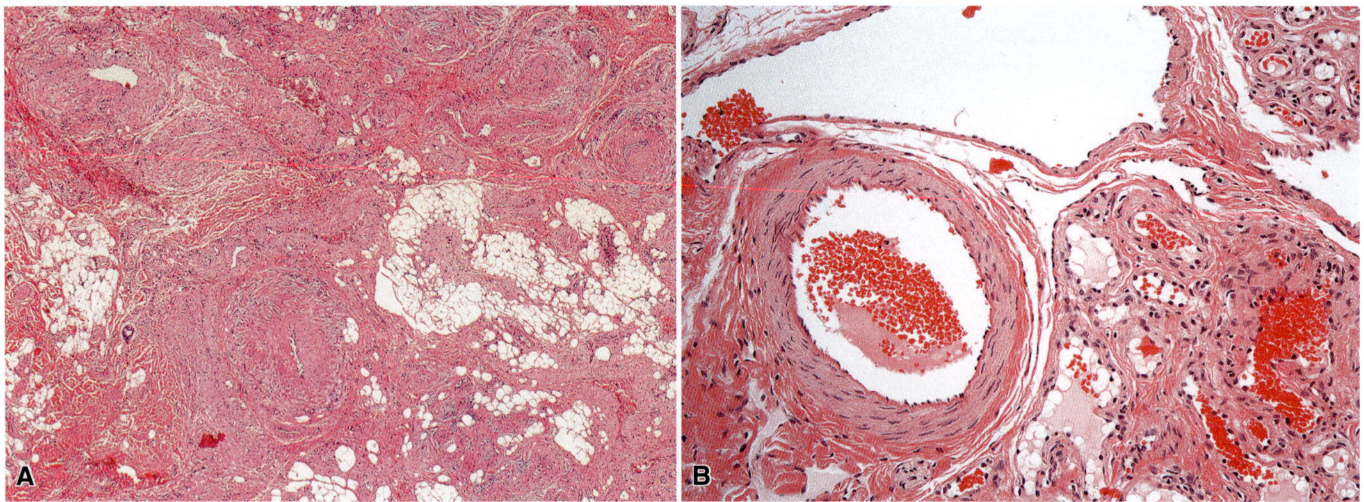

Figure 13.10 Vascular Malformation. (A) Arteriovenous malformation composed of large arteries and veins admixed with smaller caliber blood vessels. (B) Vascular malformation containing vessels of varying size and type.

The pseudopapillary appearance seen when the thin, fibrous septa of sinusoidal hemangioma are cut tangentially is reminiscent of intravascular papillary endothelial hyperplasia, but the latter is far more disorganized and has characteristic acellular, hyalinized papillae.

Arteriovenous Hemangioma and Arteriovenous Malformation

Clinical Features

Arteriovenous malformations and "arteriovenous hemangiomas" are typically readily distinguished because the latter term appears to be a misnomer and lacks a true arterial component with the resultant high intralesional blood flow. True arteriovenous malformations are defined by the presence of abnormal arterial and venous channels that are connected to each other without an intervening capillary bed.[22,100] They are most common in the head and neck region, and approximately 25% involve bone, either primarily or secondarily. Although arteriovenous malformations are occasionally evident at birth or in early childhood, in many cases, the clinical manifestations of arteriovenous shunting (e.g., localized warmth, a bruit, or a palpable thrill) do not develop until puberty. As the lesions enlarge, they may be complicated by necrosis, ulceration, hemorrhage or, rarely, high-output cardiac failure. Patients with arteriovenous malformations of the lower extremities may have acroangiodermatitis (Stewart-Bluefarb syndrome; discussed earlier).

In contrast, arteriovenous hemangiomas (also known as *cirsoid aneurysms*) typically present in middle-aged or older adults as small (<1 cm), superficial, red-purple papules or nodules.[101–104] Approximately 75% of cases arise in the head and neck region, with a predilection for the lips, perioral skin, nose, and eyelids. As discussed later, histologic evidence suggests that these may merely be arterialized venous hemangiomas.

Pathologic Features

Arteriovenous malformations are composed of varying numbers of large arteries and veins admixed with venules and capillaries in a densely fibrotic or fibromyxoid stroma (Fig. 13.10). The shunts themselves are difficult to identify without extensive serial sections, but the presence of both large arteries (recognized by their well-developed internal elastic lamina) and thick-walled veins is sufficient to establish the diagnosis. The venous channels show marked intimal hyperplasia and adventitial fibrosis because of the high rate of blood flow through the lesion. In contrast to low-flow vascular malformations, thrombosis, intravascular papillary endothelial hyperplasia, and phleboliths are not seen.

Arteriovenous hemangiomas are small, well-circumscribed, often dome-shaped, dermal lesions composed of numerous thin- and thick-walled vessels resembling veins and arteries (Fig. 13.11A). Occasionally, a minor component of capillary-sized vessels is also present.[102,104] Despite the designation *arteriovenous*, a true arterial component often cannot be seen. No well-formed internal elastic laminae are seen with elastic stains, and many of the "arterial" vessels have thick fibromuscular walls (see Fig. 13.11B) rather than concentric layers of smooth muscle.[102,104,105] Thus it is now believed that most "arteriovenous" hemangiomas are venous hemangiomas in which some vessels have undergone arterialization.[104,106] As in other venous lesions (and in contrast to true arteriovenous malformations), intravascular thrombi, papillary endothelial hyperplasia, and dystrophic calcification may be present.

Lymphangioma/Lymphatic Malformation

As with venous hemangiomas and malformations, lymphangiomas and lymphatic malformations can be difficult or impossible to distinguish. These lesions traditionally have been divided into a superficial microcystic type (lymphangioma circumscriptum) and a deep macrocystic type (cavernous lymphangioma).[107–109] It is now recognized that these distinctions are somewhat artificial because many, if not most, superficial lesions are associated with a deep component, although this component may not be clinically evident. Although both types may best be considered lymphatic malformations, the lymphangioma terminology remains widely used and is used in this chapter.

Clinical Features

Lymphangioma circumscriptum usually presents at birth or in early childhood as multiple, grouped, translucent vesicles that typically increase in number over time. The vesicles often have a pink or red tinge because of hemorrhage from adjacent capillaries, likely occurring after minor trauma, and a hyperkeratotic, verrucous surface may develop in some. The lesions are most common on the proximal extremities or limb girdles and cover an area ranging from 1 to several square centimeters. Local recurrence after excision is not infrequent, likely because of the presence of a deep cavernous lymphangioma-like component in many cases.

Cavernous lymphangiomas usually present in the first 2 years of life, although some are not recognized until adulthood because of the lack of cutaneous involvement in most cases. Approximately 50% occur in the head and neck region, with most of the remainder on the trunk

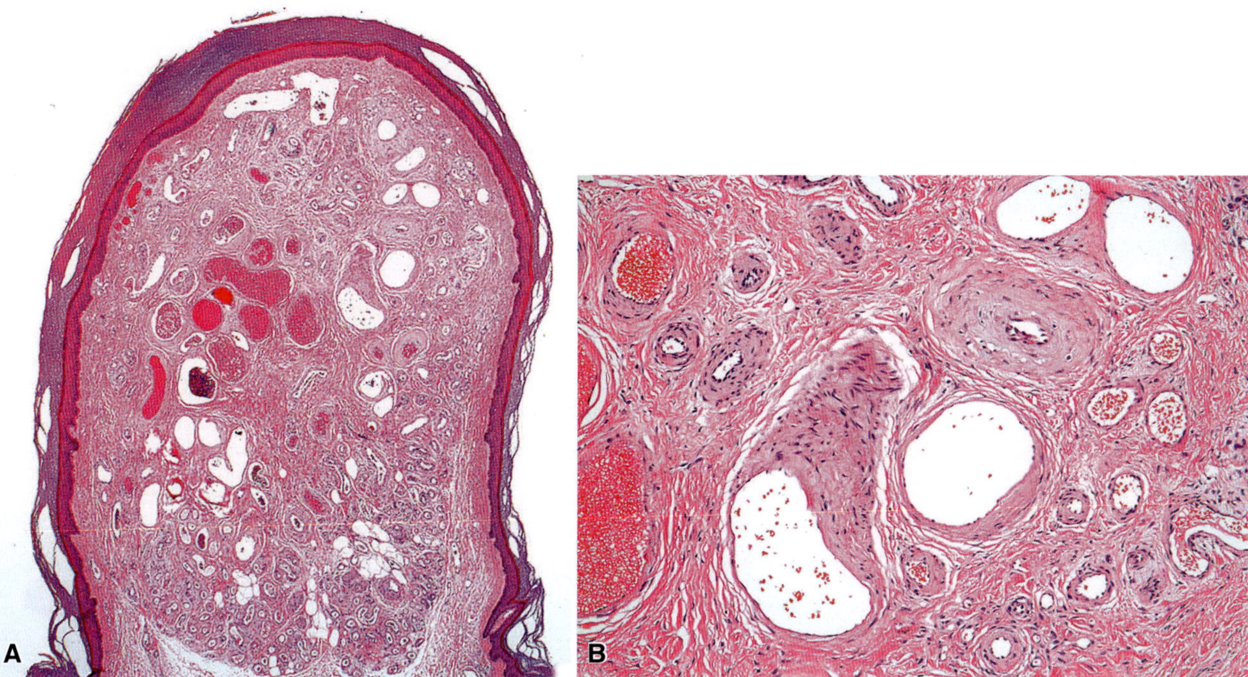

Figure 13.11 **Arteriovenous Hemangioma.** (A) Well-circumscribed dome-shaped dermal lesion. (B) Thin- and thick-walled vessels.

or extremities; 10% are intrathoracic or intraabdominal, the latter often arising in the mesentery. Intraabdominal lymphangiomas may present as an acute abdomen as a result of fluid leakage and subsequent peritonitis. The recurrence rate varies by treatment modality (sclerotherapy vs. surgery), size, and location, but even grossly excised lesions recur in 15% to 20% of cases.[110,111] Cystic hygroma (also known as *cystic lymphangioma*) is a clinical variant that presents as a large, fluid-filled mass in the neck, axilla, or groin of infants. Although more than 50% of fetal cystic hygromas detected during the first or second trimester of pregnancy are associated with chromosomal abnormalities or major congenital defects,[112,113] most of those detected at birth or in early infancy are isolated findings and have a good prognosis.

Pathologic Features

Lymphangioma circumscriptum shows markedly dilated, thin-walled lymphatic vessels immediately below an acanthotic epidermis (Fig. 13.12A). Exaggerated, papillomatous epidermal hyperplasia with thick hyperkeratosis is seen in the clinically verrucous lesions (see Fig. 13.12B). Dilated, thin-walled mid-dermal lymphatics connect the ectatic vessels in the papillary dermis to deeper, thick-walled muscular lymphatics. Elegant studies in the 1970s showed that these deep dermal muscular vessels arise from large, anomalous lymphatic cisterns lying just above the superficial fascia,[107] and failure to excise these cisterns results in recurrence of the superficial vesicles.

Cavernous lymphangiomas are composed of numerous thin-walled, irregularly shaped lymphatic channels (Fig. 13.13A) separated by a variable amount of fibrous tissue in the reticular dermis and subcutis. The stromal component is often more prominent and fibrotic in larger or long-standing lesions. Scattered lymphoid aggregates may be present (see Fig. 13.13B), and small bundles of smooth muscle are often found within the vessel walls. Intraabdominal lesions are prone to the development of reactive changes, including hemorrhage, granulation tissue, fat necrosis, and a florid myofibroblastic proliferation.[114] The superimposed reactive features may mask the underlying vascular lesion, and a high index of suspicion is required to identify the lymphatic channels. Cystic hygromas are similar but are distended by fluid in vivo and are often surrounded by a fibrous capsule.

Differential Diagnosis

The histologic diagnosis of lymphatic malformations in skin and soft tissue is straightforward. The primary differential diagnosis of intraabdominal lymphangiomas is multilocular peritoneal inclusion cysts (also known as *benign multicystic mesothelioma*).[115,116] Multilocular peritoneal inclusion cysts are lined by plump epithelioid cells that may form papillary proliferations and lack a smooth muscle component in the cyst walls. However, distinction of these cysts from cystic lymphangiomas can be difficult because the lymphatic endothelium may be plump as a result of reactive changes and smooth muscle bundles are not always identifiable. A keratin stain readily differentiates the two lesions. Intraabdominal lymphangiomas with marked superimposed reactive changes may be confused with well-differentiated liposarcoma; however, there is usually extensive fat necrosis in the former, and hyperchromatic, atypical stromal cells are absent.

Acquired Progressive Lymphangioma (Benign Lymphangioendothelioma)

Acquired progressive lymphangioma is a rare benign vascular lesion with atypical histologic features that may result in misinterpretation as angiosarcoma.[117] The term *benign lymphangioendothelioma* has also been used for these lesions.[118]

Clinical Features

Acquired progressive lymphangioma occurs in both children and adults, and it may arise at almost any cutaneous site as well as on the lip or oral mucosa.[118,119] The tumors present as solitary, erythematous, or violaceous patches or plaques that typically measure 1 to a few centimeters but can reach 10 cm or more.[118,120] Rarely, multiple lesions have been

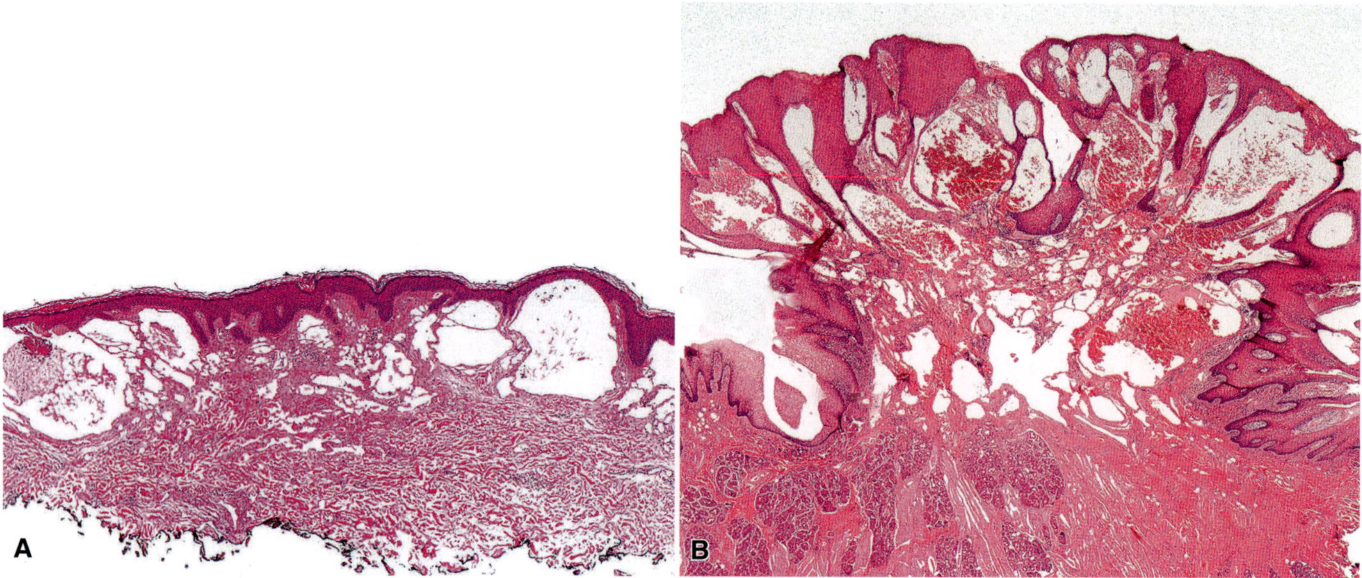

Figure 13.12 Lymphangioma Circumscriptum. (A) Dilated thin-walled lymphatic vessels immediately beneath the epidermis. (B) Clinically verrucous lesions show overlying papillomatous epidermal hyperplasia.

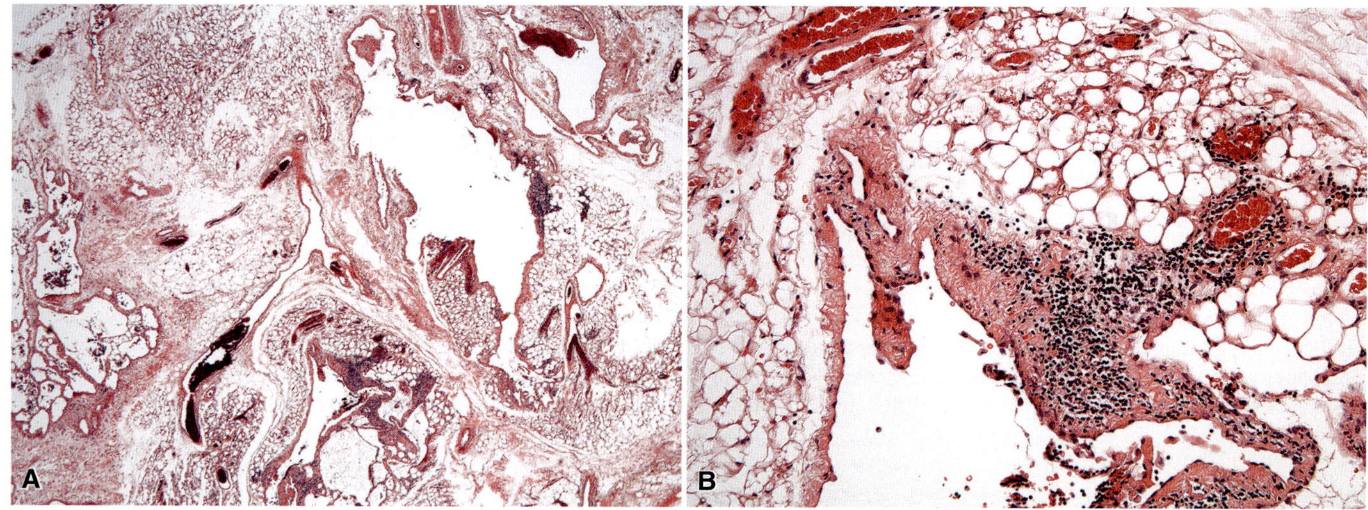

Figure 13.13 Cavernous Lymphangioma. (A) Thin-walled, irregularly shaped lymphatic channels admixed with adipose tissue. (B) Lymphoid aggregates associated with the dilated lymphatic spaces.

described.[118,120,121] There is often a long history of slow growth.[118] Local recurrence is rare after complete excision.

Pathologic Features

Histologically, acquired progressive lymphangioma can be thought of as *focal lymphangiomatosis* because the morphologic features overlap significantly with those of lymphangiomatosis of soft tissue, although these lesions affect a much smaller area (and only one tissue plane). Multiple thin-walled anastomosing channels dissect around dermal collagen bundles and adnexal structures, leaving them "floating" within apparently empty space (Fig. 13.14). This appearance has been referred to as the *hair dryer effect* because the normal dermal structures are preserved but are widely separated, as if blown apart by a hair dryer. The superficial vessels are dilated, irregular, and often oriented parallel to the epidermis, whereas those in the deep dermis are narrow and have a dissecting, pseudoangiosarcomatous growth pattern. Extension into subcutaneous tissue is infrequent.[118,120]

Small intraluminal papillary projections are common and may be so numerous as to mimic intravascular papillary endothelial hyperplasia.[118] The endothelium is typically bland, but occasionally shows focal hobnail cytomorphologic features or mild nuclear hyperchromasia. Moderate or severe cytologic atypia and endothelial multilayering are not seen, and mitoses are rare.[118] Most vascular channels appear empty, but pale pink proteinaceous material or scattered erythrocytes may be seen in occasional vessels and, infrequently, fibrin thrombi may be present. In a minority of cases an irregularly thickened, discontinuous smooth muscle layer is seen around some of the lesional vessels. An inflammatory infiltrate is usually mild or absent, and hemosiderin deposition is rare. Actin stains show that a pericytic layer is often absent, consistent with a lymphatic origin.

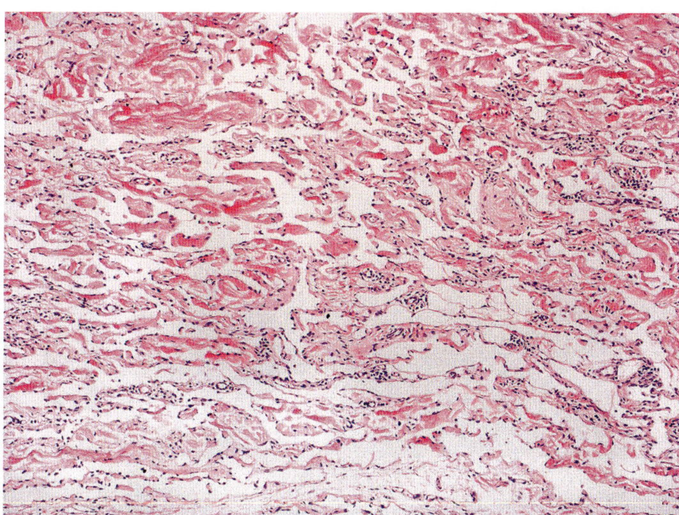

Figure 13.14 Acquired Progressive Lymphangioma (Benign Lymphangioendothelioma). Thin-walled complex anastomosing channels dissect through dermal collagen.

Differential Diagnosis

When the collapsed vascular channels are closely spaced, acquired progressive lymphangioma can closely simulate angiosarcoma. However, the lack of significant cytologic atypia, endothelial multilayering, and mitotic activity argues against a malignant diagnosis, and clinical history is helpful. Caution should be used when making the diagnosis of cutaneous angiosarcoma outside of the head and neck region in older adults unless there is a history of radiation or lymphedema.

Lymphangioma-like Kaposi sarcoma and acquired progressive lymphangioma show significant histologic overlap, but Kaposi sarcoma often has a lymphoplasmacytic infiltrate and rarely shows intraluminal papillae. The clinical presentation is also helpful because Kaposi sarcoma typically presents as multiple lesions in an immunocompromised patient or on the lower extremities of elderly men of Jewish or Mediterranean ancestry. Furthermore, the lymphangioma-like variant of Kaposi sarcoma is often associated with clinically (and histologically) typical patch, plaque, or nodular Kaposi sarcoma elsewhere. HHV-8 immunostaining can be used to confirm Kaposi sarcoma.

Hobnail hemangioma differs from acquired progressive lymphangioma by the presence of prominent hobnail endothelium in the superficial vessels and marked hemosiderin deposition within a fibrotic dermis. Postradiation atypical vascular lesions may be indistinguishable from acquired progressive lymphangioma; this distinction is best made by clinical correlation. As previously mentioned, the histologic features of acquired progressive lymphangioma are essentially identical to those of cutaneous involvement by lymphangiomatosis, and clinical information is required.

Intramuscular Angioma

Despite the name, intramuscular angiomas are generally considered vascular malformations rather than true hemangiomas. Lesions formerly reported as *infiltrating angiolipomas* are now recognized to be intramuscular angiomas.[122–124]

Clinical Features

The extremities and head and neck are the most common sites for intramuscular angiomas, and most patients present in the first three decades of life with intermittent swelling or pain on physical exertion.[125,126] However, because of their deep-seated location, some lesions do not present until adulthood, when the diagnosis may be more challenging because a vascular malformation may not be considered. A helpful clue in many cases is the presence of phleboliths on imaging studies.

Pathologic Features

Initial attempts to subclassify intramuscular angiomas by their constituent vessels proved fruitless because nearly all cases are of mixed vessel type, although one component—most often venous—typically predominates.[126,127] The histologic features are similar to those of vascular malformations in the skin and soft tissue, but more than 90% of intramuscular angiomas also contain mature adipose tissue, which may dominate the lesion (Fig. 13.15). The prominent adipocytic component may be related to atrophy of the affected muscle, which is frequently noted. Thrombi, phleboliths, and metaplastic ossification are common and may be responsible for the intermittent pain associated with these lesions.

Differential Diagnosis

The diagnosis is typically straightforward in children, but when intramuscular angiomas first come to clinical attention in adulthood, the histologic features can be misinterpreted. The most common error is interpretation of the admixed adipose tissue as neoplastic, leading to misdiagnosis as intramuscular lipoma. Closer examination of intramuscular angiomas shows an increased number of large and small vessels, some of which appear abnormal. In contrast, the vasculature in intramuscular lipomas is inconspicuous. Although both lesions are benign, the distinction is clinically relevant because the recurrence rate for intramuscular lipoma is approximately 20%, compared with at least 50% to 60% for intramuscular angioma.

Intramuscular angiomas can also mimic nonneoplastic skeletal muscle that has undergone atrophy because of disuse or compression by a long-standing adjacent mass. Atrophic skeletal muscle often has unusually prominent vessels and an increased amount of adipose tissue, and a small biopsy specimen of nonlesional tissue adjacent to a large tumor may be misinterpreted as an intramuscular angioma if the clinical history and radiologic findings are not reviewed.

Prognosis and Treatment

Because of the often extensive size and ill-defined margins of intramuscular angiomas, incomplete excision is common, resulting in clinical recurrence in up to 60% of cases.[126] Wide excision is required to prevent local recurrence but may be disfiguring. Therefore asymptomatic lesions are generally observed without treatment, and conservative therapy, such as aspirin, compressive garments, or sclerotherapy, is often preferred in symptomatic patients.[125]

Synovial Hemangioma

Clinical Features

Synovial hemangiomas are a heterogeneous group of vascular proliferations defined by their anatomic location (i.e., synovium of an intraarticular space or bursa).[128–132] Most cases present in children and young adults, and more than two-thirds of cases involve the knee joint. The typical presentation is intermittent pain or swelling, often of many years' duration. A soft, doughy mass may be palpable, and joint aspiration may show blood or blood-tinged synovial fluid. Given the young age of presentation and the histologic heterogeneity of synovial hemangiomas, it is likely that most cases would be best classified as vascular malformations, but the term *hemangioma* is in common use.

Pathologic Features

Synovial hemangiomas have a variable vascular composition, including capillary, arterial, and venous vessels, and mixed features are common.

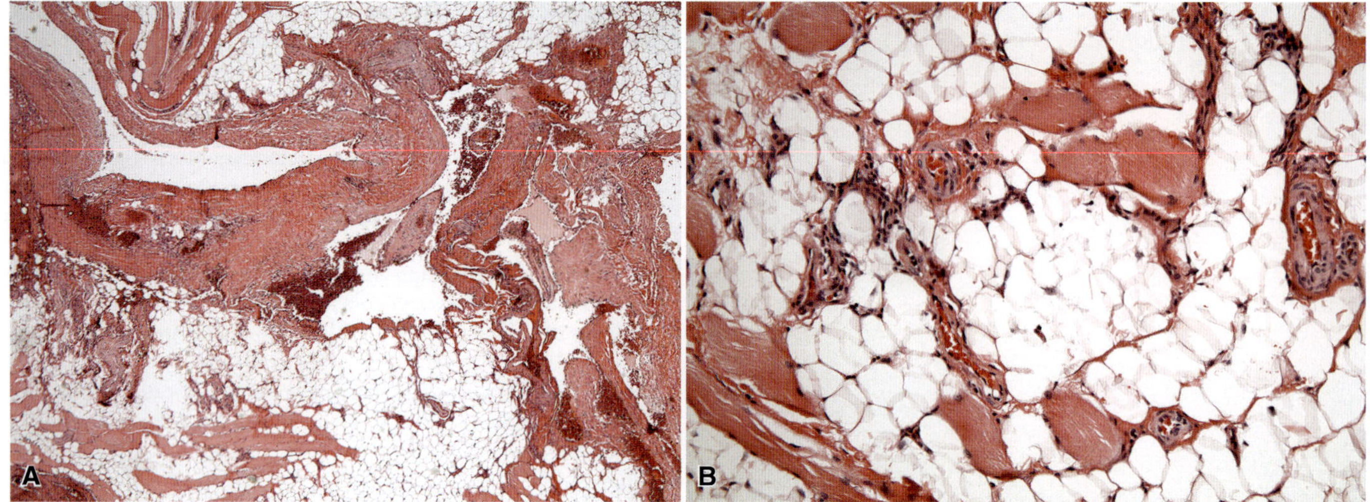

Figure 13.15 Intramuscular Angioma. (A) Lesion composed of blood vessels of varying size and caliber admixed with adipose tissue, similar to a vascular malformation. (B) Intramuscular angioma with a prominent adipocytic component infiltrating skeletal muscle fibers.

Hemosiderin deposition is often prominent, and secondary changes, including intravascular thrombosis, papillary endothelial hyperplasia, phleboliths, and partial infarction, may be seen.[130]

Differential Diagnosis

The synovium itself is a highly vascular tissue, and in reactive states, the vessels may be particularly prominent, potentially leading to misinterpretation of a synovial hyperplasia as a vascular lesion. Acute and chronic inflammation and perivascular myxoid stroma favor a reactive synovial process over synovial hemangioma.[130]

Prognosis and Treatment

Localized lesions are generally successfully treated with marginal excision. Those that diffusely involve the synovium often recur after local excision and are best treated with synovectomy.

Angiomatosis and Lymphangiomatosis

Rarely, vascular malformations may affect large areas of the body, by involving more than one tissue plane (e.g., subcutis, muscle, and bone) or multiple contiguous tissues of the same type (e.g., adjacent muscles). These lesions may be composed of either blood vessels or lymphatic channels and are referred to as *angiomatosis* or *lymphangiomatosis*, respectively.

Clinical Features

Angiomatosis of soft tissue typically presents in infancy or childhood with progressive swelling, pain, or discoloration of the affected area, most often the lower extremity or trunk.[133]

Lymphangiomatosis may be systemic or localized. The systemic form often involves the lungs, pleura, spleen, bone, and soft tissue of the mediastinum and retroperitoneum. Localized lymphangiomatosis is confined to a single anatomic region, most commonly, a lower extremity; patients come to attention in infancy or childhood because of diffuse swelling of the affected area.

Multifocal lymphangioendotheliomatosis with thrombocytopenia[134–136] (also reported as *cutaneovisceral angiomatosis with thrombocytopenia*[137]) presents at birth with multiple vascular lesions in the skin and gastrointestinal mucosa associated with thrombocytopenia. The mucocutaneous lesions increase in number during childhood and may result in recurrent gastrointestinal bleeding. Pulmonary, bone, liver, and spleen lesions have also been reported in a subset of cases.

Pathologic Features

The histologic features are similar to those of vascular malformations of soft tissue and skeletal muscle. Angiomatosis shows diffuse proliferation of variably sized blood vessels (Fig. 13.16A) accompanied by mature adipose tissue, fibrous tissue, and occasionally nerve bundles.[133,138] The vessels often show fibrointimal hyperplasia and disorganized or irregularly attenuated smooth muscle bundles. A distinctive feature is the presence of clusters of capillaries within or immediately adjacent to the walls of large veins (see Fig. 13.16B), sometimes appearing to bud off the latter.[133,138] Infrequently, angiomatosis is composed entirely of lobules of capillaries, simulating juvenile capillary hemangioma; the size and extent of the lesion distinguishes the two. Rare cases of angiomatosis with a prominent glomus cell component in the vessel walls have been designated *glomangiomatosis*.[139]

Lymphangiomatosis resembles cavernous or cystic lymphangiomas in the soft tissue and commonly shows dermal involvement, with features of acquired progressive lymphangioma (i.e., numerous anastomosing, thin-walled, empty-appearing channels dissecting around dermal collagen bundles and adnexal structures). Small intraluminal papillae may be seen in some lesional vessels.

The cutaneous lesions of multifocal lymphangioendotheliomatosis with thrombocytopenia resemble lymphangiomatosis, showing a complex network of thin-walled lymphatic channels in the dermis and often the subcutis. However, in contrast to most lymphatic malformations, the endothelium is plump to hobnailed. Intraluminal tufts or complex papillae may be present. LYVE-1 or D2-40 is usually positive in endothelial cells, supporting lymphatic differentiation.

Prognosis and Treatment

Because of the extensive nature of the lesions, complete excision of angiomatosis or lymphangiomatosis is very difficult, and the recurrence rate is high (60% to 90%).[133,138,140,141] Conservative surgery is therefore recommended because it is unlikely to be curative. Surgical reduction or medical therapy often results in symptomatic improvement. The prognosis for systemic lymphangiomatosis is poor, particularly in patients with thoracic involvement.[142]

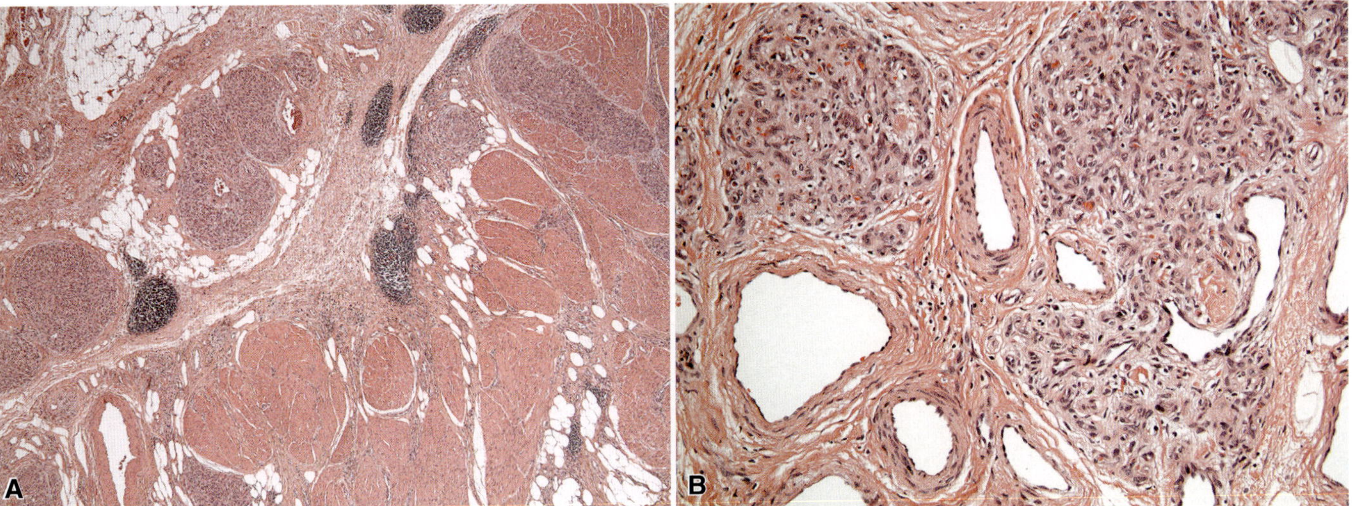

Figure 13.16 Angiomatosis. (A) Angiomatosis involving the wall of the urinary bladder showing a diffuse proliferation of variably sized blood vessels admixed with adipose tissue. (B) Clusters of capillaries admixed with veins.

Capillary Hemangioma

The term *capillary hemangioma* includes several clinically and histologically distinctive vascular neoplasms, namely, juvenile capillary hemangioma, lobular capillary hemangioma (including pyogenic granuloma), cherry angioma, verrucous angioma, and tufted angioma.

Juvenile Capillary Hemangioma (Infantile Hemangioma)

Clinical Features

Juvenile capillary hemangioma affects approximately 4% of children,[143] with a predilection for girls (female-to-male ratio, ~3 : 1); fair-skinned and premature infants are also at higher risk.[144] The vast majority of cases are sporadic, but autosomal dominant transmission has been reported in rare cases.[145] The head and neck region accounts for more than 50% of cases. Lesions present at birth or within the first few weeks of life and progress through three distinct stages: a rapid growth phase lasting 6 to 12 months; an involuting phase lasting 1 to 12 years; and an end stage, in which the skin may appear normal or show residual alteration in color or texture.[143,146]

Most lesions are limited to the skin or superficial soft tissue, but some involve skeletal muscle. Superficial lesions present as pink telangiectatic macules that thicken rapidly and become bright red during the proliferative phase, whereas deep-seated tumors are seen as soft, bluish nodules.

Pathologic Features

In the proliferative phase, well-defined lobules of tightly packed capillaries fill the dermis and often extend into the subcutis. In the earliest stage the capillaries are often poorly canalized, and the combination of inconspicuous lumina, plump endothelium, and prominent pericytes may result in a solid appearance, obscuring the vascular nature of the tumor (Fig. 13.17A and B). However, well-canalized vessels are often present at least focally, usually at the periphery of the lobules, and reticulin or actin stains may be used to highlight the vascular architecture. The capillary lobules intermingle with normal tissue, including subcutaneous fat, superficial skeletal muscle, and peripheral nerves, resulting in perineural or even endoneurial involvement in up to 10% of cases.[147] Mitotic figures are usually numerous (up to three per high-power field) in early lesions, and solid-appearing areas with loss of the characteristic lobular pattern may be focally present.[148] Mast cells are abundant in the proliferative phase.[149] A feeding artery or arteries may be identified in the adjacent soft tissue.

During the involuting phase, the capillaries dilate and the endothelial cells flatten and undergo apoptosis (see Fig. 13.17C).[150] The capillary lobules are gradually replaced by loose fibroadipose tissue, and the remaining vessels show marked basement membrane thickening. Feeding and draining vessels do not fully regress, and hypertrophied arteries and veins are often seen in end-stage lesions.[143]

Studies have shown that juvenile capillary hemangioma is clonal, supporting its classification as a neoplasm, albeit a self-limited one.[151]

Immunohistochemistry

The erythrocyte-type glucose transporter protein GLUT1 is a marker of juvenile capillary hemangioma at all stages of development, showing strong and diffuse reactivity in the endothelial cells (see Fig. 13.17D).[152,153] Normal endothelium of microvasculature with a blood-tissue barrier function, including that of the central nervous system and placenta, expresses GLUT1, but nonneoplastic cutaneous vessels, vascular malformations, and most other benign vascular neoplasms are negative for this marker. Verrucous hemangioma and rapidly involuting congenital hemangioma may show focal reactivity, in contrast to the diffuse expression in juvenile capillary hemangioma.

Differential Diagnosis

The differential diagnosis of juvenile capillary hemangioma is limited. Myopericytoma could be considered in the differential diagnosis of early cellular lesions, but these lesions are biphasic and have a hemangiopericytoma-like vascular pattern in the cellular areas. Lobular capillary hemangioma (pyogenic granuloma) differs by the presence of the following: (1) dense fibrosis rather than normal dermis between capillary lobules; (2) an epidermal collarette in many cases; (3) frequent secondary changes, including inflammation and edema; and (4) absence of GLUT1 expression.

Prognosis and Treatment

After involution, there may be telangiectasias, yellowish discoloration, atrophy, or redundant fibrofatty tissue, but this is usually not cosmetically significant. Therefore small lesions are managed by observation. Surgery,

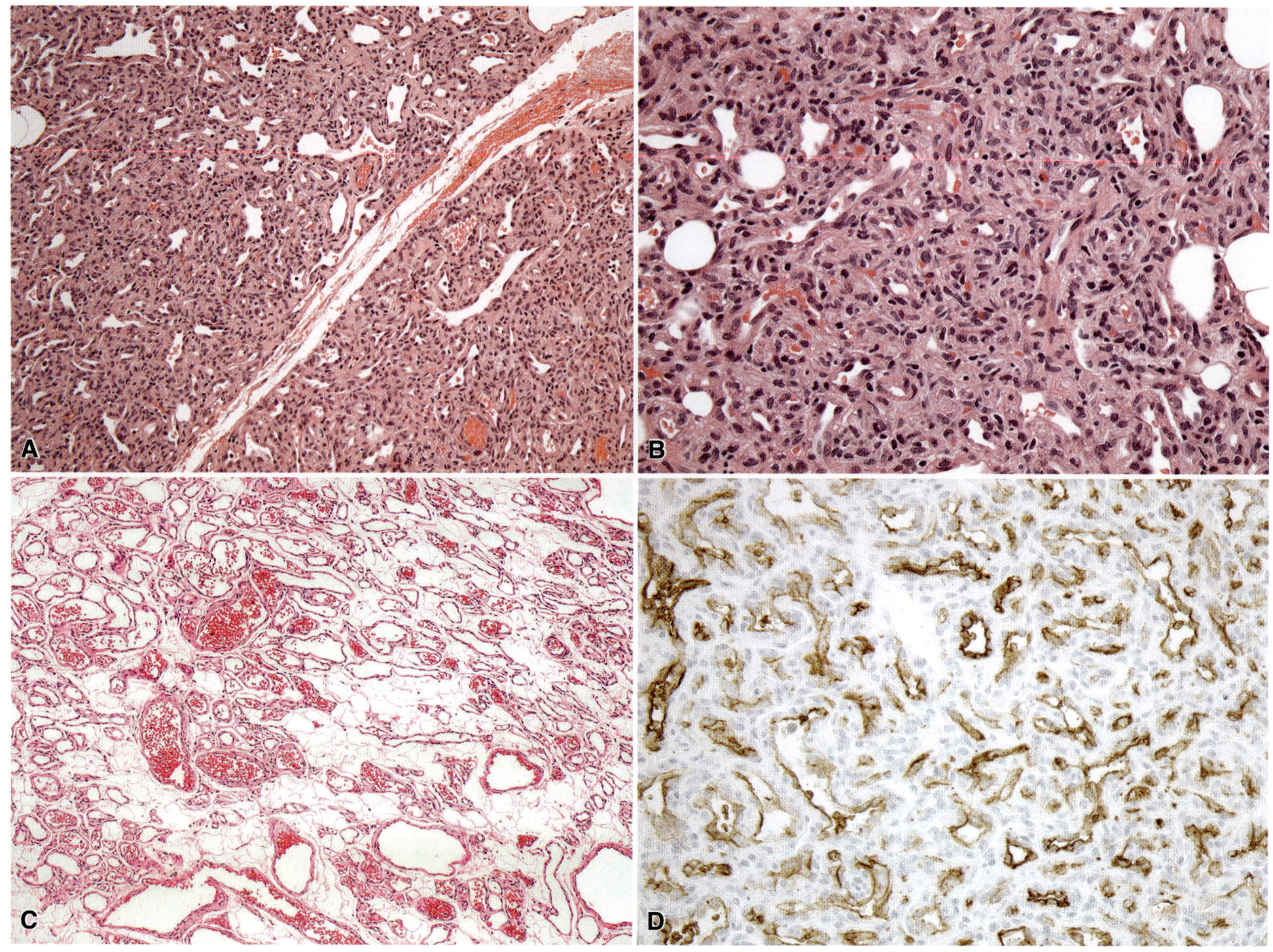

Figure 13.17 Juvenile Capillary Hemangioma. (A) Cellular lobules of tightly packed capillaries. (B) Inconspicuous lumina and prominent pericytes may result in a solid appearance. (C) Involuting juvenile capillary hemangioma showing dilated capillaries and intervening adipose tissue. (D) Diffuse reactivity for GLUT1 in the endothelial cells.

laser therapy, and medical treatment are reserved for the small subset of tumors (10% to 20%) that threaten function or are complicated by ulceration, bleeding, or infection.[22,146,154]

PRACTICE POINTS: Juvenile Capillary Hemangioma (Infantile Hemangioma)

- In the early cellular phase, juvenile capillary hemangioma may have a solid appearance, with numerous mitoses.
- Markedly thickened vascular basement membranes are a clue to late lesions.
- GLUT1 is a useful marker to distinguish juvenile capillary hemangioma from other vascular lesions, particularly in the late involuting phase, when the characteristic histologic features are absent.

Congenital Nonprogressive Hemangioma

Clinical Features

A very small proportion of hemangiomas in infants are fully developed at birth and do not undergo the characteristic growth phase of juvenile capillary hemangioma.[155] The term *congenital nonprogressive hemangioma* has been used for this group, which can be split into those that undergo rapid regression during infancy (rapidly involuting congenital hemangioma) and those that do not regress (noninvoluting congenital hemangioma).[156–158] In contrast to juvenile capillary hemangioma, these tumors affect boys and girls with equal frequency.

Pathologic Features

Clinical correlation is required to make the diagnosis because the histologic features of congenital nonprogressive hemangioma overlap with those of juvenile capillary hemangioma. However, in general, the former are less cellular than juvenile capillary hemangioma, contain prominent centrilobular draining veins, have a densely sclerotic interlobular stroma, and do not infiltrate adipose tissue or nerves.

Immunohistochemistry

Staining for GLUT1 is typically negative in congenital nonprogressive hemangiomas, but focal reactivity has been reported in rapidly involuting congenital hemangioma.[158]

Lobular Capillary Hemangioma (Pyogenic Granuloma)

Lobular capillary hemangioma was initially considered a polypoid form of granulation tissue that developed in response to a pyogenic agent, prompting the original—and still widely used—name *pyogenic granuloma*.[159] The latter term now generally refers to superficial, often ulcerated

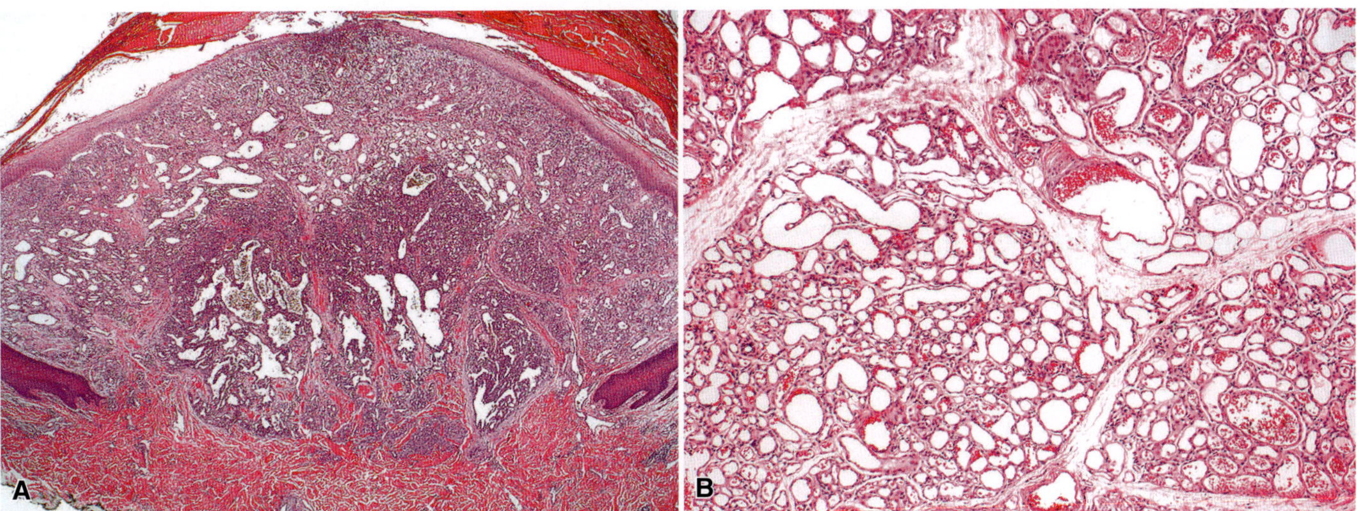

Figure 13.18 Lobular Capillary Hemangioma. (A) Pyogenic granuloma composed of superficial lobules of capillaries with an epidermal collarette. (B) Well-defined lobules of dilated capillaries.

polypoid lesions, whereas *lobular capillary hemangioma* is a more generic term that also encompasses deep and intravenous tumors.[160]

Clinical Features

Lobular capillary hemangioma arises over a wide age range, with a peak in the second and third decades. The most common sites are the head and neck, trunk, and upper extremities, particularly the fingers.[160–164] There is no sex predilection among cutaneous tumors, but mucosal lesions, which account for 10% to 15% of cases, are 2 to 3 times more common in females.[161,165] A hormonal influence seems likely for the latter lesions, particularly because gingival pyogenic granulomas are well recognized to occur in pregnancy *(granuloma gravidarum)* and were reported in association with the use of high-dose oral contraceptives in the 1970s.[166,167]

Tumors present as rapidly growing, solitary, pedunculated, or sessile red papules measuring less than 2 cm in diameter. If left untreated, the lesions become progressively fibrotic and may ultimately regress, but most are excised because of bleeding or irritation. Infrequent reports of local recurrence are usually the result of incomplete excision.[162] Rarely, multiple 1- to 5-mm red papules develop at the periphery of a previously excised lobular capillary hemangioma, sometimes in conjunction with recurrence of the primary tumor.[168] Less often, this phenomenon, known as *satellitosis*, occurs adjacent to a traumatized or irritated lesion. Exceptional cases of eruptive disseminated lobular capillary hemangioma have been reported.[169,170] These lesions typically arise in previously healthy patients and are self-limited, resolving spontaneously within several months.

Pathologic Features

The defining feature is well-defined lobules of capillaries separated by a dense fibrous stroma. In cutaneous tumors, the capillaries of superficial lobules are often more dilated than those in the deep portion of the tumor, which may be tightly packed with inconspicuous lumina. The interlobular septa contain small feeding arteries and veins. Over time, the lesion becomes less cellular as fibrosis supervenes within the capillary lobules and septa, accentuating the lobular pattern. The endothelial cells of lobular capillary hemangioma are frequently plump, and mitoses may be easily identified, particularly in densely cellular foci.[160] Rarely, nuclear hyperchromasia may be seen.[119]

The classic pyogenic granuloma is an exophytic tumor with an epidermal collarette, surface ulceration, and secondary acute inflammation and stromal edema (Fig. 13.18). In some cases, particularly nasal cavity lesions, the edema may be so marked that the lesional vessels are compressed into thin, branching cords. True granulation tissue with radially oriented capillaries may be present at the ulcerated surface, but the characteristic lobular pattern is preserved at the base of the tumor.

Subcutaneous lesions are histologically identical to those in the dermis but are surrounded by a dense, fibrous capsule and lack the secondary changes of inflammation and edema.[164] Intravascular lobular capillary hemangioma forms a polypoid nodule within the lumen of a vein and is connected to the venous wall by a thin fibrovascular stalk. In many cases the vein of origin is a small, superficial vessel that is not grossly identified by the surgeon or the pathologist. Similar to subcutaneous tumors, intravascular lesions lack secondary changes.

Differential Diagnosis

Lobular capillary hemangioma can present in infancy and, by virtue of the lobular architecture and high mitotic rate, may resemble juvenile capillary hemangioma in the proliferative phase. Typically, lobular capillary hemangiomas are small, pedunculated lesions, whereas juvenile capillary hemangiomas measure a few centimeters or more and frequently involve the entire dermis, with or without subcutaneous extension. In addition, juvenile capillary hemangiomas lack the densely fibrotic interlobular stroma of lobular capillary hemangioma and consistently express GLUT1, whereas lobular capillary hemangiomas do not.

Intranasal lobular capillary hemangioma often shows extensive secondary changes, including widely dilated vessels and marked stromal sclerosis that can result in misinterpretation as nasopharyngeal angiofibroma (see Chapter 4). However, the latter nearly always affects adolescent boys and arises posteriorly from the roof of the nasal cavity, whereas nasal lobular capillary hemangioma arises from the septum. In addition, the typical lobular pattern of lobular capillary hemangioma is identified at least focally, most often at the base of the tumor.

Some cherry angiomas are slightly elevated and may have an edematous stroma, but they usually have far fewer capillaries than even late-stage lobular capillary hemangiomas and lack a lobular architecture. Significant histologic overlap may be present in occasional cases, but

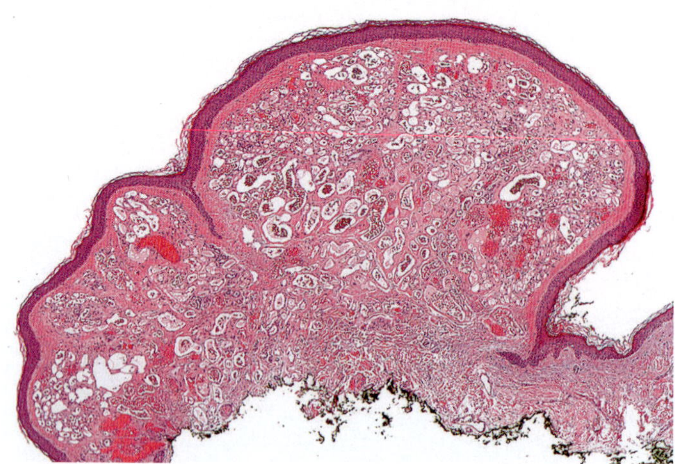

Figure 13.19 Cherry Angioma. Polypoid dermal lesion composed of dilated congested capillaries.

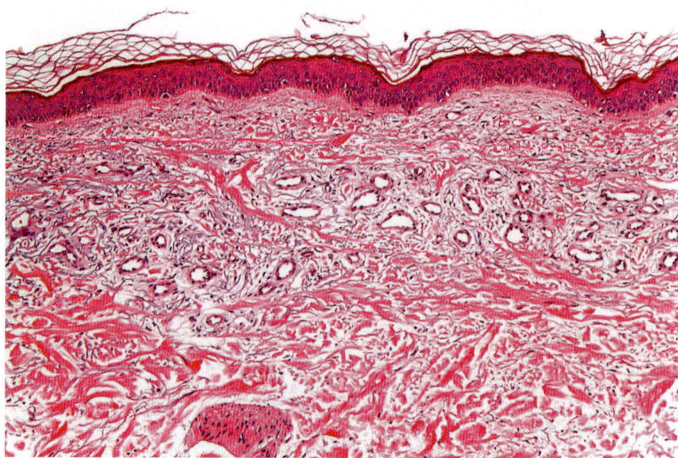

Figure 13.20 Acquired Elastotic Hemangioma. A bandlike proliferation of dilated capillaries in the dermis with background solar elastosis.

the distinction is of no clinical significance. A generic term such as *unclassified benign hemangioma* may be used for such lesions.

The differential diagnosis with bacillary angiomatosis was discussed earlier.

PRACTICE POINTS: Lobular Capillary Hemangioma (Pyogenic Granuloma)

Although lobular capillary hemangioma is generally cutaneous, identical lesions may occur in subcutaneous tissue or within blood vessels.

Intranasal tumors may show vascular dilation in addition to marked stromal edema and sclerosis, obscuring the lobular pattern.

Cherry Angioma

Clinical Features

Cherry angioma (senile angioma) is the clinical term for a very common acquired capillary hemangioma of adults. Cherry angiomas begin to appear in middle adulthood as small, red papules on the trunk and upper extremities and increase in number with age.

Pathologic Features

The superficial dermis contains a proliferation of dilated, often congested capillaries, with variably thickened walls (Fig. 13.19), sometimes associated with mild thinning of the overlying epidermis. Well-developed lesions may be polypoid, with an epidermal collarette. However, the capillary proliferation is far less exuberant than that seen in lobular capillary hemangioma (pyogenic granuloma) and typically lacks a lobular pattern.[62]

Acquired Elastotic Hemangioma

Clinical Features

Acquired elastotic hemangioma is a vascular proliferation that most commonly presents in elderly women as an irregular erythematous plaque on sun-damaged skin, particularly the dorsal forearm.[171] The clinical differential diagnosis often includes basal cell carcinoma and squamous cell carcinoma in situ.

Pathologic Features

The superficial dermis contains a horizontally arranged, bandlike proliferation of dilated capillaries, separated by a narrow grenz zone from the overlying epidermis. Significant solar elastosis is present in the area of the vascular proliferation (Fig. 13.20).

Verrucous Hemangioma

Verrucous hemangioma is a rare congenital vascular lesion named for the distinctive verrucoid clinical appearance that develops during childhood.[172] The question of whether these lesions are vascular malformations or hemangiomas has not been settled: the clinical features, including congenital onset, proportionate growth with the patient, and lack of spontaneous regression, favor a vascular malformation, whereas the uniform vessel size and only occasional focal GLUT1 reactivity suggest a hemangioma.

Clinical Features

Verrucous hemangioma presents at birth or in early infancy as a soft, bluish-red macule or papule, nearly always on a lower extremity. During childhood, the lesion slowly enlarges, ultimately measuring up to several centimeters in diameter, and the surface becomes darker, hyperkeratotic, and often verrucous, sometimes mimicking a wart or melanocytic lesion. Satellite lesions may develop at the periphery.

Pathologic Features

The fundamental lesion is a capillary hemangioma that involves the full thickness of the dermis and extends into the subcutis. Fully developed tumors show striking epidermal changes, including acanthosis, mild to marked papillomatosis, and hyperkeratosis (Fig. 13.21A). The vessels in the dermal papillae are widely dilated and congested and may appear to be intraepidermal because of envelopment by hyperplastic rete ridges. This feature may result in misdiagnosis of angiokeratoma on a superficial biopsy, and the rare reports of "angiokeratoma circumscriptum" may represent inadequately sampled verrucous hemangiomas.

The vascular proliferation in the reticular dermis and subcutis is composed of patchy, ill-defined capillary lobules (see Fig. 13.21B) that are most prominent around blood vessels and adnexal structures, leaving large areas of the reticular dermis uninvolved. Fibrosis, hemosiderin deposition, and a chronic inflammatory infiltrate are common, and purulent or hemorrhagic scale crusts may be present, leading some authors to suggest that the verrucoid epidermal changes are caused by trauma or secondary infection.[172]

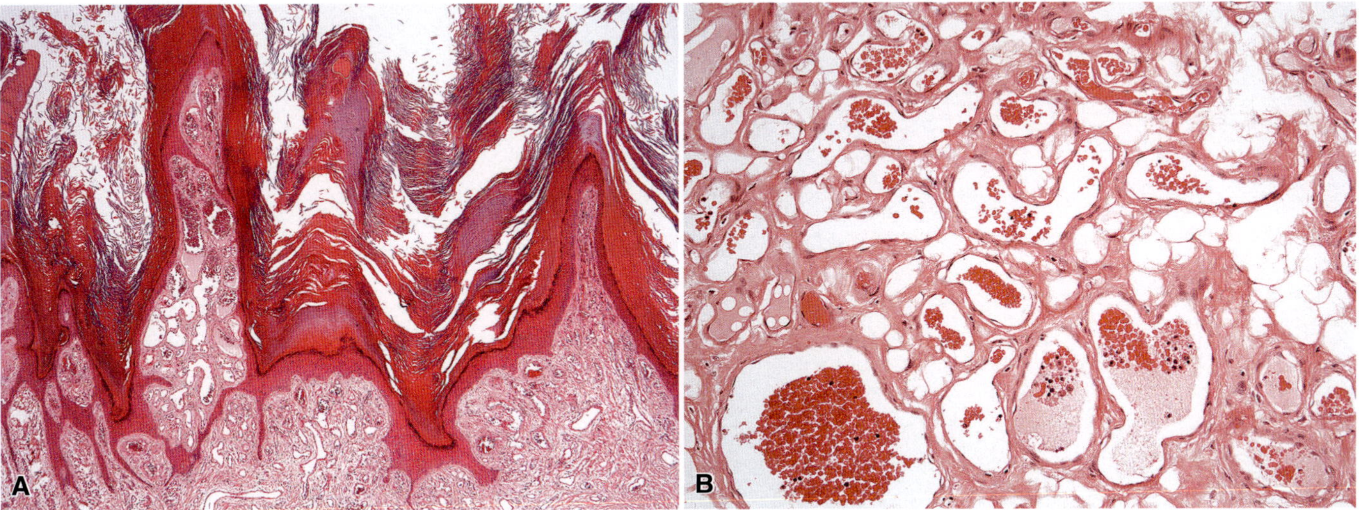

Figure 13.21 Verrucous Hemangioma. (A) Dilated dermal capillaries with striking overlying papillomatosis and hyperkeratosis. (B) The vascular proliferation extends into the subcutis.

Immunohistochemistry

By immunohistochemistry, more than half of verrucous hemangiomas express GLUT1, although reactivity is generally focal.[173]

Differential Diagnosis

The superficial portions of verrucous hemangioma and angiokeratoma are often histologically identical, but angiokeratoma does not involve the reticular dermis or subcutis. On superficial biopsy specimens, correlation with the clinical findings is helpful because angiokeratomas are acquired rather than congenital and present as solitary or multiple small (<0.5 cm) papules, in contrast to the larger, plaquelike lesions of verrucous hemangioma. Superficial lymphatic malformations (lymphangioma circumscriptum) may also be associated with verrucous epidermal changes, but the constituent vessels are readily recognized histologically as lymphatic rather than blood vascular.

Prognosis and Treatment

Because verrucous hemangiomas enlarge gradually over time, excision early in life is preferred to avoid the need for skin grafts. The vascular proliferation usually extends further laterally than is clinically evident, which may result in incomplete excision, and one-third of cases recur locally.[172,174] Because wide excision may be cosmetically disfiguring, conservative management is often preferred for large lesions.

Tufted Angioma

Clinical Features

Tufted angioma (first described in the Japanese literature as *angioblastoma*[175]) is a rare vascular neoplasm that typically affects infants or young children, although cases presenting in adulthood have been reported.[117,176,177] The most common site is the neck or upper trunk, but a significant minority of cases arise on the extremities.[178] Patients present with a dull red, indurated or nodular plaque, often with superimposed bright red papules. The lesions may be tender and infrequently are associated with hypertrichosis or hyperhidrosis.[178–180] Slow progressive enlargement is the rule, and tumors may ultimately reach 10 cm or more. Rarely, patients with congenital tufted angioma have Kasabach-Merritt syndrome, a localized consumptive coagulopathy more commonly associated with kaposiform hemangioendothelioma (discussed later).[181,182]

Pathologic Features

Small lobules of tightly packed capillaries are scattered in a characteristic "cannonball" distribution in the reticular dermis (Fig. 13.22A) and infrequently the superficial subcutis. The deep dermal lobules are often larger than those in the superficial dermis, and in some cases they coalesce to form irregular cords or aggregates. The capillaries have plump, oval to spindle-shaped endothelial cells, with numerous surrounding pericytes, and they may be poorly canalized, resulting in a solid appearance similar to that seen in early juvenile capillary hemangioma. A characteristic crescent-shaped, thin-walled vessel is often present at the periphery of the lobules (see Fig. 13.22B), and dilated lymphatic channels may be seen between the dermal capillary lobules.[177] Mitoses are uncommon, and there is no cytologic atypia.

Immunohistochemistry

Tufted angiomas are negative for GLUT1.[152] D2-40 highlights the dilated dermal lymphatics, but data on D2-40 expression within the capillary tufts are conflicting.[143,183]

Differential Diagnosis

The most challenging entity to distinguish from tufted angioma histologically is kaposiform hemangioendothelioma (Table 13.2). In contrast to tufted angioma, kaposiform hemangioendothelioma forms a solid mass with large, coalescing lobules composed of spindle cells separated by slitlike vascular spaces. Although tufted angiomas can show focal spindling of the endothelial cells, usually rounded capillaries dominate at the periphery of the lobules. The epithelioid endothelial cells and fibrin microthrombi often seen in kaposiform hemangioendothelioma are not features of tufted angioma.

The lobules of juvenile capillary hemangioma are similar to those seen in tufted angioma, but are typically larger, are not arranged in a cannonball distribution, and lack peripheral crescentic vessels. If necessary, immunohistochemistry for GLUT1 distinguishes the two neoplasms.

Occasional cases of reactive angioendotheliomatosis closely mimic tufted angioma histologically,[45] but the former usually presents as multiple lesions in adults and is often associated with systemic disease.[41]

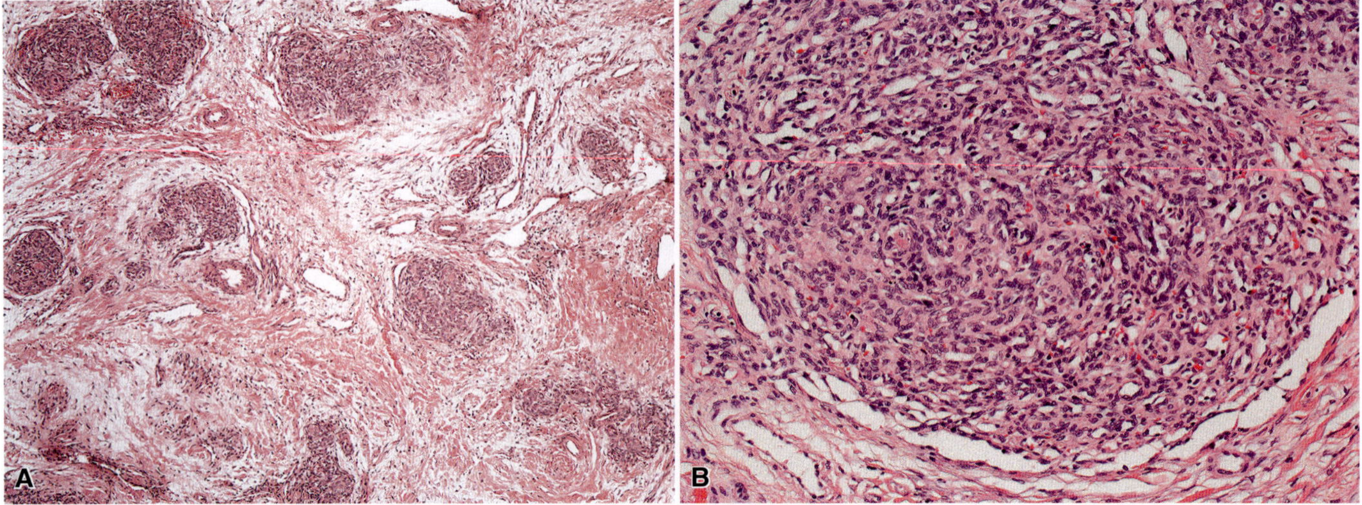

Figure 13.22 Tufted Angioma. (A) Lobules of tightly packed capillaries are scattered through the dermis in a "cannonball" distribution. (B) A lobule composed of poorly canalized capillaries and prominent pericytes. Note the crescentic thin-walled vessel at the periphery.

Table 13.2 Kaposiform Vascular Tumors

	Kaposi Sarcoma (Nodular Stage)	Kaposiform Hemangioendothelioma	Tufted Angioma
Age	Adults	Infants and young children	Children
Site	Distal extremities (rarely disseminated)	Retroperitoneum, extremities > other	Neck/upper trunk > extremities
Depth	Cutaneous	Deep soft tissue > superficial	Cutaneous; infrequent subcutaneous extension
Architecture	Typically a single circumscribed nodule	Ill-defined coalescing lobules	Small, discrete lobules
Spindle cell component	Predominant	Predominant	Absent or only focal at periphery of lobules
Vascular spaces	Slitlike	Slitlike	Rounded
Characteristic features	Lymphoplasmacytic infiltrate	Glomeruloid clusters of epithelioid cells	Dilated crescentic lymphatics at periphery of lobules

Prognosis and Treatment

Because tufted angiomas are several centimeters in size and extend into the deep dermis or subcutis, complete excision may be difficult and recurrences are not uncommon. Observation is generally preferred for large tumors unless they are symptomatic or cosmetically disfiguring.

PRACTICE POINTS: Verrucous Hemangiomas and Tufted Angioma

- Verrucous hemangioma and tufted angioma are rare variants of capillary hemangiomas that present in childhood.
- The superficial portion of verrucous hemangioma resembles angiokeratoma, but the capillary proliferation extends into the deep dermis.
- Tufted angioma is distinguished from kaposiform hemangioendothelioma by the smaller size of the capillary lobules, peripheral crescentic vessels, and lack of a prominent spindle cell component.

Symplastic Hemangioma

Clinical Features

Symplastic hemangioma is a rare hemangioma variant, with fewer than 10 cases reported to date.[184–186] The clinical features are similar to those of other superficial hemangiomas. Despite their atypical histologic features, the clinical course appears to be entirely benign.

Pathologic Features

Degenerative nuclear atypia, sometimes with multinucleation, is present in the vascular smooth muscle cells and stromal cells of an otherwise banal hemangioma (Fig. 13.23), usually an arteriovenous or capillary hemangioma. In contrast, the endothelial cells lack atypia. Other degenerative changes, including vascular thrombosis, an inflammatory infiltrate, and stromal hemorrhage and edema, are often present. Rarely, atypical mitoses may be identified.[184,186]

Microvenular Hemangioma

Clinical Features

Microvenular hemangioma is a rare benign vascular tumor with a predilection for young adults, although children and older adults can be affected.[187,188] The lesions present as red-purple nodules or plaques measuring 1 to a few centimeters and most commonly occur on the limbs.

Pathologic Features

At low power, a symmetric, often wedge-shaped proliferation of irregularly branching, compressed venules in a "chutes-and-ladders" pattern is seen within a sclerotic reticular dermis (Fig. 13.24A). A prominent pericytic layer is generally present around each vessel, and the vascular lumina may be inconspicuous (see Fig. 13.24B). Involvement of the arrector pili muscle by the neoplastic vessels is a characteristic feature. The nuclei of the endothelial cells may be plump, but atypia is absent. Actin stain highlights the presence of a well-formed layer of pericytes around each vessel.

Differential Diagnosis

The main differential diagnostic consideration is patch-stage Kaposi sarcoma. Classic features of Kaposi sarcoma, including erythrocyte extravasation, hemosiderin deposition, a perivascular lymphoplasmacytic infiltrate, a spindle cell component, and HHV-8 reactivity, are not seen in microvenular hemangioma.[189–191] In addition, the vessels in Kaposi sarcoma have thin walls, without a prominent layer of pericytes. A pericyte-predominant form of reactive angioendotheliomatosis could be considered, but the symmetric wedge shape of the vascular proliferation and the clinical setting (i.e., a solitary lesion in a healthy, often young, patient) argue against this diagnosis.

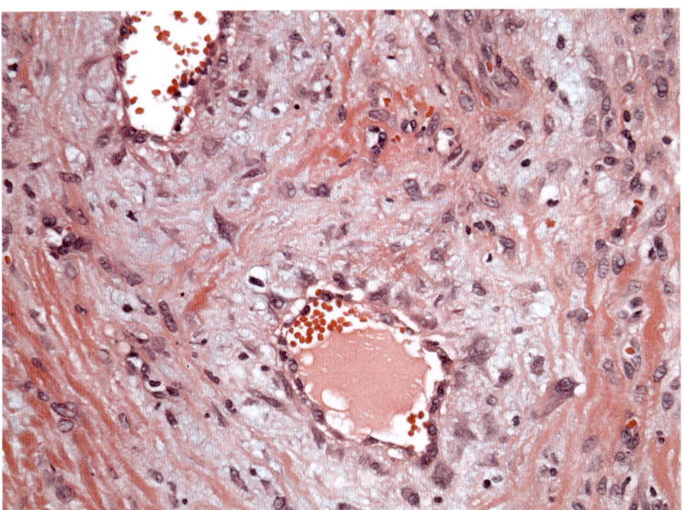

Figure 13.23 Symplastic Hemangioma. The walls of the blood vessels contain cells with degenerative nuclear atypia.

Practice Point: Microvenular Hemangioma

A "chutes-and-ladders" pattern of compressed vessels in a fibrotic dermis is characteristic of microvenular hemangioma.

Hobnail Hemangioma ("Targetoid Hemosiderotic Hemangioma")

Hobnail hemangioma was first described as *targetoid hemosiderotic hemangioma* because of the targetoid clinical appearance of some lesions.[192] However, because many hobnail hemangiomas are not clinically targetoid and other cutaneous lesions may show a targetoid pattern, the designation *hobnail hemangioma* was proposed.[192–194] Both terms remain in common use, although evidence supports lymphatic differentiation for these tumors, leading some authors to suggest that the term *hemangioma* be replaced by *angioma* or *lymphangioma*.[195]

Clinical Features

Hobnail hemangioma arises over a wide age range, with a predilection for young adults, and typically presents on the extremities or trunk, although the head and neck region, including the oral mucosa, may be involved.[192,194] In stereotypical lesions, a small violaceous papule is surrounded by a pale zone and a peripheral ecchymotic rim, resulting in a targetoid appearance. However, more commonly, the tumors present as homogeneous red-purple or brown macules or papules measuring less than 2 cm in diameter. Infrequently, the tumors may involute and recur in cycles lasting weeks to years, sometimes correlating with the menstrual cycle.[194,196–198]

Pathologic Features

Hobnail hemangiomas typically involve the superficial and deep dermis; extension into the subcutis is infrequent. The vascular proliferation is generally symmetric and wedge-shaped and has a characteristic biphasic pattern.[192,194] The superficial vessels are widely dilated and display prominent hobnail or matchsticklike endothelial cells with scant cytoplasm and an enlarged, mildly hyperchromatic nucleus that bulges into the vessel lumen (Fig. 13.25A). Polypoid or free-floating aggregates of plump endothelial cells are often seen within the lumina, and true papillae with a hyaline core lined by hobnail endothelium may be present.

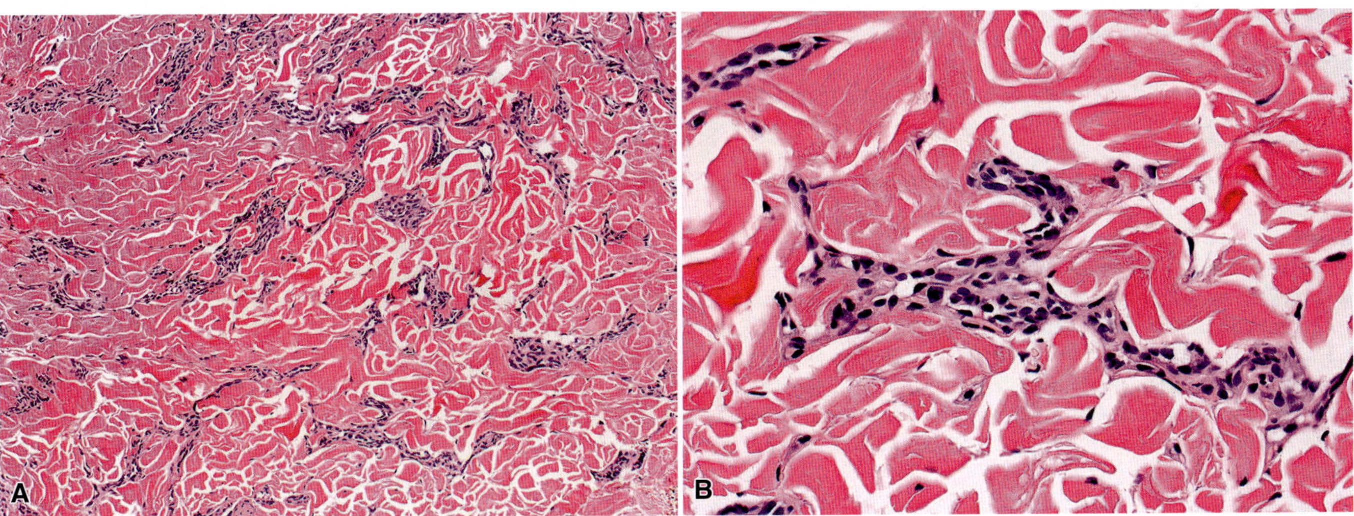

Figure 13.24 Microvenular Hemangioma. (A) The dermis contains irregularly branching compressed venules in a "chutes-and-ladders" pattern. The involved dermis is sclerotic. (B) The compressed venules often contain a prominent layer of pericytes.

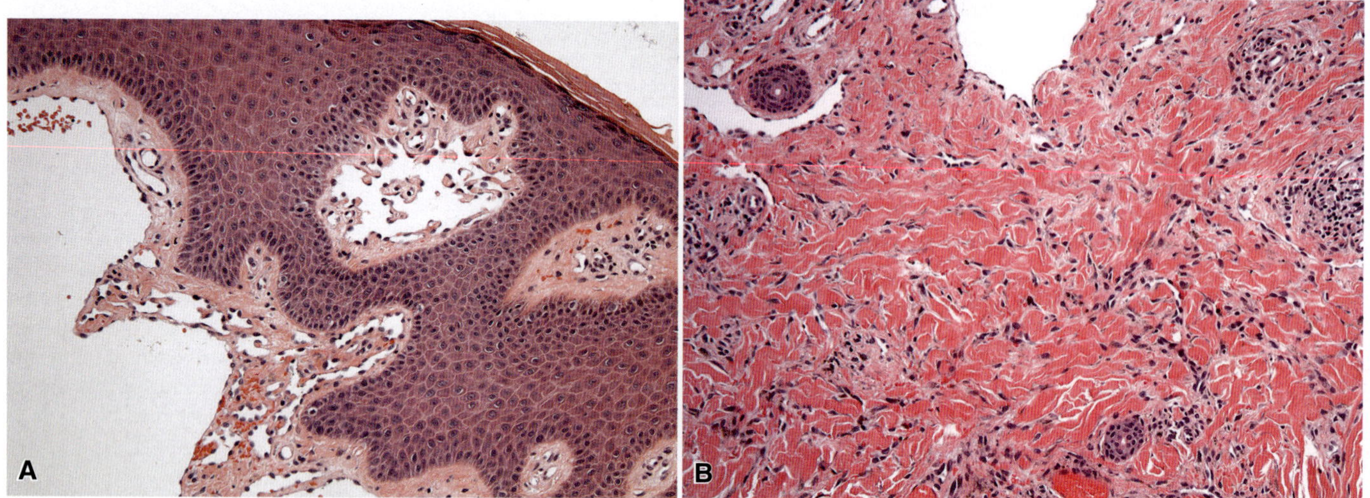

Figure 13.25 Hobnail Hemangioma. (A) Dilated superficial vessels contain "hobnail" endothelial cells with scant cytoplasm and nuclei that protrude into the lumina. Note the papillary projections. (B) The deep dermal vessels are compressed and show a dissecting growth pattern.

Table 13.3 Vascular Tumors With Hobnail Endothelium

	Hobnail Hemangioma	Papillary Intralymphatic Angioendothelioma (Dabska Tumor)	Retiform Hemangioendothelioma	Postradiation Atypical Vascular Lesion
Age	Young adults	Infants and children	Young adults	Older adults
Anatomic sites	Trunk, extremities	Wide anatomic distribution	Extremities	Any site of previous radiation (breast most common)
Depth	Dermis	Subcutis and often reticular dermis	Dermis and occasionally subcutis	Dermis
Vascular pattern	Biphasic, with dilated superficial vessels and compressed deep vessels	Cavernous, lymphangioma-like spaces with intraluminal papillae	Narrow, anastomosing channels	Variable, but often ectatic superficially; can be biphasic
Endothelial cells	Hobnail superficially, flattened deep	Flattened to hobnail	Hobnail	Flattened to hobnail
Occasional features	Small intraluminal papillae	Associated lymphatic malformation	Small intraluminal papillae	Small intraluminal papillae
Associated findings	Hemosiderin, mild lymphocytic infiltrate	Prominent lymphocytic infiltrate	Prominent lymphocytic infiltrate, hemosiderin	Patchy lymphocytic infiltrate
Margins	Symmetric, wedge shaped	Ill defined	Infiltrative	May be wedge shaped

The channels often contain erythrocytes, but occasional lymphatic-like vessels with pale eosinophilic fluid are also common.

In contrast, mid- and deep dermal vessels are compressed, have a flattened endothelial lining (see Fig. 13.25B), and show a dissecting growth pattern similar to that seen in patch-stage Kaposi sarcoma or low-grade cutaneous angiosarcoma. In some cases the dilated hobnail vascular channels predominate, and in others the narrow dissecting vessels make up nearly the entire lesion.

Cytologic atypia is generally mild or absent, but striking reactive atypia may be present adjacent to fibrin thrombi.[194,199] In addition to the hobnail endothelial cells, epithelioid endothelial cells are focally present in a minority of cases.[192,194] Mitoses are rare. Most cases show dermal fibrosis, extravasated erythrocytes, hemosiderin deposition, and a mild lymphocytic infiltrate. The targetoid clinical appearance seen in a subset of patients may be caused by a rim of extravasated erythrocytes surrounding the vascular proliferation.[192]

Immunohistochemistry

CD31 and D2-40 are typically positive, whereas CD34 is often absent or focal, suggesting lymphatic differentiation.[194,195] A minority of cases have a layer of actin-positive pericytes that is usually focal and discontinuous when present, as commonly seen in lymphatic vessels.[194,199]

Differential Diagnosis

Prominent hobnail endothelium is seen in a variety of vascular lesions, including papillary intralymphatic angioendothelioma (Dabska tumor), retiform hemangioendothelioma, and some angiosarcomas. Papillary intralymphatic angioendothelioma and retiform hemangioendothelioma are usually larger than hobnail hemangioma, are poorly circumscribed, and lack a biphasic appearance (Table 13.3). Angiosarcoma shows striking cytologic atypia and also lacks the circumscription and biphasic pattern of hobnail hemangioma; moreover, cutaneous lesions nearly always arise on the head and neck of the elderly, except in the setting of radiation therapy or lymphedema. Focal hobnail endothelial cells can be seen as a reactive phenomenon in otherwise banal hemangiomas or nonneoplastic vascular proliferations, often in association with fibrin thrombi.

Acquired progressive lymphangioma and lymphatic malformations may have dilated superficial vessels, compressed deep vessels, and small intraluminal papillae similar to those seen in hobnail hemangioma, but hobnail endothelium, extravasated erythrocytes, and hemosiderin deposition are not present. Kaposi sarcoma lacks a biphasic pattern, hobnail endothelium, and intraluminal papillae; in addition, results for HHV-8 are negative in hobnail hemangioma.[189,200]

Finally, postradiation atypical vascular lesions may show the same biphasic pattern of ectatic superficial vessels and compressed deep vessels, and the endothelial cells often have protuberant, mildly hyperchromatic nuclei. Hemosiderin deposition and extravasated erythrocytes are less common in atypical vascular lesions, but because of the significant histologic overlap with hobnail hemangioma, clinical history is essential.

PRACTICE POINTS: Hobnail Hemangioma ("Targetoid Hemosiderotic Hemangioma")

- The majority of hobnail hemangiomas lack the classic "targetoid" clinical appearance.
- A biphasic pattern is seen histologically, with hobnail endothelial cells limited to the dilated superficial vessels.
- Atypical postradiation vascular lesions can be histologically similar.

Papillary Intralymphatic Angioendothelioma (Dabska Tumor)

In 1969 Dabska reported a series of six vascular tumors in infants and children, which she termed *malignant intravascular angioendothelioma* because of the development of nodal metastases in two cases.[201] Since that time, approximately 35 additional cases have been published (although the diagnosis was questioned in some[202,203]), and no further metastases or deaths have been reported. In 1999 Fanburg-Smith and colleagues proposed changing the name to *papillary intralymphatic angioendothelioma* to emphasize the lymphatic phenotype and borderline clinical behavior.[204] Controversy remains regarding not only the biologic potential of these lesions but also their possible relationship to retiform hemangioendothelioma.[193]

Clinical Features

Although papillary intralymphatic angioendothelioma was originally considered a tumor of infants and children, more recent reports have shown that the age distribution is broader than initially believed[204]; overall, 40% of reported cases arose in adults.[205] Tumors generally arise in the superficial soft tissue, and there is no particular site predilection. Rare cases in deep soft tissue[206] and bone[207,208] have been reported. The two reported cases in visceral sites were splenic lesions[209,210]; based on the published photographs, we consider both within the histologic spectrum of splenic lymphangioma (discussed later). Papillary intralymphatic angioendothelioma typically measures 1 to several centimeters.[204]

Pathologic Features

Grossly, the tumor forms an ill-defined subcutaneous thickening, with small cystic spaces. Histologically, the dermis or subcutaneous tissue contains cavernous lymphatic-like vascular spaces, with characteristic intravascular papillae (Fig. 13.26A).[204,211] The latter vary in size from small tufts of hobnail endothelial cells that may appear to be floating within the vascular lumina, to small papillae with acellular hyaline cores (see Fig. 13.26B), to large, complex, glomeruloid structures. The papillae and many of the neoplastic vessels are lined by plump endothelial cells with prominent apical nuclei and scant to moderate amounts of basilar cytoplasm, resulting in a lymphocyte-like, hobnail, or columnar "matchstick-like" appearance. Intraluminal lymphocytes are often present and may be intimately admixed with the endothelial cells of the papillae. Intracytoplasmic vacuoles may be seen within a subset of the plump endothelial cells.

The dermis is often sclerotic, and a perivascular lymphocytic infiltrate is usually present. A significant minority of papillary intralymphatic angioendotheliomas are associated with a preexisting vascular malformation, often of lymphatic type.[204,206,207,211–214]

Mitoses are rare, and cytologic atypia is absent. Although papillary intralymphatic angioendothelioma may have some partially collapsed vascular channels, narrow anastomosing vessels with a dissecting growth pattern and solid spindle cell foci are not part of the spectrum of this entity; such cases are far more likely to represent retiform hemangioendothelioma or angiosarcoma with prominent intravascular papillae.

Immunohistochemistry

The endothelial cells are positive for CD31, VEGFR-3, and D2-40 and focally express CD34, consistent with a lymphatic phenotype.[11,204] Actin-positive pericytes may be found within the intraluminal glomeruloid structures but are absent around the neoplastic vessels. The hyaline cores of the intraluminal papillae are reactive for type IV collagen, indicating the presence of basement membrane material.[204]

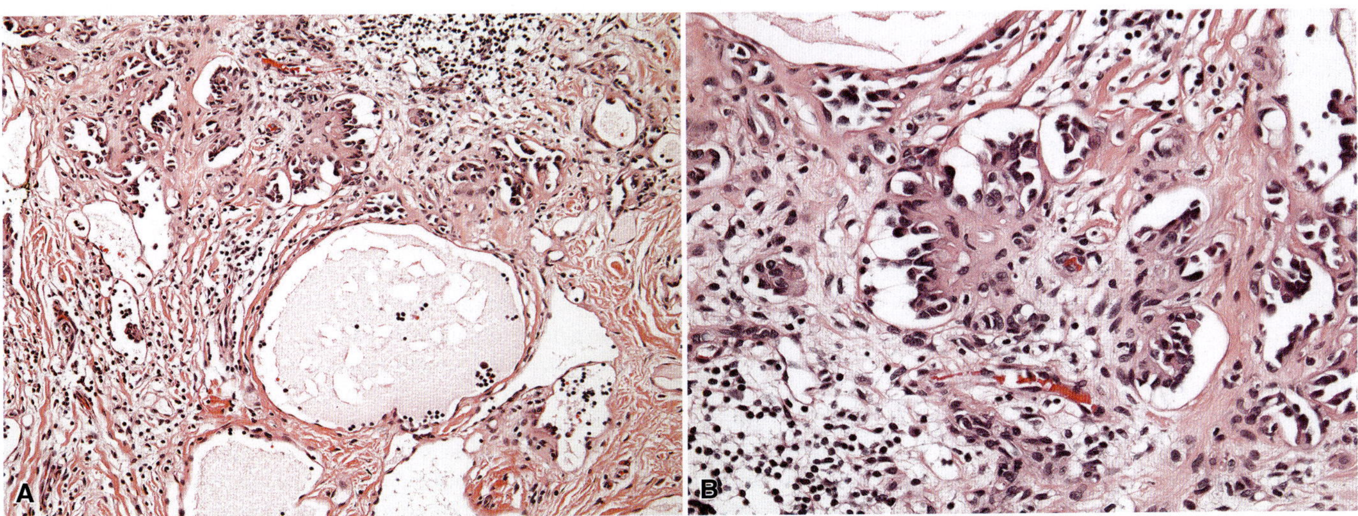

Figure 13.26 Papillary Intralymphatic Angioendothelioma (Dabska Tumor). (A) Dilated lymphatic spaces contain intravascular papillae. (B) Papillary tufts with hyaline cores lined by hobnail endothelial cells.

Differential Diagnosis

Intraluminal papillary tufts are not specific for papillary intralymphatic angioendothelioma, and they may be seen in a variety of nonneoplastic and neoplastic vascular lesions, including reactive angioendotheliomatosis, lymphatic malformations/cavernous lymphangiomas (particularly those in the spleen), retiform hemangioendothelioma, and angiosarcoma. Reactive angioendotheliomatosis (including the glomeruloid hemangioma subtype that arises in association with POEMS syndrome) lacks the consistent hobnail or matchstick appearance of the endothelium seen in papillary intralymphatic angioendothelioma and presents with multiple lesions (see Table 13.3). Cavernous lymphangiomas, particularly those in the spleen, may have focally plump endothelial cells and intraluminal papillary projections,[215,216] but in contrast to papillary intralymphatic angioendothelioma, the majority of the endothelial cells are attenuated, intravascular papillae are rarely prominent, and matchstick-like columnar endothelial cells are generally absent.

Uncommonly, angiosarcoma has intraluminal papillae lined by relatively bland hobnail endothelium.[217] In addition to distinct clinical features—cutaneous angiosarcoma is most common in the elderly and on sun-damaged skin—focal nuclear pleomorphism, mitotic activity, endothelial multilayering, and a markedly infiltrative growth pattern distinguish these tumors from papillary intralymphatic angioendothelioma.

Retiform hemangioendothelioma is the most difficult entity to differentiate from papillary intralymphatic angioendothelioma. The differential diagnosis is discussed in more detail later, but in short, the distinction is best made at low power. Papillary intralymphatic angioendothelioma has the architecture of a cavernous lymphangioma, with widely dilated vascular spaces. Retiform hemangioendothelioma is dominated by narrow anastomosing channels.

Prognosis and Treatment

The lack of well-defined diagnostic criteria for papillary intralymphatic angioendothelioma has led to a hodgepodge of lesions reported under this designation and therefore disagreement over its biologic potential. Local recurrence appears to be uncommon. In the original series, Dabska[211] reported lymph node metastases in two of six patients (one of whom ultimately died as a result of widespread pulmonary metastases[203]), but retrospective review of the slides suggested that some of these cases might be better classified as retiform hemangioendothelioma.[193] A more recent series reported a benign clinical course in all eight cases with follow-up.[204] Additional studies are needed to clarify the prognosis of this rare entity; currently, wide excision and close clinical follow-up are recommended.

PRACTICE POINTS: Papillary Intralymphatic Angioendothelioma (Dabska Tumor)

- Characteristic features of papillary intralymphatic angioendothelioma include dilated lymphatic spaces, hobnail endothelium, and intravascular papillae with acellular hyaline cores.
- Clinical behavior appears to be benign in most patients, but additional data are needed.

Retiform Hemangioendothelioma

Clinical Features

Retiform hemangioendothelioma (named for its histologic similarity to the rete testis) may present at any age but is most common in adolescence and young adulthood.[218] Approximately two-thirds of cases occur on the extremities, particularly the lower limb; the rest have a wide distribution, including the trunk, genitalia, and head and neck. Rare cases arising at a site of previous radiation or chronic lymphedema have been reported.

The tumors present as solitary, ill-defined, dermal or subcutaneous nodules or plaques measuring a few to several centimeters in diameter. Many lesions have been present for 1 year or longer, and patients often report slow growth over time.[193] Exceptionally, multiple retiform hemangioendotheliomas occur synchronously or metachronously at distant cutaneous sites.[219]

Pathologic Features

Retiform hemangioendothelioma typically involves the full thickness of the dermis. In a minority of cases, it extends into the subcutaneous tissue. The tumors are poorly circumscribed and are composed of partially compressed, anastomosing vessels lined by hobnail or matchstick endothelial cells, similar to those seen in papillary intralymphatic angioendothelioma (Fig. 13.27A). The superficial dermal vessels may be focally dilated, whereas those in the deep dermis are long and narrow (see Fig. 13.27B). The basilar cytoplasm of the endothelial cells often appears to merge imperceptibly with the adjacent dermal collagen. Infrequently, small intraluminal papillae lined by hobnail endothelium are present, and focal intracytoplasmic vacuoles are seen in the endothelial cells in rare cases.

Nearly all lesions also contain solid foci in which plump or (rarely) spindle-shaped endothelial cells form sheets or cords. On careful examination, numerous tiny vascular channels may be identified within these areas. Most cases have a prominent lymphocytic infiltrate that may partially obscure the neoplastic vessels, and intraluminal lymphocytes are commonly seen in close association with the hobnail cells. The dermis is often sclerotic and frequently shows focal hemorrhage and hemosiderin deposition.

Although the endothelial cells may appear atypical because of nuclear enlargement and hyperchromasia, they are remarkably monomorphic. In addition, nucleoli are absent and mitotic activity is rare. The only metastasizing case reported to date had predominantly solid, spindle cell morphologic features, and the metastatic tumor in the lymph node was entirely spindled, without areas of typical retiform hemangioendothelioma.[193]

Immunohistochemistry

The endothelial cells lining the vessels are positive for CD31 and CD34, and the spindle cells in the solid foci also stain with CD31, confirming their endothelial origin. Retiform hemangioendothelioma is usually negative for D2-40.[2,220] There is variable expression of VEGFR-3, but as previously mentioned, this marker is no longer considered specific for lymphatic differentiation.[9,204,220] No pericytes are seen around the neoplastic vessels or within the solid foci on actin stains.[2,193]

Differential Diagnosis

The primary differential diagnostic considerations are papillary intralymphatic angioendothelioma, angiosarcoma, and less often, hobnail hemangioma (see Table 13.3). Hobnail endothelial cells, a lymphocytic infiltrate, and intraluminal papillae are features of both retiform hemangioendothelioma and papillary intralymphatic angioendothelioma, but the latter is dominated by dilated lymphangioma-like spaces and has prominent intraluminal papillae, whereas the former is composed primarily of narrow, elongated vascular channels with only focal, if any, intraluminal papillae. The consistent D2-40 expression in papillary intralymphatic angioendothelioma and the lack of expression in retiform hemangioendothelioma imply that the two entities are not closely related.

In contrast to retiform hemangioendothelioma, angiosarcoma has at least focally significant nuclear atypia, endothelial multilayering, and occasional mitoses. Furthermore, angiosarcoma is exceptionally rare

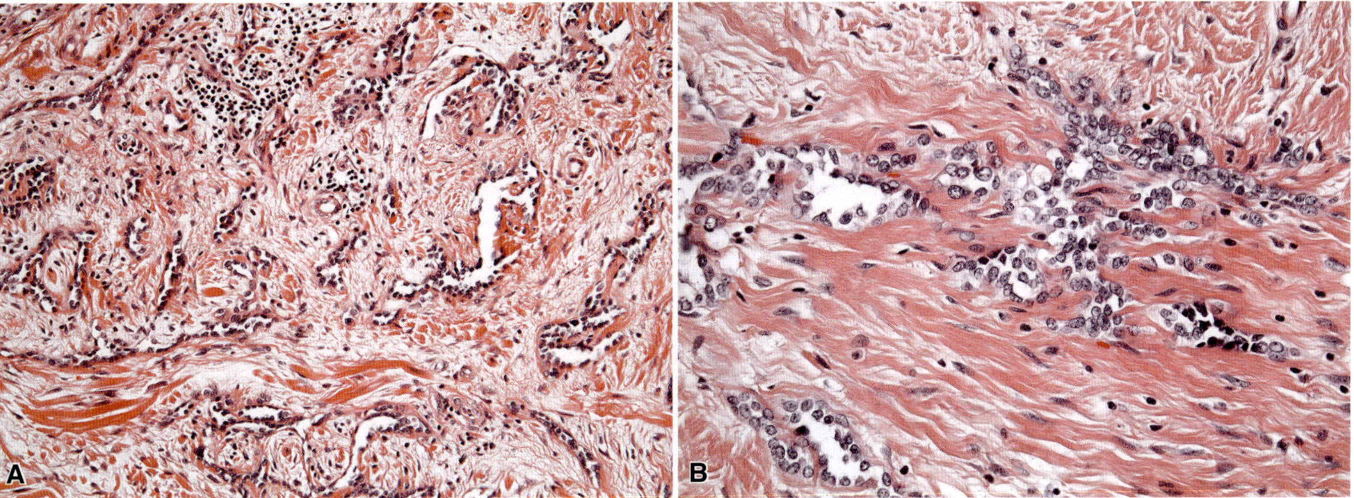

Figure 13.27 Retiform Hemangioendothelioma. (A) Branching vessels lined by hobnail endothelial cells. Note the patchy lymphocytic infiltrate. (B) Compressed vessels lined by endothelial cells with monomorphic, hyperchromatic nuclei protruding into the lumina.

on the extremities of young patients, in the absence of lymphedema or previous radiation therapy.

Hobnail hemangioma is a small, superficial lesion with a symmetric, wedge-shaped low-power appearance that contrasts with the markedly infiltrative growth pattern of retiform hemangioendothelioma. In addition, the hobnail endothelium is limited to the superficial vessels in hobnail hemangioma and is diffuse in retiform hemangioendothelioma.

Prognosis and Treatment

Retiform hemangioendothelioma is classified as a tumor of intermediate biologic potential because of its high rate of local recurrence and very low risk of metastasis. More than 50% of patients have one or more local recurrences, which may ultimately require amputation. Regional lymph node metastases have been reported in rare cases,[193] but there are no reports of distant metastasis or death. Wide local excision with close clinical follow-up is generally regarded as optimal therapy.

PRACTICE POINTS: Retiform Hemangioendothelioma

- Retiform hemangioendothelioma has a predilection for the extremities of young adults.
- Elongated, narrow vascular channels lined by hobnail endothelial cells and focal solid-appearing areas are characteristic.
- Although the margins are typically infiltrative, the cells are monomorphic and mitoses are rare.

Composite Hemangioendothelioma

Clinical Features

Composite hemangioendothelioma is a rare vascular tumor in which the histologic patterns of two or more well-described vascular neoplasms are identified in variable proportions within a single lesion.[221–223] The tumors may be cutaneous or subcutaneous, and there is a strong predilection for the distal extremities. Two cases have been reported in the oral cavity.[221,222] Many patients present in early adulthood, but there is often a history of slow growth over several years, and in a few cases the lesions were congenital.[222,223] Rare cases arising in association with lymphedema[221] or Maffucci syndrome[222] have been reported.

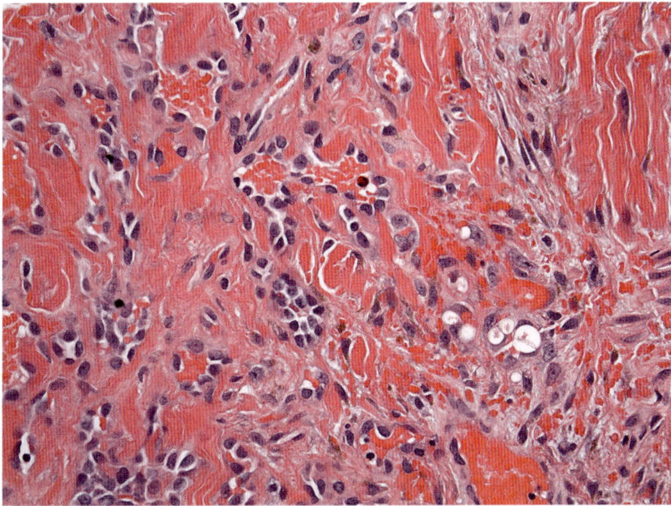

Figure 13.28 Composite Hemangioendothelioma. The tumor is heterogeneous, typically composed of areas resembling retiform hemangioendothelioma and epithelioid hemangioendothelioma. Note the cytoplasmic vacuoles *(lower right).*

Pathologic Features

The tumors are typically infiltrative within the dermis and subcutis, and, as implied by the name, they show heterogeneous architectural and cytologic features. The most common components are foci identical to those of typical retiform hemangioendothelioma, epithelioid hemangioendothelioma, and low-grade (vasoformative) angiosarcoma (Fig. 13.28). Approximately 50% of cases have areas that resemble spindle cell hemangioma, and a smaller number of cases are associated with an underlying vascular malformation. Some cases have clusters or sheets of endothelial cells, with large intracytoplasmic vacuoles that mimic lipoblasts. Rarely, high-grade angiosarcoma-like areas composed of solid sheets of atypical cells are present.[221] The different histologic components often merge imperceptibly.

Immunohistochemistry

As expected, the tumors express CD31 or CD34.[221] D2-40 is negative.

Differential Diagnosis

The combination of vascular tumor elements present in composite hemangioendothelioma distinguishes it from pure retiform hemangioendothelioma, angiosarcoma, or epithelioid hemangioendothelioma.

Prognosis and Treatment

The clinical behavior of composite hemangioendothelioma remains incompletely defined because of its rarity. Recurrence is common, and metastasis to regional lymph nodes has been reported in several cases.[221,224–226] In addition, several unpublished cases progressed to frank angiosarcoma after multiple recurrences and ultimately metastasized (C.D.M. Fletcher, personal communication).

PRACTICE POINT: Composite Hemangioendothelioma

The most common components of composite hemangioendothelioma are retiform hemangioendothelioma, epithelioid hemangioendothelioma, and low-grade angiosarcoma.

Angiosarcoma

Angiosarcoma is a rare malignancy, accounting for only 2% to 4% of soft tissue sarcomas.[227–229] More than half are cutaneous, with the remainder arising in deep soft tissue, breast, bone, or viscera, particularly the liver, spleen, and heart. The historical terms *lymphangiosarcoma* and *hemangiosarcoma* are no longer used because many angiosarcomas show features of both blood vascular and lymphatic differentiation.[4]

Clinical Features

Cutaneous Angiosarcoma. Cutaneous angiosarcoma may be sporadic or may arise in the setting of chronic lymphedema or radiation therapy. Sporadic cutaneous angiosarcoma, the most common subtype, predominantly affects the head and neck of elderly patients, with a predilection for white men.[117,230–233] Early lesions are often clinically deceptive, presenting as ill-defined, bruiselike macules measuring 1 to several centimeters. Violaceous plaques and nodules are seen in more advanced cases. At presentation, nearly half of patients have multifocal disease, which may take the form of two or more anatomically discrete lesions or small satellites around a single dominant tumor.[233,234]

Lymphedema-associated cutaneous angiosarcoma most commonly affects the upper extremity in patients who have undergone mastectomy and axillary dissection for breast cancer (Stewart-Treves syndrome). The risk of angiosarcoma in these patients is very low (0.07% to 0.45%),[235] and the incidence appears to be decreasing because of the shift toward breast-conserving surgery and sentinel lymph node biopsy.[236,237] A small number of cases arise in the setting of congenital, traumatic, filarial, or idiopathic lymphedema, and rare cases have been reported in massive localized lymphedema, a pseudotumor of morbidly obese patients.[238–241] The latency period after the onset of lymphedema averages 10 years for postmastectomy angiosarcomas and 20 years in other settings but may be 50 years or longer.[237–240] Lymphedema-associated angiosarcoma most commonly presents as one or more blue-red macules or plaques in the lymphedematous region; however, sometimes the only sign may be new-onset swelling without a visible lesion. As in sporadic cutaneous angiosarcoma, multicentricity is common.

Postradiation angiosarcoma was historically the least common subtype of cutaneous angiosarcoma,[117,242] but the incidence has increased as breast-conserving surgery with radiation therapy has become the standard of care for patients with early-stage breast cancer.[243,244] The risk of angiosarcoma in patients who have received radiation therapy for breast cancer is approximately 0.3%.[244–247] Postradiation cutaneous angiosarcoma may also occur on the anterior abdominal wall after radiation therapy for gynecologic malignancies or rarely at other sites after radiation for head and neck or penile squamous cell carcinomas, hematopoietic malignancies, and benign or nonneoplastic lesions.[248–250] Although the vast majority of postradiation angiosarcomas are cutaneous, exceptional cases arising within the mammary parenchyma, in deep soft tissue, and at visceral sites have been reported.[251] The median latency period for postradiation angiosarcoma in patients treated for breast cancer is only 5 to 6 years[245,252–255] versus 10 to 15 years for most postradiation sarcomas, including postradiation angiosarcomas at other sites.[249,256–258] The increased use of radiation to treat breast cancer has also led to the recognition of radiation-associated cutaneous atypical vascular lesions, which may have a worrisome histologic appearance but very rarely progress to angiosarcoma (discussed later).

Soft Tissue Angiosarcoma. Angiosarcoma of deep soft tissue shows a male predilection and arises over a wide age range, although children are rarely affected. The extremities and retroperitoneum are the most common sites in adults, whereas the rare soft tissue angiosarcomas in children show a predilection for the mediastinum, including the heart and pericardium.[259] Limb tumors are typically intramuscular and may arise from a large artery or, rarely, a nerve.[260,261] Patients typically present with an enlarging or painful mass. Infrequently, there may be signs and symptoms of tumor-associated hemorrhage (i.e., hematoma, hemothorax, hemorrhagic ascites, or anemia). Most soft tissue angiosarcomas are sporadic, but a small minority arise at the site of previous radiation therapy. Very rarely, they may be associated with a preexisting hemangioma, vascular malformation,[262] benign or malignant peripheral nerve sheath tumor,[260,263] or foreign body, most commonly, a vascular graft.[217,264] Interestingly, the majority of deep soft tissue angiosarcomas, as well as the rare primary angiosarcomas of the adrenal gland, thyroid, and small intestine, and the exceptionally rare angiosarcomas arising in preexisting schwannomas are the epithelioid variant.[260,261,263,265–267]

Mammary Angiosarcoma. Primary mammary parenchymal angiosarcoma is a very rare tumor with distinctive clinical characteristics, including a predilection for young women.[268,269] Secondary mammary angiosarcoma, which is nearly always cutaneous and arises after radiation therapy for breast carcinoma, is discussed earlier. Most tumors present as a palpable mass, which is often relatively large by the time of diagnosis (4 to 5 cm). Rarely, patients present with bilateral tumors.

Pathologic Features

Architecturally, angiosarcoma may be vasoformative, solid, or (often) mixed. The vasoformative areas are composed of irregular, anastomosing, thin-walled vessels with a dissecting growth pattern and infiltrative margins (Fig. 13.29A). The endothelial cells lining the neoplastic vessels have hyperchromatic, enlarged nuclei but are generally relatively uniform. Moderate or marked nuclear pleomorphism is uncommon (see Fig. 13.29B), and focally, the cells may be indistinguishable from normal endothelium.[270] Endothelial multilayering is often present (see Fig. 13.29C), and there may be small intraluminal tufts or papillae. Purely or predominantly solid angiosarcomas may have spindled or epithelioid cytomorphologic features; these are discussed later. In some cases, extensive hemorrhage obscures the tumor, mimicking a hematoma. Careful sampling may be needed to reveal malignant cells in the hemorrhagic background. Conversely, rare cases of angiosarcoma arising in a long-standing, fibrous-walled hematoma have been reported.[271]

Cutaneous angiosarcoma typically has a grenz zone and infiltrates the reticular dermis diffusely, leaving adnexal structures intact. There is often insidious radial extension of individual neoplastic vessels some distance from the primary lesion, and occasional tumors invade deeply through the subcutis, in some cases to the gala aponeurotica.[234] Many cases have a sparse or patchy lymphocytic infiltrate, with variable numbers

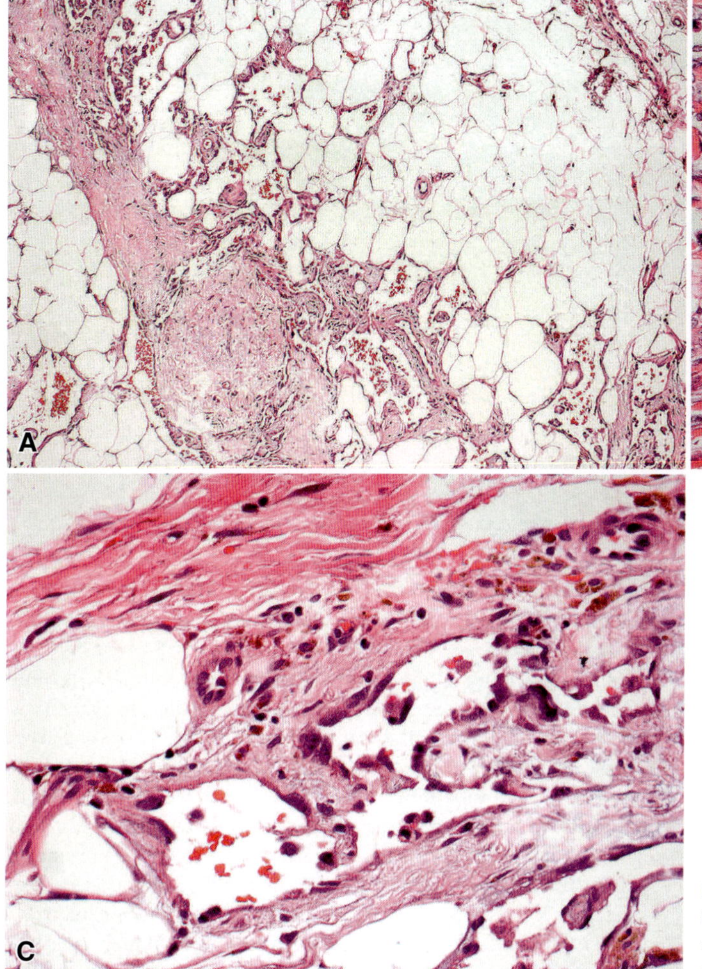

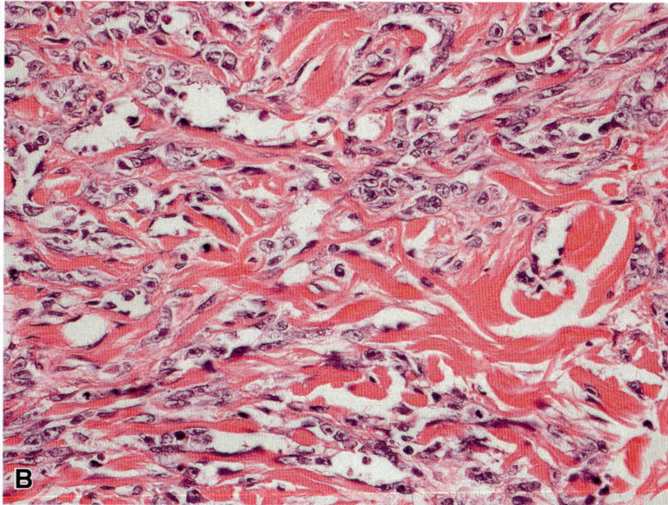

Figure 13.29 Angiosarcoma. (A) A vasoformative tumor composed of irregular thin-walled vessels with a dissecting growth pattern. (B) In this angiosarcoma, the vessels are lined by markedly atypical endothelial cells with vesicular chromatin and prominent nuclei. (C) Hyperchromatic nuclei showing tufting into the lumina.

of histiocytes, plasma cells, and eosinophils. A pseudolymphomatous pattern characterized by a dense lymphoid infiltrate containing prominent follicles and germinal centers has been reported.[242,272] Extravasated red blood cells and hemosiderin deposition are not uncommon, particularly in morphologically higher-grade tumors.

Mammary angiosarcoma is often deceptively bland in morphologically low-grade forms; the only clue to malignancy may be the insidious dissection of the neoplastic vessels through adipose tissue and around the native mammary ducts or lobules (Fig. 13.30A).[268] Intermediate-grade tumors are increasingly cellular and atypical but lack solid areas (see Fig. 13.30B). Morphologically high-grade mammary angiosarcomas show solid sheets of spindled or, less often, epithelioid cells and often show prominent hemorrhage ("blood lakes") and necrosis.

Mitoses are most prominent in solid areas but are often identifiable (albeit rare) in vasoformative foci as well. Necrosis is present in approximately 20% of cases. Intratumoral hemorrhage is common, particularly in deep soft tissue or visceral sites, and may result in an organizing hematoma with superimposed papillary endothelial hyperplasia. Although standard sarcoma grading systems, such as those developed by the National Cancer Institute and French Federation of Cancer Centers Sarcoma Group, have been applied to angiosarcoma, the traditional teaching has been that histologic grade does not correlate with prognosis.[231,233,242] However, a study suggested that assessment of two histologic features—necrosis and epithelioid cytomorphologic features—may be used to divide cutaneous angiosarcomas into prognostically relevant low- and high-risk groups; the presence of either feature defines a tumor as high risk.[230] These findings require confirmation in additional studies.

Immunohistochemistry

CD31 is positive in more than 90% of angiosarcomas, and the staining pattern is distinct and membranous, in contrast to the weak cytoplasmic staining reported in a small number of adenocarcinomas and mesotheliomas.[1] CD31 is fairly specific for endothelial differentiation, but reactivity may also be seen in megakaryocytes, platelets, some plasma cells, and macrophages; the latter can result in a misdiagnosis of angiosarcoma in a nonendothelial malignancy with numerous intratumoral macrophages.[273] CD34 is much less specific and slightly less sensitive than CD31 for poorly differentiated angiosarcoma but is a useful adjunctive marker because tumors rarely express CD34 in the absence of CD31. FLI1 shows comparable sensitivity to CD31 and CD34 and has the advantage of being a nuclear stain, but it is not specific for vascular tumors (see Table 13.1).[12] ERG is both highly sensitive and specific for angiosarcoma and also shows nuclear staining.[16] Postradiation angiosarcoma is usually positive for MYC, reflecting underlying gene amplification.[274,275] Approximately 50% of angiosarcomas express D2-40[2–4]; as previously mentioned, angiosarcomas are no longer divided into those of lymphatic versus blood vascular origin because they have similar clinical and histologic features.

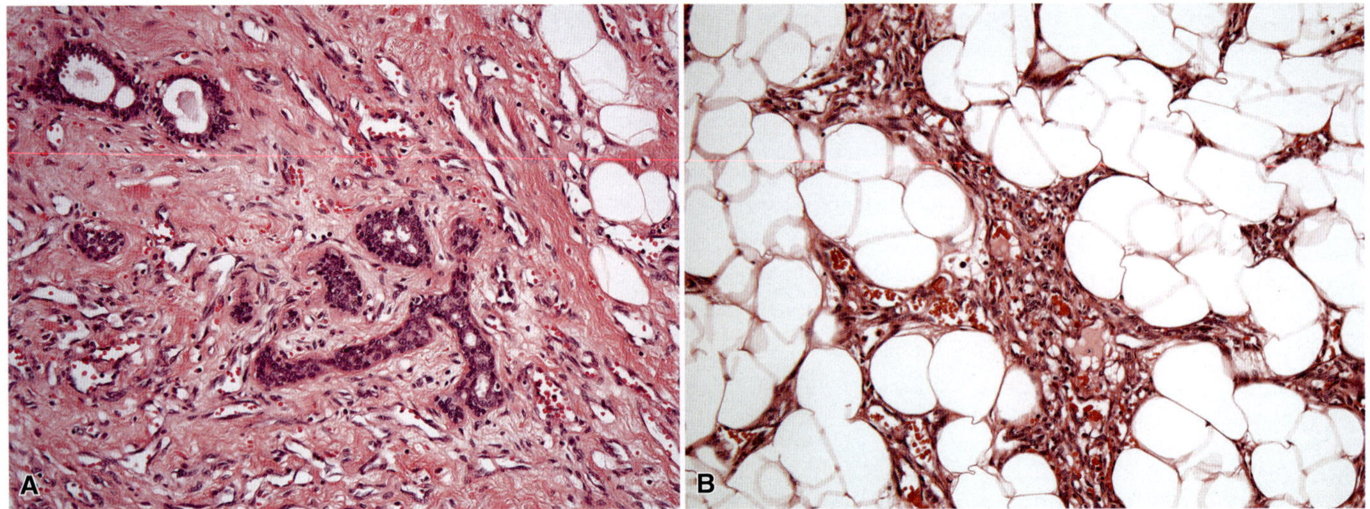

Figure 13.30 Mammary Angiosarcoma. (A) The deceptively bland lesional blood vessels show an infiltrative growth pattern around native ducts. (B) A morphologically higher-grade tumor showing increasing cellularity and atypia. Note the diffuse infiltration of adipose tissue.

Molecular Genetics

Secondary angiosarcomas (i.e., those associated with radiation or lymphedema) show amplification of the *MYC* gene by fluorescence in situ hybridization (FISH) analysis, whereas primary angiosarcomas rarely do so.[274] Importantly, *MYC* amplification is not found in postradiation atypical vascular proliferations.[275,276] Immunohistochemistry for MYC shows a strong correlation with FISH; therefore either technique may be used to aid in the differential diagnosis between postradiation angiosarcoma and postradiation atypical vascular proliferation. In histologically subtle cases of postradiation angiosarcoma, MYC immunohistochemistry can also be helpful for determining margin status.

Differential Diagnosis

The distinction between conventional angiosarcoma and specific non-neoplastic, benign, and malignant vascular tumors has been addressed previously. In general, angiosarcoma shows endothelial multilayering, a dissecting growth pattern, infiltrative margins, mitotic activity, and cytologic atypia. However, none of these features in isolation is sufficient for a malignant diagnosis, and integration of all histologic features with the clinical data is required. Conversely, low-grade angiosarcomas may be remarkably bland, and a high level of suspicion is required, particularly in the setting of head and neck lesions in elderly patients and in lesions in the mammary parenchyma. Immunostains for CD31 and ERG may be useful to highlight subtle infiltration of normal tissues, and additional levels on a biopsy specimen may help confirm the diagnosis.

Some cutaneous acantholytic (adenoid) squamous cell carcinomas have a pseudovascular pattern that can be confused with angiosarcoma.[277] Overt squamous differentiation is typically absent, but a connection to the epidermis or overlying epidermal atypia may suggest the diagnosis, and immunohistochemistry for endothelial markers is confirmatory.

Prognosis and Treatment

Angiosarcomas are aggressive, with an overall 5-year survival of approximately 35%, compared with 50% to 60% for all primary soft tissue sarcomas. The clinical setting (sporadic, postradiation, or lymphedema associated) and tumor depth (cutaneous, soft tissue, or visceral) correlate with prognosis, but this may be due in part to differences in clinical presentation and treatment options.[278] Early studies using antiangiogenic molecules, including bevacizumab (VEGF-A monoclonal antibody) and sorafenib (a broad-spectrum tyrosine-kinase inhibitor with anti-VEGFR activity), to treat soft tissue angiosarcoma have shown some promise.[279]

Sporadic cutaneous angiosarcoma of the head and neck has a poor prognosis, with long-term survival generally limited to patients who present with small (<5 cm), localized lesions.[231–233,242] Local recurrence is very common (80% to 90% of patients) because of the insidious spread of tumors into clinically normal skin as well as their frequent multifocality. Unfortunately, the accuracy of intraoperative frozen section for margin status in cutaneous angiosarcoma is low.[233] Approximately 50% of patients have metastases, most often to the lungs, cervical lymph nodes, and liver. Many patients are palliated for 1 year or longer with radiation or taxane-based chemotherapy regimens, but long-term survival is very uncommon.[229,233] The standard teaching has been that cutaneous angiosarcoma is uniformly high grade, with 5-year survival rates of 10% to 20%.[231,242] However, in a more recent study, the 5-year disease-specific survival rate was significantly better—48% for all patients combined—and classification based on histologic features (discussed earlier) resulted in clinically relevant prognostic groups, with 67% of those in the low-risk group surviving 5 years versus none of those in the high-risk group.[230]

The prognosis of lymphedema-associated cutaneous angiosarcoma is poor, with 5-year survival rates of 15% to 30%.[239–242] Patients treated with radical surgery (i.e., amputation) at the time of the initial diagnosis have the best chance of long-term survival.

The prognosis of postradiation angiosarcoma is difficult to determine because of its rarity and relatively short-term follow-up to date.[245,246,252–255] Local recurrences occur in at least 70% of cases and are often associated with the discovery of distant metastases, either synchronously or metachronously. In series with longer follow-up periods, metastatic and disease-related mortality rates ranged from 36% to 58%.[246,252,255,280] The effect of histologic grade on prognosis is controversial.

The rare cutaneous angiosarcomas that arise outside of the above three settings (i.e., sun-damaged skin of the elderly, lymphedema, and postradiation) tend to be of the epithelioid subtype and have an equally poor prognosis, with a 3-year mortality rate of 55% in a recent series.[281]

Angiosarcoma of soft tissue has a poor prognosis, with greater than 50% mortality within 1 year of diagnosis.[217] Half of patients develop metastases, most commonly to the lungs, lymph nodes, soft tissue, and bone, and 20% have local recurrences. Older age, larger tumor size, and retroperitoneal location are poor prognostic factors.

Similar to angiosarcoma of skin and soft tissue, mammary angiosarcoma is an aggressive tumor. Although early studies suggested that grading was prognostic among mammary parenchymal lesions,[269] more recent data indicated that the prognosis is uniformly poor.[268] Metastases occur in 50% to 60% of patients, and approximately 25% of patients have local recurrence. Lymph node metastases are very uncommon; therefore lymph node dissection is not indicated unless there is clinical suspicion. Mastectomy remains the treatment of choice in most cases to minimize the risk of local recurrence and subsequent distant spread.

PRACTICE POINTS: Angiosarcoma

- The clinical characteristics of angiosarcoma vary by site, but the histologic features are similar and the prognosis is uniformly poor, regardless of grade.
- In low-grade vasoformative tumors, the most helpful clues to a malignant diagnosis are diffuse infiltration of normal tissue, focal endothelial multilayering, and diffusely enlarged hyperchromatic nuclei.

Postradiation Atypical Vascular Lesion

Clinical Features

As the use of radiation in the treatment of breast carcinoma has increased, a distinct subset of radiation-induced vascular proliferations that show atypical (but not fully malignant) histologic features and generally follow a benign clinical course has been recognized.[253,282–286] These atypical vascular lesions arise a median of 3 to 5 years after radiation therapy,[253,284] overlapping with the 5- to 6-year latency period for postradiation angiosarcoma. They present clinically as solitary or multiple small (<1 cm), pink to red-brown papules or vesicles, in contrast to the large, irregular, blue-red patches, plaques, or nodules of postradiation angiosarcoma.

Pathologic Features

Histologically, atypical vascular lesions are relatively circumscribed, often wedge-shaped vascular proliferations involving the superficial and sometimes deep dermis (Fig. 13.31A).[284,286,287] Most cases have a lymphatic appearance, with thin-walled, irregular vessels that may be ectatic and superficial (see Fig. 13.31B), mimicking hobnail hemangioma or lymphangioma circumscriptum, or narrow and dissecting within the dermal collagen (see Fig. 13.31C), sometimes mimicking acquired progressive lymphangioma. Some cases have small intraluminal papillary projections. The endothelial cells may be cytologically bland or show mild nuclear atypia and hyperchromasia, but pleomorphism and prominent nucleoli are rare. A minority of atypical vascular lesions are dominated by capillary-type vessels, although a minor lymphatic component is often also present. This “vascular type” of atypical vascular lesion may show moderate nuclear atypia[287] but lacks other features of angiosarcoma, including complex anastomosing vessels with a dissecting growth pattern, endothelial multilayering, and extension into subcutaneous tissue. A patchy chronic inflammatory infiltrate is common in atypical vascular lesions.

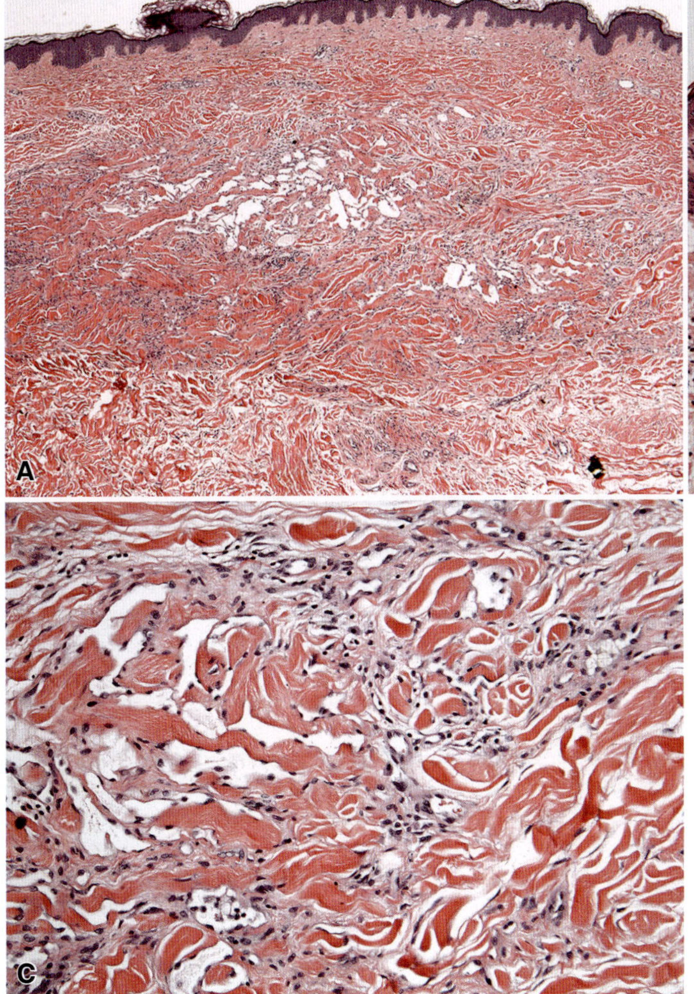

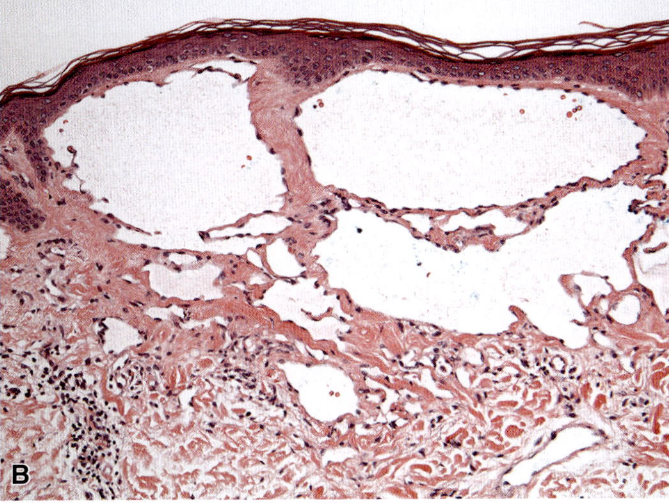

Figure 13.31 Atypical Postradiation Vascular Lesions. (A) This vascular lesion involves the mid-dermis and is wedge-shaped. (B) A superficial lesion containing widely dilated vessels, mimicking hobnail hemangioma. (C) This atypical vascular lesion shows a dissecting growth pattern through dermal collagen but lacks significant nuclear atypia or multilayering.

Table 13.4 Clinical and Histologic Features of Postradiation Atypical Vascular Lesions and Well-Differentiated Angiosarcomas

	Postradiation Atypical Vascular Lesion	Well-Differentiated Angiosarcoma
Clinical Features		
Clinical appearance	Pink-red papule(s)	Ecchymotic patches, plaques, or nodules
Size	<1 cm	>1 cm
Median latency period	3 years	6 years
Histologic Features		
Moderate to severe cytologic atypia	Absent	Present (may be focal)
Extension into subcutis	Absent	May be present
Margin	Relatively circumscribed	Diffusely infiltrative
Endothelial multilayering	Absent	Present
Mitoses	Absent	Present (infrequent to rare)
Necrosis	Absent	Uncommon

Differential Diagnosis

Atypical vascular lesions are distinguished from angiosarcoma histologically by the absence of anastomosing vessels, endothelial multilayering, mitotic activity, necrosis, and subcutaneous involvement. The features of postradiation atypical vascular lesions and cutaneous angiosarcomas are summarized in Table 13.4. The distinction between the two is generally straightforward, but occasional cases prove difficult to classify, suggesting that atypical vascular lesions and well-differentiated angiosarcoma may lie on a continuum.[269] As previously discussed under angiosarcoma, immunohistochemistry for MYC can be useful in this differential diagnosis because postradiation angiosarcomas consistently show strong nuclear reactivity and postradiation atypical vascular lesions are negative.[275]

As discussed earlier (see Table 13.3), distinguishing these lesions from hobnail hemangioma may be very difficult on histologic grounds and clinical history is crucial.

Prognosis and Treatment

Complete excision of all postradiation atypical vascular lesions is recommended (when feasible) because well-differentiated angiosarcomas frequently have foci that are histologically indistinguishable from atypical vascular lesions, and malignancy can only be excluded on examination of the entire lesion.[253,285] True local recurrence is very rare, but new atypical vascular lesions develop in approximately 20% of patients over time.[253,284,287] Development of angiosarcoma has been documented in rare cases, mandating close clinical follow-up for all patients with atypical vascular lesions.[253,287–289]

PRACTICE POINTS: Postradiation Atypical Vascular Lesion

- Atypical vascular lesions show a range of histologic features but often have a lymphangioma-like architecture.
- The endothelial cytologic features range from bland to hobnail; architectural features are most helpful in the differential diagnosis with angiosarcoma (see Table 13.4).
- The risk of angiosarcoma in patients with atypical vascular lesions appears to be very low, but complete excision and close follow-up are recommended.

Epithelioid Lesions

The family of epithelioid vascular tumors includes epithelioid hemangioma, epithelioid angiomatous nodule, epithelioid hemangioendothelioma, and epithelioid angiosarcoma. These tumors share plump, polygonal cells with abundant cytoplasm and occasional intracytoplasmic vacuoles, but their architectural and nuclear features vary markedly, allowing straightforward distinction in most cases.

The endothelial nature of epithelioid hemangioendothelioma and epithelioid angiosarcoma is often not readily apparent on routine sections; these tumors are also discussed in Chapter 6. In these cases the differential diagnosis may include epithelioid sarcoma and true epithelial tumors, particularly metastatic adenocarcinoma. Keratin expression in a minority of epithelioid vascular tumors adds to the risk of misinterpretation, but endothelial markers generally clarify the issue.

Epithelioid Hemangioma (Including Angiolymphoid Hyperplasia With Eosinophilia)

Clinical Features

Epithelioid hemangioma is most common in young to middle-aged adults and has a predilection for the head and neck region, particularly the periauricular area, followed by the distal extremities.[290–292] Most tumors involve the dermis or subcutaneous tissue, but a small proportion arise in deep soft tissue or bone.[293,294] The penis, oral mucosa, and lymph nodes are rare but well-documented sites.[295–297]

The tumors present as small subcutaneous nodules or erythematous papules that may be tender or pruritic. Up to 20% of patients have multiple lesions, typically within the same anatomic region.[292] Only 10% to 20% of patients have peripheral eosinophilia or regional lymphadenopathy,[298,299] in contrast to Kimura disease, with which epithelioid hemangioma has often been confused (discussed later).

Pathologic Features

At low power, epithelioid hemangioma is typically well circumscribed and has a lobular growth pattern, although these features tend to be more prominent in subcutaneous tumors than in those in the dermis, which have less well-defined margins. The vessels are predominantly capillary or venule sized, and the tumors often show a zonation pattern, with well-formed vessels at the periphery and compressed or poorly canalized channels in the center. In the latter areas, the endothelial cells form double-layer cords or, focally, a solid sheetlike appearance. In some examples of epithelioid hemangioma, the vessels are poorly canalized, and the lesions appear deceptively solid ("cellular epithelioid hemangioma").

The sine qua non of epithelioid hemangioma is plump cuboidal or hobnail ("tombstone") endothelial cells with abundant eosinophilic or amphophilic cytoplasm (Fig. 13.32A), plump round nuclei with fine chromatin, and occasional intracytoplasmic vacuoles. Some intratumoral vessels may be lined by flattened endothelium, but epithelioid endothelial cells predominate.

Most cases have a fibromyxoid stroma (see Fig. 13.32B), and a prominent mixed inflammatory infiltrate composed of lymphocytes and eosinophils is common, including lymphoid follicles. The infiltrate is often most pronounced at the periphery and in subcutaneous lesions may form a dense lymphoid cuff mimicking a lymph node. The designation *angiolymphoid hyperplasia with eosinophilia* has been applied to examples of epithelioid hemangioma in the head and neck in which the prominent inflammation obscures the epithelioid endothelial component[298,299]; however, neither a prominent lymphoid infiltrate nor the presence of eosinophils is required for the diagnosis, and the inflammatory component may be completely absent.

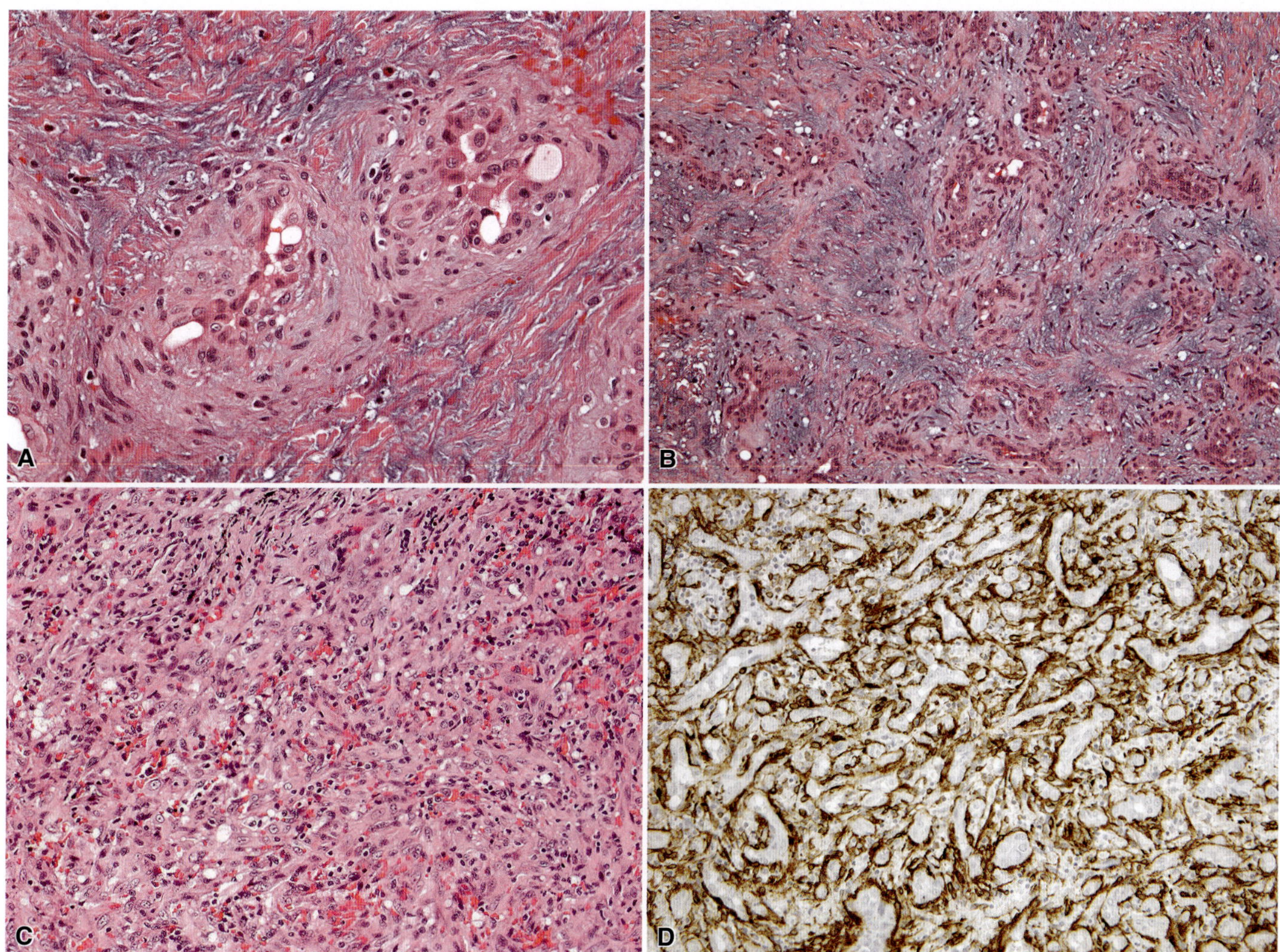

Figure 13.32 **Epithelioid Hemangioma.** (A) The lesional blood vessels contain plump endothelial cells with eosinophilic cytoplasm and occasional intracytoplasmic vacuoles. (B) Fibromyxoid stroma is common in epithelioid hemangioma. (C) Cellular epithelioid hemangioma with a solid appearance and poorly canalized vessels. (D) Immunostaining for smooth muscle actin highlights the pericytes and the vasoformative architecture.

Intimal or mural involvement of small subcutaneous muscular arteries or veins is common, and infrequently, the tumor is entirely intravascular.[298,300,301] Mitoses are rare in epithelioid hemangioma, and although mild nuclear atypia is common, nuclear pleomorphism is absent.

Immunohistochemistry

Reticulin and actin stains are useful in dissecting the architecture of the solid-appearing areas. The former highlights poorly canalized vessels with a single layer of endothelium, and the latter shows an intact layer of pericytes around compressed vessels (see Fig. 13.32C and D). True solid sheets of endothelial cells without vessel formation are not found in epithelioid hemangioma of skin and soft tissue. Keratin expression in epithelioid hemangioma has not been widely studied, but reactivity appears to be uncommon and focal (<25% of cells) when present.[295,302,303] A significant subset of epithelioid hemangiomas show nuclear staining for FOSB,[304] reflecting the presence of gene rearrangements (see next).

Molecular Genetics

FOSB gene rearrangements (usually with *ZFP36-FOSB* fusion, rarely *WWTR1-FOSB*) are found in approximately 20% of epithelioid hemangiomas.[305] Another 30% of epithelioid hemangiomas harbor *FOS* gene rearrangements (with a range of fusion partners), most often in soft tissue and bone lesions.[306,307] *FOSB* and *FOS* gene fusions appear to be more common in cellular epithelioid hemangiomas.[305,306] These gene fusions have not been identified in angiolymphoid hyperplasia with eosinophilia-type epithelioid hemangiomas evaluated thus far, suggesting that they may represent a distinct group,[306] although such tumors often show nuclear immunoreactivity for FOSB.[304]

Differential Diagnosis

Kimura disease, which has often been confused with epithelioid hemangioma, also presents as a subcutaneous mass in the head and neck region but shows a strong predilection for young Asian males and is usually associated with peripheral eosinophilia and regional lymphadenopathy.[298,308,309] Histologically, Kimura disease shows features of a reactive inflammatory process, including lymphoid follicles, a marked eosinophilic infiltrate with eosinophilic microabscesses, dense fibrosis, and proliferating high endothelial venules in the interfollicular zones. Although the endothelium may be plump and appear reactive, endothelial cells with abundant eosinophilic or amphophilic cytoplasm and intracytoplasmic vacuoles are not seen. The enlarged lymph nodes are involved by the same inflammatory process seen in the soft tissue; in contrast,

Table 13.5 Epithelioid Vascular Tumors

	Epithelioid Hemangioma	Epithelioid Angiomatous Nodule	Epithelioid Hemangioendothelioma[a]	Epithelioid Angiosarcoma
Architecture	Well-formed vessels predominate; focal cordlike or solid areas	Exophytic nodule; solid sheet of endothelial cells	Cords, strands, and single cells	Solid sheets, cleftlike spaces, and large, irregular vascular channels
Margins	Circumscribed	Circumscribed	Infiltrative	At least focally infiltrative
Cell shape	Cuboidal to hobnail	Plump, polygonal	Plump polygonal, oval, or stellate	Plump, polygonal
Cytoplasm	Eosinophilic to amphophilic	Eosinophilic to amphophilic	Pale pink, glassy	Eosinophilic to amphophilic
Intracytoplasmic vacuoles	Occasional	Occasional	Frequent	Variable
Inflammatory infiltrate	Prominent	Mild to moderate	Absent	Variable
Nuclear atypia	Absent to mild	Absent to mild	Mild to moderate	Moderate to severe
Mitotic figures	Rare	Variable	Rare/infrequent	Frequent

[a]Typical epithelioid hemangioendothelioma; features of "malignant" epithelioid hemangioendothelioma are discussed in the text.

the lymph nodes in cases of epithelioid hemangioma associated with lymphadenopathy show only reactive hyperplasia.

Despite similar nosology, epithelioid hemangioendothelioma rarely arises in the differential diagnosis for epithelioid hemangioma. Epithelioid hemangioendothelioma is composed of cords and strands of epithelioid endothelial cells, with glassy, pale pink cytoplasm in a myxohyaline stroma; vasoformative areas and an inflammatory infiltrate are typically absent (Table 13.5). Cellular epithelioid hemangiomas with solid-appearing foci may be misinterpreted as epithelioid angiosarcoma, particularly when the tumors arise at unusual sites.[295] Epithelioid angiosarcoma is often relatively monomorphic cytologically, and nuclear pleomorphism is uncommon. However, epithelioid angiosarcoma shows coarse chromatin, macronucleoli, and mitotic activity, which are not features of epithelioid hemangioma.

Inflamed lobular capillary hemangiomas and other benign vascular tumors can have markedly reactive, plump, epithelioid endothelium, but these changes are invariably focal and the intracytoplasmic vacuoles of epithelioid hemangioma are absent. Epithelioid angiomatous nodule is distinguished from epithelioid hemangioma on architectural grounds (see Table 13.5). The former is a solitary exophytic nodule composed of epithelioid endothelial cells arranged in sheets.

Prognosis and Treatment

Epithelioid hemangioma was originally considered a reactive lesion, but the presence of *FOS* and *FOSB* gene rearrangements supports a neoplastic process. Nearly one-third of lesions recur locally.

PRACTICE POINTS: Epithelioid Hemangioma

- Although epithelioid hemangioma is usually predominantly vasoformative, solid sheetlike areas may be present.
- Reticulin and actin stains can be used to highlight the poorly canalized vessels in these areas.
- *FOS* and *FOSB* gene rearrangements are found in a large subset of epithelioid hemangiomas; nuclear FOSB expression is common.

Epithelioid Angiomatous Nodule

Epithelioid angiomatous nodule is a recently described benign vascular lesion that shows morphologic overlap with epithelioid hemangioma but has distinctive clinical and histologic features.[310,311]

Clinical Features

Epithelioid angiomatous nodule presents as a solitary, red-blue exophytic papule or nodule, typically measuring less than 1 cm; multiple lesions are rare. Young to middle-aged adults are most commonly affected. The anatomic distribution is wide, and most tumors are cutaneous, but subcutaneous and mucosal lesions have also been reported.[310–312] Patients often report that the lesion developed rapidly over a period of weeks.

Pathologic Features

The tumors are well circumscribed, often exophytic, dermal nodules (Fig. 13.33A), composed predominantly of solid sheets of epithelioid cells, with occasional intracytoplasmic vacuoles (see Fig. 13.33B). Well-formed vessels lined by the epithelioid cells are also focally present. A lymphoid infiltrate, often with scattered eosinophils, is common, particularly at the periphery of the nodule. The overlying epidermis is often acanthotic and may form a collarette. A minority of tumors extend into the superficial subcutaneous tissue. Mitotic figures may be frequent and nucleoli are often prominent, but nuclear pleomorphism and necrosis are absent.

Immunohistochemistry

The epithelioid cells are positive for endothelial markers and negative for keratin.[311]

Differential Diagnosis

Although epithelioid angiomatous nodule and epithelioid hemangioma share many morphologic features, the predominantly solid architecture and absence of muscular vessel involvement in the former distinguish it from epithelioid hemangioma (see Table 13.5) epithelioid angiomatous nodules are negative for FOSB.[304]

Pyogenic granuloma lacks a sheetlike architecture and is only very rarely dominated by epithelioid endothelial cells. Epithelioid angiosarcoma is excluded by the small, well-circumscribed nature of the tumors and the absence of significant cytologic atypia.

Prognosis and Treatment

The nodules do not recur after excision, but infrequently, new lesions appear in the same anatomic region months later. Whether the lesions are reactive or neoplastic remains uncertain, but the frequently short clinical history and inflammatory infiltrate suggest a reactive etiology.

Epithelioid Hemangioendothelioma

Epithelioid hemangioendothelioma forms part of the spectrum of epithelioid vascular tumors, along with epithelioid hemangioma and epithelioid angiosarcoma.[313] Although originally described as a tumor of intermediate (borderline) malignancy, it is now classified as a malignant vascular neoplasm, albeit of lower grade than conventional angiosarcoma.[19,314] Epithelioid hemangioendothelioma is also discussed in Chapter 6.

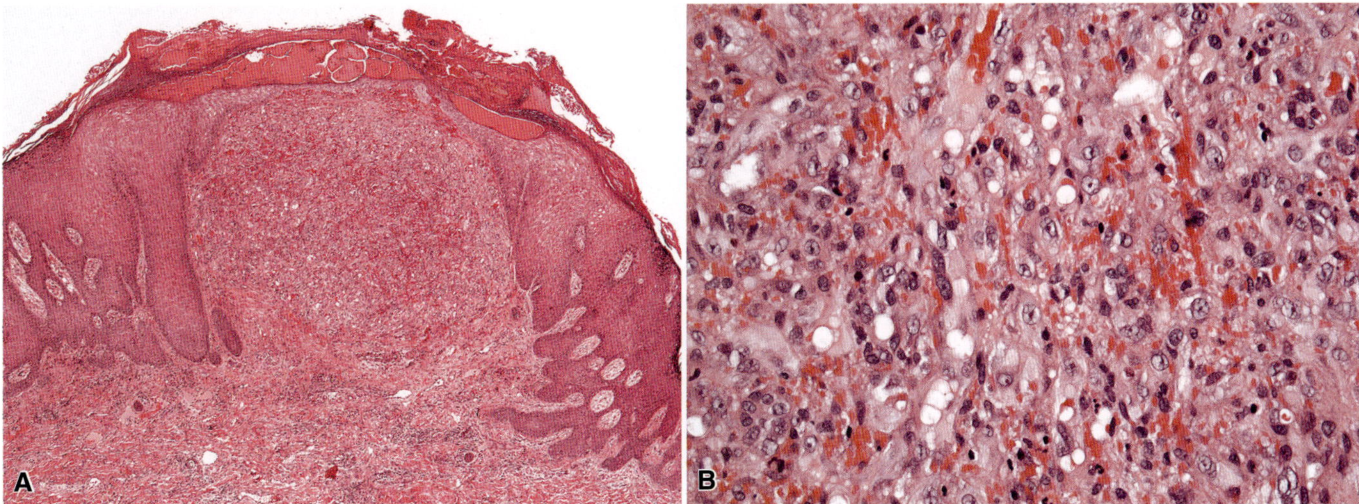

Figure 13.33 Epithelioid Angiomatous Nodule. (A) A well-circumscribed dermal nodule with adjacent epidermal hyperplasia. (B) Solid sheets of epithelioid endothelial cells with occasional intracytoplasmic vacuoles.

Table 13.6 Clinical Features of Epithelioid Hemangioendothelioma by Primary Site

	Soft Tissue	Bone	Lung	Liver
Age at presentation	Wide range; mean 48 years	Peak in second decade	Wide range; mean 40 years	Wide range; mean 40–45 years
Sex	F = M	F = M	F > M (2–3:1)	F > M (1.5:1)
Solitary vs. multifocal	Solitary	60% multifocal	90% multifocal; 75% bilateral	85% multifocal
Metastatic rate	20%–30%	20%	20%–30%	35%–45%
Mortality rate	15%	20%	40%–45%	35%–45%

F, Female; *M*, male.

Clinical Features

The most common sites for epithelioid hemangioendothelioma are somatic soft tissue,[313,314] bone,[315,316] lung,[317] and liver,[318,319] but tumors may arise at nearly any site, including the skin,[314,320] breast,[321] oral cavity,[322] brain,[323] lymph node,[297] thyroid,[324] and mediastinum.[325] The histologic features are identical, regardless of site, but the clinical presentation and prognosis are dependent on the anatomic location (Table 13.6). Epithelioid hemangioendotheliomas of skin and soft tissue are generally solitary, whereas bone and visceral tumors are often multicentric, within the same or different organs. Molecular genetic analysis has identified identical gene fusion breakpoints in multifocal epithelioid hemangioendothelioma, confirming that these are monoclonal tumors and therefore metastases rather than true multicentric disease.[326]

Epithelioid hemangioendothelioma of soft tissue affects adults of any age but is very uncommon in children.[313,314,327] There is a slight female predominance. Presenting symptoms include pain, edema, or thrombophlebitis as a result of partial occlusion of large vessels by the tumor. Tumors in deep soft tissue are somewhat more common than superficial lesions. Tumors range in size from less than 5 mm to greater than 15 cm.[314,327] Size is largely site dependent, with tumors in deep or visceral soft tissue often being very large at presentation.

Pathologic Features

In 40% to 50% of cases, soft tissue epithelioid hemangioendothelioma arises from a small to medium-sized vessel (usually a vein), which may be grossly identifiable. Histologically, the vessel wall is expanded by diffuse centrifugal growth of the tumor cells as they spread into adjacent soft tissue. Subcutaneous and deep-seated tumors often show diffuse infiltration of adjacent fat or skeletal muscle. In contrast, the rare primary cutaneous epithelioid hemangioendotheliomas are generally small and circumscribed and infrequently show involvement of a preexisting vessel.[314,320,328] Overlying epidermal hyperplasia is often seen in cutaneous tumors.

The tumor cells classically form anastomosing cords, strands, and single cells in a characteristic myxohyaline stroma (Fig. 13.34A). Occasionally, solid nests are present. Well-formed vascular channels are absent in conventional epithelioid hemangioendothelioma but may be found in the *YAP1-TFE3* variant discussed later. Intraluminal papillae with a hyaline core reminiscent of those seen in papillary intralymphatic angioendothelioma (Dabska tumor) are commonly present within the hepatic sinusoids and lymph node subcapsular sinus of hepatic and intranodal epithelioid hemangioendothelioma, respectively.[297,313,318]

Plump polygonal or stellate cells with characteristic pale pink, glassy cytoplasm dominate the tumors, although focal spindling may be seen. The nuclei are round, reniform, or folded, and they have vesicular chromatin with inconspicuous nucleoli. Intracytoplasmic vacuoles, occasionally containing an erythrocyte, are common (see Fig. 13.34B).

The myxohyaline stroma may be masked by varying degrees of stromal degeneration, including hemorrhage, cystic change, dense sclerosis, calcification, or necrosis.[314,319] Metaplastic ossification and osteoclastic giant cells are infrequent findings.[314,325] An inflammatory component is usually absent, but occasional cases show a mixed infiltrate of lymphocytes and eosinophils.

A small subset of epithelioid hemangioendotheliomas, characterized by a *YAP1-TFE3* gene fusion, has unique morphologic features. In contrast to typical epithelioid hemangioendothelioma, well-formed vascular spaces may be observed, and the endothelial cells often have voluminous eosinophilic cytoplasm and mild to moderate atypia (Fig. 13.35A).[329]

In typical epithelioid hemangioendothelioma, mitoses are very infrequent (≤1 per 10 high-power fields) and necrosis is rare. A minority of cases (approximately 10%) have worrisome histologic features and have been referred to as "malignant" epithelioid hemangioendothelioma (a misnomer as all epithelioid hemangioendotheliomas are now considered malignant).[313,314,327] In general, these tumors are

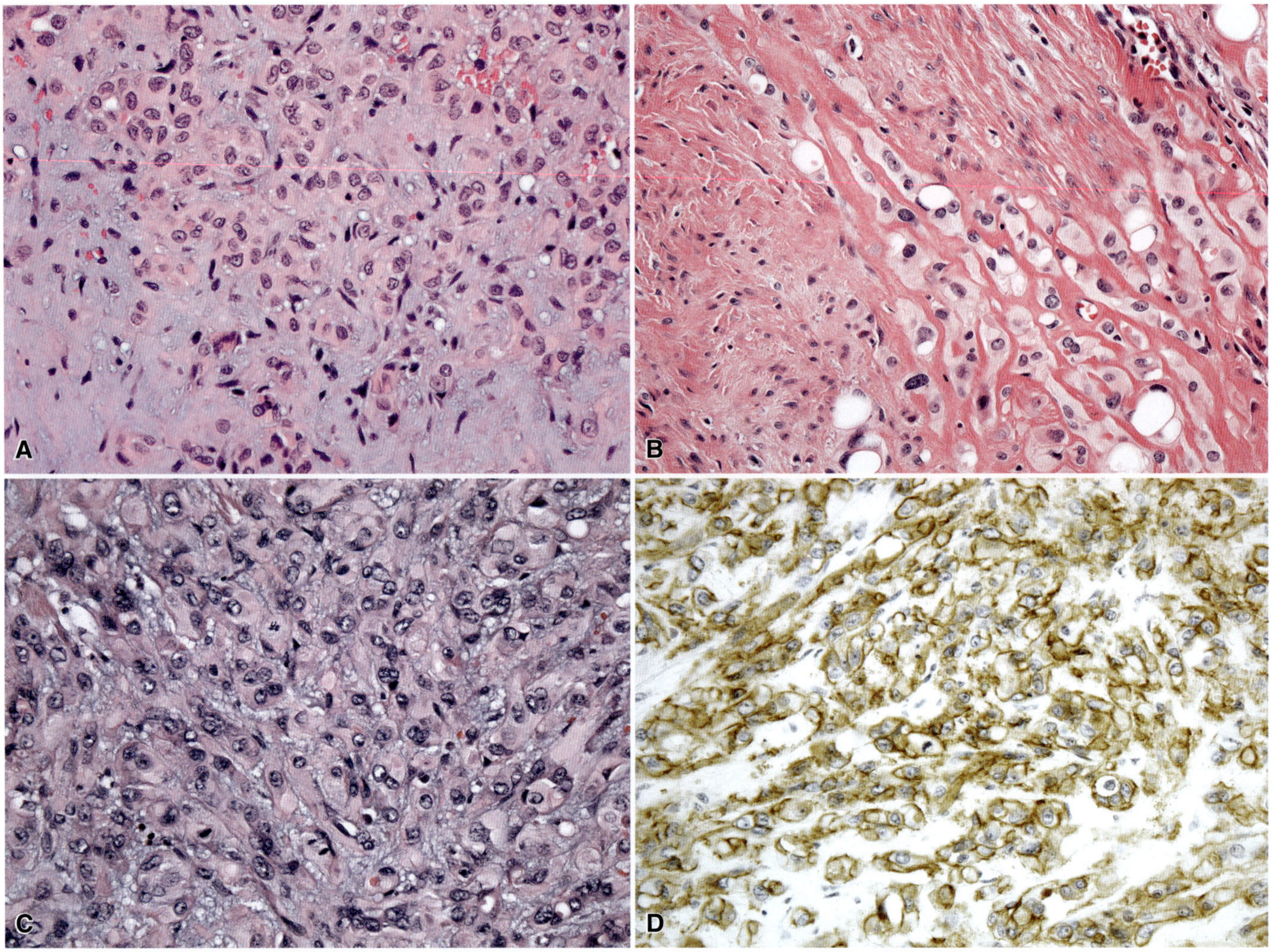

Figure 13.34 Epithelioid Hemangioendothelioma. (A) Epithelioid cells with glassy eosinophilic cytoplasm in a myxohyaline stroma. (B) Cords of epithelioid cells with pale cytoplasm and intracytoplasmic vacuoles. (C) "Malignant" epithelioid hemangioendothelioma showing more sheetlike growth, severe nuclear atypia, and a high mitotic rate. (D) CD31 is usually positive in epithelioid hemangioendothelioma.

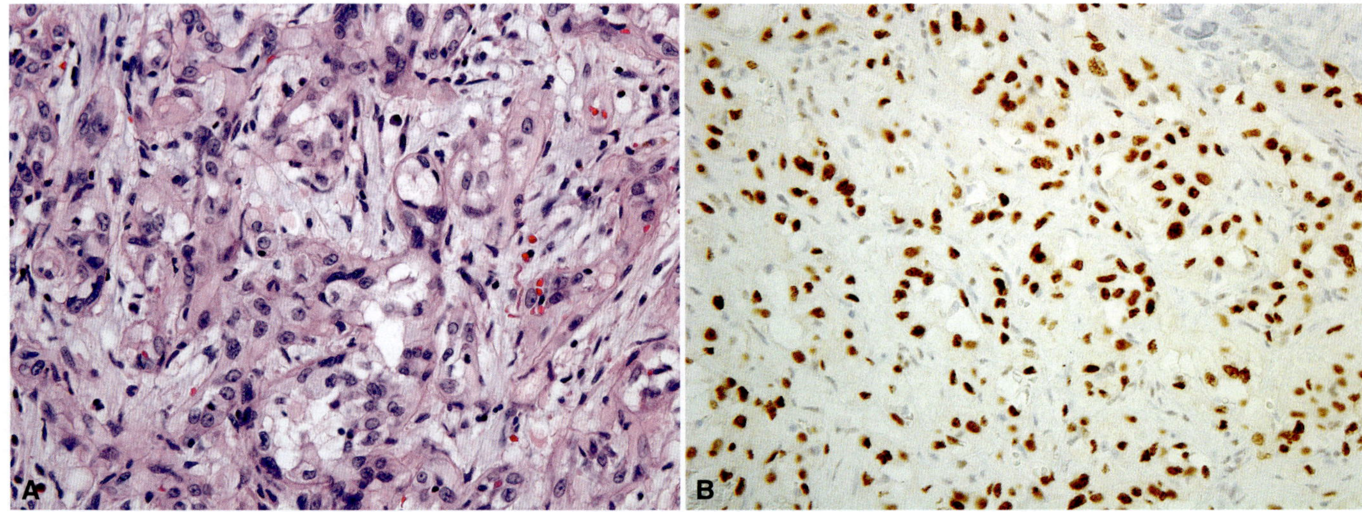

Figure 13.35 Epithelioid Hemangioendothelioma With *YAP1-TFE3* Fusion. (A) Epithelioid cells with abundant eosinophilic cytoplasm arranged in a vaguely nested architecture with occasional vascular lumens. (B) TFE3 is positive.

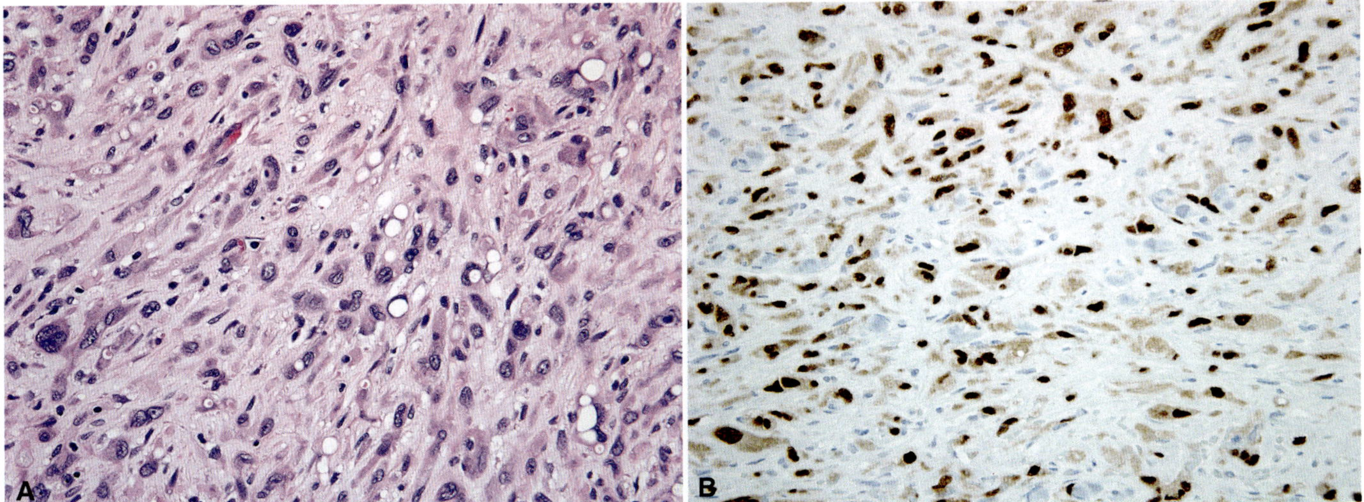

Figure 13.36 Epithelioid Hemangioendothelioma. (A) A trabecular arrangement of epithelioid cells. Note the occasional pleomorphic nuclei and intracytoplasmic vacuoles. (B) CAMTA1 is positive in 85%–90% of epithelioid hemangioendotheliomas.

characterized by solid sheetlike areas, nuclear pleomorphism, increased mitotic activity (see Fig. 13.34C), or necrosis. One study found that aggressive clinical behavior in soft tissue epithelioid hemangioendothelioma was best predicted by a mitotic rate greater than three per 50 high-power fields and tumor size greater than 3 cm.[327] "Malignant" epithelioid hemangioendothelioma is distinguished from epithelioid angiosarcoma by the presence of recognizable foci of typical epithelioid hemangioendothelioma.

Immunohistochemistry

Epithelioid hemangioendothelioma often expresses CD31 (see Fig. 13.34D), CD34, FLI1,[12] and ERG[16]; immunoreactivity in individual cases is variable and more than one vascular marker may be required. CD34 is less often positive than CD31 or ERG. Keratins are positive in 25% to 50% of tumors—and may be diffusely positive—but epithelial membrane antigen (EMA) reactivity is rare.[314,315,319,320,330] D2-40 has not been widely studied but is positive in at least a subset of epithelioid hemangioendotheliomas.[2,331] Approximately 50% of cases show actin positivity in the tumor cells.[314,320]

Immunohistochemistry directed at the recently described specific gene fusions of epithelioid hemangioendothelioma (discussed later) can be helpful to confirm the diagnosis. There is diffuse nuclear reactivity for CAMTA1 in cases with a *WWTR1-CAMTA1* fusion (85% to 90% of tumors) (Fig. 13.36), whereas cases with the *YAP1-TFE3* fusion show strong nuclear staining for TFE3 (see Fig. 13.35B).[329,332] TFE3 immunohistochemistry is less specific, as nuclear reactivity has also been reported in a subset of tumors with the *WWRT1-CAMTA1* fusion.[333]

Molecular Genetics

Two distinct subtypes of epithelioid hemangioendothelioma were recently recognized. Approximately 85% to 90% of cases, including conventional and some "malignant" epithelioid hemangioendotheliomas, have a *WWTR1-CAMTA1* fusion gene (resulting from a t(1:3) translocation).[334–336] A smaller subset (<5%) of epithelioid hemangioendotheliomas is characterized by a *YAP1-TFE3* fusion.[329,333] Tumors with the *YAP1-TFE3* fusion typically affect young adults and often show distinctive morphology, as described previously.

Differential Diagnosis

The polygonal cells with eosinophilic cytoplasm, intracytoplasmic vacuoles, and occasional keratin reactivity of epithelioid hemangioendothelioma may lead to misinterpretation as metastatic adenocarcinoma. Histologic features favoring epithelioid hemangioendothelioma over adenocarcinoma are intramural involvement of native vessels, minimal nuclear pleomorphism, and very low to absent mitotic activity. However, the distinction may be impossible without the use of immunohistochemistry for endothelial markers (e.g., CD31, CD34, and ERG).

Epithelioid hemangioendothelioma and epithelioid sarcoma can show significant histologic overlap, but the latter usually has a multinodular architecture, with central areas of necrosis or necrobiosis, and lacks the pale pink glassy cytoplasm of epithelioid hemangioendothelioma. Intracytoplasmic vacuoles and myxoid or hyalinized stroma are more common in epithelioid hemangioendothelioma but can be seen in epithelioid sarcoma. Immunohistochemistry is discriminatory: CD31 is rarely expressed in epithelioid sarcoma (although CD34 is positive in 50% of cases),[337] and EMA is invariably found in epithelioid sarcoma but is very rare in epithelioid hemangioendothelioma. CAMTA1 expression is specific for epithelioid hemangioendothelioma. SMARCB1 (INI1), a marker used in the diagnosis of epithelioid sarcoma, is also helpful: 95% of epithelioid sarcomas lose INI1 expression, whereas epithelioid hemangioendothelioma retains nuclear INI1 (as do nonneoplastic cells).[338]

High-grade myxoid liposarcoma occasionally grows in cords and trabeculae, which in conjunction with the myxoid stroma, may be reminiscent of epithelioid hemangioendothelioma. Myxoid liposarcomas are typically lobulated rather than diffusely infiltrative, and even in high-grade tumors, lipoblasts are usually identifiable, often at the periphery of the lobules, and the characteristic plexiform (crow's feet) vascular pattern is usually present. S-100 protein is frequently positive in high-grade myxoid liposarcoma, and this immunostain may also aid in the identification of lipoblasts. Furthermore, endothelial markers are uniformly negative.

Epithelioid hemangioendothelioma with a predominantly myxoid stroma may sometimes mimic extraskeletal myxoid chondrosarcoma, but the latter has a lobular architecture and is generally composed of monomorphic spindle cells with long cytoplasmic processes that form a reticular pattern. Adenomatoid tumors with a predominantly trabecular pattern may be mistaken for epithelioid hemangioendothelioma because of the presence of polygonal cells with intracytoplasmic vacuoles growing in cords and strands. However, these tumors nearly always arise in the genital tract (where epithelioid hemangioendothelioma is exceptionally rare) and they typically have tubules or cysts, sometimes with intraluminal mucin. Keratin and calretinin are uniformly positive in adenomatoid tumors, whereas endothelial markers are negative.

In most cases, epithelioid hemangioendothelioma shows little overlap with the other epithelioid vascular tumors (see Table 13.5). Epithelioid hemangioendothelioma grows in cords and strands without overtly vasoformative areas, whereas epithelioid hemangioma is predominantly vasoformative and epithelioid angiosarcoma has solid sheets of cells with focal vasoformative foci. The pale pink glassy cytoplasm and ovoid to spindled or stellate cells of epithelioid hemangioendothelioma contrast with the eosinophilic to amphophilic cytoplasm and plump polygonal cells of epithelioid hemangioma and epithelioid angiosarcoma. The latter two also lack the characteristic myxohyaline stroma of epithelioid hemangioendothelioma. However, the newly defined subset of epithelioid hemangioendotheliomas with *YAP1-TFE3* fusion often shows abundant eosinophilic cytoplasm and vasoformative areas, such that the features overlap with epithelioid hemangioma. In these cases the presence of mild-to-moderate nuclear atypia and immunoreactivity for TFE3 favor epithelioid hemangioendothelioma over epithelioid hemangioma. At the other end of the spectrum, some cases of "malignant" epithelioid hemangioendothelioma are nearly identical to epithelioid angiosarcoma, with the exception of focal typical epithelioid hemangioendothelioma-like areas. Immunohistochemistry for CAMTA1 can be invaluable for confirming the diagnosis of "malignant" epithelioid hemangioendothelioma, particularly on small biopsies.

Prognosis and Treatment

As discussed earlier, epithelioid hemangioendothelioma is now considered a sarcoma based on significant rates of metastasis and mortality.[19,295,314] Between 10% and 15% of patients with soft tissue epithelioid hemangioendothelioma have local recurrences. Metastases develop in 20% to 30% of patients, and 15% die of tumor.[314,321,327] Dividing the tumors into malignant/high-risk and conventional epithelioid hemangioendothelioma based on the criteria discussed earlier improves prognostication. The metastatic and mortality rates for malignant/high-risk epithelioid hemangioendothelioma are approximately 50% and 30%, respectively, compared with 17% and 3%, respectively, for conventional epithelioid hemangioendothelioma. Because a small proportion of cases of histologically typical epithelioid hemangioendothelioma behave in a malignant fashion and typical lesions may acquire malignant features in recurrences, long-term (>10-year) clinical follow-up is required.

The prognosis for cutaneous epithelioid hemangioendothelioma is excellent, as expected for small, superficial sarcomas. The recurrence rate is low, and no metastases or deaths have been reported.[314,320]

In contrast to most other sarcomas, epithelioid vascular tumors, including epithelioid hemangioendothelioma and epithelioid angiosarcoma, show a propensity for lymph node metastasis. Approximately 50% of metastases of epithelioid hemangioendothelioma are to regional lymph nodes, with the remainder primarily involving lungs, liver, and bone.[321,327] Rarely, patients with soft tissue epithelioid hemangioendothelioma may have synchronous or metachronous involvement of bone or visceral organs but have prolonged survival.[314]

PRACTICE POINTS: Epithelioid Hemangioendothelioma

- Although formerly classified with intermediate tumors, epithelioid hemangioendothelioma is now considered a low-grade sarcoma.
- Myxohyaline stroma, cells with glassy pink cytoplasm and intracytoplasmic vacuoles, and the absence of well-formed vessels are characteristic.
- "Malignant" epithelioid hemangioendothelioma shows frequent mitoses, significant nuclear atypia, necrosis, or solid sheetlike areas; the prognosis is significantly worse than for typical epithelioid hemangioendothelioma.
- *WWTR1-CAMTA1* fusions are found in 85% to 90% of epithelioid hemangioendotheliomas, resulting in nuclear expression of CAMTA1.
- A small subset of epithelioid hemangioendotheliomas, often with distinctive histologic features (voluminous cytoplasm, focal vasoformative architecture), harbor *YAP1-TFE3* fusions.

Epithelioid Angiosarcoma

Clinical Features

Although epithelioid cells are sometimes found as a minor component in conventional angiosarcoma, tumors in which epithelioid cytomorphologic features predominate are designated *epithelioid angiosarcoma*.[230] Most soft tissue angiosarcomas are epithelioid, as are the rare primary angiosarcomas of the adrenal gland, thyroid, and small intestine and the exceptionally rare cases of angiosarcoma arising within a benign schwannoma or chronic hematoma.[260,263,265–267,271] In contrast, epithelioid angiosarcoma is very uncommon in the skin and mammary parenchyma, with the exception of the rare pediatric cutaneous angiosarcomas, which tend to be epithelioid.[339–341] The clinical presentation is not distinctive in most cases, but a small number of patients present with signs of bleeding, including anemia, hemothorax or hemoperitoneum, a soft tissue hematoma, or gastrointestinal bleeding.

Pathologic Features

These tumors may show a nodular or lobular growth pattern and often show at least focally infiltrative margins. A solid, sheetlike arrangement is most common, but a nested or alveolar architecture simulating a carcinoma may be seen.[217] Dilated vessels lined by neoplastic cells are often focally present, particularly at the periphery.

The tumor cells are plump and round to polygonal, with a moderate amount of eosinophilic or amphophilic cytoplasm and large vesicular nuclei with coarse chromatin and prominent nucleoli (Fig. 13.37). Despite the high-grade nuclear features, significant nuclear pleomorphism is uncommon. Scattered intracytoplasmic vacuoles are typically present but may be scarce. Rarely, granular cell change has been described.[323]

Immunohistochemistry

The immunohistochemical profile is similar to that of typical angiosarcoma. Importantly, given the histologic resemblance to poorly differentiated carcinoma, 30% to 50% of epithelioid angiosarcomas express keratins and rare cases express EMA.[217,261,266,330] Approximately 10% of conventional angiosarcomas also express keratins,[330] but this rarely poses a problem because epithelial neoplasms do not enter the differential diagnosis.

A reticulin stain may outline uncanalized vascular channels in solid epithelioid areas and may show endothelial multilayering in compressed or poorly formed vessels but is now rarely used.[234,270] Actin stains may rarely show a layer of pericytes in well-differentiated, vasoformative foci, but pericytes are typically absent in the sheetlike areas.[217,234]

Differential Diagnosis

The differential diagnosis is broad because the vascular nature of the tumor may not be apparent on routine sections. Common considerations include poorly differentiated carcinoma, proximal-type epithelioid sarcoma, metastatic melanoma, epithelioid malignant peripheral nerve

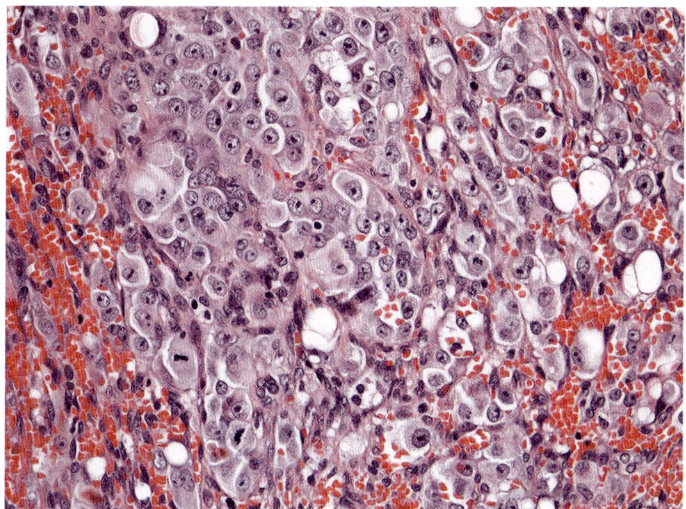

Figure 13.37 Epithelioid Angiosarcoma. Sheets of large epithelioid cells with abundant amphophilic cytoplasm, vesicular nuclei, and prominent nucleoli.

sheath tumor, and anaplastic large cell lymphoma. Keratin expression in the setting of an epithelioid neoplasm can lead to misinterpretation of epithelioid angiosarcoma as metastatic carcinoma or proximal-type epithelioid sarcoma. Histologically, focal vessel formation points to the diagnosis of angiosarcoma. Immunohistochemistry for vascular markers is discriminatory. Carcinomas do not express CD31 or CD34, and epithelioid sarcoma does not usually express CD31, although it should be noted that CD34 is positive in 50% of cases. In difficult cases, immunohistochemistry for SMARCB1 (INI1) is helpful because 95% of proximal-type epithelioid sarcomas show loss of INI1 expression, whereas epithelioid angiosarcomas show intact staining.[338]

Epithelioid malignant peripheral nerve sheath tumor and metastatic melanoma are readily differentiated by strong S-100 protein reactivity in nearly all cases. Anaplastic large cell lymphoma is distinguished by the presence of CD30 in a membranous and/or Golgi pattern.

Prognosis and Treatment

The prognosis and treatment were discussed earlier.

Spindle Cell Lesions

Vascular lesions dominated by a spindle cell pattern include kaposiform hemangioendothelioma, spindle cell hemangioma, Kaposi sarcoma, a subset of angiosarcomas, and pseudomyogenic hemangioendothelioma; the latter tumor type is discussed in Chapters 3 and 15. The vascular nature of spindle cell hemangioma is usually obvious, and the diagnosis is rarely challenging if one is familiar with the characteristic histologic features. Nonvascular tumors may enter the differential diagnosis of kaposiform hemangioendothelioma, Kaposi sarcoma, and spindle cell angiosarcoma. Compressed vascular channels, numerous extravasated erythrocytes, hemosiderin deposition, and (in angiosarcoma) intracytoplasmic vacuoles are helpful clues to endothelial differentiation, and immunohistochemical stains are confirmatory.

Spindle Cell Hemangioma

Spindle cell hemangioma was originally described as *spindle cell hemangioendothelioma*, based on the finding of frequent local recurrences (now considered multifocal lesions) and a single report of malignant transformation in a patient who had received radiation therapy.[342] The name was changed to *spindle cell hemangioma* when further data indicated a benign clinical course (discussed later).[343,344] A preexisting vascular malformation is identified in some cases.

Clinical Features

Most spindle cell hemangiomas are sporadic, but 5% to 10% arise in the setting of Maffucci syndrome (along with enchondromas), and rare cases have been reported in association with Klippel-Trénaunay syndrome, congenital lymphedema, or long-standing venous varicosities.[343–345] Patients present over a wide age range, but there is often a long clinical history, and many lesions were first noted in childhood. The tumors are most common on the distal extremities but may occur in a variety of anatomic sites, including the chest wall, genital area, head and neck, and oral cavity.[342,345–347] Rarely, spindle cell hemangioma arises in deep soft tissue or, exceptionally, at visceral sites.[343]

Approximately 50% of patients have multiple lesions, usually in the same anatomic region. However, patients with Maffucci syndrome frequently have synchronous or metachronous tumors at distant sites.[342,344,345,347] The tumors present as flesh-colored or bluish subcutaneous or deep dermal nodules, typically measuring less than 2 cm.

Pathologic Features

The tumors are multinodular within the dermis or subcutaneous tissue. The three classic histologic features, found in variable proportions in any given case, are widely dilated vascular spaces, solid spindle cell areas, and plump, rounded, or polygonal endothelial cells, with clear, often vacuolated cytoplasm (Fig. 13.38A). The cavernous vascular spaces often contain thrombi, phleboliths, or endothelial-lined fibrous papillae (in contrast to the hyaline papillae of intravascular papillary endothelial hyperplasia), which may also be found associated with organizing thrombi. The solid areas are composed of spindle cells in a haphazard or short fascicular pattern surrounding partially collapsed or poorly formed, slitlike vascular channels (see Fig. 13.38B). Small numbers of plump endothelial cells with intracytoplasmic vacuoles are found in the solid areas, either in clusters or lining the compressed vascular channels; when numerous, the vacuolated endothelial cells may mimic lipoblasts. Depending on whether angiomatous areas or solid areas predominate, the low-power appearance of spindle cell hemangioma may resemble a cavernous hemangioma or, conversely, nodular Kaposi sarcoma.

More than 50% of cases have an intravascular component, which may be mistaken for lymphovascular invasion, and 10% to 20% of spindle cell hemangiomas are entirely intravascular.[342,344,347] Significant atypia is rare, but in very rare cases, degenerative nuclear atypia may be seen in the spindle cells.[343] Mitoses are absent or scarce (≤1 per 50 high-power fields).

In many cases, the deep dermis or subcutis adjacent to the lesion contains abnormal thick-walled blood vessels that may be numerous enough to suggest a venous or arteriovenous malformation.[344,348] In addition, aberrant smooth muscle bundles may be found either adjacent to the dilated vessels or within the spindle cell areas.[344] Based on these features, some authors have suggested that spindle cell hemangioma may arise in response to a localized abnormality of blood flow, either congenital (i.e., vascular malformation) or acquired.[344]

Immunohistochemistry

Immunohistochemical and ultrastructural studies have shown that the spindle cells are predominantly fibroblasts, with a smaller population of pericytes immediately adjacent to the slitlike vessels.[348] Reticulin stains highlight the compressed vascular channels within the solid areas.

Molecular Genetics

Somatic mosaic *IDH1* mutations (or, rarely, *IDH2* mutations) have been identified in spindle cell hemangiomas (as well as enchondromas) from patients with Maffucci syndrome.[349,350] Sporadic spindle cell hemangiomas also harbor *IDH1* or *IDH2* mutations (usually *IDH1* R132C).[351]

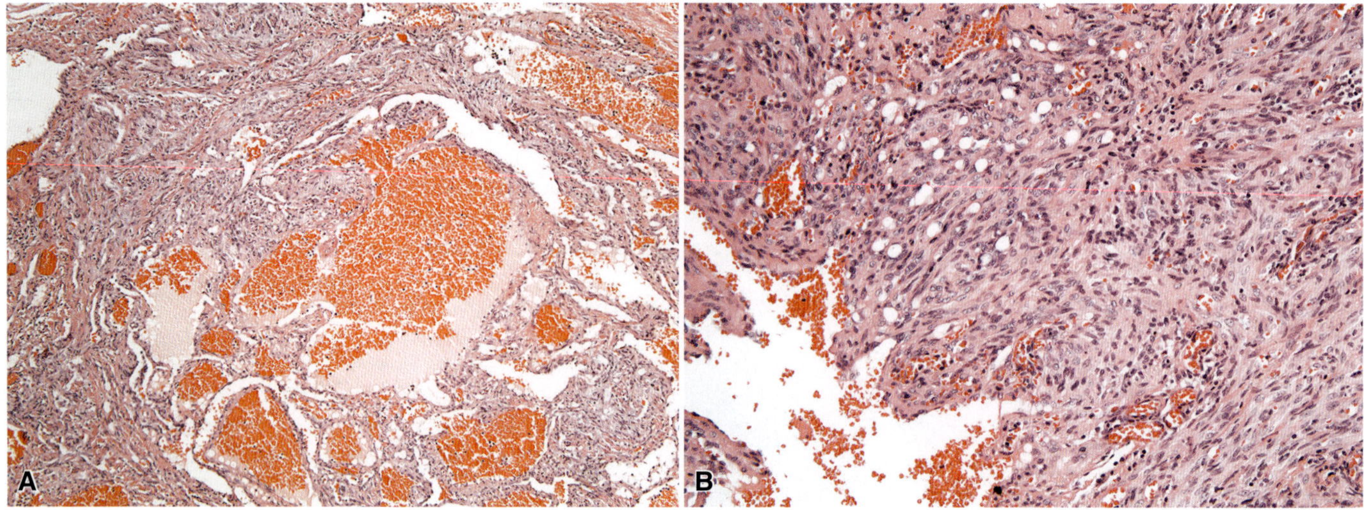

Figure 13.38 Spindle Cell Hemangioma. (A) The lesion is composed of dilated vascular spaces and solid areas of spindle cells. (B) Sheets of bland spindle cells and smaller numbers of epithelioid endothelial cells with intracytoplasmic vacuoles.

Differential Diagnosis

Although the solid areas of spindle cell hemangioma show a resemblance to nodular Kaposi sarcoma, the latter lacks cavernous vascular spaces, plump or vacuolated endothelial cells, and intravascular spread. The distinction is generally not difficult when the entire lesion is evaluated, but in the setting of a limited biopsy specimen, immunohistochemistry for HHV-8 is helpful because expression of this marker is uniformly negative in spindle cell hemangiomas.[189–191]

Entirely intravascular spindle cell hemangiomas may mimic intravascular papillary endothelial hyperplasia (Masson tumor) because of the presence of numerous intravascular papillae associated with thrombi. However, the papillae of spindle cell hemangioma are fibrous and mildly cellular rather than hyaline and acellular, as in intravascular papillary endothelial hyperplasia. Furthermore, solid spindle cell areas and vacuolated endothelial cells are not seen in intravascular papillary endothelial hyperplasia.

Prognosis and Treatment

Although more than half of patients experience local recurrences, these typically occur over decades, often arise near surgical scars rather than within them, and are most common in patients with multifocal disease at presentation.[343,344] Therefore most such "recurrences" likely represent multifocal tumors arising in the same anatomic region, perhaps because of an underlying vascular abnormality or intravascular spread of the lesion. Spindle cell hemangiomas do not metastasize; the single reported case of malignant transformation with metastasis is now considered a postradiation sarcoma.[342,343]

PRACTICE POINTS: Spindle Cell Hemangioma

- The classic features of spindle cell hemangioma are cavernous vascular spaces, solid spindled areas, and vacuolated endothelial cells.
- Tumors are frequently multifocal but are clinically benign.
- Tumors harbor mutations in *IDH1* or *IDH2*.

Kaposiform Hemangioendothelioma

Clinical Features

Kaposiform hemangioendothelioma typically occurs in infants and young children, but rare cases have been reported in adults.[352] Most tumors involve the deep soft tissue of the extremities or retroperitoneum; however, a significant minority of cases occur on the head and neck or trunk and some arise in superficial soft tissue. Very rare cases of multifocal kaposiform hemangioendothelioma have been reported.[353,354] Tumors in the deep soft tissue of the limbs may be clinically undetectable or may form an indurated mass, whereas superficial tumors present as ill-defined violaceous plaques. Patients with retroperitoneal tumors typically present with abdominal distention, jaundice, or gastrointestinal bleeding or obstruction. Approximately 20% of cases of kaposiform hemangioendothelioma arise in association with lymphangiomatosis, which may have been clinically undetected before tumor presentation and may involve distant sites, as well as the soft tissue adjacent to the lesion.[143,355]

Kaposiform hemangioendothelioma is the most common cause of Kasabach-Merritt syndrome, a potentially fatal coagulopathy in which active platelet trapping within the neoplastic vasculature leads to profound thrombocytopenia, and in some cases, microangiopathic hemolytic anemia.[181,356] The incidence of Kasabach-Merritt syndrome in patients with kaposiform hemangioendothelioma is greater than 50%, and it approaches 100% among retroperitoneal tumors.[355,357] Tufted angioma has also been reported as a cause of Kasabach-Merritt syndrome. However, in many cases the diagnosis of tufted angioma was made on a posttreatment biopsy. Because histologic overlap between tufted angioma and kaposiform hemangioendothelioma (particularly after therapy) is well recognized,[181,358,359] the true risk of Kasabach-Merritt syndrome in patients with tufted angioma is unclear.

Pathologic Features

Retroperitoneal tumors are often very infiltrative and may invade the pancreas, spleen, lymph nodes, intestines, and even the deep soft tissue of the abdominal wall.[360,361] Deep-seated somatic soft tissue tumors have similarly infiltrative margins, whereas those involving only the skin and subcutaneous tissue are often surrounded by dense fibrosis and appear relatively circumscribed.

The tumors form ill-defined lobules that coalesce into solid sheets of spindled endothelial cells (Fig. 13.39A). Within the lobules, the spindle cells form short fascicles with numerous slitlike vascular spaces containing red blood cells, mimicking Kaposi sarcoma (see Fig. 13.39B). Rounded capillaries, commonly containing fibrin microthrombi, are found at the

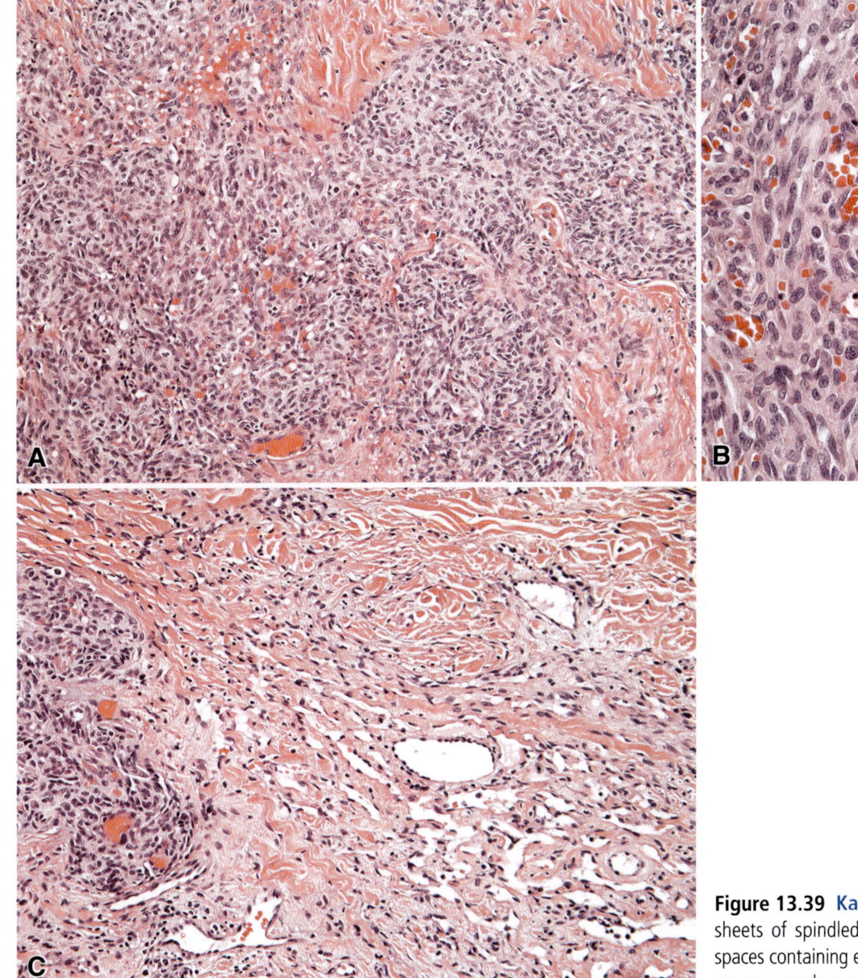

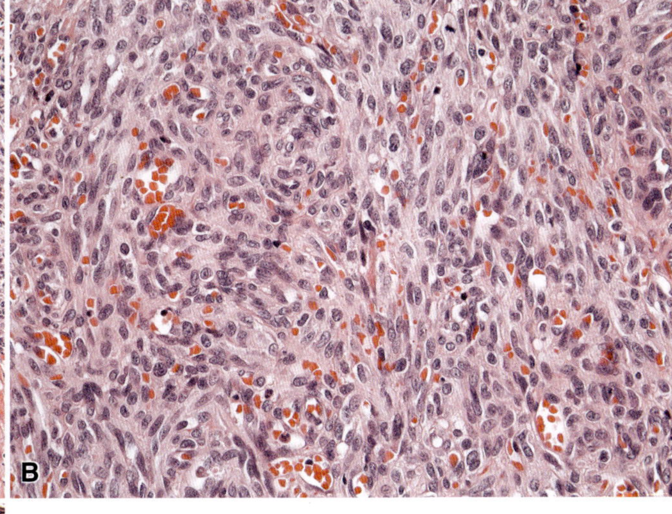

Figure 13.39 **Kaposiform Hemangioendothelioma.** (A) Coalescing lobules and sheets of spindled endothelial cells. (B) Short fascicles of spindle cells with slitlike spaces containing erythrocytes, mimicking Kaposi sarcoma. (C) Dilated lymphatic vessels are commonly seen at the periphery of kaposiform hemangioendothelioma.

periphery of lobules. Frequently, small "glomeruloid" clusters of epithelioid endothelial cells are identified within the spindled areas. Hemosiderin deposition (both stromal and intracytoplasmic) is common, and hyaline globules may be seen.[352,355] Mitoses are infrequent and cytologic atypia is absent.

Two-thirds of cases have scattered dilated lymphatic vessels or, less often, a lymphatic malformation in the soft tissue adjacent to the tumor (see Fig. 13.39C).[357] Some patients are known to have preexisting lymphangiomatosis, whereas in others, focally dilated lymphatic vessels may simply be reactive, induced by the tumor.

Immunohistochemistry

More than 90% of kaposiform hemangioendotheliomas express D2-40, LYVE-1, and VEGFR-3, consistent with lymphatic differentiation.[11,143,183,362] The well-formed capillaries at the periphery of the lobules and the glomeruloid clusters have an intact layer of actin-positive pericytes, whereas only sparse pericytic cells are found within the spindle cell areas.[352,355,357] The tumors do not express GLUT1.[357]

Differential Diagnosis

The histologic features of kaposiform hemangioendothelioma overlap significantly with those of Kaposi sarcoma (see Table 13.2). However, with the exception of the African lymphadenopathic form, Kaposi sarcoma is exceptionally rare in children. It also lacks a lobular growth pattern, well-formed capillaries with fibrin microthrombi, and epithelioid endothelial cells. Conversely, a lymphoplasmacytic infiltrate and HHV-8 reactivity are not seen in kaposiform hemangioendothelioma.[357]

It is sometimes difficult to distinguish between kaposiform hemangioendothelioma and tufted angioma, and some authors believe that the two tumors are closely related, if not identical.[143,356,357,359] Although there are undoubtedly "gray zone" cases, the two neoplasms can be distinguished in most instances. A fascicular spindle cell component is invariably present in kaposiform hemangioendothelioma and is not a feature of tufted angioma. In addition, tufted angioma is based in the dermis and the tumor nodules are more widely spaced and smaller than those of kaposiform hemangioendothelioma.

Prognosis and Treatment

Surgical excision is often contraindicated in patients with retroperitoneal kaposiform hemangioendothelioma because of severe thrombocytopenia or extensive infiltration of normal tissues. However, several centers have reported successful treatment of these lesions with combination chemotherapy regimens, including vincristine.[363,364]

Distant metastases have not been reported, but spread to regional lymph nodes or perinodal soft tissue located several centimeters from the primary mass was documented in two cases.[355,357] Mortality rates range from 10% to 25% overall and exceed 50% in patients with retroperitoneal tumors.[356,365] The most common causes of death are cerebral or intraabdominal hemorrhage secondary to thrombocytopenia, sepsis, and invasion of intraabdominal organs.

PRACTICE POINTS: Kaposiform Hemangioendothelioma

- Kaposiform hemangioendothelioma typically arises in the retroperitoneum or deep somatic soft tissue of infants and young children.
- Patients with Kasabach-Merritt syndrome (consumptive coagulopathy) have a high risk of mortality.
- Large, poorly defined lobules of fascicular spindle cells separated by slitlike spaces (mimicking Kaposi sarcoma) characterize the tumor.

Kaposi Sarcoma

Kaposi sarcoma is a multifocal, virus-induced vascular proliferation associated with HHV-8 in nearly all cases.[366] However, only a small proportion of patients seropositive for HHV-8 have Kaposi sarcoma, indicating that infection is necessary but not sufficient to induce the lesions. Whether Kaposi sarcoma represents a virus-induced endothelial hyperplasia or a neoplastic process has long been debated.[367–369] The spindle cells in Kaposi sarcoma are usually oligoclonal, and lesions at different anatomic sites in a single patient have viral episomes of different sizes, suggesting that Kaposi sarcoma is a nonneoplastic process in which multicentric lesions are independent clones rather than metastases.[370] However, based on the fulminant clinical course of some subtypes, Kaposi sarcoma is classified as a tumor of intermediate biologic potential in the WHO classification.

Clinical Features

Kaposi sarcoma is divided into four forms, based on the clinical setting: classic, African endemic, iatrogenic, and epidemic.[366,371,372] Classic Kaposi sarcoma presents as indolent cutaneous lesions in elderly persons of Eastern European or Mediterranean ancestry, with a striking male predominance (up to 15:1). The distal extremities, particularly the feet, are the initial site of predilection, and in many patients the disease remains localized to this area. Up to 10% of patients with classic Kaposi sarcoma have visceral or mucosal involvement, but the disease is very rarely a cause of death.[373–375]

The African endemic form includes three major subtypes: (1) an indolent cutaneous form that occurs predominantly in men and resembles classic Kaposi sarcoma; (2) a locally aggressive cutaneous variant that also primarily affects men and may be associated with bone involvement; and (3) an aggressive form that presents in childhood as generalized lymphadenopathy, with or without cutaneous lesions, and is often rapidly fatal.[376,377]

Iatrogenic Kaposi sarcoma is a rare complication of immunosuppression in patients who are immunocompromised because of transplantation or other reasons. As in classic Kaposi sarcoma, this form is more common among patients of Eastern European or Mediterranean descent. The clinical course depends on the degree of immunosuppression and ranges from indolent cutaneous lesions that regress on withdrawal of immunosuppressants to an aggressive disseminated disease.

Finally, epidemic Kaposi sarcoma affects patients with AIDS, with a strong predilection for homosexual men. Cutaneous lesions are typically widespread. The clinical course varies from indolent to rapidly progressive, with visceral disease.[378] As in iatrogenic Kaposi sarcoma, the prognosis depends primarily on the patient's immune status.

Regardless of the clinical subtype, Kaposi sarcoma has three clinical and histologic stages: patch, plaque, and nodular. All three are frequently present simultaneously. The earliest lesions are blue-red macules, which may become elevated over time, progressing to plaques or nodules. Older lesions may spontaneously regress, but new lesions generally appear in the same anatomic region. In patients with disseminated Kaposi sarcoma the most common extracutaneous sites of involvement are the lymph nodes, gastrointestinal tract, and lung.

Pathologic Features

Kaposi sarcoma is composed of well-formed, irregular vascular channels and spindled endothelial cells in varying proportions, depending on the stage of the lesion, as discussed later. In all forms the endothelial cells (both those lining the irregular vessels and those in the spindled fascicles) are cytologically bland. Intracellular and extracellular periodic acid–Schiff–positive (diastase-resistant) hyaline globules, believed to represent phagocytosed erythrocytes,[379] are characteristic but are neither entirely sensitive nor specific for Kaposi sarcoma.

Patch-stage Kaposi sarcoma is characterized by a subtle proliferation of thin-walled, jagged, empty-appearing vessels in the superficial and mid-reticular dermis, with a predilection for the perivascular and periadnexal regions. A helpful (but not invariably present) feature is the "promontory sign," in which the irregular vessels dissect around native dermal adnexal structures or blood vessels, leaving them partially "floating," or isolated from the rest of dermis. The spindle cell component is sparse at this stage and may be identified only after examination of multiple levels. A mild perivascular lymphoplasmacytic infiltrate is typically present, but extravasated erythrocytes, hemosiderin deposition, and hyaline globules are not prominent.

In plaque-stage Kaposi sarcoma (Fig. 13.40) the thin-walled irregular vessels involve the full thickness of the reticular dermis and may extend into the subcutaneous tissue. Irregular neoplastic vessels are still present, but a spindle cell component is readily identifiable and may dominate. The inflammatory infiltrate is generally more prominent than in patch-stage lesions, and extravasated erythrocytes, hyaline globules, and hemosiderin deposition are often conspicuous. Mitoses are sparse.

Nodular Kaposi sarcoma (Fig. 13.41A) shows a circumscribed dermal nodule composed of fascicles of spindle cells separated by slitlike vascular spaces containing extravasated erythrocytes, resulting in a sievelike appearance on cross section. Ectatic vessels with a perivascular lymphoplasmacytic infiltrate are often found at the periphery of the nodule, but a prominent vasoformative component is not seen. Hyaline globules are frequent, and mitoses are often readily identifiable.

Lymphangioma-like Kaposi sarcoma is a rare, clinically and histologically distinctive form of Kaposi sarcoma. This variant is seen in fewer than 5% of all Kaposi sarcoma biopsy specimens and is usually found in association with typical patch, plaque, or nodular lesions.[380–382] Clinically, the lesions are distinctive in that they often simulate bullae or cysts because of their compressible, spongy texture. Histologically,

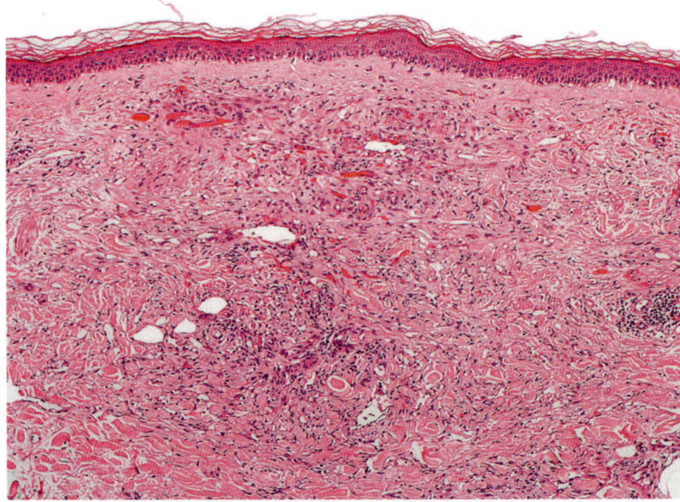

Figure 13.40 Kaposi Sarcoma. Plaque-stage Kaposi sarcoma showing thin-walled vessels and spindle cells infiltrating through the dermis.

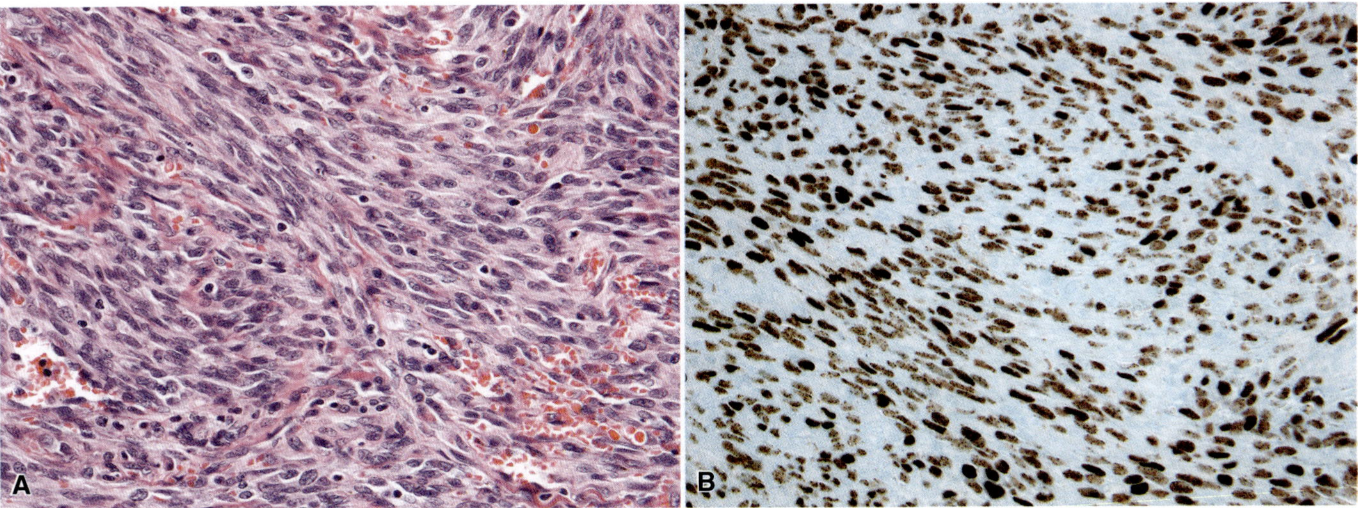

Figure 13.41 Kaposi Sarcoma. (A) Nodular Kaposi sarcoma composed of fascicles of spindle cells with slitlike vascular spaces containing extravasated erythrocytes. (B) Immunostaining for human herpesvirus 8 is useful to confirm the diagnosis of Kaposi sarcoma.

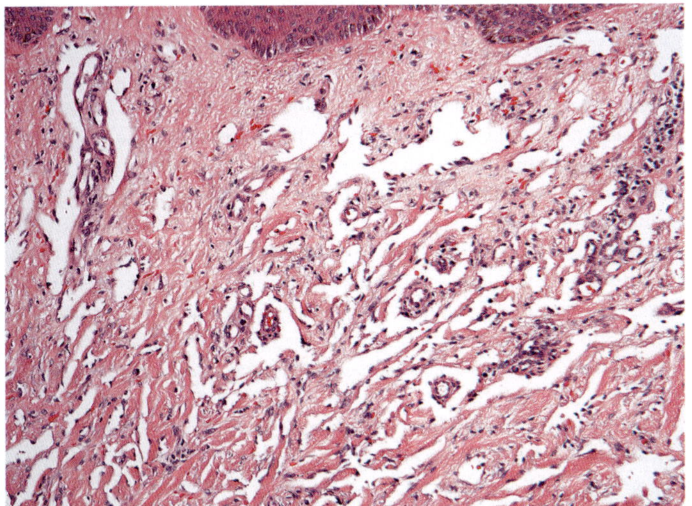

Figure 13.42 Lymphangioma-like Kaposi Sarcoma. The dilated lesional vessels have a dissecting growth pattern through the dermal collagen, mimicking acquired progressive lymphangioma.

the lesional vessels have a dissecting growth pattern through the dermal collagen, similar to patch- and plaque-stage Kaposi sarcoma, but they are widely dilated (lymphangioma-like) rather than irregular and slitlike (Fig. 13.42). A subtle increase in perivascular spindle cells may be evident on close inspection. The lymphoplasmacytic infiltrate varies from sparse to dense, and extravasated erythrocytes and hyaline globules are not seen.[382] Because many typical features of Kaposi sarcoma are absent, accurate diagnosis requires both knowledge of this unusual variant and a detailed clinical history.

In involved lymph nodes, Kaposi sarcoma characteristically involves the capsule and hilum first and subsequently extends along the sinuses, initially leaving the nodal architecture intact.[383] With extensive involvement, however, the node becomes effaced by tumor. The diagnosis is straightforward in the latter situation, but early lesions can be extremely subtle, with only a few irregular vessels associated with scattered plasma cells and spindle cells in the nodal capsule. An HHV-8 stain is helpful in these cases.

Rarely, the lesion may be entirely intravascular.[384]

Immunohistochemistry

Spindle cells of Kaposi sarcoma typically express both CD31 and CD34, but CD34 shows slightly greater sensitivity and stronger reactivity than CD31. Studies have convincingly shown lymphatic differentiation in Kaposi sarcoma. Nearly all cases express D2-40, VEGFR-3, and LYVE-1.[2,3,11,385,386] Immunohistochemistry for the HHV-8 protein latent nuclear antigen 1 (LANA-1) is very sensitive and specific for Kaposi sarcoma (see Fig. 13.41B). Vascular tumors other than Kaposi sarcoma rarely express HHV-8[189–191] (e.g., occasional cases of reactive angioendotheliomatosis[41] and two angiosarcomas arising in patients with AIDS who had a long history of Kaposi sarcoma[387]). Immunohistochemistry for HHV-8 is preferred over polymerase chain reaction-based techniques because false-positive results may occur with the latter, possibly because of the presence of HHV-8 in "bystander" peripheral blood mononuclear cells.[388]

Differential Diagnosis

Patch-stage Kaposi sarcoma may mimic an inflammatory dermatosis (i.e., superficial or superficial and deep perivascular dermatitis), but the irregular shape of the lesional vessels, the promontory sign, and the presence of numerous plasma cells suggest a diagnosis of Kaposi sarcoma.[389] In the differential diagnosis with hobnail hemangioma, a focal spindle cell component and prominent plasma cells favor Kaposi sarcoma. Clinical information is also helpful because hobnail hemangioma occurs as a solitary lesion in young to middle-aged healthy adults, whereas Kaposi sarcoma is typically multiple and arises in well-defined clinical settings. Although the lesional vessels in patch- and plaque-stage Kaposi sarcoma show a dissecting growth pattern similar to that seen in low-grade angiosarcoma, the absence of nuclear atypia, endothelial multilayering, and mitotic activity argues against the latter diagnosis.

The low-power appearance of lymphangioma-like Kaposi sarcoma overlaps significantly with that of acquired progressive lymphangioma and dermal involvement by lymphangiomatosis, but the clinical history (including the association with typical patch, plaque, or nodular lesions of Kaposi sarcoma) and the presence of a focal spindle cell component

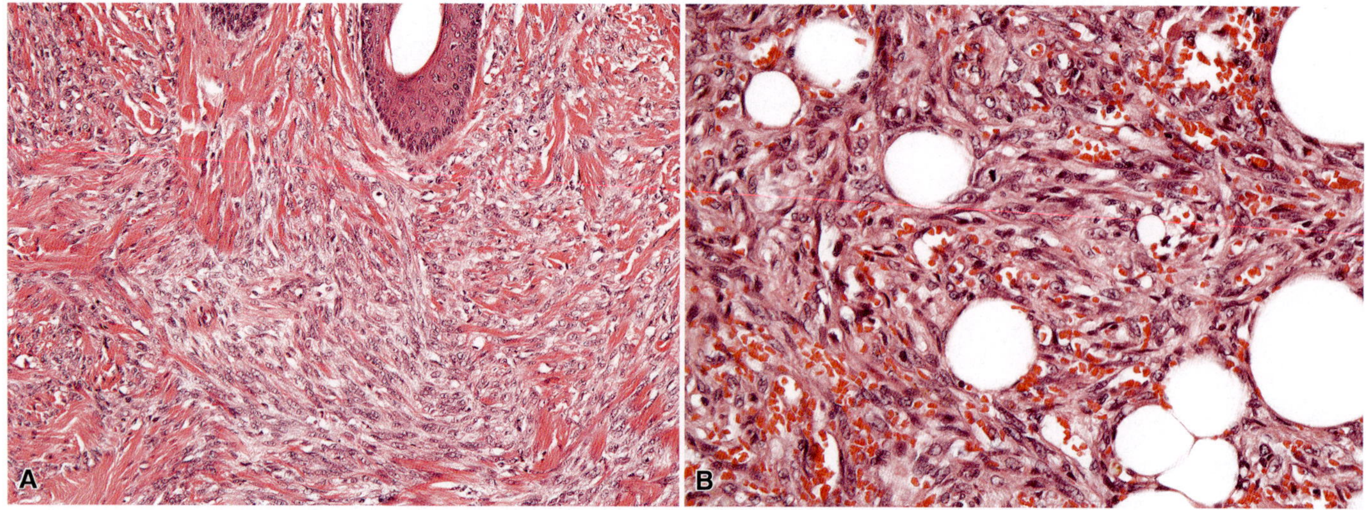

Figure 13.43 Spindle Cell Angiosarcoma. (A) Cutaneous angiosarcoma composed of short fascicles of spindle cells. (B) Sheets of spindle cells with hyperchromatic, markedly atypical nuclei. Note the prominent slitlike vascular spaces containing erythrocytes.

are clues to the diagnosis. Immunohistochemistry for HHV-8 can be very helpful in the diagnosis of subtle patch-stage or lymphangioma-like lesions or in cases in which the clinical history is unusual.

Some high-grade angiosarcomas have spindled, sievelike areas similar to those of nodular Kaposi sarcoma, but the nuclei of the spindle cells are hyperchromatic, with coarse chromatin and sometimes prominent nucleoli. HHV-8 is nearly always negative in angiosarcoma.

Prognosis and Treatment

The prognosis varies by clinical setting and was discussed earlier.

PRACTICE POINTS: Kaposi Sarcoma

- In the United States, Kaposi sarcoma is most commonly seen on the extremities of elderly patients of Mediterranean or Jewish ancestry.
- Immunosuppressed patients may present with disseminated lesions.
- The two components—irregular, thin-walled vessels and spindle cells—are present in variable proportions, depending on the stage (patch, plaque, or nodular).
- A high degree of suspicion is required to make the diagnosis of lymphangioma-like Kaposi sarcoma.
- Immunostaining for HHV-8 is very helpful for confirming the diagnosis.

Angiosarcoma (Spindle Cell)

Pathologic Features

The clinical features and prognosis were previously discussed. A subset of high-grade angiosarcomas shows purely or predominantly spindled cells. The spindle cell areas are typically composed of short fascicles (Fig. 13.43A), which often have numerous slitlike vascular channels (see Fig. 13.43B) containing erythrocytes, somewhat reminiscent of nodular Kaposi sarcoma. Rarely, long fibrosarcoma-like fascicles may be seen. The mitotic rate in these foci tends to be high, and although pleomorphism is not striking, the nuclei are hyperchromatic, with clumped chromatin. Intracytoplasmic vacuoles may be found in a minority of the cells and are a helpful clue to the diagnosis. The presence of well-formed neoplastic vessels lined by atypical cells at the periphery of the tumor is another helpful finding.

Immunohistochemical findings are similar to those discussed previously for vasoformative angiosarcoma.

Differential Diagnosis

In cutaneous tumors on the head and neck in elderly patients, the differential diagnosis of atypical spindle cell lesions typically includes spindle cell squamous cell carcinoma, spindle cell melanoma, and atypical fibroxanthoma (see Chapter 15). When the lesion is broad and diffusely infiltrative around adnexal structures, spindle cell angiosarcoma should also be considered. Immunohistochemistry is invaluable in this situation; immunostains for at least two broad-spectrum keratin antibodies, S-100 protein, CD31, and ERG should establish the diagnosis in most cases. Immunostains are also often required for the diagnosis of spindled angiosarcomas in deep soft tissue or visceral sites, where the only clues to endothelial differentiation may be focal intracytoplasmic vacuoles in a relatively monomorphic—albeit cytologically atypical—spindle cell sarcoma.

As previously discussed, spindled angiosarcomas show much greater nuclear atypia than nodular Kaposi sarcoma, and HHV-8 is nearly always negative in angiosarcoma.

References

1. Miettinen M, Lindenmayer AE, Chaubal A: Endothelial cell markers CD31, CD34, and BNH9 antibody to H- and Y-antigens: evaluation of their specificity and sensitivity in the diagnosis of vascular tumors and comparison with von Willebrand factor, *Mod Pathol* 7:82–90, 1994.
2. Fukunaga M: Expression of D2–40 in lymphatic endothelium of normal tissues and in vascular tumours, *Histopathology* 46:396–402, 2005.
3. Kahn HJ, Bailey D, Marks A: Monoclonal antibody D2–40, a new marker of lymphatic endothelium, reacts with Kaposi's sarcoma and a subset of angiosarcomas, *Mod Pathol* 15:434–440, 2002.
4. Breiteneder-Geleff S, Soleiman A, Kowalski H, et al: Angiosarcomas express mixed endothelial phenotypes of blood and lymphatic capillaries: podoplanin as a specific marker for lymphatic endothelium, *Am J Pathol* 154:385–394, 1999.
5. Achen MG, Jeltsch M, Kukk E, et al: Vascular endothelial growth factor D (VEGF-D) is a ligand for the tyrosine kinases VEGF receptor 2 (Flk1) and VEGF receptor 3 (Flt4), *Proc Natl Acad Sci USA* 95:548–553, 1998.
6. Kaipainen A, Korhonen J, Mustonen T, et al: Expression of the fms-like tyrosine kinase 4 gene becomes restricted to lymphatic endothelium during development, *Proc Natl Acad Sci USA* 92:3566–3570, 1995.
7. Banerji S, Ni J, Wang SX, et al: LYVE-1, a new homologue of the CD44 glycoprotein, is a lymph-specific receptor for hyaluronan, *J Cell Biol* 144:789–801, 1999.
8. Wigle JT, Oliver G: Prox1 function is required for the development of the murine lymphatic system, *Cell* 98:769–778, 1999.
9. Partanen TA, Alitalo K, Miettinen M: Lack of lymphatic vascular specificity of vascular endothelial growth factor receptor 3 in 185 vascular tumors, *Cancer* 86:2406–2412, 1999.
10. Evangelou E, Kyzas PA, Trikalinos TA: Comparison of the diagnostic accuracy of lymphatic endothelium markers: Bayesian approach, *Mod Pathol* 18:1490–1497, 2005.

11. Folpe AL, Veikkola T, Valtola R, et al: Vascular endothelial growth factor receptor-3 (VEGFR-3): a marker of vascular tumors with presumed lymphatic differentiation, including Kaposi's sarcoma, kaposiform and Dabska-type hemangioendotheliomas, and a subset of angiosarcomas, *Mod Pathol* 13:180–185, 2000.
12. Folpe AL, Chand EM, Goldblum JR, et al: Expression of Fli-1, a nuclear transcription factor, distinguishes vascular neoplasms from potential mimics, *Am J Surg Pathol* 25:1061–1066, 2001.
13. Folpe AL, Hill CE, Parham DM, et al: Immunohistochemical detection of FLI-1 protein expression: a study of 132 round cell tumors with emphasis on CD99-positive mimics of Ewing's sarcoma/primitive neuroectodermal tumor, *Am J Surg Pathol* 24:1657–1662, 2000.
14. Mhawech-Fauceglia P, Herrmann FR, Bshara W, et al: Friend leukaemia integration-1 expression in malignant and benign tumours: a multiple tumour tissue microarray analysis using polyclonal antibody, *J Clin Pathol* 60:694–700, 2007.
15. Rossi S, Orvieto E, Furlanetto A, et al: Utility of the immunohistochemical detection of FLI-1 expression in round cell and vascular neoplasm using a monoclonal antibody, *Mod Pathol* 17:547–552, 2004.
16. Miettinen M, Wang ZF, Paetau A, et al: ERG transcription factor as an immunohistochemical marker for vascular endothelial tumors and prostatic carcinoma, *Am J Surg Pathol* 35:432–441, 2011.
17. Poblet E, Gonzalez-Palacios F, Jimenez FJ: Different immunoreactivity of endothelial markers in well and poorly differentiated areas of angiosarcomas, *Virchows Arch* 428:217–221, 1996.
18. Kuzu I, Bicknell R, Harris AL, et al: Heterogeneity of vascular endothelial cells with relevance to diagnosis of vascular tumours, *J Clin Pathol* 45:143–148, 1992.
19. Fletcher CDM, Bridge JA, Hogendoorn PCW, et al, editors: *WHO classification of tumours of soft tissue and bone*, Lyon, 2013, IARC Press.
20. Fletcher CDM, Rubin BP, Tsang WYW: Other intermediate vascular neoplasms. In Fletcher CDM, Bridge JA, Hogendoorn PCW, et al, editors: *WHO classification of tumours of soft tissue and bone*, Lyon, 2013, IARC Press, pp 154.
21. Mulliken JB, Glowacki J: Classification of pediatric vascular lesions, *Plast Reconstr Surg* 70:120–121, 1982.
22. Enjolras O: Classification and management of the various superficial vascular anomalies: hemangiomas and vascular malformations, *J Dermatol* 24:701–710, 1997.
23. Wassef M, Blei F, Adams D, et al: Vascular anomalies classification: recommendations from the International Society for the Study of Vascular Anomalies, *Pediatrics* 136:e203–e214, 2015.
24. Masson P: Hemangioendotheliome vegetant intravasculaire, *Bull Soc Anat (Paris)* 93:517–523, 1923.
25. Clearkin KP, Enzinger FM: Intravascular papillary endothelial hyperplasia, *Arch Pathol Lab Med* 100:441–444, 1976.
26. Hashimoto H, Daimaru Y, Enjoji M: Intravascular papillary endothelial hyperplasia. A clinicopathologic study of 91 cases, *Am J Dermatopathol* 5:539–546, 1983.
27. Miyamoto H, Nagatani T, Mohri S, et al: Intravascular papillary endothelial hyperplasia, *Clin Exp Dermatol* 13:411–415, 1988.
28. Pins MR, Rosenthal DI, Springfield DS, et al: Florid extravascular papillary endothelial hyperplasia (Masson's pseudoangiosarcoma) presenting as a soft-tissue sarcoma, *Arch Pathol Lab Med* 117:259–263, 1993.
29. Reed CN, Cooper PH, Swerlick RA: Intravascular papillary endothelial hyperplasia. Multiple lesions simulating Kaposi's sarcoma, *J Am Acad Dermatol* 10:110–113, 1984.
30. Stewart M, Smoller BR: Multiple lesions of intravascular papillary endothelial hyperplasia (Masson's lesions), *Arch Pathol Lab Med* 118:315–316, 1994.
31. Inaloz HS, Patel G, Knight AG: Recurrent intravascular papillary endothelial hyperplasia developing from a pyogenic granuloma, *J Eur Acad Dermatol Venereol* 15:156–158, 2001.
32. Mentzel T, Goodlad JR, Smith MA, et al: Ancient hematoma: a unifying concept for a post-traumatic lesion mimicking an aggressive soft tissue neoplasm, *Mod Pathol* 10:334–340, 1997.
33. Okada K, Sugiyama T, Kato H, et al: Chronic expanding hematoma mimicking soft tissue neoplasm, *J Clin Oncol* 19:2971–2972, 2001.
34. Tappero JW, Koehler JE, Berger TG, et al: Bacillary angiomatosis and bacillary splenitis in immunocompetent adults, *Ann Intern Med* 118:363–365, 1993.
35. Cockerell CJ, LeBoit PE: Bacillary angiomatosis: a newly characterized, pseudoneoplastic, infectious, cutaneous vascular disorder, *J Am Acad Dermatol* 22:501–512, 1990.
36. Arias-Stella J, Lieberman PH, Erlandson RA, et al: Histology, immunohistochemistry, and ultrastructure of the verruga in Carrion's disease, *Am J Surg Pathol* 10:595–610, 1986.
37. Matteelli A, Castelli F, Spinetti A, et al: Short report: verruga peruana in an Italian traveler from Peru, *Am J Trop Med Hyg* 50:143–144, 1994.
38. Wick MR, Mills SE, Scheithauer BW, et al: Reassessment of malignant "angioendotheliomatosis." Evidence in favor of its reclassification as "intravascular lymphomatosis," *Am J Surg Pathol* 10:112–123, 1986.
39. Krell JM, Sanchez RL, Solomon AR: Diffuse dermal angiomatosis: a variant of reactive cutaneous angioendotheliomatosis, *J Cutan Pathol* 21:363–370, 1994.
40. Pasyk K: Depowski M. Proliferating systematized angioendotheliomatosis of a 5-month-old infant, *Arch Dermatol* 114:1512–1515, 1978.
41. McMenamin ME, Fletcher CD: Reactive angioendotheliomatosis: a study of 15 cases demonstrating a wide clinicopathologic spectrum, *Am J Surg Pathol* 26:685–697, 2002.
42. Kimyai-Asadi A, Nousari HC, Ketabchi N, et al: Diffuse dermal angiomatosis: a variant of reactive angioendotheliomatosis associated with atherosclerosis, *J Am Acad Dermatol* 40:257–259, 1999.
43. Requena L, Farina MC, Renedo G, et al: Intravascular and diffuse dermal reactive angioendotheliomatosis secondary to iatrogenic arteriovenous fistulas, *J Cutan Pathol* 26:159–164, 1999.
44. Rongioletti F, Rebora A: Cutaneous reactive angiomatoses: patterns and classification of reactive vascular proliferation, *J Am Acad Dermatol* 49:887–896, 2003.
45. Chu P, LeBoit PE: An eruptive vascular proliferation resembling acquired tufted angioma in the recipient of a liver transplant, *J Am Acad Dermatol* 26:322–325, 1992.
46. Al-Za'abi AM, Ghazarian D, Greenberg GR, et al: Eruptive tufted angiomas in a patient with Crohn's disease, *J Clin Pathol* 58:214–216, 2005.
47. LeBoit PE, Solomon AR, Santa Cruz DJ, et al: Angiomatosis with luminal cryoprotein deposition, *J Am Acad Dermatol* 27:969–973, 1992.
48. Bardwick PA, Zvaifler NJ, Gill GN, et al: Plasma cell dyscrasia with polyneuropathy, organomegaly, endocrinopathy, M protein, and skin changes: the POEMS syndrome. Report on two cases and a review of the literature, *Medicine (Baltimore)* 59:311–322, 1980.
49. Chan JK, Fletcher CD, Hicklin GA, et al: Glomeruloid hemangioma. A distinctive cutaneous lesion of multicentric Castleman's disease associated with POEMS syndrome, *Am J Surg Pathol* 14:1036–1046, 1990.
50. Kanitakis J, Roger H, Soubrier M, et al: Cutaneous angiomas in POEMS syndrome. An ultrastructural and immunohistochemical study, *Arch Dermatol* 124:695–698, 1988.
51. Nakanishi T, Sobue I, Toyokura Y, et al: The Crow-Fukase syndrome: a study of 102 cases in Japan, *Neurology* 34:712–720, 1984.
52. Rongioletti F, Gambini C, Lerza R: Glomeruloid hemangioma. A cutaneous marker of POEMS syndrome, *Am J Dermatopathol* 16:175–178, 1994.
53. Velez D, Delgado-Jimenez Y, Fraga J: Solitary glomeruloid haemangioma without POEMS syndrome, *J Cutan Pathol* 32:449–452, 2005.
54. Forman SB, Tyler WB, Ferringer TC, et al: Glomeruloid hemangiomas without POEMS syndrome: series of three cases, *J Cutan Pathol* 34:956–957, 2007.
55. Suurmeijer AJ, Fletcher CD: Papillary haemangioma. A distinctive cutaneous haemangioma of the head and neck area containing eosinophilic hyaline globules, *Histopathology* 51:638–648, 2007.
56. Porras-Luque JI, Fernandez-Herrera J, Dauden E, et al: Cutaneous necrosis by cold agglutinins associated with glomeruloid reactive angioendotheliomatosis, *Br J Dermatol* 139:1068–1072, 1998.
57. Yang SG, Cho KH, Bang YJ, et al: A case of glomeruloid hemangioma associated with multicentric Castleman's disease, *Am J Dermatopathol* 20:266–270, 1998.
58. Mali JW, Kuiper JP, Hamers AA: Acro-angiodermatitis of the foot, *Arch Dermatol* 92:515–518, 1965.
59. Bluefarb SM, Adams LA: Arteriovenous malformation with angiodermatitis. Stasis dermatitis simulating Kaposi's disease, *Arch Dermatol* 96:176–181, 1967.
60. Earhart RN, Aeling JA, Nuss DD, et al: Pseudo-Kaposi sarcoma. A patient with arteriovenous malformation and skin lesions simulating Kaposi sarcoma, *Arch Dermatol* 110:907–910, 1974.
61. Strutton G, Weedon D: Acro-angiodermatitis. A simulant of Kaposi's sarcoma, *Am J Dermatopathol* 9:85–89, 1987.
62. Johnson WC: Pathology of cutaneous vascular tumors, *Int J Dermatol* 15:239–270, 1976.
63. Bean WB, Walsh JR: Venous lakes, *AMA Arch Derm* 74:459–463, 1956.
64. Shovlin CL, Guttmacher AE, Buscarini E, et al: Diagnostic criteria for hereditary hemorrhagic telangiectasia (Rendu-Osler-Weber syndrome), *Am J Med Genet* 91:66–67, 2000.
65. Fuchizaki U, Miyamori H, Kitagawa S, et al: Hereditary haemorrhagic telangiectasia (Rendu-Osler-Weber disease), *Lancet* 362:1490–1494, 2003.
66. Guttmacher AE, Marchuk DA, White RI, Jr: Hereditary hemorrhagic telangiectasia, *N Engl J Med* 333:918–924, 1995.
67. Frain-Bell W: Angioma serpiginosum, *Br J Dermatol* 69:251–268, 1957.
68. Barker LP, Sachs PM: Angioma serpiginosum, a comparative study, *Arch Dermatol* 92:613–620, 1965.
69. Marriott PJ, Munro DD, Ryan T: Angioma serpiginosum—familial incidence, *Br J Dermatol* 93:701–706, 1975.
70. Imperial R, Helwig EB: Angiokeratoma. A clinicopathological study, *Arch Dermatol* 95:166–175, 1967.
71. Lynch PJ, Kosanovich M: Angiokeratoma circumscriptum, *Arch Dermatol* 96:665–668, 1967.
72. Schiller PI, Itin PH: Angiokeratomas: an update, *Dermatology* 193:275–282, 1996.
73. Jacobs AH, Walton RG: The incidence of birthmarks in the neonate, *Pediatrics* 58:218–222, 1976.
74. Calonje E, Wilson-Jones E: Vascular tumors: tumors and tumor-like conditions of blood vessels and lymphatics. In Elder DE, Elenitsas R, Johnson BL, et al, editors: *Lever's histopathology of the skin*, Philadelphia, 2004, Lippincott Williams & Wilkins, pp 1023.
75. Mills CM, Lanigan SW, Hughes J, et al: Demographic study of port wine stain patients attending a laser clinic: family history, prevalence of naevus anaemicus and results of prior treatment, *Clin Exp Dermatol* 22:166–168, 1997.
76. Klapman MH, Yao JF: Thickening and nodules in port-wine stains, *J Am Acad Dermatol* 44:300–302, 2001.
77. Tallman B, Tan OT, Morelli JG, et al: Location of port-wine stains and the likelihood of ophthalmic and/or central nervous system complications, *Pediatrics* 87:323–327, 1991.

78. Selim MM, Kelly KM, Nelson JS, et al: Confocal microscopy study of nerves and blood vessels in untreated and treated port wine stains: preliminary observations, *Dermatol Surg* 30:892–897, 2004.
79. Smoller BR, Rosen S: Port-wine stains. A disease of altered neural modulation of blood vessels?, *Arch Dermatol* 122:177–179, 1986.
80. Barsky SH, Rosen S, Geer DE, et al: The nature and evolution of port wine stains: a computer-assisted study, *J Invest Dermatol* 74:154–157, 1980.
81. Rydh M, Malm M, Jernbeck J, et al: Ectatic blood vessels in port-wine stains lack innervation: possible role in pathogenesis, *Plast Reconstr Surg* 87:419–422, 1991.
82. Finley JL, Noe JM, Arndt KA, et al: Port-wine stains. Morphologic variations and developmental lesions, *Arch Dermatol* 120:1453–1455, 1984.
83. Garzon MC, Huang JT, Enjolras O, et al: Vascular malformations. Part II: associated syndromes, *J Am Acad Dermatol* 56:541–564, 2007.
84. Mazereeuw-Hautier J, Syed S, Leisner RI, et al: Extensive venous/lymphatic malformations causing life-threatening haematological complications, *Br J Dermatol* 157:558–563, 2007.
85. Mazoyer E, Enjolras O, Laurian C, et al: Coagulation abnormalities associated with extensive venous malformations of the limbs: differentiation from Kasabach-Merritt syndrome, *Clin Lab Haematol* 24:243–251, 2002.
86. Bean WB: Blue rubber bleb nevi of the skin and gastrointestinal tract. In *Vascular spiders and related lesions of the skin*, Springfield, IL, 1958, Charles C. Thomas, pp 178–185.
87. Nahm WK, Moise S, Eichenfield LF, et al: Venous malformations in blue rubber bleb nevus syndrome: variable onset of presentation, *J Am Acad Dermatol* 50:S101–S106, 2004.
88. Labauge P, Denier C, Bergametti F, et al: Genetics of cavernous angiomas, *Lancet Neurol* 6:237–244, 2007.
89. Wood WS, Dimmick JE: Multiple infiltrating glomus tumors in children, *Cancer* 40:1680–1685, 1977.
90. Boon LM, Mulliken JB, Enjolras O, et al: Glomuvenous malformation (glomangioma) and venous malformation: distinct clinicopathologic and genetic entities, *Arch Dermatol* 140:971–976, 2004.
91. Brouillard P, Boon LM, Mulliken JB, et al: Mutations in a novel factor, glomulin, are responsible for glomuvenous malformations ("glomangiomas"), *Am J Hum Genet* 70:866–874, 2002.
92. Calonje E, Fletcher CD: Sinusoidal hemangioma. A distinctive benign vascular neoplasm within the group of cavernous hemangiomas, *Am J Surg Pathol* 15:1130–1135, 1991.
93. Hoda SA, Cranor ML, Rosen PP: Hemangiomas of the breast with atypical histological features. Further analysis of histological subtypes confirming their benign character, *Am J Surg Pathol* 16:553–560, 1992.
94. Rosen PP: Vascular tumors of the breast. V. Nonparenchymal hemangiomas of mammary subcutaneous tissues, *Am J Surg Pathol* 9:723–729, 1985.
95. Enjolras O, Mulliken JB: Vascular tumors and vascular malformations (new issues), *Adv Dermatol* 13:375–423, 1997.
96. Enjolras O, Wassef M, Brocheriou-Spelle I, et al: Sinusoidal hemangioma, *Ann Dermatol Venereol* 125:575–580, 1998.
97. Weiss SW, Goldblum JR: Benign tumors and tumor-like lesions of blood vessels. In *Enzinger and Weiss's soft tissue tumors*, 5th ed, Philadelphia, 2008, Mosby, pp 650.
98. Ide F, Obara K, Enatsu K, et al: Rare vascular proliferations of the oral mucosa, *Oral Surg Oral Med Oral Pathol Oral Radiol Endod* 97:75–78, 2004.
99. Lapertosa G, Carli C, Fulcheri E: Cavernous hemangioma of the breast (author's transl), *Pathologica* 72:255–260, 1980.
100. Kohout MP, Hansen M, Pribaz JJ, et al: Arteriovenous malformations of the head and neck: natural history and management, *Plast Reconstr Surg* 102:643–654, 1998.
101. Barrett AW, Speight PM: Superficial arteriovenous hemangioma of the oral cavity, *Oral Surg Oral Med Oral Pathol Oral Radiol Endod* 90:731–738, 2000.
102. Connelly MG, Winkelmann RK: Acral arteriovenous tumor. A clinicopathologic review, *Am J Surg Pathol* 9:15–21, 1985.
103. Girard C, Graham JH, Johnson WC: Arteriovenous hemangioma (arteriovenous shunt). A clinicopathological and histochemical study, *J Cutan Pathol* 1:73–87, 1974.
104. Koutlas IG, Jessurun J: Arteriovenous hemangioma: a clinicopathological and immunohistochemical study, *J Cutan Pathol* 21:343–349, 1994.
105. Neumann RA, Knobler RM, Schuller-Petrovic S, et al: Giant arteriovenous hemangioma (cirsoid aneurysm) of the nose, *J Dermatol Surg Oncol* 15:739–742, 1989.
106. Wade TR, Kamino H, Ackerman AB: A histologic atlas of vascular lesions, *J Dermatol Surg Oncol* 4:845–850, 1978.
107. Whimster IW: The pathology of lymphangioma circumscriptum, *Br J Dermatol* 94:473–486, 1976.
108. Peachey RD, Lim CC, Whimster IW: Lymphangioma of skin. A review of 65 cases, *Br J Dermatol* 83:519–527, 1970.
109. Flanagan BP, Helwig EB: Cutaneous lymphangioma, *Arch Dermatol* 113:24–30, 1977.
110. Hancock BJ, St-Vil D, Luks FI, et al: Complications of lymphangiomas in children, *J Pediatr Surg* 27:220–224, discussion 224–226, 1992.
111. Alqahtani A, Nguyen LT, Flageole H, et al: 25 years' experience with lymphangiomas in children, *J Pediatr Surg* 34:1164–1168, 1999.
112. Graesslin O, Derniaux E, Alanio E, et al: Characteristics and outcome of fetal cystic hygroma diagnosed in the first trimester, *Acta Obstet Gynecol Scand* 86:1442–1446, 2007.
113. Malone FD, Ball RH, Nyberg DA, et al: First-trimester septated cystic hygroma: prevalence, natural history, and pediatric outcome, *Obstet Gynecol* 106:288–294, 2005.
114. Hornick JL, Fletcher CD: Intraabdominal cystic lymphangiomas obscured by marked superimposed reactive changes: clinicopathological analysis of a series, *Hum Pathol* 36:426–432, 2005.
115. McFadden DE, Clement PB: Peritoneal inclusion cysts with mural mesothelial proliferation. A clinicopathological analysis of six cases, *Am J Surg Pathol* 10:844–854, 1986.
116. Ross MJ, Welch WR, Scully RE: Multilocular peritoneal inclusion cysts (so-called cystic mesotheliomas), *Cancer* 64:1336–1346, 1989.
117. Jones EW: Dowling oration, 1976. Malignant vascular tumours, *Clin Exp Dermatol* 1:287–312, 1976.
118. Guillou L, Fletcher CD: Benign lymphangioendothelioma (acquired progressive lymphangioma): a lesion not to be confused with well-differentiated angiosarcoma and patch stage Kaposi's sarcoma: clinicopathologic analysis of a series, *Am J Surg Pathol* 24:1047–1057, 2000.
119. Renshaw AA, Rosai J: Benign atypical vascular lesions of the lip. A study of 12 cases, *Am J Surg Pathol* 17:557–565, 1993.
120. Jones EW, Winkelmann RK, Zachary CB, et al: Benign lymphangioendothelioma, *J Am Acad Dermatol* 23:229–235, 1990.
121. Watanabe M, Kishiyama K, Ohkawara A: Acquired progressive lymphangioma, *J Am Acad Dermatol* 8:663–667, 1983.
122. Gonzalez-Crussi F, Enneking WF, Arean VM: Infiltrating angiolipoma, *J Bone Joint Surg Am* 48:1111–1124, 1966.
123. Lin JJ, Lin F: Two entities in angiolipoma. A study of 459 cases of lipoma with review of literature on infiltrating angiolipoma, *Cancer* 34:720–727, 1974.
124. Pribyl C, Burke SW, Roberts JM, et al: Infiltrating angiolipoma or intramuscular hemangioma? A report of five cases, *J Pediatr Orthop* 6:172–176, 1986.
125. Hein KD, Mulliken JB, Kozakewich HP, et al: Venous malformations of skeletal muscle, *Plast Reconstr Surg* 110:1625–1635, 2002.
126. Beham A, Fletcher CD: Intramuscular angioma: a clinicopathological analysis of 74 cases, *Histopathology* 18:53–59, 1991.
127. Allen PW, Enzinger FM: Hemangioma of skeletal muscle. An analysis of 89 cases, *Cancer* 29:8–22, 1972.
128. Schecter DC: Intra-articular hemangioma of the knee, *Am Surg* 27:638–641, 1961.
129. Bennett GE, Cobey MC: Hemangioma of joints: report of five cases, *Arch Surg* 38:487–500, 1939.
130. Devaney K, Vinh TN, Sweet DE: Synovial hemangioma: a report of 20 cases with differential diagnostic considerations, *Hum Pathol* 24:737–745, 1993.
131. Lewis RC, Jr, Coventry MB, Soule EH: Hemangioma of the synovial membrane, *J Bone Joint Surg Am* 41-A:264–271, 1959.
132. Moon NF: Synovial hemangioma of the knee joint. A review of previously reported cases and inclusion of two new cases, *Clin Orthop Relat Res* 183–190, 1973.
133. Rao VK, Weiss SW: Angiomatosis of soft tissue. An analysis of the histologic features and clinical outcome in 51 cases, *Am J Surg Pathol* 16:764–771, 1992.
134. North PE, Kahn T, Cordisco MR, et al: Multifocal lymphangioendotheliomatosis with thrombocytopenia: a newly recognized clinicopathological entity, *Arch Dermatol* 140:599–606, 2004.
135. Piggott KD, Riedel PA, Baron HI: Multifocal lymphangioendotheliomatosis with thrombocytopenia: a rare cause of gastrointestinal bleeding in the newborn period, *Pediatrics* 117:e810–e813, 2006.
136. Yeung J, Somers G, Viero S, et al: Multifocal lymphangioendotheliomatosis with thrombocytopenia, *J Am Acad Dermatol* 54:S214–S217, 2006.
137. Prasad V, Fishman SJ, Mulliken JB, et al: Cutaneovisceral angiomatosis with thrombocytopenia, *Pediatr Dev Pathol* 8:407–419, 2005.
138. Howat AJ, Campbell PE: Angiomatosis: a vascular malformation of infancy and childhood. Report of 17 cases, *Pathology* 19:377–382, 1987.
139. Folpe AL, Fanburg-Smith JC, Miettinen M, et al: Atypical and malignant glomus tumors: analysis of 52 cases, with a proposal for the reclassification of glomus tumors, *Am J Surg Pathol* 25:1–12, 2001.
140. Gomez CS, Calonje E, Ferrar DW, et al: Lymphangiomatosis of the limbs. Clinicopathologic analysis of a series with a good prognosis, *Am J Surg Pathol* 19:125–133, 1995.
141. Schultz K, Rosenberg AE, Ebb DH, et al: Lower-extremity lymphangiomatosis. A case report with a seventeen-year follow-up, *J Bone Joint Surg Am* 87:162–167, 2005.
142. Alvarez OA, Kjellin I, Zuppan CW: Thoracic lymphangiomatosis in a child, *J Pediatr Hematol Oncol* 26:136–141, 2004.
143. North PE, Waner M, Buckmiller L, et al: Vascular tumors of infancy and childhood: beyond capillary hemangioma, *Cardiovasc Pathol* 15:303–317, 2006.
144. Haggstrom AN, Drolet BA, Baselga E, et al: Prospective study of infantile hemangiomas: demographic, prenatal, and perinatal characteristics, *J Pediatr* 150:291–294, 2007.
145. Blei F, Walter J, Orlow SJ, et al: Familial segregation of hemangiomas and vascular malformations as an autosomal dominant trait, *Arch Dermatol* 134:718–722, 1998.
146. Bruckner AL, Frieden IJ: Hemangiomas of infancy, *J Am Acad Dermatol* 48:477–493, quiz 494–6, 2003.
147. Calonje E, Mentzel T, Fletcher CD: Pseudomalignant perineurial invasion in cellular ("infantile") capillary haemangiomas, *Histopathology* 26:159–164, 1995.
148. Gonzalez-Crussi F, Reyes-Mugica M: Cellular hemangiomas ("hemangioendotheliomas") in infants. Light microscopic, immunohistochemical, and ultrastructural observations, *Am J Surg Pathol* 15:769–778, 1991.

149. Glowacki J, Mulliken JB: Mast cells in hemangiomas and vascular malformations, *Pediatrics* 70:48–51, 1982.
150. Iwata J, Sonobe H, Furihata M, et al: High frequency of apoptosis in infantile capillary haemangioma, *J Pathol* 179:403–408, 1996.
151. Boye E, Yu Y, Paranya G, et al: Clonality and altered behavior of endothelial cells from hemangiomas, *J Clin Invest* 107:745–752, 2001.
152. North PE, Waner M, Mizeracki A, et al: A unique microvascular phenotype shared by juvenile hemangiomas and human placenta, *Arch Dermatol* 137:559–570, 2001.
153. North PE, Waner M, Mizeracki A, et al: GLUT1: a newly discovered immunohistochemical marker for juvenile hemangiomas, *Hum Pathol* 31:11–22, 2000.
154. Enjolras O, Gelbert F: Superficial hemangiomas: associations and management, *Pediatr Dermatol* 14:173–179, 1997.
155. Boon LM, Enjolras O, Mulliken JB: Congenital hemangioma: evidence of accelerated involution, *J Pediatr* 128:329–335, 1996.
156. North PE, Waner M, James CA, et al: Congenital nonprogressive hemangioma: a distinct clinicopathologic entity unlike infantile hemangioma, *Arch Dermatol* 137:1607–1620, 2001.
157. Enjolras O, Mulliken JB, Boon LM, et al: Noninvoluting congenital hemangioma: a rare cutaneous vascular anomaly, *Plast Reconstr Surg* 107:1647–1654, 2001.
158. Berenguer B, Mulliken JB, Enjolras O, et al: Rapidly involuting congenital hemangioma: clinical and histopathologic features, *Pediatr Dev Pathol* 6:495–510, 2003.
159. Hartzell MB: Granuloma pyogenicum, *J Cutan Dis* 22:520–523, 1904.
160. Mills SE, Cooper PH, Fechner RE: Lobular capillary hemangioma: the underlying lesion of pyogenic granuloma. A study of 73 cases from the oral and nasal mucous membranes, *Am J Surg Pathol* 4:470–479, 1980.
161. Harris MN, Desai R, Chuang TY, et al: Lobular capillary hemangiomas: an epidemiologic report, with emphasis on cutaneous lesions, *J Am Acad Dermatol* 42:1012–1016, 2000.
162. Patrice SJ, Wiss K, Mulliken JB: Pyogenic granuloma (lobular capillary hemangioma): a clinicopathologic study of 178 cases, *Pediatr Dermatol* 8:267–276, 1991.
163. Cooper PH, McAllister HA, Helwig EB: Intravenous pyogenic granuloma. A study of 18 cases, *Am J Surg Pathol* 3:221–228, 1979.
164. Cooper PH, Mills SE: Subcutaneous granuloma pyogenicum. Lobular capillary hemangioma, *Arch Dermatol* 118:30–33, 1982.
165. Angelopoulos AP: Pyogenic granuloma of the oral cavity: statistical analysis of its clinical features, *J Oral Surg* 29:840–847, 1971.
166. Mussalli NG, Hopps RM, Johnson NW: Oral pyogenic granuloma as a complication of pregnancy and the use of hormonal contraceptives, *Int J Gynaecol Obstet* 14:187–191, 1976.
167. Pearlman BA: An oral contraceptive drug and gingival enlargement; the relationship between local and systemic factors, *J Clin Periodontol* 1:47–51, 1974.
168. Warner J, Jones EW: Pyogenic granuloma recurring with multiple satellites. A report of 11 cases, *Br J Dermatol* 80:218–227, 1968.
169. Wilson BB, Greer KE, Cooper PH: Eruptive disseminated lobular capillary hemangioma (pyogenic granuloma), *J Am Acad Dermatol* 21:391–394, 1989.
170. Nappi O, Wick MR: Disseminated lobular capillary hemangioma (pyogenic granuloma). A clinicopathologic study of two cases, *Am J Dermatopathol* 8:379–385, 1986.
171. Requena L, Kutzner H, Mentzel T: Acquired elastotic hemangioma: a clinicopathologic variant of hemangioma, *J Am Acad Dermatol* 47:371–376, 2002.
172. Imperial R, Helwig EB: Verrucous hemangioma. A clinicopathologic study of 21 cases, *Arch Dermatol* 96:247–253, 1967.
173. Tennant LB, Mulliken JB, Perez-Atayde AR, et al: Verrucous hemangioma revisited, *Pediatr Dermatol* 23:208–215, 2006.
174. Chan JK, Tsang WY, Calonje E: Verrucous hemangioma: a distinct but neglected variant of cutaneous hemangioma, *Int J Surg Pathol* 2:171–176, 1995.
175. Nakagawa K: Case report of angioblastoma of the skin, *Nippon Hifuka Gakkai Zasshi* 59:92–94, 1949.
176. Alessi E, Bertani E, Sala F: Acquired tufted angioma, *Am J Dermatopathol* 8:426–429, 1986.
177. Jones EW, Orkin M: Tufted angioma (angioblastoma). A benign progressive angioma, not to be confused with Kaposi's sarcoma or low-grade angiosarcoma, *J Am Acad Dermatol* 20:214–225, 1989.
178. Wong SN, Tay YK: Tufted angioma: a report of five cases, *Pediatr Dermatol* 19:388–393, 2002.
179. Herron MD, Coffin CM, Vanderhooft SL: Tufted angiomas: variability of the clinical morphology, *Pediatr Dermatol* 19:394–401, 2002.
180. Bernstein EF, Kantor G, Howe N, et al: Tufted angioma of the thigh, *J Am Acad Dermatol* 31:307–311, 1994.
181. Enjolras O, Wassef M, Mazoyer E, et al: Infants with Kasabach-Merritt syndrome do not have "true" hemangiomas, *J Pediatr* 130:631–640, 1997.
182. Leaute-Labreze C, Bioulac-Sage P, Labbe L, et al: Tufted angioma associated with platelet trapping syndrome: response to aspirin, *Arch Dermatol* 133:1077–1079, 1997.
183. Arai E, Kuramochi A, Tsuchida T, et al: Usefulness of D2–40 immunohistochemistry for differentiation between kaposiform hemangioendothelioma and tufted angioma, *J Cutan Pathol* 33:492–497, 2006.
184. Tsang WY, Chan JK, Fletcher CD, et al: Symplastic hemangioma: a distinctive vascular neoplasm featuring bizarre stromal cells, *Int J Surg Pathol* 1:202A, 1994.
185. Kutzner H, Winzer M, Mentzel T: [Symplastic hemangioma], *Hautarzt* 51:327–331, 2000.
186. Goh SG, Dayrit JF, Calonje E: Symplastic hemangioma: report of two cases, *J Cutan Pathol* 33:735–740, 2006.
187. Hunt SJ, Santa Cruz DJ, Barr RJ: Microvenular hemangioma, *J Cutan Pathol* 18:235–240, 1991.
188. Aloi F, Tomasini C, Pippione M: Microvenular hemangioma, *Am J Dermatopathol* 15:534–538, 1993.
189. Cheuk W, Wong KO, Wong CS, et al: Immunostaining for human herpesvirus 8 latent nuclear antigen-1 helps distinguish Kaposi sarcoma from its mimickers, *Am J Clin Pathol* 121:335–342, 2004.
190. Patel RM, Goldblum JR, Hsi ED: Immunohistochemical detection of human herpes virus-8 latent nuclear antigen-1 is useful in the diagnosis of Kaposi sarcoma, *Mod Pathol* 17:456–460, 2004.
191. Robin YM, Guillou L, Michels JJ, et al: Human herpesvirus 8 immunostaining: a sensitive and specific method for diagnosing Kaposi sarcoma in paraffin-embedded sections, *Am J Clin Pathol* 121:330–334, 2004.
192. Santa Cruz DJ, Aronberg J: Targetoid hemosiderotic hemangioma, *J Am Acad Dermatol* 19:550–558, 1988.
193. Calonje E, Fletcher CD, Wilson-Jones E, et al: Retiform hemangioendothelioma. A distinctive form of low-grade angiosarcoma delineated in a series of 15 cases, *Am J Surg Pathol* 18:115–125, 1994.
194. Guillou L, Calonje E, Speight P, et al: Hobnail hemangioma: a pseudomalignant vascular lesion with a reappraisal of targetoid hemosiderotic hemangioma, *Am J Surg Pathol* 23:97–105, 1999.
195. Franke FE, Steger K, Marks A, et al: Hobnail hemangiomas (targetoid hemosiderotic hemangiomas) are true lymphangiomas, *J Cutan Pathol* 31:362–367, 2004.
196. Sahin MT, Demir MA, Gunduz K, et al: Targetoid haemosiderotic haemangioma: dermoscopic monitoring of three cases and review of the literature, *Clin Exp Dermatol* 30:672–676, 2005.
197. Carlson JA, Daulat S, Goodheart HP: Targetoid hemosiderotic hemangioma—a dynamic vascular tumor: report of 3 cases with episodic and cyclic changes and comparison with solitary angiokeratomas, *J Am Acad Dermatol* 41:215–224, 1999.
198. Morganroth GS, Tigelaar RE, Longley BJ, et al: Targetoid hemangioma associated with pregnancy and the menstrual cycle, *J Am Acad Dermatol* 32:282–284, 1995.
199. Mentzel T, Partanen TA, Kutzner H: Hobnail hemangioma ("targetoid hemosiderotic hemangioma"): clinicopathologic and immunohistochemical analysis of 62 cases, *J Cutan Pathol* 26:279–286, 1999.
200. Gutzmer R, Kaspari M, Herbst RA, et al: Absence of HHV-8 DNA in hobnail hemangiomas, *J Cutan Pathol* 29:154–158, 2002.
201. Dabska M: Malignant endovascular papillary angioendothelioma of the skin in childhood. Clinicopathologic study of 6 cases, *Cancer* 24:503–510, 1969.
202. Allen PW, Ramakrishna B, MacCormac LB: The histiocytoid hemangiomas and other controversies, *Pathol Annu* 27(Pt 2):51–87, 1992.
203. Schwartz RA, Dabski C, Dabska M: The Dabska tumor: a thirty-year retrospect, *Dermatology* 201:1–5, 2000.
204. Fanburg-Smith JC, Michal M, Partanen TA, et al: Papillary intralymphatic angioendothelioma (PILA): a report of twelve cases of a distinctive vascular tumor with phenotypic features of lymphatic vessels, *Am J Surg Pathol* 23:1004–1010, 1999.
205. Bhatia A, Nada R, Kumar Y, et al: Dabska tumor (endovascular papillary angioendothelioma) of testis: a case report with brief review of literature, *Diagn Pathol* 1:12, 2006.
206. Argani P, Athanasian E: Malignant endovascular papillary angioendothelioma (Dabska tumor) arising within a deep intramuscular hemangioma, *Arch Pathol Lab Med* 121:992–995, 1997.
207. McCarthy EF, Lietman S, Argani P, et al: Endovascular papillary angioendothelioma (Dabska tumor) of bone, *Skeletal Radiol* 28:100–103, 1999.
208. Nakayama T, Nishino M, Takasu K, et al: Endovascular papillary angioendothelioma (Dabska tumor) of bone, *Orthopedics* 27:327–328, 2004.
209. Katz JA, Mahoney DH, Shukla LW, et al: Endovascular papillary angioendothelioma in the spleen, *Pediatr Pathol* 8:185–193, 1988.
210. Rodgers B, Zeim S, Crawford B, et al: Splenic papillary angioendothelioma in a 6-year-old girl, *J Pediatr Hematol Oncol* 29:808–810, 2007.
211. Dabska M: Malignant endovascular papillary angioendothelioma of the skin in childhood. Clinicopathologic study of 6 cases, *Cancer* 24:503–510, 1969.
212. Emanuel PO, Lin R, Silver L, et al: Dabska tumor arising in lymphangioma circumscriptum, *J Cutan Pathol* 35:65–69, 2008.
213. Patterson K, Chandra RS: Malignant endovascular papillary angioendothelioma. Cutaneous borderline tumor, *Arch Pathol Lab Med* 109:671–673, 1985.
214. Quecedo E, Martinez-Escribano JA, Febrer I, et al: Dabska tumor developing within a preexisting vascular malformation, *Am J Dermatopathol* 18:302–307, 1996.
215. Kutok JL, Fletcher CD: Splenic vascular tumors, *Semin Diagn Pathol* 20:128–139, 2003.
216. Takayama A, Nakashima O, Kobayashi K, et al: Splenic lymphangioma with papillary endothelial proliferation: a case report and review of the literature, *Pathol Int* 53:483–488, 2003.
217. Meis-Kindblom JM, Kindblom LG: Angiosarcoma of soft tissue: a study of 80 cases, *Am J Surg Pathol* 22:683–697, 1998.
218. Tan D, Kraybill W, Cheney RT, et al: Retiform hemangioendothelioma: a case report and review of the literature, *J Cutan Pathol* 32:634–637, 2005.
219. Duke D, Dvorak A, Harris TJ, et al: Multiple retiform hemangioendotheliomas. A low-grade angiosarcoma, *Am J Dermatopathol* 18:606–610, 1996.
220. Parsons A, Sheehan DJ, Sangueza OP: Retiform hemangioendotheliomas usually do not express D2–40 and VEGFR-3, *Am J Dermatopathol* 30:31–33, 2008.

221. Nayler SJ, Rubin BP, Calonje E, et al: Composite hemangioendothelioma: a complex, low-grade vascular lesion mimicking angiosarcoma, *Am J Surg Pathol* 24:352–361, 2000.
222. Fukunaga M, Suzuki K, Saegusa N, et al: Composite hemangioendothelioma: report of 5 cases including one with associated Maffucci syndrome, *Am J Surg Pathol* 31:1567–1572, 2007.
223. Reis-Filho JS, Paiva ME, Lopes JM: Congenital composite hemangioendothelioma: case report and reappraisal of the hemangioendothelioma spectrum, *J Cutan Pathol* 29:226–231, 2002.
224. Requena L, Luis Díaz J, Manzarbeitia F, et al: Cutaneous composite hemangioendothelioma with satellitosis and lymph node metastasis, *J Cutan Pathol* 35:225–230, 2008.
225. Aydingöz IE, Demirkesen C, Serdar ZA, et al: Composite haemangioendothelioma with lymph-node metastasis: an unusual presentation at an uncommon site, *Clin Exp Dermatol* 34:e802–e806, 2009.
226. Mahmoudizad R, Samrao A, Bentow JJ, et al: Composite hemangioendothelioma: An unusual presentation of a rare vascular tumor, *Am J Clin Pathol* 141:732–736, 2014.
227. Ross JA, Severson RK, Davis S, et al: Trends in the incidence of soft tissue sarcomas in the United States from 1973 through 1987, *Cancer* 72:486–490, 1993.
228. Toro JR, Travis LB, Wu HJ, et al: Incidence patterns of soft tissue sarcomas, regardless of primary site, in the surveillance, epidemiology and end results program, 1978–2001: an analysis of 26,758 cases, *Int J Cancer* 119:2922–2930, 2006.
229. Fata F, O'Reilly E, Ilson D, et al: Paclitaxel in the treatment of patients with angiosarcoma of the scalp or face, *Cancer* 86:2034–2037, 1999.
230. Deyrup AT, McKenney JK, Tighiouart M, et al: Sporadic cutaneous angiosarcomas: a proposal for risk stratification based on 69 cases, *Am J Surg Pathol* 32:72–77, 2008.
231. Holden CA, Spittle MF, Jones EW: Angiosarcoma of the face and scalp, prognosis and treatment, *Cancer* 59:1046–1057, 1987.
232. Morgan MB, Swann M, Somach S, et al: Cutaneous angiosarcoma: a case series with prognostic correlation, *J Am Acad Dermatol* 50:867–874, 2004.
233. Pawlik TM, Paulino AF, McGinn CJ, et al: Cutaneous angiosarcoma of the scalp: a multidisciplinary approach, *Cancer* 98:1716–1726, 2003.
234. Rosai J, Sumner HW, Kostianovsky M, et al: Angiosarcoma of the skin. A clinicopathologic and fine structural study, *Hum Pathol* 7:83–109, 1976.
235. Janse AJ, van Coevorden F, Peterse H, et al: Lymphedema-induced lymphangiosarcoma, *Eur J Surg Oncol* 21:155–158, 1995.
236. Heitmann C, Ingianni G: Stewart-Treves syndrome: lymphangiosarcoma following mastectomy, *Ann Plast Surg* 44:72–75, 2000.
237. Brady MS, Garfein CF, Petrek JA, et al: Post-treatment sarcoma in breast cancer patients, *Ann Surg Oncol* 1:66–72, 1994.
238. Alessi E, Sala F, Berti E: Angiosarcomas in lymphedematous limbs, *Am J Dermatopathol* 8:371–378, 1986.
239. Sordillo PP, Chapman R, Hajdu SI, et al: Lymphangiosarcoma, *Cancer* 48:1674–1679, 1981.
240. Woodward AH, Ivins JC, Soule EH: Lymphangiosarcoma arising in chronic lymphedematous extremities, *Cancer* 30:562–572, 1972.
241. Shon W, Ida CM, Boland-Froemming JM, et al: Cutaneous angiosarcoma arising in massive localized lymphedema of the morbidly obese: a report of five cases and review of the literature, *J Cutan Pathol* 38:560–564, 2011.
242. Maddox JC, Evans HL: Angiosarcoma of skin and soft tissue: a study of forty-four cases, *Cancer* 48:1907–1921, 1981.
243. Mark RJ, Poen JC, Tran LM, et al: Angiosarcoma. A report of 67 patients and a review of the literature, *Cancer* 77:2400–2406, 1996.
244. West JG, Qureshi A, West JE, et al: Risk of angiosarcoma following breast conservation: a clinical alert, *Breast J* 11:115–123, 2005.
245. Strobbe LJ, Peterse HL, van Tinteren H, et al: Angiosarcoma of the breast after conservation therapy for invasive cancer, the incidence and outcome. An unforseen sequela, *Breast Cancer Res Treat* 47:101–109, 1998.
246. Marchal C, Weber B, de Lafontan B, et al: Nine breast angiosarcomas after conservative treatment for breast carcinoma: a survey from French comprehensive Cancer Centers, *Int J Radiat Oncol Biol Phys* 44:113–119, 1999.
247. Kiss K, Andreasen S, Talman MM, et al: The incidence of radiotherapy-induced angiosarcoma in the skin after treatment for breast cancer in Denmark. A population-based study, *Mod Pathol* 30:132A, 2017.
248. Chen KT, Hoffman KD, Hendricks EJ: Angiosarcoma following therapeutic irradiation, *Cancer* 44:2044–2048, 1979.
249. Cafiero F, Gipponi M, Peressini A, et al: Radiation-associated angiosarcoma: diagnostic and therapeutic implications—two case reports and a review of the literature, *Cancer* 77:2496–2502, 1996.
250. Nanus DM, Kelsen D, Clark DG: Radiation-induced angiosarcoma, *Cancer* 60:777–779, 1987.
251. Policarpio-Nicolas ML, Nicolas MM, Keh P, et al: Postradiation angiosarcoma of the small intestine: a case report and review of literature, *Ann Diagn Pathol* 10:301–305, 2006.
252. Billings SD, McKenney JK, Folpe AL, et al: Cutaneous angiosarcoma following breast-conserving surgery and radiation: an analysis of 27 cases, *Am J Surg Pathol* 28:781–788, 2004.
253. Brenn T, Fletcher CD: Radiation-associated cutaneous atypical vascular lesions and angiosarcoma: clinicopathologic analysis of 42 cases, *Am J Surg Pathol* 29:983–996, 2005.
254. Rao J, Dekoven JG, Beatty JD, et al: Cutaneous angiosarcoma as a delayed complication of radiation therapy for carcinoma of the breast, *J Am Acad Dermatol* 49:532–538, 2003.
255. Vorburger SA, Xing Y, Hunt KK, et al: Angiosarcoma of the breast, *Cancer* 104:2682–2688, 2005.
256. Wiklund TA, Blomqvist CP, Raty J, et al: Postirradiation sarcoma. Analysis of a nationwide cancer registry material, *Cancer* 68:524–531, 1991.
257. Sheppard DG, Libshitz HI: Post-radiation sarcomas: a review of the clinical and imaging features in 63 cases, *Clin Radiol* 56:22–29, 2001.
258. Laskin WB, Silverman TA, Enzinger FM: Postradiation soft tissue sarcomas. An analysis of 53 cases, *Cancer* 62:2330–2340, 1988.
259. Deyrup AT, Miettinen M, North PE, et al: Angiosarcomas arising in the viscera and soft tissue of children and young adults: a clinicopathologic study of 15 cases, *Am J Surg Pathol* 33:264–269, 2009.
260. Mentzel T, Katenkamp D: Intraneural angiosarcoma and angiosarcoma arising in benign and malignant peripheral nerve sheath tumours: clinicopathological and immunohistochemical analysis of four cases, *Histopathology* 35:114–120, 1999.
261. Fletcher CD, Beham A, Bekir S, et al: Epithelioid angiosarcoma of deep soft tissue: a distinctive tumor readily mistaken for an epithelial neoplasm, *Am J Surg Pathol* 15:915–924, 1991.
262. Rossi S, Fletcher CD: Angiosarcoma arising in hemangioma/vascular malformation: report of four cases and review of the literature, *Am J Surg Pathol* 26:1319–1329, 2002.
263. McMenamin ME, Fletcher CD: Expanding the spectrum of malignant change in schwannomas: epithelioid malignant change, epithelioid malignant peripheral nerve sheath tumor, and epithelioid angiosarcoma: a study of 17 cases, *Am J Surg Pathol* 25:13–25, 2001.
264. Jennings TA, Peterson L, Axiotis CA, et al: Angiosarcoma associated with foreign body material. A report of three cases, *Cancer* 62:2436–2444, 1988.
265. Eusebi V, Carcangiu ML, Dina R, et al: Keratin-positive epithelioid angiosarcoma of thyroid. A report of four cases, *Am J Surg Pathol* 14:737–747, 1990.
266. Wenig BM, Abbondanzo SL, Heffess CS: Epithelioid angiosarcoma of the adrenal glands. A clinicopathologic study of nine cases with a discussion of the implications of finding "epithelial-specific" markers, *Am J Surg Pathol* 18:62–73, 1994.
267. Lee FY, Wen MC, Wang J: Epithelioid angiosarcoma arising in a deep-seated plexiform schwannoma: a case report and literature review, *Hum Pathol* 38:1096–1101, 2007.
268. Nascimento AF, Raut CP, Fletcher CD: Primary angiosarcoma of the breast: clinicopathologic analysis of 49 cases, suggesting that grade is not prognostic, *Am J Surg Pathol* 32:1896–1904, 2008.
269. Rosen PP, Kimmel M, Ernsberger D: Mammary angiosarcoma. The prognostic significance of tumor differentiation, *Cancer* 62:2145–2151, 1988.
270. Cooper PH: Angiosarcomas of the skin, *Semin Diagn Pathol* 4:2–17, 1987.
271. Burgert-Lon CE, Riddle ND, Lackman RD, et al: Angiosarcoma arising in chronic expanding hematoma: five cases of an underrecognized association, *Am J Surg Pathol* 39:1540–1547, 2015.
272. Requena L, Santonja C, Stutz N, et al: Pseudolymphomatous cutaneous angiosarcoma: a rare variant of cutaneous angiosarcoma readily mistaken for cutaneous lymphoma, *Am J Dermatopathol* 29:342–350, 2007.
273. McKenney JK, Weiss SW, Folpe AL: CD31 expression in intratumoral macrophages: a potential diagnostic pitfall, *Am J Surg Pathol* 25:1167–1173, 2001.
274. Manner J, Radlwimmer B, Hohenberger P, et al: MYC high level gene amplification is a distinctive feature of angiosarcomas after irradiation or chronic lymphedema, *Am J Pathol* 176:34–39, 2010.
275. Mentzel T, Schildhaus HU, Palmedo G, et al: Postradiation cutaneous angiosarcoma after treatment of breast carcinoma is characterized by MYC amplification in contrast to atypical vascular lesions after radiotherapy and control cases: clinicopathological, immunohistochemical and molecular analysis of 66 cases, *Mod Pathol* 25:75–85, 2012.
276. Guo T, Zhang L, Chang NE, et al: Consistent MYC and FLT4 gene amplification in radiation-induced angiosarcoma but not in other radiation-associated atypical vascular lesions, *Genes Chromosomes Cancer* 50:25–33, 2011.
277. Nappi O, Wick MR, Pettinato G, et al: Pseudovascular adenoid squamous cell carcinoma of the skin. A neoplasm that may be mistaken for angiosarcoma, *Am J Surg Pathol* 16:429–438, 1992.
278. Albores-Saavedra J, Schwartz AM, Henson DE, et al: Cutaneous angiosarcoma. Analysis of 434 cases from the Surveillance, Epidemiology, and End Results Program, 1973-2007, *Ann Diagn Pathol* 15:93–97, 2011.
279. Young RJ, Brown NJ, Reed MW, et al: Angiosarcoma, *Lancet Oncol* 11:983–991, 2010.
280. Hodgson NC, Bowen-Wells C, Moffat F, et al: Angiosarcomas of the breast: a review of 70 cases, *Am J Clin Oncol* 30:570–573, 2007.
281. Suchak R, Thway K, Zelger B, et al: Primary cutaneous epithelioid angiosarcoma: a clinicopathologic study of 13 cases of a rare neoplasm occurring outside the setting of conventional angiosarcomas and with a predilection for the limbs, *Am J Surg Pathol* 35:60–69, 2011.
282. Fineberg S, Rosen PP: Cutaneous angiosarcoma and atypical vascular lesions of the skin and breast after radiation therapy for breast carcinoma, *Am J Clin Pathol* 102:757–763, 1994.
283. Brenn T, Fletcher CD: Postradiation vascular proliferations: an increasing problem, *Histopathology* 48:106–114, 2006.
284. Gengler C, Coindre JM, Leroux A, et al: Vascular proliferations of the skin after radiation therapy for breast cancer: clinicopathologic analysis of a series in favor of a benign process: a study from the French Sarcoma Group, *Cancer* 109:1584–1598, 2007.
285. Mattoch IW, Robbins JB, Kempson RL, et al: Post-radiotherapy vascular proliferations in mammary skin: a clinicopathologic study of 11 cases, *J Am Acad Dermatol* 57:126–133, 2007.
286. Requena L, Kutzner H, Mentzel T, et al: Benign vascular proliferations in irradiated skin, *Am J Surg Pathol* 26:328–337, 2002.

287. Patton KT, Deyrup AT, Weiss SW: Atypical vascular lesions after surgery and radiation of the breast: a clinicopathologic study of 32 cases analyzing histologic heterogeneity and association with angiosarcoma, *Am J Surg Pathol* 32:943–950, 2008.
288. Di Tommaso L, Fabbri A: Cutaneous angiosarcoma arising after radiotherapy treatment of a breast carcinoma. Description of a case and review of the literature, *Pathologica* 95:196–202, 2003.
289. Feigenberg SJ, Mendenhall NP, Reith JD, et al: Angiosarcoma after breast-conserving therapy: experience with hyperfractionated radiotherapy, *Int J Radiat Oncol Biol Phys* 52:620–626, 2002.
290. Olsen TG, Helwig EB: Angiolymphoid hyperplasia with eosinophilia. A clinicopathologic study of 116 patients, *J Am Acad Dermatol* 12:781–796, 1985.
291. Peters E, Altini M, Kola AH: Oral angiolymphoid hyperplasia with eosinophilia, *Oral Surg Oral Med Oral Pathol* 61:73–79, 1986.
292. Fetsch JF, Weiss SW: Observations concerning the pathogenesis of epithelioid hemangioma (angiolymphoid hyperplasia), *Mod Pathol* 4:449–455, 1991.
293. Buchanan R, Sworn MJ, Mousley JM: Angiolymphoid hyperplasia with eosinophilia involving skeletal muscle, *Histopathology* 4:197–204, 1980.
294. O'Connell JX, Kattapuram SV, Mankin HJ, et al: Epithelioid hemangioma of bone. A tumor often mistaken for low-grade angiosarcoma or malignant hemangioendothelioma, *Am J Surg Pathol* 17:610–617, 1993.
295. Fetsch JF, Sesterhenn IA, Miettinen M, et al: Epithelioid hemangioma of the penis: a clinicopathologic and immunohistochemical analysis of 19 cases, with special reference to exuberant examples often confused with epithelioid hemangioendothelioma and epithelioid angiosarcoma, *Am J Surg Pathol* 28:523–533, 2004.
296. Bartralot R, Garcia-Patos V, Hueto J, et al: Angiolymphoid hyperplasia with eosinophilia affecting the oral mucosa: report of a case and a review of the literature, *Br J Dermatol* 134:744–748, 1996.
297. Chan JK, Frizzera G, Fletcher CD, et al: Primary vascular tumors of lymph nodes other than Kaposi's sarcoma. Analysis of 39 cases and delineation of two new entities, *Am J Surg Pathol* 16:335–350, 1992.
298. Chan JK, Hui PK, Ng CS, et al: Epithelioid haemangioma (angiolymphoid hyperplasia with eosinophilia) and Kimura's disease in Chinese, *Histopathology* 15:557–574, 1989.
299. Tsang WY, Chan JK: The family of epithelioid vascular tumors, *Histol Histopathol* 8:187–212, 1993.
300. Rosai J, Akerman LR: Intravenous atypical vascular proliferation. A cutaneous lesion simulating a malignant blood vessel tumor, *Arch Dermatol* 109:714–717, 1974.
301. Koubaa W, Verdier M, Perez M, et al: Intra-arterial angiolymphoid hyperplasia with eosinophilia, *J Cutan Pathol* 35:495–498, 2008.
302. Gray MH, Rosenberg AE, Dickersin GR, et al: Cytokeratin expression in epithelioid vascular neoplasms, *Hum Pathol* 21:212–217, 1990.
303. Sun ZJ, Zhang L, Zhang WF, et al: Epithelioid hemangioma in the oral mucosa: a clinicopathological study of seven cases and review of the literature, *Oral Oncol* 42:441–447, 2006.
304. Hung HP, Fletcher CD, Hornick JL: FOSB is a useful diagnostic marker for pseudomyogenic hemangioendothelioma, *Am J Surg Pathol* 41:596–606, 2017.
305. Antonescu CR, Chen HW, Zhang L, et al: ZFP36-FOSB fusion defines a subset of epithelioid hemangioma with atypical features, *Genes Chromosomes Cancer* 53:951–959, 2014.
306. Huang SC, Zhang L, Sung YS, et al: Frequent FOS gene rearrangements in epithelioid hemangioma: A molecular study of 58 cases with morphologic reappraisal, *Am J Surg Pathol* 39:1313–1321, 2015.
307. van IJzendoorn DG, de Jong D, Romagosa C, et al: Fusion events lead to truncation of FOS in epithelioid hemangioma of bone, *Genes Chromosomes Cancer* 54:565–574, 2015.
308. Rosai J, Gold J, Landy R: The histiocytoid hemangiomas. A unifying concept embracing several previously described entities of skin, soft tissue, large vessels, bone, and heart, *Hum Pathol* 10:707–730, 1979.
309. Urabe A, Tsuneyoshi M, Enjoji M: Epithelioid hemangioma versus Kimura's disease. A comparative clinicopathologic study, *Am J Surg Pathol* 11:758–766, 1987.
310. Sangueza OP, Walsh SN, Sheehan DJ, et al: Cutaneous epithelioid angiomatous nodule: a case series and proposed classification, *Am J Dermatopathol* 30:16–20, 2008.
311. Brenn T, Fletcher CD: Cutaneous epithelioid angiomatous nodule: a distinct lesion in the morphologic spectrum of epithelioid vascular tumors, *Am J Dermatopathol* 26:14–21, 2004.
312. Misago N, Inoue T, Narisawa Y: Subcutaneous epithelioid angiomatous nodule: a variant of epithelioid hemangioma, *J Dermatol* 33:73–74, 2006.
313. Weiss SW, Enzinger FM: Epithelioid hemangioendothelioma: a vascular tumor often mistaken for a carcinoma, *Cancer* 50:970–981, 1982.
314. Mentzel T, Beham A, Calonje E, et al: Epithelioid hemangioendothelioma of skin and soft tissues: clinicopathologic and immunohistochemical study of 30 cases, *Am J Surg Pathol* 21:363–374, 1997.
315. Kleer CG, Unni KK, McLeod RA: Epithelioid hemangioendothelioma of bone, *Am J Surg Pathol* 20:1301–1311, 1996.
316. Tsuneyoshi M, Dorfman HD, Bauer TW: Epithelioid hemangioendothelioma of bone. A clinicopathologic, ultrastructural, and immunohistochemical study, *Am J Surg Pathol* 10:754–764, 1986.
317. Bhagavan BS, Dorfman HD, Murthy MS, et al: Intravascular bronchiolo-alveolar tumor (IVBAT): A low-grade sclerosing epithelioid angiosarcoma of lung, *Am J Surg Pathol* 6:41–52, 1982.
318. Ishak KG, Sesterhenn IA, Goodman ZD, et al: Epithelioid hemangioendothelioma of the liver: a clinicopathologic and follow-up study of 32 cases, *Hum Pathol* 15:839–852, 1984.
319. Makhlouf HR, Ishak KG, Goodman ZD: Epithelioid hemangioendothelioma of the liver: a clinicopathologic study of 137 cases, *Cancer* 85:562–582, 1999.
320. Quante M, Patel NK, Hill S, et al: Epithelioid hemangioendothelioma presenting in the skin: a clinicopathologic study of eight cases, *Am J Dermatopathol* 20:541–546, 1998.
321. Weiss SW, Ishak KG, Dail DH, et al: Epithelioid hemangioendothelioma and related lesions, *Semin Diagn Pathol* 3:259–287, 1986.
322. Chi AC, Weathers DR, Folpe AL, et al: Epithelioid hemangioendothelioma of the oral cavity: report of two cases and review of the literature, *Oral Surg Oral Med Oral Pathol Oral Radiol Endod* 100:717–724, 2005.
323. Nora FE, Scheithauer BW: Primary epithelioid hemangioendothelioma of the brain, *Am J Surg Pathol* 20:707–714, 1996.
324. Siddiqui MT, Evans HL, Ro JY, et al: Epithelioid haemangioendothelioma of the thyroid gland: a case report and review of literature, *Histopathology* 32:473–476, 1998.
325. Suster S, Moran CA, Koss MN: Epithelioid hemangioendothelioma of the anterior mediastinum. Clinicopathologic, immunohistochemical, and ultrastructural analysis of 12 cases, *Am J Surg Pathol* 18:871–881, 1994.
326. Errani C, Sung YS, Zhang L, et al: Monoclonality of multifocal epithelioid hemangioendothelioma of the liver by analysis of WWTR1-CAMTA1 breakpoints, *Cancer Genet* 205:12–17, 2012.
327. Deyrup AT, Tighiouart M, Montag AG, et al: Epithelioid hemangioendothelioma of soft tissue: a proposal for risk stratification based on 49 cases, *Am J Surg Pathol* 32:924–927, 2008.
328. Clarke LE, Lee R, Militello G, et al: Cutaneous epithelioid hemangioendothelioma, *J Cutan Pathol* 35:236–240, 2008.
329. Antonescu CR, Le Loarer F, Mosquera JM, et al: Novel YAP1-TFE3 fusion defines a distinct subset of epithelioid hemangioendothelioma, *Genes Chromosomes Cancer* 52:775–784, 2013.
330. Miettinen M, Fetsch JF: Distribution of keratins in normal endothelial cells and a spectrum of vascular tumors: implications in tumor diagnosis, *Hum Pathol* 31:1062–1067, 2000.
331. Fujii T, Zen Y, Sato Y, et al: Podoplanin is a useful diagnostic marker for epithelioid hemangioendothelioma of the liver, *Mod Pathol* 21:125–130, 2008.
332. Doyle LA, Fletcher CD, Hornick JL: Nuclear expression of CAMTA1 distinguishes epithelioid hemangioendothelioma from histologic mimics, *Am J Surg Pathol* 40:94–102, 2016.
333. Flucke U, Vogels RJ, de Saint Aubain Somerhausen N, et al: Epithelioid hemangioendothelioma: clinicopathologic, immunhistochemical, and molecular genetic analysis of 39 cases, *Diagn Pathol* 9:131–142, 2014.
334. Mendlick MR, Nelson M, Pickering D, et al: Translocation t(1;3)(p36.3;q25) is a nonrandom aberration in epithelioid hemangioendothelioma, *Am J Surg Pathol* 25:684–687, 2001.
335. Tanas MR, Sboner A, Oliveira AM, et al: Identification of a disease-defining gene fusion in epithelioid hemangioendothelioma, *Sci Transl Med* 3:98ra82, 2011.
336. Errani C, Zhang L, Sung YS, et al: A novel WWTR1-CAMTA1 gene fusion is a consistent abnormality in epithelioid hemangioendothelioma of different anatomic sites, *Genes Chromosomes Cancer* 50:644–653, 2011.
337. Miettinen M, Fanburg-Smith JC, Virolainen M, et al: Epithelioid sarcoma: an immunohistochemical analysis of 112 classical and variant cases and a discussion of the differential diagnosis, *Hum Pathol* 30:934–942, 1999.
338. Hornick JL, Dal Cin P, Fletcher CDM: Loss of INI1 expression is characteristic of both conventional and proximal-type epithelioid sarcoma, *Am J Surg Pathol* 33:542–550, 2009.
339. Marrogi AJ, Hunt SJ, Cruz DJ: Cutaneous epithelioid angiosarcoma, *Am J Dermatopathol* 12:350–356, 1990.
340. Prescott RJ, Banerjee SS, Eyden BP, et al: Cutaneous epithelioid angiosarcoma: a clinicopathological study of four cases, *Histopathology* 25:421–429, 1994.
341. Deyrup AT, Miettinen M, North PE, et al: Pediatric cutaneous angiosarcomas: a clinicopathologic study of 10 cases, *Am J Surg Pathol* 35:770–775, 2011.
342. Weiss SW, Enzinger FM: Spindle cell hemangioendothelioma. A low-grade angiosarcoma resembling a cavernous hemangioma and Kaposi's sarcoma, *Am J Surg Pathol* 10:521–530, 1986.
343. Perkins P, Weiss SW: Spindle cell hemangioendothelioma. An analysis of 78 cases with reassessment of its pathogenesis and biologic behavior, *Am J Surg Pathol* 20:1196–1204, 1996.
344. Fletcher CD, Beham A, Schmid C: Spindle cell haemangioendothelioma: a clinicopathological and immunohistochemical study indicative of a non-neoplastic lesion, *Histopathology* 18:291–301, 1991.
345. Fanburg JC, Meis-Kindblom JM, Rosenberg AE: Multiple enchondromas associated with spindle-cell hemangioendotheliomas. An overlooked variant of Maffucci's syndrome, *Am J Surg Pathol* 19:1029–1038, 1995.
346. Tosios K, Koutlas IG, Kapranos N, et al: Spindle-cell hemangioendothelioma of the oral cavity. A case report, *J Oral Pathol Med* 24:379–382, 1995.
347. Scott GA, Rosai J: Spindle cell hemangioendothelioma. Report of seven additional cases of a recently described vascular neoplasm, *Am J Dermatopathol* 10:281–288, 1988.
348. Ding J, Hashimoto H, Imayama S, et al: Spindle cell haemangioendothelioma: probably a benign vascular lesion not a low-grade angiosarcoma. A clinicopathological, ultrastructural and immunohistochemical study, *Virchows Arch A Pathol Anat Histopathol* 420:77–85, 1992.
349. Pansuriya TC, van Eijk R, d'Adamo P, et al: Somatic mosaic IDH1 and IDH2 mutations are associated with enchondroma and spindle cell hemangioma in Ollier disease and Maffucci syndrome, *Nat Genet* 43:1256–1261, 2011.

350. Amary MF, Damato S, Halai D, et al: Ollier disease and Maffucci syndrome are caused by somatic mosaic mutations of IDH1 and IDH2, *Nat Genet* 43:1262–1265, 2011.
351. Kurek KC, Pansuriya TC, van Ruler MA, et al: R132C IDH1 mutations are found in spindle cell hemangiomas and not in other vascular tumors or malformations, *Am J Pathol* 182:1494–1500, 2013.
352. Mentzel T, Mazzoleni G, Dei Tos AP, et al: Kaposiform hemangioendothelioma in adults. Clinicopathologic and immunohistochemical analysis of three cases, *Am J Clin Pathol* 108:450–455, 1997.
353. Deraedt K, Vander Poorten V, Van Geet C, et al: Multifocal kaposiform haemangioendothelioma, *Virchows Arch* 448:843–846, 2006.
354. Gianotti R, Gelmetti C, Alessi E: Congenital cutaneous multifocal kaposiform hemangioendothelioma, *Am J Dermatopathol* 21:557–561, 1999.
355. Zukerberg LR, Nickoloff BJ, Weiss SW: Kaposiform hemangioendothelioma of infancy and childhood. An aggressive neoplasm associated with Kasabach-Merritt syndrome and lymphangiomatosis, *Am J Surg Pathol* 17:321–328, 1993.
356. Sarkar M, Mulliken JB, Kozakewich HP, et al: Thrombocytopenic coagulopathy (Kasabach-Merritt phenomenon) is associated with Kaposiform hemangioendothelioma and not with common infantile hemangioma, *Plast Reconstr Surg* 100:1377–1386, 1997.
357. Lyons LL, North PE, Mac-Moune Lai F, et al: Kaposiform hemangioendothelioma: a study of 33 cases emphasizing its pathologic, immunophenotypic, and biologic uniqueness from juvenile hemangioma, *Am J Surg Pathol* 28:559–568, 2004.
358. Alvarez-Mendoza A, Lourdes TS, Ridaura-Sanz C, et al: Histopathology of vascular lesions found in Kasabach-Merritt syndrome: review based on 13 cases, *Pediatr Dev Pathol* 3:556–560, 2000.
359. Enjolras O, Mulliken JB, Wassef M, et al: Residual lesions after Kasabach-Merritt phenomenon in 41 patients, *J Am Acad Dermatol* 42:225–235, 2000.
360. Niedt GW, Greco MA, Wieczorek R, et al: Hemangioma with Kaposi's sarcoma-like features: report of two cases, *Pediatr Pathol* 9:567–575, 1989.
361. Tsang WY, Chan JK, Fletcher CD: Recently characterized vascular tumours of skin and soft tissues, *Histopathology* 19:489–501, 1991.
362. Debelenko LV, Perez-Atayde AR, Mulliken JB, et al: D2–40 immunohistochemical analysis of pediatric vascular tumors reveals positivity in kaposiform hemangioendothelioma, *Mod Pathol* 18:1454–1460, 2005.
363. Haisley-Royster C, Enjolras O, Frieden IJ, et al: Kasabach-merritt phenomenon: a retrospective study of treatment with vincristine, *J Pediatr Hematol Oncol* 24:459–462, 2002.
364. Hauer J, Graubner U, Konstantopoulos N, et al: Effective treatment of kaposiform hemangioendotheliomas associated with Kasabach-Merritt phenomenon using four-drug regimen, *Pediatr Blood Cancer* 49:852–854, 2007.
365. el Dessouky M, Azmy AF, Raine PA, et al: Kasabach-Merritt syndrome, *J Pediatr Surg* 23:109–111, 1988.
366. Geraminejad P, Memar O, Aronson I, et al: Kaposi's sarcoma and other manifestations of human herpesvirus 8, *J Am Acad Dermatol* 47:641–655, 2002.
367. Costa J, Rabson AS: Generalised Kaposi's sarcoma is not a neoplasm, *Lancet* 1:58, 1983.
368. Gill PS, Tsai YC, Rao AP, et al: Evidence for multiclonality in multicentric Kaposi's sarcoma, *Proc Natl Acad Sci USA* 95:8257–8261, 1998.
369. Rabkin CS, Janz S, Lash A, et al: Monoclonal origin of multicentric Kaposi's sarcoma lesions, *N Engl J Med* 336:988–993, 1997.
370. Duprez R, Lacoste V, Briere J, et al: Evidence for a multiclonal origin of multicentric advanced lesions of Kaposi sarcoma, *J Natl Cancer Inst* 99:1086–1094, 2007.
371. Antman K, Chang Y: Kaposi's sarcoma, *N Engl J Med* 342:1027–1038, 2000.
372. Chor PJ, Santa Cruz DJ: Kaposi's sarcoma. A clinicopathologic review and differential diagnosis, *J Cutan Pathol* 19:6–20, 1992.
373. Iscovich J, Boffetta P, Franceschi S, et al: Classic kaposi sarcoma: epidemiology and risk factors, *Cancer* 88:500–517, 2000.
374. Weissmann A, Linn S, Weltfriend S, et al: Epidemiological study of classic Kaposi's sarcoma: a retrospective review of 125 cases from Northern Israel, *J Eur Acad Dermatol Venereol* 14:91–95, 2000.
375. Stratigos JD, Potouridou I, Katoulis AC, et al: Classic Kaposi's sarcoma in Greece: a clinico-epidemiological profile, *Int J Dermatol* 36:735–740, 1997.
376. Taylor JF, Templeton AC, Vogel CL, et al: Kaposi's sarcoma in Uganda: a clinico-pathological study, *Int J Cancer* 8:122–135, 1971.
377. Templeton AC, Bhana D: Prognosis in Kaposi's sarcoma, *J Natl Cancer Inst* 55:1301–1304, 1975.
378. Gottlieb GJ, Ackerman AB: Kaposi's sarcoma: an extensively disseminated form in young homosexual men, *Hum Pathol* 13:882–892, 1982.
379. Fukunaga M, Silverberg SG: Hyaline globules in Kaposi's sarcoma: a light microscopic and immunohistochemical study, *Mod Pathol* 4:187–190, 1991.
380. Ronchese F, Kern AB: Lymphangioma-like tumors in Kaposi's sarcoma, *AMA Arch Derm* 75:418–427, 1957.
381. Leibowitz MR, Dagliotti M, Smith E, et al: Rapidly fatal lymphangioma-like Kaposi's sarcoma, *Histopathology* 4:559–566, 1980.
382. Cossu S, Satta R, Cottoni F, et al: Lymphangioma-like variant of Kaposi's sarcoma: clinicopathologic study of seven cases with review of the literature, *Am J Dermatopathol* 19:16–22, 1997.
383. Cox FH, Helwig EB: Kaposi's sarcoma, *Cancer* 12:289–298, 1959.
384. Luzar B, Antony F, Ramdial PK, et al: Intravascular Kaposi's sarcoma—a hitherto unrecognized phenomenon, *J Cutan Pathol* 34:861–864, 2007.
385. Yu H, Gibson JA, Pinkus GS, et al: Podoplanin (D2–40) is a novel marker for follicular dendritic cell tumors, *Am J Clin Pathol* 128:776–782, 2007.
386. Xu H, Edwards JR, Espinosa O, et al: Expression of a lymphatic endothelial cell marker in benign and malignant vascular tumors, *Hum Pathol* 35:857–861, 2004.
387. Naresh KN, Francis N, Sarwar N, et al: Expression of human herpesvirus 8 (HHV-8), latent nuclear antigen 1 (LANA1) in angiosarcoma in acquired immunodeficiency syndrome (AIDS)—a report of two cases, *Histopathology* 51:861–864, 2007.
388. Hammock L, Reisenauer A, Wang W, et al: Latency-associated nuclear antigen expression and human herpesvirus-8 polymerase chain reaction in the evaluation of Kaposi sarcoma and other vascular tumors in HIV-positive patients, *Mod Pathol* 18:463–468, 2005.
389. Ackerman AB: Subtle clues to diagnosis by conventional microscopy. The patch stage of Kaposi's sarcoma, *Am J Dermatopathol* 1:165–172, 1979.

14

Cartilaginous and Osseous Soft Tissue Lesions

Jodi M. Carter, MD, PhD, and André M. Oliveira, MD, PhD

Soft tissue tumors and other mass-forming lesions exhibiting osteocartilaginous differentiation are commonly encountered in diagnostic soft tissue pathology. They comprise diverse entities with distinct clinicopathologic features and clinical behaviors. However, it is important to remember that, occasionally, nonmesenchymal tumors may also display osseous and cartilaginous differentiation. Hence, to avoid diagnostic errors, a systematic approach to such tumors is advisable. The following simple four-step algorithm can be helpful (Box 14.1).

Step 1. Confirm the presence of osteocartilaginous differentiation. It is not unusual to confuse hyalinized collagen with osteoid or a myxoid matrix with cartilage. Admittedly where one draws the line between hyalinized collagen and osteoid at the histologic level is a subjective and highly controversial matter, especially considering that both matrices are primarily composed of type I collagen. Some subtle histologic clues may be helpful. The identification of calcification (with a basophilic appearance) rather than a purely eosinophilic matrix or the presence of plump plasmacytoid cells (osteoblasts) surrounding this eosinophilic matrix supports the presence of osteoid or bone formation. Nonetheless it is worth noting that plump osteoblasts are primarily seen in association with metaplastic bone (e.g., fracture callus) and not with neoplastic bone (e.g., osteosarcoma). SATB2 is a nuclear transcription factor required for osteoblast lineage commitment. Recent studies have demonstrated that immunohistochemistry for SATB2 may be useful to confirm osteoblastic differentiation in soft tissue tumors; however, nuclear staining for SATB2 is not entirely specific.[1] In addition, chondrocytes express S-100 protein, and immunohistochemistry for S-100 protein is useful for the confirmation of cartilaginous differentiation, although this marker is also expressed by other cell types.

Step 2. Exclude a primary bone tumor extending into surrounding soft tissue. In most cases, this can easily be assessed by reviewing radiologic studies or obtaining additional clinical information. Furthermore, some bone tumors have unique histologic features that can easily be differentiated from primary soft tissue tumors.

Step 3. Exclude a nonmesenchymal tumor showing osteocartilaginous differentiation. For example, heterologous osseous or cartilaginous differentiation can be seen in a subset of metaplastic carcinomas of the breast and other anatomic sites. In addition, osteocartilaginous differentiation is common in myoepithelial and mixed epithelial-myoepithelial tumors (e.g., pleomorphic adenoma of salivary gland; chondroid syringoma). In such instances, recognition of the (myo) epithelial component by morphologic or immunohistochemical analysis is necessary.

Step 4. Distinguish primary osseous and cartilaginous soft tissue tumors from soft tissue tumors showing secondary (heterologous) osteocartilaginous differentiation. The latter tumor types are discussed in detail elsewhere in this book; the most important considerations for differential diagnosis are briefly mentioned at the end of this chapter. For example, a retroperitoneal sarcoma showing osseous or cartilaginous differentiation is most likely a dedifferentiated liposarcoma. This chapter provides a detailed discussion of primary soft tissue tumors and lesions with osteocartilaginous differentiation.

Myositis Ossificans and Heterotopic Ossification

Clinical Features

Myositis ossificans, also known as *myositis ossificans circumscripta*, is an apparently nonneoplastic soft tissue lesion that occurs more commonly during the second and third decades of life, usually in physically active individuals.[2] These lesions show a male predilection and most commonly occur within the skeletal muscles of the lower extremities, especially

Box 14.1 Approach to Tumors Exhibiting Osteocartilaginous Differentiation

Confirm that there is indeed bone or cartilaginous differentiation. Hyalinized collagen and myxoid matrix with retraction artifact may simulate bone and cartilage, respectively.
Exclude an underlying bone lesion with secondary soft tissue involvement (review radiologic studies if appropriate).
Exclude a nonmesenchymal tumor showing heterologous osteocartilaginous differentiation.
Differentiate between primary soft tissue tumors with osteocartilaginous differentiation and soft tissues tumors in which osteocartilaginous differentiation is a secondary phenomenon.

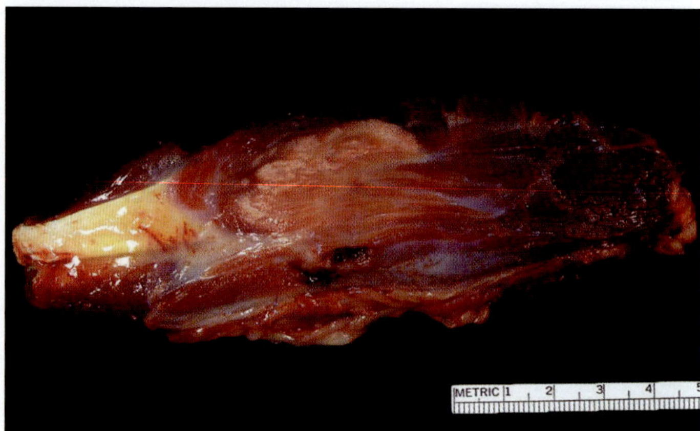

Figure 14.1 **Gross Appearance of Myositis Ossificans.** The typical peripheral ossification is evident on macroscopic inspection.

the thighs and buttocks (Fig. 14.1). However, similar processes can also occur in adipose tissue (panniculitis ossificans) or fascia (fasciitis ossificans). In more than 50% of cases, a history of trauma is elicited; pain is a common and early complaint. A lesion indistinguishable from myositis ossificans has also been reported in the mesentery.[3]

Heterotopic ossification is considered by some a synonym for myositis ossificans, perhaps a more mature, later phase of the latter process. Others consider heterotopic ossification an aberrant chondro-ossification of soft tissues caused by a variety of distinct disorders. McCarthy and Sundaram have provided a comprehensive review of the subject.[4]

Pathologic Features

Histologically, myositis ossificans is a generally well-circumscribed lesion characterized by a central cellular spindle cell area, composed of (myo) fibroblasts with nodular fasciitis–like features associated with immature woven bone formation (Fig. 14.2). Toward the periphery, the lesion displays more organized and mature lamellar bone formation (Fig. 14.3). This progressive maturation from the center to the periphery is classically known as a "zoning" phenomenon and is essentially diagnostic of myositis ossificans. Foci of cartilage undergoing endochondral ossification are also commonly seen. Other findings include cystic degeneration, hemorrhage, and the presence of multinucleated osteoclast-like giant cells as well as other chronic inflammatory cells. The histologic features are nicely mirrored by the radiologic findings, which show a characteristic shell of bone with ring-like features and central lucency (Fig. 14.4),[4] usually after 3 to 4 weeks of evolution. As such, myositis ossificans is usually diagnosed at the radiologic level. Histologic analysis is typically required for sizable lesions or lesions with unusual radiologic features or clinical evolution.

Immunohistochemistry and Molecular Genetics

Currently there is no role for immunohistochemistry or genetic analysis for the diagnosis of myositis ossificans. By immunohistochemistry, the spindle cell component can express muscle-specific actin or smooth muscle actin.

Differential Diagnosis

The most important differential diagnosis for myositis ossificans is extraskeletal osteosarcoma. In contrast to myositis ossificans, extraskeletal osteosarcoma tends to occur in older patients and does not exhibit a "zoning" phenomenon; bone formation in extraskeletal osteosarcoma is more randomly distributed. Furthermore, marked nuclear pleomorphism and hyperchromasia are typical of extraskeletal osteosarcoma and should not be seen in myositis ossificans. Cystic degeneration and hemorrhage in myositis ossificans simulate the histologic features of soft tissue aneurysmal bone cyst.[5] Fracture callus can occasionally be mistaken for myositis ossificans. This problem can easily be solved by good radiologic correlation (see earlier discussion).

Prognosis and Treatment

Myositis ossificans is a benign and self-limited condition. Surgery is usually not necessary except when secondary complications arise. Malignant transformation in myositis ossificans has been reported but remains a debatable subject.

PRACTICE POINTS: Myositis Ossificans

Typically found in younger individuals.
Tends to contain areas similar to nodular fasciitis in the lesional center and progressive bone formation and maturation toward the periphery ("zoning" phenomenon).
Review radiologic studies; they are diagnostic in most instances.
Exclude extraskeletal osteosarcoma, which is highly atypical and pleomorphic, does not show the "zoning" phenomenon, and is primarily found in older adults.

Fibro-Osseous Pseudotumor of the Digits

Clinical Features

Fibro-osseous pseudotumor of the digits (FOPD), also known as *florid reactive periostitis* or a form of bone surface heterotopic ossification, is a poorly understood condition that closely simulates myositis ossificans.[6,7] FOPD more commonly occurs around the proximal phalanx of the fingers of young women. Toes can sometimes be affected. Whether FOPD is reactive or neoplastic in nature remains controversial. Clinically, FOPD presents as a painful swelling of the subcutaneous tissues of the involved digit that simulates a neoplasm.

Pathologic Features

Histologically, FOPD is composed of a cytologically bland spindle cell proliferation with nodular fasciitis–like features associated with immature woven bone formation in a somewhat disorganized fashion (Fig. 14.5). No zoning pattern is seen. Some authorities believe that the lesion is related to bizarre parosteal osteochondromatous proliferation (BPOP), which is among the most important differential diagnoses (see section "Differential Diagnosis").

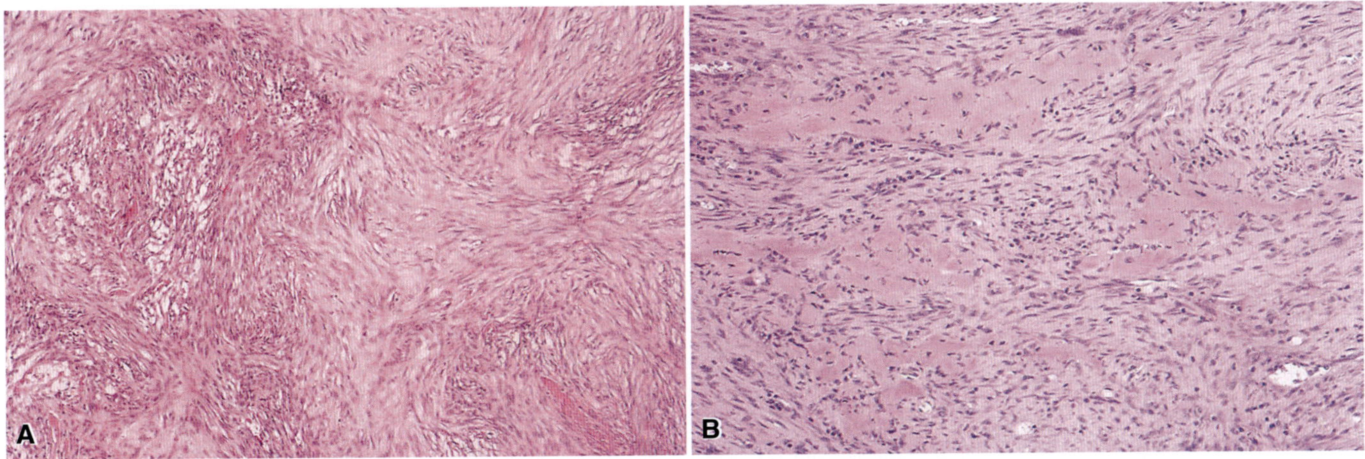

Figure 14.2 Myositis Ossificans. Histologically, the central area of myositis ossificans closely simulates nodular fasciitis (A). Focal formation of immature bone can be seen within the proliferation of spindle cells (B).

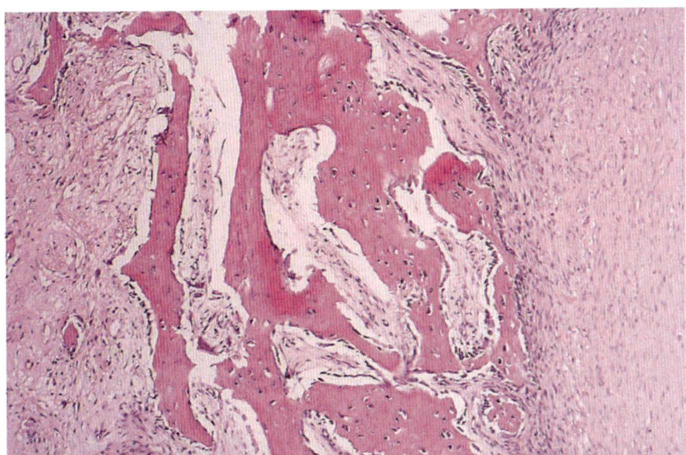

Figure 14.3 Myositis Ossificans. A later phase of myositis ossificans shows peripheral formation of mature bone.

Immunohistochemistry and Molecular Genetics

FOPD has no distinctive immunohistochemical or molecular genetic signature.

Differential Diagnosis

The most important differential diagnosis for FOPD is BPOP, which is also attached to the bone surface and has recently been shown to be neoplastic in nature.[8,9] In contrast to FOPD, BPOP is characterized by a hypercellular cartilaginous cap that matures into trabecular bone. The chondrocytes are enlarged and can be atypical, closely simulating the atypical chondrocytes in chondrosarcoma.[10,11] However, a typical feature of BPOP is the presence of a peculiar basophilic calcification similar to that seen in aneurysmal bone cyst ("blue bone") at the junction between the cartilaginous cap and the trabecular bone. Osteosarcoma (skeletal and extraskeletal) is another important diagnostic consideration but shows a much higher degree of cytologic atypia and pleomorphism. In addition, osteosarcoma is rare in the distal extremities. Subungual exostosis shows characteristic radiologic features and often displays a cartilaginous component that matures into trabecular-like bone.

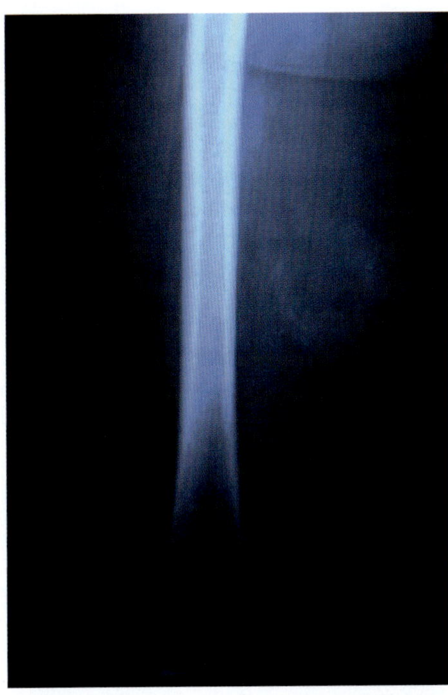

Figure 14.4 Myositis Ossificans. The characteristic central lucency and peripheral bone sclerosis of myositis ossificans is visible on a plain radiograph.

Prognosis and Treatment

FOPD follows a benign clinical course but can recur locally.[6,7,12] Surgical excision is the primary treatment.

PRACTICE POINTS: Fibro-Osseous Pseudotumor of the Digits

- As its name implies, FOPD is primarily located in the distal extremities.
- FOPD shows nodular fasciitis–like features and disorganized metaplastic bone formation.
- FOPD should be differentiated from bizarre parosteal osteochondromatous proliferation. Radiologic studies are paramount.

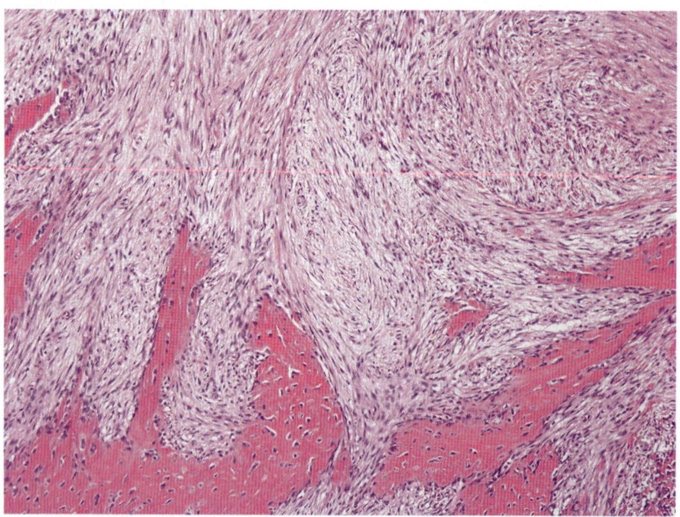

Figure 14.5 Fibro-osseous Pseudotumor of the Digits. A nodular fasciitis–like bland proliferation of spindle cells associated with the formation of immature bone is characteristic of fibro-osseous pseudotumor of the digits. No "zoning" is apparent (unlike in myositis ossificans).

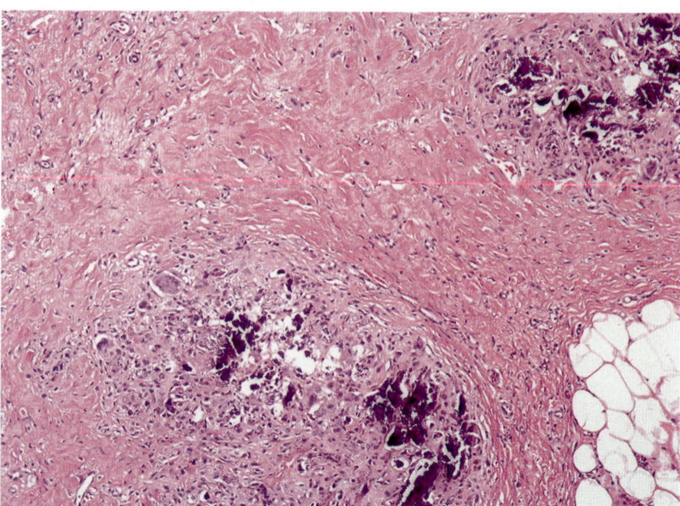

Figure 14.6 Tumoral Calcinosis. Nodules of amorphous calcified deposits surrounded by multinucleated giant cells and other inflammatory cells are characteristic of tumoral calcinosis. Note the granulomatous appearance of the lesion.

Fibrodysplasia Ossificans Progressiva

Clinical Features

Fibrodysplasia ossificans progressiva (FOP) is a rare autosomal dominant disorder characterized by several skeletal malformations and progressive extraskeletal aberrant chondro-ossification.[13,14] The clinical onset of FOP commonly occurs before the fifth year of life. The progressive soft tissue chondro-ossification develops initially around the upper paraspinal muscles and progresses distally and centripetally to the extremities.

Pathologic Features

The histologic features of FOP are relatively nonspecific and characterized by an initial fibroblastic proliferative phase that evolves over time to an aberrant ossification of muscles, adipose tissue, fascia, tendons, and other structures.

Molecular Genetics

FOP has recently been found to be caused by a constitutive activating mutation of the activin A receptor gene (*ACVR1*; R206H), which encodes for bone morphogenetic protein type I receptor.[15] This leads to aberrant signaling of this pathway and resultant progressive ectopic soft tissue osteochondrogenesis. Recently, hypoxic signaling via HIF-1α has been implicated in the development of both FOP and nonsyndromic heterotopic ossification.[16]

Differential Diagnosis

The differential diagnosis of FOP is varied and includes any benign soft tissue osteocartilaginous lesion. A high degree of suspicion and a detailed clinical history are among the most important tools for reaching the correct diagnosis of FOP.

Prognosis and Treatment

Currently there is no specific treatment for FOP, and various attempts at pharmacologic approaches have shown limited success. The disease is progressive and ultimately leads to respiratory insufficiency and death due to involvement of the thoracic cage.

Tumoral Calcinosis and Tumoral Calcinosis–Like Lesions

Despite the fact that tumoral calcinosis is not primarily a bone- or cartilage-forming lesion, it is included in this chapter because it closely simulates osteocartilaginous tumors.

Clinical Features

Tumoral calcinosis is a nonneoplastic condition characterized by periarticular tumor-like calcium deposits most commonly surrounding the major joints, especially the hips, shoulders, and elbows.[17,18] Unfortunately the nomenclature regarding tumoral calcinosis is confusing, and different authors adopt different classification schemes. Overall, tumoral calcinosis can be familial or sporadic, or it may occur as a secondary manifestation of a number of diseases or conditions (discussed further on). In the latter situation, the deposits can be referred to as tumoral calcinosis–like lesions to differentiate them from primary or familial tumoral calcinosis. Patients typically present during the first two decades of life and the lesions are often multicentric and bilateral. Tumor calcinosis is more common in black males.

Pathologic Features

Histologically, tumoral calcinosis is characterized by lobular deposits of amorphous calcium crystals, eliciting a chronic inflammatory response, typically with numerous foreign body–type multinucleated giant cells that impart a "granulomatous" appearance (Fig. 14.6).

Molecular Genetics

Familial tumoral calcinosis has several subtypes, including a hyperphosphatemic variant and a normophosphatemic variant. Hyperphosphatemic familial tumor calcinosis is an autosomal recessive disease characterized by germline mutations of *GALNT3*, *FGF23*, and *KL* (*alpha-Klotho*), which all impair fibroblast growth factor 23 (FGF23) signaling, a circulating factor involved in phosphorus homeostasis.[19-21] A recent review by Folsom et al. provides a comprehensive review of the disease biology.[22]

Differential Diagnosis

Tumor calcinosis–like lesions, which have also been indiscriminately labeled *tumoral calcinosis*, occur in a variety of anatomic locations and are commonly associated with diseases causing metabolic calcium-phosphate imbalances such as renal insufficiency, milk-alkali syndrome, and hypervitaminosis D. Laskin and colleagues have described histologically similar lesions in the distal extremities.[20]

The differential diagnosis for tumoral calcinosis is broad and includes all tumoral calcinosis–like lesions or processes that lead to abnormal ectopic calcium deposition in the soft tissues. However, in routine clinical practice, an underlying metabolic disorder secondary to renal insufficiency should be the first consideration when a tumoral calcinosis–like lesion is encountered.

Prognosis and Treatment

Surgical excision is the primary treatment for symptomatic lesions irrespective of the underlying etiology. Familial tumoral calcinosis is treated with targeted therapies to reduce intestinal absorption and/or promote renal excretion of phosphate. In the setting of tumoral calcinosis–like lesions, therapeutic modalities target the underlying causative disease.

PRACTICE POINTS: Tumoral Calcinosis

- Often multifocal.
- An underlying metabolic disorder of calcium-phosphate metabolism, especially renal insufficiency, should be excluded.
- Solitary lesions in the distal extremities are often sporadic ("tumoral calcinosis–like lesions").
- Tumoral calcinosis and tumoral calcinosis–like lesions have similar histologic features—soft tissue nodules showing ectopic calcification associated with a granulomatous reaction.

Soft Tissue Chondroma

Clinical Features

Soft tissue chondroma is a benign hyaline cartilage neoplasm that most often involves the soft tissues of the distal extremities, including the digits, hands and feet, with the fingers being the most common location.[23,24] By definition, soft tissue chondroma (or chondroma of soft parts) does not involve bone or joint spaces. As such, a primary intraosseous, bone surface, or intraarticular hyaline cartilage lesion must be excluded by reviewing radiologic studies. Occasionally soft tissue chondroma can appear at more proximal anatomic sites, including the trunk, head, and neck. However, in these instances other entities should be excluded (see Differential Diagnosis). Clinically, patients typically present with a long-standing, painless solitary mass; however, pain and paresthesias are occasionally reported.

Pathologic Features

Soft tissue chondroma is a well-circumscribed, often multilobulated hyaline cartilaginous tumor (Figs. 14.7 and 14.8). Secondary dystrophic calcification is rather common and may obscure the cartilaginous nature of the neoplasm. Myxoid change, cystic degeneration, and hemorrhage are not uncommon and may be quite extensive. Occasional examples may show an epithelioid appearance, which can lead to the erroneous impression of an epithelial neoplasm. Other cases tend to be more spindled, and the questionable terminology "immature" chondroma is occasionally used. A soft tissue chondroma variant histologically similar to chondroblastoma has also been described (Fig. 14.9).[25] Chondrocytes in soft tissue chondroma exhibit a mild to moderate degree of cytologic atypia, but mitoses are not typically seen; cellularity is usually increased when compared with normal hyaline cartilage but chondrocyte clustering is often maintained (Fig. 14.10).

Immunohistochemistry

Soft tissue chondroma is virtually always positive for S-100 protein. However, immunohistochemical analysis is rarely required for the diagnosis except for the more diagnostically challenging morphologic variants previously described.

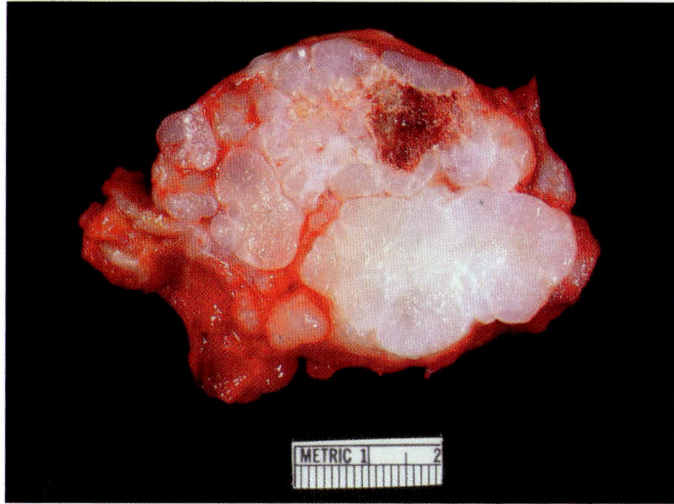

Figure 14.7 Soft Tissue Chondroma. A soft tissue chondroma is grossly well circumscribed and often multilobulated.

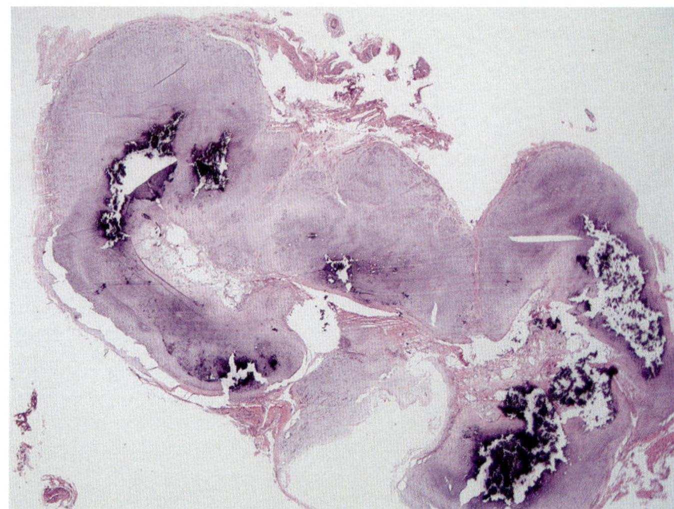

Figure 14.8 Soft Tissue Chondroma. Histologically, soft tissue chondroma is a well-circumscribed hyaline cartilaginous lesion.

Molecular Genetics

In contrast to enchondromas,[26] only a few cases of soft tissue chondroma have been characterized at the genetic level. Rearrangements of *HMGA2* on chromosome 12q15 are common, with one case harboring a *HMGA2-LPP* fusion.[27] Mutations in isocitrate dehydrogenase (*IDH1*), which frequently occur in both benign and malignant intraosseous and periosteal hyaline cartilage tumors, are not present in soft tissue chondromas.[28]

Differential Diagnosis

The most important considerations in the differential diagnosis are periosteal (surface or juxtacortical) chondroma and enchondroma (intraosseous chondroma). Radiologic studies should easily resolve the matter. Synovial chondromatosis overlaps histologically with soft tissue chondroma but is primarily seen in association with large joints and should be strongly considered if multiple lesions are present. Tumoral calcinosis–like lesions, as described earlier, should be considered in heavily calcified tumors, where the cartilaginous nature of the process

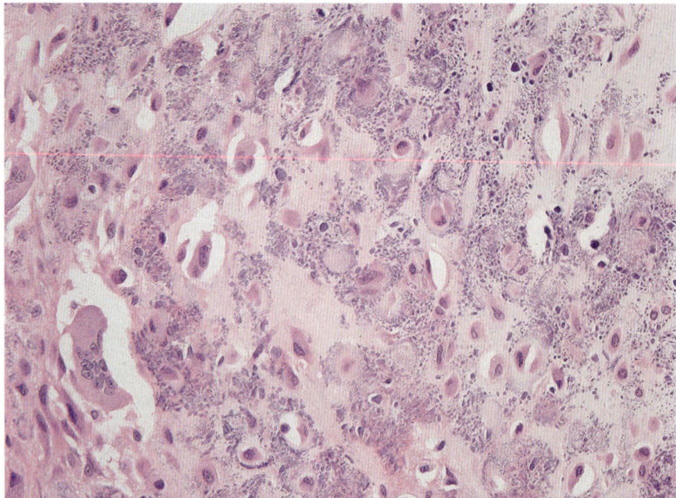

Figure 14.9 Chondroblastoma-Like Soft Tissue Chondroma. Note the large epithelioid cells, delicate pattern of calcification, and osteoclast-like giant cells.

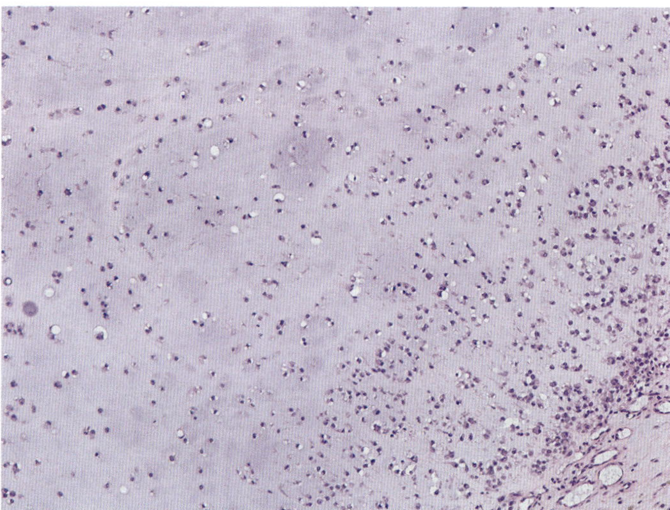

Figure 14.10 Soft Tissue Chondroma. The chondrocytes in soft tissue chondroma exhibit mild to moderate cytologic atypia and tend to conglomerate at the periphery of the cartilaginous nodules.

is not apparent. Lipomas with chondroid metaplasia or chondroid lipoma are also potential confounders (see Chapter 12). Careful histologic examination helps in these instances. The rare skeletal chondrosarcomas of the hands and feet that extend into the surrounding soft tissues should also be excluded. However, as underscored previously, radiologic studies are indispensable in this scenario.

Prognosis and Treatment

Soft tissue chondroma is primarily treated by surgical excision. Lesions may recur locally in up to 20% of cases; however, this number is based on large consultation-based series, which may have overestimated their true biologic potential. Malignant transformation is exceedingly rare (if it occurs at all) and should raise the possibility of a skeletal chondrosarcoma with secondary soft tissue involvement that was initially misdiagnosed as soft tissue chondroma.

PRACTICE POINTS: Soft Tissue Chondroma

- Primarily located in the distal extremities; the fingers are the most common location.
- Review radiologic studies to exclude a primary periosteal or intraosseous hyaline cartilage tumor extending into soft tissue.
- Consider synovial chondromatosis if located near major joints.
- May display moderate cytologic atypia, increased cellularity, and myxoid change, simulating chondrosarcoma.

Synovial Chondromatosis

Clinical Features

Synovial chondromatosis is a synovial-based cartilaginous neoplasm that most often involves the knee, followed by the hip and elbow joints.[29,30] Occasionally, other anatomic sites may be affected. Until recently, the disease was considered reactive in nature, but cytogenetic studies have strongly supported its neoplastic, clonal nature (see later discussion). Synovial chondromatosis most often affects middle-aged adults, with a male predominance. The most common clinical symptom is pain, but joint effusion and stiffness are also observed. Radiologically, synovial chondromatosis is characterized by the presence of calcified soft tissue masses around the affected joints, better visualized by magnetic resonance imaging.

Pathologic Features

Grossly, synovial chondromatosis is composed of numerous glistening nodules of cartilage within synovial soft tissue (Fig. 14.11). Histologically, the presence of multiple hyaline cartilaginous nodules, often lined by synovium, is typical (Fig. 14.12A). The chondrocytes tend to be clustered in small aggregates surrounded by the hyaline cartilaginous matrix, which is of diagnostic relevance; nuclear hyperchromasia, mild cytologic atypia, and binucleation are also rather common (see Fig. 14.12B).[31] Mitoses are rarely seen. Dystrophic calcification is common, but ossification is unusual.

Immunohistochemistry

Synovial chondromatosis consistently expresses S-100 protein, but immunohistochemistry is not required for diagnosis.

Molecular Genetics

Cytogenetically, synovial chondromatosis exhibits recurrent abnormalities of chromosome 6,[32] but other chromosomal abnormalities have also been encountered. Dysregulation of the hedgehog signaling pathway may be involved in the pathogenesis of synovial chondromatosis.[33]

Differential Diagnosis

The most important differential diagnostic considerations are loose bodies associated with osteoarthritis, soft tissue chondroma, and chondrosarcoma. Osteoarthritis (degenerative joint disease) occurs in older individuals and displays distinct radiologic features. Soft tissue chondroma occurs primarily in association with small joints and is localized.

Synovial chondrosarcoma, which may arise de novo or as malignant transformation of synovial chondromatosis, is exceedingly rare. Most of these tumors appear to arise from pre-existing synovial chondromatosis, with a transformation rate of approximately 5%.[34,35]

Synovial chondrosarcoma most often resembles and behaves as a low-grade chondrosarcoma (i.e., grade 1 chondrosarcoma). As such, the histologic features of malignancy can be subtle and the diagnosis can be very challenging. Typically, there is increased cellularity with loss of chondrocyte clustering, a higher degree of cytologic atypia, and

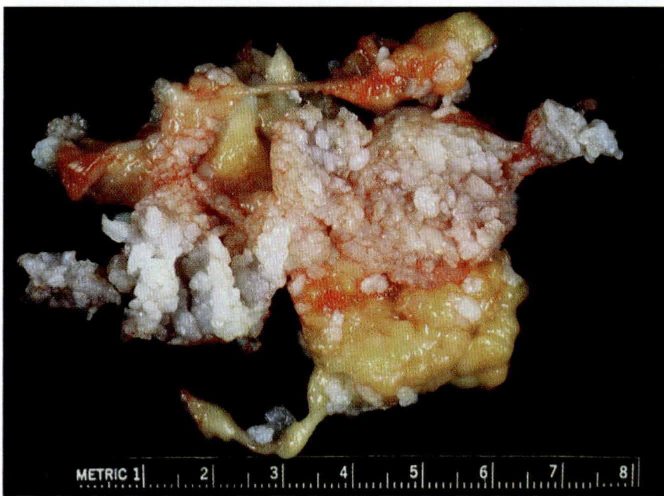

Figure 14.11 **Synovial Chondromatosis.** Synovial chondromatosis is grossly characterized by numerous cartilaginous nodules.

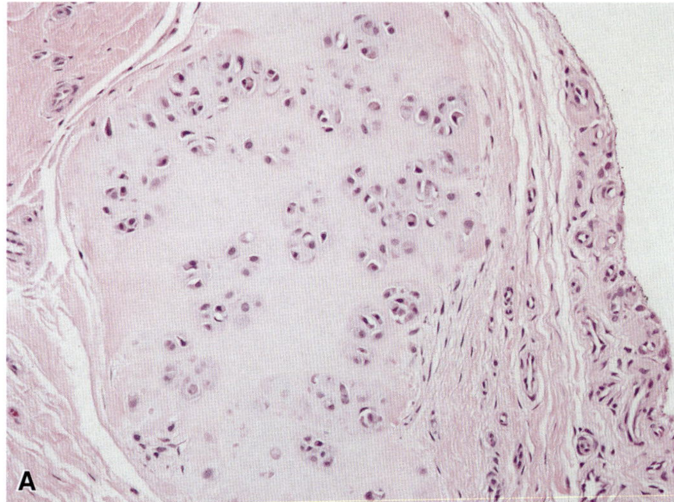

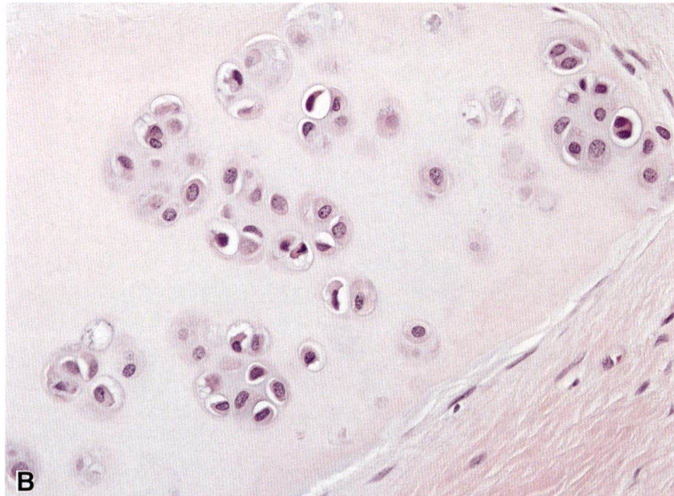

Figure 14.12 **Synovial Chondromatosis.** Histologically, in synovial chondromatosis the chondrocytes tend to be clustered in small aggregates surrounded by the hyaline matrix. The synovial lining can be seen on the right side of the field (A). Note the atypical cytology and occasional binucleation (B).

myxoid change. Radiologic studies may show aggressive features, including extension into underlying bone, which can be a helpful diagnostic clue. In this setting, a primary chondrosarcoma of bone extending into the soft tissues should be radiologically excluded.

Prognosis and Treatment

Synovectomy, total or partial, is the usual treatment for synovial chondromatosis, but total joint arthroplasty is sometimes performed, especially for recurrent disease. The disease can recur locally and occasionally follows a more locally aggressive course. Malignant transformation to synovial chondrosarcoma most often occurs after a protracted clinical course with multiple prior interventions for recurrent disease. Although synovial chondrosarcoma most often behaves as a low-grade conventional chondrosarcoma, pulmonary metastases have been reported in a subset of cases.[31]

PRACTICE POINTS: Synovial Chondromatosis

- Typically seen in association with large joints, most commonly the knee and hip.
- Radiologic studies are often helpful.
- Clustering of atypical chondrocytes and synovial lining around some of the cartilaginous nodules are characteristic features.

Soft Tissue Aneurysmal Bone Cyst

Clinical Features

Aneurysmal bone cyst (ABC) has traditionally been seen as a reactive bone lesion. However, studies have shown that not only can ABC occur outside the skeleton but it can be a neoplastic, clonal process.[36-38] Indeed, lesions indistinguishable from skeletal ABC can also occur in the soft tissues.[38] Like its skeletal counterpart, soft tissue ABC also occurs in young patients. Radiologically, the lesion may simulate myositis ossificans.

Pathologic Features

Soft tissue ABC shows the same histologic features as skeletal ABC. The tumor is generally well circumscribed and characterized by blood-filled spaces separated by a loose, bland, mitotically active spindle cell proliferation (Fig. 14.13). At most, cytologic atypia is mild. Multinucleated osteoclast-like giant cells are seen throughout the lesion but tend to be unevenly clustered. Occasionally, giant cells may be absent. Metaplastic bone formation or even osteoid formation is common; a peculiar form of calcification associated with bone formation, so-called blue bone, is of diagnostic relevance. Occasionally ABC lacks a cystic appearance, in which case it is designated "solid" ABC (Fig. 14.14).

Molecular Genetics

Many cases of ABC have been characterized cytogenetically or at the molecular level.[37,40] They commonly show rearrangements of *USP6* on chromosome 17p13. The most common fusion gene is *CDH11-USP6*, which results in the aberrant transcriptional upregulation of *USP6* driven by the strong *CDH11* promoter.[37] Several other fusion genes have also been described.[40]

Differential Diagnosis

The most important differential diagnosis is myositis ossificans, which can be quite challenging at the histologic level.[38] No single histologic feature is unique to either of these lesions, but the presence of typical "blue bone" favors ABC. In this regard, a prolonged clinical history of a case initially diagnosed as myositis ossificans should raise the

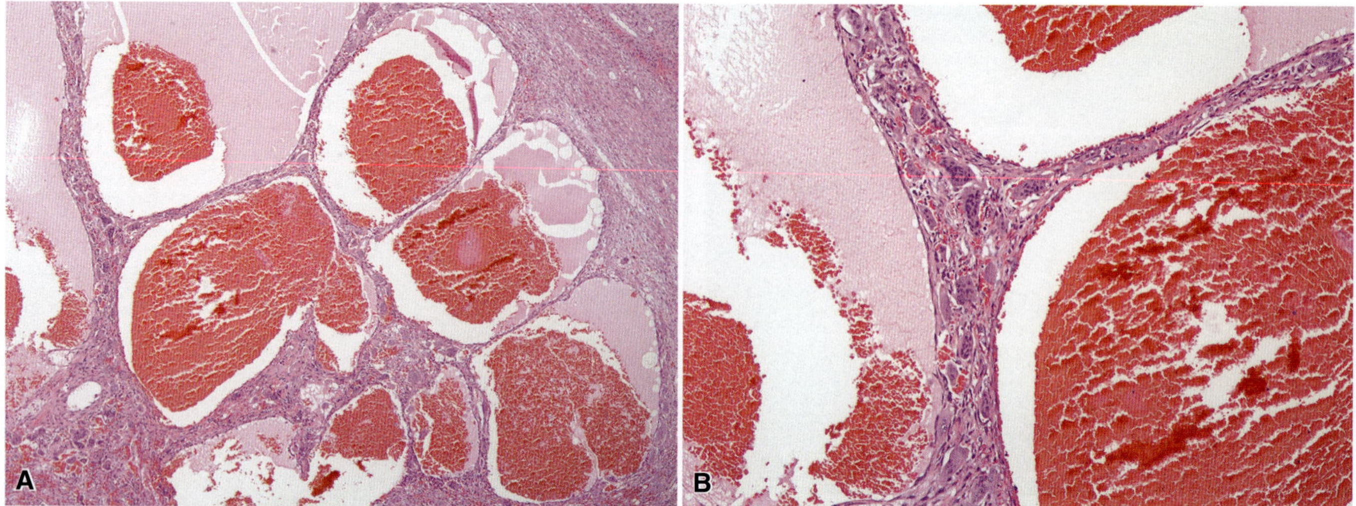

Figure 14.13 **Soft Tissue Aneurysmal Bone Cyst.** In a soft tissue aneurysmal bone cyst, blood-filled cystic spaces (A) separated by a loose proliferation of spindle cells with prominent multinucleated osteoclast-like giant cells (B) are characteristic.

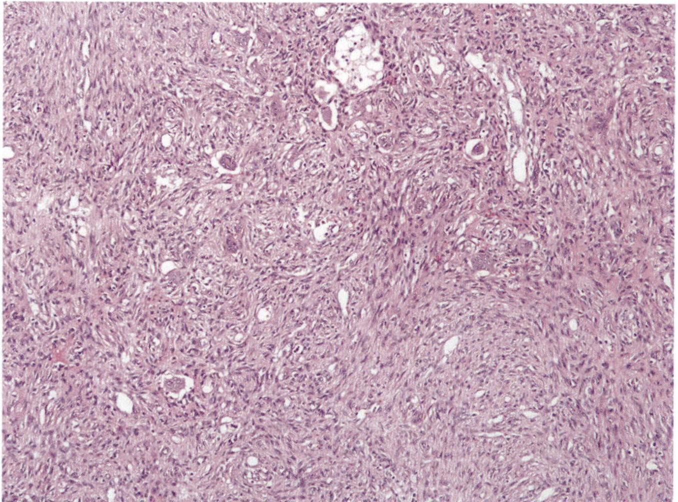

Figure 14.14 **Soft Tissue Aneurysmal Bone Cyst.** In some cases, a soft tissue aneurysmal bone cyst shows a more solid appearance and may vaguely simulate nodular fasciitis.

possibility of soft tissue ABC. Extraskeletal osteosarcoma showing telangiectatic features is another diagnostic consideration. However, these tumors are highly atypical and pleomorphic and usually occur in older adults.

Prognosis and Treatment

The recommended treatment for soft tissue ABC is simple excision, but experience is limited when compared with its skeletal counterpart.[38] The lesion may recur locally, similar to what is observed in bone.

PRACTICE POINTS: Soft Tissue Aneurysmal Bone Cyst

- Closely simulates myositis ossificans.
- Histologic features include blood-filled cystic spaces separated by a bland, mitotically active spindle cell proliferation with clusters of osteoclast-like giant cells.
- Prolonged clinical history suggests aneurysmal bone cyst over myositis ossificans.
- Presence of "blue bone" favors aneurysmal bone cyst.
- One should not see significant cytologic atypia in a soft tissue aneurysmal bone cyst; extraskeletal osteosarcoma should be excluded if this is the case.

Extraskeletal Myxoid Chondrosarcoma

Extraskeletal myxoid chondrosarcoma, previously also known as *chordoid sarcoma*, is a rare type of sarcoma of uncertain lineage.[41-43] Despite initial claims of its putative chondroid origin or differentiation, more recent findings have challenged this idea,[43,44] and today extraskeletal myxoid chondrosarcoma is classified as a tumor of uncertain differentiation according to the World Health Organization classification.[41] See Chapter 5 for a detailed discussion of extraskeletal myxoid chondrosarcoma.

Extraskeletal Mesenchymal Chondrosarcoma

Clinical Features

Extraskeletal mesenchymal chondrosarcoma is an exceedingly rare soft tissue sarcoma with histologic features analogous to those of its skeletal counterpart.[45,46] The tumor most commonly occurs in younger individuals, especially during the second and third decades of life, and has a female predominance. The head and neck and thigh are by far the most commonly involved anatomic sites.[46,47]

Pathologic Features

Grossly, mesenchymal chondrosarcoma is well circumscribed, with a fleshy appearance and foci of variably calcified cartilage (Fig. 14.15). Histologically, mesenchymal chondrosarcoma is characterized by a primitive-appearing cellular round-to-ovoid cell proliferation exhibiting a hemangiopericytoma-like vascular architecture (Fig. 14.16A), very similar to the morphology of synovial sarcoma. Amid this cellular proliferation, areas of mature hyaline cartilage are identified (see Fig. 14.16B and C). These areas can be focal or more diffuse, and secondary dystrophic calcification and even ossification are occasionally seen.

Immunohistochemistry

S-100 expression is observed in the cartilaginous areas but not in the more primitive areas. CD99 is commonly expressed by these neoplasms, usually in a membranous pattern. NKX2-2 (a nuclear transcription factor expressed in Ewing sarcoma) is often positive in mesenchymal chondrosarcoma.[48] Focal expression of myogenic markers, such as desmin, has occasionally been reported.

Molecular Genetics

Most mesenchymal chondrosarcomas harbor the *HEY1-NCOA2* fusion.[49] A single example harboring the alternate fusion *IRF2BP2-CDX1* has been described.[50]

Differential Diagnosis

The most important differential diagnostic considerations are synovial sarcoma, extraskeletal Ewing sarcoma, malignant solitary fibrous tumor, and small cell osteosarcoma. Synovial sarcoma expresses keratins, epithelial membrane antigen, and transducin-like enhancer of split 1 (TLE1), and it shows a specific translocation t(X;18), which is not seen in mesenchymal chondrosarcoma. Synovial sarcoma also lacks cartilaginous differentiation. Similar to mesenchymal chondrosarcoma, extraskeletal Ewing sarcoma is a small round cell sarcoma that consistently expresses CD99 and NKX2-2, but does not display cartilaginous differentiation or a hemangiopericytoma-like vascular pattern. In difficult cases or with limited biopsy material, molecular testing for *HEY1-NCOA2* fusion transcripts can be useful. Malignant solitary fibrous tumor also typically contains hemangiopericytoma-like vessels but usually shows less uniform cellularity and architecture, lacks cartilaginous differentiation, and expresses CD34 and STAT6. Extraskeletal small cell osteosarcoma is exceedingly rare and characteristically shows lace-like osteoid formation.

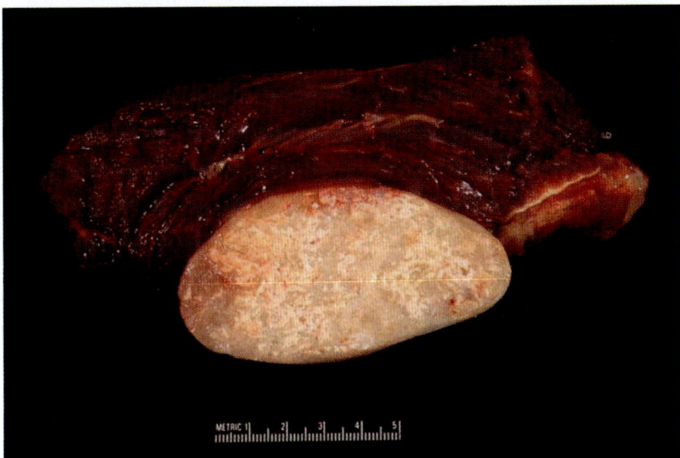

Figure 14.15 Gross Appearance of Mesenchymal Chondrosarcoma. Note the flesh-like features of the tumor and areas of calcified cartilage.

Prognosis and Treatment

Mesenchymal chondrosarcoma is a highly aggressive sarcoma that often metastasizes to the lungs. The 5- and 10-year overall survival rates are approximately 50% and 40%, respectively.[51,52] Treatment involves radical surgery, radiation therapy, and chemotherapy, although the latter is of limited benefit.

PRACTICE POINTS: Extraskeletal Mesenchymal Chondrosarcoma

- Quite rare and commonly seen in younger individuals.
- Cellular small, round- to ovoid-cell neoplasm with a hemangiopericytoma-like vascular pattern and islands of hyaline cartilage.
- Synovial sarcoma and Ewing sarcoma should be excluded.

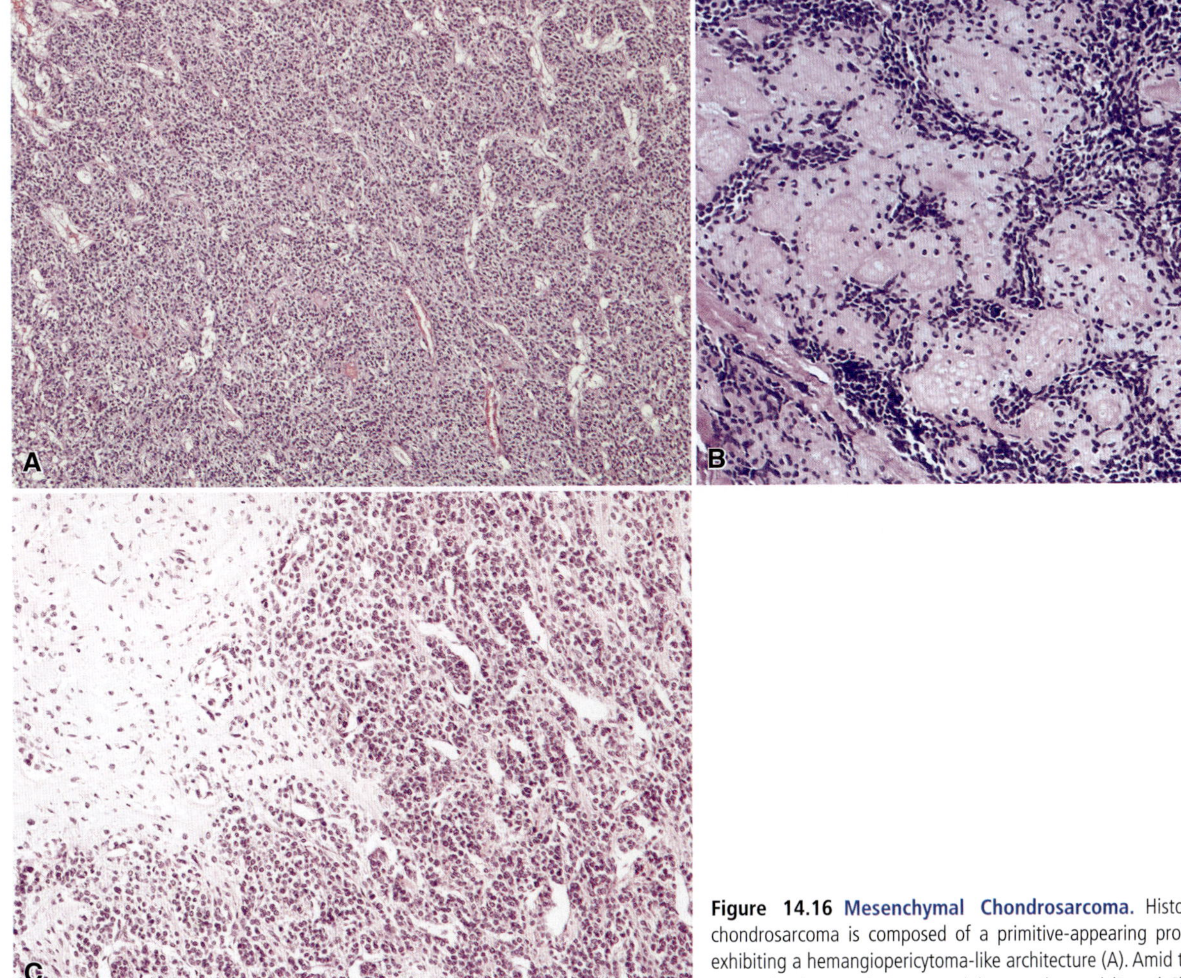

Figure 14.16 Mesenchymal Chondrosarcoma. Histologically, mesenchymal chondrosarcoma is composed of a primitive-appearing proliferation of round cells exhibiting a hemangiopericytoma-like architecture (A). Amid this cellular proliferation, mature hyaline cartilaginous nodules are observed (B and C).

Extraskeletal Osteosarcoma

Clinical Features

Extraskeletal osteosarcoma is defined as a malignant mesenchymal neoplasm that arises in the soft tissues and shows osteoblastic differentiation. It is a rare entity and represents less than 1% of all soft tissue sarcomas. The tumor primarily occurs in the deep soft tissues of the lower extremities, especially the thigh, as well as the retroperitoneum.[53-55] In contrast to its skeletal counterpart, extraskeletal osteosarcoma typically occurs in older adults, usually after the sixth decade of life. Men seem to be more commonly affected than women. In approximately 5% of cases, a history of previous radiation is elicited. Trauma has also been claimed to be a predisposing factor in up to 5% to 10% of cases, but this association is highly controversial.

Pathologic Features

Grossly, extraskeletal osteosarcoma is typically a well-circumscribed, large fleshy tumor with areas of hemorrhage and necrosis (Fig. 14.17). Histologically, extraskeletal osteosarcoma almost always shows a high-grade spindle cell and pleomorphic morphology, similar to high-grade undifferentiated pleomorphic sarcomas (Fig. 14.18A); however, it may show a variety of histologic appearances, including epithelioid, telangiectatic, chondroblastic, small cell, and giant cell–rich patterns, or a combination of these. Osteoid formation is the sine qua non for the diagnosis (see Fig. 14.18B); osteoid may be diffuse or focal, solid or lace-like, and tends to be more centrally located in the lesion, in contrast to myositis ossificans ("reverse zoning" phenomenon). Multinucleated giant cells, hemorrhage, and necrosis are also commonly observed. Extraskeletal osteosarcoma is also discussed in Chapter 7 (in the context of pleomorphic sarcomas) and briefly in Chapter 11 (in the context of giant cell–rich tumors).

Immunohistochemistry

Immunohistochemical analysis is usually not needed for the diagnosis of osteosarcoma except to exclude other tumor types (before osteoid has been identified). As briefly mentioned at the beginning of the chapter, immunohistochemistry for SATB2 may be helpful as a more objective means of confirming osteoblastic differentiation, when it is difficult to make the distinction between osteoid and sclerotic collagen (Fig. 14.19).[1]

Molecular Genetics

Cytogenetic studies usually show complex karyotypes with extensive numeric and structural chromosomal abnormalities. A recent study of genomewide DNA copy number and targeted sequencing in a large series of extraskeletal osteosarcomas identified frequent copy-number losses of genes encoding cell-cycle checkpoint regulators such as *CDKN2A*, *RB1*, and *TP53*, as well as mutations in genes affecting methylation/demethylation, chromatin remodeling, and the WNT/SHH pathway.[56]

Differential Diagnosis

The differential diagnosis includes other high-grade pleomorphic sarcomas and myositis ossificans. Histologic analysis and immunohistochemistry help differentiate extraskeletal osteosarcoma from other pleomorphic sarcomas (see Chapter 7). As discussed previously, myositis ossificans does not display the degree of pleomorphism and cytologic atypia of extraskeletal osteosarcoma.

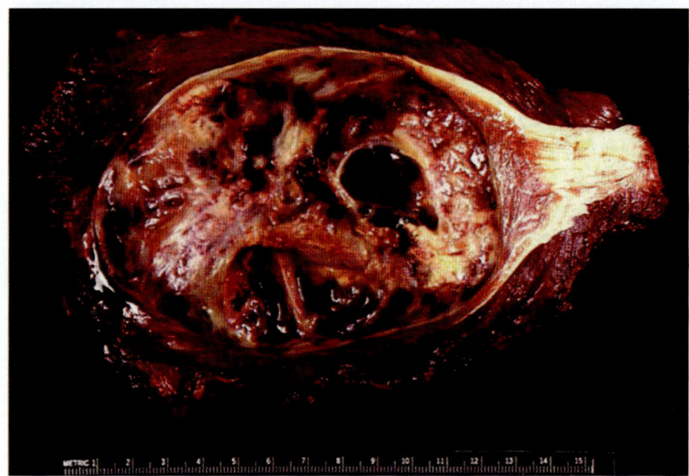

Figure 14.17 Gross Appearance of Extraskeletal Osteosarcoma. Note the areas of hemorrhage and cystic degeneration.

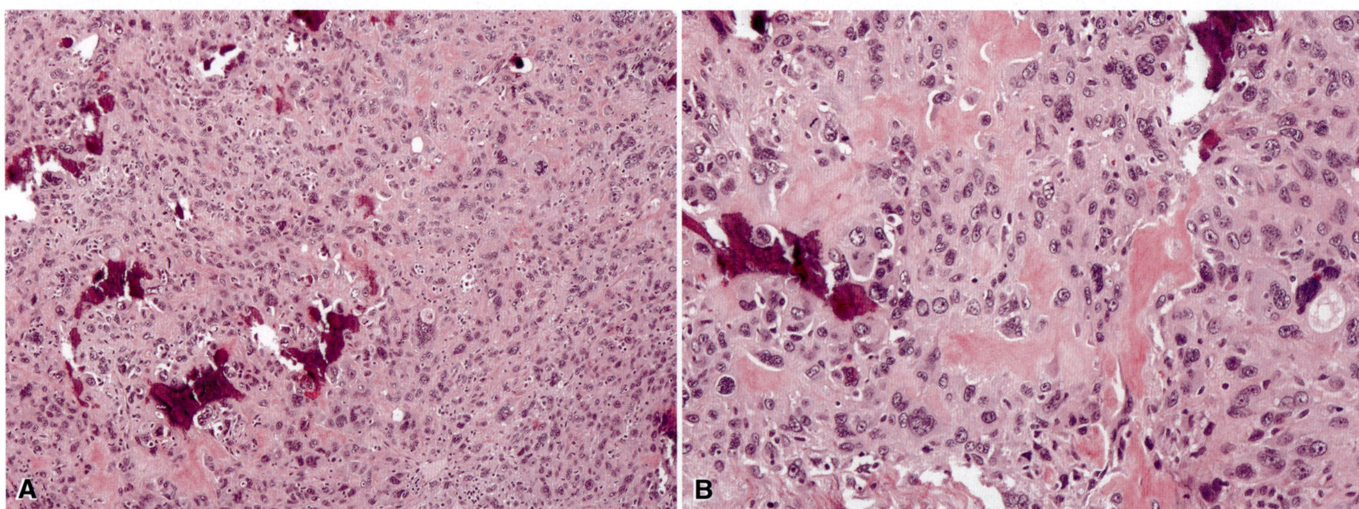

Figure 14.18 Extraskeletal Osteosarcoma. Histologically, extraskeletal osteosarcoma is composed of pleomorphic cells intermixed with immature bone formation (A). Atypical mitoses are often easily seen. Note the partial calcification of the osteoid material (B).

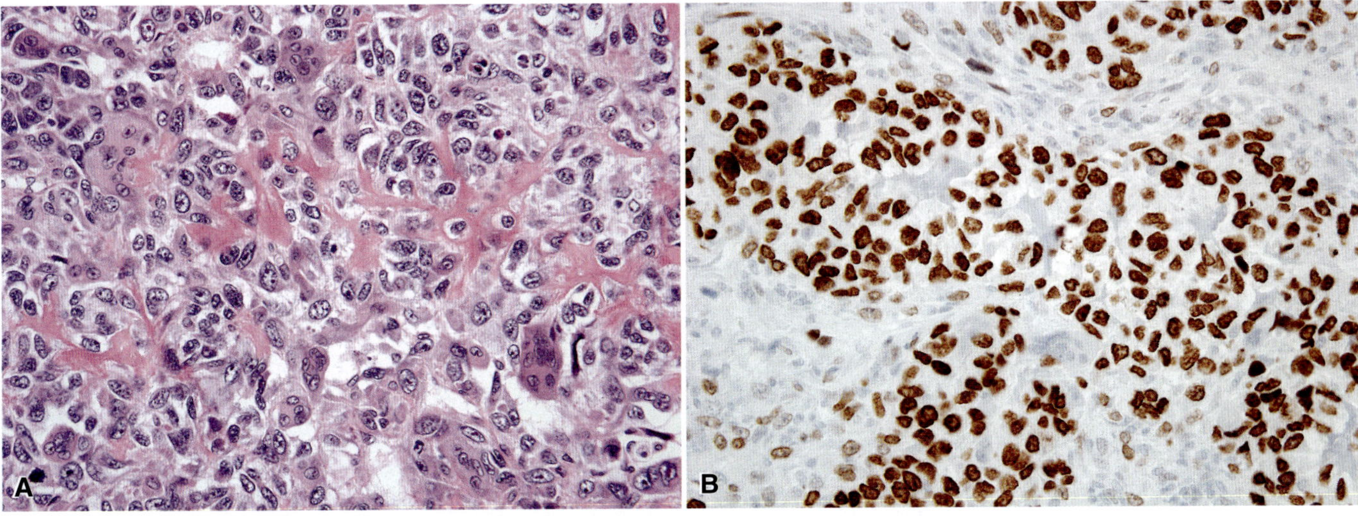

Figure 14.19 Extraskeletal Osteosarcoma. Extraskeletal osteosarcoma with limited osteoid matrix (A). Note the occasional osteoclast-like giant cells. It may be difficult to distinguish sclerotic collagen from osteoid; nuclear staining for SATB2 can help confirm osteoblastic differentiation (B).

Prognosis and Treatment

Clinically, extraskeletal osteosarcomas behave in a very aggressive fashion, with local recurrence, metastasis, and death rates of approximately 50%, 60%, and 60% to 80%, respectively.[54,55,57] The lungs are the most common metastatic sites. The treatment of extraskeletal osteosarcoma is similar to that of other high-grade pleomorphic sarcomas and commonly involves a combination of radical surgery, chemotherapy, and radiation therapy. In contrast to skeletal osteosarcomas diagnosed in children, extraskeletal osteosarcoma tends to be highly resistant to chemotherapy protocols.

PRACTICE POINTS: Extraskeletal Osteosarcoma

- Primarily seen in older adults.
- The presence of marked cytologic atypia and pleomorphism helps exclude the possibility of myositis ossificans.
- May be difficult to distinguish from other high-grade spindle cell and pleomorphic sarcomas.
- Careful histologic examination is the most important step for the correct identification of osteoid.

Neoplasms Showing Heterologous Osteocartilaginous Differentiation

A wide range of benign and malignant mesenchymal neoplasms may on occasion show osseous or cartilaginous differentiation as a secondary phenomenon. Some of the tumors in which this phenomenon is most commonly seen include lipoma (chondrolipoma or osseous lipoma),[58,59] giant cell tumor of soft tissues,[60] myoepithelial tumors of soft tissue,[61] ossifying fibromyxoid tumor,[62,63] phosphaturic mesenchymal tumor,[64] malignant peripheral nerve sheath tumor, and well-differentiated and dedifferentiated liposarcomas.[65,66] These tumors are described in detail elsewhere in this book. In addition, a subset of epithelial and epithelial-myoepithelial tumors can show osseous or cartilaginous differentiation. For example, sarcomatoid differentiation in a poorly differentiated carcinoma may contain heterologous chondroblastic or osteoblastic differentiation. Typical examples include metaplastic spindle cell carcinoma of the breast and cartilaginous differentiation in pleomorphic adenoma. Finally, there are a number of cutaneous lesions that are defined by metaplastic bone or cartilage formation (e.g., osteoma cutis) or show secondary osteocartilaginous differentiation (e.g., pilomatricoma, melanocytic nevi). A discussion of these entities is beyond the scope of this chapter.

In all of these scenarios, when the surgical pathologist is confronted with a tumor showing osteocartilaginous differentiation, the four-step algorithm described at the beginning of this chapter should help discriminate correctly among these entities.

References

1. Conner JR, Hornick JL: SATB2 is a novel marker of osteoblastic differentiation in bone and soft tissue tumours, *Histopathology* 63:36–49, 2013.
2. Kransdorf MJ, Meis JM, Jelinek JS: Myositis ossificans: MR appearance with radiologic-pathologic correlation, *AJR Am J Roentgenol* 157:1243–1248, 1991.
3. Patel RM, Weiss SW, Folpe AL: Heterotopic mesenteric ossification: a distinctive pseudosarcoma commonly associated with intestinal obstruction, *Am J Surg Pathol* 30:119–122, 2006.
4. McCarthy EF, Sundaram M: Heterotopic ossification: a review, *Skeletal Radiol* 34:609–619, 2005.
5. Sukov WR, Franco MF, Erickson-Johnson M, et al: Frequency of USP6 rearrangements in myositis ossificans, brown tumor, and cherubism: molecular cytogenetic evidence that a subset of "myositis ossificans-like lesions" are the early phases in the formation of soft-tissue aneurysmal bone cyst, *Skeletal Radiol* 37:321–327, 2008.
6. Dupree WB, Enzinger FM: Fibro-osseous pseudotumor of the digits, *Cancer* 58:2103–2109, 1986.
7. Spjut HJ, Dorfman HD: Florid reactive periostitis of the tubular bones of the hands and feet. A benign lesion which may simulate osteosarcoma, *Am J Surg Pathol* 5:423–433, 1981.
8. Zambrano E, Nose V, Perez-Atayde AR, et al: Distinct chromosomal rearrangements in subungual (Dupuytren) exostosis and bizarre parosteal osteochondromatous proliferation (Nora lesion), *Am J Surg Pathol* 28:1033–1039, 2004.
9. Nilsson M, Domanski HA, Mertens F, et al: Molecular cytogenetic characterization of recurrent translocation breakpoints in bizarre parosteal osteochondromatous proliferation (Nora's lesion), *Hum Pathol* 35:1063–1069, 2004.
10. Meneses MF, Unni KK, Swee RG: Bizarre parosteal osteochondromatous proliferation of bone (Nora's lesion), *Am J Surg Pathol* 17:691–697, 1993.
11. Nora FE, Dahlin DC, Beabout JW: Bizarre parosteal osteochondromatous proliferations of the hands and feet, *Am J Surg Pathol* 7:245–250, 1983.
12. Chaudhry IH, Kazakov DV, Michal M, et al: Fibro-osseous pseudotumor of the digit: a clinicopathological study of 17 cases, *J Cutan Pathol* 37:323–329, 2010.
13. Gannon FH, Valentine BA, Shore EM, et al: Acute lymphocytic infiltration in an extremely early lesion of fibrodysplasia ossificans progressiva, *Clin Orthop Relat Res* 346:19–25, 1998.
14. Kaplan FS, Glaser DL, Pignolo RJ, et al: A new era for fibrodysplasia ossificans progressiva: a druggable target for the second skeleton, *Expert Opin Biol Ther* 7:705–712, 2007.
15. Shore EM, Xu M, Feldman GJ, et al: A recurrent mutation in the BMP type I receptor ACVR1 causes inherited and sporadic fibrodysplasia ossificans progressiva, *Nat Genet* 38:525–527, 2006.

16. Agarwal S, Loder S, Brownley C, et al: Inhibition of Hif1α prevents both trauma-induced and genetic heterotopic ossification, *Proc Natl Acad Sci USA* 113:E338–E347, 2016.
17. Pakasa NM, Kalengayi RM: Tumoral calcinosis: a clinicopathological study of 111 cases with emphasis on the earliest changes, *Histopathology* 31:18–24, 1997.
18. McKee PH, Liomba NG, Hutt MS: Tumoral calcinosis: a pathological study of fifty-six cases, *Br J Dermatol* 107:669–674, 1982.
19. Juppner H: Novel regulators of phosphate homeostasis and bone metabolism, *Ther Apher Dial* 11(Suppl 1):S3–S22, 2007.
20. Laskin WB, Miettinen M, Fetsch JF: Calcareous lesions of the distal extremities resembling tumoral calcinosis (tumoral calcinosis-like lesions): clinicopathologic study of 43 cases emphasizing a pathogenesis-based approach to classification, *Am J Surg Pathol* 31:15–25, 2007.
21. Larsson T, Yu X, Davis SI, et al: A novel recessive mutation in fibroblast growth factor-23 causes familial tumoral calcinosis, *J Clin Endocrin Metabol* 90:2424–2427, 2005.
22. Folsom LJ, Imel EA: Hyperphosphatemic familial tumoral calcinosis: genetic models of deficient FGF23 action, *Curr Osteoporos Rep* 13:78–87, 2015.
23. Dahlin DC, Salvador AH: Cartilaginous tumors of the soft tissues of the hands and feet, *Mayo Clin Proc* 49:721–726, 1974.
24. Chung EB, Enzinger FM: Chondroma of soft parts, *Cancer* 41:1414–1424, 1978.
25. Cates JM, Rosenberg AE, O'Connell JX, et al: Chondroblastoma-like chondroma of soft tissue: an underrecognized variant and its differential diagnosis, *Am J Surg Pathol* 25:661–666, 2001.
26. Sandberg AA, Bridge JA: Updates on the cytogenetics and molecular genetics of bone and soft tissue tumors: chondrosarcoma and other cartilaginous neoplasms, *Cancer Genet Cytogenet* 143:1–31, 2003.
27. Dahlen A, Mertens F, Rydholm A, et al: Fusion, disruption, and expression of HMGA2 in bone and soft tissue chondromas, *Mod Pathol* 16:1132–1140, 2003.
28. Damato S, Alorjani M, Bonar F, et al: *IDH1* mutations are not found in cartilaginous tumours other than central and periosteal chondrosarcomas and enchondromas, *Histopathology* 60:363–365, 2012.
29. Sciot R, Bridge JA: Synovial chondromatosis. In Fletcher CD, Bridge JA, Hogendoorn PCW, et al, editors: *WHO classification of tumours of soft tissue and bone*, Lyon, France, 2013, IARC Press.
30. Sviland L, Malcolm AJ: Synovial chondromatosis presenting as painless soft tissue mass—a report of 19 cases, *Histopathology* 27:275–279, 1995.
31. Unni K, Inwards C, Bridge J, et al: *Tumors of the bones and joints*, Washington, DC, 2005, Armed Forces Institute of Pathology.
32. Buddingh EP, Krallman P, Neff JR, et al: Chromosome 6 abnormalities are recurrent in synovial chondromatosis, *Cancer Genet Cytogenet* 140:18–22, 2003.
33. Hopyan S, Nadesan P, Yu C, et al: Dysregulation of hedgehog signalling predisposes to synovial chondromatosis, *J Pathol* 206:143–150, 2005.
34. McCarthy C, Anderson WJ, Vlychou M, et al: Primary synovial chondromatosis: a reassessment of malignant potential in 155 cases, *Skeletal Radiol* 45:755–762, 2016.
35. Evans S, Boffano M, Chaudhry S, et al: Synovial chondrosarcoma arising in synovial chondromatosis, *Sarcoma* 2014:647939, 2014.
36. Oliveira AM, Chou MM, Perez-Atayde AR, et al: Aneurysmal bone cyst: a neoplasm driven by upregulation of the USP6 oncogene, *J Clin Oncol* 24:e1, 2006.
37. Oliveira AM, Perez-Atayde AR, Inwards CY, et al: USP6 and CDH11 oncogenes identify the neoplastic cell in primary aneurysmal bone cysts and are absent in so-called secondary aneurysmal bone cysts, *Am J Pathol* 165:1773–1780, 2004.
38. Nielsen GP, Fletcher CD, Smith MA, et al: Soft tissue aneurysmal bone cyst: a clinicopathologic study of five cases, *Am J Surg Pathol* 26:64–69, 2002.
39. Oliveira AM, Hsi BL, Weremowicz S, et al: USP6 (Tre2) fusion oncogenes in aneurysmal bone cyst, *Cancer Res* 64:1920–1923, 2004.
40. Oliveira AM, Perez-Atayde AR, Dal CP, et al: Aneurysmal bone cyst variant translocations upregulate USP6 transcription by promoter swapping with the ZNF9, COL1A1, TRAP150, and OMD genes, *Oncogene* 24:3419–3426, 2005.
41. Lucas DR, Stenman G: Extraskeletal myxoid chondrosarcoma. In Fletcher CD, Bridge JA, Hogendoorn PCW, et al, editors: *WHO classification of tumours of soft tissue and bone*, Lyon, France, 2013, IARC Press.
42. Meis-Kindblom JM, Bergh P, Gunterberg B, et al: Extraskeletal myxoid chondrosarcoma: a reappraisal of its morphologic spectrum and prognostic factors based on 117 cases, *Am J Surg Pathol* 23:636–650, 1999.
43. Aigner T, Oliveira AM, Nascimento AG: Extraskeletal myxoid chondrosarcomas do not show a chondrocytic phenotype, *Mod Pathol* 17:214–221, 2004.
44. Hisaoka M, Hashimoto H: Extraskeletal myxoid chondrosarcoma: updated clinicopathological and molecular genetic characteristics, *Pathol Int* 55:453–463, 2005.
45. Guccion JG, Font RL, Enzinger FM, et al: Extraskeletal mesenchymal chondrosarcoma, *Arch Pathol* 95:336–340, 1973.
46. Nakashima Y, Unni KK, Shives TC, et al: Mesenchymal chondrosarcoma of bone and soft tissue. A review of 111 cases, *Cancer* 57:2444–2453, 1986.
47. Naumann S, Krallman PA, Unni KK, et al: Translocation der(13;21)(q10;q10) in skeletal and extraskeletal mesenchymal chondrosarcoma, *Mod Pathol* 15:572–576, 2002.
48. Hung YP, Fletcher CD, Hornick JL: Evaluation of NKX2-2 expression in round cell sarcomas and other tumors with EWSR1 rearrangement: imperfect specificity for Ewing sarcoma, *Mod Pathol* 29:370–380, 2016.
49. Wang L, Motoi T, Khanin R, et al: Identification of a novel, recurrent HEY1-NCOA2 fusion in mesenchymal chondrosarcoma based on a genome-wide screen of exon-level expression data, *Genes Chromosomes Cancer* 51:127–139, 2012.
50. Nyquist KB, Panagopoulos I, Thorsen J, et al: Whole-transcriptome sequencing identifies novel IRF2BP2-CDX1 fusion gene brought about by translocation t(1;5)(q42;q32) in mesenchymal chondrosarcoma, *PLoS ONE* 7:e49705, 2012.
51. Schneiderman BA, Kliethermes SA, Nystrom LM: Survival in mesenchymal chondrosarcoma varies based on age and tumor location: a survival analysis of the SEER database, *Clin Orthop Relat Res* 475:799–805, 2017.
52. Xu J, Li D, Xie L, et al: Mesenchymal chondrosarcoma of bone and soft tissue: a systematic review of 107 patients in the past 20 years, *PLoS ONE* 10:e0122216, 2015.
53. Allan CJ, Soule EH: Osteogenic sarcoma of the somatic soft tissues. Clinicopathologic study of 26 cases and review of literature, *Cancer* 27:1121–1133, 1971.
54. Chung EB, Enzinger FM: Extraskeletal osteosarcoma, *Cancer* 60:1132–1142, 1987.
55. Lee JS, Fetsch JF, Wasdhal DA, et al: A review of 40 patients with extraskeletal osteosarcoma, *Cancer* 76:2253–2259, 1995.
56. Jour G, Wang L, Middha S, et al: The molecular landscape of extraskeletal osteosarcoma: a clinicopathological and molecular biomarker study, *J Pathol Clin Res* 2:9–20, 2015.
57. Bane BL, Evans HL, Ro JY, et al: Extraskeletal osteosarcoma. A clinicopathologic review of 26 cases, *Cancer* 65:2762–2770, 1990.
58. Ohtsuka H: Chondrolipoma of the popliteal fossa and Japanese reports, *J Dermatol* 33:202–206, 2006.
59. Turkoz HK, Varnali Y, Comunoglu C: [A case of osteolipoma of the head and neck area], *Kulak Burun Bogaz Ihtis Derg* 13:84–86, 2004.
60. Oliveira AM, Dei Tos AP, Fletcher CD, et al: Primary giant cell tumor of soft tissues: a study of 22 cases, *Am J Surg Pathol* 24:248–256, 2000.
61. Hornick JL, Fletcher CD: Myoepithelial tumors of soft tissue: a clinicopathologic and immunohistochemical study of 101 cases with evaluation of prognostic parameters, *Am J Surg Pathol* 27:1183–1196, 2003.
62. Enzinger FM, Weiss SW, Liang CY: Ossifying fibromyxoid tumor of soft parts. A clinicopathological analysis of 59 cases, *Am J Surg Pathol* 13:817–827, 1989.
63. Miettinen M: Ossifying fibromyxoid tumor of soft parts. Additional observations of a distinctive soft tissue tumor, *Am J Clin Pathol* 95:142–149, 1991.
64. Folpe AL, Fanburg-Smith JC, Billings SD, et al: Most osteomalacia-associated mesenchymal tumors are a single histopathologic entity: an analysis of 32 cases and a comprehensive review of the literature, *Am J Surg Pathol* 28:1–30, 2004.
65. Nascimento AG, Kurtin PJ, Guillou L, et al: Dedifferentiated liposarcoma: a report of nine cases with a peculiar neurallike whorling pattern associated with metaplastic bone formation, *Am J Surg Pathol* 22:945–955, 1998.
66. Yoshida A, Ushiku T, Motoi T, et al: Well-differentiated liposarcoma with low-grade osteosarcomatous component: an underrecognized variant, *Am J Surg Pathol* 34:1361–1366, 2010.

15

Cutaneous Mesenchymal Tumors

Thomas Brenn, MD, PhD, FRCPath, and Jason L. Hornick, MD, PhD

Cutaneous mesenchymal tumors are considered separately in this chapter because many of the tumors are either unique to or predominate in the skin or show specific features when presenting in the skin.

The morphologic spectrum of cutaneous soft tissue tumors is wide and varied, and it includes spindle cell, epithelioid, myxoid, and pleomorphic patterns, in addition to clear cell features. The largest morphologic category is that of spindle cell tumors, with benign fibrous histiocytoma being the most common cutaneous mesenchymal tumor overall.

The diagnosis of cutaneous mesenchymal tumors may be challenging due to the significant morphologic overlap between tumors. Furthermore, although the vast majority of cutaneous mesenchymal tumors are benign, distinction from malignant tumors may be difficult because distinguishing features may be subtle and difficult to assess, especially on limited samples (e.g., shave or punch biopsies). Conversely, tumors with histologic features of malignancy may behave in an entirely benign fashion when confined to the dermis (e.g., cutaneous atypical smooth muscle tumors and atypical fibroxanthoma [AFX]). Of particular importance is the consideration of melanocytic tumors and poorly differentiated squamous cell carcinoma in the differential diagnosis of cutaneous mesenchymal neoplasms. It is imperative to pay attention to subtle clinical as well as morphologic clues, in addition to the inclusion of markers of melanocytic and epithelial differentiation in an immunohistochemical panel. Desmoplastic and neurotropic melanoma as well as desmoplastic and spindle cell or sarcomatoid squamous cell carcinoma should always enter the differential diagnosis of tumors presenting on sun-exposed skin of the elderly. They are notoriously difficult to diagnose, and often multiple immunohistochemical markers are necessary to detect their line of differentiation. The presence of S-100 protein (Table 15.1) and, to a lesser extent, keratin

Table 15.1 Cutaneous Tumors Characterized by Immunohistochemical Expression of S-100 Protein

	Clinical Presentation	Histologic Features	Immunohistochemistry
Melanoma	Increasing incidence with age Wide anatomic distribution Clinically pigmented	Junctional activity/in situ component Melanin pigment Cytologic atypia and pleomorphism Expansile growth	S-100 + Melan A + HMB-45 +
Cutaneous myoepithelioma	Young adults Extremities, but wide anatomic distribution Small papule/nodule	Dermal-based Lack of junctional activity Wide morphologic spectrum with epithelioid, spindle cell, plasmacytoid, and myxoid features Distinctive syncytial variant with abundant palely eosinophilic cytoplasm	S-100 + Keratin ± EMA + GFAP + SMA + Calponin + Desmin – p63 ± SOX10 +
Dermal nerve sheath myxoma	Adults Distal extremities Nodule (few cm)	Multilobular growth within dermis and subcutis Sharply demarcated and encapsulated tumor lobules Myxoid matrix	S-100 + GFAP + EMA + (capsule)
Granular cell tumor	Adults Wide anatomic distribution Nodule or plaque	Dermal-based tumor with infiltrative growth into subcutis Large polygonal tumor cells with abundant granular cytoplasm	S-100 + NKI-C3 + NSE + CD68 +
Solitary circumscribed neuroma	Adulthood Central face Small papule	Well-circumscribed tumor within dermis Schwannian differentiation Numerous intralesional axons Partial perineurial capsule	S-100 + NFP + EMA + (capsule)
Neurofibroma	Wide age range Wide anatomic distribution Small papule	Well-circumscribed but unencapsulated tumor Based in dermis or subcutis Short spindle cells with wavy nuclei Lack of cytologic atypia Presence of mast cells	S-100 + NFP + (axons) CD34 +
Malignant peripheral nerve sheath tumor	Adults Wide anatomic distribution Usually deep-seated tumor Rare cutaneous presentation Frequently associated with neurofibromatosis type 1	Atypical spindle cells with varying cellularity Myxoid stromal change Perivascular condensation of tumor cells Heterologous differentiation possible	S-100 + (50%) GFAP + (40%) SOX10 + (40%) Loss of H3K27me3 (30% low grade; 90% high grade)
Clear cell sarcoma	Young adults Distal lower extremities Deep-seated mass	Infiltrative tumor Deep soft tissue Nests and fascicles of short spindle cells with eosinophilic to clear cytoplasm Wreathlike multinucleated giant cells	S-100 + HMB-45 + SOX10 +
Langerhans cell histiocytosis	Multiorgan disease Children and young adults	Dermal-based tumor Sheetlike arrangement Epidermotropism and Pautrier-like intraepidermal aggregates Small uniform cells with abundant pale cytoplasm and reniform or bean shaped nuclei characteristic of Langerhans cells Inflammatory cell infiltrate with conspicuous eosinophils	S-100 + CD1a + Langerin +
Rosai-Dorfman disease	Systemic vs. primary cutaneous Solitary or multiple plaques and nodules Wide anatomic distribution	Well-circumscribed but unencapsulated dermal tumor Possible involvement of subcutis Characteristic large polygonal histiocytes with abundant palely eosinophilic cytoplasm and vesicular nuclei containing eosinophilic nucleoli Emperipolesis Mixed inflammatory cell infiltrate	S-100 + CD68 +

EMA, Epithelial membrane antigen; *GFAP,* glial fibrillary acidic protein; *H3K27me3,* histone H3 with trimethylated lysine 27.

expression may also be seen in various cutaneous mesenchymal tumors, further complicating the issue. In contrast to deep-seated soft tissue tumors, cutaneous tumors less frequently display specific diagnostically helpful cytogenetic or molecular genetic findings.

In keeping with the overall structure of this book, tumors in this chapter are organized according to histologic patterns rather than lines of differentiation. Exceptions are cutaneous adipocytic tumors, which are addressed separately in brief at the end of the chapter, as well as cutaneous vascular tumors, which are discussed together with vascular tumors at other sites in Chapter 13. The differential diagnosis of cutaneous mesenchymal tumors according to histologic pattern is further emphasized in accompanying tables.

PRACTICE POINTS: Considerations When Diagnosing Cutaneous Mesenchymal Tumors

- Wide morphologic spectrum of cutaneous mesenchymal tumors
- Significant morphologic overlap between cutaneous mesenchymal tumors
- Subtle features of malignancy, especially on partial and superficial samples (shave or punch biopsy)
- Histologic features of malignancy are not necessarily associated with aggressive clinical behavior in certain tumors when confined to dermis
- Melanoma and poorly differentiated squamous cell carcinoma should always be considered in the differential diagnosis
- Clinical features and presentation warrant attention
- Careful interpretation of immunohistochemical findings

Spindle Cell Tumors

Benign Fibrous Histiocytoma (Dermatofibroma) and Variants

Fibrous histiocytomas are the most common mesenchymal tumors arising in the skin. They show a wide morphologic spectrum, and multiple variants are recognized (Table 15.2). Awareness of and familiarity with these variants of fibrous histiocytoma are important because their morphologic features can easily be mistaken for other lesions, including tumors with more sinister prognoses (Table 15.3). Furthermore, some of the morphologic variants are associated with specific clinical features and behavior. Epithelioid fibrous histiocytoma is described later in the chapter in the section "Epithelioid Tumors." A deep variant has also been described in soft tissue and is discussed separately in Chapter 3. On a molecular level, fusion genes, mainly involving protein kinase C (PKC) isoforms or the *ALK* gene have been identified in a subset of these tumors.[1-3] Although PKC fusion genes are seen across the morphologic variants of fibrous histiocytoma, *ALK* gene rearrangements are most prevalent in the epithelioid variant.

Clinical Features

Dermal benign fibrous histiocytoma (dermatofibroma) occurs over a wide age range but shows a predilection for adults in the third and fourth decades. Women are more frequently affected, and the extremities are favored sites, followed by the trunk. Head and neck involvement is rare. The clinical presentation is of a solitary, relatively

Table 15.2 Variants of Benign Fibrous Histiocytoma

	Clinical Presentation	Histology	Behavior
Dermatofibroma	Young adults Female predilection Extremities and trunk Red to brown papule or plaque	Circumscribed dermal-based tumor Ovoid spindle cells in haphazard arrangement Admixed foam cells and giant cells Overlying epidermal hyperplasia and basal layer hyperpigmentation	Simple excision curative
Hemosiderotic FH	Bluish to black papule or plaque Otherwise same as dermatofibroma	Same as dermatofibroma but abundant hemosiderin-laden histiocytes and giant cells	Simple excision curative
Atrophic FH	Same as dermatofibroma	Same as dermatofibroma but less cellular and prominent stromal hyalinization	Simple excision curative
Clear cell FH	Same as dermatofibroma	Same as dermatofibroma but abundant clear cell change of tumor cells	Simple excision curative
Granular cell FH	Same as dermatofibroma	Same as dermatofibroma but abundant granular cell change of tumor cells	Simple excision curative
Palisading FH	Predilection for acral sites Otherwise same as dermatofibroma	Same as dermatofibroma but striking nuclear palisading of tumor cells reminiscent of Verocay bodies	Simple excision curative
Epithelioid FH	Adults Lower extremities Red polypoid nodule	Polypoid architecture often with epidermal collarette Polygonal epithelioid cells with abundant eosinophilic cytoplasm, vesicular nuclei, and small eosinophilic nucleoli Occasional binucleated cells	Simple excision curative
Lipidized FH	Predilection for ankle Otherwise same as dermatofibroma	Same as dermatofibroma but marked lipidization of tumor cells with prominent surrounding stromal hyalinization	Simple excision curative
Cellular FH	Young adults Male predominance Extremities, head and neck Larger nodule (few cm)	Highly cellular center composed of longer and more tapered spindle cells arranged in fascicles More typical features of dermatofibroma at periphery	Local nondestructive recurrence in 20% Distant metastasis exceptional
Aneurysmal FH	Adults Female predominance Extremities and trunk Bluish to black nodule	Same as dermatofibroma and cellular fibrous histiocytoma but central blood-filled cystic space and abundant hemosiderin deposition	Local nondestructive recurrence in 20% Distant metastasis exceptional
Atypical FH	Adults Extremities Larger nodule (few cm)	Same as dermatofibroma but presence of marked nuclear pleomorphism and hyperchromasia	Local nondestructive recurrence in 20% Distant metastasis exceptional

FH, Fibrous histiocytoma.

Table 15.3 Differential Diagnosis of Benign Fibrous Histiocytoma

	Clinical Presentation	Histologic Features	Immunohistochemistry
Dermatomyofibroma	Adults Shoulder girdle Plaque with discoloration	Dermal-based lesion Involvement of superficial subcutis Plaquelike growth Uniform spindle cells in fascicles No cytologic atypia No mitotic activity	SMA + Desmin – S-100 –
Pilar leiomyoma	Young adults Extremities and trunk Nodule or plaque	Dermal-based lesion Ill-defined lesion Fascicles of uniform spindle cells ramifying between dermal collagen Scattered cytologic atypia No mitotic activity	SMA + Desmin + h-Caldesmon + Keratin ±
Myofibroma	Children and young adults Head and neck, but wide anatomic distribution Nodule (few cm)	Well-circumscribed and nodular growth Dermis and/or subcutis Biphasic cell population: spindle cells in fascicles; small primitive round to ovoid cells around branching vessels No cytologic atypia	SMA + Desmin –
Neurofibroma	Wide age range Wide anatomic distribution Papule or nodule	Dermal-based lesion Subcutaneous extension Circumscribed but unencapsulated Uniform spindle cells with wavy nuclei	S-100 + CD34 + NFP + (axons)
Scar	History of prior trauma	Uniform and bland spindle cells oriented parallel to skin surface Vertically oriented vessels	SMA ± Desmin – S-100 –
Sclerosing blue nevus	Young adults Wide anatomic distribution Papule or plaque with bluish discoloration	Uniform and bland short spindle cells in abundant collagenous stroma Pigmented dendritic melanocytes	S-100 ± Melan A + HMB-45 +
Spindle cell atypical fibroxanthoma	Elderly Sun-exposed skin (scalp) Ulcerated nodule	Dermal-based tumor Well-circumscribed lesion Epidermal ulceration Epidermal collarette Pleomorphic spindle cells Fascicular growth Abundant mitoses	S-100 – Melan A – Keratin – EMA – SMA ± Desmin –
Kaposi sarcoma	Purplish plaque Distinct clinical settings: Classic endemic affecting elderly males from Mediterranean region and Ashkenazi Jewish descent HIV-related Immunosuppression-associated Endemic Africans	Dermal-based lesion Infiltrative growth Uniform spindle cells No cytologic atypia Slitlike spaces Hemosiderin deposition Plasma cell–rich inflammatory cell infiltrate	CD34 + CD31 + HHV-8 +
Spindle cell hemangioma	Young adults Extremities Single or multiple bluish nodules	Poorly circumscribed Dermal and subcutaneous involvement Thin-walled, dilated cavernous vessels Uniform spindle cells in short fascicles Occasional cells with cytoplasmic vacuoles	CD34 + CD31 + HHV-8 –
Dermatofibrosarcoma protuberans	Young adults Wide anatomic distribution Large plaque/tumor	Dermal-based tumor Diffusely infiltrative growth Subcutaneous involvement in honeycomb pattern Bland spindle cells, storiform architecture Rare mitoses	CD34 + S-100 – SMA – Desmin –
Spindle cell angiosarcoma	Large tumor Distinct clinical settings: Sun-exposed area of elderly Radiation-associated Lymphedema-associated	Dermal-based tumor Subcutaneous involvement Diffusely infiltrative growth Spindle cells in sheets and fascicles Vasoformation Cytologic atypia Mitotic activity	CD34 + CD31 + ERG +

Table 15.3 Differential Diagnosis of Benign Fibrous Histiocytoma—cont'd

	Clinical Presentation	Histologic Features	Immunohistochemistry
Leiomyosarcoma	Adults Wide anatomic distribution Plaque or nodule	Dermal-based lesion Subcutaneous involvement Infiltrative growth Spindle cells with eosinophilic cytoplasm Fascicular growth Cytologic atypia and pleomorphism Mitotic activity	SMA + Desmin + h-Caldesmon + S-100 – Keratin ±
Malignant peripheral nerve sheath tumor	Adults Wide anatomic distribution Deep-seated tumor Rare cutaneous presentation Frequently associated with neurofibromatosis type 1	Atypical spindle cells with varying cellularity Myxoid stromal change Perivascular condensation of tumor cells Heterologous differentiation possible	S-100 + (50%) GFAP + (40%) SOX10 + (40%) Loss of H3K27me3 (30% low grade; 90% high grade)
Spindle cell and desmoplastic melanoma	Adults; increasing incidence with age Sun-exposed skin Pigmented plaque or nodule	Dermal-based lesion Subcutaneous involvement ± Junctional activity Infiltrative growth Spindle cells in fascicles and nests ± Desmoplastic stroma Cytologic atypia Mitotic activity	S-100 + SOX10 + Melan A ±
Spindle cell squamous cell carcinoma	Elderly Sun-exposed skin Plaque or exophytic tumor	Dermal-based lesion Subcutaneous involvement ± Squamous cell carcinoma in situ or actinic keratosis Infiltrative growth Spindle cells in fascicles and nests ± Desmoplastic stroma Cytologic atypia Mitotic activity	Keratins + p63/p40 + EMA ± SMA ± Desmin – S-100 –

EMA, Epithelial membrane antigen; *HHV-8*, human herpesvirus 8; *H3K27me3*, histone H3 with trimethylated lysine 27; *SMA*, smooth muscle actin.

circumscribed and well-demarcated firm papule or plaque measuring less than 1 cm in diameter. Dermatofibromas are often hyperpigmented or red and may occasionally appear bluish or black. They are rarely multiple. An eruptive variant has been reported in association with immunosuppression.

Pathologic Features

Dermatofibroma is a relatively circumscribed dermal-based tumor with a vaguely nodular appearance (Fig. 15.1). It is composed of short spindle cells in a haphazard arrangement. Tumor cellularity is higher toward the center of the lesion and reduced at its periphery, where tumor cells surround individual collagen bundles, also referred to as *entrapment of dermal collagen* (Fig. 15.2). A storiform growth pattern may be a focal feature. Varying numbers of foamy histiocytes and multinucleated (including Touton) giant cells may be present (Fig. 15.3), and an accompanying admixed chronic inflammatory infiltrate composed of lymphocytes and plasma cells is frequently seen. Hemosiderin deposition may be present within histiocytes and can be extensive in the hemosiderotic variant ("sclerosing hemangioma") (Fig. 15.4). Dermatofibroma is centered in and largely confined to the dermis, but focal extension into superficial subcutis is not unusual due to growth along preexisting fibrous septa (Fig. 15.5).[4] A pushing growth pattern into superficial subcutis is less frequently observed. Dermatofibroma typically spares the papillary dermis, and hyperplasia of the overlying epidermis often also showing basal cell layer hyperpigmentation is a characteristic feature (Fig. 15.6). A basaloid proliferation reminiscent of immature hair follicles or trichoblastoma may also be seen (Fig. 15.7). Rarely, tumor cells show extensive clear cell change (clear cell fibrous histiocytoma).[5] Nuclear

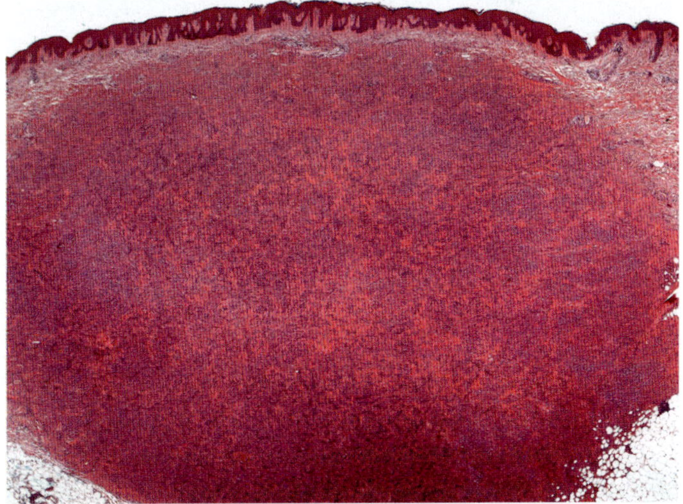

Figure 15.1 Benign Fibrous Histiocytoma. This nodular and well-circumscribed tumor is centered within the dermis and shows only focal involvement of the superficial aspect of the subcutis. Also note the sparing of the papillary dermis and hyperplasia of the overlying epidermis.

palisading reminiscent of Verocay bodies has been reported to occur predominantly in tumors of acral locations and is referred to as the *palisading variant* (Fig. 15.8).[6] Extensive granular cell change may rarely be seen (granular cell dermatofibroma) (Fig. 15.9).[7] Prominent lipidization of tumor cells with surrounding stromal hyalinization is a feature seen

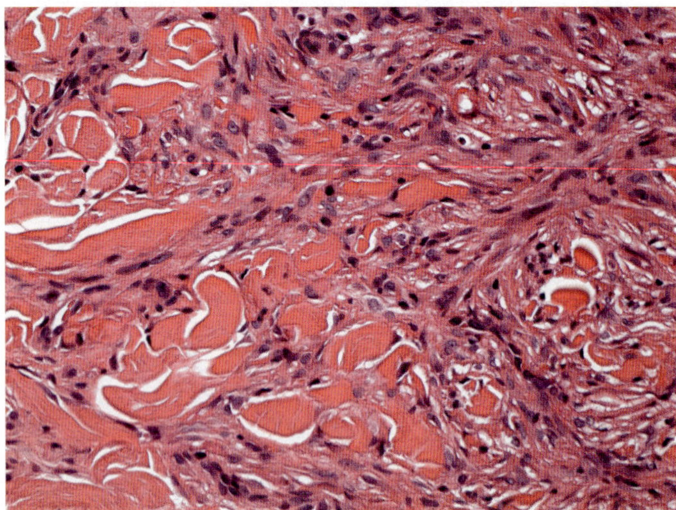

Figure 15.2 **Benign Fibrous Histiocytoma.** The tumor is composed of short spindle cells in a haphazard arrangement. Cellularity is decreased toward the periphery of the tumor, with spindle cells surrounding individual preexisting collagen fibers.

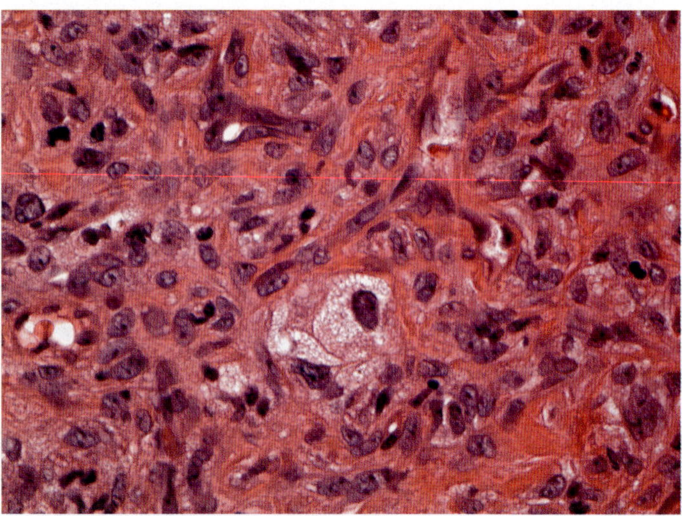

Figure 15.3 **Benign Fibrous Histiocytoma.** Lipidized cells are admixed within a population of spindle cells.

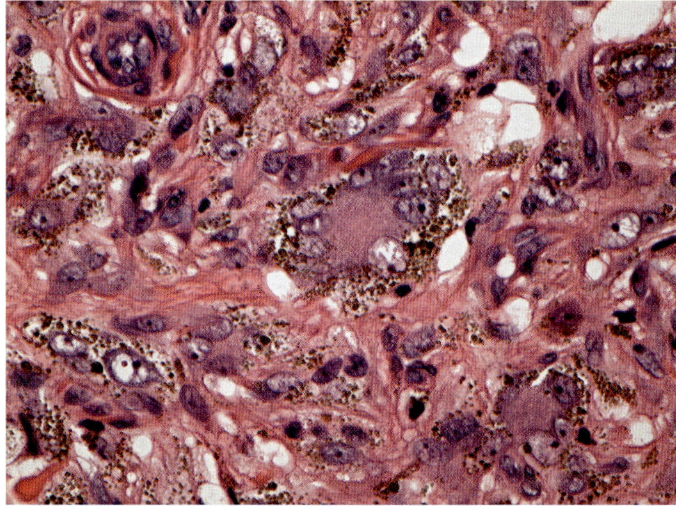

Figure 15.4 **Benign Fibrous Histiocytoma.** The hemosiderotic variant is characterized by abundant hemosiderin deposition within histiocytes and multinucleate giant cells.

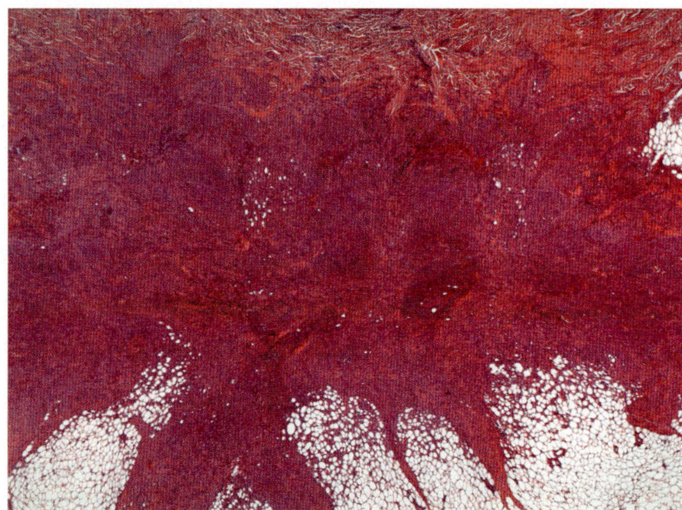

Figure 15.5 **Benign Fibrous Histiocytoma.** Although tumors are largely confined to the dermis, involvement of superficial subcutis and extension along preexisting fibrous septa may occasionally be identified.

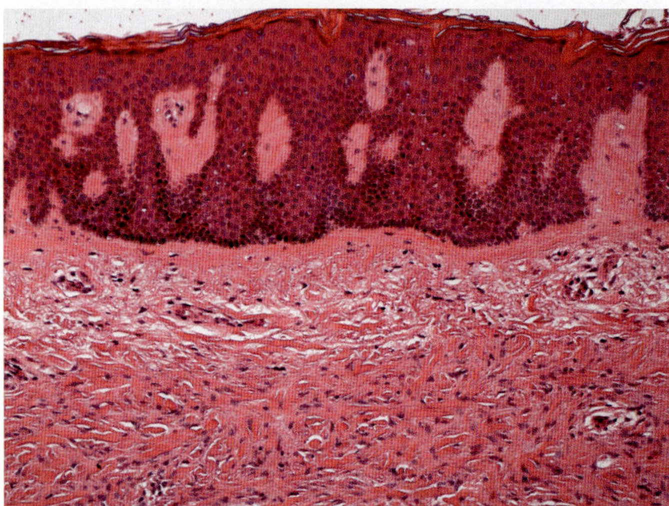

Figure 15.6 **Benign Fibrous Histiocytoma.** A characteristic feature is the presence of regular hyperplasia of the overlying epidermis, frequently also showing basal cell layer hyperpigmentation.

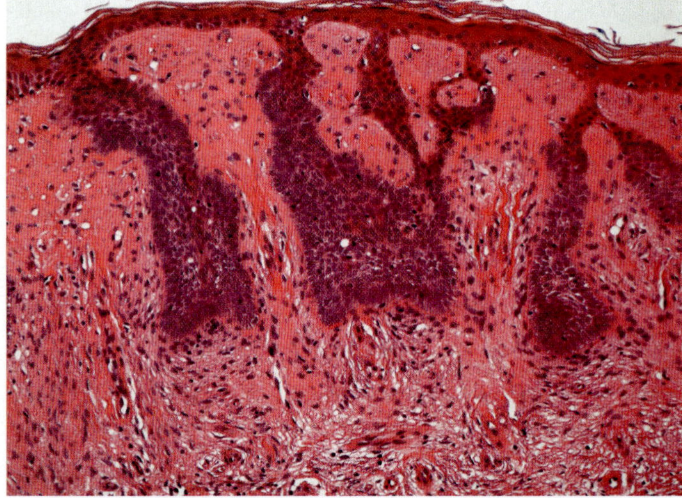

Figure 15.7 **Benign Fibrous Histiocytoma.** A basaloid proliferation reminiscent of trichoblastoma may occasionally be seen to arise from the overlying epidermis.

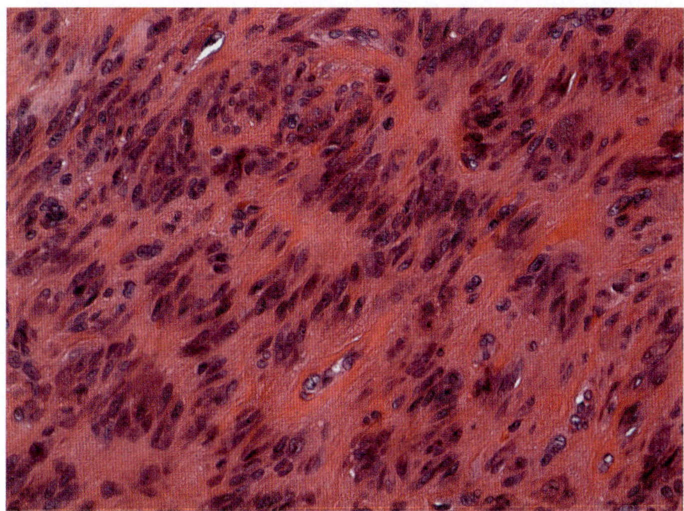

Figure 15.8 **Benign Fibrous Histiocytoma.** Nuclear palisading reminiscent of Verocay bodies is observed in the palisading variant.

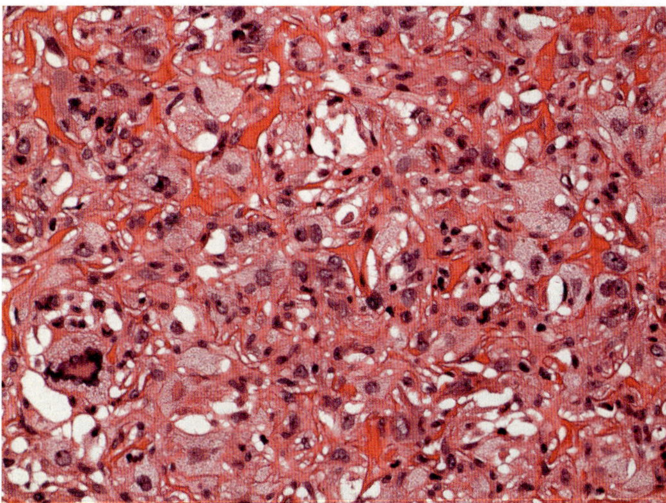

Figure 15.10 **Benign Fibrous Histiocytoma.** Extensive lipidization of tumor cells separated by hyalinized stromal collagen is seen in the lipidized or ankle-type variant.

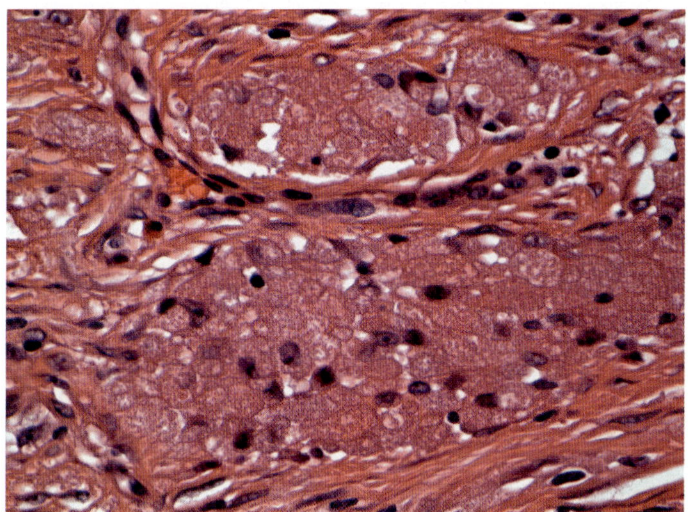

Figure 15.9 **Benign Fibrous Histiocytoma.** Marked cytoplasmic granular cell change characterizes the granular cell variant.

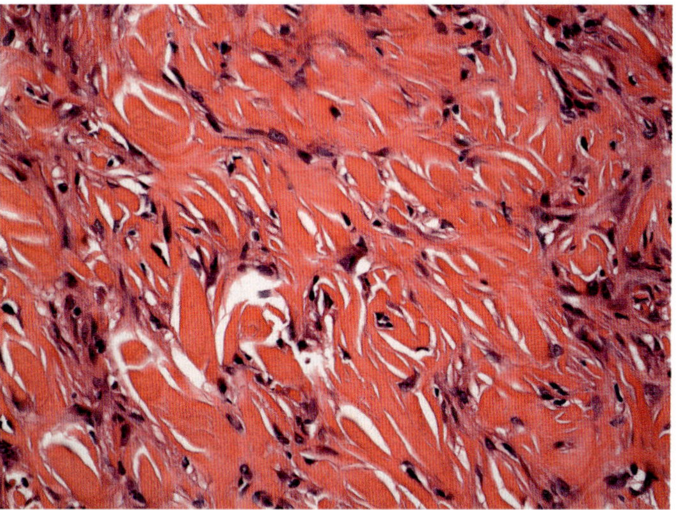

Figure 15.11 **Benign Fibrous Histiocytoma.** Marked stromal hyalinization and hypocellularity are the characteristic features of the atrophic variant.

predominantly in tumors arising on the lower extremity, particularly the ankle ("lipidized" or "ankle-type" fibrous histiocytoma) (Fig. 15.10).[8] Due to the extensive lipid accumulation, these tumors have a yellowish clinical appearance. Long-standing lesions are characterized by hypocellularity and stromal hyalinization, predominantly affecting the center of the lesion (atrophic variant) (Fig. 15.11).[9]

Immunohistochemistry

By immunohistochemistry, smooth muscle actin (SMA) or muscle-specific actin expression is seen in a significant subset of tumors (Fig. 15.12A). Expression of CD34 is a rare phenomenon present in approximately 5% of tumors, but S-100 protein or desmin expression is not a feature. Tumors are often populated by S-100 protein or factor XIIIa–positive dendritic cells (see Fig. 15.12B).

Differential Diagnosis

By far the most important differential diagnosis is dermatofibrosarcoma protuberans (DFSP). In contrast to dermatofibroma, the tumor cells in DFSP appear more monotonous and show a more pronounced storiform arrangement. Although CD34 positivity and extension into subcutis may be a particular pitfall in dermatofibroma, subcutaneous involvement is only focal and superficial and does not show the characteristic honeycomb infiltration of adipose tissue as seen in DFSP. Dermatofibroma can be mistaken for a scar, but the horizontal fibrosis containing vertically oriented vessels are histologic clues to the latter diagnosis. The clinical history may also be helpful in this distinction. Pilar leiomyoma and dermatomyofibroma also show some morphologic overlap with dermatofibroma. Dermatofibromas show a more haphazard rather than fascicular arrangement of tumor cells. In addition, leiomyoma expresses desmin and h-caldesmon by immunohistochemistry. Dermatomyofibroma forms a plaque composed of long fascicles aligned in parallel with the overlying epidermis. Myofibroma/myopericytoma typically shows biphasic morphology with primitive-appearing cells as well as nodules of more myoid spindle cells. The tumors are more cellular and well circumscribed, and they often show a distinctive perivascular growth pattern. Neurofibromas show a better demarcated growth pattern and contain characteristic uniform spindle cells with wavy nuclei, which are positive for S-100 protein by immunohistochemistry. The

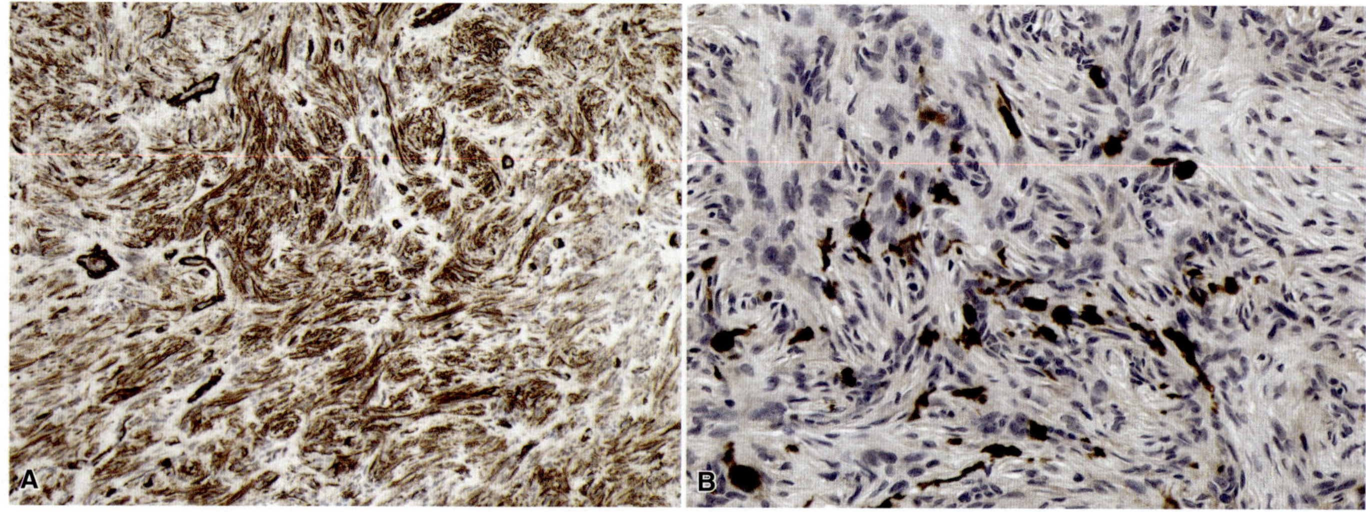

Figure 15.12 Benign Fibrous Histiocytoma. Expression of smooth muscle actin is observed in a significant subset of tumors (A). Tumors may be colonized by S-100–positive dendritic cells (B).

hemosiderotic variant can be mistaken for sclerosing blue nevi, as well as patch- or plaque-stage Kaposi sarcoma. Sclerosing blue nevi are characterized by the presence of pigmented dendritic melanocytes, which can be confirmed by the presence of melanin pigment and S-100 protein and/or HMB-45 immunohistochemistry. Kaposi sarcoma is an ill-defined and infiltrative tumor. Spindle cells are positive for endothelial markers as well as human herpesvirus 8.

Prognosis and Treatment

Fibrous histiocytomas are benign mesenchymal tumors. Except for specific variants (see subsequent discussion), excision is curative and recurrences are exceptional. However, cellular, aneurysmal, and atypical fibrous histiocytoma are associated with an approximately 20% risk of nondestructive local recurrence if incompletely removed. Metastases are exceptionally rare.

PRACTICE POINTS: Fibrous Histiocytoma

- Fibrous histiocytoma is the most common cutaneous mesenchymal neoplasm
- Fibrous histiocytoma shows a wide histologic spectrum, and multiple variants are recognized
- All variants (except epithelioid) share characteristic histologic features, including lateral collagen entrapment and overlying epidermal hyperplasia
- Infiltration of superficial subcutis is not uncommon and does not affect prognosis
- Clinical behavior is benign, but some variants (cellular, aneurysmal, and atypical) are associated with nondestructive local recurrence in 20% of cases

Cellular Benign Fibrous Histiocytoma

Cellular benign fibrous histiocytoma is an uncommon variant, representing approximately 5% of all fibrous histiocytomas. It shows a predilection for males and occurs predominantly on the extremities as well as on the head and neck. The tumor presents as a nodule. Tumors are frequently larger than typical dermatofibromas. They have a tendency for local recurrence in 20% of cases, and very rare distant metastases have been reported.[10,11]

Histologically, cellular benign fibrous histiocytomas are characterized by increased cellularity in the central aspect (Fig. 15.13). They are composed of longer and more tapering spindle cells containing larger amounts of eosinophilic cytoplasm (Fig. 15.14). Tumor cells show a fascicular growth pattern, and mitotic figures may be apparent. Extension

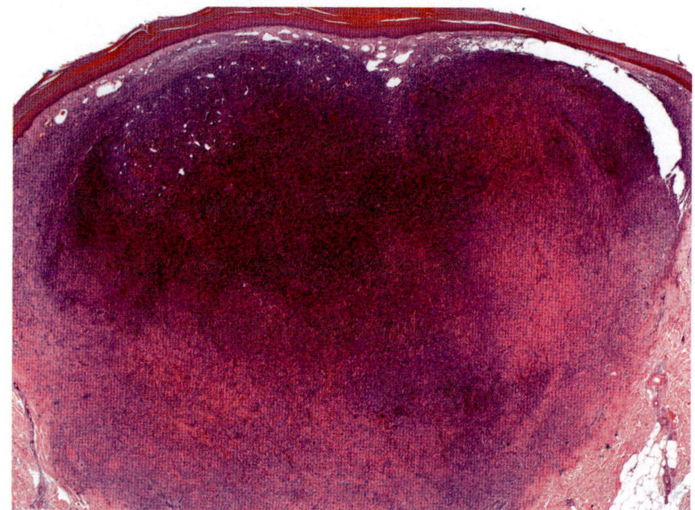

Figure 15.13 Cellular Benign Fibrous Histiocytoma. The cellular variant is frequently larger, showing increased tumor cellularity.

into superficial subcutis is frequently observed, and central necrosis may be observed in approximately 10% of cases.[10] As in common dermatofibroma, tumor cellularity is reduced toward the periphery, where it shows the characteristic entrapment of dermal collagen bundles, which is an important histologic clue to the correct diagnosis. However, hyperplasia of the overlying epidermis is a less consistent finding in cellular benign fibrous histiocytoma. By immunohistochemistry, tumor cells show variable staining for SMA in nearly all cases. Focal desmin expression may be seen in 32% of cases, but expression of CD34 is rare (5%).[12] S-100 protein is consistently negative.

Due to their fascicular growth pattern, differentiation from the fibrosarcomatous variant of DFSP or an atypical intradermal smooth muscle neoplasm (AISMN) may be difficult. The presence of peripheral entrapment of collagen bundles, lack of invasion of deeper subcutis, and the absence of CD34 staining help distinguish cellular benign fibrous histiocytoma from DFSP. Furthermore, tumor cells in cellular benign fibrous histiocytoma lack the brightly eosinophilic cytoplasm and cigar-shaped nuclei characteristic of smooth muscle tumors. Limited

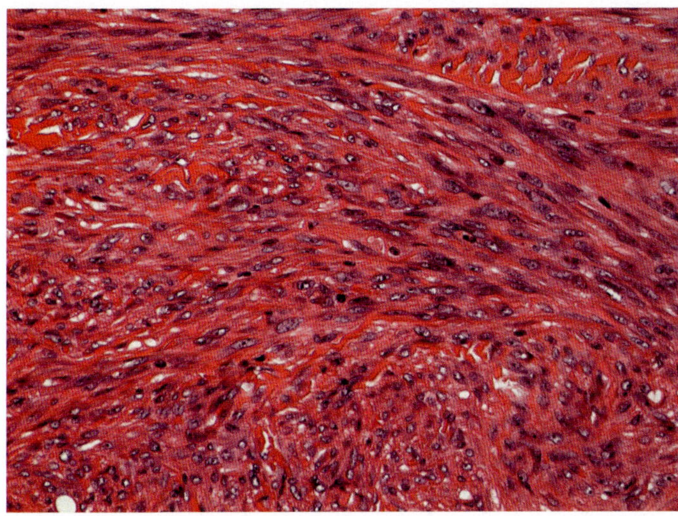

Figure 15.14 Cellular Benign Fibrous Histiocytoma. The cellular variant is composed of spindle cells containing larger amounts of eosinophilic cytoplasm. Tumor cells are arranged in a fascicular pattern.

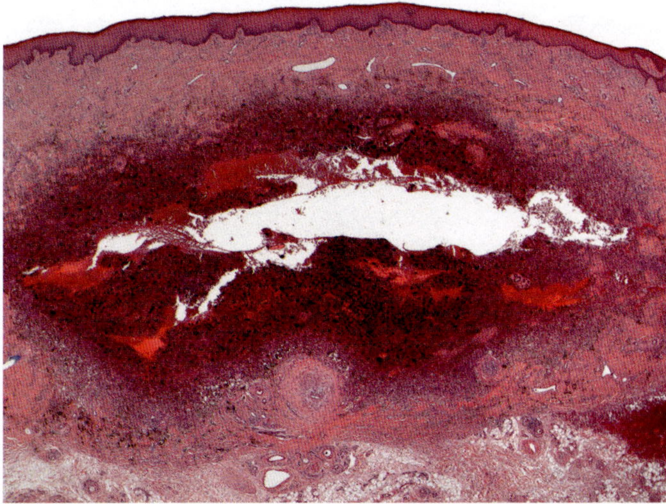

Figure 15.15 Aneurysmal Benign Fibrous Histiocytoma. This circumscribed dermal-based tumor shows a central blood-filled space characteristic of the aneurysmal variant.

(if any) desmin expression and the lack of h-caldesmon further exclude smooth muscle differentiation. Other cellular spindle cell tumors such as spindle cell melanoma and spindle cell squamous cell carcinoma should also be considered. Immunohistochemistry for S-100 protein and keratins easily resolves this diagnostic problem. Clues to a diagnosis of nodular fasciitis include a short clinical history as well as specific morphologic features such as myxoid stromal change and erythrocyte extravasation.

Aneurysmal Benign Fibrous Histiocytoma

Aneurysmal benign fibrous histiocytoma presents as a brown to bluish nodule with a predilection for the extremities and trunk of middle-aged adults, with a slight female predominance.[13] Tumors can measure several centimeters in size, and there may be a history of rapid growth. Clinically, they can easily be mistaken for melanoma or hemangioma. Analogous to cellular benign fibrous histiocytoma, the aneurysmal variant shows a tendency for local recurrence (in 20% of cases), but metastases are exceptional.[11,13]

The characteristic histologic finding is the presence of blood-filled cystic and cleftlike spaces within the center of the tumor (Fig. 15.15). The surrounding solid aspects show the typical features of fibrous histiocytoma, often resembling the cellular variant. Hemorrhage and hemosiderin deposition are prominent features, and mitotic activity is often present.[13]

The most important differential diagnosis includes vascular tumors such as spindle cell angiosarcoma and nodular Kaposi sarcoma. Immunohistochemistry allows for straightforward separation because the spindle cells in aneurysmal benign fibrous histiocytoma lack expression of endothelial markers such as CD34, CD31, and ERG, although admixed histiocytes may be CD31 positive. Furthermore, both cutaneous angiosarcoma and Kaposi sarcoma occur in distinct clinical settings. Due to the prominent pigmentation, aneurysmal benign fibrous histiocytoma may also be mistaken for melanoma. Inspection of the periphery of the tumor, absence of an overlying in situ component, and a lack of S-100 protein expression readily resolve this diagnostic dilemma.

Atypical (Pseudosarcomatous) Fibrous Histiocytoma

Atypical fibrous histiocytoma is a rare neoplasm that has previously also been referred to as *pseudosarcomatous fibrous histiocytoma* or *dermatofibroma with monster cells*. The tumor shows a predilection for the extremities of young to middle-aged adults.[14,15] It presents as a polypoid or nodular tumor and may be significantly larger than common fibrous histiocytomas. Local recurrence can be a complication (in ~20% of cases), and distant metastasis with associated mortality has very rarely been documented.[15]

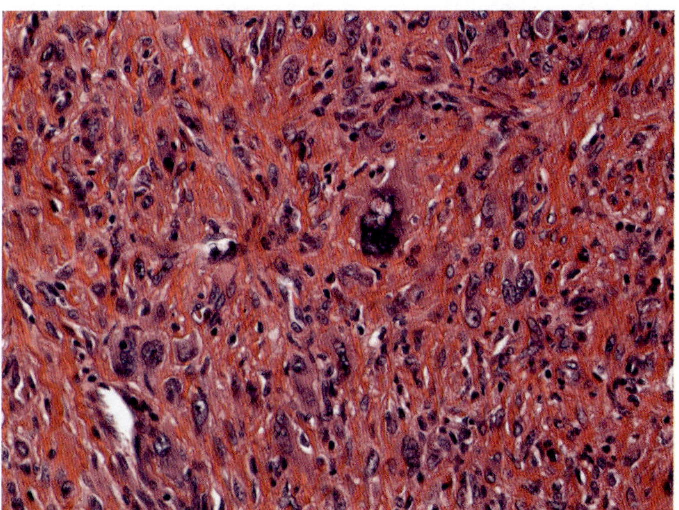

Figure 15.16 Atypical Fibrous Histiocytoma. Features of the atypical variant include marked nuclear pleomorphism and hyperchromasia in the background of an otherwise typical fibrous histiocytoma.

The characteristic histologic feature is the presence of pleomorphic spindle cells showing nuclear hyperchromasia and often bizarre nuclei in a background of an otherwise typical fibrous histiocytoma (Fig. 15.16). Pleomorphic multinucleated cells may also be present. Mitotic activity is often high and may include atypical forms. Involvement of superficial subcutis and central necrosis are additional features, similar to cellular benign fibrous histiocytoma.

The main differential diagnostic considerations are AFX and undifferentiated pleomorphic dermal sarcoma. Histologic distinction may be difficult. In contrast to atypical fibrous histiocytoma, AFX arises on sun-damaged skin of the elderly. Although the histologic features show significant overlap, AFX typically extends to the epidermis without a

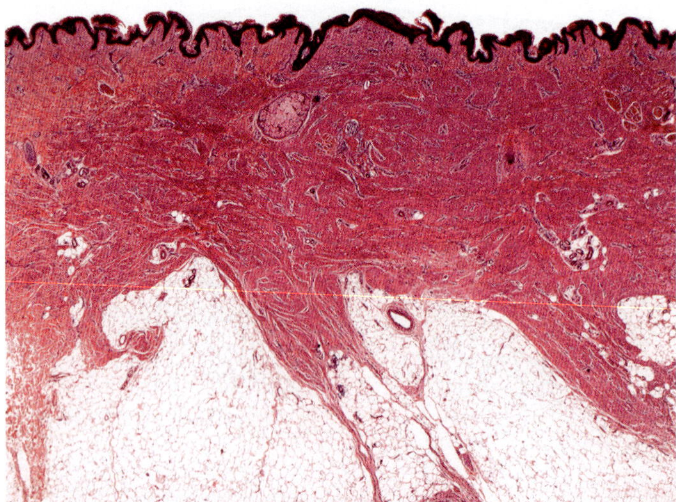

Figure 15.17 **Dermatomyofibroma.** A plaquelike growth pattern within dermis and only focal involvement of superficial subcutis are typical of this tumor type.

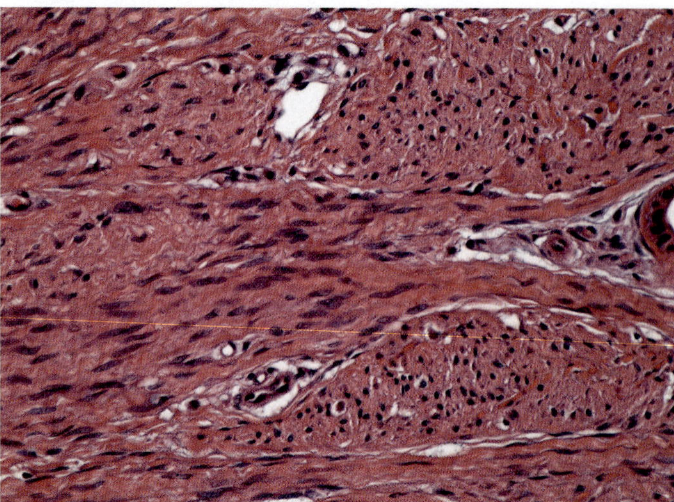

Figure 15.18 **Dermatomyofibroma.** The tumor is composed of bland-appearing spindle cells arranged in fascicles oriented parallel to the skin surface.

grenz zone, and epidermal ulceration is common. AFX by definition is confined to the dermis. Undifferentiated pleomorphic dermal sarcomas usually occur in older adults, and they lack the peripheral collagen entrapment and epidermal hyperplasia seen in atypical fibrous histiocytoma. The differential diagnosis also includes other sarcomas with pleomorphic features such as leiomyosarcoma, as well as melanoma and carcinoma. These tumors can usually be separated by immunohistochemistry for desmin, S-100 protein, and keratins.

Dermatomyofibroma

Dermatomyofibroma, previously also known as *plaquelike dermal fibromatosis,* is a rare distinctive benign cutaneous tumor showing myofibroblastic differentiation.

Clinical Features

The tumor occurs as an occasionally discolored plaque measuring a few centimeters in size with a strong predilection for the shoulder girdle, neck, and upper arm of young female adults.[16-19] Children may also be affected.

Pathologic Features

Dermatomyofibroma is based in the reticular dermis, where it grows in a plaquelike pattern (Fig. 15.17). The papillary dermis is spared, but focal extension into superficial subcutis may be seen. The tumor is composed of bland and uniform spindle cells in a fascicular arrangement, oriented parallel to the skin surface (Fig. 15.18). Infrequent mitoses may be seen, but cytologic atypia is not a feature.[16–18,20]

Immunohistochemistry

By immunohistochemistry, most cases show expression of SMA and muscle-specific actin, but desmin is negative, supporting myofibroblastic differentiation. CD34 is also focally positive in a subset of cases.[20]

Differential Diagnosis

The main differential diagnosis includes plaque-type DFSP, fibroblastic connective tissue nevus, and neurofibroma. In contrast to dermatomyofibroma, plaque-type DFSP shows strong and diffuse CD34 expression. Fibroblastic connective tissue nevus lacks the uniform plaquelike architecture of dermatomyofibroma, instead being composed of disorderly bundles of bland spindle cells in the dermis and subcutaneous tissue

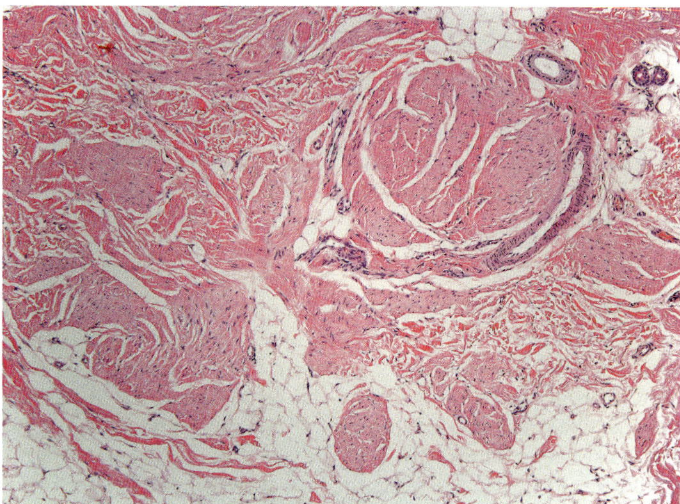

Figure 15.19 **Connective Tissue Nevus.** The lesion is composed of haphazardly arranged bundles of spindle cells in the dermis and subcutis.

(Fig. 15.19); CD34 is usually positive, and SMA expression is at most weak and focal. Neurofibroma can be separated by immunohistochemistry for S-100 protein. Rare hemorrhagic cases mimic plaque-stage Kaposi sarcoma, which would, however, show positive staining for endothelial markers and human herpesvirus 8.[21]

Prognosis and Treatment

The clinical behavior is benign. Local excision is curative.

Pilar Leiomyoma

The spectrum of superficial benign smooth muscle tumors includes pilar leiomyoma and angioleiomyoma, in addition to leiomyomas of genital sites and the nipple and areola. Only pilar leiomyoma is discussed in this section. Genital smooth muscle tumors are discussed in Chapter 17.

Clinical Features

Pilar leiomyoma usually affects young adults. Lesions may be multiple or less frequently solitary. Multiple pilar leiomyomas affect the limbs

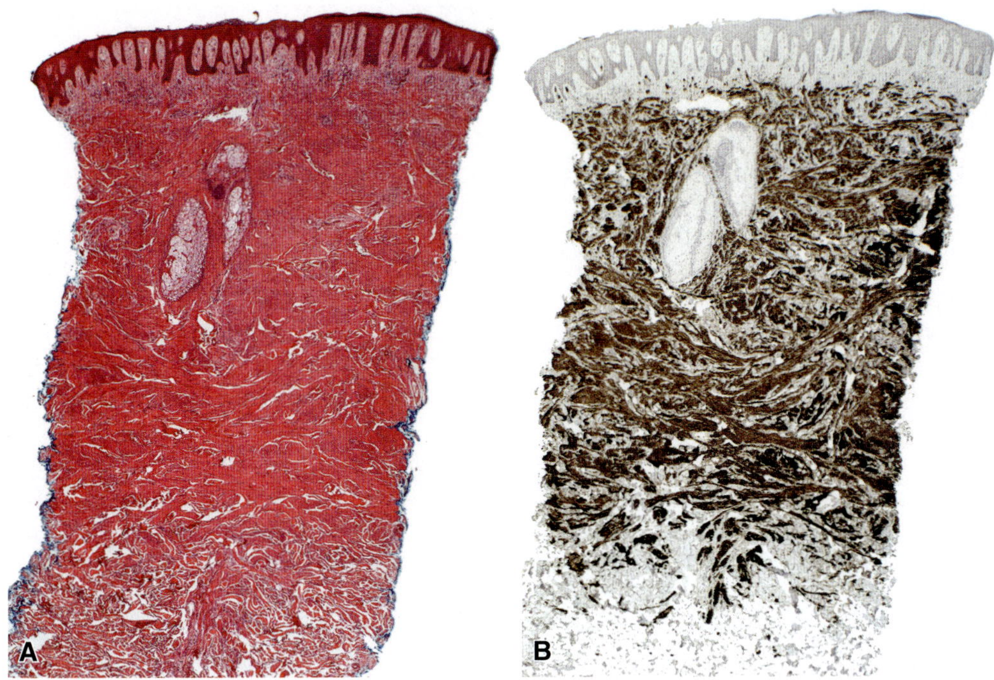

Figure 15.20 Pilar Leiomyoma. This cellular neoplasm is confined to the dermis (A). Tumor cells are diffusely positive for desmin (B).

and trunk. Lesions often present as painful papules measuring less than 1 cm in diameter.[22] A positive family history with an autosomal dominant trait can be elucidated in a minority of patients, and females may also develop multiple uterine leiomyomas. The familial disorder may be complicated by the development of papillary renal cell carcinoma (hereditary leiomyomatosis and renal cell cancer syndrome [HLRCC]).[23,24] In contrast, solitary pilar leiomyomas show a strong predilection for the limbs. They present as larger plaques with a predilection for males.[22]

Pathologic Features

Pilar leiomyoma is a dermal-based tumor (Fig. 15.20A), but focal involvement of the superficial subcutis may occasionally be seen. Tumors are ill-defined and composed of interweaving fascicles of spindle cells containing blunt-ended, cigar-shaped nuclei with brightly eosinophilic cytoplasm characteristic of smooth muscle differentiation (Fig. 15.21). At the periphery, tumor cells merge with surrounding collagen bundles. A nodular and well-circumscribed growth pattern is less frequently observed. Mitotic activity is scarce, but scattered cells showing degenerative nuclear atypia reminiscent of symplastic uterine leiomyoma may be seen. The overlying epidermis may be hyperplastic.

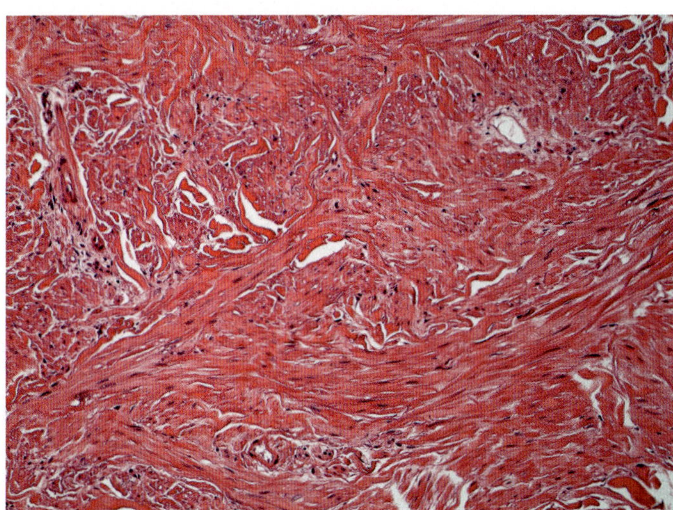

Figure 15.21 Pilar Leiomyoma. The tumor is composed of bland-appearing spindle cells containing abundant eosinophilic cytoplasm arranged in interweaving fascicles.

Immunohistochemistry

Tumor cells show strong, diffuse reactivity for SMA, desmin, and h-caldesmon (see Fig. 15.20B).

Molecular Genetics

The autosomal dominant syndrome of multiple pilar and uterine leiomyomas as well as papillary renal cell carcinoma (HLRCC) is caused by germline mutations in the fumarate hydratase *(FH)* gene on chromosome 1q42.3–43. Although involved in the tricarboxylic acid (Krebs) cycle, this gene also functions as a tumor suppressor gene in this context.[23,24]

Differential Diagnosis

AISMNs are characterized by the presence of cytologic atypia and increased mitotic activity (see later discussion). Metastatic leiomyosarcoma to the skin is typically well circumscribed, and nuclear atypia and a high mitotic rate are diagnostic features. DFSP lacks the fascicular architecture and cytoplasmic eosinophilia of pilar leiomyoma, and CD34 and desmin staining resolves this diagnostic consideration.

Prognosis and Treatment

Local excision is curative. Recurrence is exceptional.

Atypical Intradermal Smooth Muscle Neoplasm

AISMN is often referred to as *cutaneous leiomyosarcoma*.[25,26] However, when the tumors are confined to the dermis, they may recur locally but do not metastasize.[25,26] The "sarcoma" designation is therefore inappropriate unless there is invasion of subcutaneous tissue.

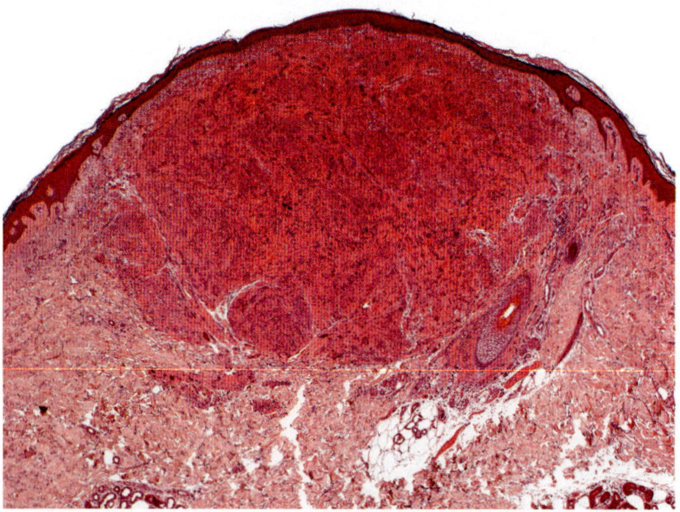

Figure 15.22 Atypical Intradermal Smooth Muscle Neoplasm. The tumor is limited to the dermis and shows a mixed nodular and infiltrative growth pattern.

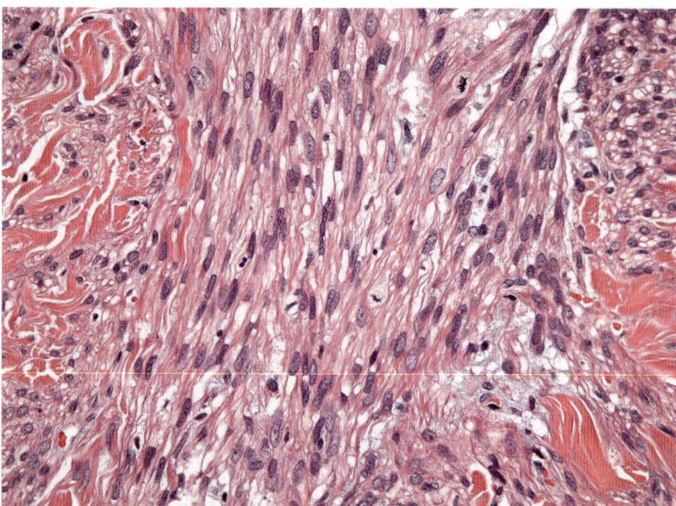

Figure 15.24 Atypical Intradermal Smooth Muscle Neoplasm. The tumor cells show nuclear atypia and mitotic activity. Note the well-defined cell borders.

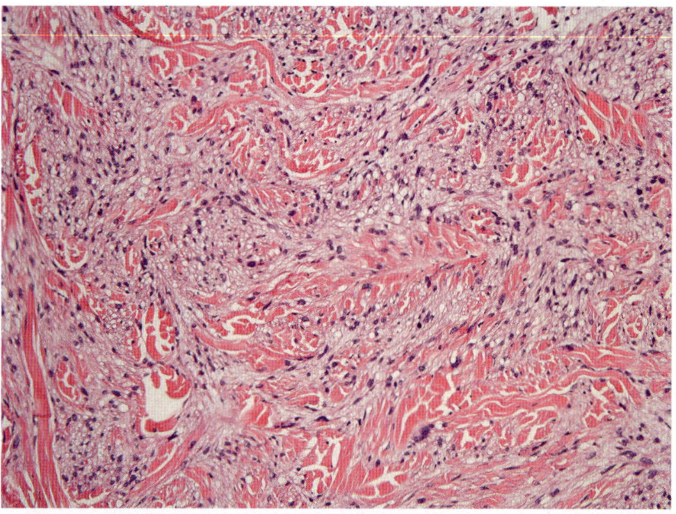

Figure 15.23 Atypical Intradermal Smooth Muscle Neoplasm. Like pilar leiomyoma, bundles of tumor cells ramify through the dermis.

Clinical Features

AISMN affects middle-aged to elderly adults, with a striking male predilection (male-to-female ratio of nearly 5:1).[25,26] The trunk and lower limbs are most often involved. Most tumors range from 1 to 2 cm in size. AISMN typically presents as a slowly growing, occasionally painful nodule or mass.

Pathologic Features

Similar to pilar leiomyoma, AISMN is based in the dermis and usually shows a predominantly infiltrative growth pattern, with fascicles of spindle cells ramifying between dermal collagen bundles (Figs. 15.22 and 15.23). In areas, a nodular architecture may be seen (see Fig. 15.22). Only very limited involvement of the superficial subcutis with a pushing border is acceptable for the designation AISMN.[25,26] The spindle cells contain blunt-ended (cigar-shaped) nuclei and brightly eosinophilic cytoplasm, with well-defined cell borders, typical of smooth muscle cells. The presence of nuclear atypia, which is usually mild to moderate, and mitotic activity distinguish AISMN from conventional pilar leiomyoma (Fig. 15.24). Epithelioid cytomorphology is rare. Necrosis is uncommon. Recurrent tumors more often show a nodular growth pattern, marked nuclear atypia, a higher mitotic rate, and necrosis.[25] Overlying epidermal hyperplasia may be seen.

Immunohistochemistry

Nearly all tumors are positive for SMA, desmin, and h-caldesmon. Focal staining for keratin is observed in approximately 50% of cases.[25] CD34, S-100 protein, HMB-45, and melan A are consistently negative.

Differential Diagnosis

The main differential diagnosis includes pilar leiomyoma, metastatic leiomyosarcoma, cellular benign fibrous histiocytoma, and atypical fibrous histiocytoma. In contrast to pilar leiomyoma, which often presents as multiple lesions, AISMN is solitary. Pilar leiomyoma lacks nuclear atypia and more than occasional mitotic figures. Metastatic leiomyosarcoma shows a well-circumscribed growth pattern without the infiltrative margins of primary intradermal smooth muscle tumors. Cellular benign fibrous histiocytoma may share expression of SMA and desmin by immunohistochemistry, but it lacks the well-defined bundles, blunt-ended nuclei, nuclear atypia, and bright cytoplasmic eosinophilia of AISMN. Atypical fibrous histiocytoma contains scattered cells with nuclear atypia and pleomorphism but, in contrast to AISMN, generally shows a mixed fascicular and storiform architecture, and the tumor cells are more heterogeneous with pale cytoplasm. Strong desmin and h-caldesmon expression distinguish smooth muscle tumors from atypical fibrous histiocytoma. The rare tumors that arise on the head and neck should be distinguished from spindle cell squamous cell carcinoma and malignant melanoma. A search for overlying epidermal dysplasia or a junctional component is warranted in this context. Similar to squamous cell carcinoma, AISMN is often at least focally positive for keratins, and spindle cell squamous cell carcinoma can be focally positive for SMA, although desmin and h-caldesmon are not expressed; p63 expression favors spindle cell squamous cell carcinoma over AISMN. Staining for S-100 protein and other melanocytic markers can distinguish melanoma from AISMN.

Prognosis and Treatment

AISMN recurs locally in 20% to 30% of cases.[25] Margin status is the only predictor of local recurrence. Complete excision with negative

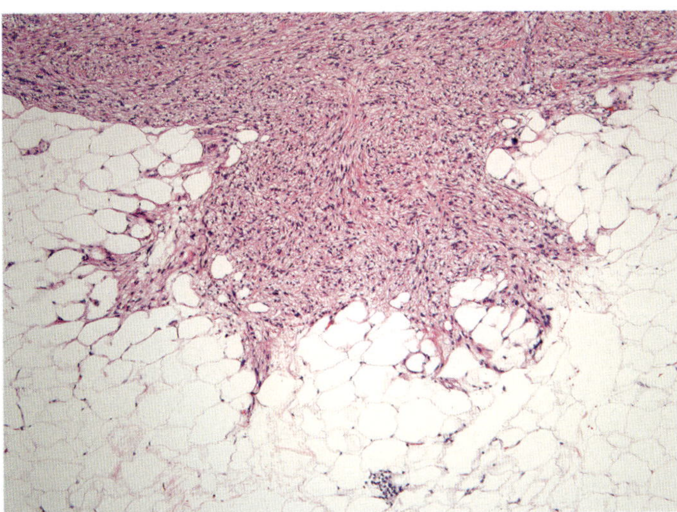

Figure 15.25 Cutaneous Leiomyosarcoma. Tumors that infiltrate subcutaneous adipose tissue should be designated cutaneous leiomyosarcoma.

margins is therefore appropriate therapy. Tumors confined to the dermis do not metastasize.[25,26] Tumors showing invasion into the subcutaneous adipose tissue warrant the designation "cutaneous leiomyosarcoma" (Fig. 15.25) because they may rarely metastasize.[26]

PRACTICE POINTS: Atypical Intradermal Smooth Muscle Neoplasm

- When confined to the dermis, has no metastatic potential (sarcoma designation inappropriate)
- Distinctive growth pattern with bundles irregularly ramifying through dermal collagen
- Distinguished from pilar leiomyoma by the presence of nuclear atypia, pleomorphism, and mitotic activity
- Positive for SMA, desmin, h-caldesmon, and often keratins
- Minimal extension into superficial subcutis with a pushing border is acceptable
- When infiltrates subcutaneous adipose tissue, there is a small risk of metastasis; the designation "cutaneous leiomyosarcoma" is appropriate

Storiform Collagenoma

Clinical Features

Storiform collagenoma (sclerotic fibroma) classically occurs as a solitary nodule of less than 1 cm. It has a wide anatomic distribution. Young to middle-aged adults of both genders are affected. The occurrence of multiple tumors or oral involvement may be an indicator of Cowden syndrome (PTEN hamartoma tumor syndrome).[27,28] Recognition of this association is important for early detection and treatment of associated visceral malignancies, mainly affecting the breast, thyroid, and endometrium.[29,30]

Pathologic Features

The histologic appearances of storiform collagenoma are distinctive. Tumors present as well-circumscribed nodules within the dermis (Fig. 15.26). Composed of hyalinized collagen bundles separated by prominent clefts, they contain bland-appearing spindle cells arranged in a storiform pattern (Fig. 15.27).[31] Similar tumors containing bizarre-shaped multinucleated giant cells have been referred to as *giant cell collagenoma.*[32]

Immunohistochemistry

Spindle cells may be positive for CD34 but are negative for smooth muscle markers, S-100 protein, and epithelial membrane antigen (EMA) (Fig. 15.28).[27,31]

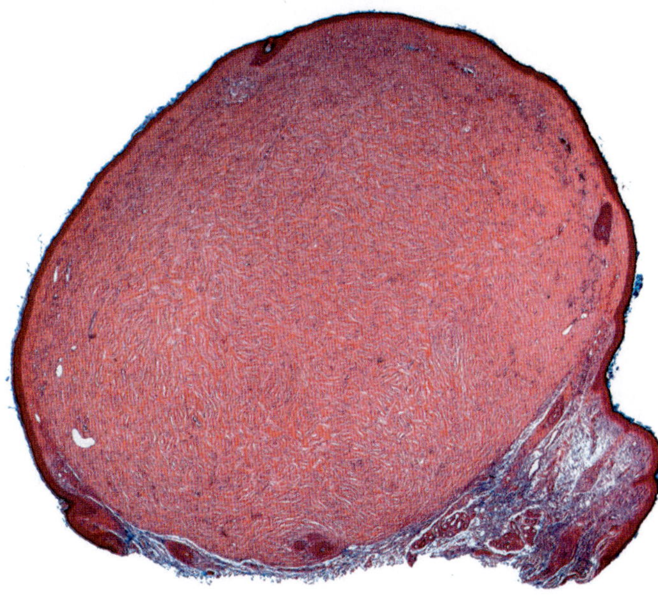

Figure 15.26 Storiform Collagenoma. This polypoid and well-circumscribed tumor is located within the dermis.

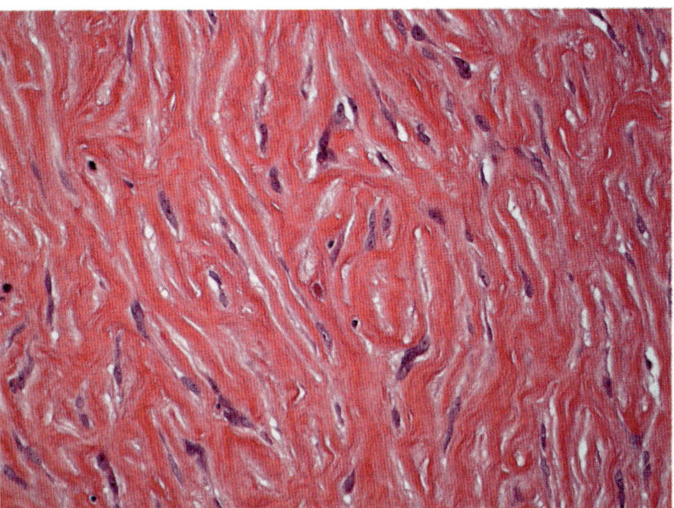

Figure 15.27 Storiform Collagenoma. Sclerotic collagen bundles are separated by prominent clefts containing short spindle cells.

Differential Diagnosis

The main differential diagnosis includes perineurioma, which can be excluded by a lack of EMA expression in storiform collagenoma. Investigators have reported histologic features reminiscent of storiform collagenoma following inflammatory conditions such as folliculitis, and some examples of storiform collagenoma may represent long-standing dermatofibromas.

Prognosis and Treatment

The behavior of storiform collagenoma is entirely benign. Simple excision is curative.

Solitary Circumscribed Neuroma

Solitary circumscribed neuroma was initially reported as palisaded encapsulated neuroma. However, the former designation is preferred because it more accurately reflects the features of this benign neural

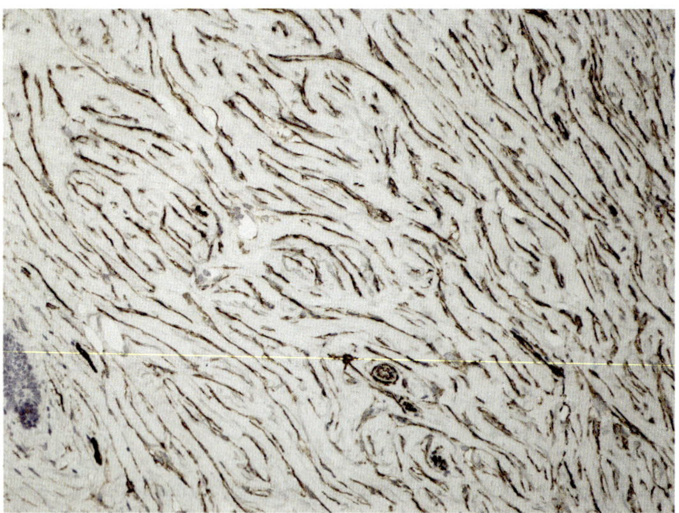

Figure 15.28 **Storiform Collagenoma.** Spindle cells express CD34 strongly and diffusely.

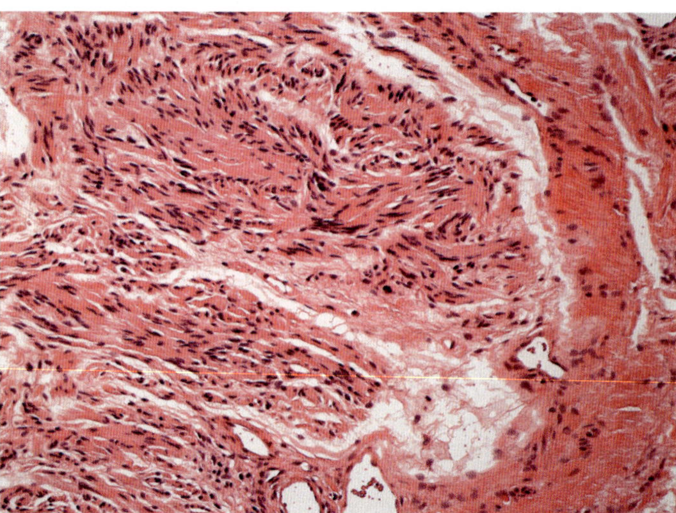

Figure 15.30 **Solitary Circumscribed Neuroma.** The tumor is composed of uniform spindle cells only focally showing vague nuclear palisading.

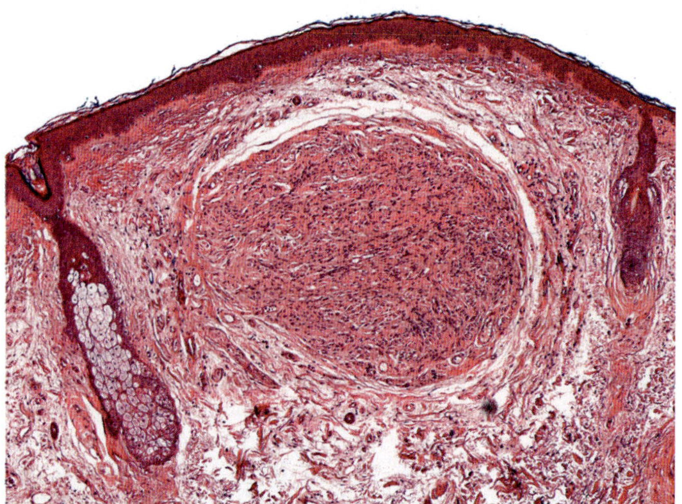

Figure 15.29 **Solitary Circumscribed Neuroma.** Presentation as a circumscribed tumor within superficial dermis is characteristic.

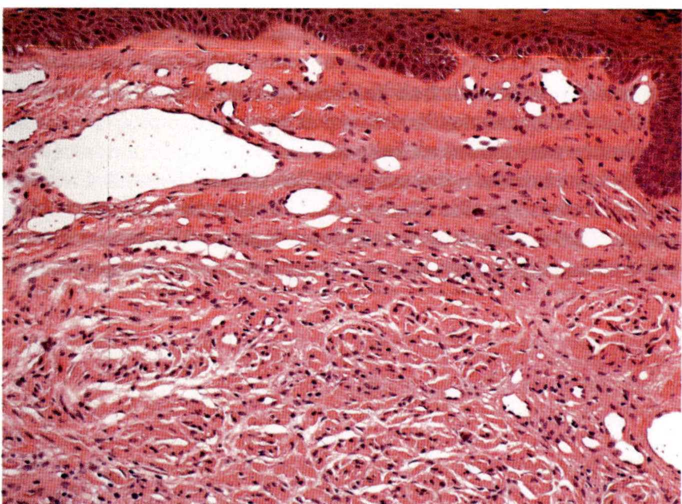

Figure 15.31 **Solitary Circumscribed Neuroma.** In areas, the tumor lacks encapsulation and merges with the surrounding dermis.

tumor, which shows only variable nuclear palisading and is at most only partially encapsulated.

Clinical Features

Solitary circumscribed neuroma is not uncommon, with a strong predilection for the central face of middle-aged adults with an equal gender distribution.[33-35] The lips and oral cavity may also be affected. It presents as a solitary, skin-colored papule measuring up to 0.5 cm in diameter. It is not associated with neurofibromatosis or other inherited syndromes.

Pathologic Features

Solitary circumscribed neuroma is located within the dermis and presents as a well-circumscribed tumor composed of spindle cells showing schwannian differentiation and numerous intratumoral axons (Fig. 15.29). Spindle cells are arranged in short fascicles and contain wavy nuclei lacking atypia (Fig. 15.30). Nuclear palisading reminiscent of Verocay bodies may occasionally be observed. Encapsulation is at most partial, and in particular the superficial aspect of the tumor appears to merge with the surrounding dermis (Fig. 15.31).[33-36] Plexiform growth and epithelioid cytomorphology have been reported but are rare.

Immunohistochemistry

Spindle cells are diffusely positive for S-100 protein, and numerous intratumoral axons are highlighted by neurofilament protein (Fig. 15.32A and B). The partial capsule contains EMA-positive perineurial cells (see Fig. 15.32C).[33-36]

Differential Diagnosis

The clinical and histologic features are quite characteristic. Schwannoma may occasionally present as a dermal tumor. However, schwannomas are encapsulated, with hypocellular, myxoid areas and hyalinized blood vessels, and they are largely devoid of intratumoral axons. Neurofibromas are not as sharply circumscribed, and tumor cells show a less fascicular architecture. Solitary circumscribed neuroma may be mistaken for a smooth muscle neoplasm. It can easily be distinguished by S-100 protein and desmin immunostains.

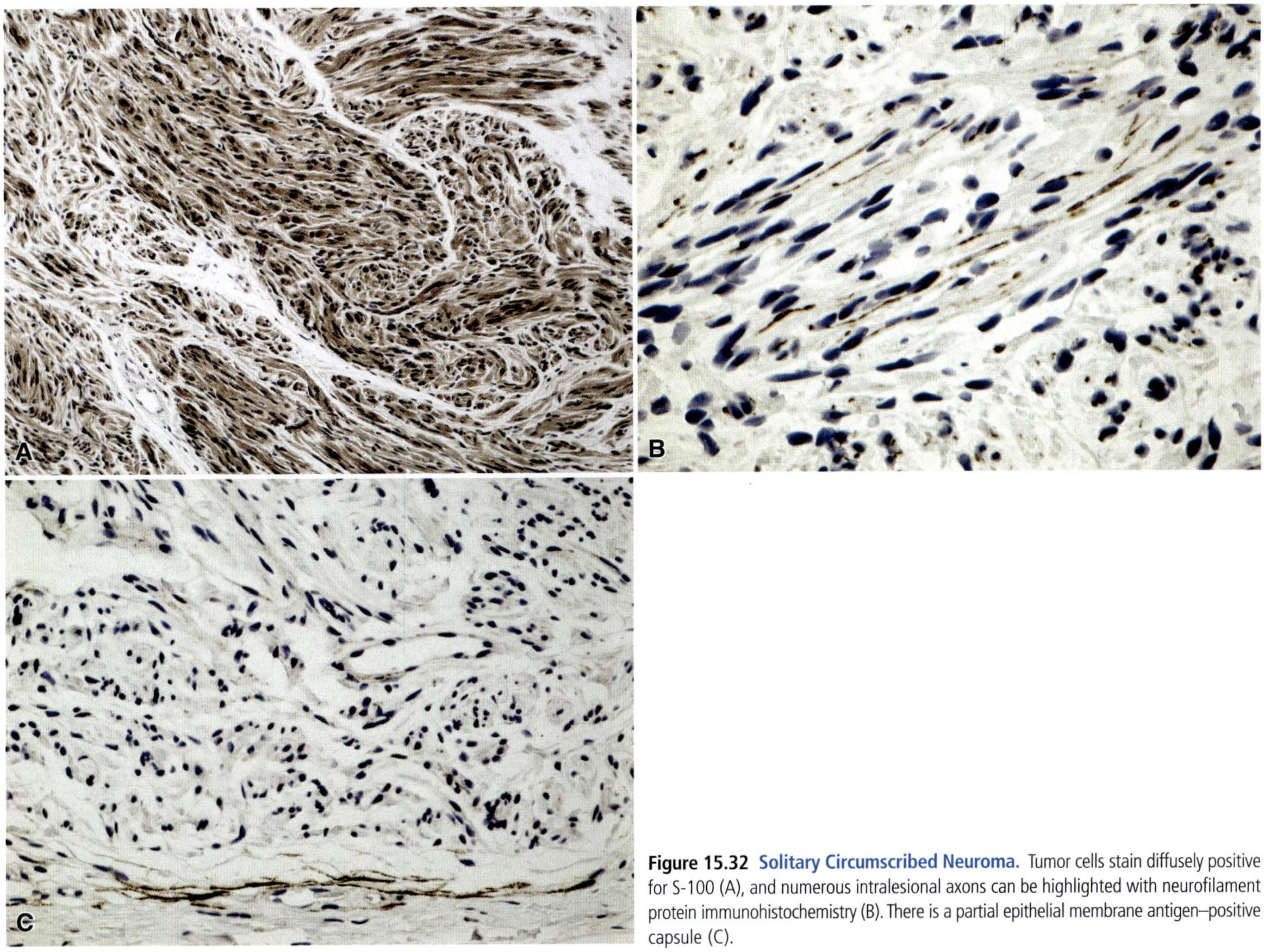

Figure 15.32 Solitary Circumscribed Neuroma. Tumor cells stain diffusely positive for S-100 (A), and numerous intralesional axons can be highlighted with neurofilament protein immunohistochemistry (B). There is a partial epithelial membrane antigen–positive capsule (C).

Prognosis and Treatment

The clinical behavior is entirely benign. This tumor does not recur.

Dermatofibrosarcoma Protuberans

DFSP is a locally aggressive tumor with significant potential for local recurrence but no metastatic risk in its conventional form. It shows a morphologic spectrum; in particular, recognition of the fibrosarcomatous variant is important because it is associated with acquisition of metastatic potential. Furthermore, DFSP is closely related to giant cell fibroblastoma (see subsequent discussion). This notion is supported by the finding that both histologic patterns can be found in a single tumor, and both tumors show identical immunohistochemical as well as cytogenetic findings.

Clinical Features

DFSP is a rare neoplasm with an incidence of two to four new cases per million per year.[37,38] Young adults in the second to fourth decade are predominantly affected,[38] but presentation in childhood and congenital onset have been documented.[39,40] There is a slight male predominance. Tumors show a predilection for the trunk and extremities,[38,41] and the head and neck area is less frequently affected. The characteristic clinical presentation is of a large, multinodular tumor measuring several centimeters in diameter and showing red to bluish discoloration. Tumors are slow growing, and frequently there is a history of a long-standing plaque (>10 years) prior to the development of nodular areas.[38]

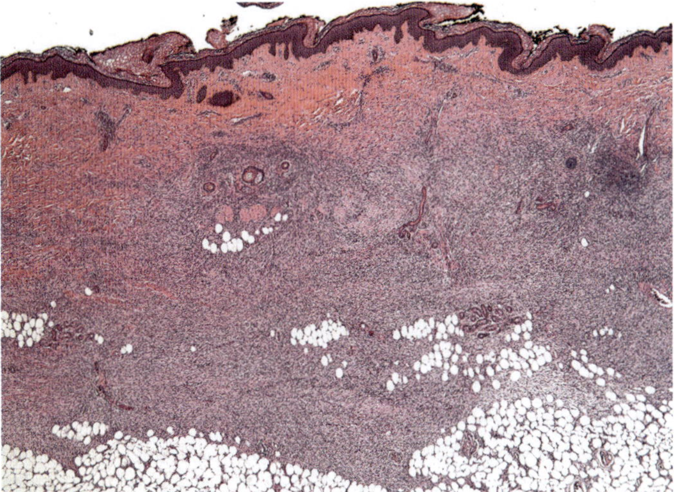

Figure 15.33 Dermatofibrosarcoma Protuberans. The tumor has infiltrative margins through the dermis and subcutis. Note the lack of epidermal hyperplasia.

Pathologic Features

DFSP is an ill-defined and diffusely infiltrative tumor of the dermis and subcutis (Fig. 15.33). The tumor is centered within the dermis and may extend to the overlying epidermis, which does not typically show the characteristic hyperplasia associated with benign fibrous histiocytoma.

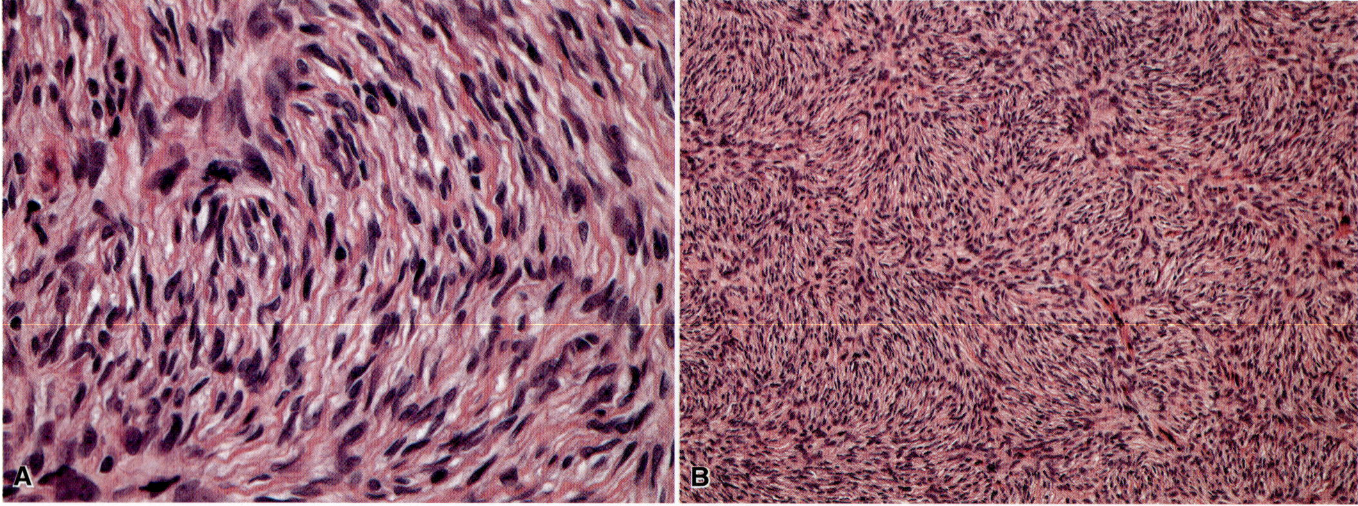

Figure 15.34 Dermatofibrosarcoma Protuberans. The classic variant is characterized by a population of monotonous spindle cells showing only rare mitotic activity (A). The cells are arranged in tight whorls (B).

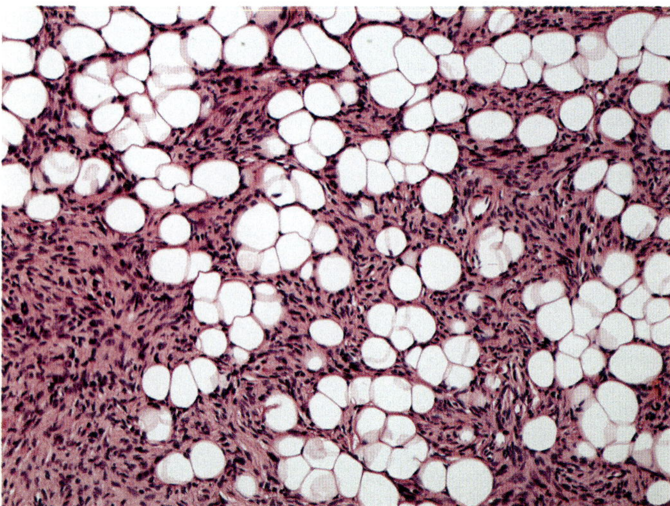

Figure 15.35 Dermatofibrosarcoma Protuberans. The tumor diffusely infiltrates subcutaneous adipose tissue, leaving behind intact adipocytes and giving rise to the characteristic honeycomb pattern.

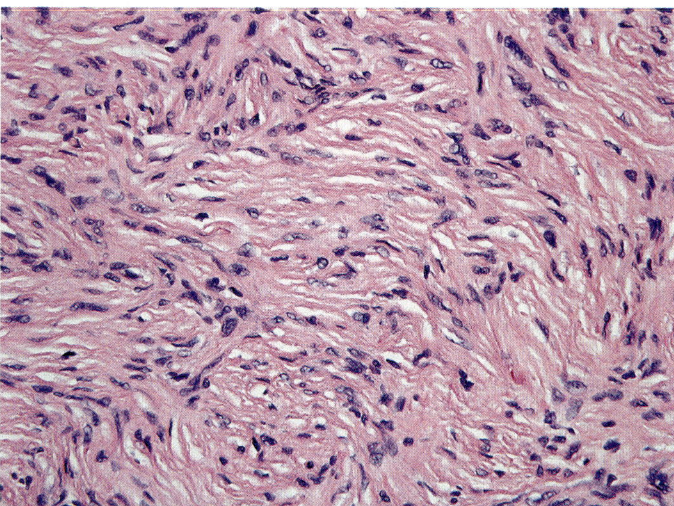

Figure 15.36 Dermatofibrosarcoma Protuberans. Some tumors show marked stromal hyalinization and have a deceptively bland appearance. Such tumors may be mistaken for soft tissue perineurioma.

The tumor is composed of a uniform population of slender spindle cells; nuclear pleomorphism is absent (Fig. 15.34A). Tumor cells are arranged in a monotonous storiform pattern, often forming tight whorls (see Fig. 15.34B). At the periphery of the tumor, spindle cells are frequently arranged singly, which mimics entrapment of preexisting collagen bundles seen in benign fibrous histiocytoma. The tumor shows a characteristic pattern of invasion of subcutaneous tissue. Tumor cells percolate through adipose tissue in narrow strands, leaving behind intact adipocytes and thereby creating a lacelike or honeycomb appearance (Fig. 15.35). Mitotic activity in DFSP is low, usually less than 5 mitoses per 10 high-power fields. Necrosis is uncommon. Some cases show marked stromal hyalinization, which can give the tumor a deceptively bland appearance (Fig. 15.36). DFSP may show a number of characteristic histologic patterns. It is important to remember that multiple morphologic patterns may be present in a single tumor and that recurrences may show different morphologic features. Furthermore, recognition of the fibrosarcomatous variant is particularly important because it is associated with adverse outcomes.

- Fibrosarcomatous DFSP is composed of spindle cells in a fascicular arrangement with a characteristic herringbone appearance, usually in a background of more classical storiform DFSP (Fig. 15.37). Tumor cells in fibrosarcomatous areas show more pronounced nuclear atypia, and mitotic activity is often high (10 to 20 mitoses per 10 high-power fields) (Fig. 15.38). Tumor necrosis may be found.[42–44] Areas of pleomorphic sarcoma may rarely be identified.[42,45,46]
- Myxoid DFSP is characterized by the presence of extensive myxoid stromal change, which may involve large parts of or even the entire tumor.[20,47,48] Although the tumor maintains the infiltrative growth of conventional DFSP, individual tumor cells appear bland and may have a predominantly stellate morphology (Fig. 15.39). They show a haphazard arrangement with loss of the typical storiform pattern. Within the tumor stroma, thin-walled vessels may be prominent (see Fig. 15.39).
- Pigmented DFSP (Bednar tumor) shows colonization of an otherwise classic DFSP by pigmented dendritic cells.[49,50]

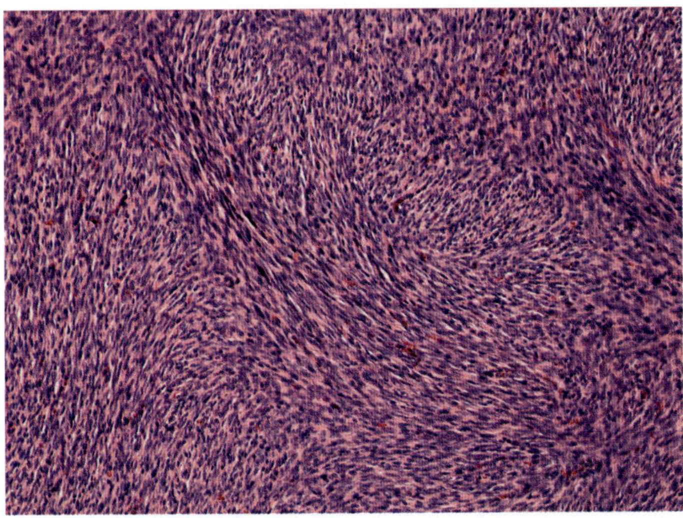

Figure 15.37 Dermatofibrosarcoma Protuberans. The fibrosarcomatous variant is highly cellular and has a fascicular arrangement reminiscent of a herringbone pattern.

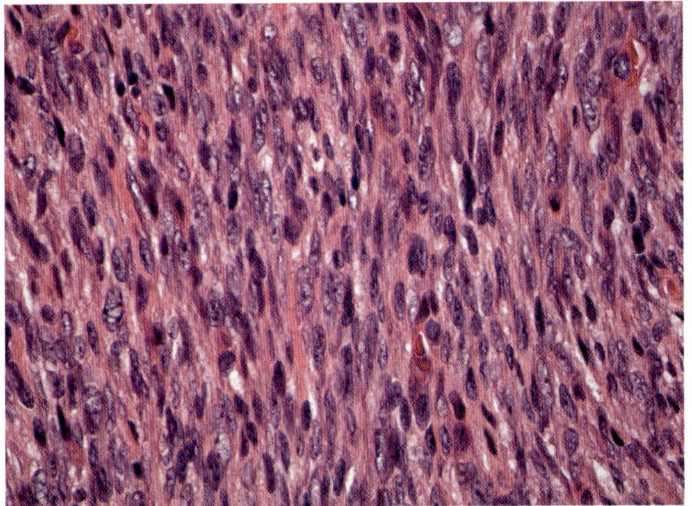

Figure 15.38 Dermatofibrosarcoma Protuberans. Tumor cells of the fibrosarcomatous variant show spindle cell morphology with more vesicular chromatin.

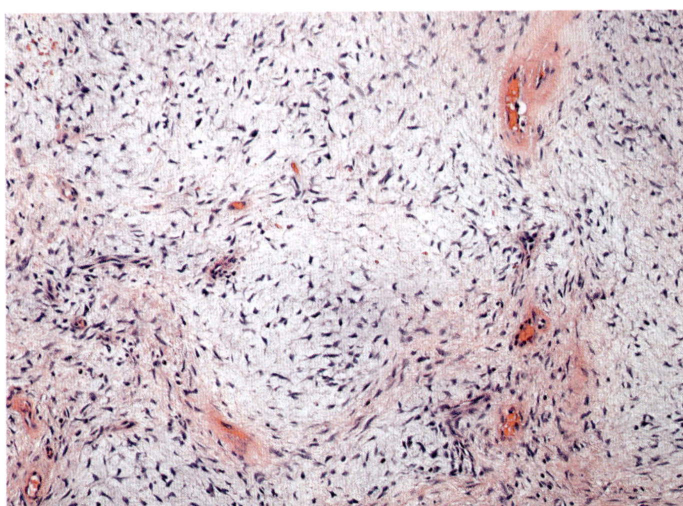

Figure 15.39 Dermatofibrosarcoma Protuberans. In the myxoid variant, stellate cells are loosely arranged within a myxoid stroma. Also note the background of prominent thin-walled vessels.

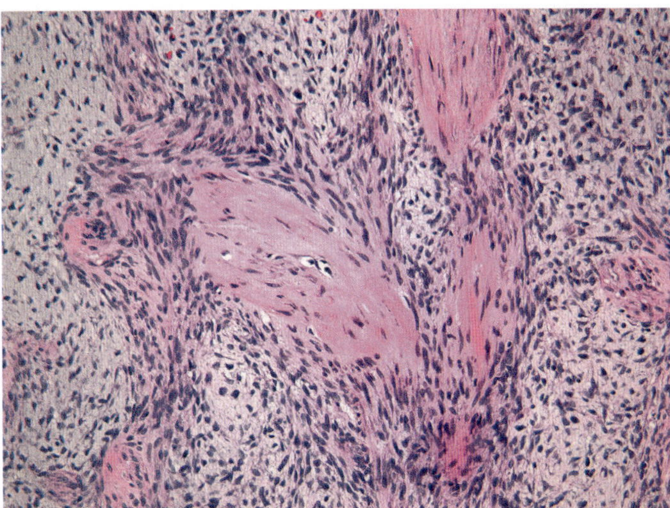

Figure 15.40 Dermatofibrosarcoma Protuberans. Myoid nodules are most often seen in the fibrosarcomatous variant. Note the association with blood vessel walls.

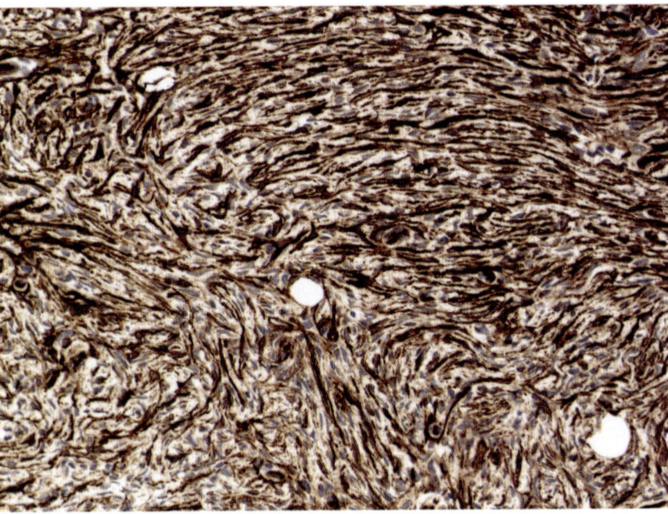

Figure 15.41 Dermatofibrosarcoma Protuberans. Tumor cells are strongly and diffusely positive for CD34.

- DFSP with myoid nodules often, but not exclusively, occurs in association with fibrosarcomatous transformation. It is characterized by the presence of nodules and bundles of eosinophilic spindle cells showing myofibroblastic differentiation, often adjacent to or involving the walls of blood vessels (Fig. 15.40).[51,52]
- Giant cell fibroblastoma and DFSP are regarded as a morphologic spectrum of the same tumor. Areas of giant cell fibroblastoma are not infrequently identified within otherwise classic DFSP.[53-56]

Granular cell change and nuclear palisading reminiscent of Verocay body formation are rarely observed.[57,58]

Immunohistochemistry

Tumor cells are strongly and diffusely positive for CD34 (Fig. 15.41).[59] CD34 expression may be weaker or even absent in areas of fibrosarcomatous change and is also absent in myoid nodules, which display SMA expression in keeping with their myofibroblastic phenotype. S-100 protein and desmin are not expressed in DFSP.

Molecular Genetics

The characteristic finding in the large majority of patients with DFSP as well as giant cell fibroblastoma is a chromosomal translocation t(17;22)(q22;q13). The translocation is most frequently present in the form of a supernumerary ring chromosome, particularly in adults, whereas a linear translocation is predominantly observed in children.[60] The t(17;22) translocation results in a fusion gene involving the collagen type 1 alpha 1 *(COL1A1)* gene on chromosome 17 and the platelet-derived growth factor β *(PDGFB)* gene on chromosome 22,[61–64] thereby placing *PDGFB* expression under the control of the *COL1A1* promoter. This finding explains susceptibility of the tumor to treatment with the receptor tyrosine kinase inhibitor imatinib mesylate.[60,65–67]

Differential Diagnosis

The main differential diagnosis is benign fibrous histiocytoma (dermatofibroma), especially the cellular variant. This becomes a particular issue on superficial samples (e.g., shave biopsies), when adequate evaluation for invasion of subcutis is not possible. However, benign fibrous histiocytoma generally lacks the monotonous appearances of DFSP and overall appears better circumscribed. CD34 immunohistochemistry solves the problem in most cases. Perineurioma may show features reminiscent of DFSP, particularly when hyalinized and in small and superficial biopsies. However, perineuriomas are usually well circumscribed and composed of slender spindle cells showing characteristic long bipolar cytoplasmic processes. The characteristic immunohistochemical finding is expression of EMA, although expression of CD34 is also often observed. Dermatomyofibroma is composed of bundles of myofibroblastic spindle cells characterized by SMA positivity and lack of CD34 expression in most cases, oriented perpendicular to the skin surface, and involvement of subcutis is not a prominent feature. Superficial DFSP is difficult to distinguish from a rare CD34-positive dermal spindle cell neoplasm that has been referred to as *medallion-like dermal dendrocyte hamartoma*[68,69] and *plaquelike CD34-positive dermal fibroma.*[70] This tumor type is composed of a bandlike proliferation of uniform fibroblastic spindle cells showing a storiform growth pattern in the dermis (Fig. 15.42). Although both DFSP and plaquelike dermal fibroma are CD34 positive, the latter is well circumscribed and does not infiltrate subcutaneous tissue. In difficult cases, detection of the *COL1A1-PDGFB* gene fusion by reverse transcriptase polymerase chain reaction (RT-PCR) or fluorescence in situ hybridization (FISH) can be used to confirm DFSP.[70]

The diagnosis of fibrosarcomatous DFSP depends on the recognition of areas of more classic DFSP. If only fibrosarcomatous areas are present on a biopsy, the differential diagnosis is broad and includes spindle cell carcinoma, spindle cell melanoma, as well as various spindle cell sarcomas (including malignant peripheral nerve sheath tumor [MPNST] and monophasic synovial sarcoma, in particular). Melanoma and carcinoma can be excluded by negativity for S-100 protein or keratins. Due to CD34 positivity, spindle cell angiosarcoma merits diagnostic consideration. The clinical presentation and absence of the specific risk factors in addition to lack of vascular channel formation make this an unlikely diagnosis. MPNST very rarely affects the dermis and subcutis (mostly in patients with neurofibromatosis type 1) and is positive for S-100 protein, glial fibrillary acidic protein (GFAP), and/or SOX10 in approximately 50% of cases. Synovial sarcoma shows focal staining for EMA and keratins, and nuclear reactivity for transducin-like enhancer of split 1 (TLE1) is observed in most cases, whereas this marker is usually negative in fibrosarcomatous DFSP. Additional tumor sampling to identify areas of conventional DFSP or FISH for *PDGFB* is helpful for a definitive diagnosis.

The prominent myxoid change in myxoid DFSP may lead to confusion with neural tumors. Myxoid neurofibroma in particular may be a challenging differential diagnosis. Clues to the correct diagnosis include the more wavy rather than stellate nuclei in neurofibroma and lack of the diffusely infiltrative growth pattern, with the exception of diffuse neurofibroma. In addition, neurofibroma is positive for S-100 protein by immunohistochemistry. Superficial angiomyxoma may show significant morphologic overlap with myxoid DFSP, especially on superficial biopsies. This includes the stellate cellular morphology, as well as the presence of prominent thin-walled vessels and CD34 expression. However, in contrast to myxoid DFSP superficial angiomyxoma is less cellular, shows a more lobulated architecture, and lacks the characteristic honeycomb infiltration of subcutaneous adipose tissue. Myxoid liposarcoma can be distinguished by the presence of univacuolated and bivacuolated lipoblasts and abundant delicate branching ("crow's feet") vessels. Low-grade myxofibrosarcoma shows a more lobular growth pattern, contains distinctive curvilinear blood vessels, and is characterized by more pronounced nuclear atypia and pleomorphism. Low-grade fibromyxoid

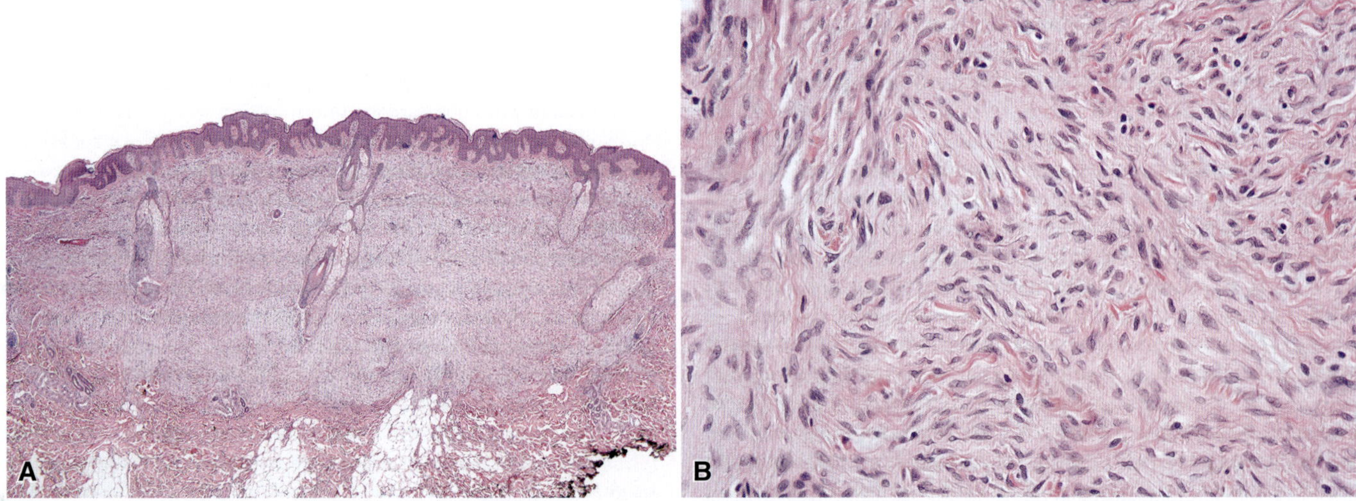

Figure 15.42 **Plaquelike Dermal Fibroma.** This rare tumor has a plaquelike growth pattern and is limited to the dermis (A). Its storiform architecture and bland spindle cell morphology (B) resemble dermatofibrosarcoma.

sarcoma may be a particularly challenging differential diagnosis. However, these tumors usually arise in deeper tissues rather than dermis. Sharply demarcated myxoid and fibrous areas and a whorled growth pattern are characteristic features. EMA is often positive in low-grade fibromyxoid sarcoma, whereas CD34 is usually negative. MUC4 is a specific marker for this tumor type.[71] MPNST may show similar histologic features but can be distinguished by immunohistochemical positivity for S-100 protein, GFAP, or SOX10 and location in deep soft tissue rather than the superficial location of DFSP.

Due to the presence of pigmented melanocytes, pigmented DFSP could be mistaken for spindle cell or desmoplastic melanoma. However, immunohistochemistry for S-100 protein reveals positive staining in the scattered dendritic cells only.

Prognosis and Treatment

Classic DFSP is characterized by a significant potential for local recurrence but does not metastasize. The reported rate of local recurrence is variable and ranges from 20% to 40%.[41,72,73] The local recurrence rate is largely influenced by adequacy of surgical excision, and wide local excision with excision margins greater than 4 cm appears to be most effective in preventing local recurrence.[74] Mohs micrographic surgery has also been proposed more recently in the treatment of DFSP and may be beneficial at anatomically sensitive sites where wide margins cannot be achieved without significant morbidity or loss of function. Published data appear promising, especially when combined with evaluation of margins on paraffin-embedded sections (modified Mohs micrographic surgery).[75–79] Treatment with imatinib mesylate can result in partial or complete tumor regression, which is helpful in anatomic sites where surgical excision with negative margins is difficult.[66,67,80]

Although the clinical behavior of variants such as myxoid and pigmented DFSP are comparable to conventional DFSP, the presence of fibrosarcomatous change is associated with an adverse prognosis. Fibrosarcomatous DFSP is associated with a higher risk of local recurrence (up to 60%), as well as a small risk of distant metastasis (10% to 15%) and death from disease.[42,44]

PRACTICE POINTS: Dermatofibrosarcoma Protuberans

- Locally aggressive and destructive tumor with a specific translocation t(17;22)
- Tumor extent is often much greater than clinically appreciable
- Treatment of choice is wide local excision
- Distinctive morphologic variants are recognized
- Different morphologic patterns can occur in a single tumor
- Recurrences may show different morphologic features
- Giant cell fibroblastoma is a closely related tumor that shares the same immunohistochemical features and translocation as DFSP
- Although conventional DFSP does not metastasize, the fibrosarcomatous variant is associated with a 10% to 15% risk of distant metastasis

Giant Cell Fibroblastoma

Giant cell fibroblastoma is a rare tumor that predominantly affects children younger than 10 years of age, with a male predominance of 2:1.[81–83] However, the tumor affects people of all ages, and presentation in adults may occasionally be observed. The tumor presents as a slow-growing painless mass often measuring several centimeters. The anatomic distribution is wide, but there is a predilection for the trunk and extremities.[81,82] The clinical course is characterized by a high rate of local recurrence of up to 50%, although no distant metastases have been reported to date.[83,84] Similar to DFSP, treatment is therefore surgical, with wide local excision or Mohs micrographic surgery at anatomically sensitive sites.

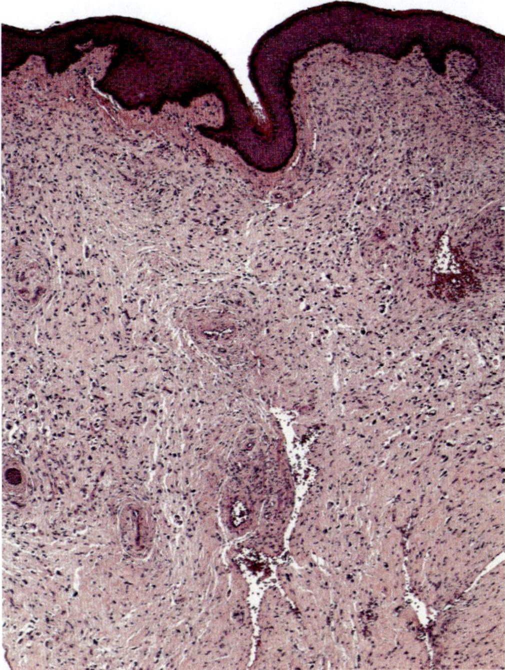

Figure 15.43 Giant Cell Fibroblastoma. This dermal-based tumor shows prominent myxoid stromal change.

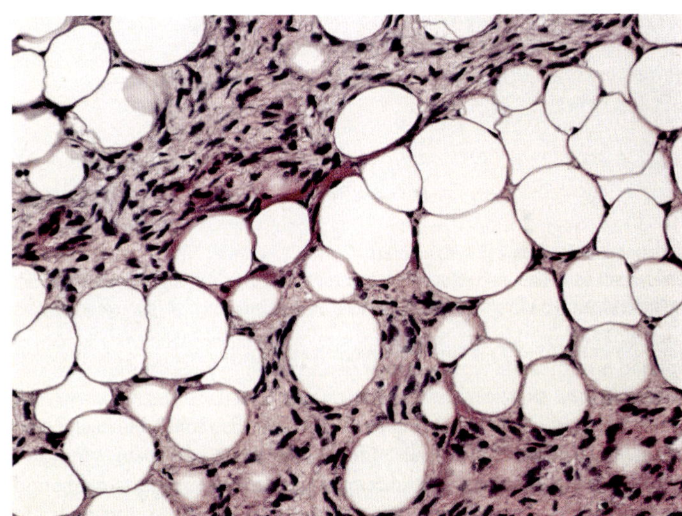

Figure 15.44 Giant Cell Fibroblastoma. The pattern of invasion into subcutaneous adipose tissue is similar to that seen in dermatofibrosarcoma protuberans.

Histologically, giant cell fibroblastoma is a poorly marginated tumor based within the dermis (Fig. 15.43) and extending into subcutis, often giving rise to a honeycomb appearance (Fig. 15.44). The tumor is composed of mildly pleomorphic, hyperchromatic spindle cells within a variably myxoid stromal background (Fig. 15.45). Cellularity is variable, with hypercellular to hypocellular areas showing stromal hyalinization. The characteristic feature is the presence of large, irregularly shaped pseudovascular spaces lined by multinucleated giant cells (Fig. 15.46). Mitotic activity is low, and necrosis is uncommon.

By immunohistochemistry, tumor cells express CD34 but are negative for other endothelial markers or S-100 protein.

Analogous to DFSP, there is a recurrent translocation t(17;22)(q22;q13) involving the *PDGFB* and *COL1A1* genes.

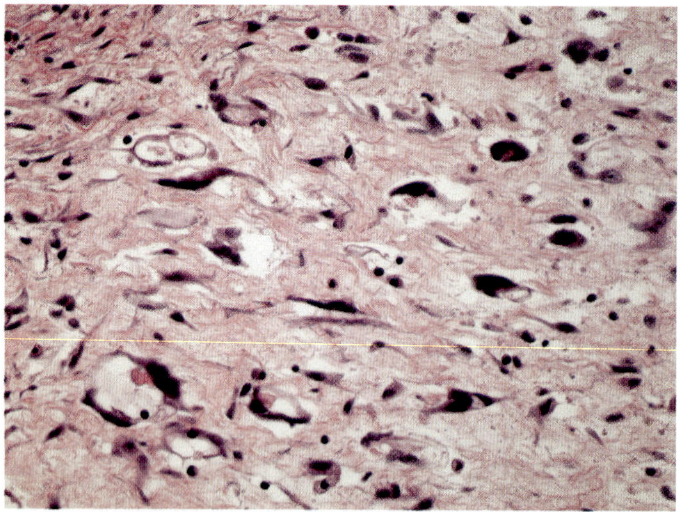

Figure 15.45 Giant Cell Fibroblastoma. Tumor cells are characterized by nuclear pleomorphism and hyperchromasia. Also note the myxoid stromal background.

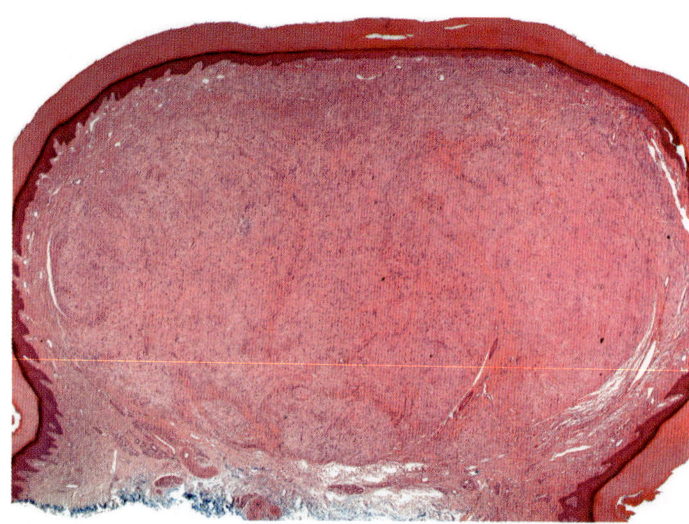

Figure 15.47 Perineurioma. This nodular tumor is well circumscribed.

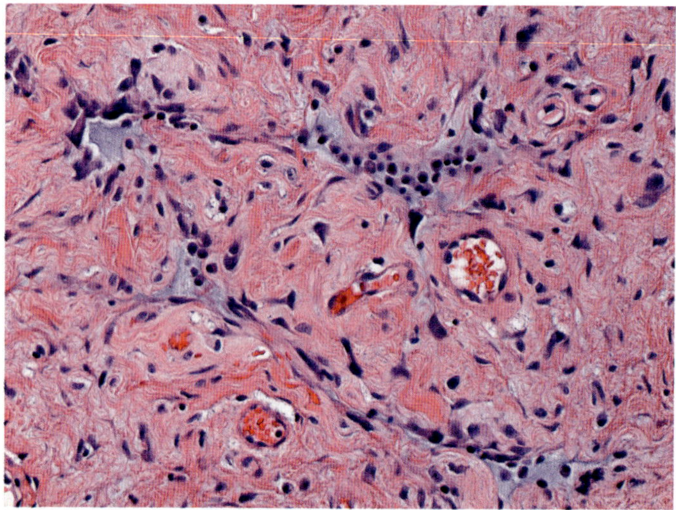

Figure 15.46 Giant Cell Fibroblastoma. A characteristic feature is the presence of irregularly shaped pseudovascular channels lined by tumor cells.

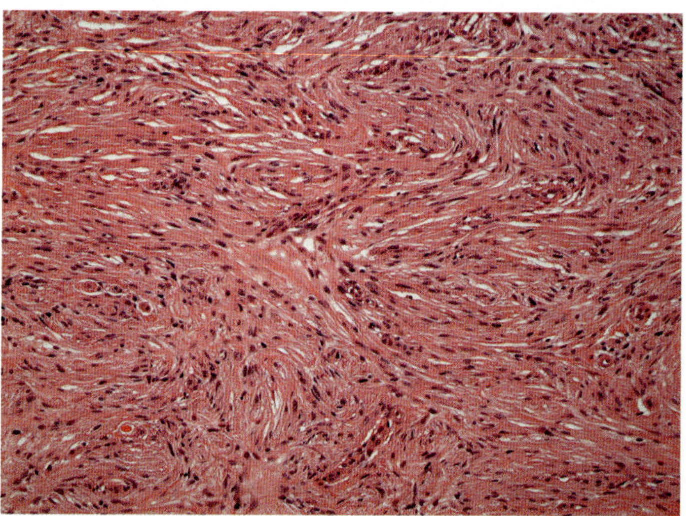

Figure 15.48 Perineurioma. A storiform to whorled growth pattern is typical.

Perineurioma

Soft tissue perineurioma is an uncommon benign peripheral nerve sheath tumor composed of perineurial cells.[85] Approximately 10% to 20% of soft tissue perineuriomas arise primarily in the dermis.[85-88] Soft tissue perineurioma is discussed in detail in Chapter 3.

Clinical Features

Cutaneous perineurioma usually presents as a painless nodule. There is no gender predilection, and patients over a wide age range may be affected, with a peak in middle-aged adults.[85] Lower limbs are most commonly involved, followed by the upper limbs and trunk. Most tumors are between 0.5 and 1.5 cm in diameter.

Pathologic Features

Perineuriomas are well-circumscribed but unencapsulated tumors and may extend to the epidermis (Fig. 15.47). The tumors are composed of bland ovoid to spindled cells with slender nuclei arranged in a storiform to whorled architecture (Fig. 15.48).[85,86] The tumor cells contain elongated cytoplasmic processes (Fig. 15.49A). The stroma may be collagenous or myxoid. Mitotic activity is low, and necrosis is absent.

Immunohistochemistry

Perineuriomas are characteristically positive for EMA (see Fig. 15.49B), although staining may be focal and weak.[85] CD34 is also positive in most cases[85,88] and may be more extensive than EMA. Both EMA and CD34 often highlight the delicate cytoplasmic processes. A subset of cases shows reactivity for the tight junction–associated protein claudin-1.[85] SMA may be focally positive in occasional cases. S-100 protein, GFAP, and desmin are consistently negative.

Differential Diagnosis

The main differential diagnostic consideration for perineurioma is DFSP, especially in superficial shave biopsies. Although both tumor types show a storiform architecture and express CD34, perineuriomas are well circumscribed and are positive for EMA.

Prognosis and Treatment

Cutaneous perineuriomas are benign and do not recur.

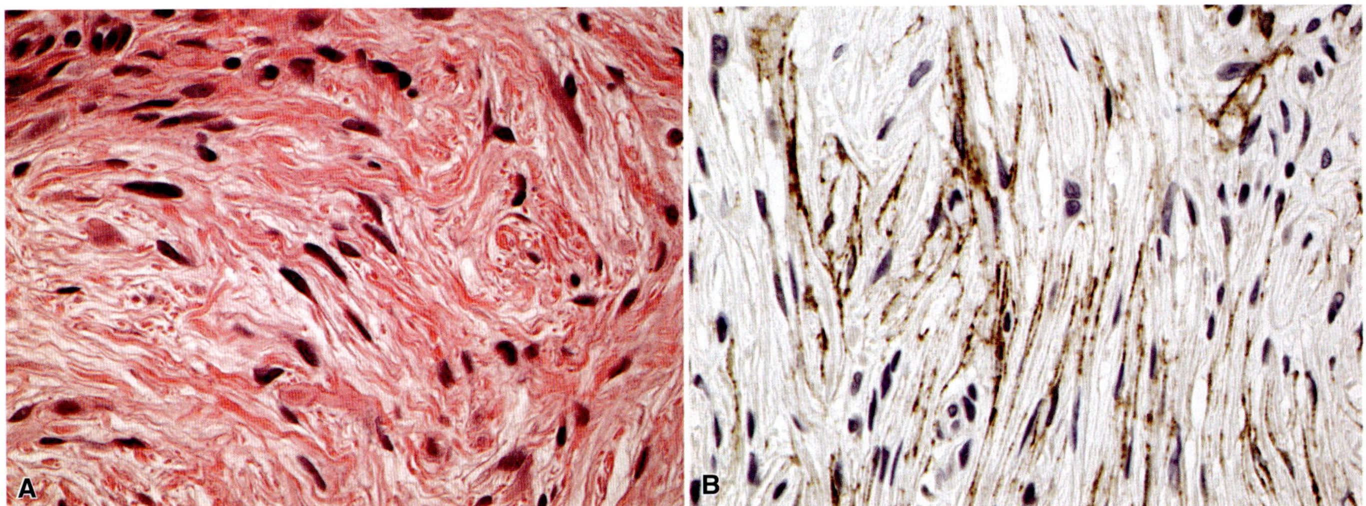

Figure 15.49 **Perineurioma.** The slender tumor cells contain elongated cytoplasmic processes (A), which are positive for epithelial membrane antigen (B).

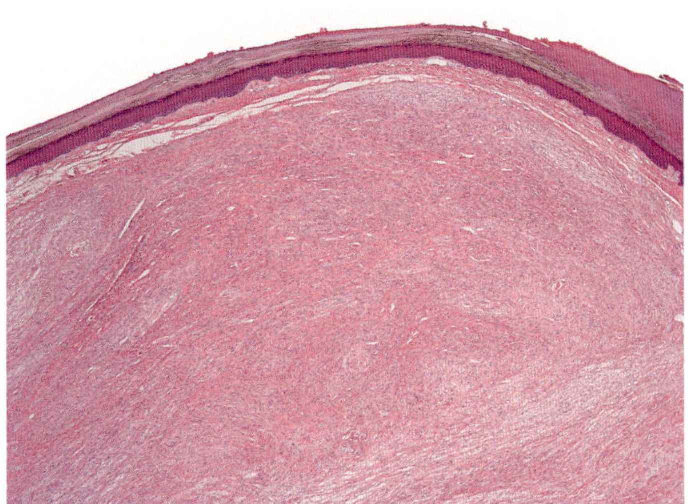

Figure 15.50 **Hybrid Schwannoma/Perineurioma.** This well-circumscribed tumor involves the dermis and has a whorled growth pattern.

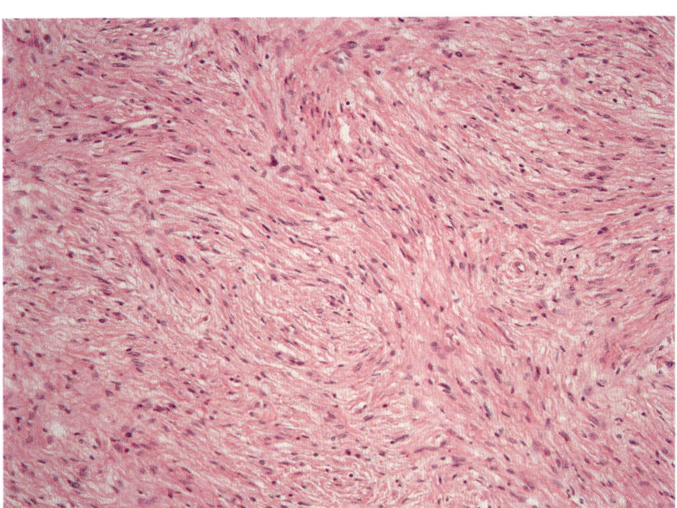

Figure 15.51 **Hybrid Schwannoma/Perineurioma.** The tumor shows a storiform and whorled architecture.

Hybrid Schwannoma/Perineurioma

In recent years, benign nerve sheath tumors composed of an intimate admixture of Schwann cells and perineurial cells have been recognized.[89,90] Most hybrid schwannoma/perineuriomas involve superficial soft tissues.[89] These tumors are not associated with neurofibromatosis type 1.

Clinical Features

Hybrid schwannoma/perineurioma affects patients in a wide age range, with a peak in young to middle-aged adults, and has an equal gender distribution. Patients present with a painless nodule or mass. The tumors occur over a wide anatomic distribution.[89] Most tumors are between 1 and 5 cm in size.

Pathologic Features

Histologically, hybrid schwannoma/perineurioma is well circumscribed but unencapsulated (Fig. 15.50). The tumor is composed of plump spindle cells with tapering nuclei and palely eosinophilic cytoplasm, in a storiform, whorled, and lamellar architecture (Fig. 15.51).[89] Under high magnification, a subset of cells with more slender nuclei and delicate cytoplasmic processes can be appreciated (Fig. 15.52). The tumor may show degenerative nuclear atypia, similar to ancient schwannoma.[89] Mitotic activity is scarce.

Immunohistochemistry

S-100 protein is positive in the Schwann cells (Fig. 15.53A), which usually constitute 60% to 70% of cells in hybrid schwannoma/perineuriomas, whereas EMA and CD34 are positive in perineurial cells (see Fig. 15.53B).[89] Most tumors also express GFAP and claudin-1.

Differential Diagnosis

The differential diagnosis includes other benign nerve sheath tumors and low-grade MPNST. Schwannomas typically show alternating hypercellular and hypocellular areas with perivascular hyalinization, and they are diffusely positive for S-100 protein. Schwannomas are encapsulated; the perineurial capsule is positive for EMA, but EMA is negative within the tumor, in contrast to hybrid schwannoma/perineurioma. Neurofibromas lack the storiform to whorled growth pattern of hybrid schwannoma/perineurioma and are less uniformly cellular. Both tumor types show extensive staining for S-100 protein, but neurofibromas are generally negative for EMA or at most show focal staining and contain scattered neurofilament protein–positive axons. Soft tissue perineurioma is the closest histologic mimic, showing similar architectural features, but is composed of a pure population of EMA-positive perineurial cells and lacks the plumper S-100 protein–positive Schwann cells. MPNST often shows varying cellularity with accentuation around blood vessels, nuclear atypia, and mitotic activity. MPNST rarely shows strong, diffuse staining for S-100 protein, and EMA is usually negative.

Prognosis and Treatment

Hybrid schwannoma/perineurioma is benign and only rarely recurs locally. It does not metastasize.

Dendritic Cell Neurofibroma

In 2001 Michal and colleagues reported 18 distinctive benign cutaneous nerve sheath tumors as dendritic cell neurofibroma with pseudorosettes.[91] Very few cases have been reported subsequently, most by the same authors.[92,93] The relationship with conventional neurofibroma is uncertain.[94] Although most cases arise in the sporadic setting, one reported case has occurred in a patient with presumed type 1 neurofibromatosis.[95]

Clinical Features

Dendritic cell neurofibroma affects adults with a wide age range and anatomic distribution, and it has no gender predilection.[91] Patients present with a painless, dome-shaped cutaneous nodule. Most lesions are between 0.5 and 1 cm in size.

Pathologic Features

Dendritic cell neurofibroma is usually situated in the superficial dermis, is well circumscribed, and has a multinodular, plexiform growth pattern, particularly in the deeper aspects of the lesion (Fig. 15.54). The tumor is dominated by small round hyperchromatic cells with irregular nuclei

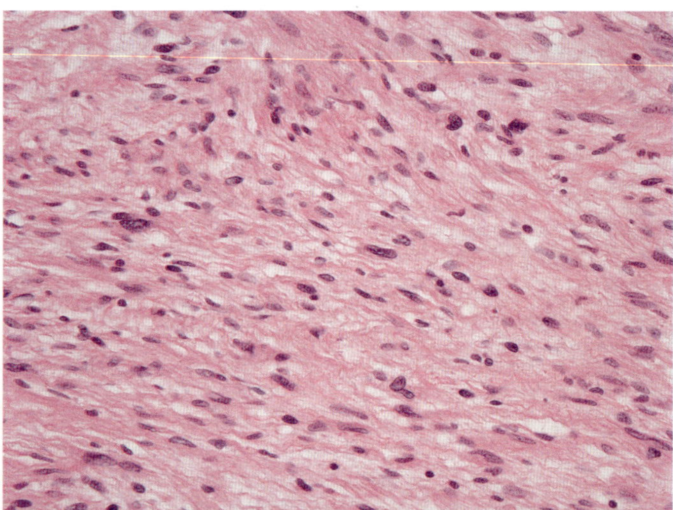

Figure 15.52 Hybrid Schwannoma/Perineurioma. The tumor is composed of an admixture of plump spindle cells with tapering nuclei and smaller cells with slender nuclei and delicate cytoplasmic processes. Note the focal nuclear atypia.

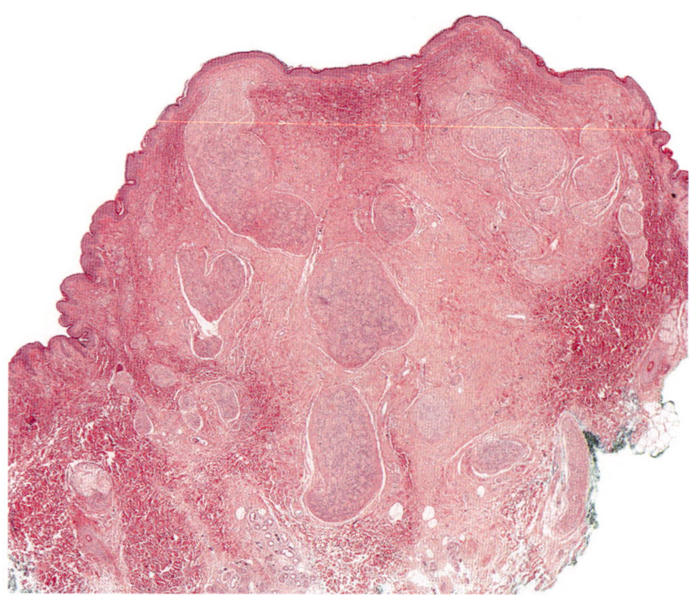

Figure 15.54 Dendritic Cell Neurofibroma. This dermal tumor shows a multinodular architecture.

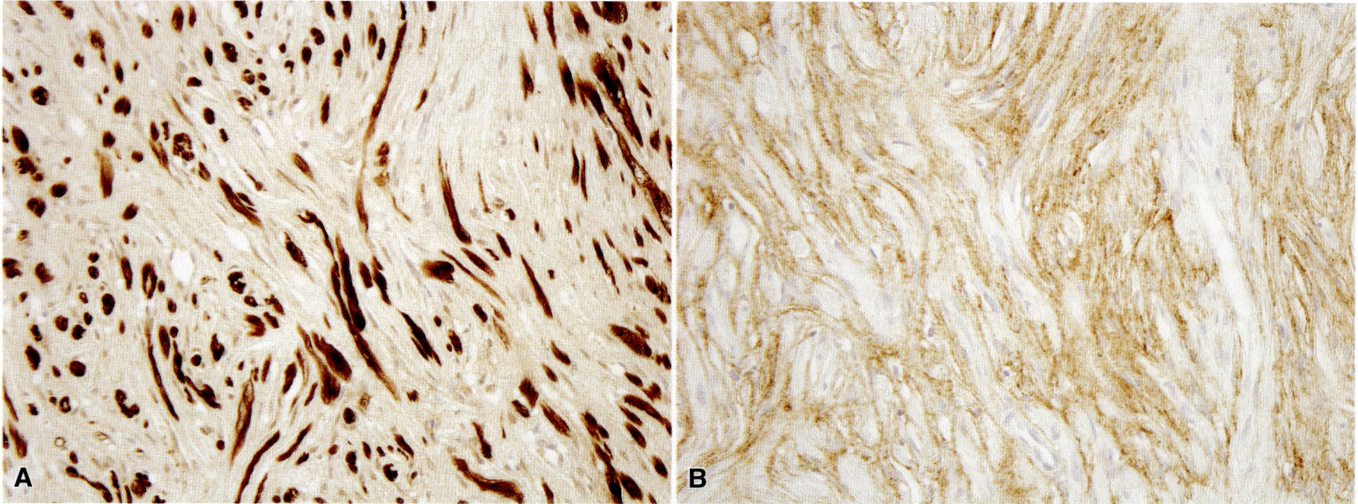

Figure 15.53 Hybrid Schwannoma/Perineurioma. Immunohistochemistry shows an admixture of S-100 protein–positive Schwann cells (A) and epithelial membrane antigen–positive perineurial cells (B).

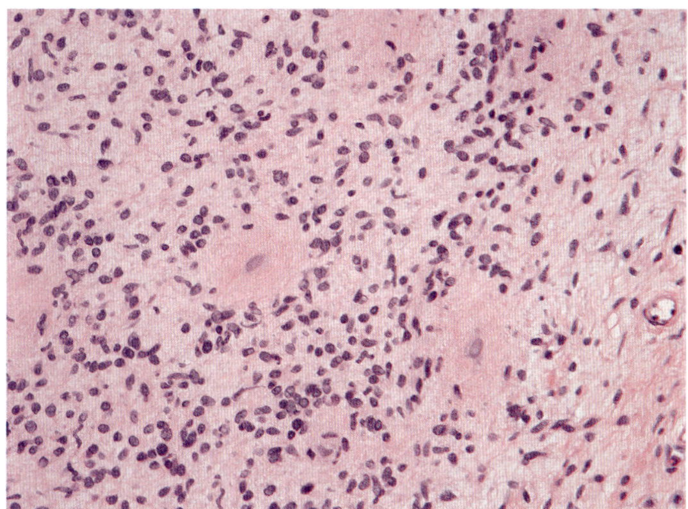

Figure 15.55 Dendritic Cell Neurofibroma. Small round to short spindled cells are arranged around larger cells with vesicular nuclei and abundant pale cytoplasm.

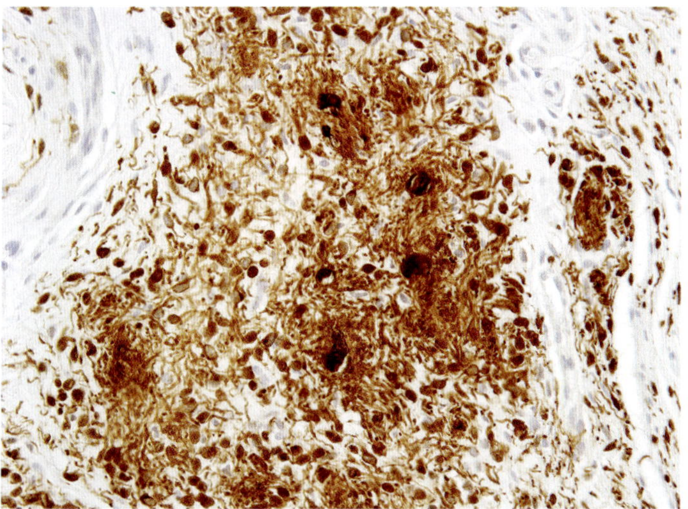

Figure 15.56 Dendritic Cell Neurofibroma. S-100 protein is positive in both cell types and highlights dendritic cell processes in the larger cells.

and inconspicuous cytoplasm, resembling lymphocytes. There is a minor second population of larger cells with vesicular nuclei, inconspicuous nucleoli, and abundant pale eosinophilic cytoplasm, around which the small cells are concentrically arranged in pseudorosettes (Fig. 15.55). No nuclear atypia or mitotic activity is evident.

Immunohistochemistry

Both cell types are diffusely positive for S-100 protein, more intensively staining the larger cells. S-100 protein highlights characteristic dendritic cell processes in the large cells (Fig. 15.56).[91] EMA occasionally stains a partial perineurial capsule. The tumor cells are negative for GFAP, HMB-45, chromogranin, synaptophysin, SMA, desmin, and keratin.[91]

Differential Diagnosis

After the distinctive histologic features of dendritic cell neurofibroma are recognized, there is no realistic differential diagnosis.

Prognosis and Treatment

Dendritic cell neurofibroma is entirely benign. It does not recur.

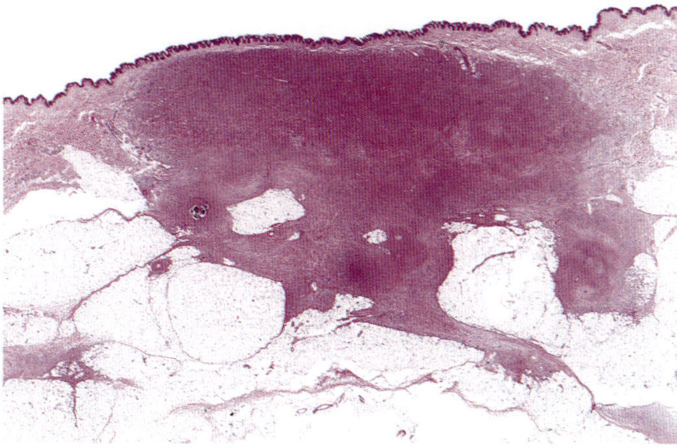

Figure 15.57 Pseudomyogenic Hemangioendothelioma. The tumor has infiltrative margins through the dermis. Note the overlying epidermal hyperplasia.

Pseudomyogenic Hemangioendothelioma

Originally reported as the fibroma-like variant of epithelioid sarcoma,[96] pseudomyogenic hemangioendothelioma is a distinctive endothelial neoplasm of intermediate biologic potential that often presents as multiple discontiguous lesions in different tissue planes of a limb and histologically mimics a myoid tumor.[97] Most patients (75%) present with cutaneous nodules.[97] This tumor type has also been referred to as *epithelioid sarcoma-like hemangioendothelioma*.[98] Pseudomyogenic hemangioendothelioma is also discussed in Chapter 3.

Clinical Features

Patients with pseudomyogenic hemangioendothelioma present with a single nodule or multiple cutaneous nodules, which may be painless or painful. Approximately 50% of affected patients also have intramuscular lesions, and 20% have lesions in bone.[97] The limbs and limb girdles are most often involved (especially lower extremities). There is a striking male predominance, nearly 5:1. The peak incidence occurs in the second and third decades of life; this tumor type is rare in adults older than 50 years.[97] Most tumors range from 1 to 2 cm in size.

Pathologic Features

Pseudomyogenic hemangioendothelioma shows infiltrative margins. Overlying epidermal hyperplasia is common in tumors involving the dermis (Fig. 15.57), and ulceration may be present. The tumor is composed of sheets and loose fascicles of relatively uniform, plump spindle cells with vesicular nuclei, usually small nucleoli, and abundant brightly eosinophilic cytoplasm, which may mimic rhabdomyoblasts (Fig. 15.58).[97] A subset of tumors contains a prominent neutrophilic inflammatory infiltrate. Extensive infiltration of the subcutaneous adipose tissue may be seen (Fig. 15.59). Mitotic activity is usually low, and nuclear atypia is generally mild.

Immunohistochemistry

Tumors are diffusely positive for keratin AE1/AE3 and show extensive nuclear staining for FLI1 and ERG (Fig. 15.60).[97] Nearly all tumors show nuclear expression of FOSB (see Fig. 15.60C), reflecting the presence of *FOSB* gene fusions (see later).[99] Approximately 50% of tumors are positive for CD31. EMA and keratin MNF116 are usually negative. Although SMA may be focally positive, desmin is not expressed. CD34 and S-100 protein are consistently negative. All tumors show intact expression of SMARCB1 (INI1).[97]

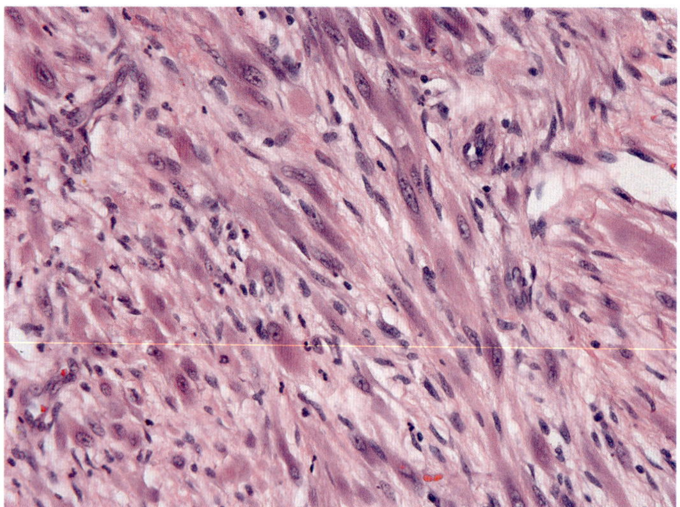

Figure 15.58 Pseudomyogenic Hemangioendothelioma. The tumor is composed of loose fascicles of plump spindle cells with abundant brightly eosinophilic cytoplasm. Note the stromal neutrophils.

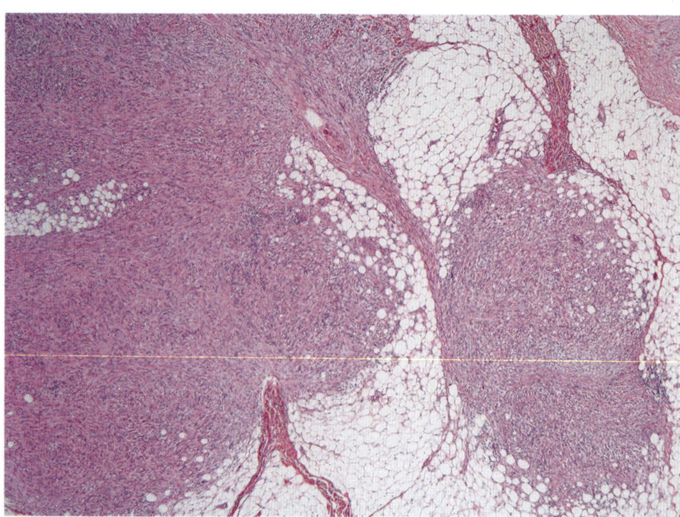

Figure 15.59 Pseudomyogenic Hemangioendothelioma. The tumor often infiltrates subcutaneous adipose tissue.

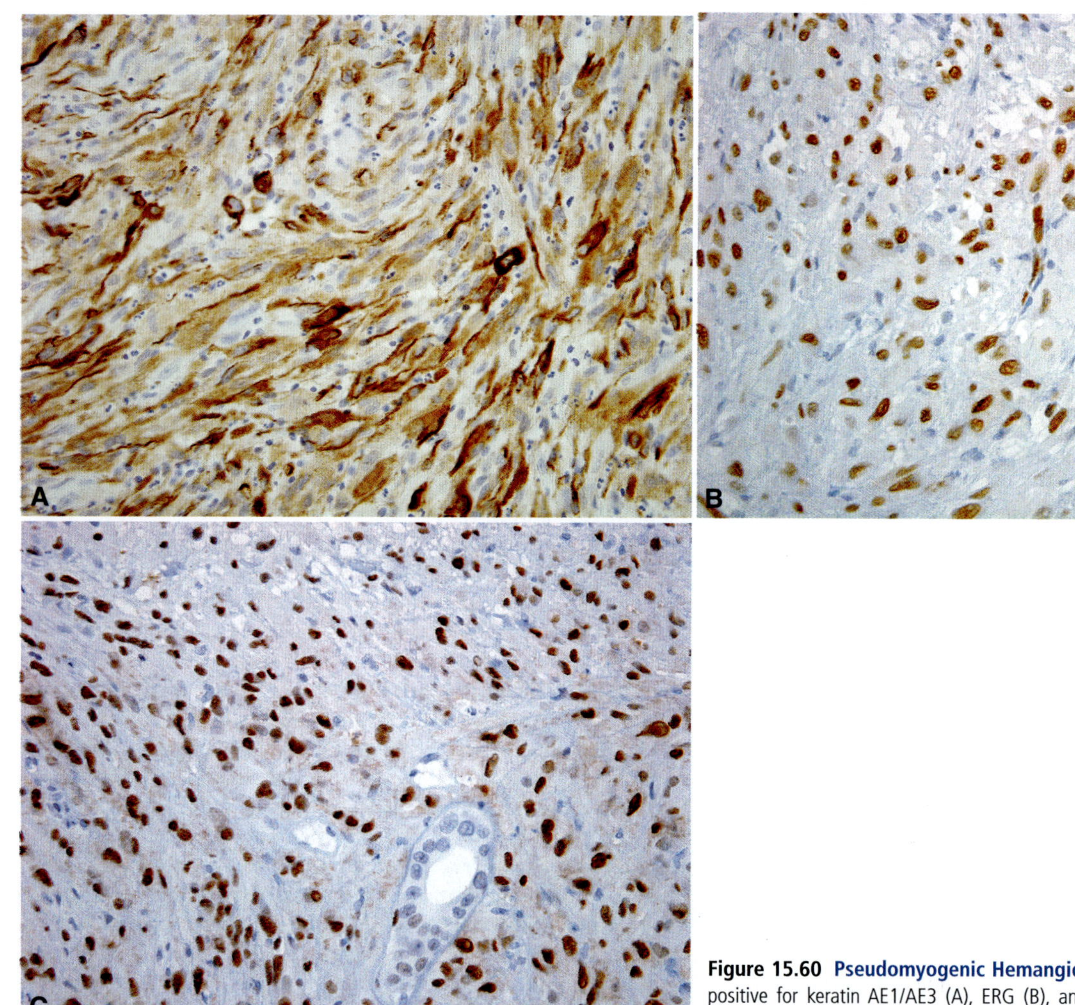

Figure 15.60 Pseudomyogenic Hemangioendothelioma. The tumor cells are positive for keratin AE1/AE3 (A), ERG (B), and FOSB (C), the latter reflecting the presence of *FOSB* gene rearrangement.

Molecular Genetics

A t(7;19)(q22;q13) translocation, resulting in a *SERPINE1-FOSB* fusion gene, has recently been identified as a recurrent alteration in pseudomyogenic hemangioendothelioma; some tumors harbor *FOSB* rearrangements without *SERPINE1* involvement.[99,100]

Differential Diagnosis

The differential diagnosis for pseudomyogenic hemangioendothelioma includes spindle cell squamous cell carcinoma, cellular benign fibrous histiocytoma, epithelioid sarcoma, and myofibroblastic or smooth muscle tumors. Spindle cell squamous cell carcinoma arises in sun-damaged skin of older adults. In contrast to pseudomyogenic hemangioendothelioma, spindle cell squamous cell carcinoma is often positive for keratin MNF116, and ERG, FOSB, and CD31 are negative. Although both pseudomyogenic hemangioendothelioma and cellular benign fibrous histiocytoma are often associated with epidermal hyperplasia, fibrous histiocytomas do not contain plump cells with brightly eosinophilic cytoplasm and are negative for keratins. Epithelioid sarcoma shows a nodular growth pattern and is composed of small epithelioid cells, in contrast to the sheetlike architecture and plump spindle cell morphology of pseudomyogenic hemangioendothelioma. Unlike pseudomyogenic hemangioendothelioma, epithelioid sarcoma is usually positive for EMA, consistently shows loss of SMARCB1 (INI1) expression, and 50% of tumors express CD34.[101,102] Smooth muscle and myofibroblastic tumors can be excluded by negative staining for desmin and at most focal staining for SMA.

Prognosis and Treatment

More than 50% of patients with pseudomyogenic hemangioendothelioma experience local recurrences or develop additional cutaneous nodules in the same anatomic region.[97] Despite the ominous multifocal clinical presentation, distant metastases are rare. Conservative surgery (when feasible) seems to be the best therapeutic approach.

PRACTICE POINTS: Pseudomyogenic Hemangioendothelioma

- Originally reported as "fibroma-like" variant of epithelioid sarcoma
- Marked predilection for the limbs of young men
- Distinctive clinical presentation with multiple discontiguous cutaneous nodules
- May also present with separate nodules in muscle and bone
- Histologically mimics a myoid tumor
- Positive for keratin AE1/AE3, ERG, FOSB, 50% for CD31; negative for keratin MNF116 and CD34
- Intact expression of SMARCB1 (INI1) (unlike epithelioid sarcoma)
- Local recurrences or development of new nodules in same anatomic region common
- Despite ominous presentation, distant metastases are rare

Myxoid Tumors

Superficial Acral Fibromyxoma

Clinical Features

Superficial acral fibromyxoma, which has also been referred to as *digital fibromyxoma,* is a recently described entity showing a strong predilection for the fingers and toes.[103–105] Occasionally, other acral sites such as the palm and heel may also be affected, and tumors rarely arise at nonacral sites. The vast majority of cases arise in proximity to the nail bed.[103–105] The typical presentation is of a solitary and frequently exophytic nodule averaging 2 cm in diameter. Although this lesion affects individuals of varying ages, it is typically a tumor of adults, with presentation around the fifth decade, and a male predominance.[103,104] A similar tumor reported as cellular digital fibroma may represent part of the spectrum of superficial acral fibromyxoma.[106]

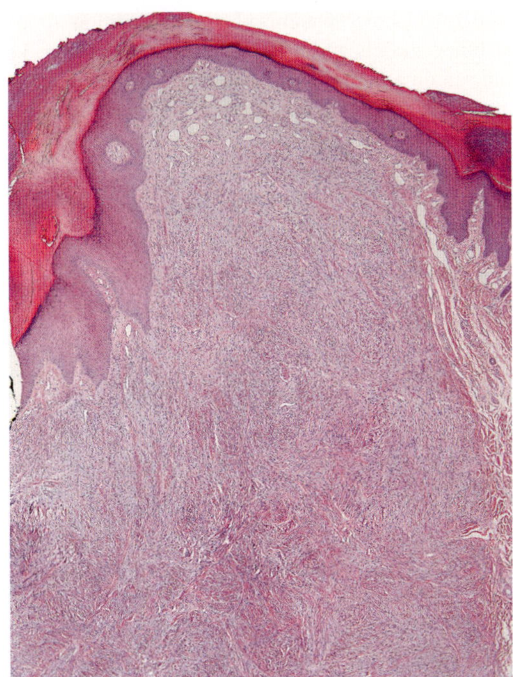

Figure 15.61 Superficial Acral Fibromyxoma. This dermal tumor arises near the nail bed and often extends to the overlying epidermis.

Pathologic Features

Superficial acral fibromyxoma is a dermal-based, well-circumscribed tumor that may extend to the epidermis (Fig. 15.61). Subcutaneous involvement may be observed, but extension into deeper tissue such as fascia or bone is rare. The tumor is composed of bland stellate or spindle cells arranged in loose fascicles or a more storiform pattern within a myxoid to collagenous stroma (Fig. 15.62). Mitotic activity is low or absent. Occasionally, there is verrucous hyperplasia of the overlying epidermis.

Immunohistochemistry

Tumor cells often express CD34. In addition, EMA and SMA are focally positive in a small subset of cases. Most tumors show loss of nuclear staining for RB1.[107] Immunohistochemistry for S-100 protein and desmin is negative.

Differential Diagnosis

Cutaneous tumors with prominent myxoid stroma are summarized in Table 15.4. Superficial acral fibromyxoma closely resembles myxoid neurofibroma, which is easily excluded by lack of S-100 protein expression. Superficial angiomyxoma shows a predilection for the head and neck and trunk rather than acral sites, shows a lobulated, infiltrative growth pattern with more prominent blood vessels, and often contains stromal neutrophils. Digital mucous cysts lack the deep extension of superficial acral fibromyxoma and are markedly less cellular. Perineurioma must be considered, especially in view of significant immunohistochemical overlap with CD34 and EMA expression. Superficial acral fibromyxoma lacks the whorled growth pattern and bipolar cytoplasmic processes characteristic of perineurioma. Myxoid DFSP is an important consideration, because both tumors express CD34. The distinction may be particularly difficult on superficial biopsies. Superficial acral fibromyxoma is better circumscribed and lacks the honeycomb pattern of subcutaneous adipose tissue infiltration. Furthermore, DFSP only rarely occurs on acral sites and shows the characteristic t(17;22) translocation.

Myxofibrosarcoma shows pleomorphism in addition to prominent curvilinear blood vessels and a lobulated growth pattern. Low-grade fibromyxoid sarcoma is usually deep seated and shows a predilection for more proximal aspects of the limbs. Expression of MUC4 and the t(7;16) translocation involving *FUS* are typical findings.

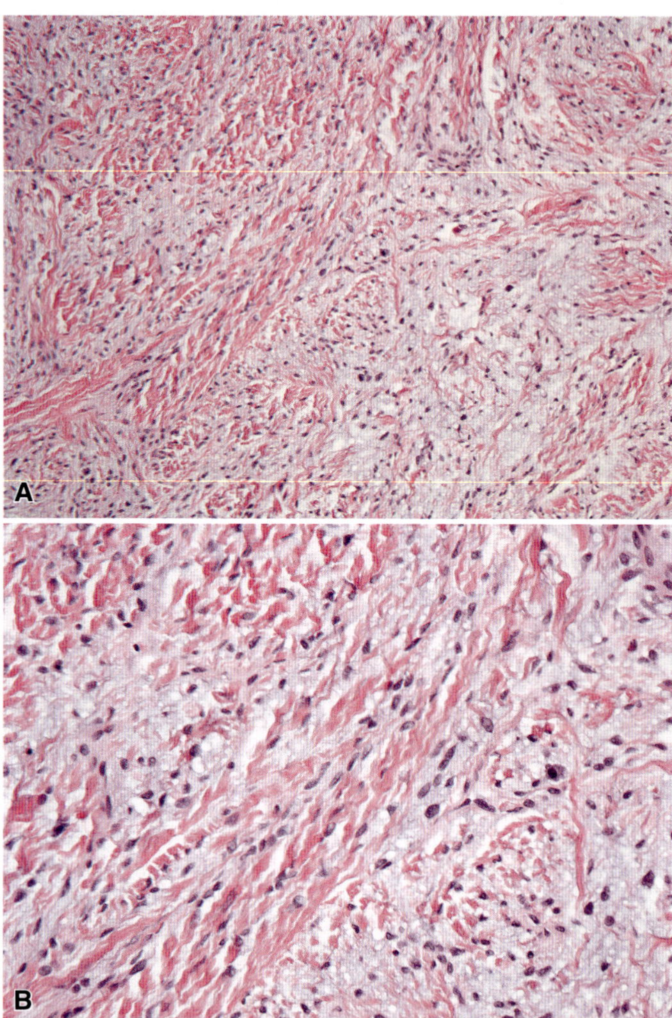

Figure 15.62 Superficial Acral Fibromyxoma. The tumor has a loose fascicular architecture (A) and is composed of bland spindle cells in a collagenous to myxoid stroma (B).

Prognosis and Treatment

Superficial acral fibromyxoma is benign, with a local recurrence rate of approximately 20%. Distant metastases do not occur.

Superficial Angiomyxoma

Clinical Features

Superficial angiomyxoma is usually sporadic but may be associated with the Carney complex. Sporadic tumors present as solitary papules or nodules sometimes showing polypoid growth that measure 2 to 3 cm.[108] They show a predilection for the head and neck area as well as the trunk, and they may also involve genital sites.[108,109] Involvement of the extremities is less frequent. The tumor affects individuals over a wide age range, including children, and congenital presentation has also been documented.[108] The median age at presentation is 45 years, and there is a male predominance.[108] The "cutaneous myxoma" described in Carney complex represents superficial angiomyxoma.[108] Superficial angiomyxomas in Carney complex are often multiple and show a predilection for the eyelids, ear, and nipple.[110] Carney complex is an autosomal dominant disorder also characterized by myxomas of the heart; multiple facial lentigines with a predilection for the lips and conjunctiva; epithelioid blue nevi; endocrine abnormalities, including primary pigmented nodular adrenocortical disease; pituitary adenoma; large cell calcifying Sertoli cell tumor; and psammomatous melanotic schwannoma.[111-113] Recognition of the cutaneous markers of this syndrome is important to allow early detection of cardiac myxomas, which are associated with a high mortality rate if undetected. Superficial angiomyxoma is also discussed in Chapter 5.

Pathologic Features

Superficial angiomyxoma is a poorly delineated tumor located within the reticular dermis, frequently extending into the subcutis. The tumor has a lobulated or multinodular growth pattern, often infiltrating surrounding tissues (Fig. 15.63). It is characterized by abundant myxoid stroma that contains spindled to stellate fibroblast-like cells with varying cellularity (Fig. 15.64). Cytologic atypia is absent, and mitotic activity is low. In addition, there is a background of small, thin-walled blood vessels with a focally arborizing pattern (Fig. 15.65). Scattered stromal neutrophils may be seen in approximately 50% of cases, which is a helpful clue to the diagnosis. An additional and occasionally prominent finding is the presence of an epithelial proliferation, which is frequently related to entrapped skin adnexal structures such as hair follicular units (Fig. 15.66). These epithelial structures encompass a spectrum ranging from epithelial strands to basaloid buds and cysts.

Table 15.4 Cutaneous Tumors With Prominent Myxoid Stroma

	Clinical Features	Histology	Immunohistochemistry
Superficial angiomyxoma	Adults Wide anatomic distribution Papule or nodule (few cm) Association with Carney complex when multiple	Lobulated tumor Dermis and subcutis Infiltrative growth Abundant myxoid stroma Uniform stellate and spindle cells No cytologic atypia Intralesional neutrophils Epithelial proliferation related to hair follicle	CD34 ± SMA – Desmin – S-100 –
Superficial acral fibromyxoma	Adults Fingers and toes, near nail bed Nodule (few cm)	Well-demarcated tumor Dermal-based tumor Frequent involvement of subcutis Uniform stellate to spindle cells in loose fascicles Myxoid to collagenous stroma No cytologic atypia	CD34 + EMA ± SMA – Desmin – S-100 –

Table 15.4 Cutaneous Tumors With Prominent Myxoid Stroma—cont'd

	Clinical Features	Histology	Immunohistochemistry
Cellular neurothekeoma	Young adults Head and neck, upper trunk and shoulder Papule or nodule (1 cm)	Poorly demarcated Dermal-based lesions Possible subcutaneous involvement Micronodular Nests and short fascicles Epithelioid cells with abundant cytoplasm Scattered cytologic atypia Mitotic activity Varying amounts of myxoid change	NKI-C3 + NSE + SMA ± S-100 –
Myoepithelioma	Adults Wide anatomic distribution Nodule (few cm)	Dermal-based tumor Lobulated or sheetlike growth Variable cytology: uniform ovoid spindle cells with indistinct cell borders; epithelioid cells with stromal sclerosis; plasmacytoid cells; spindle cells in myxoid stroma No significant cytologic atypia Occasional mitoses	S-100 + GFAP + EMA + Keratin ± SMA + Calponin + Desmin – p63 ±
Dermal nerve sheath myxoma	Adults Distal extremities Nodule (few cm)	Multinodular dermal-based tumor Well-demarcated, encapsulated tumor lobules Abundant myxoid stroma Uniform stellate to spindle cells	S-100 + GFAP + EMA + (capsule)
Myxoid neurofibroma	Adults Wide anatomic distribution Papule or nodule	Classic features of neurofibroma with prominent myxoid stromal change	S-100 + CD34 +
Cutaneous focal mucinosis	Adults Wide anatomic distribution Papule or nodule	Nodular but unencapsulated lesion Dermal-based lesion Myxoid stroma Cleftlike spaces Uniform stellate to spindle cells No cytologic atypia	CD34 ±
Digital mucous cyst	Adults Fingers and toes Nodule	Similar to cutaneous focal mucinosis	CD34 ±
Deep (aggressive) angiomyxoma	Adults Pelvic/perineal area Large mass	Diffusely infiltrative growth Bland stellate to spindle cells in abundant myxoid stroma Prominent vascular pattern Smooth muscle cells spilling off vessels	SMA + Desmin + S-100 –
Myxoid dermatofibrosarcoma	Young adults Wide anatomic distribution Large plaque/tumor	Dermal-based lesion Diffusely infiltrative growth Subcutaneous involvement in honeycomb pattern Bland stellate to spindle cells Rare mitoses Often associated with more typical dermatofibrosarcoma protuberans	CD34 + S-100 – SMA – Desmin –
Low-grade myxofibrosarcoma	Elderly adults Extremities Slowly enlarging mass	Infiltrative and multinodular growth Varying cellularity and pleomorphism Myxoid stroma Curvilinear thin-walled vessels	SMA ± Desmin – S-100 – CD34 ±
Myxoinflammatory fibroblastic sarcoma	Adults Hands and feet Tumor (few cm)	Infiltrative and multinodular Dermis and subcutis Myxoid and sclerotic areas Scattered pleomorphic and multinucleated tumor cells Mixed inflammatory cell infiltrate	CD34 ± S-100 –
Myxoid melanoma	Increasing incidence with age Wide anatomic distribution Pigmented tumor	Atypical epithelioid, spindle, or stellate cells in abundant myxoid stroma Junctional activity Presence of more typical melanoma	S-100 + SOX10 + Melan A + HMB-45 ±

EMA, Epithelial membrane antigen; *GFAP*, glial fibrillary acidic protein; *SMA*, smooth muscle actin.

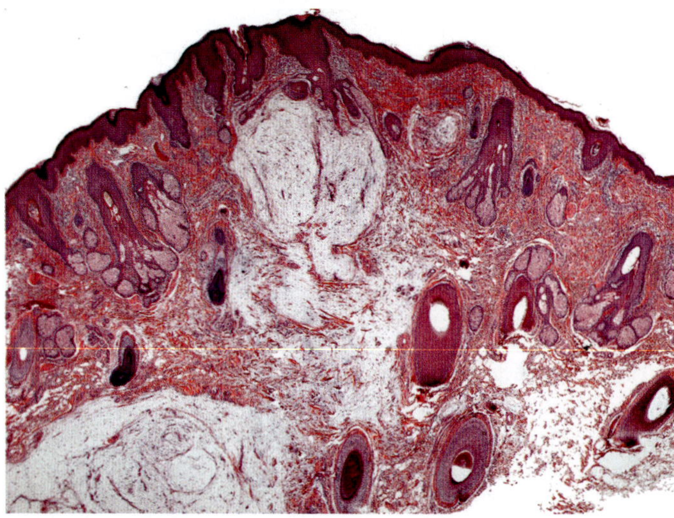

Figure 15.63 Superficial Angiomyxoma. Note the lobulated architecture and infiltrative growth pattern.

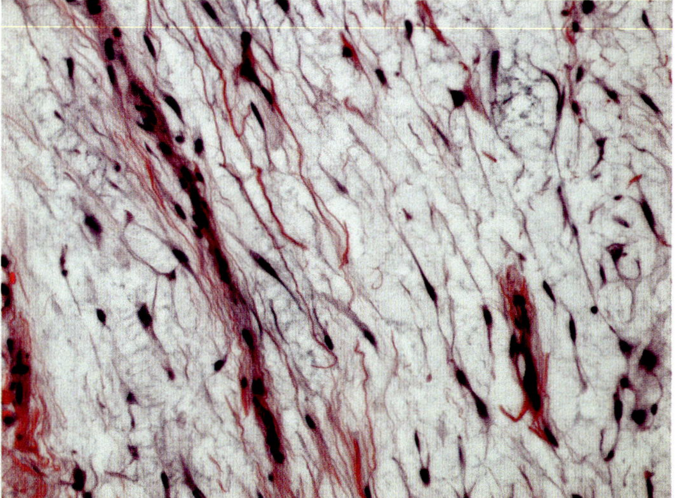

Figure 15.64 Superficial Angiomyxoma. Stellate- to spindle-shaped cells are found within a myxoid matrix.

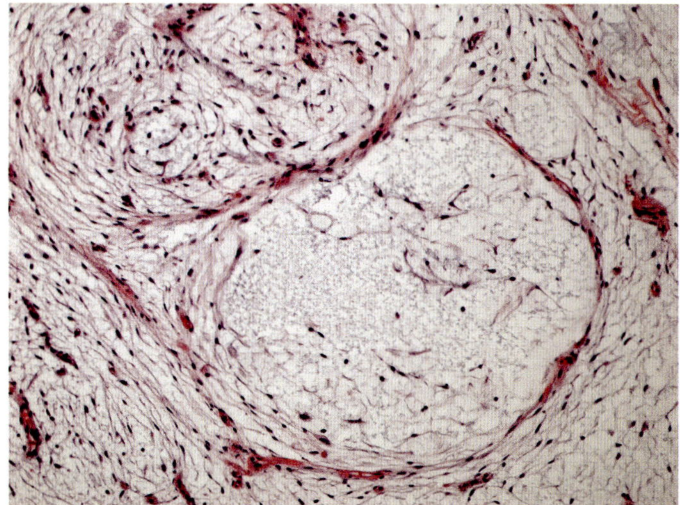

Figure 15.65 Superficial Angiomyxoma. A background of thin-walled curvilinear vessels is a characteristic feature.

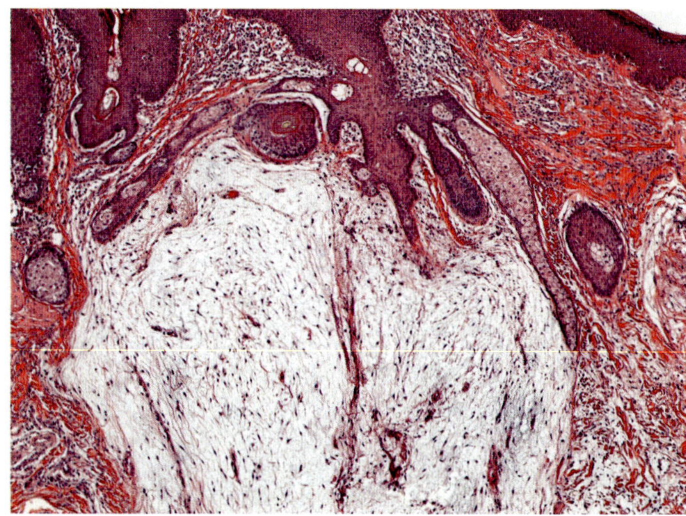

Figure 15.66 Superficial Angiomyxoma. An abnormally formed hair follicle is found in association with this tumor.

Immunohistochemistry

Tumor cells may focally express CD34, but they are negative for SMA, desmin, and S-100 protein.

Differential Diagnosis

Digital mucous cyst is markedly hypocellular and occurs predominantly on the fingers. Nerve sheath myxoma is a multinodular neoplasm composed of more sharply demarcated lobules showing less infiltrative growth and strong, diffuse expression of S-100 protein. Deep (aggressive) angiomyxoma enters the differential diagnosis because of the relatively high incidence of superficial angiomyxoma in the genital area. However, deep angiomyxoma is more deeply situated (as the name implies) and shows a more diffusely infiltrative growth pattern, in addition to the characteristic bundles of smooth muscle cells spinning off blood vessels. Low-grade myxofibrosarcoma usually affects elderly adults and contains scattered pleomorphic cells and distinctive curvilinear blood vessels, which are not seen in superficial angiomyxoma. Low-grade fibromyxoid sarcoma is usually deep seated with a more collagenous stroma, hypercellular areas showing a whorled arrangement, and consistent expression of MUC4.

Prognosis and Treatment

Superficial angiomyxoma is characterized by local, nondestructive recurrence in 30% to 40% of cases, but no adverse outcomes have been reported.

Digital Mucous Cyst (Cutaneous Myxoid Cyst)

Digital mucous cysts present in adults as solitary, dome-shaped nodules with a strong predilection for the dorsum of the finger, typically at the base of the nail. The toes are significantly less frequently affected.[114,115]

Digital mucous cysts are hypocellular lesions containing stellate to spindle cells in an abundant myxoid matrix (Fig. 15.67). No epithelial elements are present, and digital mucous cysts are not true cysts. Overall, the histologic features closely resemble those of cutaneous focal mucinosis.

Cutaneous Focal Mucinosis

Cutaneous focal mucinosis classically occurs as a solitary skin-colored papule or nodule showing a wide anatomic distribution with sparing of the joints of the hands and feet.[114,116,117] There is no gender predilection,

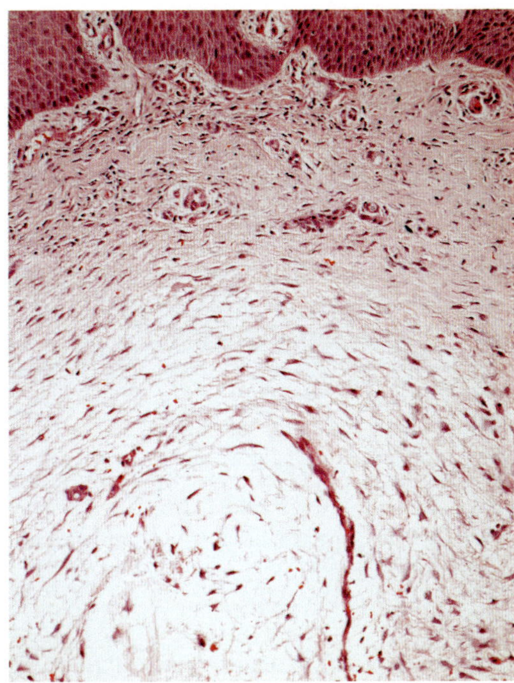

Figure 15.67 Digital Mucous Cyst. This hypocellular nodular tumor is located within the superficial dermis and shows prominent myxoid change.

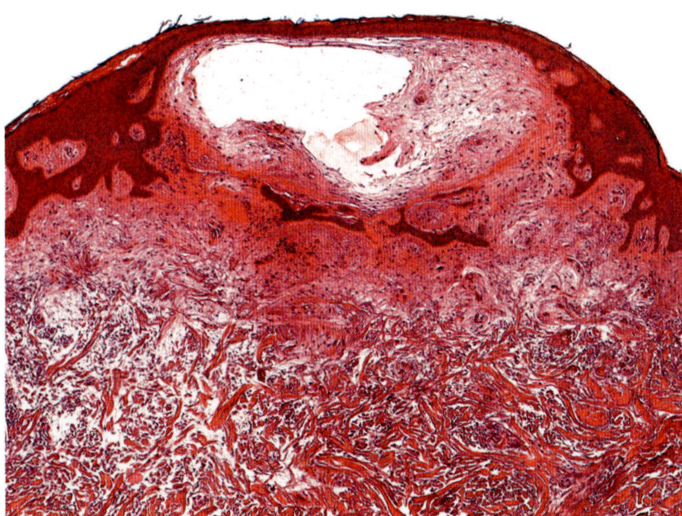

Figure 15.68 Cutaneous Focal Mucinosis. The well-circumscribed lesion shows myxoid stromal change and cleftlike spaces.

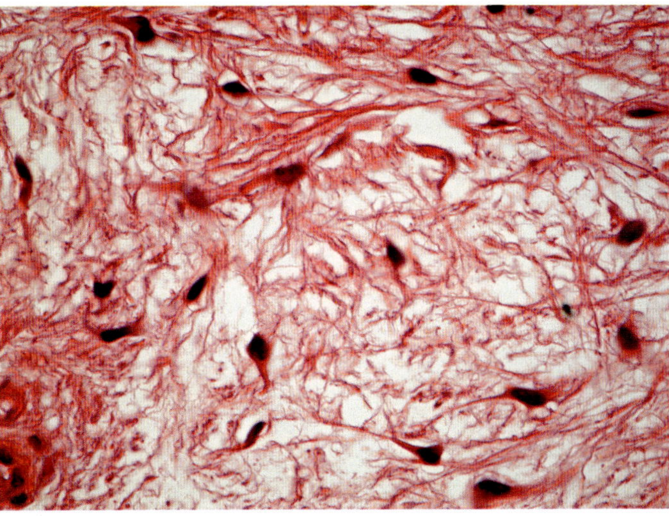

Figure 15.69 Cutaneous Focal Mucinosis. Within abundant myxoid matrix are stellate fibroblast-like cells.

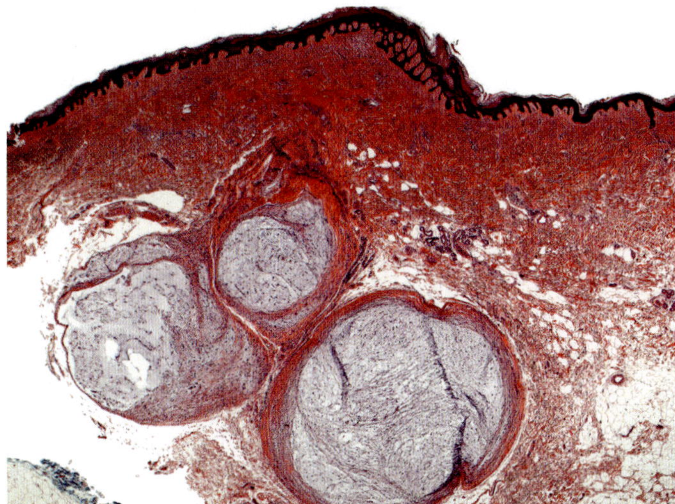

Figure 15.70 Dermal Nerve Sheath Myxoma. This tumor shows a multinodular growth pattern within the dermis.

and the age range is wide. However, presentation in adulthood is typical. Cutaneous focal mucinosis is thought to be a reactive rather than neoplastic process, and its behavior is entirely benign.

Histologically, focal cutaneous mucinosis is a nodular lesion within the superficial dermis, giving rise to a dome-shaped appearance. The characteristic finding is the presence of abundant myxoid stromal change, with stellate to spindle cells in varying numbers and occasional cleftlike spaces (Figs. 15.68 and 15.69). Cellularity is low and often increased at the periphery of the lesion.

Inconsistent expression of factor XIIIa and CD34 may be observed by immunohistochemistry.

Dermal Nerve Sheath Myxoma

Dermal nerve sheath myxoma was previously also known as *myxoid neurothekeoma*. Although cellular neurothekeoma may show myxoid stromal change, these tumor types are unrelated.[118] Dermal nerve sheath myxoma is also discussed in Chapter 5.

Clinical Features

Dermal nerve sheath myxoma affects individuals over a wide age range, although it has a predilection for adults in the fourth decade, with an equal gender distribution.[119] The tumor occurs as a slow-growing mass measuring between 0.5 and 2.5 cm in diameter. There is a strong predilection for the extremities, in particular the fingers and the hand.

Pathologic Features

The tumors show a characteristic multinodular growth pattern, frequently involving both dermis and subcutis (Fig. 15.70). Individual tumor nodules are sharply demarcated and contain an abundant myxoid matrix (Fig. 15.71). Tumor cells range from small, hyperchromatic epithelioid

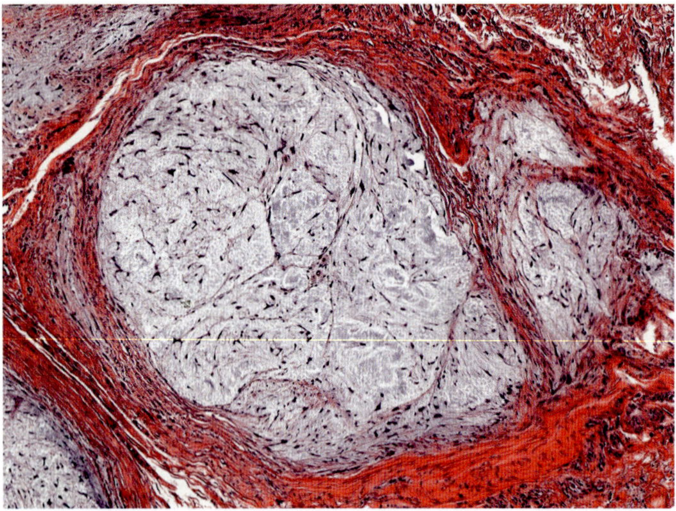

Figure 15.71 Dermal Nerve Sheath Myxoma. Individual tumor lobules are well circumscribed and contain abundant myxoid stroma.

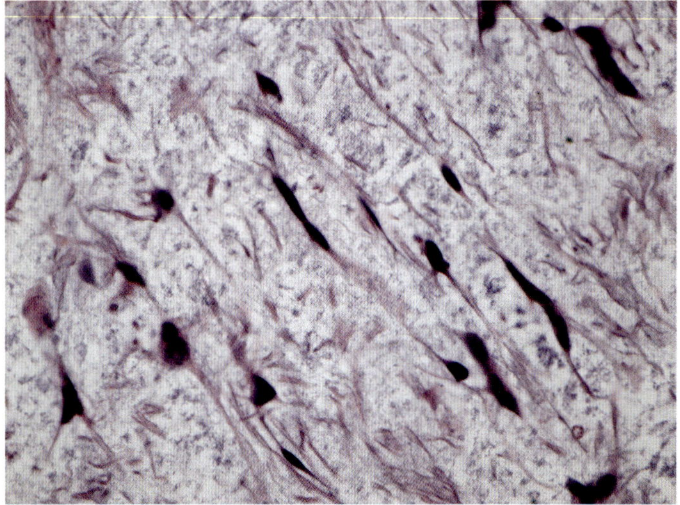

Figure 15.72 Dermal Nerve Sheath Myxoma. Within a myxoid stroma are bland multinucleated as well as stellate and spindle cells.

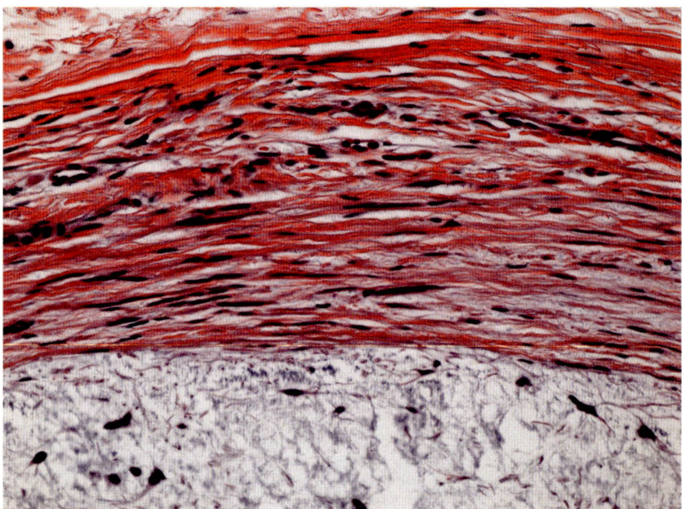

Figure 15.73 Dermal Nerve Sheath Myxoma. Myxoid tumor lobules are surrounded by a fibrous capsule containing spindle cells.

cells arranged in cords, nests, or ringlike configurations to spindled or stellate cells (Fig. 15.72). The tumor nodules are surrounded by a thin capsule containing spindled perineurial cells (Fig. 15.73). Cytologic atypia and mitotic activity are not prominent features.

Immunohistochemistry

Tumor cells diffusely express S-100 protein and GFAP.[119] Positive staining for EMA is often observed in spindled perineurial cells at the periphery of tumor lobules.

Differential Diagnosis

The histologic features of dermal nerve sheath myxoma are rather characteristic and distinctive. Cellular neurothekeoma may show extensive myxoid change and therefore mimic dermal nerve sheath myxoma. The diagnosis can easily be established by recognition of more typical areas of cellular neurothekeoma with a micronodular growth pattern and syncytial epithelioid cells with palely eosinophilic cytoplasm and lack of S-100 protein expression. Myoepithelioma may also show a lobular architecture and reticular growth pattern with myxoid stroma. In addition, tumor cells may express both S-100 protein and GFAP. However, extensive myxoid stroma is a feature observed predominantly in myoepithelioma of soft tissue rather than skin, and myoepitheliomas lack the sharply demarcated lobules of dermal nerve sheath myxoma. Recognition of other histologic patterns of myoepithelioma and positivity for keratins and/or EMA are helpful findings. Superficial angiomyxoma shows a more infiltrative growth pattern and tumor lobules are less well circumscribed. These tumors do not express S-100 protein. Dermal nerve sheath myxoma is distinguished from low-grade myxofibrosarcoma by a lack of significant atypia and more uniform cellularity. Low-grade fibromyxoid sarcoma usually arises in deep soft tissue, lacks well-developed and circumscribed tumor lobules, and expresses MUC4. Furthermore, both of these myxoid sarcomas are negative for S-100 protein.

Prognosis and Treatment

Dermal nerve sheath myxoma shows a tendency for nondestructive local recurrence if inadequately excised, in up to 50% of cases.[119] No further adverse outcomes have been reported.

Epithelioid Tumors

Granular Cell Tumor

Clinical Features

Granular cell tumor is not uncommon and involves a wide range of anatomic locations. It shows a particular predilection for the tongue, trunk, and arms, but any site can be affected, including deep soft tissue and visceral locations.[120] Tumors occur most frequently in adults, and there is a female predilection.[121,122] In approximately 10% of cases, tumors are multiple, and exceptional tumors have been found to be familial.[120] Tumors occur as raised nodules and plaques usually measuring less than 2 cm in diameter. They frequently have a verrucous appearance. Granular cell tumor is also discussed in Chapter 6.

Pathologic Features

Granular cell tumors are poorly demarcated and infiltrative neoplasms (Fig. 15.74). In the skin, they are centered in the dermis but frequently extend into deeper tissues. The tumor is arranged in sheets, nests of varying sizes, and trabeculae composed of large polygonal epithelioid cells with indistinct cell borders containing granular eosinophilic cytoplasm and small uniform nuclei (Fig. 15.75).[121,122] Mitotic figures

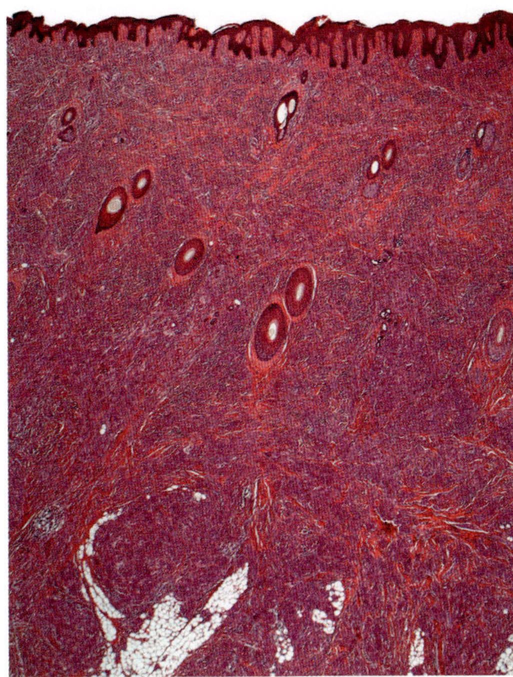

Figure 15.74 **Granular Cell Tumor.** This large dermal-based tumor shows infiltrative growth into subcutaneous tissue.

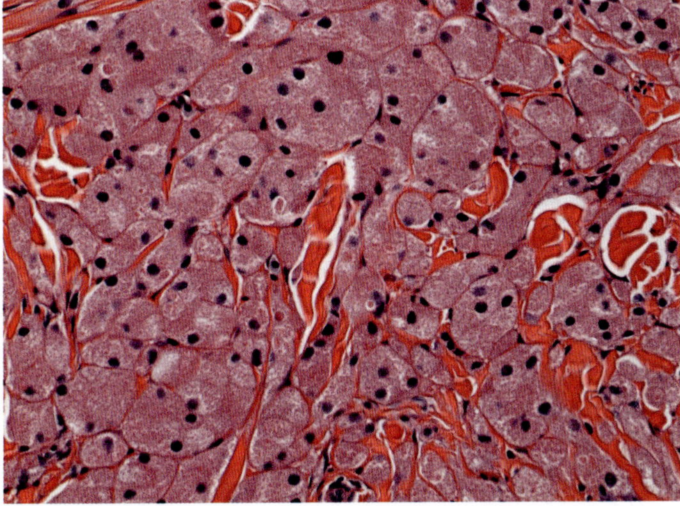

Figure 15.75 **Granular Cell Tumor.** The tumor is composed of large epithelioid to polygonal cells having abundant granular cytoplasm and small uniform nuclei lacking significant pleomorphism. Tumor cells are arranged in nests and trabeculae.

may be identified, and scattered cells showing nuclear pleomorphism with hyperchromatic or vesicular nuclei may occasionally be seen. Perineural growth is common and may prompt an erroneous diagnosis of malignancy (Fig. 15.76).[120,123] A further distinctive feature is the presence of marked (pseudoepitheliomatous) epidermal hyperplasia, which can easily be mistaken for squamous cell carcinoma on a superficial biopsy.

Immunohistochemistry

Tumor cells are positive for S-100 protein, reflecting schwannian differentiation (Fig. 15.77).[124] In addition, tumor cells express NKI-C3, neuron-specific enolase (NSE), and CD68, markers commonly associated with numerous lysosomes and granular cell change.[123,125]

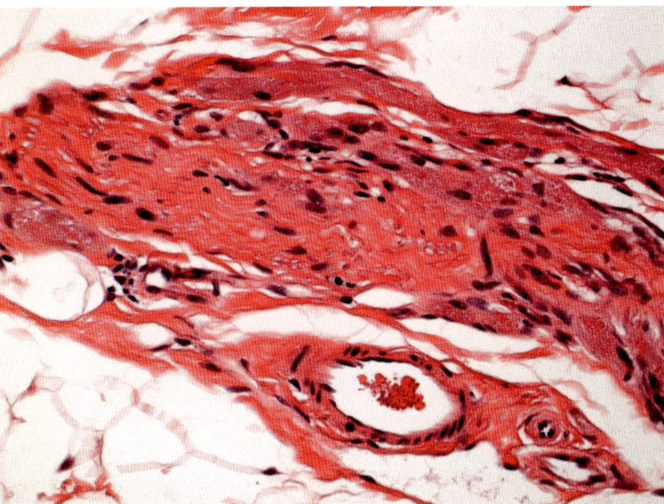

Figure 15.76 **Granular Cell Tumor.** Perineural infiltration is a frequent finding and is not associated with malignant behavior.

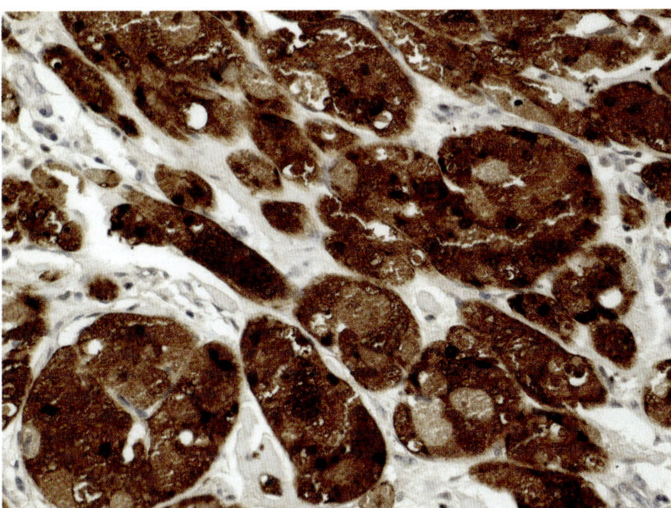

Figure 15.77 **Granular Cell Tumor.** S-100 expression is diffuse in tumor cells.

Differential Diagnosis

The histologic features of granular cell tumor are quite distinctive. The chief differential diagnostic consideration is melanoma, which can on occasion show granular cell change and is also diffusely positive for S-100 protein. Absence of an overlying in situ component and the diffuse granular cell change are clues to the correct diagnosis. Furthermore, the bland cytology appears incongruous with the infiltrative growth pattern, and HMB-45 and melan A expression is absent in granular cell tumors.[123] Mesenchymal neoplasms may rarely show granular cell change, in particular smooth muscle tumors. This diagnostic dilemma is easily solved by immunohistochemistry for desmin or other smooth muscle markers.

Prognosis and Treatment

The vast majority of granular cell tumors are benign, and recurrences are uncommon, even following incomplete excision. The rare malignant granular cell tumors are mostly large tumors in deep soft tissue and are particularly rare in the skin. The precise criteria for malignancy are only poorly defined. Factors predicting adverse outcome include large tumor size, tumor necrosis, a high mitotic rate, spindle cell morphology,

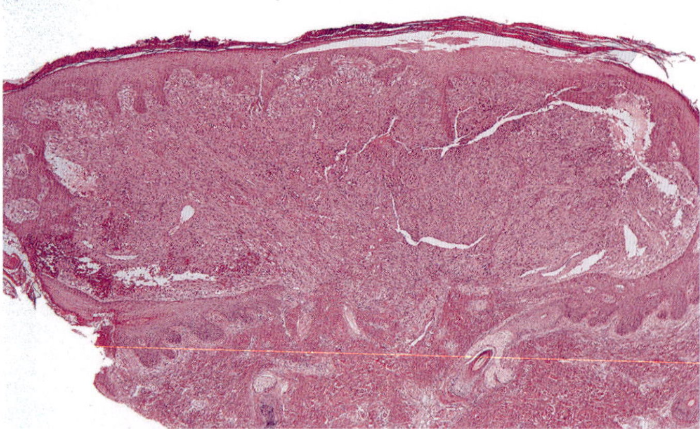

Figure 15.78 Nonneural Granular Cell Tumor. This dermal tumor often shows a polypoid appearance. Note the epidermal collarette.

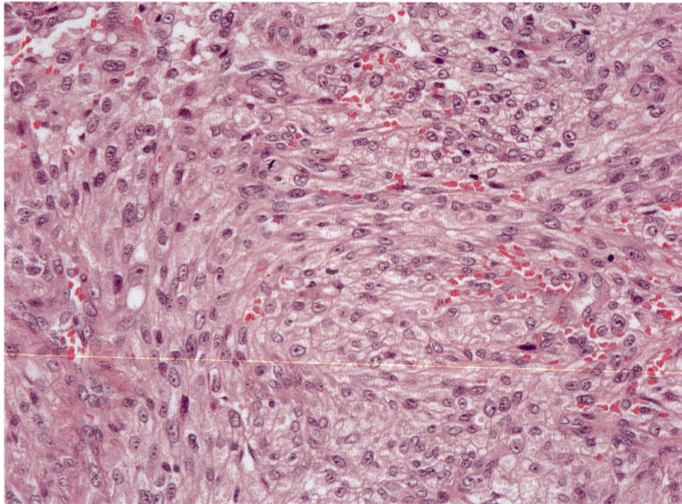

Figure 15.79 Nonneural Granular Cell Tumor. The tumor is composed of plump spindled to epithelioid cells with vesicular nuclei and abundant granular cytoplasm. Note the presence of mild nuclear atypia.

and vesicular nuclei with prominent nucleoli (see Chapter 6).[120] Malignant granular cell tumors have significant metastatic potential and poor survival.

Nonneural Granular Cell Tumor

Nonneural granular cell tumor is a rare benign cutaneous neoplasm showing some histologic features reminiscent of conventional granular cell tumor but lacking neural differentiation by immunohistochemistry.[126,127] This tumor type was originally described by LeBoit and associates as primitive polypoid granular cell tumor.[128]

Clinical Features

Nonneural granular cell tumor shows a wide anatomic distribution and an equal gender distribution. It affects individuals of varying ages, with a peak incidence in young adults.[126–128] Tumors are usually smooth, nontender cutaneous nodules measuring approximately 1 cm in diameter.

Pathologic Features

Nonneural granular cell tumor is a well-demarcated dermal-based neoplasm. Extension into superficial subcutis may occasionally be seen. Superficially located tumors often show a polypoid configuration with a surrounding epidermal collarette (Fig. 15.78). Tumor cells grow in a sheetlike arrangement. They are typically predominantly spindled and focally more epithelioid and contain vesicular nuclei with mild atypia, small eosinophilic nucleoli, and abundant granular eosinophilic cytoplasm (Fig. 15.79). Mitotic activity may occasionally be conspicuous, including rare atypical forms.[126,127]

Immunohistochemistry

Tumor cells are positive for NKI-C3, CD68, and NSE, reflecting the presence of abundant lysosomes. In contrast to conventional granular cell tumor, S-100 protein is negative, and no expression of SMA, desmin, EMA, or keratin is apparent.[126,127]

Differential Diagnosis

Nonneural granular cell tumor is a diagnosis of exclusion because many tumors can show granular cell change. The differential diagnosis therefore includes conventional granular cell tumor, which is characterized by positivity for S-100 protein. Melanoma must always be considered, but the absence of markers of melanocytic differentiation argues against this possibility. Smooth muscle tumors may occasionally show granular cell change, and, in light of the mitotic activity, one could consider primary or even metastatic leiomyosarcoma. The absence of a fascicular architecture, lack of the typical broad, cigar-shaped nuclei, and lack of reactivity for SMA and desmin argue against this diagnosis. AFX shows a significant degree of cytologic atypia and pleomorphism and is restricted to the sun-damaged skin of the elderly. Cellular neurothekeoma shows some similarities, including abundant palely eosinophilic cytoplasm, spindled to epithelioid cytomorphology, and staining for lysosomal markers. However, tumor cells are arranged in a more nested, micronodular pattern, and tumors are less well circumscribed.

Prognosis and Treatment

Although experience with this rare tumor is limited, to date no recurrences have been reported after simple excision. Rare cases have been associated with regional lymph node metastasis, but distant metastases or an adverse outcome have not been reported.[127,129]

Epithelioid Fibrous Histiocytoma

Epithelioid fibrous histiocytoma is characterized clinically by a nodular and polypoid appearance, often showing red-brown discoloration. It shows a predilection for the extremities and typically affects young to middle-aged adults. It has a benign clinical behavior, and recurrence is exceptional.[130] The relationship to conventional benign fibrous histiocytoma has been questioned.[131]

Histologically, epithelioid fibrous histiocytoma differs from conventional benign fibrous histiocytoma in that the tumor is well circumscribed and polypoid, often with an epidermal collarette (Fig. 15.80). Tumor cells are epithelioid and contain eosinophilic cytoplasm and vesicular nuclei with small nucleoli, including occasional binucleated forms (Figs. 15.81 and 15.82). Approximately 60% of tumors show at least focal reactivity for EMA.[131] The majority of tumors demonstrate *ALK* gene rearrangements by FISH, resulting in ALK overexpression with diffuse cytoplasmic staining by immunohistochemistry (see Fig. 15.82B).[132]

Epithelioid fibrous histiocytoma can easily be mistaken for Spitz nevus or spitzoid melanoma (a subset of which also harbors *ALK* rearrangements), but the lack of immunoreactivity for S-100 protein excludes a melanocytic tumor. Cutaneous myoepithelioma could also be considered, but again the absence of S-100 protein expression resolves this diagnostic problem.

Cutaneous Myoepithelioma

Histologically similar to their salivary gland counterparts, myoepithelial tumors of the skin and soft tissues have recently been recognized.[133–138] Myoepithelial tumors of the skin include chondroid syringoma (mixed tumor), cutaneous myoepithelioma,[133,135,136] and their rare malignant counterparts.[137,139,140] Although cutaneous myoepitheliomas may show similar features as examples arising in soft tissue, the majority of cutaneous myoepitheliomas represent a distinctive syncytial variant.[133,134,137] Myoepithelial tumors of soft tissue are discussed in Chapters 5 and 6. Mixed tumor is discussed in Chapter 9.

Clinical Features

Cutaneous myoepitheliomas affect patients over a broad age range, with a 3:1 male predominance.[133,134,141] The extremities are most often affected, although the anatomic distribution is wide. The clinical presentation is of a long-standing painless nodule. Tumors range in size from 0.5 to 3 cm (mean, 1 cm).

Pathologic Features

Histologically, cutaneous myoepitheliomas are poorly marginated with irregular borders (Fig. 15.83). Most tumors are confined to the dermis. Overlying epidermal hyperplasia is relatively common, and an epidermal collarette may occasionally be observed. Syncytial cutaneous myoepitheliomas are composed of sheets of histiocytoid, ovoid, or epithelioid cells with palely eosinophilic cytoplasm and usually minimal intervening stroma (Fig. 15.84).[137] Focal areas of myxoid stroma may be present, and adipocytic differentiation is occasionally seen. The nuclei are typically bland and uniform with fine chromatin and inconspicuous nuclei. Mitotic activity is scarce. Some cutaneous myoepitheliomas resemble their soft tissue counterparts, with a lobulated architecture, a reticular, trabecular, or nested growth pattern, prominent myxoid stroma, and epithelioid, spindled, or plasmacytoid cytomorphology (see Chapters 5 and 6).[133,138] Rarely, cutaneous myoepithelial tumors may exhibit cytologic features of malignancy, in the form of coarse chromatin, prominent nucleoli,

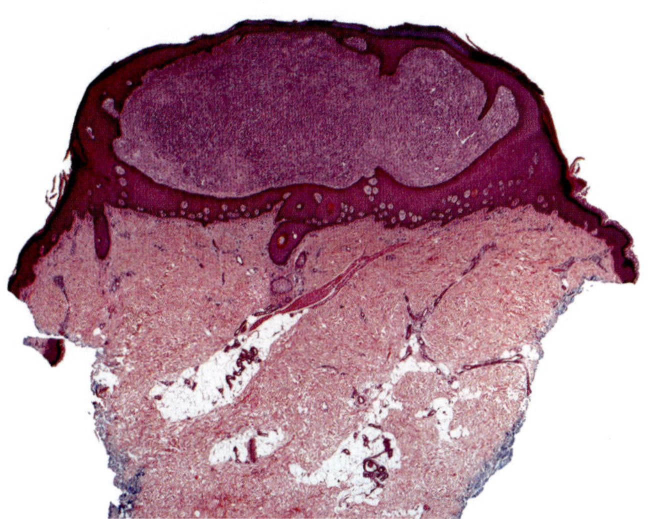

Figure 15.80 Epithelioid Fibrous Histiocytoma. The epithelioid variant is well circumscribed, and a surrounding epidermal collarette is a distinctive feature.

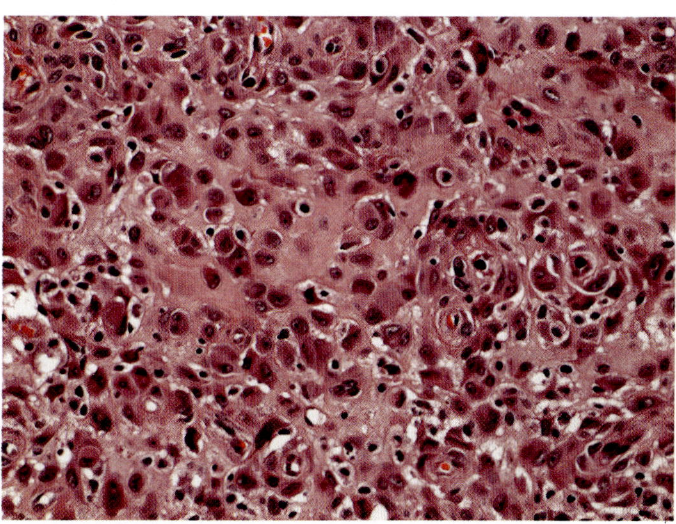

Figure 15.81 Epithelioid Fibrous Histiocytoma. The epithelioid variant is composed of epithelioid cells with abundant eosinophilic cytoplasm containing vesicular nuclei and small eosinophilic nucleoli.

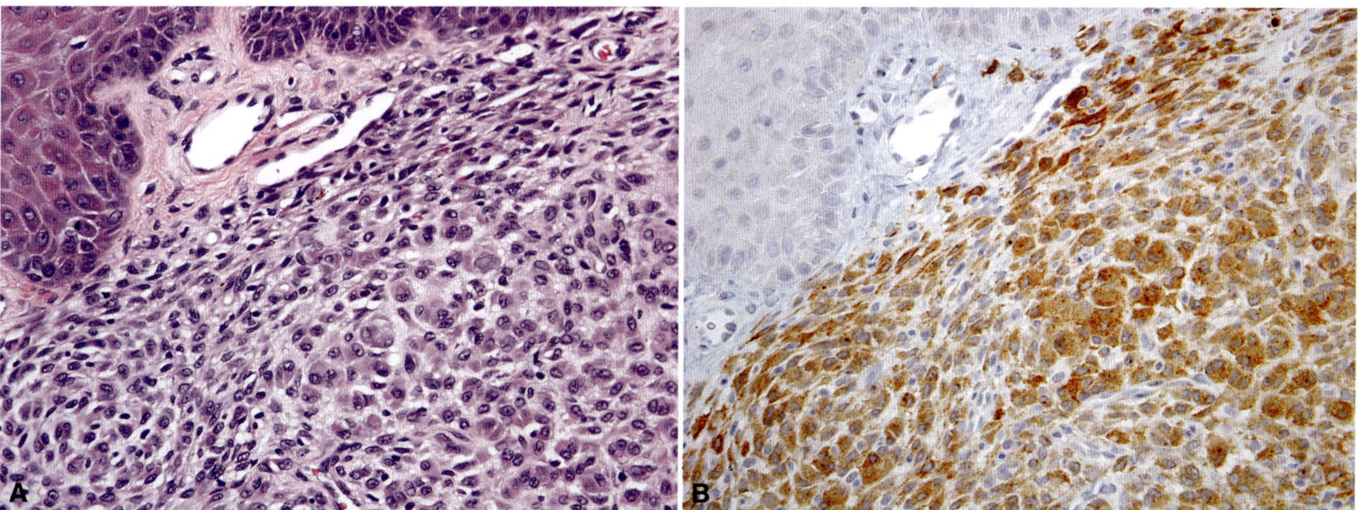

Figure 15.82 Epithelioid Fibrous Histiocytoma. Note the well-circumscribed margin and occasional binucleate cells (A). Diffuse expression of ALK is characteristic (B), correlating with the presence of *ALK* gene fusions.

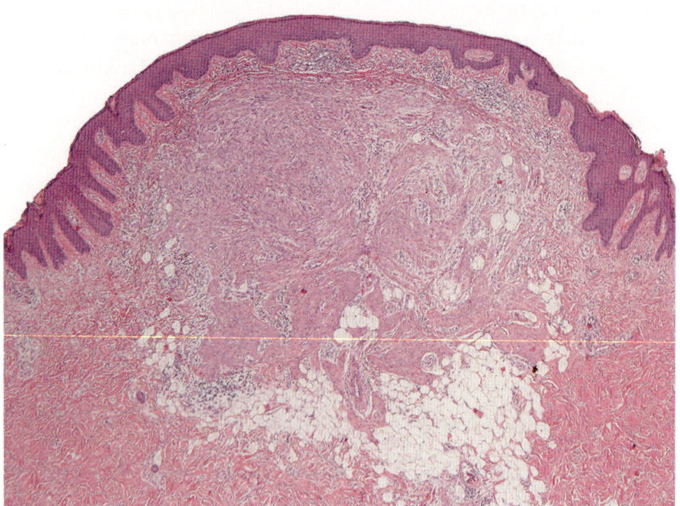

Figure 15.83 Cutaneous Myoepithelioma, Syncytial Variant. The tumor has irregular borders and overlying epidermal hyperplasia.

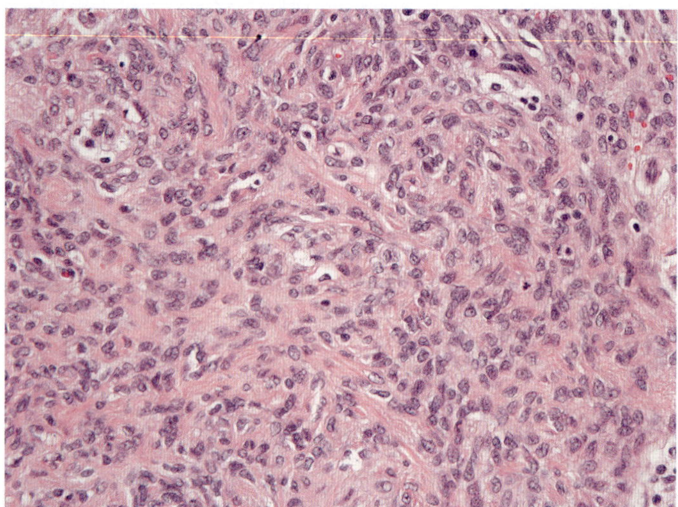

Figure 15.84 Cutaneous Myoepithelioma, Syncytial Variant. The tumor is composed of sheets of ovoid cells with palely eosinophilic cytoplasm and indistinct cell borders.

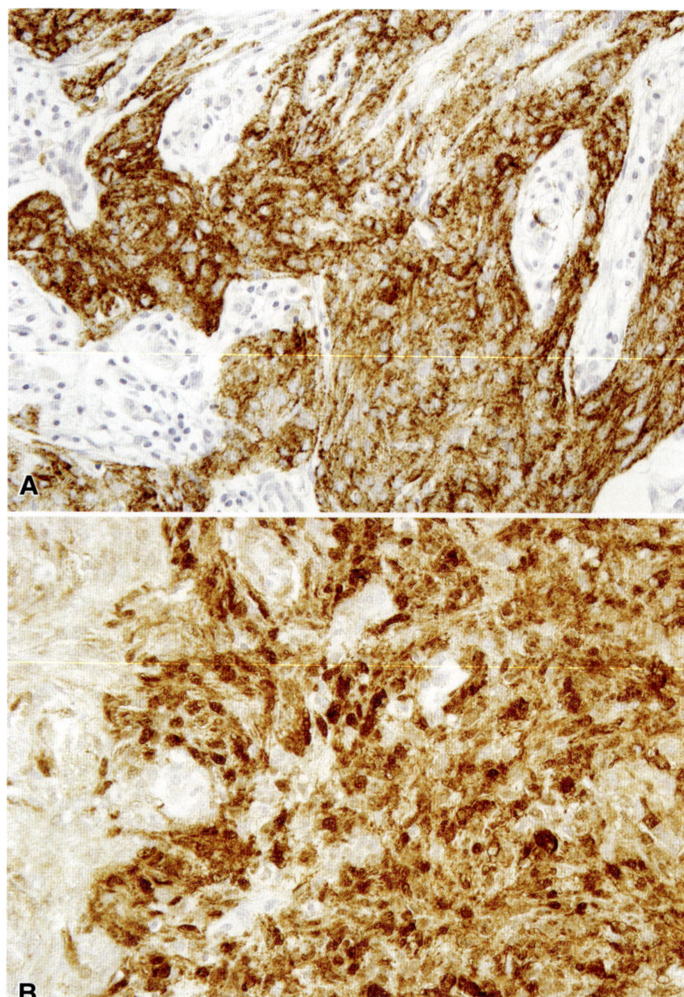

Figure 15.85 Cutaneous Myoepithelioma, Syncytial Variant. The tumor cells characteristically coexpress epithelial membrane antigen (A) and S-100 protein (B).

pleomorphism, and a high mitotic rate.[133,137,138,140] As few such cases have been reported, the minimal criteria for diagnosing a cutaneous myoepithelial carcinoma have not been established, but tumors with clear-cut malignant features behave in an aggressive fashion (see later discussion).

Immunohistochemistry

Cutaneous syncytial myoepitheliomas are diffusely positive for both S-100 protein and EMA (Fig. 15.85), and a large subset of tumors are also positive for GFAP and SOX10.[133,142] Unlike conventional myoepitheliomas of soft tissue, keratin expression is usually absent. Immunoreactivity for calponin and SMA may also be observed. Desmin, HMB-45, and melan A are negative.

Molecular Genetics

More than 80% of syncytial cutaneous myoepitheliomas show rearrangements of the *EWSR1* gene by FISH (with as yet unidentified fusion partners), whereas *PLAG1* gene rearrangement is detected in tumors with ductal differentiation (mixed tumors).[141,143]

Differential Diagnosis

The differential diagnosis for conventional myoepitheliomas of soft tissue is discussed in Chapters 5 and 6. The differential diagnosis for cutaneous syncytial myoepithelioma is summarized in Table 15.5; these tumors may be mistaken for epithelioid fibrous histiocytoma, "early" juvenile xanthogranuloma (JXG) (without lipidization), and a melanocytic tumor, especially Spitz nevus. Epithelioid fibrous histiocytoma often shows a polypoid appearance and an epidermal collarette, similar to cutaneous myoepithelioma. However, epithelioid fibrous histiocytoma usually contains scattered binucleated cells and more intervening stroma between tumor cells. Both tumor types can show staining for EMA, but epithelioid fibrous histiocytoma is positive for ALK and negative for S-100 protein and GFAP. "Early" JXG often lacks the characteristic multinucleated giant cells and lipidization helpful for proper recognition. JXG usually contains scattered inflammatory cells (lymphocytes and eosinophils), shows a marked predilection for young children, and is negative for EMA and S-100 protein. Spitz nevi lack the sheetlike syncytial architecture of cutaneous myoepithelioma, instead showing a nested appearance with decreasing cellularity with depth. Both tumors are positive for S-100 protein, but Spitz nevi are also positive for melan A and are consistently negative for EMA and GFAP.

Table 15.5 Differential Diagnosis of Cutaneous Myoepithelioma, Syncytial Variant

	Clinical Presentation	Histologic Features	Immunohistochemistry
Cutaneous myoepithelioma, syncytial variant	Young adults Extremities, but wide anatomic distribution Small papule/nodule	Dermal-based lesion Nodular growth Lack of junctional activity Ovoid to epithelioid cells with syncytial cell borders No significant cytologic atypia Occasional mitotic activity	S-100 + Keratin ± EMA + GFAP + SMA + Calponin + Desmin – p63 ±
Spitz nevus	Children and young adults Wide anatomic range Small papule/nodule	Dermal-based lesion Wedge-shaped architecture Lesional symmetry Junctional component Epithelioid to spindle cells No significant cytologic atypia Rare mitotic activity Cytologic and architectural "maturation" with depth	S-100 + Melan A + Keratin – EMA – GFAP –
Spitzoid melanoma	Adults Wide anatomic distribution Papule/nodule	Dermal-based lesion ± subcutaneous involvement Lesional asymmetry Expansile growth Junctional component Epithelioid to spindle cells Cytologic atypia Mitotic activity	S-100 + Melan A + Keratin – EMA – GFAP –
Epithelioid fibrous histiocytoma	Adults Extremities Nodule	Dermal-based lesion Polypoid and nodular growth Epidermal collarette No junctional activity Epithelioid cells with occasional binucleated forms No significant cytologic atypia Occasional mitotic activity	ALK + S-100 – Keratin – EMA ± GFAP –

EMA, epithelial membrane antigen; *GFAP,* glial fibrillary acidic protein; *SMA,* smooth muscle actin.

Prognosis and Treatment

Cutaneous myoepitheliomas exhibit nondestructive local recurrences in 20% of cases[133,134]; complete excision with negative margins is therefore indicated. Regional lymph node metastases are rare, and adverse outcomes for cytologically benign cutaneous myoepitheliomas have not been observed, even for those patients with lymph node involvement. Cutaneous myoepithelial carcinomas pursue an aggressive clinical course with a significant potential for distant metastasis and death.[137,139,140]

Cellular Neurothekeoma

In the past, cellular neurothekeoma was thought to fall on a spectrum with "myxoid" neurothekeoma (now known as *dermal nerve sheath myxoma*), and "mixed-type" neurothekeoma, because cellular neurothekeomas may contain variably prominent myxoid stroma.[144,145] However, it is now known that dermal nerve sheath myxomas are schwannian in nature (and are diffusely positive for S-100 protein),[119] whereas cellular neurothekeomas are not nerve sheath tumors at all, although they continue to carry this confusing name.[118,146,147] The line of differentiation exhibited by these distinctive tumors is not entirely certain, although a fibroblastic/myofibroblastic lineage seems most likely.[118,147]

Clinical Features

Cellular neurothekeoma has a peak incidence in the first three decades of life (mean age, 25 years). The tumor commonly affects young children, with a 2:1 female predominance.[146,147] The most common anatomic sites are the head and neck (especially the face), shoulder, and upper extremities. The typical clinical presentation is of a painless nodule or mass. Most tumors are between 0.5 and 2 cm in diameter.

Pathologic Features

Cellular neurothekeomas may be limited to the dermis or extend into the subcutis. Histologically, cellular neurothekeoma shows a micronodular or lobulated architecture and irregular borders with the surrounding dermis or adipose tissue (Fig. 15.86A). The tumors are composed of nests or bundles of predominantly plump epithelioid and occasionally more spindled cells containing abundant palely eosinophilic cytoplasm, often separated by dense sclerotic collagen (Figs. 15.86B and 15.87). Approximately 30% of cellular neurothekeomas contain focally myxoid stroma (Fig. 15.88),[146,147] which occasionally predominates. The tumor cells typically have round to ovoid nuclei with fine chromatin and small nucleoli and abundant cytoplasm with ill-defined cell borders with a syncytial appearance (see Fig. 15.86B). The mitotic rate is usually low. Some cellular neurothekeomas contain pleomorphic cells with large nuclei and prominent nucleoli,[147–149] and they may occasionally show a high mitotic rate, including rare atypical mitotic figures. Such examples have previously been known as "atypical" cellular neurothekeomas,[148] although the presence of atypical histologic features has no clinical significance (see subsequent discussion). Occasional osteoclast-like giant cells may be present.

Immunohistochemistry

Cellular neurothekeomas have no specific immunophenotype, although both NKI-C3 and NSE are virtually always diffusely positive and therefore

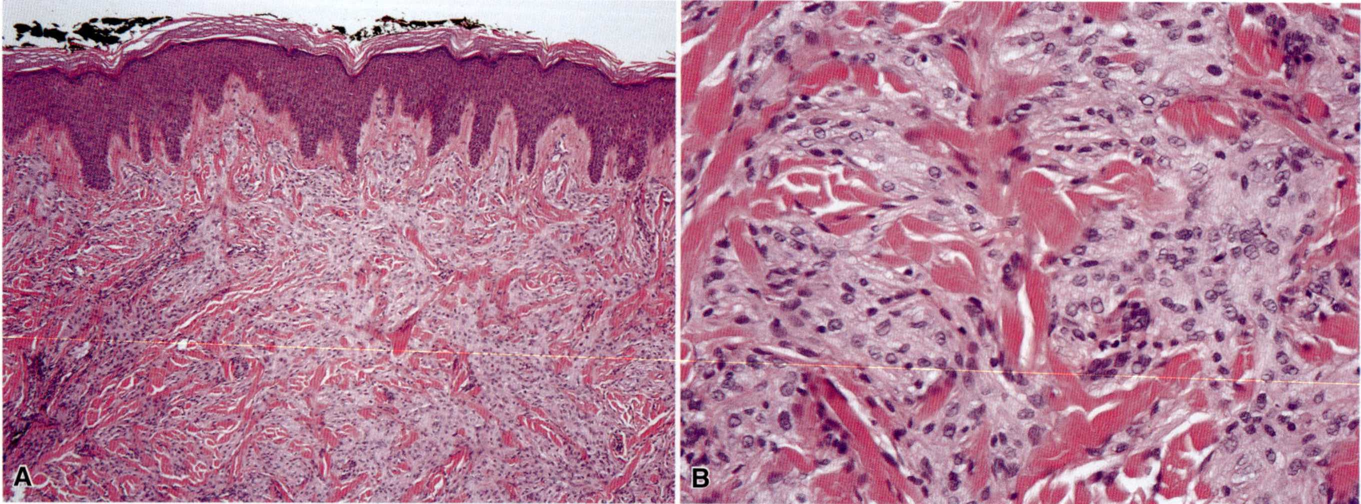

Figure 15.86 Cellular Neurothekeoma. This dermal-based tumor shows an infiltrative architecture (A). The epithelioid tumor cells contain abundant palely eosinophilic cytoplasm (B).

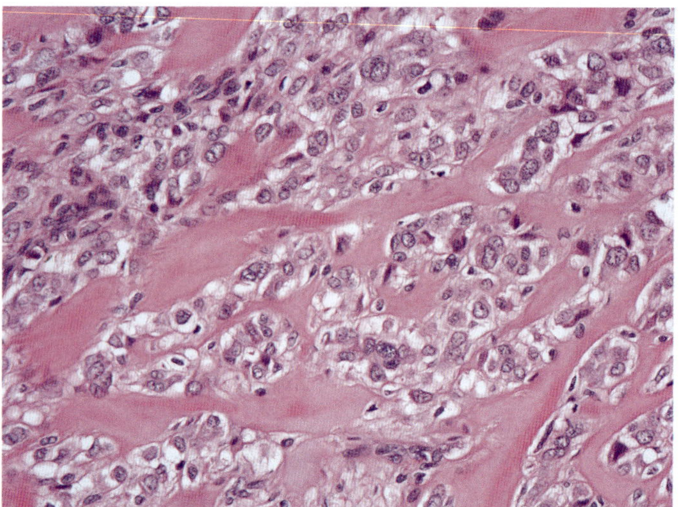

Figure 15.87 Cellular Neurothekeoma. The tumor is composed of nests of epithelioid cells. Note the dense sclerotic collagen and mild nuclear atypia.

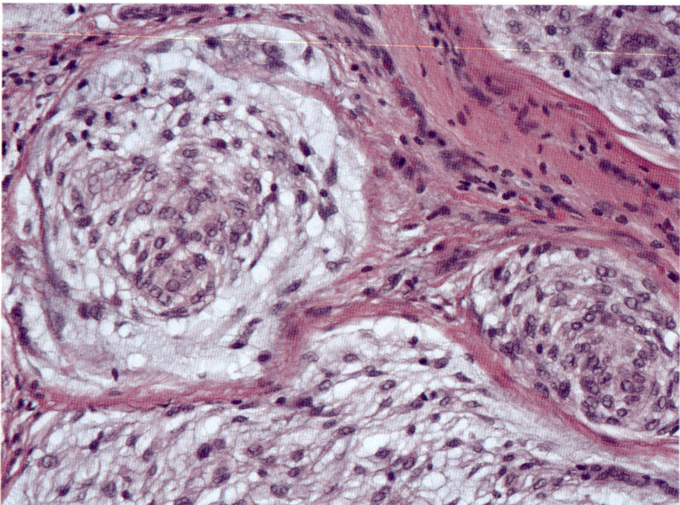

Figure 15.88 Cellular Neurothekeoma. Some tumors contain prominent myxoid stroma. Note the lobulated growth pattern and pale cytoplasm.

can be used to support the diagnosis in the appropriate context.[147] Focal or diffuse staining for SMA is observed in approximately 60% of cases, and the tumors usually express microphthalmia transcription factor (MITF) and p63.[150–152] S-100 protein, SOX10, HMB-45, melan A, and desmin are negative.

Differential Diagnosis

The main differential diagnosis for cellular neurothekeoma is a melanocytic tumor (especially Spitz nevus), dermal nerve sheath myxoma, pilar leiomyoma, and plexiform fibrohistiocytic tumor (the latter for cellular neurothekeomas that infiltrate subcutaneous fat). Spitz nevi also occur on the head and neck of children and young adults and show a nested architecture and epithelioid to spindle cell morphology. However, cellular neurothekeomas lack a junctional component and the downward maturation typical of Spitz nevus. NKI-C3 and NSE can both be positive in melanocytic tumors. Immunoreactivity for S-100 protein and melan A can distinguish Spitz nevus from cellular neurothekeoma. When cellular neurothekeomas contain extensive myxoid stroma, they may mimic dermal nerve sheath myxoma. Unlike cellular neurothekeoma, dermal nerve sheath myxoma usually arises on the distal extremities (especially hands) and only rarely on the face. Dermal nerve sheath myxoma is composed of large, sharply demarcated lobules and lacks the infiltrative margins of cellular neurothekeoma. Expression of S-100 protein and GFAP confirms the diagnosis of dermal nerve sheath myxoma. Cellular neurothekeoma showing prominent spindle cell morphology, fascicular architecture, and infiltrative growth through sclerotic dermal collagen can resemble pilar leiomyoma. However, pilar leiomyomas contain more brightly eosinophilic cytoplasm and broader (cigar-shaped) nuclei. Positive staining for desmin is only seen in pilar leiomyoma. Plexiform fibrohistiocytic tumor shows a similar age and anatomic distribution as cellular neurothekeoma, although the distal extremities are more often involved. In contrast to cellular neurothekeoma, which is composed of uniform epithelioid cells, plexiform fibrohistiocytic tumor shows a biphasic appearance, with nodules of mononuclear histiocytoid cells and osteoclast-like giant cells, interconnected by fascicles of fibromatosis-like myofibroblastic spindle cells (see Chapter 11).

Prognosis and Treatment

Cellular neurothekeomas are benign and occasionally recur in a non-destructive fashion (in at most 10% of cases), generally following incomplete excision.[146,147] Tumors on the face seem to have the highest recurrence rate, likely attributable to conservative surgery. Atypical histologic features (large tumor size, pleomorphism, or a high mitotic rate) do not affect the rate of local recurrence.[147] Cellular neurothekeomas only very rarely metastasize to regional lymph nodes.

PRACTICE POINTS: Cellular Neurothekeoma

- No relationship to dermal nerve sheath myxoma ("myxoid neurothekeoma")
- Not a nerve sheath tumor
- Most common in head and neck, shoulder, and upper arms of children and young adults
- Micronodular architecture with irregular borders
- Some cases contain variably prominent myxoid stroma
- Nuclear atypia, pleomorphism, and mitotic activity of no clinical significance
- No specific immunophenotype, although positive for NKI-C3, NSE, and often SMA
- Local recurrences uncommon following incomplete excision

Perivascular Epithelioid Cell Tumor

Perivascular epithelioid cell tumors (PEComas) are distinctive mesenchymal tumors composed of cells showing a mixed melanocytic and smooth muscle phenotype.[153–155] PEComas most commonly arise in the retroperitoneum and pelvis and at visceral sites and more rarely in somatic soft tissues and skin.[156,157] Cutaneous PEComas are rare, representing approximately 5% of all PEComas.[157,158] PEComas of soft tissue and visceral sites are discussed in Chapters 6 and 16.

Clinical Features

Cutaneous PEComas usually affect female patients; the female-to-male ratio is 5:1. Individuals of varying ages are affected, with the peak occurring in middle age.[156,157] The limbs are most often involved. The typical presentation is a slow-growing painless nodule. Most tumors range from 1 to 2 cm in size. Cutaneous PEComas do not appear to be associated with tuberous sclerosis complex.

Pathologic Features

Cutaneous PEComas are centered in the dermis and often extend into subcutaneous tissue, either with a pushing border or infiltrative margins. There is usually a grenz zone between the tumor and the epidermis. Histologically, cutaneous PEComa is composed of nests, trabeculae, and sheets of predominantly epithelioid cells with variably clear to granular eosinophilic cytoplasm (Fig. 15.89). Focally more spindled cells may be present. The nests are surrounded by delicate thin-walled blood vessels (Fig. 15.90). The tumor cells contain rounded nuclei with vesicular chromatin and small nucleoli. Occasional multinucleated tumor cells may be seen. Mitotic activity is typically scant.

Immunohistochemistry

Cutaneous PEComas are typically at least focally positive for HMB-45 (Fig. 15.91), and melan A is also often focally positive. Nuclear staining for MITF is usually extensive. Approximately 50% of cutaneous PEComas are positive for desmin, but SMA expression is rare.[157] S-100 protein may be focally positive in occasional cases. EMA and keratins are negative. In contrast to a subset of their visceral counterparts, cutaneous PEComas do not express TFE3, and no *TFE3* gene rearrangements have been identified.[150,159]

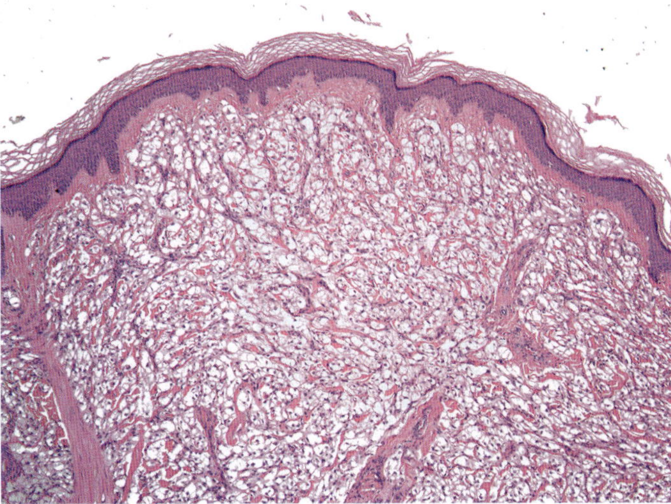

Figure 15.89 Cutaneous Perivascular Epithelioid Cell Tumor (PEComa). This dermal tumor is composed of sheets and nests of epithelioid cells with abundant clear cytoplasm.

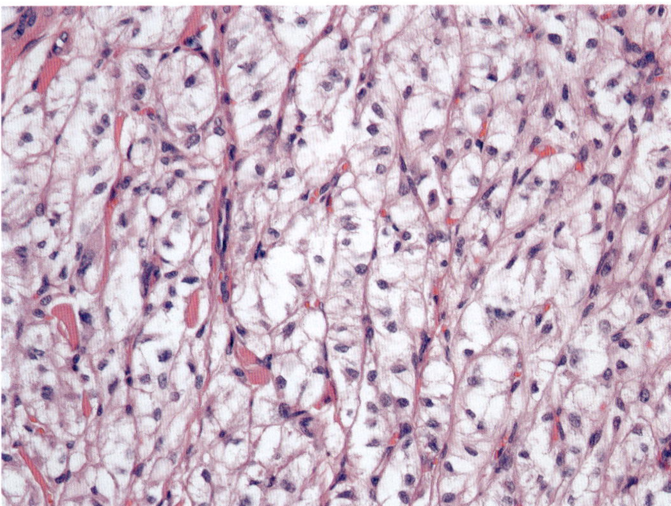

Figure 15.90 Cutaneous Perivascular Epithelioid Cell Tumor (PEComa). The tumor nests are surrounded by delicate thin-walled vessels. Note the bland nuclei and abundant granular to clear cytoplasm.

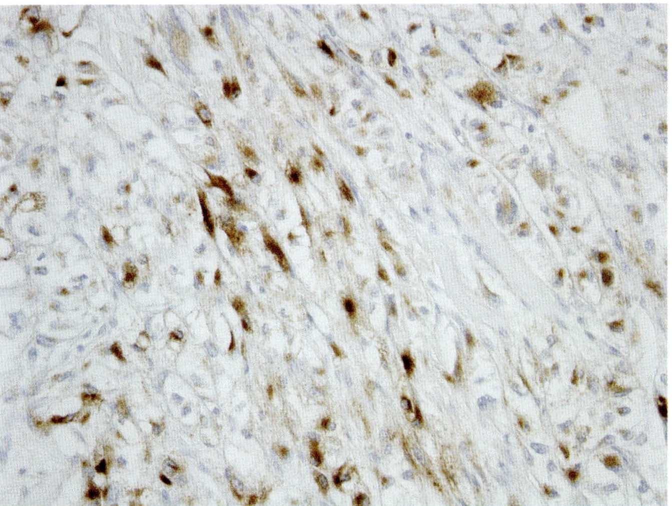

Figure 15.91 Cutaneous Perivascular Epithelioid Cell Tumor (PEComa). Scattered tumor cells are positive for HMB-45.

Table 15.6 Cutaneous Tumors Showing Clear Cell Features

	Clinical Features	Histologic Features	Immunohistochemistry
Perivascular epithelioid cell tumor (PEComa)	Adults Extremities and trunk Small plaque or nodule	Dermal-based tumor with involvement of subcutis Nested and trabecular growth Epithelioid and spindle cells with clear to granular eosinophilic cytoplasm No pleomorphism Infrequent mitotic activity Background of delicate thin-walled vessels	HMB-45 + Melan A + Desmin ± SMA ± S-100 – Keratin –
Distinctive dermal clear cell mesenchymal neoplasm	Adults Extremities Nodules	Dermal-based tumor with extension into subcutis Nodular growth with slightly infiltrative margins Large polygonal cells with clear to granular cytoplasm Rare pleomorphism Rare mitotic activity Background of thin walled vessels	NKI-C3 + CD68 + S-100 – HMB-45 – Melan A – Keratin – EMA –
Clear cell fibrous histiocytoma	Adults Extremities and trunk Small papule or plaque	Abundant clear cell change in otherwise typical dermatofibroma	S-100 – SMA ± Desmin – CD34 –
Clear cell AFX	Elderly adults Head and neck Rapidly growing exophytic nodule	Abundant clear cell change in otherwise typical AFX	S-100 – SMA ± Desmin – CD34 – Keratin –
Clear cell sarcoma	Young adults Distal lower extremities Deep-seated mass	Infiltrative tumor Deep soft tissue Nests and fascicles Short spindle cells with eosinophilic to clear cytoplasm Wreathlike multinucleated giant cells	S-100 + HMB-45 + SOX10 +
Balloon cell/clear cell melanoma	Increasing incidence with age Wide anatomic distribution Pigmented tumor	Abundant clear cell change in otherwise typical melanoma	S-100 + Melan A + HMB-45 ± SOX10 +
Clear cell squamous cell carcinoma	Elderly adults Head and neck Plaque or exophytic tumor	Abundant clear cell change in otherwise typical squamous cell carcinoma	Keratin + p63/p40 + SMA ± S-100 –
Eccrine tumors (e.g., hidradenoma, poroma and their malignant counterparts)	Adults Extremities Plaque or nodule	Dermal-based tumor ± Epidermal connection Ductal differentiation	Keratin + EMA + CEA + S-100 –
Hair follicular tumors (e.g., trichilemmal carcinoma)	Elderly adults Head and neck, hands Plaque or nodule	Dermal-based tumor Connection with epidermis and/or follicular structures Pushing borders Peripheral palisading Trichilemmal keratinization Variable pleomorphism Mitotic activity	Keratin + S-100 –
Metastatic carcinoma, particularly RCC	Underlying visceral malignancy	Nodular tumor Prominent vascular pattern	Keratin + EMA + PAX8 + RCC antigen ± S-100 –

AFX, Atypical fibroxanthoma; *EMA*, epithelial membrane antigen; *RCC*, renal cell carcinoma; *SMA*, smooth muscle actin.

Differential Diagnosis

The differential diagnosis includes other superficial tumors with clear cell features (Table 15.6), such as balloon cell (or clear cell) melanoma, clear cell benign fibrous histiocytoma, clear cell sarcoma, metastatic clear cell (renal cell) carcinoma, and the distinctive dermal clear cell neoplasm.[160] Balloon cell melanoma typically contains a junctional component and shows pagetoid spread, which are not observed in cutaneous PEComa. Strong expression of S-100 protein favors a melanocytic tumor, whereas desmin expression favors PEComa. Benign fibrous histiocytomas rarely show clear cell features. However, in contrast to cutaneous PEComa, benign fibrous histiocytomas show epidermal hyperplasia and lack expression of HMB-45 and melan A. Clear cell sarcoma usually involves deep soft tissues and rarely extends into the dermis. Expression of both S-100 protein and melanocytic markers is typical of clear cell sarcoma, whereas cutaneous PEComas are usually negative for S-100 protein. Detection of *EWSR1* gene rearrangement by FISH can be used to confirm the diagnosis of clear cell sarcoma. Metastatic renal cell carcinoma can be distinguished by expression of EMA, keratins, and PAX8, as well as negativity for melanocytic markers. The distinctive dermal clear cell neoplasm shows very similar histologic features as cutaneous PEComa but lacks expression of melanocytic markers.

Prognosis and Treatment

Cutaneous PEComas are benign. They do not recur.

Distinctive Dermal Clear Cell Mesenchymal Neoplasm

This dermal-based tumor of uncertain differentiation has only recently been reported. Its behavior appears to be benign, but experience with this likely mesenchymal neoplasm is limited.[160]

Clinical Features

Distinctive dermal clear cell mesenchymal neoplasm is a tumor of adults with equal gender distribution. It presents as a small cutaneous nodule measuring up to 2.5 cm with a strong predilection for the lower extremities.[160]

Pathologic Features

Tumors are dermal based with nodular outlines but somewhat infiltrative margins, and focal infiltration of subcutis is often present.[160] They are composed of large ovoid to polygonal cells containing abundant clear-to-pale granular cytoplasm and vesicular nuclei (Fig. 15.92). Tumor cells are arranged in sheets, and intratumoral thin-walled vessels may be present. Scattered cells with nuclear pleomorphism may occasionally be observed, but mitotic activity is scarce.

Immunohistochemistry

Tumor cells are positive for the lysosomal markers NKI-C3 and CD68 but are negative for S-100 protein, melan A, HMB-45, keratins, EMA, and CD34.

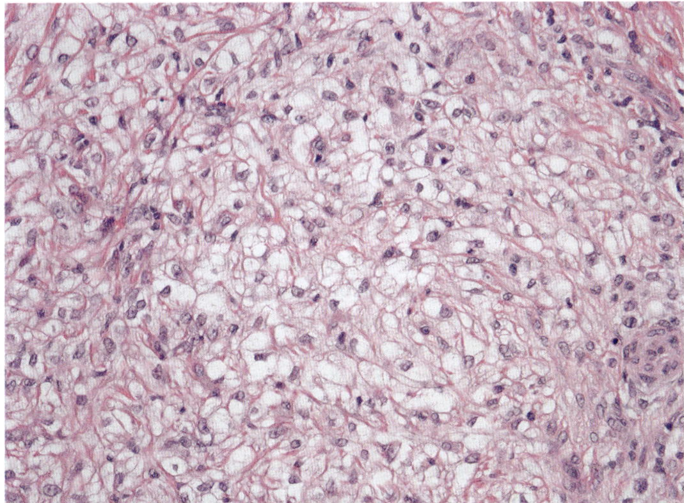

Figure 15.92 Distinctive Dermal Clear Cell Mesenchymal Neoplasm. The tumor is composed of sheets of epithelioid cells with clear cytoplasm, closely mimicking perivascular epithelioid cell tumor (PEComa).

Differential Diagnosis

The differential diagnosis includes other neoplasms with prominent clear cell features (see Table 15.6). In particular, skin adnexal tumors such as eccrine hidradenoma, clear cell hidradenocarcinoma, eccrine poroma, and eccrine porocarcinoma, as well as trichilemmal carcinoma and sebaceous tumors merit consideration, all of which can be excluded using keratin immunohistochemistry. Further histologic clues include ductal differentiation in eccrine tumors, trichilemmal keratinization in trichilemmal carcinoma, and the presence of vacuolated cytoplasm in sebaceous tumors. Balloon cell or clear cell melanoma is excluded by the absence of an overlying in situ component, as well as lack of expression of melanocytic markers. Clear cell AFX presents on sun-damaged skin of the head and neck, particularly the scalp, of the elderly and is characterized by marked cytologic atypia and mitotic activity. The very rare clear cell benign fibrous histiocytoma shows the typical entrapment of surrounding collagen bundles, in addition to hyperplasia of the overlying epidermis. Cutaneous PEComa shows many morphologic and clinical similarities. In contrast to distinctive dermal clear cell mesenchymal neoplasm, cutaneous PEComa is positive for HMB-45 and often for desmin. Clear cell sarcoma usually arises in deep soft tissue but may rarely involve the skin. It is organized in small nests and fascicles with expression of S-100 protein and melanocytic markers by immunohistochemistry. Metastatic clear cell renal cell carcinoma is another close morphologic mimic. Clinical history, the rich vascularization, and expression of EMA, keratins, and PAX8 in renal cell carcinoma easily solve this diagnostic dilemma.

Prognosis and Treatment

Experience with this rare tumor is limited. So far, behavior appears to be benign.

Epithelioid Schwannoma

Epithelioid schwannoma is an uncommon variant that usually arises in skin and subcutaneous tissue. It may easily be mistaken for other tumor types.[161,162]

Clinical Features

Epithelioid schwannoma has a wide age distribution, with a peak in middle-aged adults, and an approximately equal gender distribution. Although the anatomic distribution is broad, the extremities are most often involved. The clinical presentation is of a painless nodule. Most tumors are between 0.5 and 3 cm in size. Nearly 90% of tumors arise in subcutaneous tissue and skin.[163,164]

Pathologic Features

Epithelioid schwannoma is well circumscribed and usually encapsulated (Fig. 15.93). The tumors often show a multinodular appearance and are composed of sheets, nests, cords, and trabeculae of uniform epithelioid cells with vesicular nuclei, small central nucleoli, and eosinophilic cytoplasm, in a collagenous stroma (Fig. 15.94A).[161–164] Mild nuclear atypia may be present. Variably prominent myxoid stroma is a common feature (see Fig. 15.94B). A minor component of more typical spindle-shaped Schwann cells is often observed. Mitotic activity is scant.

Immunohistochemistry

The tumor cells are diffusely positive for S-100 protein and SOX10 and often also for GFAP. NFP-positive axons are absent. Around 40% of epithelioid schwannomas show loss of SMARCB1 (INI1) expression.[164] EMA and keratins are negative in tumor cells, although EMA often highlights the perineurial capsule. HMB-45 and melan A are not expressed.

Differential Diagnosis

The main differential diagnostic considerations are myoepithelioma, epithelioid MPNST, and a melanocytic neoplasm. Myoepitheliomas also often show a multinodular growth pattern, myxoid stroma, and a nested and trabecular architecture, although myoepitheliomas are usually positive for EMA and keratins, which are not expressed by epithelioid schwannoma. Epithelioid MPNST may present in dermis and subcutis, and malignant transformation in epithelioid schwannoma may rarely occur. Epithelioid MPNST is characterized by increased cellularity and significant nuclear atypia with large nucleoli.[165] Unlike conventional spindle cell MPNST, epithelioid MPNST is diffusely positive for S-100 protein and SOX10, similar to epithelioid schwannoma. In addition, both tumor types may show loss of SMARCB1 (INI1) expression. However, epithelioid MPNST usually lacks an EMA-positive capsule. In contrast to epithelioid schwannoma, melanocytic tumors are unencapsulated and usually express HMB-45 and melan A.

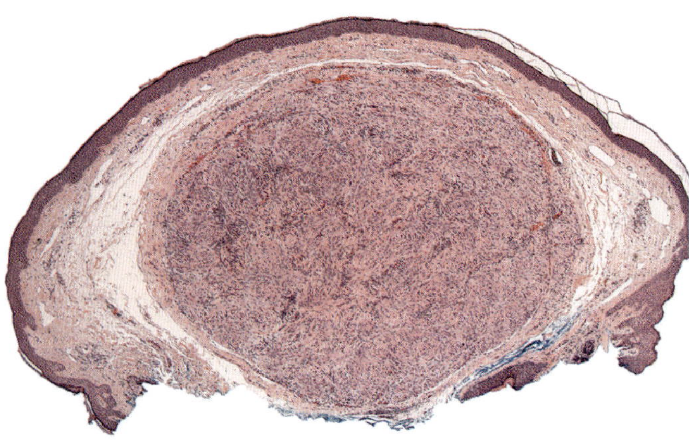

Figure 15.93 Epithelioid Schwannoma. This well-circumscribed dermal tumor is composed of sheets of epithelioid cells.

Prognosis and Treatment

Epithelioid schwannomas are benign. They only occasionally recur locally in a nondestructive fashion following incomplete excision,[161] and metastases do not occur.

Sclerosing Perineurioma

Perineuriomas include soft tissue, intraneural, and sclerosing variants.[85,166] Although approximately 10% of soft tissue perineuriomas arise in the dermis, the distinctive sclerosing variant is nearly exclusive to the skin and subcutaneous tissue of the fingers and hands.[166]

Clinical Features

Sclerosing perineurioma typically affects young adults, with a male predominance. Nearly all tumors arise in the fingers or palms. The typical presentation is a long-standing painless nodule. Tumor size ranges from 0.5 to 3 cm.

Pathologic Features

Sclerosing perineurioma usually involves the dermis or subcutis and is relatively circumscribed but unencapsulated. Histologically, the tumor is composed of rounded to epithelioid cells arranged in cords and trabeculae, within a densely hyalinized collagenous stroma (Fig. 15.95). The typical cytomorphology of perineurial cells is usually inconspicuous on histologic examination.[166]

Immunohistochemistry

Tumor cells show strong, diffuse expression of EMA (Fig. 15.96), which often highlights delicate elongated cytoplasmic processes.[166] Occasional tumors may be focally positive for keratins or SMA. The tight junction–associated protein claudin-1 is expressed in a subset of cases. S-100 protein, GFAP, and desmin are negative.

Differential Diagnosis

After the distinctive histologic features and anatomic site are recognized, diagnosing sclerosing perineurioma is generally straightforward. However, the differential diagnosis may include fibroma of tendon sheath, giant cell tumor of tendon sheath (localized-type tenosynovial giant cell tumor), storiform collagenoma (sclerotic fibroma), glomus tumor, an adnexal neoplasm, and epithelioid hemangioendothelioma. Fibroma of tendon sheath also arises on the fingers of young adults

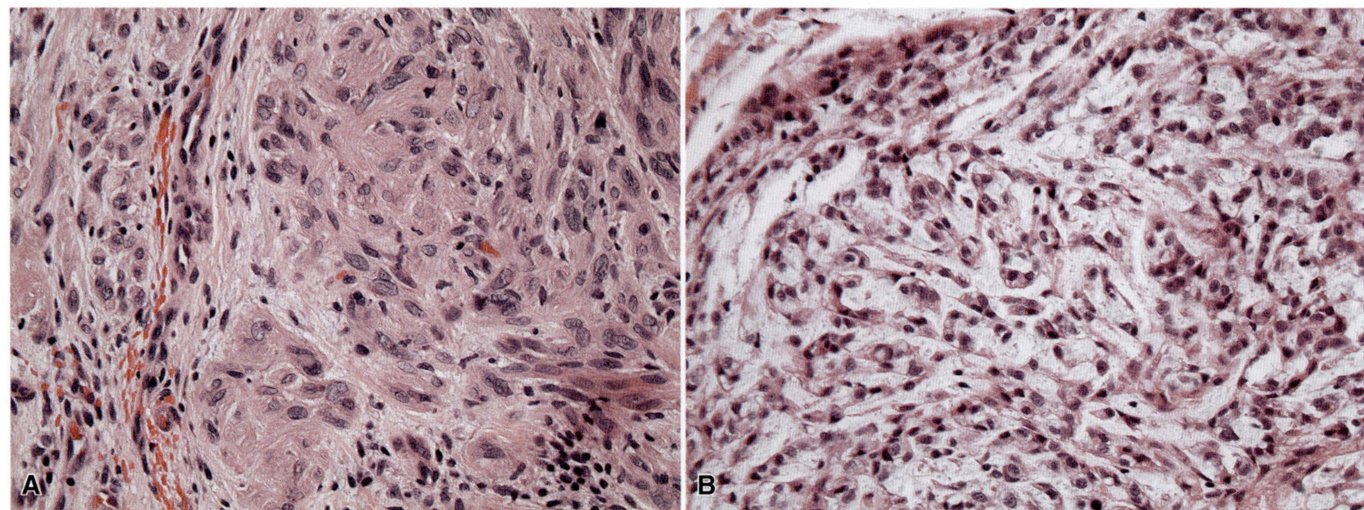

Figure 15.94 Epithelioid Schwannoma. The tumor is composed of bland epithelioid to polygonal cells with fibrillary eosinophilic cytoplasm (A). Some tumors show prominent myxoid stroma. Note the trabecular growth pattern (B).

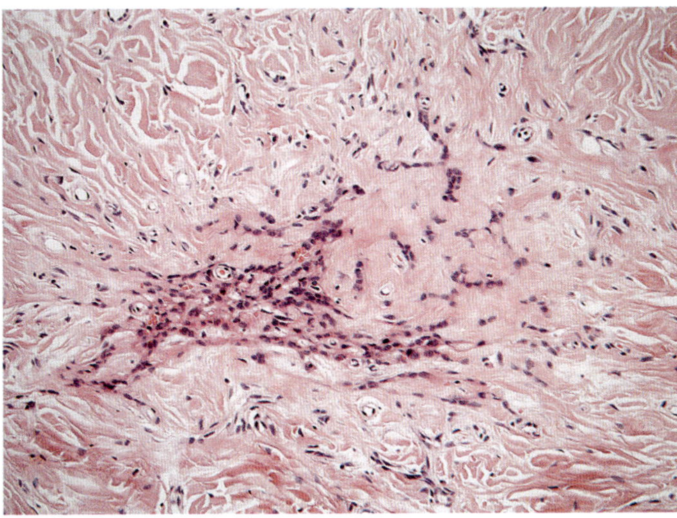

Figure 15.95 Sclerosing Perineurioma. The tumor is composed of cords of rounded cells in a dense collagenous stroma.

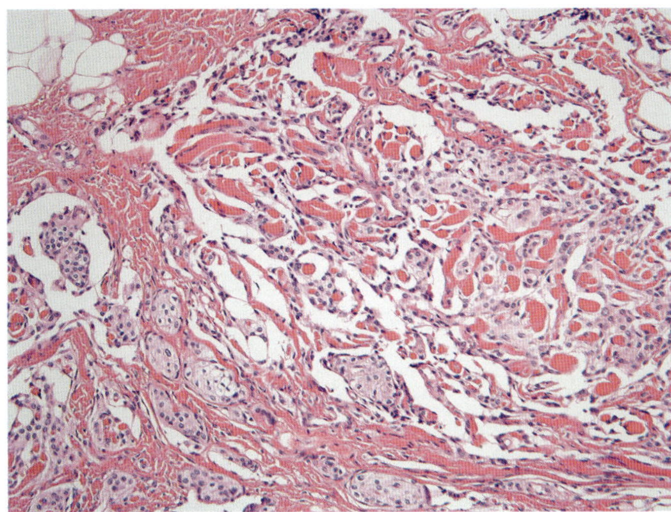

Figure 15.97 Cutaneous Meningioma. The tumor is composed of lobules of ovoid cells and shows infiltrative margins.

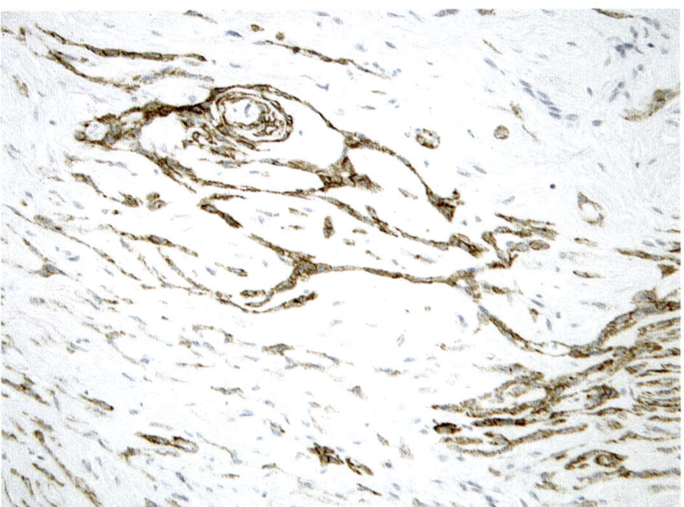

Figure 15.96 Sclerosing Perineurioma. The tumor cells are positive for epithelial membrane antigen.

but involves deep (tendinous) tissue rather than the dermis. In contrast to the epithelioid cytomorphology of sclerosing perineurioma, fibroma of tendon sheath is composed of cellular fascicles of short spindle cells that are negative for EMA. Tenosynovial giant cell tumors also involve the fingers and may show extensive stromal hyalinization. However, giant cell tumor of tendon sheath is typically deep seated and contains sheets of small mononuclear histiocytoid cells, as well as occasional foam cells and osteoclastic giant cells. Storiform collagenoma is a well-circumscribed dermal nodule consisting of a storiform arrangement of small, bland spindle cells in a collagenous stroma with cleftlike spaces. Multiple lesions are a typical feature of Cowden syndrome. Storiform collagenoma lacks the epithelioid morphology and EMA expression of sclerosing perineurioma. Glomus tumors may sometimes contain collagenous stroma and show rounded to epithelioid cytomorphology, similar to sclerosing perineurioma. However, glomus tumors usually show sheetlike areas with cells within the walls of blood vessels and are strongly positive for SMA and negative for EMA. Adnexal tumors also express EMA but often show focal ductal differentiation, and they are typically positive for keratins. Epithelioid hemangioendothelioma is also composed of cords of epithelioid cells but usually contains a characteristic myxohyaline stroma, is negative for EMA, and consistently shows expression of CD31, ERG, and CAMTA1.

Prognosis and Treatment

Sclerosing perineuriomas are benign. They do not recur.[166]

Cutaneous Meningioma and Ectopic Meningothelial Hamartoma

Meningiomas indistinguishable from primary dural tumors rarely occur in the skin and subcutaneous tissue.[167-169] In such cases, extension from an underlying intracranial tumor should be excluded. A distinctive meningothelial lesion known as *ectopic meningothelial hamartoma* may mimic angiosarcoma.[170] Extracranial meningioma is also discussed in Chapter 6.

Clinical Features

Cutaneous meningiomas typically occur on the scalp of infants and young children, although adolescents and young adults may occasionally be affected.[167–168] The typical clinical presentation is of a painless nodule. Tumors may be up to several centimeters in size. Ectopic meningothelial hamartomas have similar clinical features.[170]

Pathologic Features

Many cutaneous meningiomas show similar histologic features as primary dural meningiomas being composed of lobules and sheets of uniform ovoid, epithelioid, or spindle cells in a whorled architecture. An infiltrative growth pattern through the dermis and subcutaneous tissue is common (Fig. 15.97). Ectopic meningothelial hamartoma is composed of uniform cuboidal to epithelioid cells showing a complex, infiltrative growth pattern between dermal structures, around blood vessels, and within adipose and deeper connective tissues (Figs. 15.98 and 15.99).[170] Dilated pseudovascular channels and microcystic architecture are typical features (see Fig. 15.98).

Immunohistochemistry

Like conventional meningioma, the lesional cells in cutaneous meningioma and ectopic meningothelial hamartoma are positive for EMA (Fig. 15.100) but are negative for S-100 protein, CD34, and CD31.

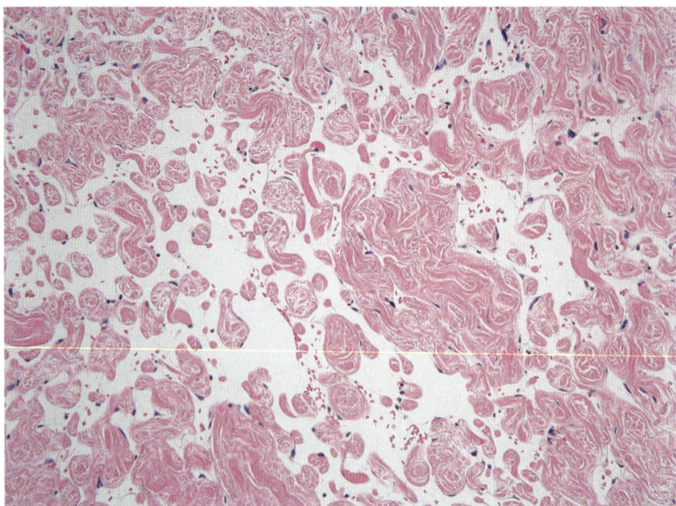

Figure 15.98 Ectopic Meningothelial Hamartoma. The lesion shows an infiltrative architecture with dilated pseudovascular spaces.

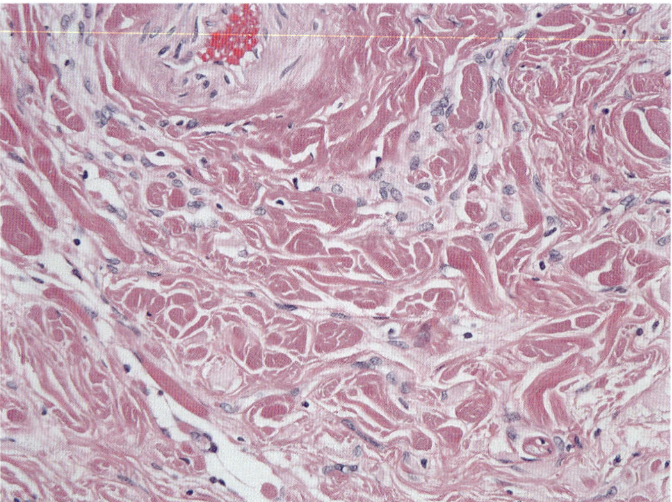

Figure 15.99 Ectopic Meningothelial Hamartoma. The lesional cells are uniform and rounded with pale cytoplasm. Note the infiltrative growth pattern.

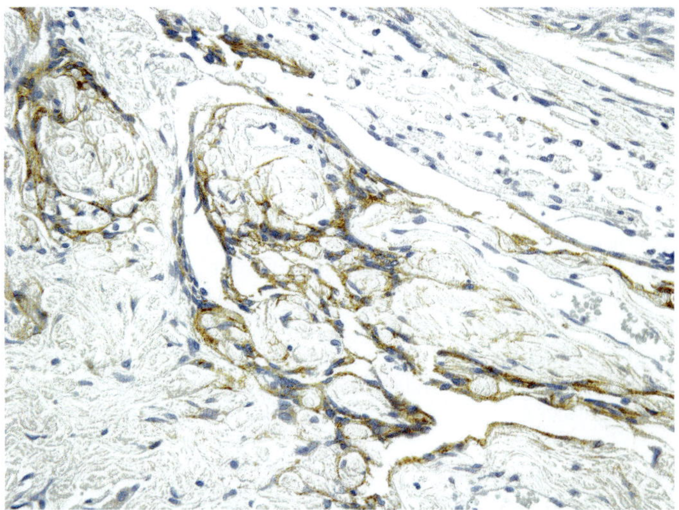

Figure 15.100 Ectopic Meningothelial Hamartoma. The cells are positive for epithelial membrane antigen.

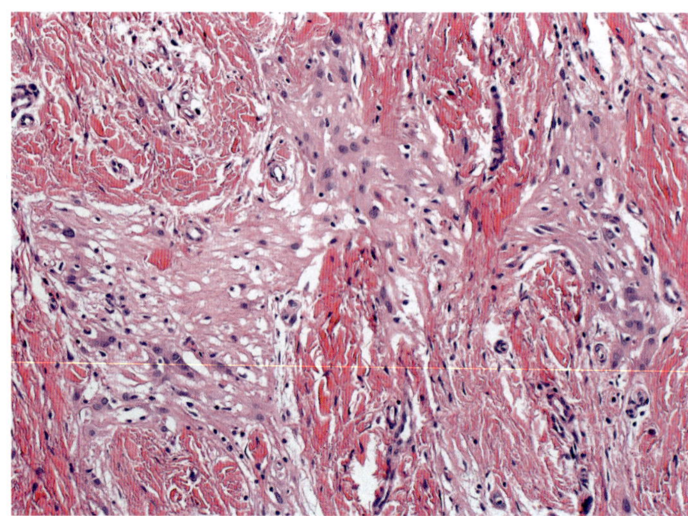

Figure 15.101 Nasal Glioma. The tumor is composed of nests of large cells with abundant fibrillary cytoplasm in a fibrotic stroma.

Differential Diagnosis

Before diagnosing cutaneous meningioma, extension from an intracranial tumor should be excluded. Soft tissue perineurioma shows similar cytoarchitectural features but usually lacks the lobulated growth pattern and infiltrative margins of cutaneous meningioma. Both tumor types express EMA; diffuse staining for CD34 favors perineurioma. Ectopic meningothelial hamartoma may be confused with a vascular neoplasm, especially angiosarcoma, given the pseudoinfiltrative architecture. However, endothelial neoplasms are negative for EMA but consistently show expression of CD31 and ERG.

Prognosis and Treatment

Cutaneous meningioma and ectopic meningothelial hamartoma are benign lesions. They do not recur.

Nasal Glioma (Nasal Glial Heterotopia)

Rarely, heterotopic glial tissue can present clinically as a mass lesion, most commonly in the nasal cavity but occasionally on the bridge or elsewhere on the nose in subcutaneous tissue or dermis. Although these lesions are known as *nasal glioma*, they are likely heterotopic in nature.[168] Patients typically present in infancy or early childhood, with lesions ranging in size from 1 to 5 cm. Histologic appearances are those of normal glial tissue containing astrocytes and neurofibrillary matrix (Fig. 15.101). Immunohistochemistry for S-100 protein and GFAP is strongly positive (Figs. 15.102 and 15.103). After the nature of the tissue is recognized, diagnosis is straightforward. Recurrence is rare following surgical excision.

Juvenile Xanthogranuloma and Related Disorders

The clinical and histologic spectrum of non-Langerhans cell histiocytoses is broad, and the literature on this topic is confusing. Many different entities in this disease group have been reported, often only as single case reports, reflecting the rarity of most of these disorders. We favor a unifying concept suggesting that there is a disease spectrum, with JXG being the most frequent and prototypical disease.[171,172] Other entities such as reticulohistiocytoma, multicentric reticulohistiocytosis, spindle cell xanthogranuloma, scalloped cell xanthogranuloma, benign cephalic histiocytosis, generalized eruptive histiocytoma, papular xanthoma, and xanthoma disseminatum show some distinctive clinical and histologic features, but most, if not all, of these lesions show significant overlap with JXG. Only JXG, reticulohistiocytoma, and multicentric reticulohistiocytosis will be covered in detail in this chapter.

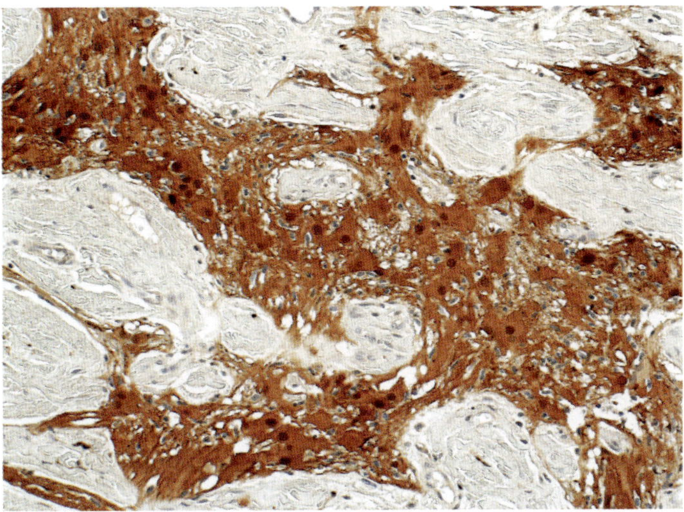

Figure 15.102 **Nasal Glioma.** S-100 is strongly positive in lesional cells.

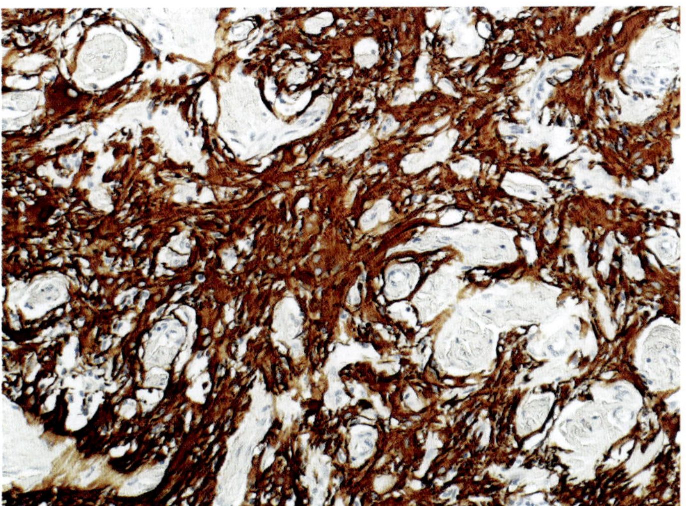

Figure 15.103 **Nasal Glioma.** The lesional cells also express glial fibrillary acidic protein.

Clinical Features

JXG is an uncommon disease that predominantly affects young children and infants. It has a slight male predominance.[173,174] A congenital presentation is seen in approximately one-third of patients. Adolescents and adults may also be affected (xanthogranuloma).

Tumors are predominantly solitary, and the skin is the most frequently affected organ. JXG shows a predilection for the head and neck, as well as the trunk.[173,174] Presentation in adolescents or adults is usually as solitary cutaneous tumors, whereas multicentric disease and involvement of deep soft tissue and visceral organs is largely restricted to infants and young children.[173,174] Cutaneous lesions occur as firm papules or plaques measuring less than 1 cm and showing erythematous to yellowish discoloration.[173,174] In contrast, soft tissue tumors are typically larger, measuring less than 3 cm in subcutis, but typically more than 4 cm in deep soft tissue.

Pathologic Features

Cutaneous JXG is centered within the dermis as a relatively circumscribed tumor with a nodular or multinodular growth pattern (Fig. 15.104). Focal extension into subcutis may be seen. Tumors are characteristically composed of an admixture of mononuclear histiocytes,

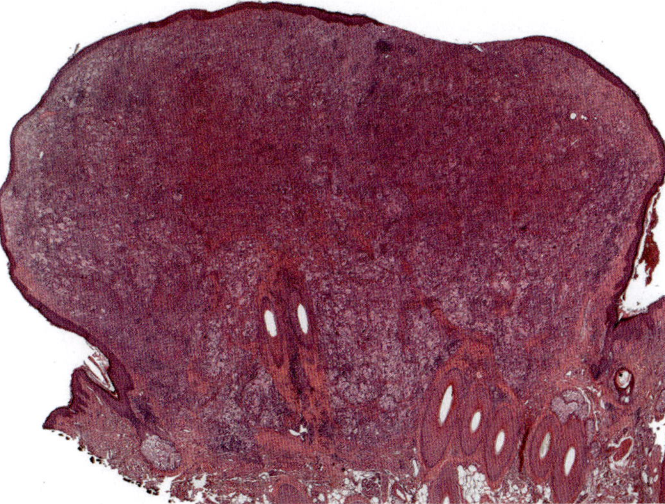

Figure 15.104 **Juvenile Xanthogranuloma.** This dermal-based tumor shows a nodular and polypoid growth pattern.

multinucleated giant cells, and spindle cells in varying numbers and showing varying degrees of lipidization (Fig. 15.105). An admixed inflammatory cell infiltrate composed of neutrophils, lymphocytes, plasma cells, and eosinophils may also be present. The classic lesions of JXG show abundant mononuclear histiocytes with moderate amounts of eosinophilic to vacuolated cytoplasm and round to ovoid nuclei, in addition to conspicuous multinucleated giant cells, which are predominantly of the Touton type, characterized by a central core of eosinophilic cytoplasm surrounded by a peripheral ring of multiple nuclei and an outermost layer of vacuolated foamy cytoplasm (Fig. 15.106). Other multinucleated giant cells, including foreign body–type giant cells and Langhans-type giant cells, may also be present. Engulfing of inflammatory cells by multinucleated giant cells (emperipolesis) may occasionally be observed. Early lesions show a predominance of the mononuclear histiocytes with more eosinophilic and less vacuolated cytoplasm. Lipidization is less pronounced, and Touton-type giant cells are sparse or absent. Mitotic activity is often more conspicuous than in classic lesions. Occasionally, spindle cells predominate, and stromal fibrosis may be present in older lesions. The overlying epidermis is uninvolved and often atrophic and flattened. Epidermal ulceration may be observed. There are no significant morphologic differences between cutaneous lesions arising in childhood or in adulthood. Deep-seated tumors are often well circumscribed but may show infiltration into adjacent tissues. Their appearance is more frequently monomorphous, and lipidization is less pronounced.

Immunohistochemistry

Mononuclear histiocytes show strong, diffuse expression of CD68, CD163, and CD4 and are often positive for factor XIIIa. Focal and scattered reactivity for S-100 protein may be observed in a minority of cases, but no expression of CD1a or langerin is seen. Spindle cells may be positive for SMA.

Differential Diagnosis

The fully developed classic lesions of JXG rarely present a diagnostic dilemma. More problematic are early lesions with abundant mononuclear histiocytes, lack of Touton-type giant cells, and little or no lipidization. Melanocytic tumors are excluded immunohistochemically by absence of S-100 protein, HMB-45, and melan A expression, and carcinoma is excluded by lack of keratin expression. Distinction from Langerhans cell histiocytosis (Fig. 15.107) can be made by lack of epidermotropism

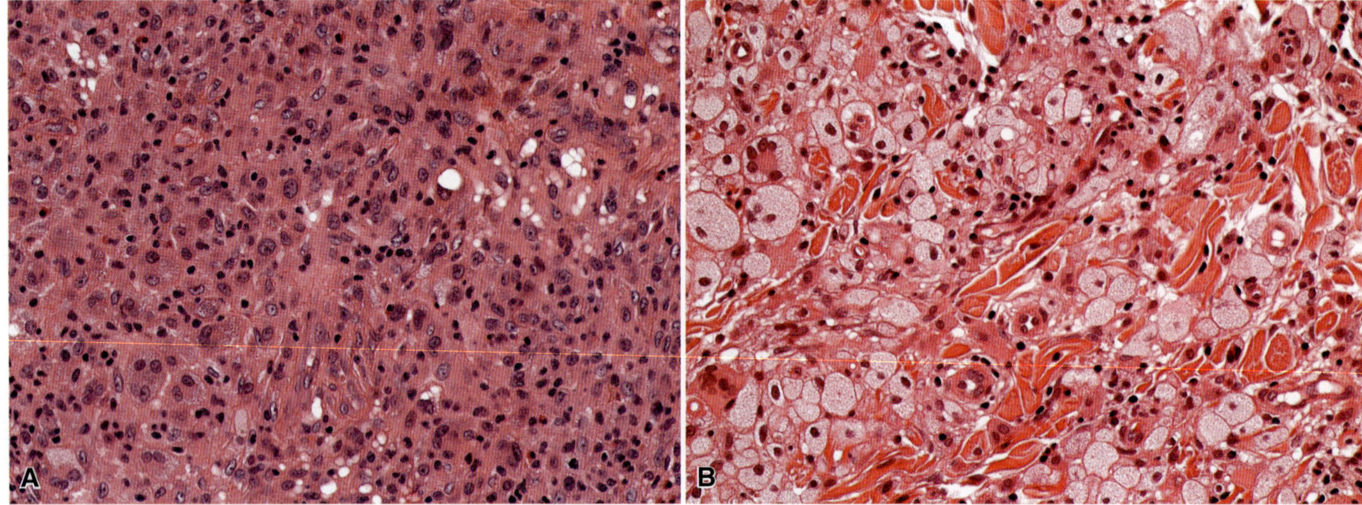

Figure 15.105 Juvenile Xanthogranuloma. The tumor is composed of sheets of small epithelioid cells (A). In areas, xanthomatous cells predominate (B).

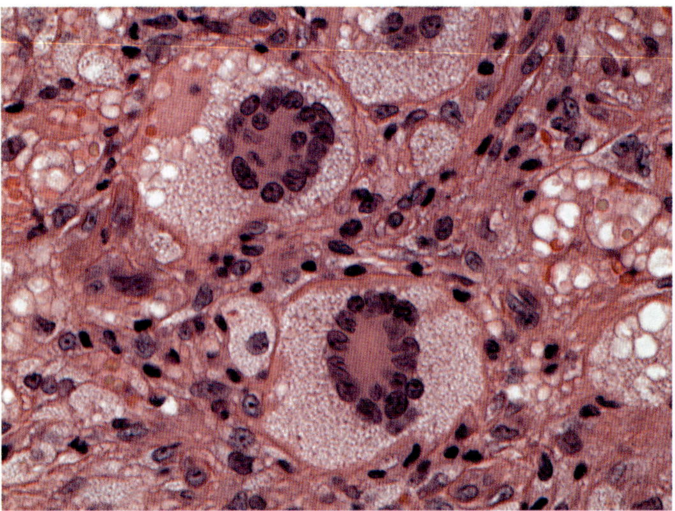

Figure 15.106 Juvenile Xanthogranuloma. The presence of Touton-type giant cells is a characteristic feature.

and absence of S-100 protein, CD1a (see Fig. 15.107C), and langerin expression. Xanthoma shows uniform lipidization and lacks admixed inflammatory cells and the characteristic multinucleated giant cells. JXG showing extensive stromal fibrosis may resemble benign fibrous histiocytoma, but the latter shows epidermal hyperplasia, peripheral collagen entrapment, and a more heterogeneous composition. Cutaneous Rosai-Dorfman disease is characterized by the presence of characteristic large S-100 protein–positive histiocytes with round, vesicular nuclei and prominent nucleoli. Distinction from other non–Langerhans cell histiocytoses may be difficult. As discussed earlier, these entities are closely related to JXG and may represent part of a clinicopathologic spectrum. Reticulohistiocytoma and multicentric reticulohistiocytosis are briefly discussed later.

Prognosis and Treatment

The prognosis in children is very good; there is a tendency for spontaneous regression and resolution. Simple excision is curative for solitary cutaneous tumors. Mortality is very rare and due to visceral involvement with subsequent organ failure.

Reticulohistiocytoma

Reticulohistiocytoma is a rare lesion presenting as a small solitary cutaneous papule or nodule measuring less than 1 cm in diameter.[175] Individuals over a wide age range may be affected, but the lesion classically presents in early adulthood (20 to 40 years) and has a slight male predominance.[176] The anatomic distribution is broad and includes the oral cavity.[175] However, the digits and face appear largely to be spared. Simple excision is curative. Histologically, reticulohistiocytoma is a relatively circumscribed, nodular tumor within the dermis with possible extension into superficial subcutis. It is composed of characteristic mononuclear and multinucleated epithelioid histiocytes with abundant brightly eosinophilic, glassy-appearing cytoplasm containing bland round to ovoid nuclei (Fig. 15.108). Mild nuclear pleomorphism and rare mitotic activity may be present. An admixed inflammatory infiltrate composed of lymphocytes, plasma cells, eosinophils, and neutrophils in varying proportions is typical. The lesional histiocytes are positive for CD68 and CD163 by immunohistochemistry. Rare and focal staining for S-100 protein but not CD1a may be observed.

Multicentric Reticulohistiocytosis

Multicentric reticulohistiocytosis is a multisystem disease affecting adults, with a mean age of 50 years.[177] In contrast to reticulohistiocytoma, with which it shares many histologic features, there is a female predominance and a predilection for the hands followed by the face, extremities, and trunk.[176,177] Mucosal lesions, which predominantly affect the oral cavity, are present in approximately 30% of cases.[177] Cutaneous lesions are multiple and symmetrical papules and nodules, ranging from several millimeters to a few centimeters. These are frequently accompanied by a progressive, symmetrical erosive arthritis, which often is the presenting symptom.[177] The joints of the hand, wrist, and knee are predominantly affected, followed by the shoulder and ankles. The clinical course is characterized by remission and relapse, most often resulting in a disfiguring and crippling arthritis.[177] The disease is frequently accompanied by generalized systemic symptoms, such as weight loss, fever, malaise, myalgia, and lymphadenopathy. Occasionally, there may be an underlying malignancy or associated autoimmune disease.[177,178] Histologically, multicentric reticulohistiocytosis is characterized by a circumscribed collection of histiocytes reminiscent of but usually smaller than those of

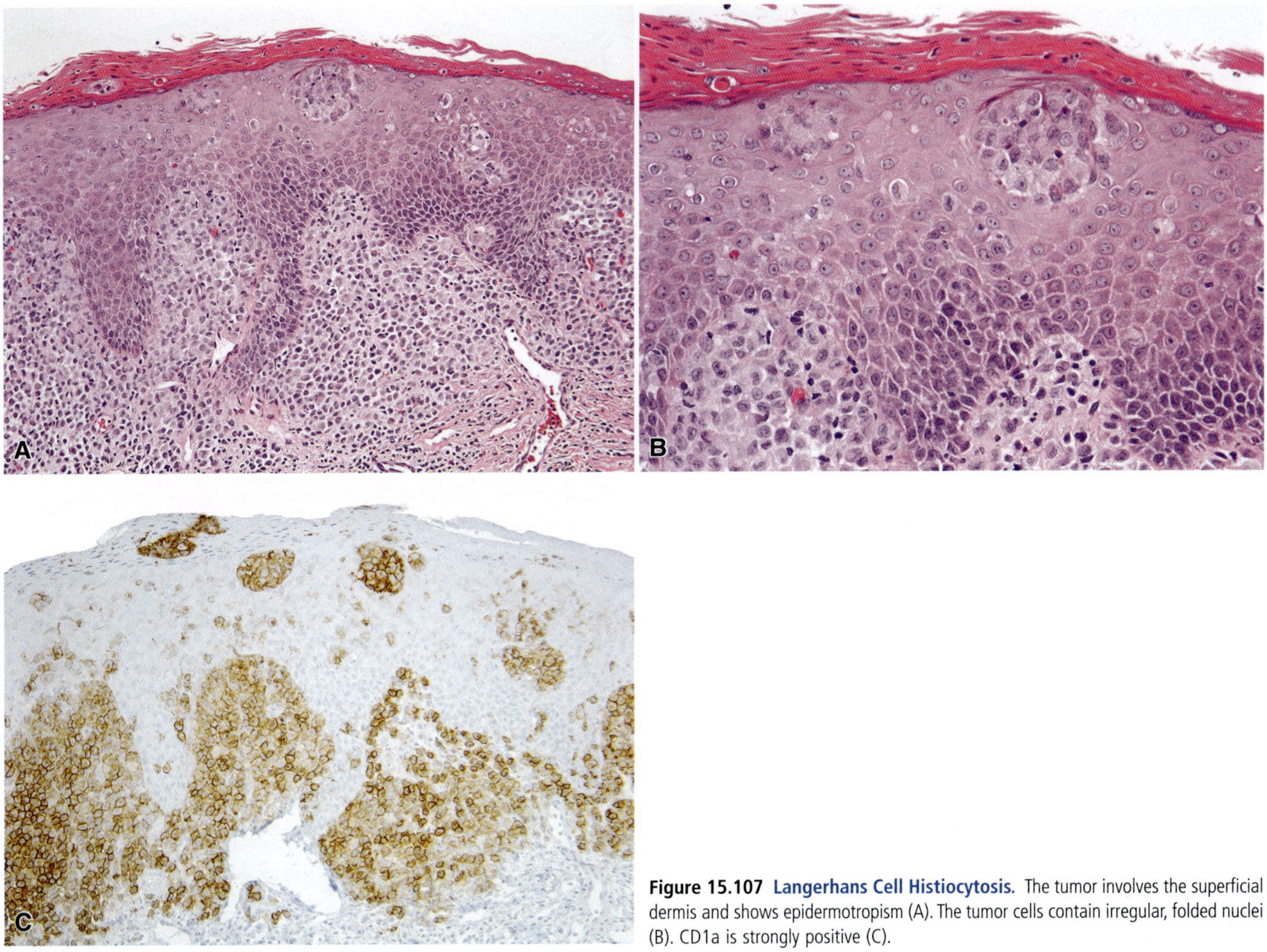

Figure 15.107 **Langerhans Cell Histiocytosis.** The tumor involves the superficial dermis and shows epidermotropism (A). The tumor cells contain irregular, folded nuclei (B). CD1a is strongly positive (C).

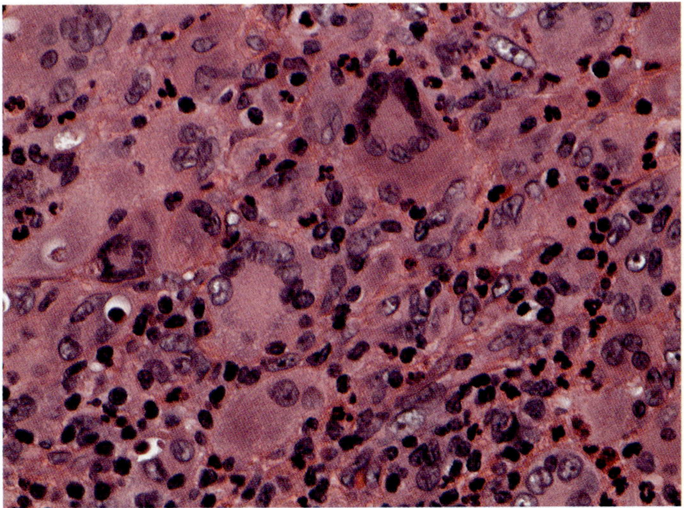

Figure 15.108 **Reticulohistiocytoma.** Tumor cells are mononucleated or multinucleated with abundant eosinophilic, "glassy" cytoplasm. There is a background of inflammatory cells.

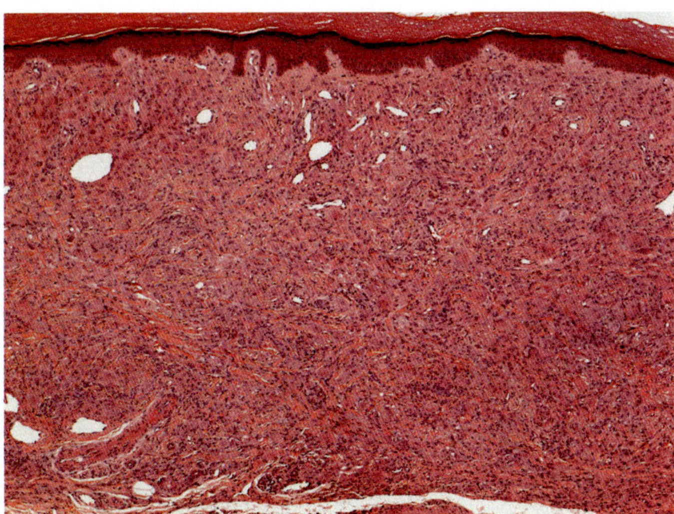

Figure 15.109 **Multicentric Reticulohistiocytosis.** This dermal-based tumor shows a plaquelike growth pattern.

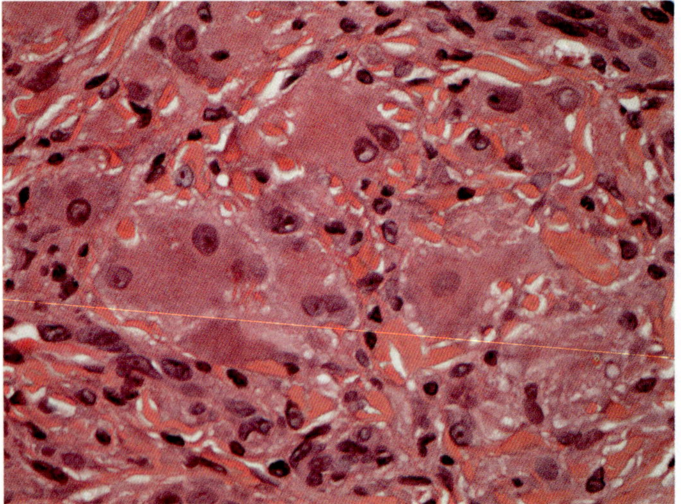

Figure 15.110 **Multicentric Reticulohistiocytosis.** Histiocytes show cytologic features similar to those seen in reticulohistiocytoma.

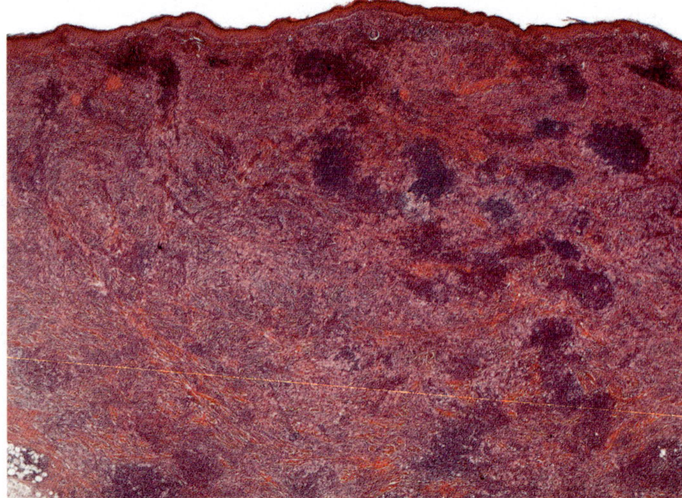

Figure 15.111 **Cutaneous Rosai-Dorfman Disease.** A nodular growth centered within the dermis is the typical presentation.

reticulohistiocytoma (Figs. 15.109 and 15.110). In addition, these lesions may appear more lipidized. The immunohistochemical phenotype is that of histiocytes, identical to reticulohistiocytoma.

Cutaneous Rosai-Dorfman Disease

Sinus histiocytosis with massive lymphadenopathy or Rosai-Dorfman disease is also discussed in Chapter 10. Extranodal involvement is seen in more than 40% of patients, and the skin is among the most frequently affected sites. In additions, Rosai-Dorfman disease can show purely extranodal manifestations. Disease confined to the skin (cutaneous Rosai-Dorfman disease) is not an uncommon clinical presentation, which shows distinct clinicopathologic features.

In contrast to its nodal counterpart, cutaneous Rosai-Dorfman disease shows a predilection for females and predominantly affects middle-aged adults of Caucasian and Asian descent.[179–183] The disease is frequently multifocal with a clinical presentation as plaques and nodules showing discoloration. There is no predilection for specific anatomic regions. The disease course is chronic and characterized by persistence of lesions, spontaneous resolution, and recurrences.

The histologic hallmark is the presence of the characteristic S-100 protein–positive histiocytes within the lesion, often in a sheetlike arrangement. These distinctive histiocytes are large polygonal cells containing abundant palely eosinophilic cytoplasm and large, round, vesicular nuclei with prominent nucleoli. A mixed inflammatory infiltrate containing lymphocytes, plasma cells, eosinophils, and neutrophils is typically present in varying amounts. Individual or clusters of inflammatory cells may be engulfed by the histiocytes, a finding also referred to as *emperipolesis,* which is a helpful diagnostic clue. Lesions of cutaneous Rosai-Dorfman disease have a nodular appearance with somewhat infiltrative margins (Fig. 15.111). They are centered within the dermis, but subcutaneous involvement may also be evident. Occasionally, the lesions show a sclerotic stromal response, making the diagnosis challenging. The differential diagnosis includes JXG and reticulohistiocytoma. The presence of the characteristic pale histiocytes with voluminous cytoplasm, emperipolesis, and expression of S-100 protein by immunohistochemistry is diagnostic (Figs. 15.112 and 15.113).

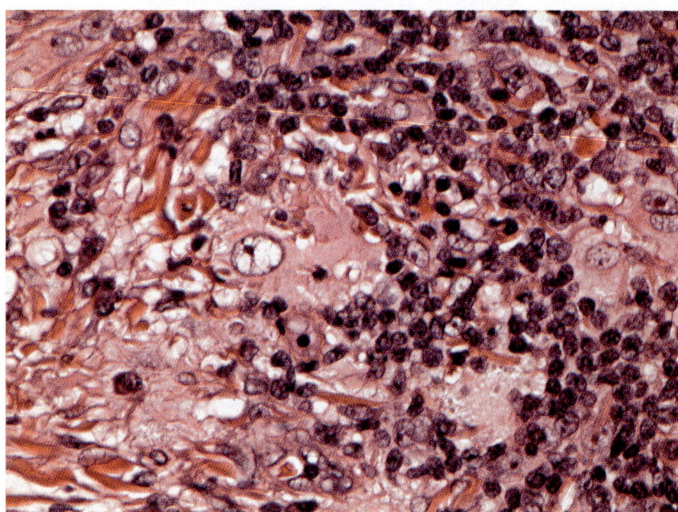

Figure 15.112 **Cutaneous Rosai-Dorfman Disease.** Large polygonal histiocytes containing abundant palely eosinophilic cytoplasm and large vesicular nuclei with eosinophilic nucleoli are pathognomonic. Also note the presence of an admixed chronic inflammatory infiltrate.

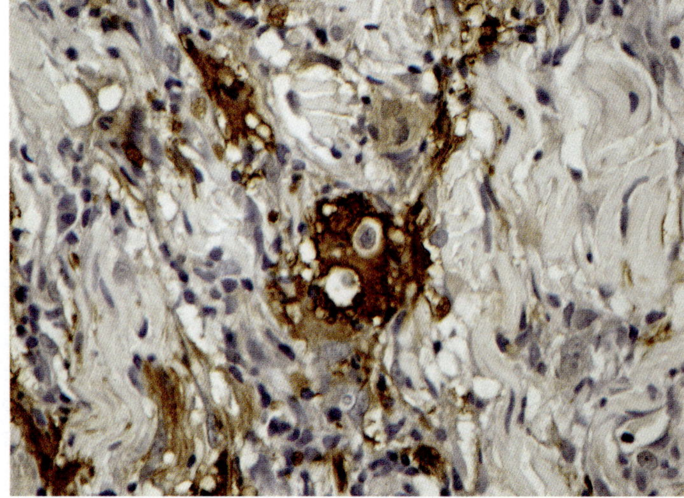

Figure 15.113 **Cutaneous Rosai-Dorfman Disease.** Histiocytes express S-100 by immunohistochemistry. This also highlights emperipolesis.

Epithelioid Sarcoma

This tumor type is discussed in Chapter 6.

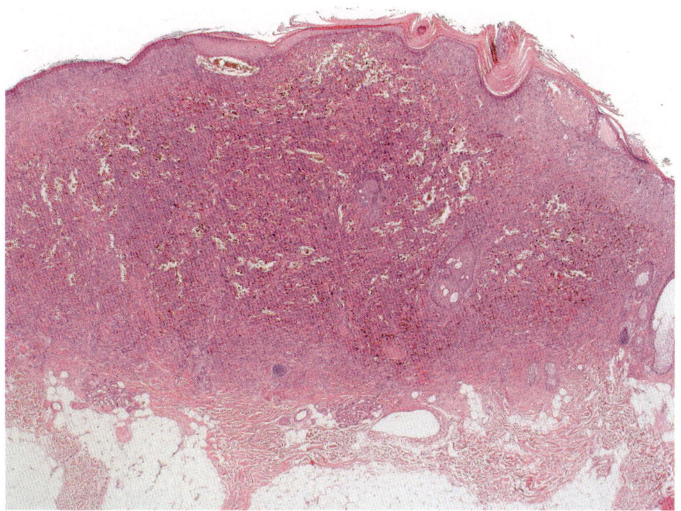

Figure 15.114 **Atypical Fibroxanthoma.** This well-circumscribed tumor has pushing rather than infiltrative borders and is confined to the dermis.

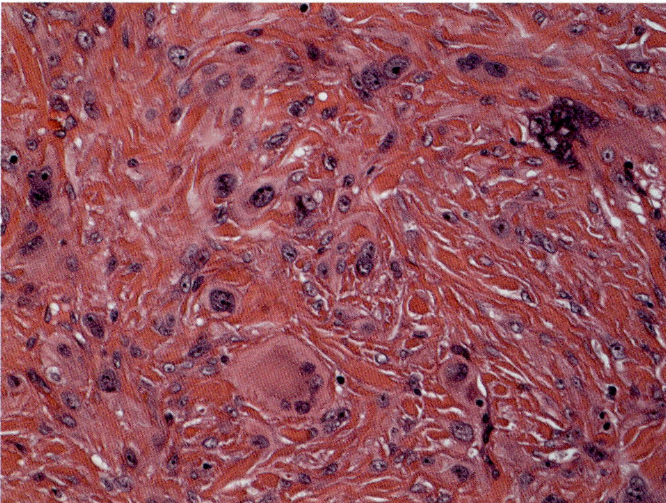

Figure 15.115 **Atypical Fibroxanthoma.** The tumor is composed of pleomorphic epithelioid, multinucleate, and xanthomatous cells.

Pleomorphic Tumors

Atypical Fibroxanthoma

AFX is an unusual dermal tumor occurring in a well-defined clinical setting. AFX is a diagnosis of exclusion, and its clinical behavior is entirely benign if strict diagnostic criteria are applied. Similar tumors showing invasion of subcutis or deeper structures or other features of malignancy such as tumor necrosis or lymphovascular and perineural invasion are characterized by locally destructive growth and have the potential for local recurrence and rarely distant metastasis. These tumors are best regarded as pleomorphic dermal sarcoma (see subsequent discussion).[184] The designation "superficial variant of malignant fibrous histiocytoma" has also been applied as a synonym for AFX; however, this term should be avoided because it implies the biologic potential of a high-grade sarcoma with the possibility of significant overtreatment (see also Chapter 7).

Clinical Features

AFX invariably presents on sun-exposed and actinically damaged skin of the head and neck area of elderly patients. Peak incidence occurs in the seventh to eighth decade.[185–187] Tumors appear relatively circumscribed and nodular, measuring a few centimeters in diameter. There is typically a short history of rapid growth, and ulceration is common. Occasionally, tumors appear pigmented due to extensive hemosiderin deposition.[188] Like other neoplasms arising on sun-damaged skin, AFX has been observed in younger patients with xeroderma pigmentosum.

Pathologic Features

Tumors are characteristically well demarcated with pushing rather than infiltrative borders (Fig. 15.114).[185,189] They frequently show a polypoid appearance with a surrounding epidermal collarette. The tumor abuts the overlying epidermis, and ulceration is common. By definition, AFX is confined to the dermis, but focal extension into the very superficial subcutis with a pushing border is acceptable. In its classic form, AFX is composed of an admixture of pleomorphic spindle and epithelioid cells, as well as multinucleate giant cells and xanthomatous cells (Fig. 15.115). The nuclei are frequently hyperchromatic and appear bizarre, and mitotic figures including atypical forms are easily found (Fig. 15.116). Hemosiderin deposition is a frequent and occasionally prominent finding (hemosiderotic variant).[188] Furthermore, intratumoral hemorrhage and blood-filled spaces may be observed (pseudoangiomatous variant) (Fig. 15.117).[190] Clear cell change, granular cell change, a keloidal stromal reaction, or osteoclast-like

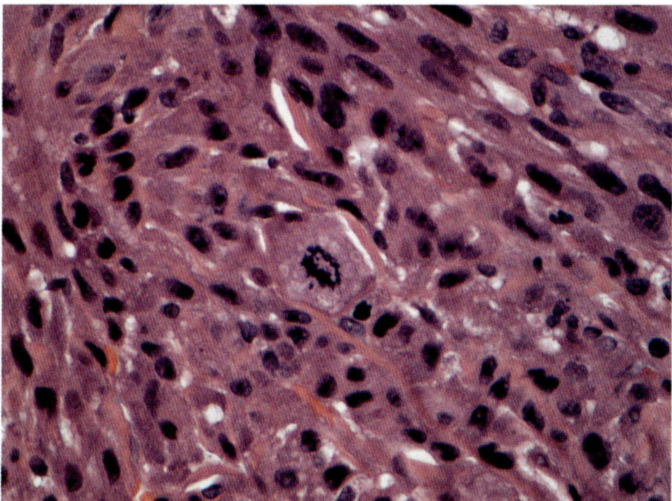

Figure 15.116 **Atypical Fibroxanthoma.** Atypical mitotic figures are easily identified.

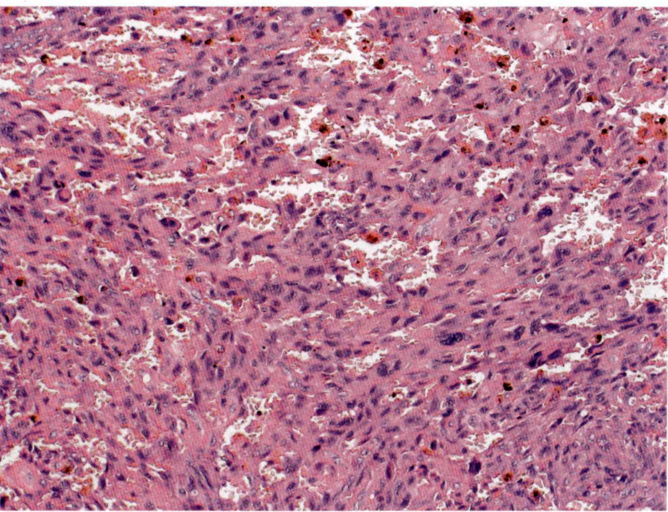

Figure 15.117 **Atypical Fibroxanthoma.** Hemorrhage and pseudovascular spaces may mimic angiosarcoma.

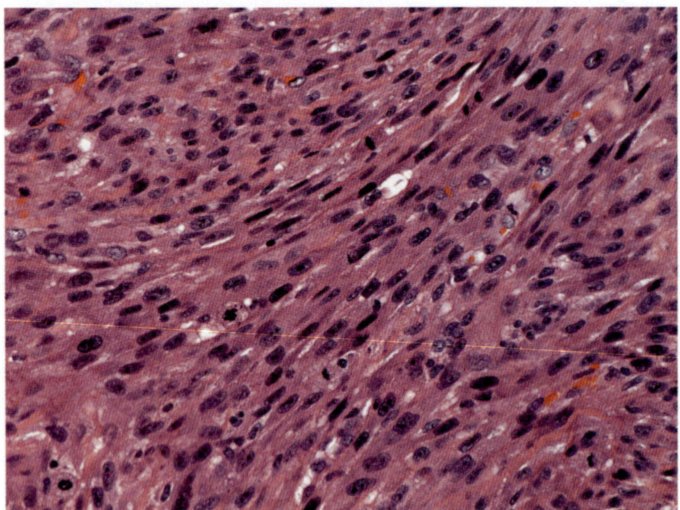

Figure 15.118 **Atypical Fibroxanthoma.** The spindle cell variant is characterized by the presence of atypical spindle cells in a fascicular arrangement.

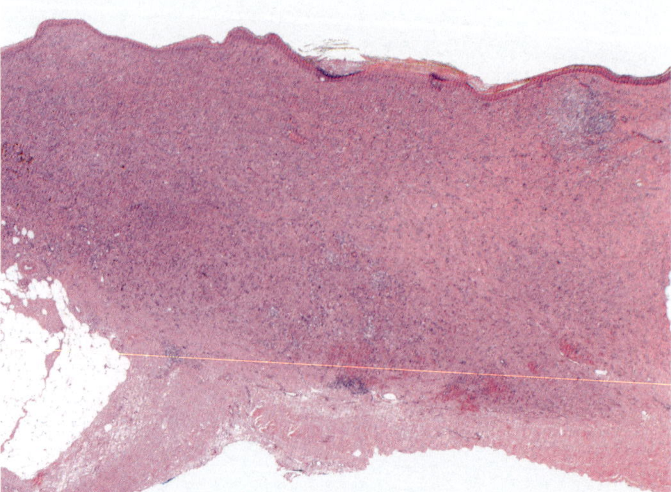

Figure 15.119 **Pleomorphic Dermal Sarcoma.** These poorly demarcated tumors are based within dermis and invade into subcutaneous fat and underlying fibrous tissue.

giant cells may be present in varying amounts.[187,188,191–193] The spindle cell variant is not uncommon and is characterized by a relatively monomorphic population of atypical spindle cells (Fig. 15.118).[185,194] Solar elastosis of the adjacent or underlying dermis and nearby squamous dysplasia are often present in association with AFX.

Immunohistochemistry

Tumor cells are often focally positive for SMA and calponin, as well as CD10, CD68, CD99, and procollagen I.[195–198] These markers lack specificity and play no real role in diagnosis. Importantly, tumor cells do not express keratins, S-100 protein, desmin, or h-caldesmon. However, colonization of the tumor by S-100 protein–positive dendritic cells may be seen and may lead to misinterpretation of S-100 protein expression in tumor cells.[195,199] A small subset of tumors shows melan A expression in multinucleated giant cells.[200] CD31 expression is rarely observed. When present, it is weak and granular, similar to the staining pattern observed in histiocytes and unlike the strong membranous staining in endothelial cells.[189]

Molecular Genetics

Studies have identified the classic ultraviolet (UV)-induced *TP53* mutations and *TERT* promoter mutations confirming sun exposure as an etiologic mechanism in tumor development.[201–204] *HRAS* and *PIK3CA* are rarely mutated, but no mutations have been detected in the *KRAS* or *NRAS* genes in AFX.[204,205]

Differential Diagnosis

AFX is a diagnosis of exclusion. Important considerations include other tumors with a predilection for sun-exposed skin of the elderly. These include melanoma, poorly differentiated or spindle cell squamous cell carcinoma, and angiosarcoma. Epidermal origin, the presence of better-differentiated areas, and keratin, p63 and p40 expression by immunohistochemistry support a diagnosis of squamous cell carcinoma. However, it is important to note that keratin expression in poorly differentiated squamous cell carcinoma may be focal; often, multiple antibodies against keratins need to be used to confirm the diagnosis. Spindle cell melanoma should be entertained when junctional melanocytic activity or outright melanoma in situ is present. The presence of S-100 protein expression is further support for this diagnosis. Of note, other melanocytic markers such as HMB-45 and melan A are often negative in spindle cell melanomas. Spindle cell angiosarcoma can be recognized by the identification of vasoformative elements, in addition to the expression of endothelial markers such as CD31, CD34, and ERG by tumor cells.

Cutaneous leiomyosarcoma, either metastatic or primary, may also enter the differential diagnosis. These tumors are characterized by fascicles of spindle cells containing brightly eosinophilic cytoplasm and plump, cigar-shaped nuclei. Smooth muscle differentiation can be confirmed using desmin and h-caldesmon immunohistochemistry. Atypical fibrous histiocytoma is another histologic mimic. However, presentation on the head and neck of the elderly would be unusual for fibrous histiocytoma. Furthermore, evaluation of the periphery of the tumor for the typical pattern of collagen entrapment and identification of more conventional areas of fibrous histiocytoma are helpful in this instance.

Prognosis and Treatment

If strict diagnostic criteria are applied, AFX is a benign tumor with essentially no potential for local recurrence or metastasis.[185] Complete excision to allow assessment of the entire tumor and its deepest extent is critical to confirm:

- Lack of infiltration of subcutis
- Absence of perineural or lymphovascular invasion
- Absence of tumor necrosis

The presence of any of these features is not compatible with a diagnosis of AFX and confers the potential for recurrence and uncommon distant metastasis.[185,206] These tumors should then be regarded as dermal sarcomas (Fig. 15.119).[184] Therefore the diagnosis of AFX cannot be made reliably on a shave or other superficial biopsy. Provided the requisite markers (several keratins and S-100 protein) are negative, in such a biopsy, a diagnosis of *atypical intradermal spindle cell neoplasm* is appropriate, with a comment that complete excision is advised before a definitive diagnosis of AFX can be rendered.

PRACTICE POINTS: Histologic Criteria for the Diagnosis of Atypical Fibroxanthoma

Tumor circumscription
Lack of infiltrative growth
Lack of subcutaneous involvement
Lack of perineural or lymphovascular invasion
Lack of tumor necrosis
Lack of melanocytic, epithelial, or muscle differentiation by immunohistochemistry

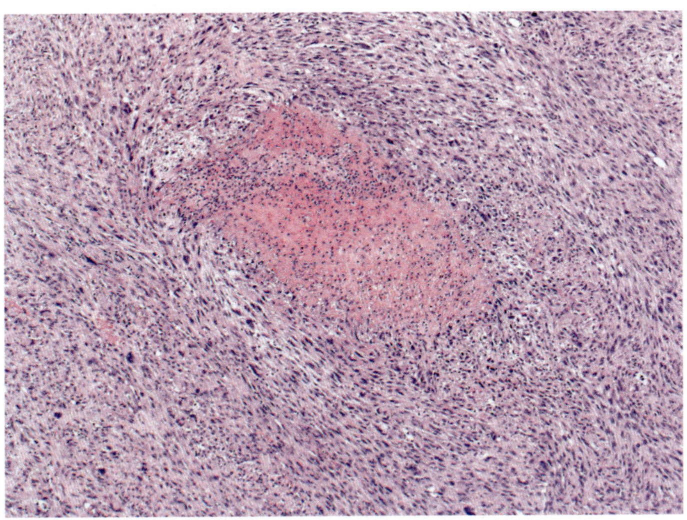

Figure 15.120 **Pleomorphic Dermal Sarcoma.** Tumor necrosis is present.

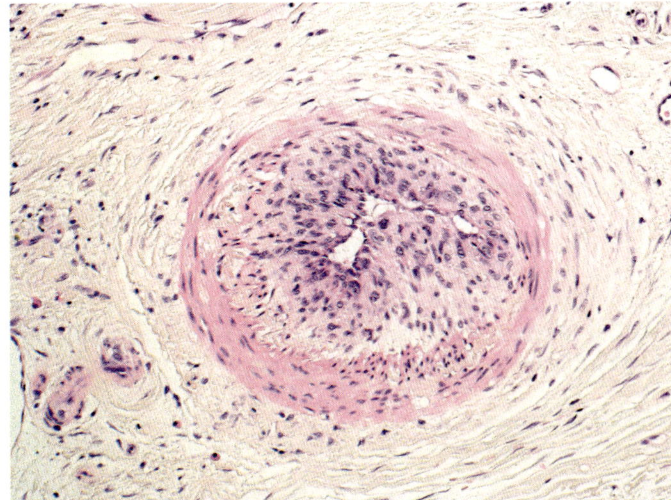

Figure 15.121 **Pleomorphic Dermal Sarcoma.** A focus of lymphovascular invasion is noted.

Pleomorphic Dermal Sarcoma

Pleomorphic dermal sarcoma, also referred to as undifferentiated pleomorphic sarcoma of the skin, is a tumor with similar clinical presentation, morphology, and immunohistochemical profile to AFX. However, the additional presence of subcutaneous tissue infiltration, lymphovascular or perineural invasion, or tumor necrosis confers potential for aggressive behavior.[184]

Clinical Features

The tumors present as large nodules and plaques with a median diameter of 2.5 cm. They occur exclusively on sun-damaged skin and show a strong predilection for the scalp of elderly males.[184]

Pathologic Features

Pleomorphic dermal sarcoma is a large and frequently ill-defined dermal-based tumor (see Fig. 15.119). It extends to the overlying epidermis, which may be ulcerated. The tumor commonly invades subcutaneous adipose tissue and may extend into underlying skeletal muscle, fascia, or galea. Tumor necrosis, lymphovascular invasion, or perineural infiltration may also be noted (Figs. 15.120 and 15.121).[184] Similar to AFX, the tumor cells are large, polygonal, and frequently multinucleated, with abundant and occasionally frothy cytoplasm (Fig. 15.122). Atypical spindle cells are admixed in varying proportions. Mitotic activity is brisk, and atypical mitoses are present (Fig. 15.123). Pleomorphic dermal sarcoma shows a wide morphologic spectrum, including spindle cell–predominant tumors, myxoid, keloidal or desmoplastic stromal change, and a pseudoangiomatous or storiform growth pattern (Fig. 15.124).[184]

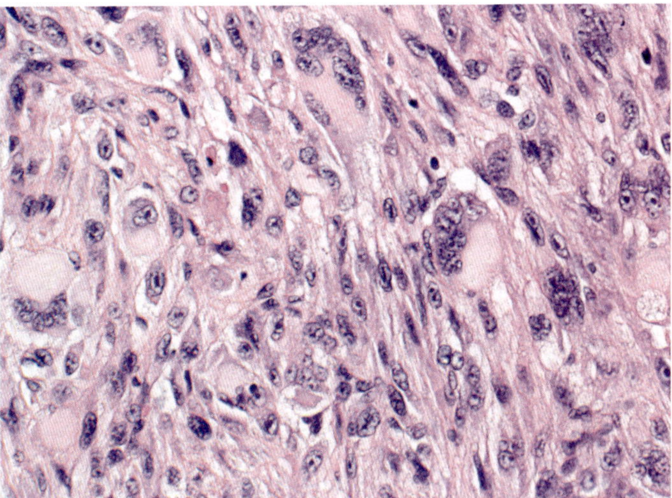

Figure 15.122 **Pleomorphic Dermal Sarcoma.** The tumor cells are large epithelioid and polygonal with abundant cytoplasm. Multinucleated forms are admixed.

Immunohistochemistry

The immunohistochemical profile is identical to that of AFX, and there are no specific diagnostic markers. The tumors express CD10 and are consistently negative for S-100 protein, kertatins, desmin, and CD34.[184] SMA expression is commonly found in the spindle cells, whereas very limited melan A and EMA are seen in a small subset of tumors.[184,200] CD31 expression may be focally encountered as weak granular cytoplasmic staining.[184,190]

Molecular Genetics

Analogous to AFX, pleomorphic dermal sarcoma shows UV signature mutations in the *TP53* gene, as well as *TERT* promoter gene mutations.[203,204]

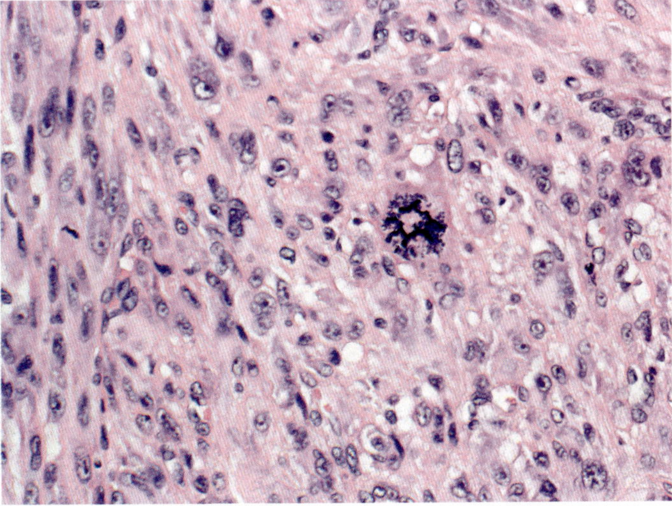

Figure 15.123 **Pleomorphic Dermal Sarcoma.** Atypical mitoses are a frequent finding.

Differential Diagnosis

Pleomorphic dermal sarcoma is separated from AFX by the presence of at least one of the following findings: invasive tumor growth beyond the dermis, tumor necrosis, lymphovascular invasion, or perineural infiltration. Melanoma is excluded by lack of S-100 protein, and spindle cell or desmoplastic squamous cell carcinoma can be ruled out by the lack of keratin expression and the absence of better differentiated areas of squamous cell carcinoma. The absence of desmin expression argues against a diagnosis of leiomyosarcoma. The most reliable way of excluding cutaneous angiosarcoma is by immunohistochemistry for CD31 and ERG. ERG is consistently negative in pleomorphic dermal sarcoma, and CD31 is at most focal, weak and granular cytoplasmic, unlike the strong membranous staining in vascular tumors.

Prognosis and Treatment

Pleomorphic dermal sarcoma has an approximately 30% risk for local recurrence and a 10% risk for distant metastasis.[184] The lung, lymph nodes, skin, and soft tissue are preferred metastatic sites.[184,207] The behavior of these tumors may be more aggressive than appreciated because long-term follow-up is difficult to obtain in view of the advanced age at presentation, the high rate of comorbidities, and mortality due to unrelated causes. The presence of metastasis is associated with high mortality.[208]

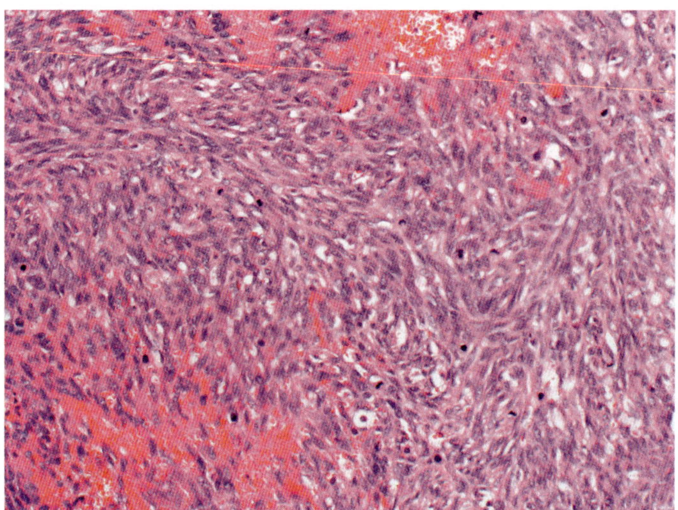

Figure 15.124 Pleomorphic Dermal Sarcoma. Hemorrhage and pseudovascular spaces are characteristic of the pseudoangiomatous variant, mimicking angiosarcoma.

Pleomorphic Fibroma

"Pleomorphic fibroma" is a designation that has been applied to hypocellular polypoid cutaneous lesions containing scattered atypical pleomorphic cells.[209] Most examples of pleomorphic fibroma likely represent fibroepithelial polyps showing nuclear pleomorphism as a result of degenerative nuclear atypia, analogous to pseudosarcomatous fibroepithelial stromal polyps of the vulvovaginal region,[210] whereas a similar histologic pattern may also occasionally be seen in other long-standing dermal lesions with degenerative atypia. Pleomorphic fibroma shows a wide anatomic and age distribution in adults.[209] It presents as a dome-shaped cutaneous nodule containing scattered pleomorphic cells within a hypocellular collagenous background (Fig. 15.125). The lesion lacks a discrete margin and often extends to the epidermis. By immunohistochemistry, the lesional cells are positive for CD34,[211] similar to other dermal fibroblasts. These lesions do not recur.

Adipocytic Tumors

Dermal Lipoma and Nevus Lipomatosus Superficialis

The presence of mature adipose tissue within dermal collagen bundles can be seen in two distinct clinical settings: dermal lipoma and nevus lipomatosus superficialis.

Clinical Features

Dermal lipoma is not uncommon and presents as a solitary, circumscribed, often exophytic tumor that clinically resembles a skin tag or fibroepithelial polyp. This lesion shows a wide age range and anatomic distribution.

In contrast, nevus lipomatosus superficialis is rare. The disorder shows a predilection for the pelvic girdle. It frequently presents at birth or develops within the first two decades of life as a large plaque composed of multiple individual papules frequently in a linear or zonal arrangement (Fig. 15.126).[212,213] More extensive involvement of skin folds has also been reported as having a "Michelin tire" appearance.[214,215] Individuals of both genders are equally affected.

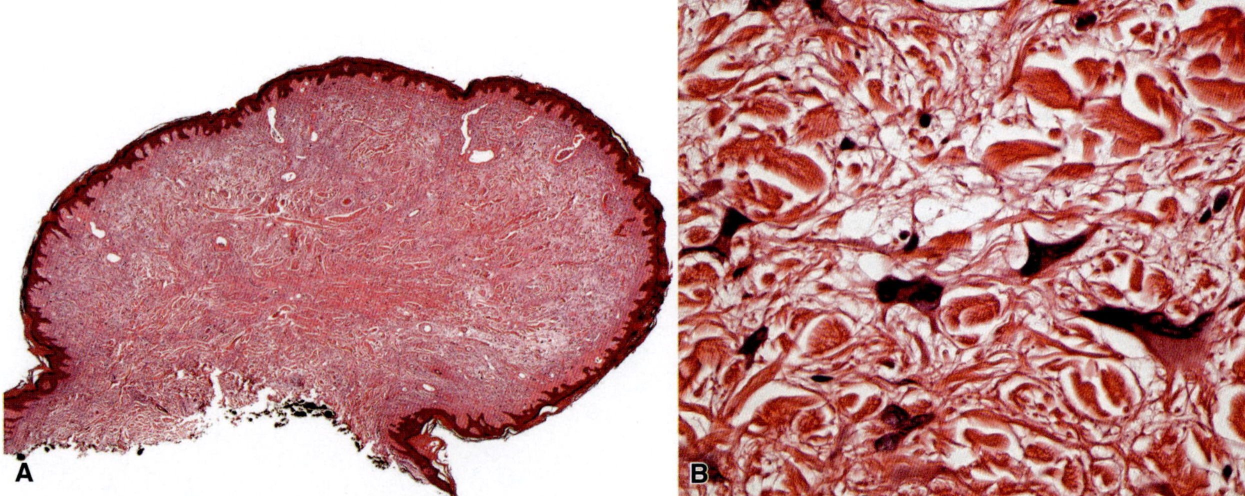

Figure 15.125 Pleomorphic Fibroma. This fibroepithelial polyp (A) contains scattered pleomorphic cells in a hypocellular collagenous background (B).

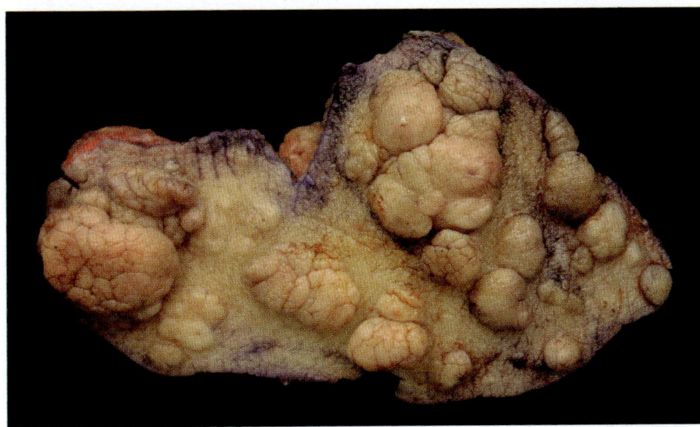

Figure 15.126 **Nevus Lipomatosus Superficialis.** Some examples have a dramatic clinical appearance. Note the multiple papules and cauliflower-like protrusions from the skin. The lesions were excised for cosmetic reasons.

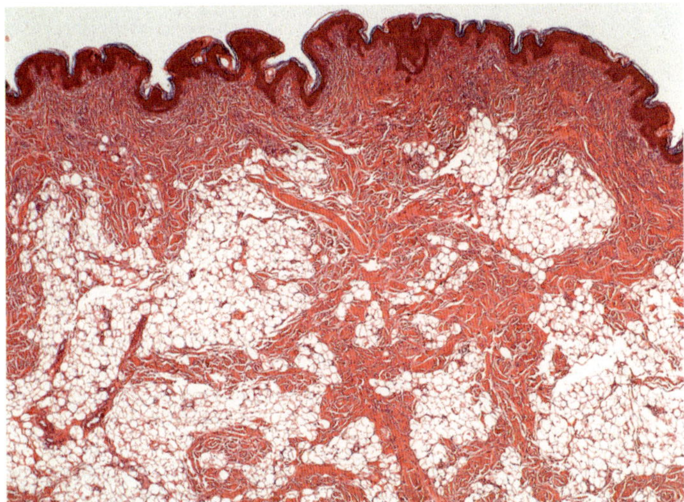

Figure 15.127 **Dermal Lipoma.** Note the presence of mature adipose tissue within reticular dermis.

Pathologic Features

The characteristic finding in dermal lipoma is the permeation of dermal collagen by mature adipocytes (Fig. 15.127). The tumors are typically less well demarcated than lipomas arising in the subcutis.

Nevus lipomatosus superficialis shows similar histologic findings to dermal lipoma. In addition, abnormalities in other connective tissues elements may be present, such as increased vasculature, increased loose fibrous tissue, and decreased elastic tissue.

Prognosis and Treatment

Treatment is cosmetic. Simple excision is curative.

Dermal Spindle Cell Lipoma and Pleomorphic Lipoma

Although spindle cell lipoma and pleomorphic lipoma are covered in detail in Chapter 12, they are also mentioned in this chapter because they display some unique clinical and histologic features when they present in the skin. In contrast to its more deeply seated counterpart, dermal spindle cell lipoma shows a predilection for females and a broader anatomic distribution.[216] Tumors present as soft, painless, slowly growing nodules measuring less than 4 cm in diameter and affecting the head and neck region, as well as the limbs, trunk, and genital area.[216–218]

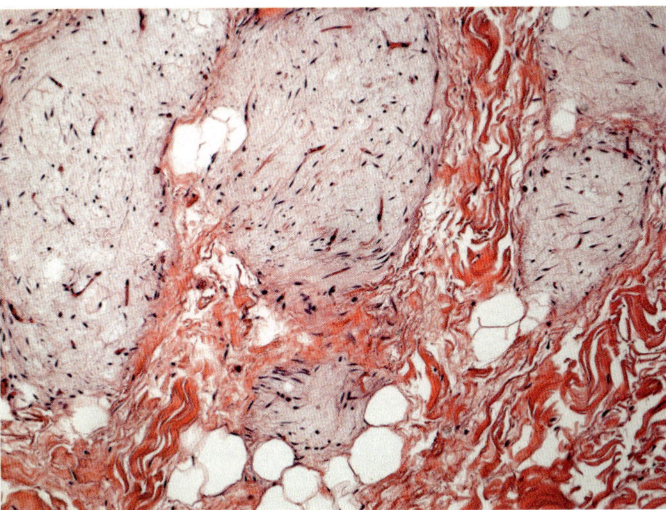

Figure 15.128 **Dermal Spindle Cell Lipoma.** The tumor has an infiltrative growth pattern within reticular dermal collagen bundles.

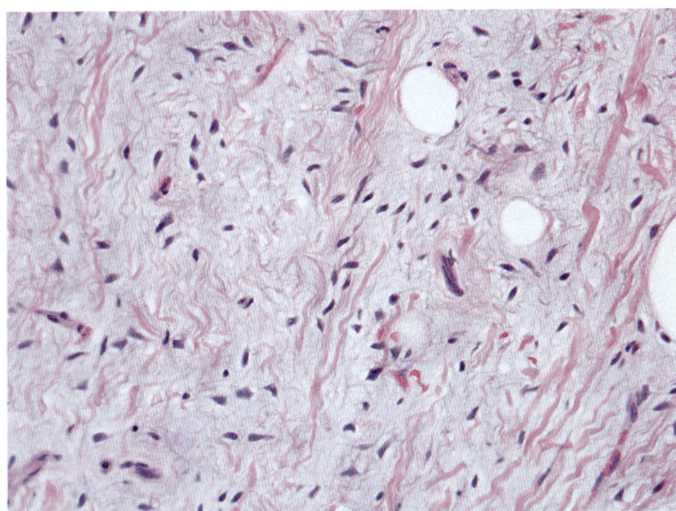

Figure 15.129 **Dermal Spindle Cell Lipoma.** The tumor is composed of bland, short spindle cells within a myxoid stroma, also containing ropy collagen bundles.

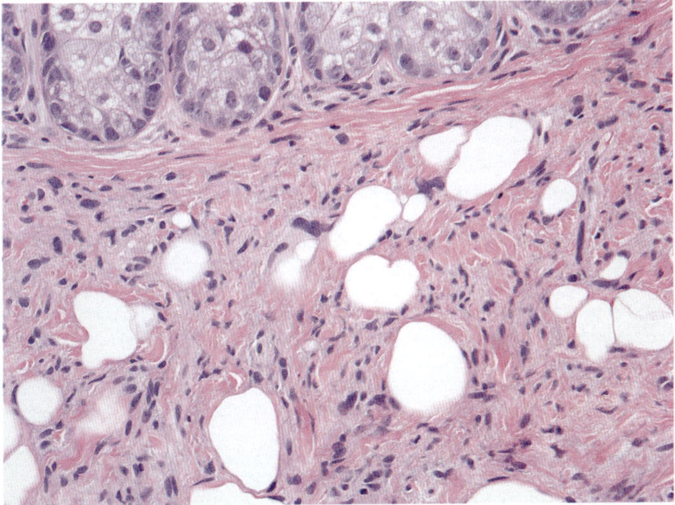

Figure 15.130 **Dermal Pleomorphic Lipoma.** The tumor contains scattered pleomorphic multinucleated cells. Note the admixed adipocytes and short spindle cells.

Histologically, they show the typical features of spindle cell lipoma, being composed of short ovoid spindle cells often in a myxoid matrix containing ropy collagen bundles and admixed adipocytes in varying amounts (Figs. 15.128 and 15.129). Elements of pleomorphic lipoma may also be identified (Fig. 15.130). In contrast to subcutaneous tumors, dermal spindle cell lipoma is poorly marginated and shows infiltrative growth among dermal collagen bundles (see Fig. 15.128). Dermal spindle cell lipoma is characterized by benign clinical behavior with only rare local recurrences.[216]

References

1. Panagopoulos I, Gorunova L, Bjerkehagen B, et al: LAMTOR1-PRKCD and NUMA1-SFMBT1 fusion genes identified by RNA sequencing in aneurysmal benign fibrous histiocytoma with t(3;11)(p21;q13), *Cancer Genet* 208:545–551, 2015.
2. Walther C, Hofvander J, Nilsson J, et al: Gene fusion detection in formalin-fixed paraffin-embedded benign fibrous histiocytomas using fluorescence in situ hybridization and RNA sequencing, *Lab Invest* 95:1071–1076, 2015.
3. Płaszczyca A, Nilsson J, Magnusson L, et al: Fusions involving protein kinase C and membrane-associated proteins in benign fibrous histiocytoma, *Int J Biochem Cell Biol* 53:475–481, 2014.
4. Kamino H, Jacobson M: Dermatofibroma extending into the subcutaneous tissue. Differential diagnosis from dermatofibrosarcoma protuberans, *Am J Surg Pathol* 14:1156–1164, 1990.
5. Wambacher-Gasser B, Zelger B, Zelger BG, et al: Clear cell dermatofibroma, *Histopathology* 30:64–69, 1997.
6. Schwob VS, Santa Cruz DJ: Palisading cutaneous fibrous histiocytoma, *J Cutan Pathol* 13:403–407, 1986.
7. Zelger BG, Steiner H, Kutzner H, et al: Granular cell dermatofibroma, *Histopathology* 31:258–262, 1997.
8. Iwata J, Fletcher CD: Lipidized fibrous histiocytoma: clinicopathologic analysis of 22 cases, *Am J Dermatopathol* 22:126–134, 2000.
9. Zelger BW, Ofner D, Zelger BG: Atrophic variants of dermatofibroma and dermatofibrosarcoma protuberans, *Histopathology* 26:519–527, 1995.
10. Calonje E, Mentzel T, Fletcher CD: Cellular benign fibrous histiocytoma. Clinicopathologic analysis of 74 cases of a distinctive variant of cutaneous fibrous histiocytoma with frequent recurrence, *Am J Surg Pathol* 18:668–676, 1994.
11. Guillou L, Gebhard S, Salmeron M, et al: Metastasizing fibrous histiocytoma of the skin: a clinicopathologic and immunohistochemical analysis of three cases, *Mod Pathol* 13:654–660, 2000.
12. Volpicelli ER, Fletcher CD: Desmin and CD34 positivity in cellular fibrous histiocytoma: an immunohistochemical analysis of 100 cases, *J Cutan Pathol* 39:747–752, 2012.
13. Calonje E, Fletcher CD: Aneurysmal benign fibrous histiocytoma: clinicopathological analysis of 40 cases of a tumour frequently misdiagnosed as a vascular neoplasm, *Histopathology* 26:323–331, 1995.
14. Beham A, Fletcher CD: Atypical 'pseudosarcomatous' variant of cutaneous benign fibrous histiocytoma: report of eight cases, *Histopathology* 17:167–169, 1990.
15. Kaddu S, McMenamin ME, Fletcher CD: Atypical fibrous histiocytoma of the skin: clinicopathologic analysis of 59 cases with evidence of infrequent metastasis, *Am J Surg Pathol* 26:35–46, 2002.
16. Colome MI, Sanchez RL: Dermatomyofibroma: report of two cases, *J Cutan Pathol* 21:371–376, 1994.
17. Kamino H, Reddy VB, Gero M, et al: Dermatomyofibroma. A benign cutaneous, plaque-like proliferation of fibroblasts and myofibroblasts in young adults, *J Cutan Pathol* 19:85–93, 1992.
18. Mentzel T, Calonje E, Fletcher CD: Dermatomyofibroma: additional observations on a distinctive cutaneous myofibroblastic tumour with emphasis on differential diagnosis, *Br J Dermatol* 129:69–73, 1993.
19. Mentzel T, Kutzner H: Dermatomyofibroma: clinicopathologic and immunohistochemical analysis of 56 cases and reappraisal of a rare and distinct cutaneous neoplasm, *Am J Dermatopathol* 31:44–49, 2009.
20. Mentzel T, Scharer L, Kazakov DV, et al: Myxoid dermatofibrosarcoma protuberans: clinicopathologic, immunohistochemical, and molecular analysis of eight cases, *Am J Dermatopathol* 29:443–448, 2007.
21. Mentzel T, Kutzner H: Haemorrhagic dermatomyofibroma (plaque-like dermal fibromatosis): clinicopathological and immunohistochemical analysis of three cases resembling plaque-stage Kaposi's sarcoma, *Histopathology* 42:594–598, 2003.
22. Raj S, Calonje E, Kraus M, et al: Cutaneous pilar leiomyoma: clinicopathologic analysis of 53 lesions in 45 patients, *Am J Dermatopathol* 19:2–9, 1997.
23. Alam NA, Bevan S, Churchman M, et al: Localization of a gene (MCUL1) for multiple cutaneous leiomyomata and uterine fibroids to chromosome 1q42.3-q43, *Am J Hum Genet* 68:1264–1269, 2001.
24. Chuang GS, Martinez-Mir A, Engler DE, et al: Multiple cutaneous and uterine leiomyomata resulting from missense mutations in the fumarate hydratase gene, *Clin Exp Dermatol* 31:118–121, 2006.
25. Kraft S, Fletcher CD: Atypical intradermal smooth muscle neoplasms: clinicopathologic analysis of 84 cases and a reappraisal of cutaneous "leiomyosarcoma", *Am J Surg Pathol* 35:599–607, 2011.
26. Massi D, Franchi A, Alos L, et al: Primary cutaneous leiomyosarcoma: clinicopathological analysis of 36 cases, *Histopathology* 56:251–262, 2010.
27. Alawi F, Freedman PD: Sporadic sclerotic fibroma of the oral soft tissues, *Am J Dermatopathol* 26:182–187, 2004.
28. Al-Daraji WI, Ramsay HM, Ali RB: Storiform collagenoma as a clue for Cowden disease or PTEN hamartoma tumour syndrome, *J Clin Pathol* 60:840–842, 2007.
29. Chapman MS, Perry AE, Baughman RD: Cowden's syndrome, Lhermitte-Duclos disease, and sclerotic fibroma, *Am J Dermatopathol* 20:413–416, 1998.
30. Fistarol SK, Anliker MD, Itin PH: Cowden disease or multiple hamartoma sy drome—cutaneous clue to internal malignancy, *Eur J Dermatol* 12:411–421, 2002.
31. Hanft VN, Shea CR, McNutt NS, et al: Expression of CD34 in sclerotic ("plywood") fibromas, *Am J Dermatopathol* 22:17–21, 2000.
32. Rudolph P, Schubert C, Harms D, et al: Giant cell collagenoma: a benign dermal tumor with distinctive multinucleate cells, *Am J Surg Pathol* 22:557–563, 1998.
33. Fletcher CD: Solitary circumscribed neuroma of the skin (so-called palisaded, encapsulated neuroma). A clinicopathologic and immunohistochemical study, *Am J Surg Pathol* 13:574–580, 1989.
34. Dakin MC, Leppard B, Theaker JM: The palisaded, encapsulated neuroma (solitary circumscribed neuroma), *Histopathology* 20:405–410, 1992.
35. Megahed M: Palisaded encapsulated neuroma (solitary circumscribed neuroma). A clinicopathologic and immunohistochemical study, *Am J Dermatopathol* 16:120–125, 1994.
36. Albrecht S, Kahn HJ, From L: Palisaded encapsulated neuroma: an immunohistochemical study, *Mod Pathol* 2:403–406, 1989.
37. Criscione VD, Weinstock MA: Descriptive epidemiology of dermatofibrosarcoma protuberans in the United States, 1973 to 2002, *J Am Acad Dermatol* 56:968–973, 2007.
38. Monnier D, Vidal C, Martin L, et al: Dermatofibrosarcoma protuberans: a population-based cancer registry descriptive study of 66 consecutive cases diagnosed between 1982 and 2002, *J Eur Acad Dermatol Venereol* 20:1237–1242, 2006.
39. McKee PH, Fletcher CD: Dermatofibrosarcoma protuberans presenting in infancy and childhood, *J Cutan Pathol* 18:241–246, 1991.
40. Jafarian F, McCuaig C, Kokta V, et al: Dermatofibrosarcoma protuberans in childhood and adolescence: report of eight patients, *Pediatr Dermatol* 25:317–325, 2008.
41. Fletcher CD, Evans BJ, MacArtney JC, et al: Dermatofibrosarcoma protuberans: a clinicopathological and immunohistochemical study with a review of the literature, *Histopathology* 9:921–938, 1985.
42. Mentzel T, Beham A, Katenkamp D, et al: Fibrosarcomatous ("high-grade") dermatofibrosarcoma protuberans: clinicopathologic and immunohistochemical study of a series of 41 cases with emphasis on prognostic significance, *Am J Surg Pathol* 22:576–587, 1998.
43. Connelly JH, Evans HL: Dermatofibrosarcoma protuberans. A clinicopathologic review with emphasis on fibrosarcomatous areas, *Am J Surg Pathol* 16:921–925, 1992.
44. Abbott JJ, Oliveira AM, Nascimento AG: The prognostic significance of fibrosarcomatous transformation in dermatofibrosarcoma protuberans, *Am J Surg Pathol* 30:436–443, 2006.
45. Goldblum JR, Reith JD, Weiss SW: Sarcomas arising in dermatofibrosarcoma protuberans: a reappraisal of biologic behavior in eighteen cases treated by wide local excision with extended clinical follow up, *Am J Surg Pathol* 24:1125–1130, 2000.
46. Swaby MG, Evans HL, Fletcher CD, et al: Dermatofibrosarcoma protuberans with unusual sarcomatous transformation: a series of 4 cases with molecular confirmation, *Am J Dermatopathol* 33:354–360, 2011.
47. Reimann JD, Fletcher CD: Myxoid dermatofibrosarcoma protuberans: a rare variant analyzed in a series of 23 cases, *Am J Surg Pathol* 31:1371–1377, 2007.
48. Frierson HF, Cooper PH: Myxoid variant of dermatofibrosarcoma protuberans, *Am J Surg Pathol* 7:445–450, 1983.
49. Fletcher CD, Theaker JM, Flanagan A, et al: Pigmented dermatofibrosarcoma protuberans (Bednar tumour): melanocytic colonization or neuroectodermal differentiation? A clinicopathological and immunohistochemical study, *Histopathology* 13:631–643, 1988.
50. Dupree WB, Langloss JM, Weiss SW: Pigmented dermatofibrosarcoma protuberans (Bednar tumor). A pathologic, ultrastructural, and immunohistochemical study, *Am J Surg Pathol* 9:630–639, 1985.
51. Zamecnik M: Myoid cells in the fibrosarcomatous variant of dermatofibrosarcoma protuberans, *Histopathology* 36:186, 2000.
52. Calonje E, Fletcher CD: Myoid differentiation in dermatofibrosarcoma protuberans and its fibrosarcomatous variant: clinicopathologic analysis of 5 cases, *J Cutan Pathol* 23:30–36, 1996.
53. Terrier-Lacombe MJ, Guillou L, Maire G, et al: Dermatofibrosarcoma protuberans, giant cell fibroblastoma, and hybrid lesions in children: clinicopathologic comparative analysis of 28 cases with molecular data—a study from the French Federation of Cancer Centers Sarcoma Group, *Am J Surg Pathol* 27:27–39, 2003.

54. Sigel JE, Bergfeld WF, Goldblum JR: A morphologic study of dermatofibrosarcoma protuberans: expansion of a histologic profile, *J Cutan Pathol* 27:159–163, 2000.
55. Harvell JD, Kilpatrick SE, White WL: Histogenetic relations between giant cell fibroblastoma and dermatofibrosarcoma protuberans. CD34 staining showing the spectrum and a simulator, *Am J Dermatopathol* 20:339–345, 1998.
56. Beham A, Fletcher CD: Dermatofibrosarcoma protuberans with areas resembling giant cell fibroblastoma: report of two cases, *Histopathology* 17:165–167, 1990.
57. Banerjee SS, Harris M, Eyden BP, et al: Granular cell variant of dermatofibrosarcoma protuberans, *Histopathology* 17:375–378, 1990.
58. Llatjos R, Fernandez-Figueras MT, Diaz-Cascajo C, et al: Palisading and verocay body-prominent dermatofibrosarcoma protuberans: a report of three cases, *Histopathology* 37:452–455,2000.
59. Kutzner H: Expression of the human progenitor cell antigen CD34 (HPCA-1) distinguishes dermatofibrosarcoma protuberans from fibrous histiocytoma in formalin-fixed, paraffin-embedded tissue, *J Am Acad Dermatol* 28:613–617, 1993.
60. Sirvent N, Maire G, Pedeutour F: Genetics of dermatofibrosarcoma protuberans family of tumors: from ring chromosomes to tyrosine kinase inhibitor treatment, *Genes Chromosomes Cancer* 37:1–19, 2003.
61. Abbott JJ, Erickson-Johnson M, Wang X, et al: Gains of COL1A1-PDGFB genomic copies occur in fibrosarcomatous transformation of dermatofibrosarcoma protuberans, *Mod Pathol* 19:1512–1518, 2006.
62. Naeem R, Lux ML, Huang SF, et al: Ring chromosomes in dermatofibrosarcoma protuberans are composed of interspersed sequences from chromosomes 17 and 22, *Am J Pathol* 147:1553–1558, 1995.
63. Pedeutour F, Simon MP, Minoletti F, et al: Translocation, t(17;22)(q22;q13), in dermatofibrosarcoma protuberans: a new tumor-associated chromosome rearrangement, *Cytogenet Cell Genet* 72:171–174, 1996.
64. Takahira T, Oda Y, Tamiya S, et al: Detection of COL1A1-PDGFB fusion transcripts and PDGFB/PDGFRB mRNA expression in dermatofibrosarcoma protuberans, *Mod Pathol* 20:668–675, 2007.
65. Abrams TA, Schuetze SM: Targeted therapy for dermatofibrosarcoma protuberans, *Curr Oncol Rep* 8:291–296, 2006.
66. McArthur GA, Demetri GD, van Oosterom A, et al: Molecular and clinical analysis of locally advanced dermatofibrosarcoma protuberans treated with imatinib: Imatinib Target Exploration Consortium Study B2225, *J Clin Oncol* 23:866–873, 2005.
67. Rutkowski P, Van Glabbeke M, Rankin CJ, et al: Imatinib mesylate in advanced dermatofibrosarcoma protuberans: pooled analysis of two phase II clinical trials, *J Clin Oncol* 28:1772–1779, 2010.
68. Marque M, Bessis D, Pedeutour F, et al: Medallion-like dermal dendrocyte hamartoma: the main diagnostic pitfall is congenital atrophic dermatofibrosarcoma, *Br J Dermatol* 160:190–193, 2009.
69. Rodriguez-Jurado R, Palacios C, Duran-McKinster C, et al: Medallion-like dermal dendrocyte hamartoma: a new clinically and histopathologically distinct lesion, *J Am Acad Dermatol* 51:359–363, 2004.
70. Kutzner H, Mentzel T, Palmedo G, et al: Plaque-like CD34-positive dermal fibroma ("medallion-like dermal dendrocyte hamartoma"): clinicopathologic, immunohistochemical, and molecular analysis of 5 cases emphasizing its distinction from superficial, plaque-like dermatofibrosarcoma protuberans, *Am J Surg Pathol* 34:190–201, 2010.
71. Doyle LA, Möller E, Dal Cin P, et al: MUC4 is a highly sensitive and specific marker for low-grade fibromyxoid sarcoma, *Am J Surg Pathol* 35:733–741, 2011.
72. Roses DF, Valensi Q, LaTrenta G, et al: Surgical treatment of dermatofibrosarcoma protuberans, *Surg Gynecol Obstet* 162:449–452, 1986.
73. Rutgers EJ, Kroon BB, Albus-Lutter CE, et al: Dermatofibrosarcoma protuberans: treatment and prognosis, *Eur J Surg Oncol* 18:241–248, 1992.
74. Kimmel Z, Ratner D, Kim JY, et al: Peripheral excision margins for dermatofibrosarcoma protuberans: a meta-analysis of spatial data, *Ann Surg Oncol* 14:2113–2120, 2007.
75. Wacker J, Khan-Durani B, Hartschuh W: Modified Mohs micrographic surgery in the therapy of dermatofibrosarcoma protuberans: analysis of 22 patients, *Ann Surg Oncol* 11:438–444, 2004.
76. Gloster HM, Jr, Harris KR, Roenigk RK: A comparison between Mohs micrographic surgery and wide surgical excision for the treatment of dermatofibrosarcoma protuberans, *J Am Acad Dermatol* 35:82–87, 1996.
77. Yu W, Tsoukas MM, Chapman SM, et al: Surgical treatment for dermatofibrosarcoma protuberans: the Dartmouth experience and literature review, *Ann Plast Surg* 60:288–293, 2008.
78. DuBay D, Cimmino V, Lowe L, et al: Low recurrence rate after surgery for dermatofibrosarcoma protuberans: a multidisciplinary approach from a single institution, *Cancer* 100:1008–1016, 2004.
79. Snow SN, Gordon EM, Larson PO, et al: Dermatofibrosarcoma protuberans: a report on 29 patients treated by Mohs micrographic surgery with long-term follow-up and review of the literature, *Cancer* 101:28–38, 2004.
80. Thomison J, McCarter M, McClain D, et al: Hyalinized collagen in a dermatofibrosarcoma protuberans after treatment with imatinib mesylate, *J Cutan Pathol* 35:1003–1006, 2008.
81. Jha P, Moosavi C, Fanburg-Smith JC: Giant cell fibroblastoma: an update and addition of 86 new cases from the Armed Forces Institute of Pathology, in honor of Dr. Franz M. Enzinger, *Ann Diagn Pathol* 11:81–88, 2007.
82. Dymock RB, Allen PW, Stirling JW, et al: Giant cell fibroblastoma. A distinctive, recurrent tumor of childhood, *Am J Surg Pathol* 11:263–271, 1987.
83. Shmookler BM, Enzinger FM, Weiss SW: Giant cell fibroblastoma. A juvenile form of dermatofibrosarcoma protuberans, *Cancer* 64:2154–2161, 1989.
84. Fletcher CD: Giant cell fibroblastoma of soft tissue: a clinicopathological and immunohistochemical study, *Histopathology* 13:499–508, 1988.
85. Hornick JL, Fletcher CD: Soft tissue perineurioma: clinicopathologic analysis of 81 cases including those with atypical histologic features, *Am J Surg Pathol* 29:845–858, 2005.
86. Robson AM, Calonje E: Cutaneous perineurioma: a poorly recognized tumour often misdiagnosed as epithelioid histiocytoma, *Histopathology* 37:332–339, 2000.
87. Smith K, Skelton H: Cutaneous fibrous perineurioma, *J Cutan Pathol* 25:333–337, 1998.
88. Fox MD, Gleason BC, Thomas AB, et al: Extra-acral cutaneous/soft tissue sclerosing perineurioma: an under-recognized entity in the differential of CD34-positive cutaneous neoplasms, *J Cutan Pathol* 37:1053–1056, 2010.
89. Hornick JL, Bundock EA, Fletcher CD: Hybrid schwannoma/perineurioma: clinicopathologic analysis of 42 distinctive benign nerve sheath tumors, *Am J Surg Pathol* 33:1554–1561, 2009.
90. Kazakov DV, Pitha J, Sima R, et al: Hybrid peripheral nerve sheath tumors: Schwannoma-perineurioma and neurofibroma-perineurioma. A report of three cases in extradigital locations, *Ann Diagn Pathol* 9:16–23, 2005.
91. Michal M, Fanburg-Smith JC, Mentzel T, et al: Dendritic cell neurofibroma with pseudorosettes: a report of 18 cases of a distinct and hitherto unrecognized neurofibroma variant, *Am J Surg Pathol* 25:587–594, 2001.
92. Kazakov DV, Mukensnabl P, Zamecnik M, et al: Intraneural dendritic cell neurofibroma with pseudorosettes, *Am J Dermatopathol* 26:72–75, 2004.
93. Kazakov DV, Vanecek T, Sima R, et al: Dendritic cell neurofibroma with pseudorosettes lacks mutations in exons 1–15 of the neurofibromatosis type 2 gene, *Am J Dermatopathol* 27:286–289, 2005.
94. Woodruff JM, Busam KJ: Histologically benign cutaneous dendritic cell tumor with pseudorosettes, *Am J Surg Pathol* 26:1644–1645, author reply 5–8, 2002.
95. Simpson RH, Seymour MJ: Dendritic cell neurofibroma with pseudorosettes: two tumors in a patient with evidence of neurofibromatosis, *Am J Surg Pathol* 25:1458–1459, 2001.
96. Mirra JM, Kessler S, Bhuta S, et al: The fibroma-like variant of epithelioid sarcoma. A fibrohistiocytic/myoid cell lesion often confused with benign and malignant spindle cell tumors, *Cancer* 69:1382–1395, 1992.
97. Hornick JL, Fletcher CD: Pseudomyogenic hemangioendothelioma: a distinctive, often multicentric tumor with indolent behavior, *Am J Surg Pathol* 35:190–201, 2011.
98. Billings SD, Folpe AL, Weiss SW: Epithelioid sarcoma-like hemangioendothelioma, *Am J Surg Pathol* 27:48–57, 2003.
99. Hung YP, Fletcher CD, Hornick JL: FOSB is a useful diagnostic marker for pseudomyogenic hemangioendothelioma, *Am J Surg Pathol* 41:596–606, 2017
100. Walther C, Tayebwa J, Lilljebjörn H, et al: A novel SERPINE1-FOSB fusion gene results in transcriptional up-regulation of FOSB in pseudomyogenic haemangioendothelioma, *J Pathol* 232:534–540, 2014.
101. Hornick JL, Dal Cin P, Fletcher CD: Loss of INI1 expression is characteristic of both conventional and proximal-type epithelioid sarcoma, *Am J Surg Pathol* 33:542–550, 2009.
102. Orrock JM, Abbott JJ, Gibson LE, et al: INI1 and GLUT-1 expression in epithelioid sarcoma and its cutaneous neoplastic and nonneoplastic mimics, *Am J Dermatopathol* 31:152–156, 2009.
103. Fetsch JF, Laskin WB, Miettinen M: Superficial acral fibromyxoma: a clinicopathologic and immunohistochemical analysis of 37 cases of a distinctive soft tissue tumor with a predilection for the fingers and toes, *Hum Pathol* 32:704–714, 2001.
104. Al-Daraji WI, Miettinen M: Superficial acral fibromyxoma: a clinicopathological analysis of 32 tumors including 4 in the heel, *J Cutan Pathol* 35:1020–1026, 2008.
105. Hollmann TJ, Bovée JV, Fletcher CD: Digital fibromyxoma (superficial acral fibromyxoma): a detailed characterization of 124 cases, *Am J Surg Pathol* 36:789–798, 2012.
106. McNiff JM, Subtil A, Cowper SE, et al: Cellular digital fibromas: distinctive CD34-positive lesions that may mimic dermatofibrosarcoma protuberans, *J Cutan Pathol* 32:413–418, 2005.
107. Agaimy A, Michal M, Giedl J, et al: Superficial acral fibromyxoma: clinicopathologic, immunohistochemical and molecular study of 11 cases highlighting frequent Rb1 loss/deletions, *Hum Pathol* 60:192–198, 2017
108. Calonje E, Guerin D, McCormick D, et al: Superficial angiomyxoma: clinicopathologic analysis of a series of distinctive but poorly recognized cutaneous tumors with tendency for recurrence, *Am J Surg Pathol* 23:910–917, 1999.
109. Fetsch JF, Laskin WB, Tavassoli FA: Superficial angiomyxoma (cutaneous myxoma): a clinicopathologic study of 17 cases arising in the genital region, *Int J Gynecol Pathol* 16:325–334, 1997.
110. Ferreiro JA, Carney JA: Myxomas of the external ear and their significance, *Am J Surg Pathol* 18:274–280, 1994.
111. Carney JA, Gordon H, Carpenter PC, et al: The complex of myxomas, spotty pigmentation, and endocrine overactivity, *Medicine (Baltimore)* 64:270–283, 1985.
112. Carney JA, Ferreiro JA: The epithelioid blue nevus. A multicentric familial tumor with important associations, including cardiac myxoma and psammomatous melanotic schwannoma, *Am J Surg Pathol* 20:259–272, 1996.

113. Carney JA: Differences between nonfamilial and familial cardiac myxoma, *Am J Surg Pathol* 9:53–55, 1985.
114. Rongioletti F, Rebora A: Cutaneous mucinoses: microscopic criteria for diagnosis, *Am J Dermatopathol* 23:257–267, 2001.
115. Johnson WC, Graham JH, Helwig EB: Cutaneous myxoid cyst. A clinicopathological and histochemical study, *JAMA* 191:15–20, 1965.
116. Wilk M, Schmoeckel C: Cutaneous focal mucinosis—a histopathological and immunohistochemical analysis of 11 cases, *J Cutan Pathol* 21:446–452, 1994.
117. Johnson WC, Helwig EB: Cutaneous focal mucinosis. A clinicopathological and histochemical study, *Arch Dermatol* 93:13–20, 1966.
118. Sheth S, Li X, Binder S, et al: Differential gene expression profiles of neurothekeomas and nerve sheath myxomas by microarray analysis, *Mod Pathol* 24:343–354, 2011.
119. Fetsch JF, Laskin WB, Miettinen M: Nerve sheath myxoma: a clinicopathologic and immunohistochemical analysis of 57 morphologically distinctive, S-100 protein and GFAP-positive, myxoid peripheral nerve sheath tumors with a predilection for the extremities and a high local recurrence rate, *Am J Surg Pathol* 29:1615–1624, 2005.
120. Fanburg-Smith JC, Meis-Kindblom JM, Fante R, et al: Malignant granular cell tumor of soft tissue: diagnostic criteria and clinicopathologic correlation, *Am J Surg Pathol* 22:779–794, 1998.
121. Ordonez NG: Granular cell tumor: a review and update, *Adv Anat Pathol* 6:186–203, 1999.
122. Khansur T, Balducci L, Tavassoli M: Granular cell tumor. Clinical spectrum of the benign and malignant entity, *Cancer* 60:220–222, 1987.
123. Gleason BC, Nascimento AF: HMB-45 and Melan-A are useful in the differential diagnosis between granular cell tumor and malignant melanoma, *Am J Dermatopathol* 29:22–27, 2007.
124. Ordonez NG, Mackay B: Granular cell tumor: a review of the pathology and histogenesis, *Ultrastruct Pathol* 23:207–222, 1999.
125. Le BH, Boyer PJ, Lewis JE, et al: Granular cell tumor: immunohistochemical assessment of inhibin-alpha, protein gene product 9.5, S100 protein, CD68, and Ki-67 proliferative index with clinical correlation, *Arch Pathol Lab Med* 128:771–775, 2004.
126. Chaudhry IH, Calonje E: Dermal non-neural granular cell tumour (so-called primitive polypoid granular cell tumour): a distinctive entity further delineated in a clinicopathological study of 11 cases, *Histopathology* 47:179–185, 2005.
127. Lazar AJ, Fletcher CD: Primitive nonneural granular cell tumors of skin: clinicopathologic analysis of 13 cases, *Am J Surg Pathol* 29:927–934, 2005.
128. LeBoit PE, Barr RJ, Burall S, et al: Primitive polypoid granular-cell tumor and other cutaneous granular-cell neoplasms of apparent nonneural origin, *Am J Surg Pathol* 15:48–58, 1991.
129. Al Habeeb A, Weinreb I, Ghazarian D: Primitive non-neural granular cell tumour with lymph node metastasis, *J Clin Pathol* 62:847–849, 2009.
130. Singh Gomez C, Calonje E, Fletcher CD: Epithelioid benign fibrous histiocytoma of skin: clinico-pathological analysis of 20 cases of a poorly known variant, *Histopathology* 24:123–129, 1994.
131. Doyle LA, Fletcher CD: EMA positivity in epithelioid benign fibrous histiocytoma—a potential diagnostic pitfall, *J Cutan Pathol* 38:697–703, 2011.
132. Doyle LA, Mariño-Enriquez A, Fletcher CD, et al: ALK rearrangement and overexpression in epithelioid fibrous histiocytoma, *Mod Pathol* 28:904–912, 2015.
133. Hornick JL, Fletcher CD: Cutaneous myoepithelioma: a clinicopathologic and immunohistochemical study of 14 cases, *Hum Pathol* 35:14–24, 2004.
134. Kutzner H, Mentzel T, Kaddu S, et al: Cutaneous myoepithelioma: an under-recognized cutaneous neoplasm composed of myoepithelial cells, *Am J Surg Pathol* 25:348–355, 2001.
135. Mentzel T, Requena L, Kaddu S, et al: Cutaneous myoepithelial neoplasms: clinicopathologic and immunohistochemical study of 20 cases suggesting a continuous spectrum ranging from benign mixed tumor of the skin to cutaneous myoepithelioma and myoepithelial carcinoma, *J Cutan Pathol* 30:294–302, 2003.
136. Michal M, Miettinen M: Myoepitheliomas of the skin and soft tissues. Report of 12 cases, *Virchows Arch* 434:393–400, 1999.
137. Gleason BC, Hornick JL: Myoepithelial tumours of skin and soft tissue: an update, *Diagn Histopathol* 14:552–560, 2008.
138. Hornick JL, Fletcher CD: Myoepithelial tumors of soft tissue: a clinicopathologic and immunohistochemical study of 101 cases with evaluation of prognostic parameters, *Am J Surg Pathol* 27:1183–1196, 2003.
139. Law RM, Viglione MP, Barrett TL: Metastatic myoepithelial carcinoma in a child, *J Cutan Pathol* 35:779–781, 2008.
140. Tanahashi J, Kashima K, Daa T, et al: A case of cutaneous myoepithelial carcinoma, *J Cutan Pathol* 34:648–653, 2007.
141. Jo VY, Antonescu CR, Zhang L, et al: Cutaneous syncytial myoepithelioma: clinicopathologic characterization in a series of 38 cases, *Am J Surg Pathol* 37:710–718, 2013.
142. Naujokas A, Charli-Joseph Y, Ruben BS, et al: SOX-10 expression in cutaneous myoepitheliomas and mixed tumors, *J Cutan Pathol* 41:353–363, 2014.
143. Antonescu CR, Zhang L, Shao SY, et al: Frequent PLAG1 gene rearrangements in skin and soft tissue myoepithelioma with ductal differentiation, *Genes Chromosomes Cancer* 52:675–682, 2013.
144. Argenyi ZB, LeBoit PE, Santa Cruz D, et al: Nerve sheath myxoma (neurothekeoma) of the skin: light microscopic and immunohistochemical reappraisal of the cellular variant, *J Cutan Pathol* 20:294–303, 1993.
145. Laskin WB, Fetsch JF, Miettinen M: The "neurothekeoma": immunohistochemical analysis distinguishes the true nerve sheath myxoma from its mimics, *Hum Pathol* 31:1230–1241, 2000.
146. Fetsch JF, Laskin WB, Hallman JR, et al: Neurothekeoma: an analysis of 178 tumors with detailed immunohistochemical data and long-term patient follow-up information, *Am J Surg Pathol* 31:1103–1114, 2007.
147. Hornick JL, Fletcher CD: Cellular neurothekeoma: detailed characterization in a series of 133 cases, *Am J Surg Pathol* 31:329–340, 2007.
148. Busam KJ, Mentzel T, Colpaert C, et al: Atypical or worrisome features in cellular neurothekeoma: a study of 10 cases, *Am J Surg Pathol* 22:1067–1072, 1998.
149. Stratton J, Billings SD: Cellular neurothekeoma: analysis of 37 cases emphasizing atypical histologic features, *Mod Pathol* 27:701–710, 2014.
150. Fox MD, Billings SD, Gleason BC, et al: Expression of MiTF may be helpful in differentiating cellular neurothekeoma from plexiform fibrohistiocytic tumor (histiocytoid predominant) in a partial biopsy specimen, *Am J Dermatopathol* 34:157–160, 2012.
151. Fried I, Sitthinamsuwan P, Muangsomboon S, et al: SOX-10 and MiTF expression in cellular and 'mixed' neurothekeoma, *J Cutan Pathol* 41:640–645, 2014.
152. Jo VY, Fletcher CD: p63 immunohistochemical staining is limited in soft tissue tumors, *Am J Clin Pathol* 136:762–766, 2011.
153. Hornick JL, Fletcher CD: PEComa: what do we know so far?, *Histopathology* 48:75–82, 2006.
154. Folpe AL, Kwiatkowski DJ: Perivascular epithelioid cell neoplasms: pathology and pathogenesis, *Hum Pathol* 41:1–15, 2010.
155. Folpe AL, Mentzel T, Lehr HA, et al: Perivascular epithelioid cell neoplasms of soft tissue and gynecologic origin: a clinicopathologic study of 26 cases and review of the literature, *Am J Surg Pathol* 29:1558–1575, 2005.
156. Mentzel T, Reisshauer S, Rutten A, et al: Cutaneous clear cell myomelanocytic tumour: a new member of the growing family of perivascular epithelioid cell tumours (PEComas). Clinicopathological and immunohistochemical analysis of seven cases, *Histopathology* 46:498–504, 2005.
157. Liegl B, Hornick JL, Fletcher CD: Primary cutaneous PEComa: distinctive clear cell lesions of skin, *Am J Surg Pathol* 32:608–614, 2008.
158. Walsh SN, Sangueza OP: PEComas: a review with emphasis on cutaneous lesions, *Semin Diagn Pathol* 26:123–130, 2009.
159. Llamas-Velasco M, Mentzel T, et al: Cutaneous PEComa does not harbour TFE3 gene fusions: immunohistochemical and molecular study of 17 cases, *Histopathology* 63:122–129, 2013.
160. Lazar AJ, Fletcher CD: Distinctive dermal clear cell mesenchymal neoplasm: clinicopathologic analysis of five cases, *Am J Dermatopathol* 26:273–279, 2004.
161. Laskin WB, Fetsch JF, Lasota J, et al: Benign epithelioid peripheral nerve sheath tumors of the soft tissues: clinicopathologic spectrum of 33 cases, *Am J Surg Pathol* 29:39–51, 2005.
162. Kindblom LG, Meis-Kindblom JM, Havel G, et al: Benign epithelioid schwannoma, *Am J Surg Pathol* 22:762–770, 1998.
163. Hart J, Gardner JM, Edgar M, et al: Epithelioid schwannomas: an analysis of 58 cases including atypical variants, *Am J Surg Pathol* 40:704–713, 2016.
164. Jo VY, Fletcher CDM: SMARCB1/INI1 loss in epithelioid schwannoma: a clinicopathologic and immunohistochemical study of 65 cases, *Am J Surg Pathol* 41:1013–1022, 2017.
165. Jo VY, Fletcher CD: Epithelioid malignant peripheral nerve sheath tumor: clinicopathologic analysis of 63 cases, *Am J Surg Pathol* 39:673–682, 2015.
166. Fetsch JF, Miettinen M: Sclerosing perineurioma: a clinicopathologic study of 19 cases of a distinctive soft tissue lesion with a predilection for the fingers and palms of young adults, *Am J Surg Pathol* 21:1433–1442, 1997.
167. Lopez DA, Silvers DN, Helwig EB: Cutaneous meningiomas—a clinicopathologic study, *Cancer* 34:728–744, 1974.
168. Argenyi ZB: Cutaneous neural heterotopias and related tumors relevant for the dermatopathologist, *Semin Diagn Pathol* 13:60–71, 1996.
169. Theaker JM, Fletcher CD, Tudway AJ: Cutaneous heterotopic meningeal nodules, *Histopathology* 16:475–479, 1990.
170. Suster S, Rosai J: Hamartoma of the scalp with ectopic meningothelial elements. A distinctive benign soft tissue lesion that may simulate angiosarcoma, *Am J Surg Pathol* 14:1–11, 1990.
171. Zelger BW, Cerio R: Xanthogranuloma is the archetype of non-Langerhans cell histiocytoses, *Br J Dermatol* 145:369–371, 2001.
172. Zelger BW, Sidoroff A, Orchard G, et al: Non-Langerhans cell histiocytoses. A new unifying concept, *Am J Dermatopathol* 18:490–504, 1996.
173. Janssen D, Harms D: Juvenile xanthogranuloma in childhood and adolescence: a clinicopathologic study of 129 patients from the kiel pediatric tumor registry, *Am J Surg Pathol* 29:21–28, 2005.
174. Dehner LP: Reawakening to the existence of juvenile xanthogranuloma, *Am J Surg Pathol* 29:119–120, 2005.
175. Miettinen M, Fetsch JF: Reticulohistiocytoma (solitary epithelioid histiocytoma): a clinicopathologic and immunohistochemical study of 44 cases, *Am J Surg Pathol* 30:521–528, 2006.
176. Zelger B, Cerio R, Soyer HP, et al: Reticulohistiocytoma and multicentric reticulohistiocytosis. Histopathologic and immunophenotypic distinct entities, *Am J Dermatopathol* 16:577–584, 1994.
177. Luz FB, Gaspar TAP, Kalil-Gaspar N, et al: Multicentric reticulohistiocytosis, *J Eur Acad Dermatol Venereol* 15:524–531, 2001.

178. Oliver GF, Umbert I, Winkelmann RK, et al: Reticulohistiocytoma cutis—review of 15 cases and an association with systemic vasculitis in two cases, *Clin Exp Dermatol* 15:1–6, 1990.
179. Kong YY, Kong JC, Shi DR, et al: Cutaneous Rosai-Dorfman disease: a clinical and histopathologic study of 25 cases in China, *Am J Surg Pathol* 31:341–350, 2007.
180. Wang KH, Chen WY, Liu HN, et al: Cutaneous Rosai-Dorfman disease: clinicopathological profiles, spectrum and evolution of 21 lesions in six patients, *Br J Dermatol* 154:277–286, 2006.
181. Lu CI, Kuo TT, Wong WR, et al: Clinical and histopathologic spectrum of cutaneous Rosai-Dorfman disease in Taiwan, *J Am Acad Dermatol* 51:931–939, 2004.
182. Brenn T, Calonje E, Granter SR, et al: Cutaneous Rosai-Dorfman disease is a distinct clinical entity, *Am J Dermatopathol* 24:385–391, 2002.
183. Chu P, LeBoit PE: Histologic features of cutaneous sinus histiocytosis (Rosai-Dorfman disease): study of cases both with and without systemic involvement, *J Cutan Pathol* 19:201–206, 1992.
184. Miller K, Goodlad JR, Brenn T: Pleomorphic dermal sarcoma: adverse histologic features predict aggressive behavior and allow distinction from atypical fibroxanthoma, *Am J Surg Pathol* 36:1317–1326, 2012.
185. Mirza B, Weedon D: Atypical fibroxanthoma: a clinicopathological study of 89 cases, *Australas J Dermatol* 46:235–238, 2005.
186. Leong AS, Milios J: Atypical fibroxanthoma of the skin: a clinicopathological and immunohistochemical study and a discussion of its histogenesis, *Histopathology* 11:463–475, 1987.
187. Beer TW, Drury P, Heenan PJ: Atypical fibroxanthoma: a histological and immunohistochemical review of 171 cases, *Am J Dermatopathol* 32:533–540, 2010.
188. Diaz-Cascajo C, Borghi S: Bonczkowitz M. Pigmented atypical fibroxanthoma, *Histopathology* 33:537–541, 1998.
189. Luzar B, Calonje E: Morphological and immunohistochemical characteristics of atypical fibroxanthoma with a special emphasis on potential diagnostic pitfalls: a review, *J Cutan Pathol* 37:301–309, 2010.
190. Thum C, Husain EA, Mulholland K, et al: Atypical fibroxanthoma with pseudoangiomatous features: a histological and immunohistochemical mimic of cutaneous angiosarcoma, *Ann Diagn Pathol* 17:502–507, 2013.
191. Requena L, Sangueza OP, Sanchez Yus E, et al: Clear-cell atypical fibroxanthoma: an uncommon histopathologic variant of atypical fibroxanthoma, *J Cutan Pathol* 24:176–182, 1997.
192. Crowson AN, Carlson-Sweet K, Macinnis C, et al: Clear cell atypical fibroxanthoma: a clinicopathologic study, *J Cutan Pathol* 29:374–381, 2002.
193. Rudisaile SN, Hurt MA, Santa Cruz DJ: Granular cell atypical fibroxanthoma, *J Cutan Pathol* 32:314–317, 2005.
194. Calonje E, Wadden C, Wilson-Jones E, et al: Spindle-cell non-pleomorphic atypical fibroxanthoma: analysis of a series and delineation of a distinctive variant, *Histopathology* 22:247–254, 1993.
195. Longacre TA, Smoller BR, Rouse RV: Atypical fibroxanthoma. Multiple immunohistologic profiles, *Am J Surg Pathol* 17:1199–1209, 1993.
196. Jensen K, Wilkinson B, Wines N, et al: Procollagen 1 expression in atypical fibroxanthoma and other tumors, *J Cutan Pathol* 31:57–61, 2004.
197. Hartel PH, Jackson J, Ducatman BS, et al: CD99 immunoreactivity in atypical fibroxanthoma and pleomorphic malignant fibrous histiocytoma: a useful diagnostic marker, *J Cutan Pathol* 33(Suppl 2):24–28, 2006.
198. de Feraudy S, Mar N, McCalmont TH: Evaluation of CD10 and procollagen 1 expression in atypical fibroxanthoma and dermatofibroma, *Am J Surg Pathol* 32:1111–1122, 2008.
199. Ricci A, Jr, Cartun RW, Zakowski MF: Atypical fibroxanthoma. A study of 14 cases emphasizing the presence of Langerhans' histiocytes with implications for differential diagnosis by antibody panels, *Am J Surg Pathol* 12:591–598, 1988.
200. Thum C, Hollowood K, Birch J, et al: Aberrant Melan-A expression in atypical fibroxanthoma and undifferentiated pleomorphic sarcoma of the skin, *J Cutan Pathol* 38:954–960, 2011.
201. Dei Tos AP, Maestro R, Doglioni C, et al: Ultraviolet-induced p53 mutations in atypical fibroxanthoma, *Am J Pathol* 145:11–17, 1994.
202. Sakamoto A, Oda Y, Itakura E, et al: Immunoexpression of ultraviolet photoproducts and p53 mutation analysis in atypical fibroxanthoma and superficial malignant fibrous histiocytoma, *Mod Pathol* 14:581–588, 2001.
203. Griewank KG, Schilling B, Murali R, et al: TERT promoter mutations are frequent in atypical fibroxanthomas and pleomorphic dermal sarcomas, *Mod Pathol* 27:502–508, 2014.
204. Helbig D, Ihle MA, Pütz K, et al: Oncogene and therapeutic target analyses in atypical fibroxanthomas and pleomorphic dermal sarcomas, *Oncotarget* 7:21763–21774, 2016.
205. Sakamoto A, Oda Y, Itakura E, et al: H-, K-, and N-ras gene mutation in atypical fibroxanthoma and malignant fibrous histiocytoma, *Hum Pathol* 32:1225–1231, 2001.
206. Dettrick A, Strutton G: Atypical fibroxanthoma with perineural or intraneural invasion: report of two cases, *J Cutan Pathol* 33:318–322, 2006.
207. Tardío JC, Pinedo F, Aramburu JA, et al: Pleomorphic dermal sarcoma: a more aggressive neoplasm than previously estimated, *J Cutan Pathol* 43:101–112, 2016.
208. Wang WL, Torres-Cabala C, Curry JL, et al: Metastatic atypical fibroxanthoma: a series of 11 cases including with minimal and no subcutaneous involvement, *Am J Dermatopathol* 37:455–461, 2015.
209. Kamino H, Lee JY, Berke A: Pleomorphic fibroma of the skin: a benign neoplasm with cytologic atypia. A clinicopathologic study of eight cases, *Am J Surg Pathol* 13:107–113, 1989.
210. Nucci MR, Young RH, Fletcher CD: Cellular pseudosarcomatous fibroepithelial stromal polyps of the lower female genital tract: an underrecognized lesion often misdiagnosed as sarcoma, *Am J Surg Pathol* 24:231–240, 2000.
211. Rudolph P, Schubert C, Zelger BG, et al: Differential expression of CD34 and Ki-M1p in pleomorphic fibroma and dermatofibroma with monster cells, *Am J Dermatopathol* 21:414–419, 1999.
212. Mehregan AH, Tavafoghi V, Ghandchi A: Nevus lipomatosus cutaneus superficialis (Hoffmann-Zurhelle), *J Cutan Pathol* 2:307–313, 1975.
213. Jones EW, Marks R, Pongsehirun D: Naevus superficialis lipomatosus. A clinicopathological report of twenty cases, *Br J Dermatol* 93:121–133, 1975.
214. Ross CM: Generalized folded skin with an underlying lipomatous nevus. "The Michelin tire baby.", *Arch Dermatol* 100:320–333, 1969.
215. Burgdorf WH, Doran CK, Worret WI: Folded skin with scarring: Michelin tire baby syndrome?, *J Am Acad Dermatol* 7:90–93, 1982.
216. French CA, Mentzel T, Kutzner H, et al: Intradermal spindle cell/pleomorphic lipoma: a distinct subset, *Am J Dermatopathol* 22:496–502, 2000.
217. Reis-Filho JS, Milanezi F, Soares MF, et al: Intradermal spindle cell/pleomorphic lipoma of the vulva: case report and review of the literature, *J Cutan Pathol* 29:59–62, 2002.
218. Mentzel T, Rütten A, Hantschke M, et al: S-100 protein expressing spindle cells in spindle cell lipoma: a diagnostic pitfall, *Virchows Arch* 469:435–438, 2016.

16

Mesenchymal Tumors of the Gastrointestinal Tract

Brian P. Rubin, MD, PhD, and Jason L. Hornick, MD, PhD

Epithelial neoplasms predominate in the gastrointestinal (GI) tract, as they do in all parenchymal organs and organ systems. However, a wide array of mesenchymal neoplasms also arises in the GI tract, some of which are exclusive or nearly exclusive to such sites. Other mesenchymal tumors that also arise in somatic soft tissue have distinctive features in the GI tract. Most mesenchymal neoplasms are uncommon or rare, and many have overlapping histologic features; therefore, they may be difficult to classify accurately. The purpose of this chapter is to discuss the clinical and pathologic features of the most common mesenchymal tumors of the tubal GI tract, as well as more recently recognized and rarer tumor types. This chapter also focuses on applications of immunohistochemistry and (when relevant) molecular genetics with an emphasis on differential diagnosis. Screening colonoscopy is widely used today, and distinctive colorectal polyps containing spindle cell proliferations are increasingly being recognized; these polyps are also covered in some detail to allow for proper diagnosis.

When confronted with a spindle cell neoplasm in the GI tract, it is necessary to ask two major questions. The first question is whether it is possible that the tumor is an epithelial neoplasm masquerading as a mesenchymal neoplasm (Box 16.1). Just because a neoplasm is composed largely of spindle-shaped cells does not mean that it is not a carcinoma. Remember that carcinomas are many times more common than mesenchymal neoplasms in the GI tract. Immunohistochemical staining for keratins is helpful in this context, because the majority of mesenchymal neoplasms are negative for keratins, whereas even spindle cell (sarcomatoid) and pleomorphic carcinomas are almost always at least focally positive for keratins. When sarcomatoid carcinoma is suspected, at least two keratins should be used; AE1/AE3 and CAM5.2 are excellent screening keratins in this context, which should "unmask" most sarcomatoid carcinomas. Careful histologic examination is critical, and submission of additional tissue sections may also be useful, because there may be focal areas of epithelial dysplasia or a component of conventional adenocarcinoma or squamous cell carcinoma, recognition of which can confirm the diagnosis.

The second question to ask is whether the tumor is a gastrointestinal stromal tumor (GIST). GISTs compose up to 90% of clinically significant mesenchymal neoplasms of the GI tract; thus, this tumor type should always be considered in the differential diagnosis of mural spindle cell (or epithelioid) neoplasms. Although GIST can have a variety of histologic patterns, immunohistochemistry for KIT (CD117) and DOG1 has made the diagnosis relatively straightforward in most cases.

It is also important to appreciate that the distribution and frequency of different mesenchymal neoplasms vary considerably within different anatomic regions of the GI tract. For instance, a spindle cell neoplasm of the esophageal wall is more likely to be a leiomyoma than a GIST, whereas this situation is reversed in the stomach and small intestine. The distribution of the most common mesenchymal neoplasms according to anatomic location is summarized in Box 16.2. It is important to know whether the lesion involves the mucosa, the wall, the mesentery, or the serosa. Mesenchymal tumors often have a characteristic depth of involvement in the tubal gut. For example, GIST usually involves the wall of the GI tract, whereas desmoid fibromatosis typically arises in the mesentery with secondary invasion into the bowel wall.

Once the basic information previously discussed has been determined, histologic features should be considered (Box 16.3). Is the lesion monomorphic or pleomorphic? Is it composed predominantly of

Box 16.1 Important Questions to Ask When Faced With a Mesenchymal Lesion of the Gastrointestinal Tract

Could the lesion be an epithelial neoplasm masquerading as a mesenchymal neoplasm?
Is the lesion a gastrointestinal stromal tumor?
Where is the lesion located?
Does the lesion involve the serosa, wall, or mucosa?
Does the lesion predominantly contain epithelioid or spindle-shaped cells?
Is there a principal architectural arrangement of the cells?
What does the cytoplasm look like? Quality? Color?
Is the lesion mitotically active?
Are there atypical mitotic figures?
Are there any distinctive features?

Box 16.2 Most Common Locations of Various Mesenchymal Neoplasms of the Gastrointestinal Tract

Esophagus

Leiomyoma
Granular cell tumor

Stomach

Gastrointestinal stromal tumor
Schwannoma
Inflammatory fibroid polyp
Glomus tumor
Plexiform fibromyxoma

Small Intestine

Gastrointestinal stromal tumor
Desmoid fibromatosis (mesentery)
Inflammatory fibroid polyp
Clear cell sarcoma-like tumor

Colon

Leiomyoma of the muscularis mucosae
Mucosal perineurioma
Polypoid ganglioneuroma
Perivascular epithelioid cell tumor (PEComa)

Box 16.3 Histologic Patterns

Spindle Cell

GIST
Schwannoma
Leiomyoma
Leiomyosarcoma
Desmoid fibromatosis
Inflammatory fibroid polyp
Plexiform fibromyxoma
Clear cell sarcoma-like tumor

Epithelioid

GIST (especially *PDGFRA*-mutant and succinate dehydrogenase-deficient gastric GIST)
Granular cell tumor
Glomus tumor
Clear cell sarcoma-like tumor
PEComa

Myxoid

GIST (especially *PDGFRA*-mutant epithelioid GIST)
Plexiform fibromyxoma

Pleomorphic

Leiomyosarcoma
Dedifferentiated liposarcoma

GIST, Gastrointestinal stromal tumor; *PDGFRA*, platelet-derived growth factor receptor A; *PEComa*, perivascular epithelioid cell tumor.

epithelioid cells or spindle-shaped cells? Is there a predominant architectural pattern such as nested for epithelioid neoplasms or fascicular for spindle cell neoplasms? What do the nuclei look like? What about the cytoplasm? How about the stroma—is it myxoid? Is the lesion mitotically active? Are there atypical mitotic figures? Are there any other distinctive features such as vacuolated cytoplasm or nuclear palisading? The discussions of the neoplasms in this chapter will examine each of these questions, with emphasis on approaches to differential diagnosis. Once a differential diagnosis has been generated based on site, depth, and histologic pattern, a specific diagnosis can be confirmed with a carefully chosen panel of immunohistochemical markers, in some cases supplemented with molecular studies.

This chapter does not attempt to be absolutely comprehensive. Submucosal lipomas are relatively common in the colon, but diagnosis is usually straightforward, and these lesions are therefore not discussed. Well-differentiated and dedifferentiated liposarcomas may involve the wall of the GI tract; these tumor types are discussed in detail in Chapter 12 and will not be covered in this chapter, except in differential diagnosis when appropriate. Vascular lesions (other than vascular malformations) are rare in the GI tract and are histologically similar to their counterparts arising at other anatomic sites; these lesions are discussed in detail in Chapter 13.

Gastrointestinal Stromal Tumor

GISTs are the most common clinically significant mesenchymal neoplasm of the GI tract.[1,2] Historically, these lesions were classified as smooth muscle tumors under the names leiomyoma, leiomyosarcoma, or leiomyoblastoma (the latter for epithelioid examples). However, it is now recognized that these tumors are not true smooth muscle neoplasms and must be distinguished from leiomyoma and leiomyosarcoma. Perhaps the most important message of this section is to exclude the diagnosis of GIST, especially in the stomach and small intestine, before considering other less common diagnoses.

GIST has gained considerable clinical importance; it has become the "poster child" for targeted therapy in solid tumors (see the section "Prognosis and Treatment"). GIST therapies target KIT and platelet-derived growth factor receptor A (PDGFRA), which are constitutively activated by mutation and drive cellular proliferation in most GISTs. Because effective systemic therapies for GIST are available, proper diagnosis is critically important. The finding of KIT activation in GIST also led to the realization that GISTs arise from interstitial cells of Cajal or precursors to such cells. Interstitial cells of Cajal are distinctive mesenchymal cells within the stomach and bowel wall that are involved in peristalsis. GIST is one of the few mesenchymal neoplasms for which the normal cellular counterpart has been identified.

Clinical Features

GIST can develop at any age but is most common in middle-aged to elderly adults; the median age is 58 years.[1–3] It occurs approximately equally in males and females. GIST can be seen at any site along the GI tract, including unusual sites such as the gallbladder, pancreas, and appendix, but is most common in the stomach (60%) and small intestine (30%). Rarely, GISTs appear to arise from extragastrointestinal soft tissues within the abdomen (mesentery or omentum), pelvis, or retroperitoneum; collectively, such tumors are known as extragastrointestinal GISTs.[4–6] However, careful analysis of such lesions indicates that a major subset originates from the GI musculature, grow in an exophytic manner, and subsequently lose their attachment to the GI tract.[7] True extragastrointestinal GISTs are exceedingly rare.

GIST has a tendency to ulcerate the mucosa; it typically presents with GI bleeding, anemia, or intestinal obstruction. Affected patients may present with a palpable mass. Massive intraabdominal hemorrhage is uncommon. Some tumors are identified incidentally by radiography, whereas other cases are found incidentally during endoscopy or surgery for unrelated reasons. Small, clinically insignificant tumors known as microGISTs are very common in the stomach, and are present in up to 35% of middle-aged to elderly adults.[8–10]

Aggressive GISTs have a propensity for dissemination throughout the surfaces of the abdominal cavity and metastasis to the liver. Although GISTs are capable of metastasizing outside of the abdomen, primarily to lung and bone, this is a rare occurrence. Importantly, in contrast to carcinomas, GISTs rarely metastasize to lymph nodes (with notable exceptions; see subsequent discussion), making compulsory lymph node dissection unnecessary.

Rarely, GISTs occur in children (1%–2%), mainly in girls.[11–13] Such tumors arise in the stomach, often as multifocal lesions, and commonly metastasize to lymph nodes. Gastric GISTs are also a major feature of two tumor syndromes: Carney triad (along with pulmonary chondroma and paraganglioma) and Carney-Stratakis syndrome (along with paraganglioma).[14–16] Pediatric GISTs, the GISTs in patients with Carney triad and Carney-Stratakis syndrome, and up to 10% of gastric GISTs in adults outside of these syndromes have distinctive histologic features, clinical behavior, and molecular pathogenesis, and are now referred to collectively as succinate dehydrogenase (SDH)-deficient GISTs. GISTs are also a less common tumor type of type 1 neurofibromatosis (NF1); when present, such tumors typically arise as multiple lesions in the small intestine.[17,18]

Pathologic Features

GISTs range from incidental minute lesions no more than 1 mm in size to large masses more than 40 cm in greatest dimension.[19] The median size for clinically significant GISTs is 6 cm in the stomach, 4.5 cm in the duodenum, and 7 cm in the jejunum/ileum.[13,20,21] Lesions are usually centered in the bowel wall with frequent mucosal ulceration (Fig. 16.1). On cut section, they may be either fibrous or fleshy with central degeneration (see Fig. 16.1). Some GISTs are almost entirely cystic, whereas others are gelatinous or extensively necrotic.

GISTs range from pure spindle cell neoplasms (Fig. 16.2) to pure epithelioid neoplasms (Fig. 16.3). A subset of tumors contains both

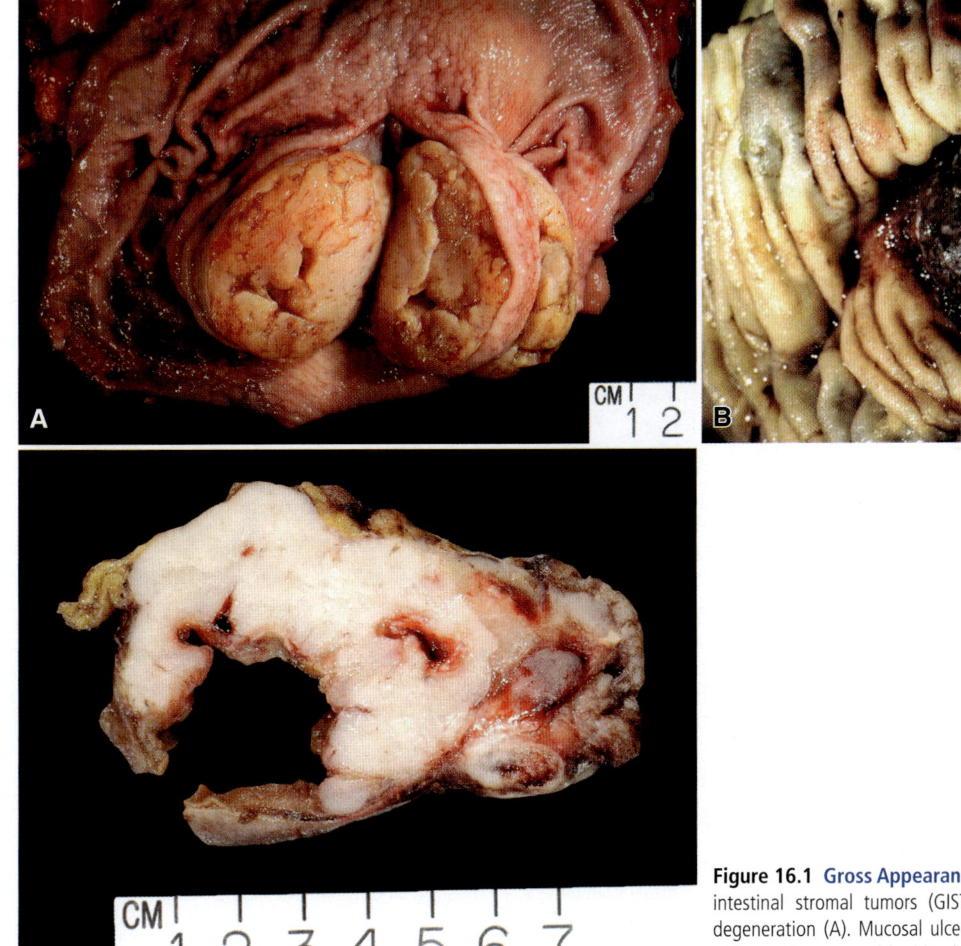

Figure 16.1 Gross Appearances of Gastrointestinal Stromal Tumors. Gastrointestinal stromal tumors (GIST) showing typical fleshy appearance with central degeneration (A). Mucosal ulceration is common, as seen in this small bowel GIST with an ulcer capped by blood and granulation tissue (B). This aggressive GIST has replaced the wall of the small bowel (C).

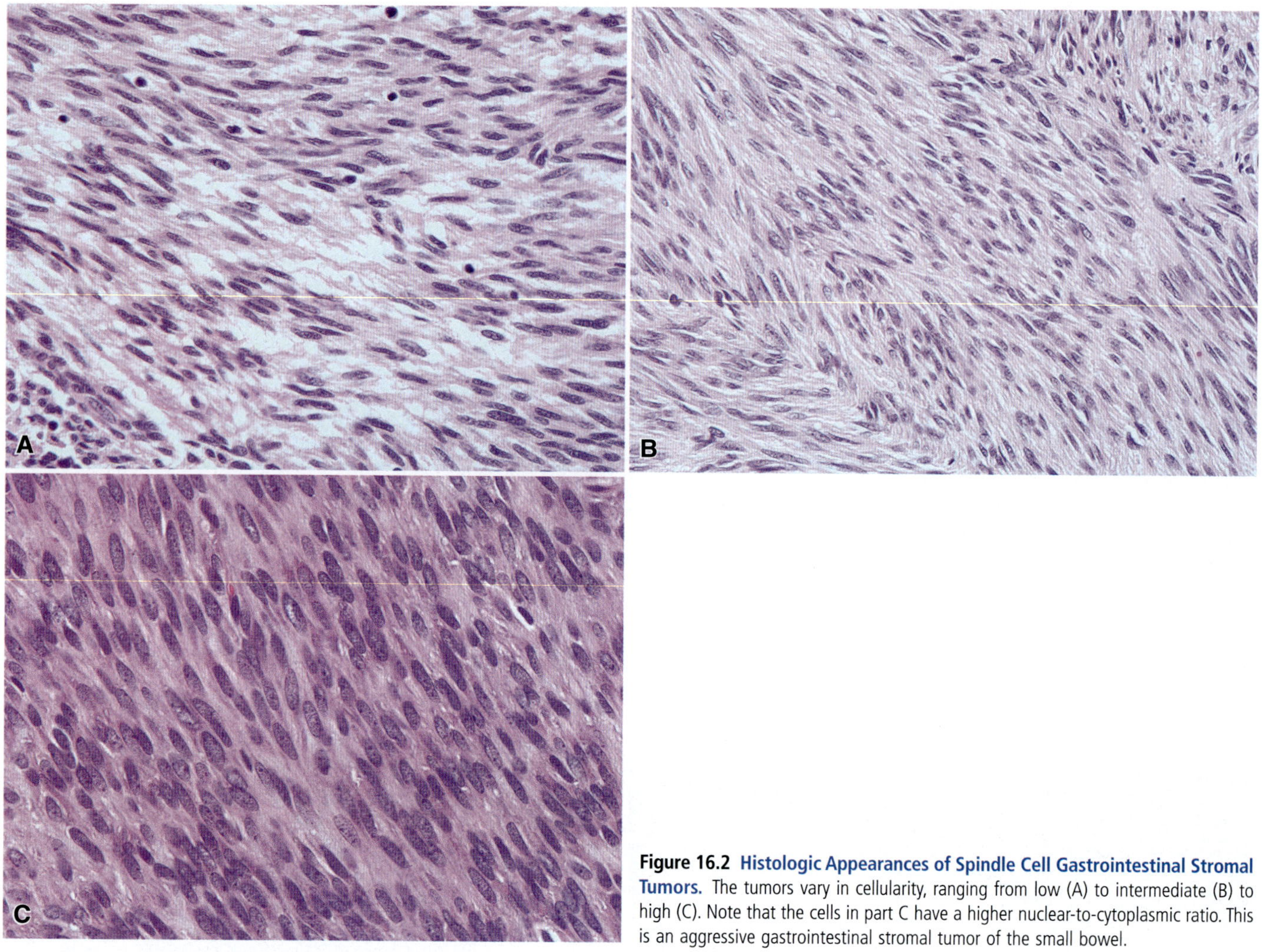

Figure 16.2 **Histologic Appearances of Spindle Cell Gastrointestinal Stromal Tumors.** The tumors vary in cellularity, ranging from low (A) to intermediate (B) to high (C). Note that the cells in part C have a higher nuclear-to-cytoplasmic ratio. This is an aggressive gastrointestinal stromal tumor of the small bowel.

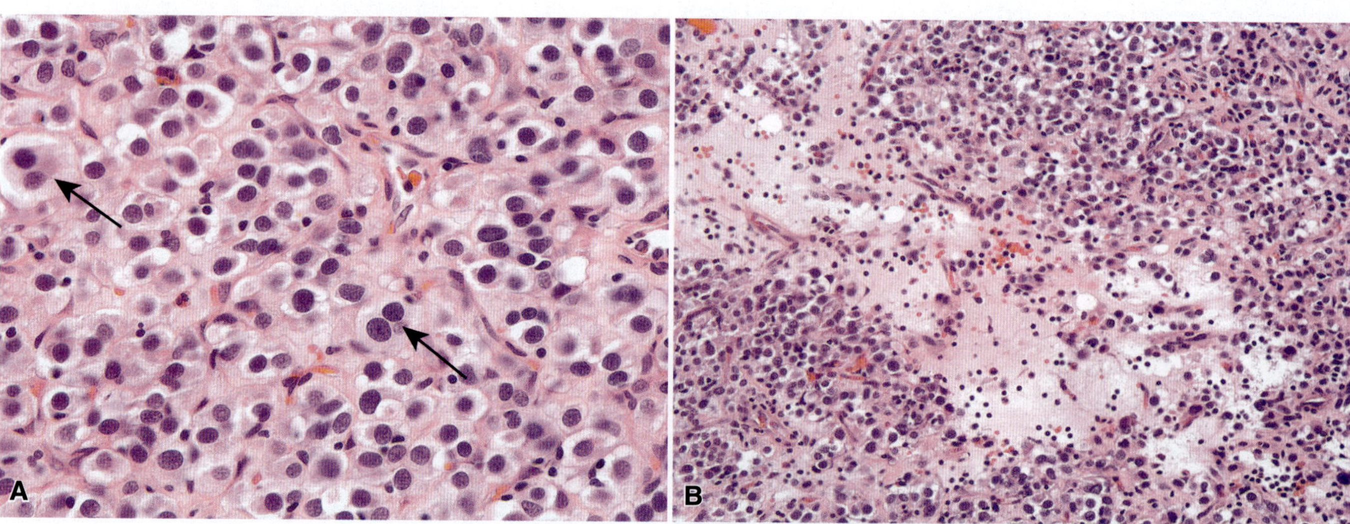

Figure 16.3 **Histologic Appearances of Epithelioid Gastrointestinal Stromal Tumors.** The tumor is composed of nests of epithelioid cells with abundant eosinophilic cytoplasm, variably sized nucleoli, and frequent binucleation (A, *arrows*). Epithelioid gastrointestinal stromal tumors often have areas of myxoid stroma (B).

spindle cells and epithelioid cells. Lesions vary considerably in terms of cellularity. Less-cellular neoplasms are generally smaller, tend to have hyalinized stroma, and may exhibit dystrophic calcifications (Fig. 16.4). Spindle cell GISTs contain elongated nuclei with vesicular chromatin, inconspicuous nucleoli, and moderate amounts of fibrillary palely eosinophilic cytoplasm (Fig. 16.5). The spindle cells are usually arranged in short fascicles. Nuclear palisading and paranuclear vacuolization are not unusual (Fig. 16.6); the latter is a feature of gastric tumors. The vasculature may be minimal or prominent, hyalinized, or hemangiopericytoma-like, but there are no characteristic vascular features. A sparse chronic inflammatory component may be observed, most often scattered lymphocytes. So-called skeinoid fibers, variably sized collections of collagen fibrils, can also be found in the stroma of GISTs; this is seen almost exclusively in the small bowel (Fig. 16.7).[20,21] Epithelioid GISTs contain round nuclei, vesicular chromatin, variably prominent nucleoli, and abundant eosinophilic cytoplasm with ill-defined cell borders or clear cytoplasm with distinct cell borders (Fig. 16.8). Binucleation is not unusual. The epithelioid cells are arranged in sheets or nests. When tumor cells are arranged in nests, this may impart a paraganglioma-like appearance. Myxoid stroma is more common in epithelioid GISTs (Fig. 16.9).

A distinctive multinodular or plexiform architecture is observed in SDH-deficient GISTs (Fig. 16.10).[14,22–24] This histologic pattern is characterized by coarse lobules of tumor separated by bands of normal smooth muscle or small nodules with irregular margins extending from the main tumor (Fig. 16.11A). Such a growth pattern should raise the possibility of this unusual subset of GISTs, because they show distinct clinical behavior. These tumors nearly always have epithelioid or mixed epithelioid and spindle cell morphology (see Fig. 16.11B).[22,23]

Mitotic activity is usually low in both epithelioid and spindle cell GISTs; the mitotic rate must be determined in 5 mm^2 to perform risk stratification (see the section "Prognosis and Treatment"). Furthermore,

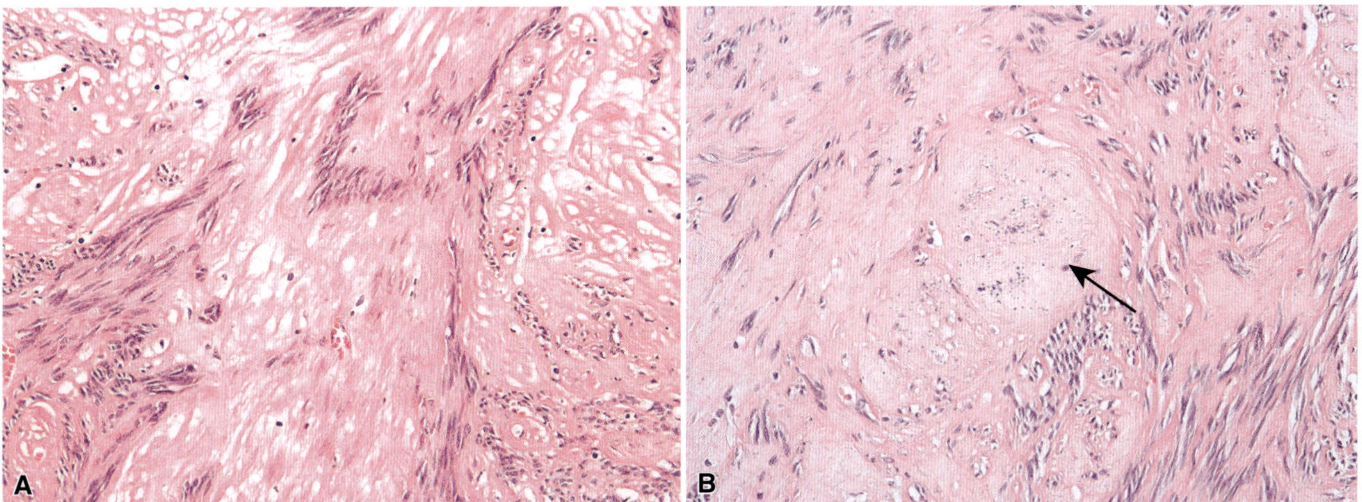

Figure 16.4 Hypocellular Gastrointestinal Stromal Tumor. The tumor contains hyalinized stroma (A) and dystrophic calcifications (B, *arrow*).

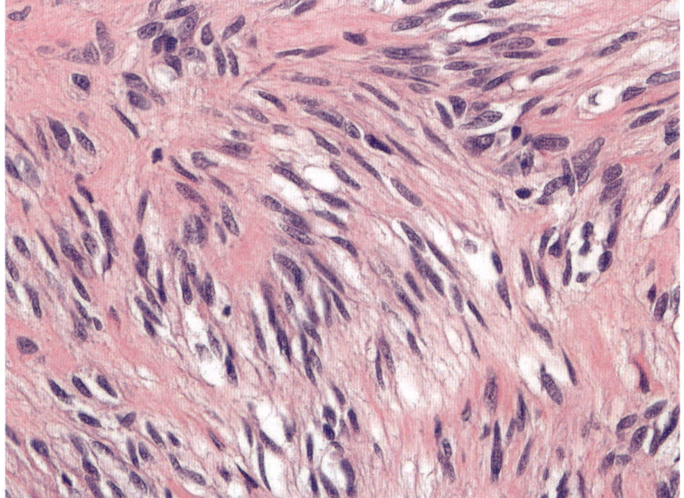

Figure 16.5 Spindle Cell Gastrointestinal Stromal Tumor. The tumor is composed of uniform, bland spindle cells with elongated nuclei and palely eosinophilic, fibrillary cytoplasm.

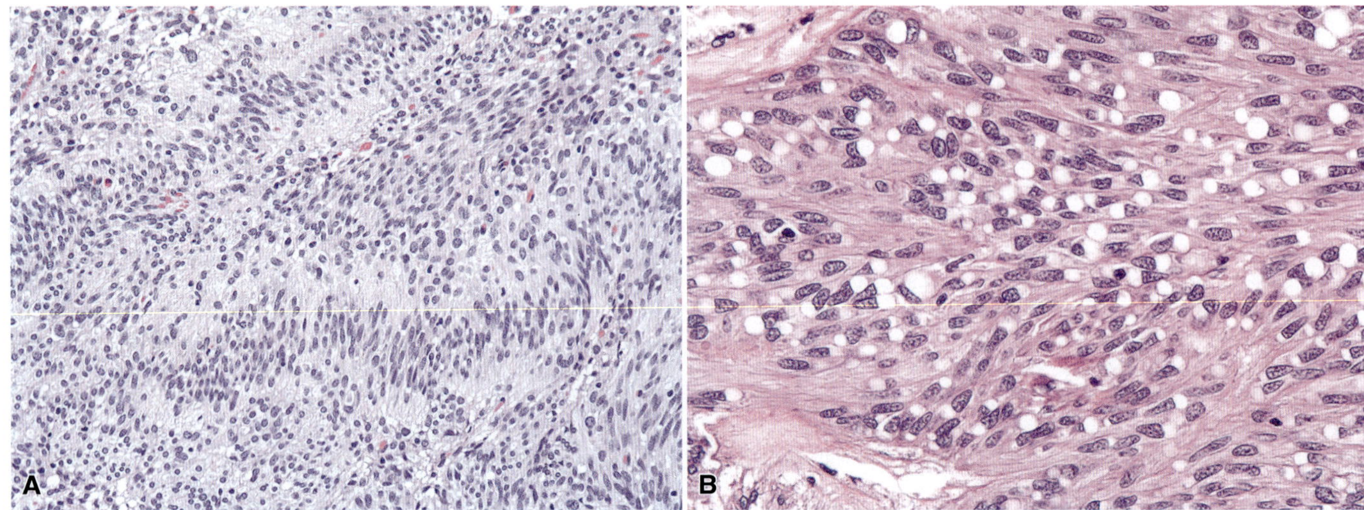

Figure 16.6 Spindle Cell Gastrointestinal Stromal Tumor. Some tumors show nuclear palisading (A) or paranuclear vacuolization (B).

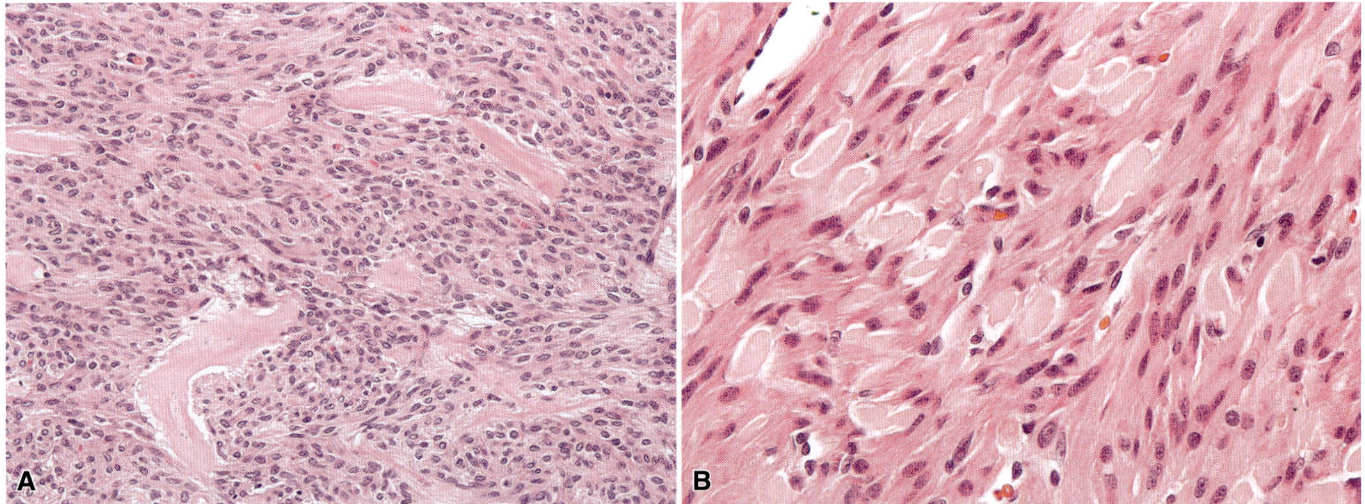

Figure 16.7 Spindle Cell Gastrointestinal Stromal Tumor. (A and B) Skeinoid fibers in two different spindle cell gastrointestinal stromal tumors of the small bowel.

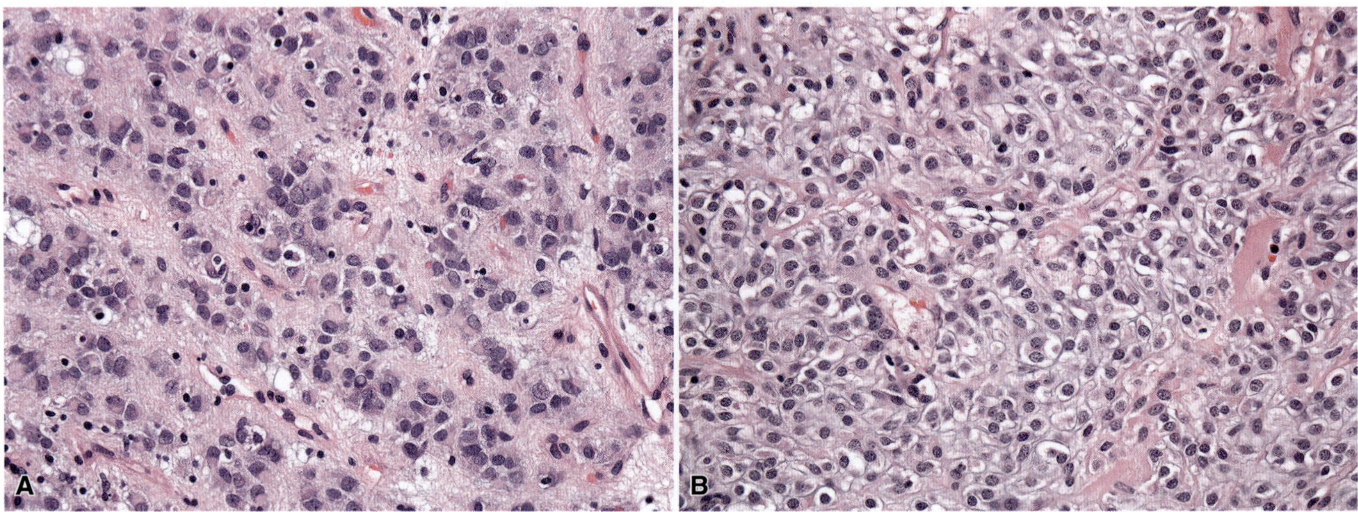

Figure 16.8 Epithelioid Gastrointestinal Stromal Tumor. The tumor may be composed of rounded cells with eosinophilic, fibrillary cytoplasm (A) or clear cells with well-defined cell borders (B).

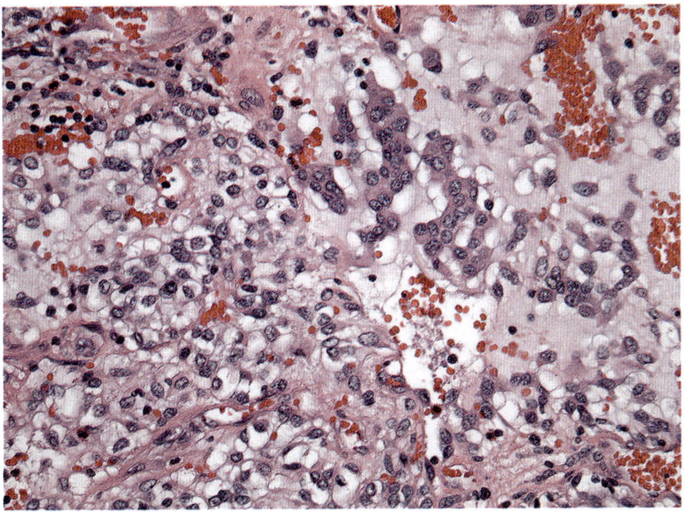

Figure 16.9 Epithelioid Gastrointestinal Stromal Tumor. Some tumors contain prominent myxoid stroma.

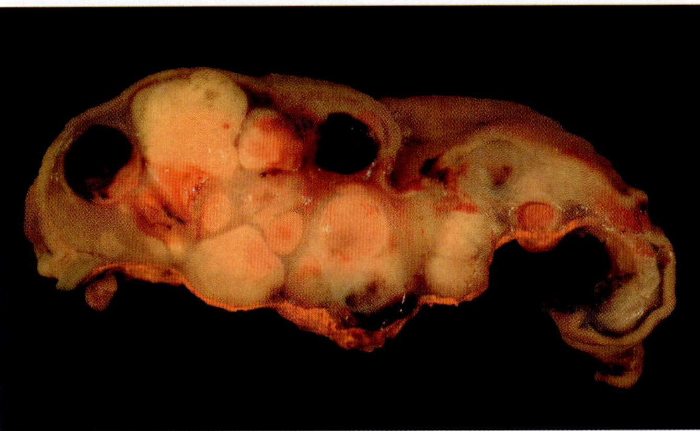

Figure 16.10 Gross Appearance of Succinate Dehydrogenase-Deficient Gastrointestinal Stromal Tumor. The tumor infiltrates the wall of the stomach as multiple nodules.

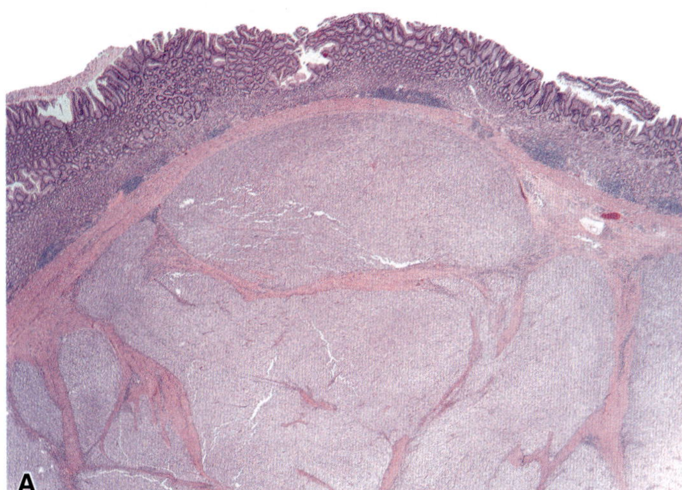

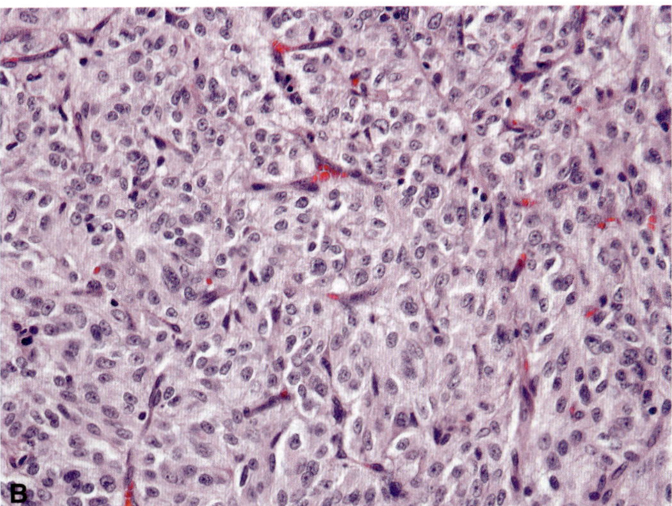

Figure 16.11 Succinate Dehydrogenase-Deficient Gastrointestinal Stromal Tumor. These tumors show a multinodular and plexiform architecture (A). Most succinate dehydrogenase-deficient gastrointestinal stromal tumors show epithelioid morphology (B).

atypical mitotic figures are very rare. Nuclear pleomorphism is also highly unusual in GIST, observed in no more than 2% of tumors. More often than not, cytologic pleomorphism suggests the diagnosis of other sarcomas such as leiomyosarcoma. One notable exception is the very rare dedifferentiated GIST.[25] Analogous to dedifferentiated liposarcoma, dedifferentiated GIST is defined by a transition from morphologically and immunohistochemically typical GIST to an anaplastic sarcomatous appearance that lacks the histologic features of GIST, as well as KIT and DOG1 expression (Fig. 16.12). The dedifferentiated component may show a wide range of histologic appearances, ranging from a fascicular spindle cell appearance to wildly pleomorphic or resembling "inflammatory malignant fibrous histiocytoma."

Immunohistochemistry

Approximately 95% of GISTs are strongly positive for KIT (CD117).[2,3] KIT immunoreactivity is usually diffuse and cytoplasmic but may occasionally show a membranous or a dot-like (Golgi) pattern (Fig. 16.13). The membranous pattern is the least common. Interestingly, KIT-negative GISTs tend to have epithelioid morphology, arise in the stomach, and harbor *PDGFRA* mutations.[26] All other GIST genotypes usually express KIT diffusely and strongly. Approximately 70% of GISTs are positive for CD34, 30% for smooth muscle actin (SMA), and 5% for S-100. Desmin or keratin expression is observed in 2% and less than 1% of tumors, respectively. However, up to 20% of duodenal GISTs can be immunoreactive for S-100,[20] usually focally, and 10%–15% of gastric epithelioid GISTs are focally positive for desmin. The smooth muscle marker h-caldesmon is positive in about 80% of GISTs; this marker therefore cannot be used to distinguish between GISTs and smooth muscle tumors.[27] DOG1 (also known as ANO1, anoctamin 1) has been developed as an additional immunohistochemical marker.[28,29] DOG1 is sensitive and relatively specific for GIST, and is diffusely and strongly positive in 98% of GISTs (see Fig. 16.13D). It is especially

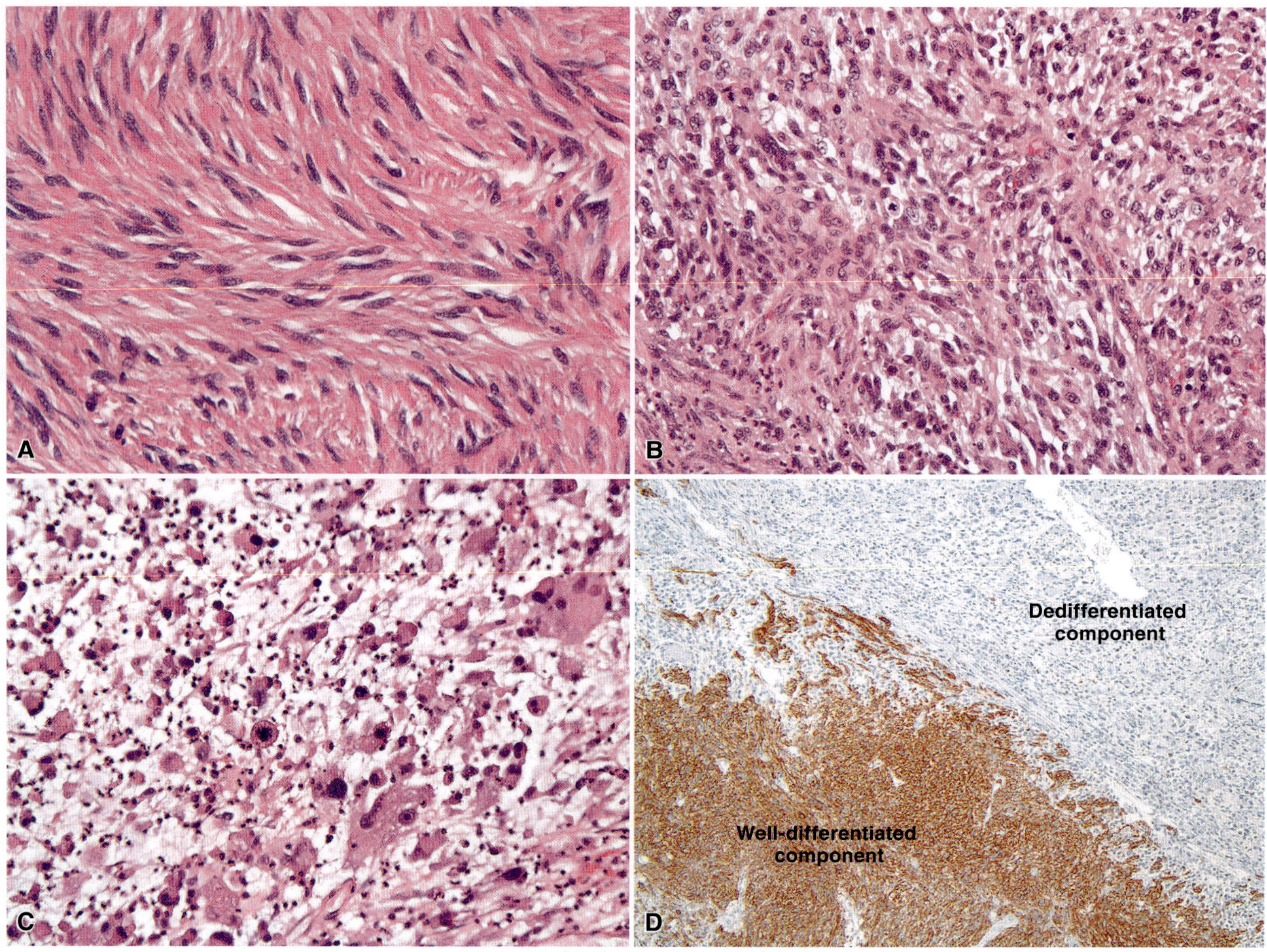

Figure 16.12 **Dedifferentiated Gastrointestinal Stromal Tumor.** Well-differentiated spindle cell gastrointestinal stromal tumor (GIST) (A) with a transition to a poorly differentiated neoplasm with round cell morphology and scant myxoid stroma (B). In areas, the tumor cells are pleomorphic, contain atypical mitotic figures, and include large bizarre cells (C). Immunohistochemistry for KIT is positive in the well-differentiated GIST and negative in the dedifferentiated component (D).

useful in the diagnosis of KIT-negative GISTs and GISTs with only limited KIT expression (Fig. 16.14).[30]

One warning regarding KIT staining: it is important to maintain good controls. Overzealous antigen retrieval or inadequate dilution may occasionally result in false positive staining. Mast cells, which are nearly always present in sections of bowel wall, show strong membranous staining for KIT and thus serve as an excellent internal control (Fig. 16.15). The muscle wall should be entirely negative. When antigen retrieval is used, gastric glands may show weak nonspecific cytoplasmic staining for KIT. No such staining is seen without antigen retrieval.

Immunohistochemistry for the mitochondrial protein succinate dehydrogenase subunit B (SDHB) can be used to identify SDH-deficient GISTs.[22,24,31] These distinctive gastric GISTs show loss of SDHB expression (irrespective of the underlying mutation), whereas conventional adult GISTs show normal granular cytoplasmic (mitochondrial) staining (Fig. 16.16).[22] SDH-deficient GISTs with *SDHA* mutations (see below) show loss of SDHA expression as well as SDHB; SDHA can therefore be used to identify *SDHA*-mutant tumors.[32,33]

Molecular Genetics

About 80% of advanced GISTs contain activating *KIT* mutations.[34-36] There are four mutation "hotspots," which makes identification of mutations relatively straightforward (Fig. 16.17). In about 65% of GISTs, *KIT* mutations are identified in exon 11, 10% in exon 9, and approximately 1% each in exons 13 and 17. Activating mutations in *PDGFRA* are identified in 5%–10% of advanced GISTs (see Fig. 16.17).[37] The most common "hotspot" in *PDGFRA* is exon 18 (nearly always the D842V substitution), followed by exons 12 and 14. *PDGFRA* mutations are found predominantly in gastric and omental GISTs with epithelioid cytomorphology.[26,38] *KIT* or *PDGFRA* mutations are found in the smallest, subcentimeter microGISTs and thus are thought to constitute the earliest molecular events in most GISTs.[39] *KIT* and *PDGFRA* mutations are mutually exclusive. All of the mutant forms of *KIT* and *PDGFRA* encode virtually full-length, constitutively activated KIT and PDGFRA, which drive cellular proliferation. Inhibition of KIT or PDGFRA has a dramatic therapeutic effect in GIST. Those GISTs without identifiable *KIT* or *PDGFRA* mutations are known as wild-type GISTs. This

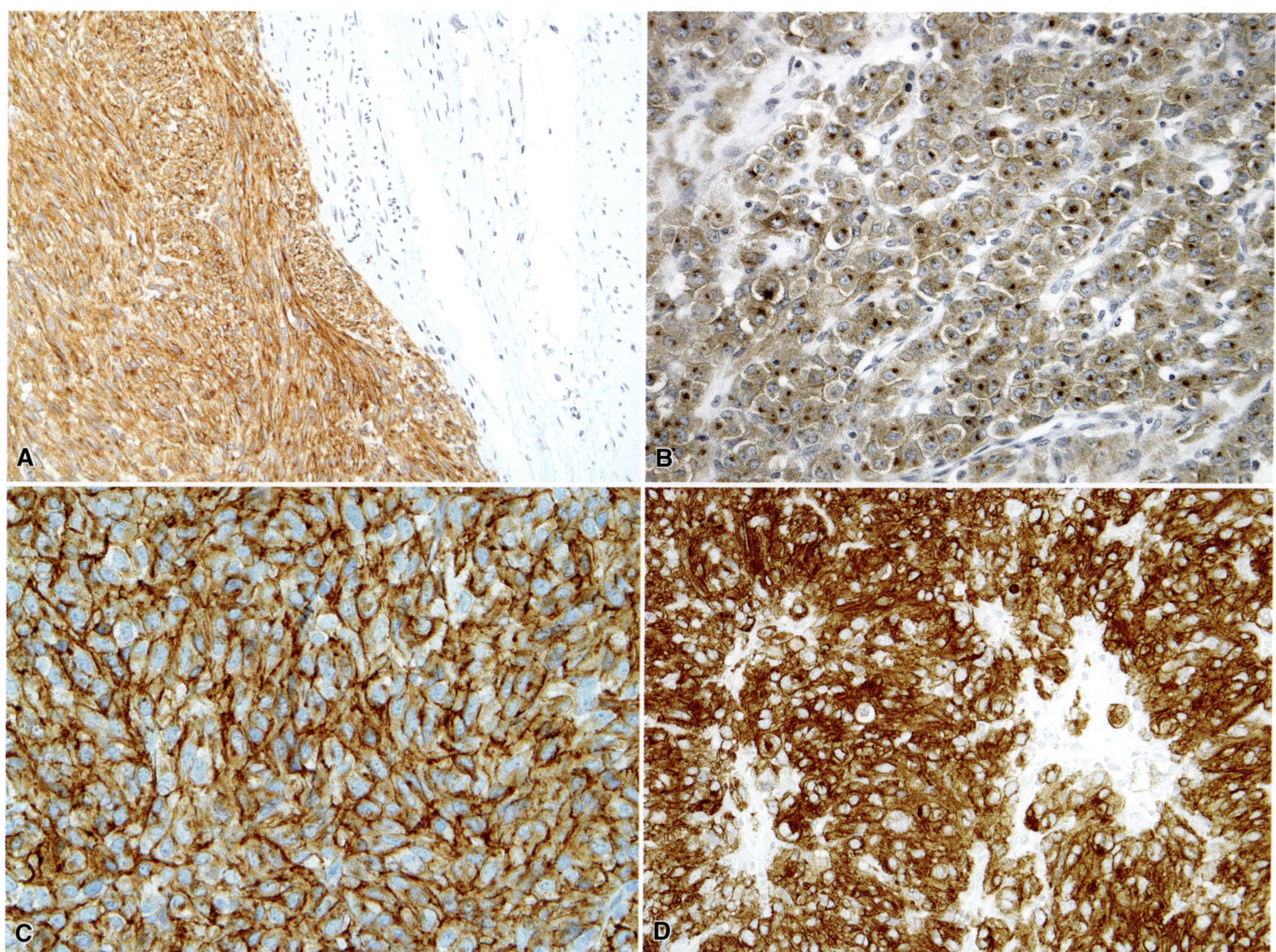

Figure 16.13 Immunohistochemistry for KIT and DOG1 in Gastrointestinal Stromal Tumor. A diffuse, cytoplasmic pattern of KIT staining is most common (A). Some (predominantly epithelioid) tumors show a dot-like (Golgi) pattern of KIT staining (B). A membranous pattern of KIT staining is rare (C). DOG1 typically shows a membranous staining pattern (D).

group is comprised predominantly of SDH-deficient GISTs (5% of all GISTs), *BRAF* V600E-mutant GISTs (1% of all GISTs; Fig. 16.18), and *NF1*-mutant GISTs (1% of all GISTs).[35,36,40–42] Very recently, extremely rare gene fusions involving *FGFR1* and *NTRK3* have been identified in GISTs.[43,44] Finally, there is still a group of exceedingly rare, truly wild-type GISTs known as quadruple-wild-type GISTs that do not have any apparent oncogenic driver mutations.[45] The genetics of GISTs is also discussed in Chapter 18.

Multiple families have been identified with familial GIST.[46] Affected patients harbor germline mutations in *KIT* or *PDGFRA* of exactly the same types that are found in sporadic GISTs. Patients who harbor germline *KIT* or *PDGFRA* mutations develop GIST with nearly 100% penetrance. As mentioned earlier, GIST is also associated with several tumor syndromes. Approximately 7% of patients with NF1 develop GISTs. NF1-associated GISTs typically arise in the small intestine as multiple small tumors.[17,18] GIST is also associated with Carney-Stratakis syndrome, which is characterized by paraganglioma and gastric GIST.[15] Similar to familial paraganglioma, patients with Carney-Stratakis harbor germline mutations in the SDH subunit genes *SDHB, SDHC,* or *SDHD.*[47] Sporadic (non-syndromic) SDH-deficient GISTs also harbor germline or less commonly somatic mutations in *SDHA, SDHB, SDHC,* or *SDHD.*[48–50] Overall, *SDHA* mutations are the most common alterations in this group of tumors, found in 35%–40% of SDH-deficient GISTs.[32,33] As mentioned previously, pediatric GISTs, similar gastric GISTs in adults, and GISTs in patients with Carney triad and Carney-Stratakis syndrome show loss of SDHB protein expression by immunohistochemistry and SDH function, irrespective of whether they have germline mutations in SDH subunit genes (or which particular gene is mutated).[22,24,31,48] Patients with Carney triad develop epithelioid gastric GIST, pulmonary chondroma, and extraadrenal paraganglioma.[16] The genetic basis of Carney triad has recently been elucidated; in most cases, this syndrome is due to hypermethylation of the *SDHC* promoter, which also leads to loss of SDHB expression.[51,52] Mutational analysis for *KIT* and *PDGFRA* is recommended if imatinib therapy is initiated for unresectable or metastatic disease (see later discussion).[53] Mutational analysis should also be performed for patients with primary localized disease, when tumors are intermediate or high risk; adjuvant imatinib therapy prevents recurrence in such patients. This analysis is straightforward and does not require frozen tissue; the genomic "hotspots" can be amplified from DNA derived from paraffin-embedded tissue.

It is taken for granted that *KIT* or *PDGFRA* mutation is the initiating event in the pathogenesis of most GISTs. However, not as much is

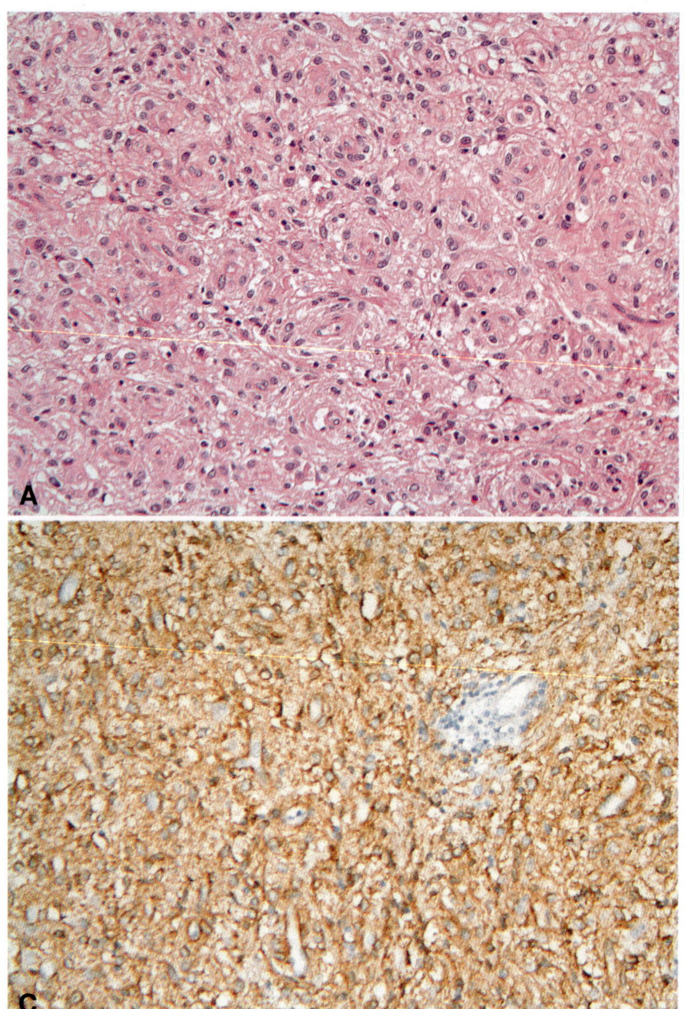

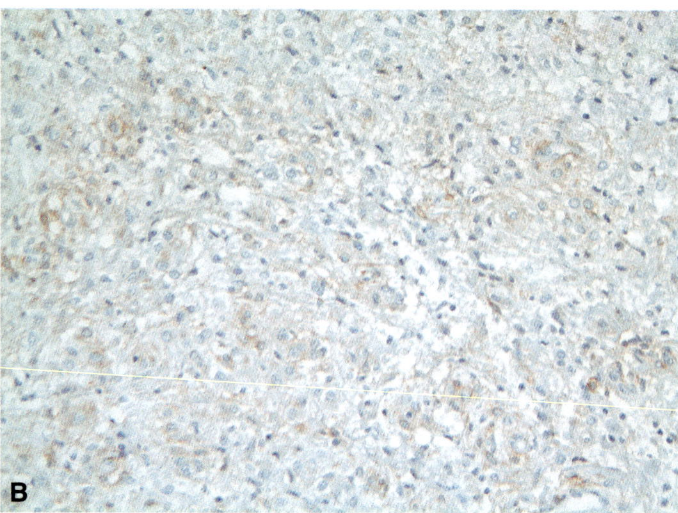

Figure 16.14 *PDGFRA*-Mutant Gastrointestinal Stromal Tumor. Epithelioid morphology is common in gastrointestinal stromal tumors with *PDGFRA* mutations (A). There is very limited (weak and focal) KIT expression (B). However, the tumor is diffusely and strongly positive for DOG1 (C).

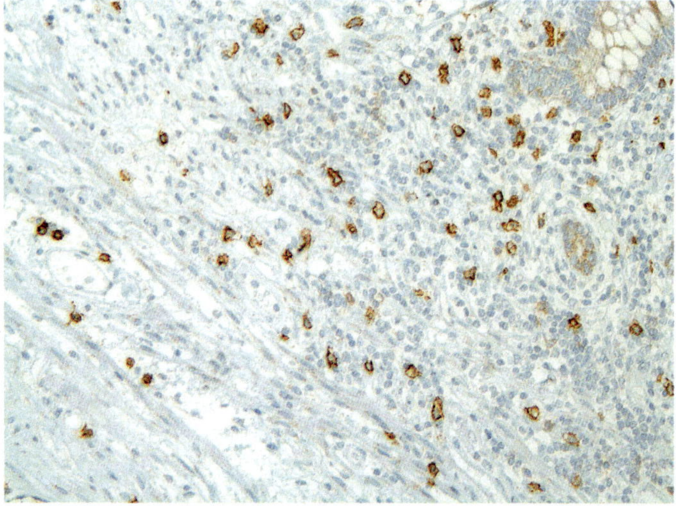

Figure 16.15 KIT Immunoreactivity in Mast Cells. Shown here are numerous KIT-positive mast cells in the lamina propria of the small bowel. Note the membranous staining pattern, which is a clue that the positive cells are mast cells.

known about the secondary events involved in malignant progression. The accumulated data from cytogenetic and comparative genomic hybridization analysis indicate that losses at chromosomes 14q and 22q are very frequent and are not believed to contribute to malignant behavior. However, losses at 1p, 9p/9q, 11p, and 15q, as well as gains at 5p, 8q, 17q, and 20q, are reported more often in clinically aggressive GISTs.[54] In general, greater numbers of genetic changes correlate with more aggressive behavior.

Loss of 9p is associated with an aggressive clinical course and appears to represent loss of the *CDKN2A* locus.[55] The *CDKN2A* locus encodes two distinct tumor suppressor genes, *p16* (*INK4A*) and *p14* (*ARF*). Loss of both transcripts contributes to the aggressive phenotype.[56]

Differential Diagnosis

The differential diagnosis for GIST is broad, but it is important to remember that GISTs are the most common mesenchymal neoplasms of the GI tract. Therefore when confronted with a mesenchymal neoplasm that involves the tubal gut, especially the stomach and small intestine, the diagnosis is very likely to be GIST. However, other tumor types can mimic GIST: leiomyoma, leiomyosarcoma, schwannoma, and desmoid fibromatosis, among others. Fortunately, immunohistochemistry is very

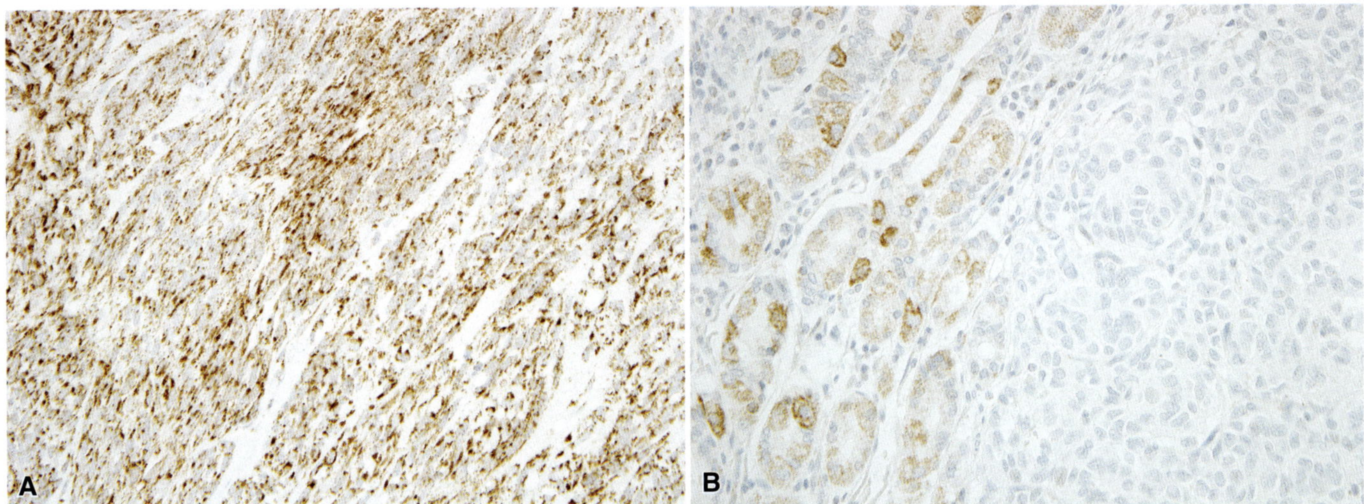

Figure 16.16 **Immunohistochemistry for Succinate Dehydrogenase Subunit B in Gastrointestinal Stromal Tumor.** Normal granular cytoplasmic staining for succinate dehydrogenase subunit B (SDHB) in a typical *KIT*-mutant gastrointestinal stromal tumor (GIST) (A). Loss of SDHB staining in a succinate dehydrogenase-deficient GIST (B). Note the positive staining in the adjacent gastric mucosa.

Table 16.1 Differential Diagnosis of Common Mesenchymal Tumors of the Gastrointestinal Tract

Diagnosis	KIT and DOG1	Desmin	S-100
GIST	+++ (95%–98%)	— (2%)	— (5%)
Leiomyoma	—	+++ (100%)	—
Leiomyosarcoma	—	++ (50%)	—
Schwannoma	—	—	+++ (100%)
Desmoid fibromatosis	—	—	—

GIST, Gastrointestinal stromal tumor.

helpful in resolving this differential diagnosis (Table 16.1). Mural leiomyomas are most common in the esophagus, whereas polypoid leiomyomas of the muscularis mucosae arise in the colorectum; at both of these sites, leiomyoma is more common than GIST. In contrast to GIST, leiomyoma is composed of fascicles of spindle cells with blunt-ended (cigar-shaped) nuclei, brightly eosinophilic cytoplasm, and well-defined cell borders. Leiomyoma is invariably diffusely and strongly positive for SMA and desmin, and negative for KIT and DOG1. Of note, esophageal leiomyomas often contain numerous KIT-positive mast cells and interstitial cells of Cajal, which can be a diagnostic pitfall if mistakenly interpreted as positive staining in tumor cells.[57] Primary leiomyosarcomas of the GI tract are very rare, vastly outnumbered by GISTs. In contrast to GIST, leiomyosarcomas usually have prominent cytologic pleomorphism and a high mitotic rate, including atypical mitotic figures. Leiomyosarcoma is usually positive for SMA, very often positive for desmin, and negative for KIT. In the GI tract, schwannomas are most common in the stomach, and in this location, they tend to have prominent peripheral lymphoid aggregates. Gastric schwannomas generally lack the varying cellularity (Antoni A and B zonation), Verocay bodies, and hyalinized vessels typical of schwannomas of peripheral nerves. GI schwannomas have a greater degree of cytologic variability than GIST and often contain prominent stromal collagen. Schwannomas are invariably positive for S-100 and negative for KIT. Desmoid fibromatosis usually involves the mesentery with secondary invasion into the bowel wall. Desmoid tumors are composed of long fascicles of spindle cells often with prominent stromal collagen. These tumors are focally positive for SMA but are negative for KIT and DOG1. About 80% of desmoid tumors show aberrant nuclear staining for β-catenin, which can be used to confirm the diagnosis.

Epithelioid GIST should be distinguished from well-differentiated neuroendocrine (carcinoid) tumor, poorly differentiated adenocarcinoma, and glomus tumor. Carcinoid tumors often have a predominantly trabecular or nested architecture, and the uniform tumor cells contain scant cytoplasm and finely granular ("salt and pepper") chromatin. Keratin and chromogranin are strongly positive, whereas KIT and DOG1 are negative. Poorly differentiated adenocarcinomas of the stomach frequently have signet-ring–cell morphology with eccentric nuclei and a single mucin-containing cytoplasmic vacuole, and they are positive for broad-spectrum keratins, often for CK20 and CDX-2, and usually negative for KIT and DOG1 of note, a subset of gastric adenocarcinomas is positive for DOG1, which is a potential diagnostic pitfall. Glomus tumors rarely develop in the GI tract, most often in the wall of the stomach. Like a subset of epithelioid gastric GISTs, glomus tumors are composed of sheets of uniform rounded to epithelioid cells with sharply demarcated cytoplasmic borders. A helpful diagnostic clue is subendothelial growth within blood vessel walls, often most easily appreciated at the periphery of the tumor. Glomus tumors are strongly positive for SMA and caldesmon but negative for KIT and DOG1.

Prognosis and Treatment

GISTs range from those with essentially no risk of metastasis to those with a high risk of aggressive behavior.[58] The system of risk stratification most commonly used is based on anatomic site, tumor size, and mitotic activity (Table 16.2).[58] Importantly, this risk stratification system does not apply to SDH-deficient GISTs; tumor size and mitotic rate do not predict progression in these tumors.[59] There are three Food and Drug

Table 16.2 Risk Stratification of Primary Gastrointestinal Stromal Tumor by Mitotic Index, Size, and Site

Mitotic Index (per 5 mm²)[a]	Size (cm)	Risk of Progressive Disease[a]			
		Stomach	Duodenum	Jejunum/Ileum	Rectum
≤5	≤2	None (0%)	None (0%)	None (0%)	None (0%)
≤5	>2–5	Very low (1.9%)	Low (8.3%)	Low (4.3%)	Low (8.5%)
≤5	>5–10	Low (3.6%)	Insufficient data	Moderate (24%)	Insufficient data
≤5	>10	Moderate (10%)	High (34%)	High (52%)	High (57%)
>5	≤2	None; small number of cases	Insufficient data	High; small number of cases	High (54%)
>5	>2–5	Moderate (16%)	High (50%)	High (73%)	High (52%)
>5	>5–10	High (55%)	Insufficient data	High (85%)	Insufficient data
>5	>10	High (86%)	High (86%)	High (90%)	High (71%)

[a]Defined as metastasis or tumor-related death. Field diameter should be determined for individual microscopes. On most modern microscopes, 5 mm² is equivalent to approximately 20 high-power (40×) fields. Data are based on long-term follow-up of 1055 gastric, 629 small intestinal, 144 duodenal, and 111 rectal GISTs.

Adapted from Demetri GD, von Mehren M, Antonescu CR, et al. NCCN Task Force report: update on the management of patients with gastrointestinal stromal tumors. *J Natl Compr Canc Netw* 8(suppl 2):S1–S41, 2010; and Miettinen M, Lasota J. Gastrointestinal stromal tumors: pathology and prognosis at different sites. *Semin Diagn Pathol* 23:70–83, 2006.

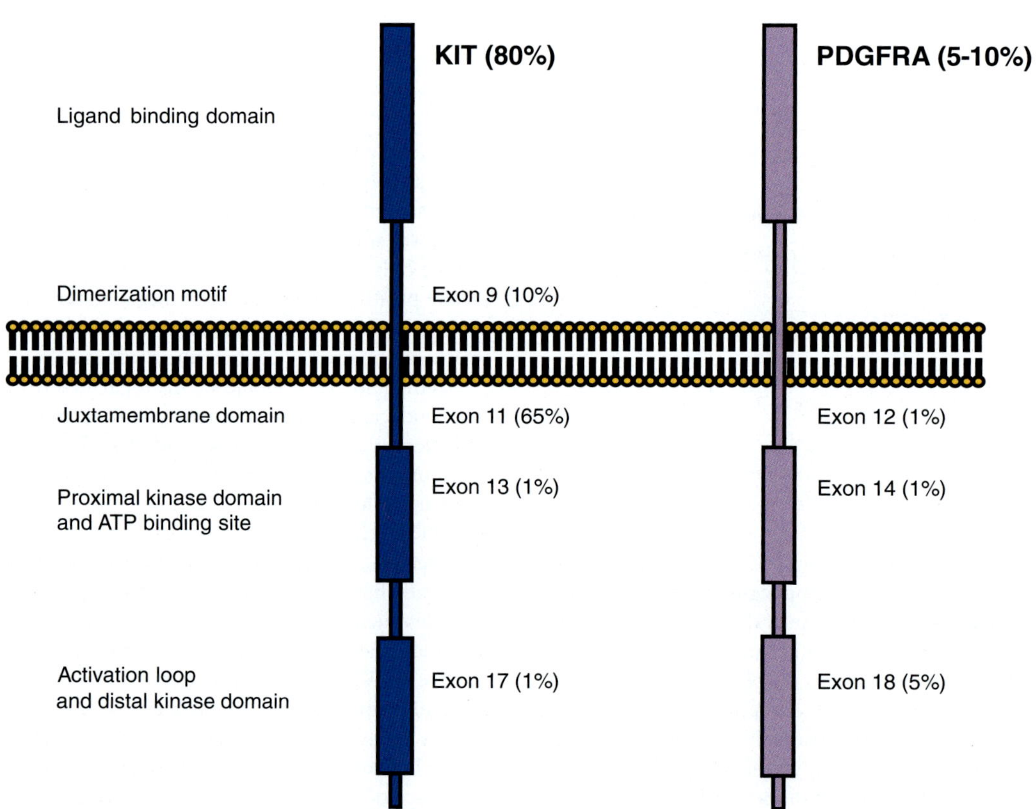

Figure 16.17 Distribution of *KIT* and platelet-derived growth factor receptor A *(PDGFRA)* mutations in gastrointestinal stromal tumor.

Administration–approved targeted therapies for GIST. Imatinib mesylate, sunitinib malate, and regorafenib are small molecule inhibitors that directly target KIT and PDGFRA.[53] Imatinib is used as first-line therapy primarily in the setting of metastatic or unresectable GIST, and sunitinib is used in patients who do not tolerate imatinib or have progressed on imatinib therapy. Regorafenib is used primarily in patients who fail both imatinib and sunitinib. Interestingly, although patients with most tumors respond well to imatinib, some genetic subsets do not respond as well or at all.[60] As is expected, GISTs associated with NF1, SDH-deficient GISTs, and *BRAF*-mutant GISTs do not respond to KIT/PDGFRA inhibitors. *KIT* exon 9 mutant tumors tend to respond less well; increasing the daily dose of imatinib from 400 to 800 mg can overcome the lack of response in *KIT* exon 9 mutant tumors.[61,62] GIST patients with the most common *PDGFRA* mutation, D842V, do not respond to any of the FDA-approved GIST therapies and should be enrolled in clinical trials with experimental agents. Secondary resistance

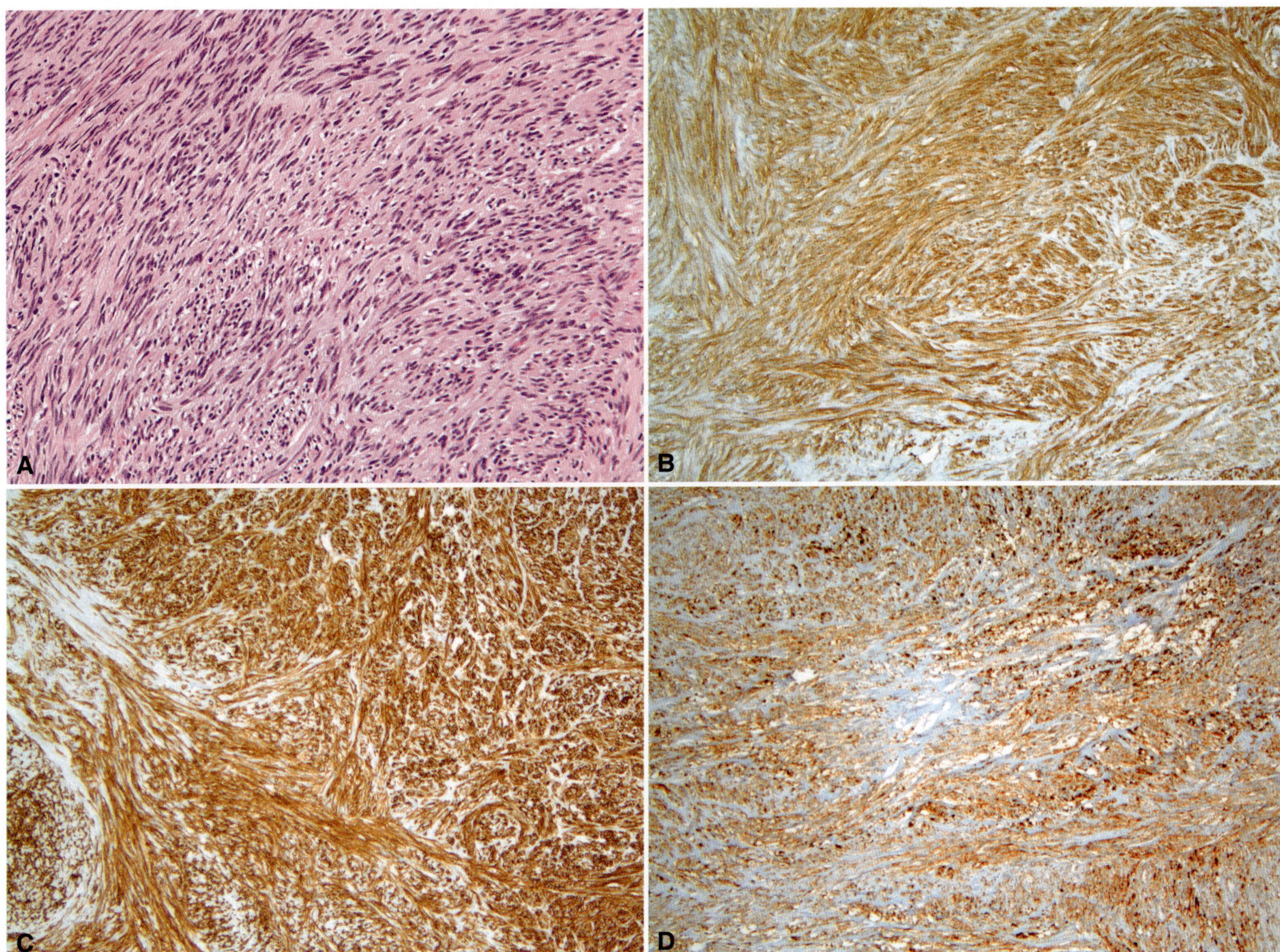

Figure 16.18 ***BRAF*-Mutant Gastrointestinal Stromal Tumor.** The tumor shows a fascicular architecture and uniform spindle cell morphology (A). By immunohistochemistry, the tumor cells are diffusely and strongly positive for KIT (B), DOG1 (C), and BRAF V600E (D).

to imatinib, defined as those GISTs that initially respond to imatinib but after a period of 6 months or more show tumor progression on therapy, is seen within 2 years in about 50% of patients with GIST.[53] Secondary resistance is usually due to second-site intraallelic mutations in *KIT*, which abrogate binding to imatinib.[35] Patients who develop secondary resistance to imatinib can benefit from treatment with sunitinib and regorafenib. Interestingly, although only few cases have been reported, GISTs with *BRAF* V600E mutations appear to respond to BRAF inhibitors.[63]

Occasionally, GISTs are resected after treatment with targeted therapies. Although changes such as hypocellularity, hyalinosis, myxoid stroma, and necrosis have been described, these changes do not appear to correlate reliably with clinical response.[64] It is reasonable to note the histologic appearance of treated GISTs in pathology reports; however, evaluating treatment response histologically does not play a role in the current management of patients with GIST. Occasionally, treated GISTs may show morphologic changes, such as a shift from spindle cell to epithelioid morphology or the development of pleomorphism,[65,66] and rare GISTs lose KIT expression or otherwise change their immunophenotype, such as acquiring expression of smooth muscle markers.[65] A very rare form of tumor progression in GISTs following tyrosine kinase inhibitor therapy is the development of heterologous rhabdomyosarcomatous differentiation, indistinguishable from embryonal or pleomorphic rhabdomyosarcoma.[67] This unusual form of clonal evolution is associated with extremely aggressive clinical behavior.

GISTs rarely recur at anastomotic sites, and relatively narrow surgical margins are therefore adequate to achieve local control (e.g., wedge resection or partial gastrectomy for gastric tumors). The one notable exception is SDH-deficient GISTs, which often recur locally in the stomach, sometimes years or even decades following primary excision.[14,22]

Leiomyoma

Leiomyoma is the second most common mesenchymal tumor of the GI tract, after GIST. It is difficult to obtain accurate numbers as to what proportion of mesenchymal tumors are leiomyomas due to referral bias in most large series, but a single institution series estimated that they composed 32% of all mesenchymal neoplasms of the GI tract.[68] GIST accounted for 54% of these tumors, so both tumor types combined represented 86% of all mesenchymal neoplasms of the GI tract.

Clinical Features

Leiomyomas are most common in the colorectal region.[69] Approximately 80% of leiomyomas occur in this area, where they almost always present as small submucosal polyps that arise from the muscularis mucosae (Fig. 16.19). The second most common site for leiomyoma is the esophagus.[70] Approximately 10% of leiomyomas are found in this location.

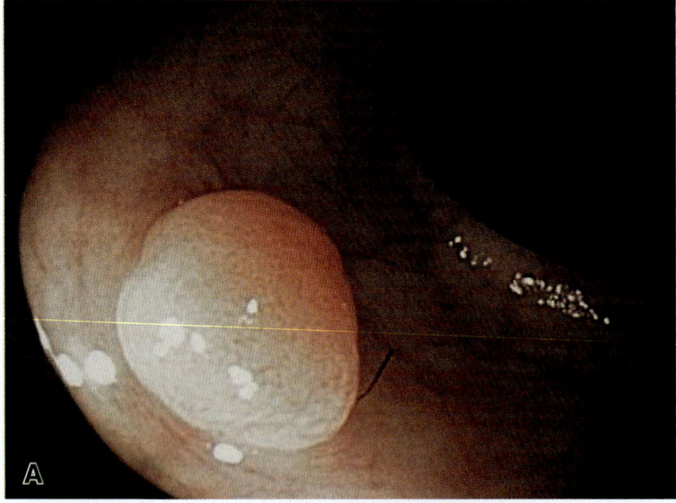

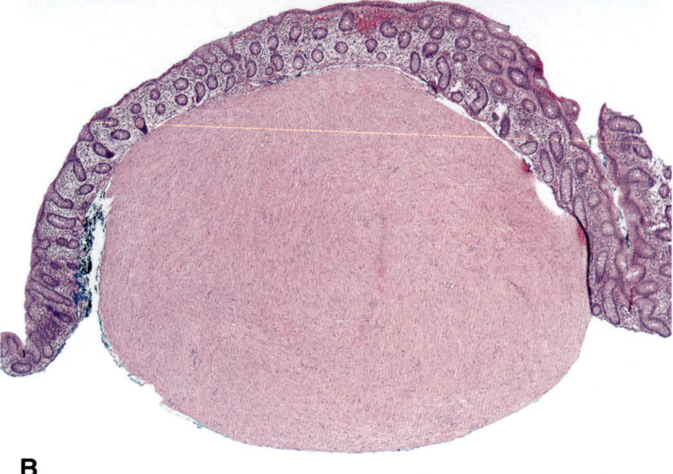

Figure 16.19 Leiomyoma of the Muscularis Mucosae. Endoscopic appearance of a colonic polypoid leiomyoma (A). This submucosal nodule is covered by intact mucosa. Low-power view of a sigmoid colonic leiomyoma of the muscularis mucosae (B). Note the sharply circumscribed nodule protruding into the submucosa.

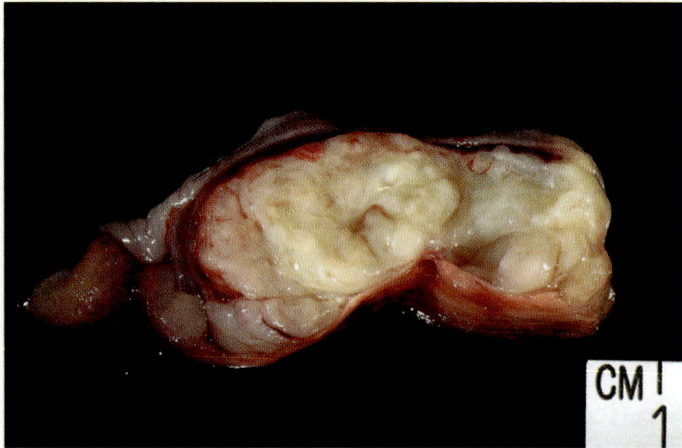

Figure 16.20 Mural Leiomyoma. Gross appearance of an esophageal leiomyoma.

Esophageal leiomyomas usually arise from the muscularis propria, where they form intramural masses, but may rarely occur as polyps. Intramural leiomyomas tend to form much larger masses than polypoid leiomyomas. Leiomyomas of the stomach and small intestine are rare and predominantly intramural.

Leiomyomas are more common in men, with a 2.4:1 male-to-female ratio in the colorectal region and a 2:1 ratio in the esophagus.[69,70] Leiomyomas can occur over a wide age range.[69,70] In the colon, they are more common in middle-aged to elderly adults with a median age of 62 years, whereas in the esophagus they occur in a younger population with a median age of 35 years.

Presenting symptoms depend on location. In the esophagus, patients present with dysphagia, cough, or GI bleeding, or tumors can present as incidental masses.[70] On occasion, they can mimic mediastinal masses. In the colorectal region, leiomyomas are most often identified incidentally during screening colonoscopy.[69]

Pathologic Features

Leiomyomas present in the colorectal region as small polyps, ranging in size from 1 to 22 mm (median, 4 mm; see Fig. 16.19).[69] Mural leiomyomas of the esophagus are larger, ranging in size from 1 to 18 cm (median, 5 cm; Fig. 16.20). Leiomyomas are well circumscribed but unencapsulated and are often lobulated, with a firm consistency. On cut section, the tumors are white to tan with a whorled, fibrous appearance.

Histologically, leiomyomas are composed of fascicles of spindle cells with brightly eosinophilic cytoplasm and elongated, broad (cigar-shaped) nuclei with tapering or blunt ends (Fig. 16.21). Cytologic atypia is rare, but degenerative nuclear atypia has been described in several cases that contained bizarre cells similar to symplastic leiomyoma of the uterus.[69] Mitotic activity is very low or absent, usually less than 1 per 50 high-power fields. Necrosis is not seen. Epithelioid leiomyomas of the GI tract have not been described.

As is seen in GIST, if a concerted effort is made to detect clinically inapparent leiomyomas, they are actually quite common. In one study, 150 esophagogastric resection specimens that were removed for carcinomas were examined in detail with an average of 30 sections per case.[10] Small (mean, 1.7 mm) esophageal leiomyomas were identified in 47% of patients. Interestingly, many patients had multiple lesions with a mean of three leiomyomas (one patient had 13 individual lesions).

Immunohistochemistry

All leiomyomas are uniformly positive for SMA, desmin, and caldesmon (see Fig. 16.21D and E).[69,70] They are negative for CD34, KIT, DOG1, and S-100. Esophageal mural leiomyomas often contain numerous KIT-positive mast cells (see Fig. 16.21F), as well as KIT- and DOG1-positive interstitial cells of Cajal.[29,57]

Molecular Genetics

Very limited data are available regarding the molecular features of GI leiomyomas. Deletion of *COL4A5* and *COL4A6* at Xq22, encoding collagen type IV alpha 5 and alpha 6, has been reported in a single case of esophageal leiomyoma.[71] This gene region is also lost in diffuse esophageal leiomyomatosis, which is characterized by replacement of the esophageal muscularis propria by an abnormal nodular smooth muscle proliferation.[72] Diffuse leiomyomatosis predominantly affects children and adolescents but can occur at any age. Leiomyomatosis can occur sporadically or as a familial syndrome, usually associated with Alport syndrome, which is characterized by an inherited nephropathy. One case of a large discrete leiomyoma has been described in the setting of familial diffuse leiomyomatosis.[73]

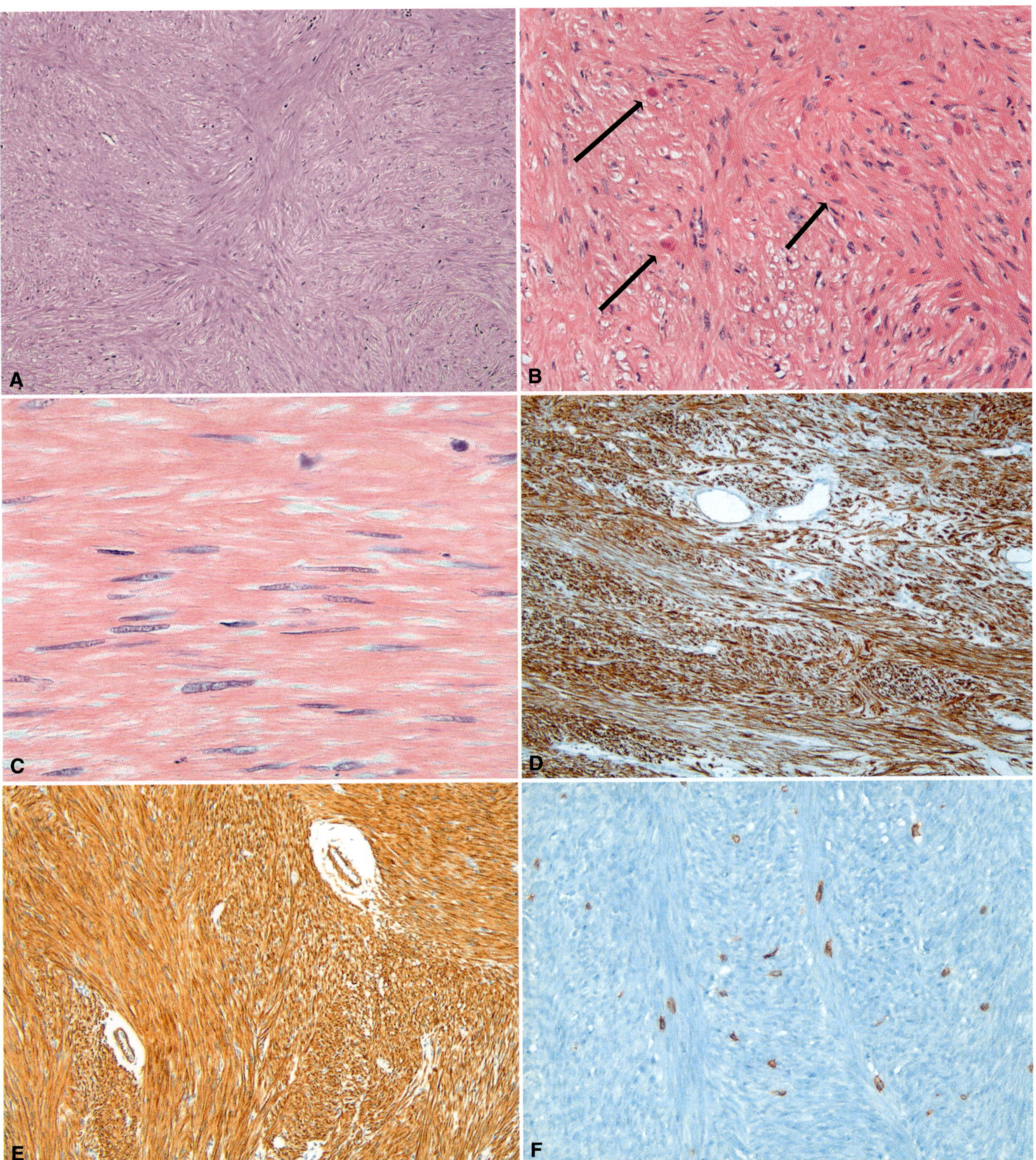

Figure 16.21 Histologic Appearances of Lei omyoma. Low-power view of a colorectal leiomyoma showing a relatively hypocellular neoplasm composed of fascicles of spindle-shaped cells with brightly eosinophilic cytoplasm (A). Medium-power view of an esophageal leiomyoma with occasional eosinophilic globules *(arrows)*, which are sometimes seen in benign smooth muscle tumors (B). High-power view of esophageal leiomyoma (C). Note that the tumor cells have elongated nuclei with tapering or blunt ends. By immunohistochemistry, leiomyomas are diffusely and strongly positive for smooth muscle actin, desmin (D), and h-caldesmon (E). Numerous KIT-positive mast cells in an esophageal leiomyoma (F).

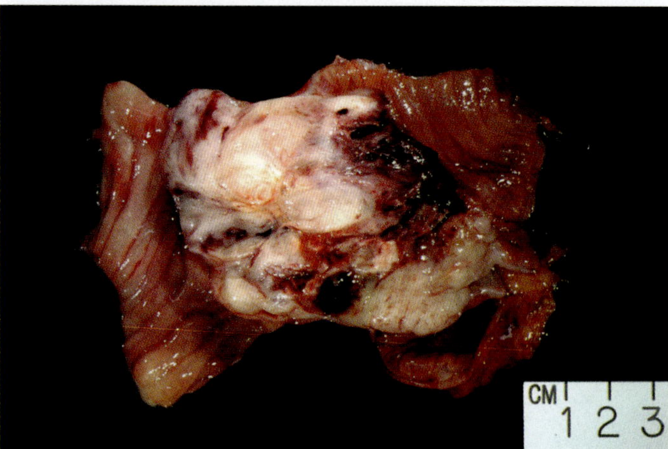

Figure 16.22 Gross Appearance of a Leiomyosarcoma of the Small Bowel. The tumor is fleshy with areas of hemorrhage.

Differential Diagnosis

The differential diagnosis of leiomyoma primarily includes GIST and to some extent schwannoma. It is important to remember that clinically apparent leiomyomas occur in an inverse anatomic distribution compared with GIST. Leiomyomas are more common than GIST in the esophagus and colorectal region, whereas GISTs are vastly more common in the stomach and small intestine. Schwannomas are rare in the GI tract and occur most often in the stomach. Leiomyomas are generally less cellular and more brightly eosinophilic than GIST, lack mitotic activity, and in contrast to GIST, are diffusely and strongly positive for desmin and negative for KIT and DOG1. In contrast to leiomyomas, schwannomas are negative for desmin and diffusely and strongly positive for S-100. As previously mentioned, numerous KIT-positive mast cells can be seen in leiomyomas (as well as schwannomas), which is a potential diagnostic pitfall.[57]

Prognosis and Treatment

Leiomyomas are universally benign.[69,70] Colorectal polypoid leiomyomas are treated by polypectomy alone, whereas intramural leiomyomas can be excised by myomectomy or segmental resection.

Leiomyosarcoma

True leiomyosarcomas of the GI tract are extremely rare.[20,68–70,74,75] It is difficult to estimate the precise incidence of such tumors, but in a large study of 262 mesenchymal tumors of the GI tract, there were only three bona fide leiomyosarcomas, amounting to scarcely more than 1% of the total.[68]

Clinical Features

Leiomyosarcomas can occur at any site within the GI tract but are most common in the small intestine and colon.[20,68–70,74,75] Patients may present with anemia, GI bleeding, dysphagia, or bowel obstruction, depending on the anatomic location. For instance, individuals with esophageal leiomyosarcomas are more likely to present with dysphagia, whereas those with leiomyosarcomas of the small intestine are more likely to present with obstruction.[70,75] Leiomyosarcomas can develop over a broad age range but tend to predominate in middle-aged to elderly adults, and the tumors are slightly more common in men.

Pathologic Features

Grossly, GI leiomyosarcomas are usually large (Fig. 16.22). In one report of leiomyosarcomas of the duodenum, the five lesions ranged from 10 to 19 cm (median, 13 cm).[20] The tumors generally involve the full-thickness of the bowel wall, including the mucosa, which is often ulcerated, as well as the serosal surface. Leiomyosarcomas can also occur as ulcerated intraluminal polypoid masses.[20] These tumors may be lobulated, and on cut section they are gray, pink, or tan fleshy masses, often with areas of necrosis.

Histologically, GI leiomyosarcomas are similar to leiomyosarcomas elsewhere. They are composed of fascicles of spindle cells with elongated nuclei with blunt or tapering ends and brightly eosinophilic cytoplasm (Fig. 16.23). Nuclear pleomorphism is often prominent and can be extensive. Mitotic activity is usually very high, often more than 10 per 10 high-power fields. Nuclear palisading, paranuclear vacuoles, and skeinoid fibers (features of GIST) are not present. Coagulative necrosis is common. Epithelioid cytomorphology is exceedingly rare. Due to the rarity of primary GI leiomyosarcomas and the relatively recent separation of true smooth muscle tumors from GIST, the minimal criteria for malignancy have not been established. However, any mitotically active smooth muscle neoplasm of the bowel wall with nuclear atypia should be regarded as at least low-grade malignant.[75] If in doubt about whether a given lesion is malignant, the designation "smooth muscle tumor of uncertain malignant potential" (STUMP) may be used.

Immunohistochemistry

Leiomyosarcomas are usually diffusely and strongly positive for SMA. Expression of desmin and caldesmon is more variable and can be focal or diffuse. CD34 can be positive in smooth muscle tumors, including leiomyosarcomas.[70] Broad-spectrum keratins are often at least focally positive. GI leiomyosarcomas are negative for S-100, KIT, and DOG1.

Molecular Genetics

Leiomyosarcomas are characterized by complex genetic changes and do not possess *KIT* or *PDGFRA* mutations.

Differential Diagnosis

The differential diagnosis primarily includes GIST, leiomyoma, and schwannoma. Bright cytoplasmic eosinophilia and prominent nuclear pleomorphism distinguish leiomyosarcomas from GISTs. Furthermore, in contrast to leiomyosarcomas, GISTs are rarely positive for desmin and almost always positive for KIT and DOG1. GI leiomyomas lack cytologic pleomorphism and mitotic activity. Generally, distinguishing between GI leiomyomas and leiomyosarcomas is straightforward, because leiomyosarcomas usually show striking mitotic activity and marked nuclear atypia. However, occasionally, GI leiomyosarcomas are well differentiated with only focal cytologic atypia and a low mitotic rate.[75] GI schwannomas usually arise in the stomach, an especially rare primary site for leiomyosarcomas. Unlike leiomyosarcomas, schwannomas have a peripheral lymphoid cuff and lack significant pleomorphism. Schwannomas are negative for desmin, and they are diffusely and strongly positive for S-100.

Prognosis and Treatment

Leiomyosarcomas exhibit locally aggressive behavior and a high rate of distant metastasis. Leiomyosarcomas have a tendency to metastasize to intraabdominal surfaces and the liver, and they less often spread to the lungs and bone. GI leiomyosarcomas can also spread to regional lymph nodes, but this is rare.[76] Many GI leiomyosarcomas ultimately lead to patient death. Aggressive multimodal therapy is required.

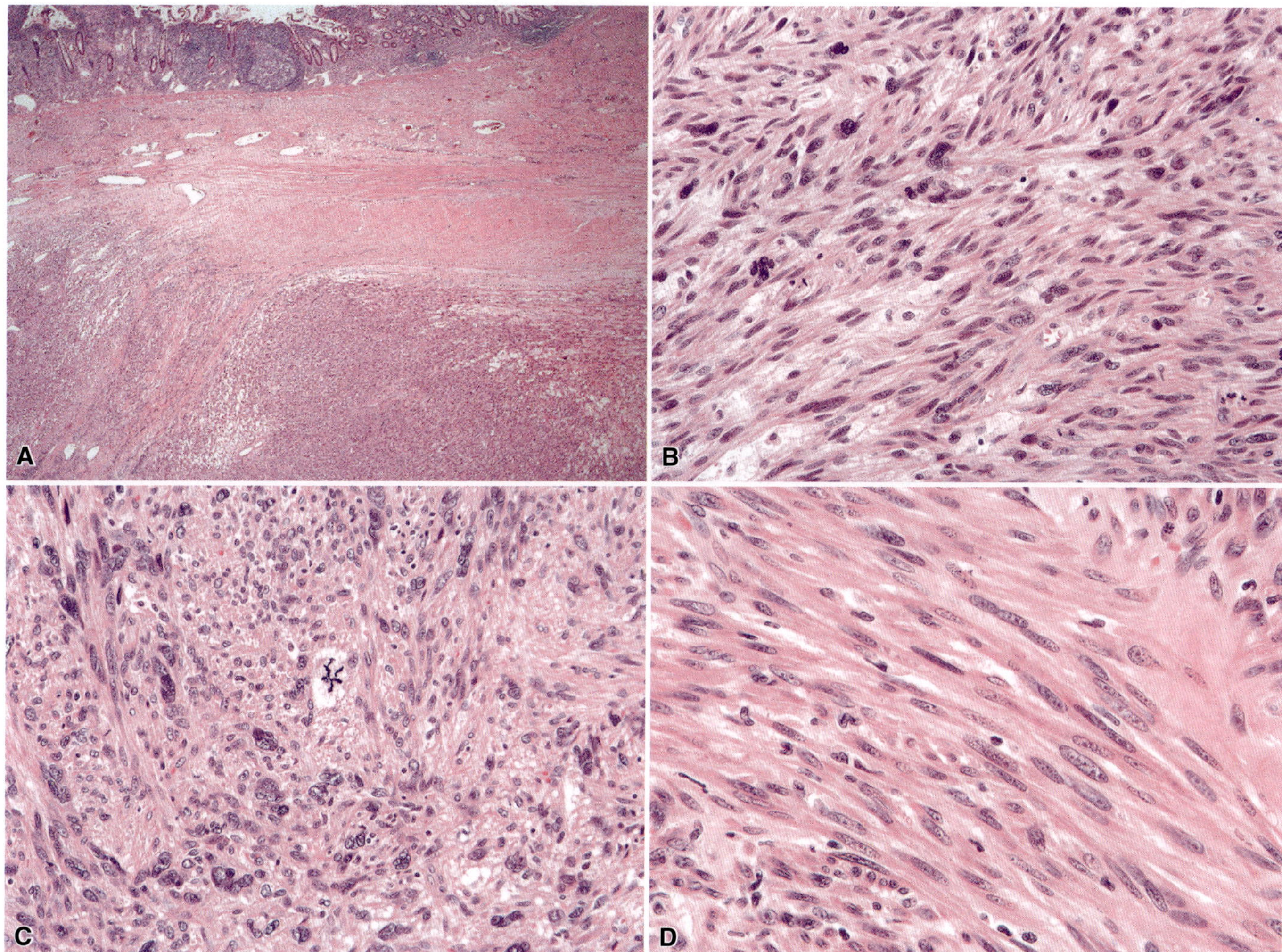

Figure 16.23 Histologic Appearances of Leiomyosarcoma. Low-power view of a leiomyosarcoma of the small bowel, infiltrating through the muscularis propria (A). Leiomyosarcomas are typically composed of fascicles of spindle-shaped cells with nuclear pleomorphism and dense eosinophilic cytoplasm (B). Nuclear pleomorphism can be prominent, and atypical mitotic figures are not unusual (C). High-power view of a leiomyosarcoma showing characteristic cytologic features (D). The tumor cells have broad, elongated nuclei and brightly eosinophilic cytoplasm.

Schwannoma

Schwannoma is a rare neoplasm of the GI tract, accounting for approximately 3% of all GI mesenchymal tumors.

Clinical Features

Schwannoma can occur anywhere in the GI tract but is most common in the stomach, followed by the colon and rectum. The esophagus and small intestine are rarely affected.[77–81] There is an equal sex predilection. Schwannomas develop in patients over a wide age range (18–87 years), with a median between 53 and 68 years.[78,80]

Presenting symptoms depend on location. Patients with gastric schwannomas present with dyspepsia, indigestion, abdominal pain, a mass, or GI bleeding; those with colorectal schwannomas present with rectal bleeding, obstruction, constipation, or abdominal pain; and those with esophageal schwannomas present with chest pain or dysphagia. Schwannomas are generally located within the muscularis propria or submucosa with bulging into the lumen. The overlying mucosa is prone to ulceration. Interestingly, colorectal schwannomas have a tendency to appear as ulcerated polypoid lesions.[80]

Pathologic Features

Grossly, most GI schwannomas are circumscribed, mural tumors (Fig. 16.24A). They range in size from 0.5 to 12 cm, with a median of 3–5 cm. On cut section, they are homogenous, firm or rubbery, and usually yellow. Hemorrhage, cystic change, or necrosis is not typically seen.

GI schwannomas differ histologically from conventional schwannomas of peripheral nerves. They are circumscribed but unencapsulated and usually surrounded by a dense lymphoplasmacytic cuff, often with germinal centers (see Fig. 16.24B). They have overall pushing borders, but it is not unusual to see tumor cells infiltrate among the muscle bundles at the periphery. The vast majority of GI schwannomas are moderately cellular lesions composed of spindle cells with a variably prominent collagenous stroma (see Fig. 16.24C). The lesional cells are admixed with lymphocytes and arranged in short bundles. In contrast to conventional schwannomas, Verocay bodies, nuclear palisading, perivascular hyalinization, or foamy histiocytes are not typically evident. The spindle cells contain elongated nuclei with tapering ends and a single inconspicuous nucleolus (see Fig. 16.24D). There is often

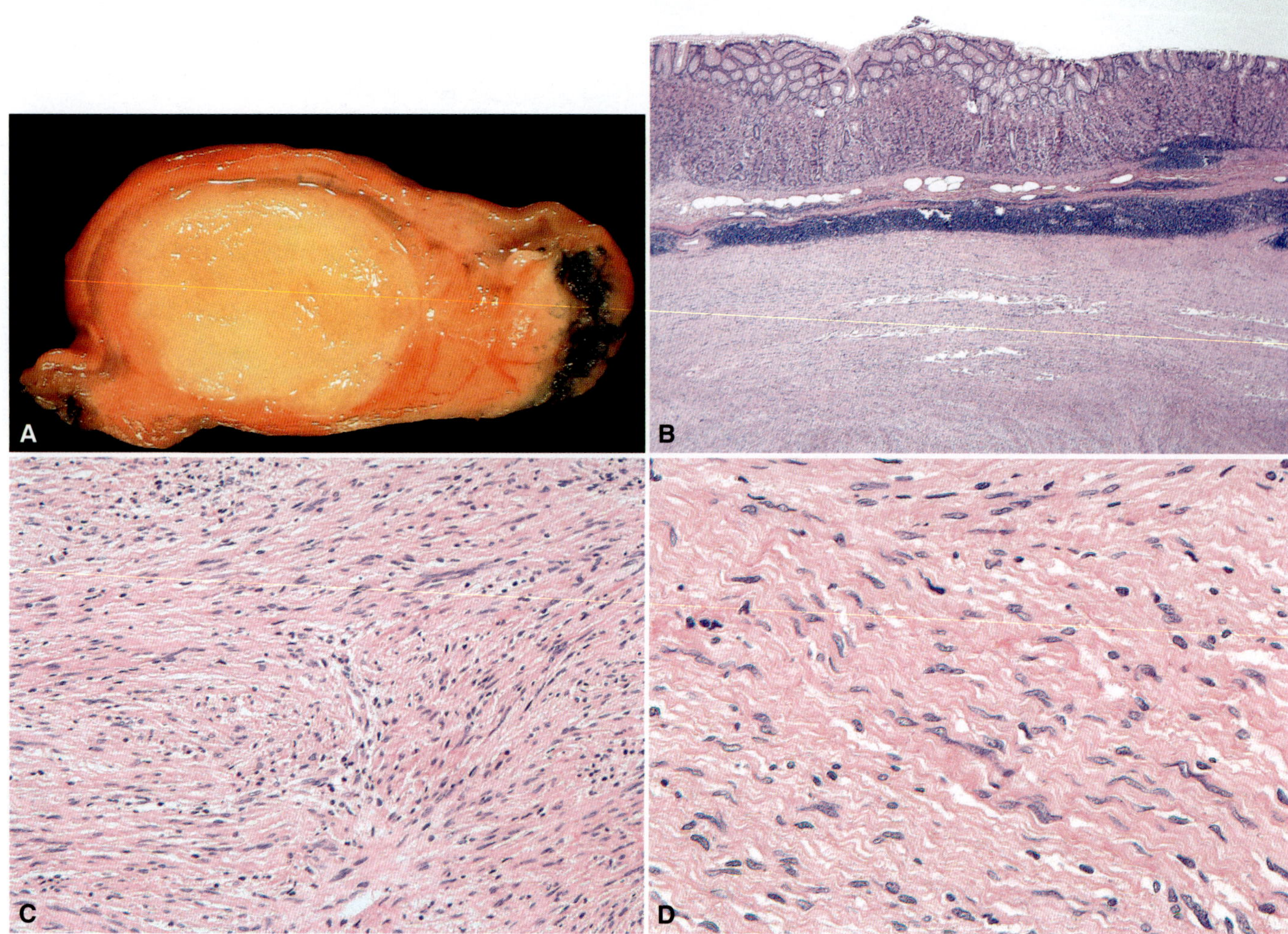

Figure 16.24 Gastric Schwannoma. Gross appearance of a gastric schwannoma (A). Note the circumscription and yellow cut surface. Histologic appearances of gastric schwannoma. There is usually a dense lymphocytic infiltrate at the periphery of the tumor (B). Gastric schwannomas are moderately cellular tumors composed of fascicles of spindle-shaped cells admixed with lymphocytes (C). The spindle cells typically have wavy nuclei and fibrillary eosinophilic cytoplasm (D).

scattered mild nuclear atypia with hyperchromasia. Mitotic figures are usually absent or rare. Atypical mitotic figures are not identified.

Rarely, GI schwannoma can have epithelioid cytomorphology, similar to epithelioid schwannoma of the superficial soft tissues (see Chapter 15). The epithelioid cells are usually arranged in sheets or cords and sometimes in a pseudoglandular pattern. In a series of colorectal schwannomas, all four epithelioid examples were located in the descending or sigmoid colon, three of which were submucosal.[80]

A rare variant of schwannoma referred to as *microcystic/reticular schwannoma* appears to have a predilection for the GI tract.[82] In the largest reported series, 5 of the 10 tumors arose in the GI tract, 4 in the submucosa. These lesions had the typical clinical features of GI schwannoma but distinctive histologic features. All were circumscribed and unencapsulated, but none were surrounded by a lymphoid cuff. As their name implies, the lesional cells are arranged in a striking microcystic and reticular growth pattern composed of anastomosing spindle cells set in a myxoid, fibrillary, or collagenous stroma (Fig. 16.25). Of note, the microcystic pattern may display a pseudoglandular appearance suggestive of mucinous adenocarcinoma. A case of signet-ring–cell schwannoma of the stomach has also been described; the appearance is similar to those tumors described as microcystic/reticular schwannoma.[38]

Immunohistochemistry

GI schwannomas are diffusely and strongly positive for S-100 (Fig. 16.26) and glial fibrillary acidic protein (GFAP),[77–81] but they are negative for KIT, desmin, and SMA. CD34 may be focally positive. Unlike conventional schwannomas, an epithelial membrane antigen (EMA)–positive perineurial capsule is absent.

Molecular Genetics

GI schwannomas are sporadic tumors that are not associated with either NF1 or NF2. In contrast to conventional schwannoma, loss of heterozygosity at 22q12, the region of *NF2*, is unusual.[83] Loss of heterozygosity at 17q11.2, the region of the *NF1* gene that encodes neurofibromin, is more common, being present in 50% of cases, which is similar to neurofibromas.

Differential Diagnosis

The main differential diagnosis of the most common spindle cell variant of schwannoma includes GIST, leiomyoma, inflammatory myofibroblastic tumor (IMT), and metastatic melanoma. Immunohistochemistry is helpful in distinguishing among different lesions in the differential diagnosis (see Table 16.1). GIST usually has a more hypercellular, syncytial

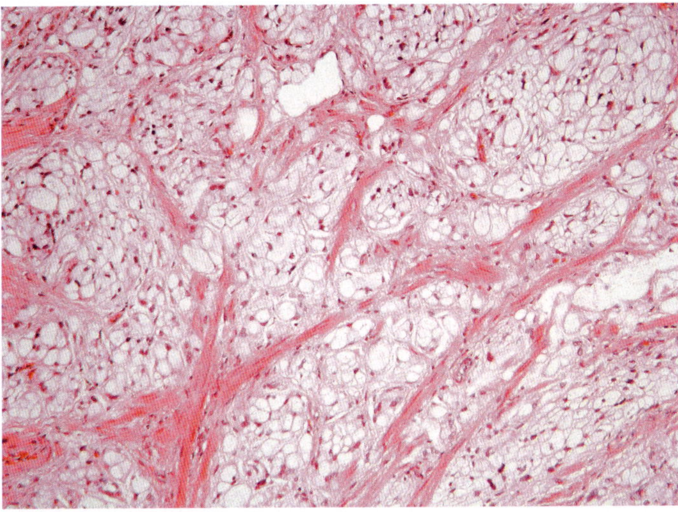

Figure 16.25 **Microcystic/Reticular Schwannoma.** Note the anastomosing strands of spindle cells and hyalinized stroma.

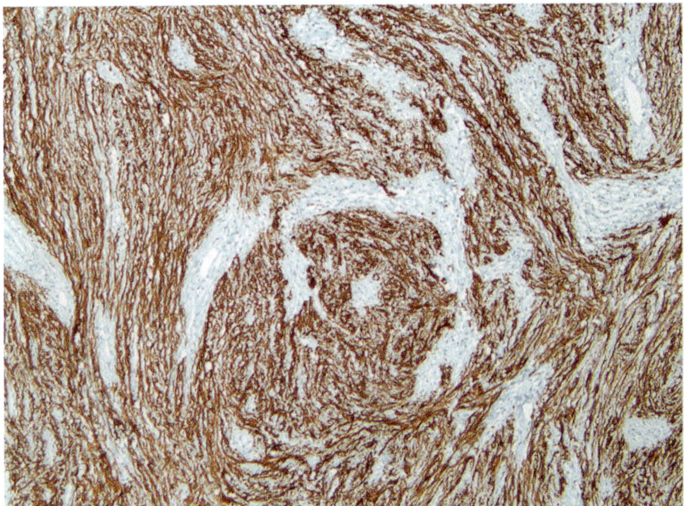

Figure 16.26 **Gastric Schwannoma.** The tumors are uniformly positive for S-100.

appearance with minimal stroma and remarkably uniform cytology, and it lacks the distinctive peripheral lymphoid cuff of GI schwannoma. In contrast to schwannoma, GIST is positive for KIT and DOG1, and it is negative for S-100 in most cases. Leiomyoma has a uniformly fascicular architecture and bright cytoplasmic eosinophilia, and is negative for S-100 and diffusely and strongly positive for SMA, desmin, and caldesmon. IMT is composed of loose fascicles of plump spindle cells admixed with predominantly chronic inflammatory cells. IMT shows variable expression of SMA and desmin, and 50% for anaplastic lymphoma kinase (ALK), but it is consistently negative for S-100. Finally, metastatic melanoma also typically has extensive S-100 immunoreactivity. However, in contrast to schwannoma, these lesions may be positive for other melanocytic markers, including HMB-45 and melan A, and they usually have marked mitotic activity and striking nuclear atypia with prominent nucleoli.

Prognosis and Treatment

GI schwannomas are invariably benign. Conservative excision is adequate therapy.

PRACTICE POINTS: Gastrointestinal Schwannomas

- Most common in stomach (mural mass), followed by colon and rectum (polypoid mass)
- Well circumscribed but unencapsulated
- Surrounded by dense lymphoplasmacytic cuff
- Unlike conventional schwannoma, usually no Verocay bodies, Antoni A and B zonation, or perivascular hyalinization
- S-100 diffusely positive, KIT and DOG1 negative

Gastrointestinal Clear Cell Sarcoma-like Tumor

Clear cell sarcoma (CCS) is a rare translocation-associated soft tissue neoplasm that generally involves the tendons and aponeuroses of the distal extremities. However, a CCS-like tumor has also been described in the GI tract.[84–87] GI CCS-like tumors, which have also been referred to as *osteoclast-rich tumors of the GI tract with features resembling CCS of soft parts*[88–90] and more recently as *malignant gastrointestinal neuroectodermal tumor* (GNET),[91] have distinctive histologic and immunophenotypic features, leading to the conclusion that such tumors are not in fact simply GI tract examples of conventional CCS, but instead represent a unique tumor type with similar cytogenetic findings.[89–91] Conventional CCS is discussed in Chapter 3.

Clinical Features

About 50 CCS-like tumors involving the tubal gut have been reported and are increasingly being recognized.[87,88,90–92] The tumors show an approximately equal gender distribution. The small intestine is the most common site (~75% of tumors), and the stomach, colon, and pancreas are rarely affected.[90] The age distribution is broad, with a peak in young to middle-aged adults (median, about 40 years of age). Patients present with partial small bowel obstruction, abdominal pain, diarrhea, fever, or nausea.

Pathologic Features

The tumors range from 1.8 to 15 cm in size (median, 5 cm). They usually show transmural involvement of the bowel wall, often with mucosal ulceration and extension to the serosa. There is also a tendency to invade into mesentery or adjacent organs. On cut section, the lesions are firm or fleshy and white with infiltrative borders.

Most GI CCS-like tumors have histologic features quite different from conventional CCS of soft tissue. The neoplastic cells in such cases usually display a nodular architecture through the bowel wall with infiltration into normal tissues at the tumor periphery (Fig. 16.27). A sheet-like architecture often predominates, with a distinctive pseudopapillary or alveolar appearance, at least focally (Fig. 16.28). The pseudopapillary architecture may mimic papillary adenocarcinoma. A nested growth pattern may also be seen, typically at the infiltrating border of the tumor (see Fig. 16.28). The lesional cells range from small to medium sized and are usually predominantly rounded, epithelioid, or ovoid (Fig. 16.29); spindle cell morphology may be focally observed in a subset of cases (see Fig. 16.28). The nuclei have round to slightly irregular contours and variably prominent nucleoli, usually small, but occasionally large and eosinophilic. The cytoplasm can be either palely eosinophilic, or, more rarely, clear. A single case has been described with oncocytic cytoplasm.[93] Although the cytologic features are usually uniform, rare cases have been described with moderate to severe cytologic

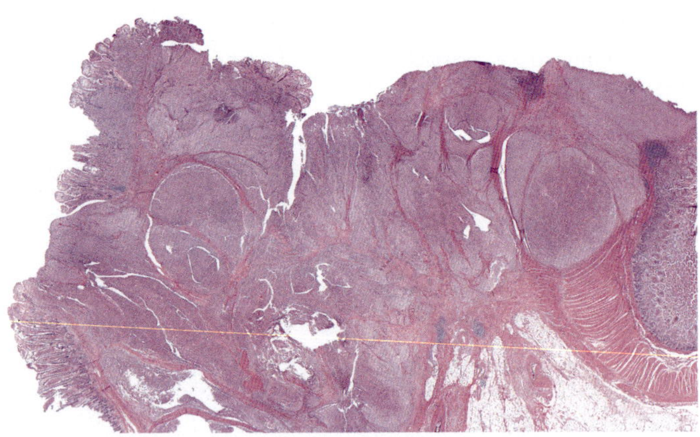

Figure 16.27 Clear Cell Sarcoma-Like Tumor of the Gastrointestinal Tract. The tumor shows a nodular, infiltrative growth pattern through the wall of the small bowel.

atypia and nuclear pleomorphism.[92] Osteoclast-like giant cells are common and may be focally numerous (see Fig. 16.29); this type of giant cell is not seen in conventional CCS at other anatomic locations, which instead typically have wreath-like giant cells. Mitotic activity is variable and may be high. Necrosis can be seen focally. A small subset of cases has histologic features indistinguishable from conventional CCS of somatic soft tissue, being composed of nests and fascicles of uniform epithelioid to spindle cells with eosinophilic to clear cytoplasm, distinct nucleoli, occasional wreath-like giant cells, and melanocytic differentiation in the form of melanin pigment or immunohistochemical reactivity for melanocytic markers such as HMB-45. A proposal has been made to refer to such lesions as conventional CCS and to distinguish these lesions from CCS-like tumors of the GI tract.[91]

Immunohistochemistry and Ultrastructure

GI CCS-like tumors are diffusely and strongly positive for S-100 and SOX10 (Fig. 16.30).[87,88,90,91] However, melanocytic markers (HMB-45 and melan A) are negative.[87,88,90,91] Neuron-specific enolase (45%), synaptophysin (56%), CD56 (70%), NB84 (50%), and neurofilament protein (NFP; 14%) are reported to be positive.[91] GI CCS-like tumors are uniformly negative for KIT, CD34, SMA, desmin, and keratins.

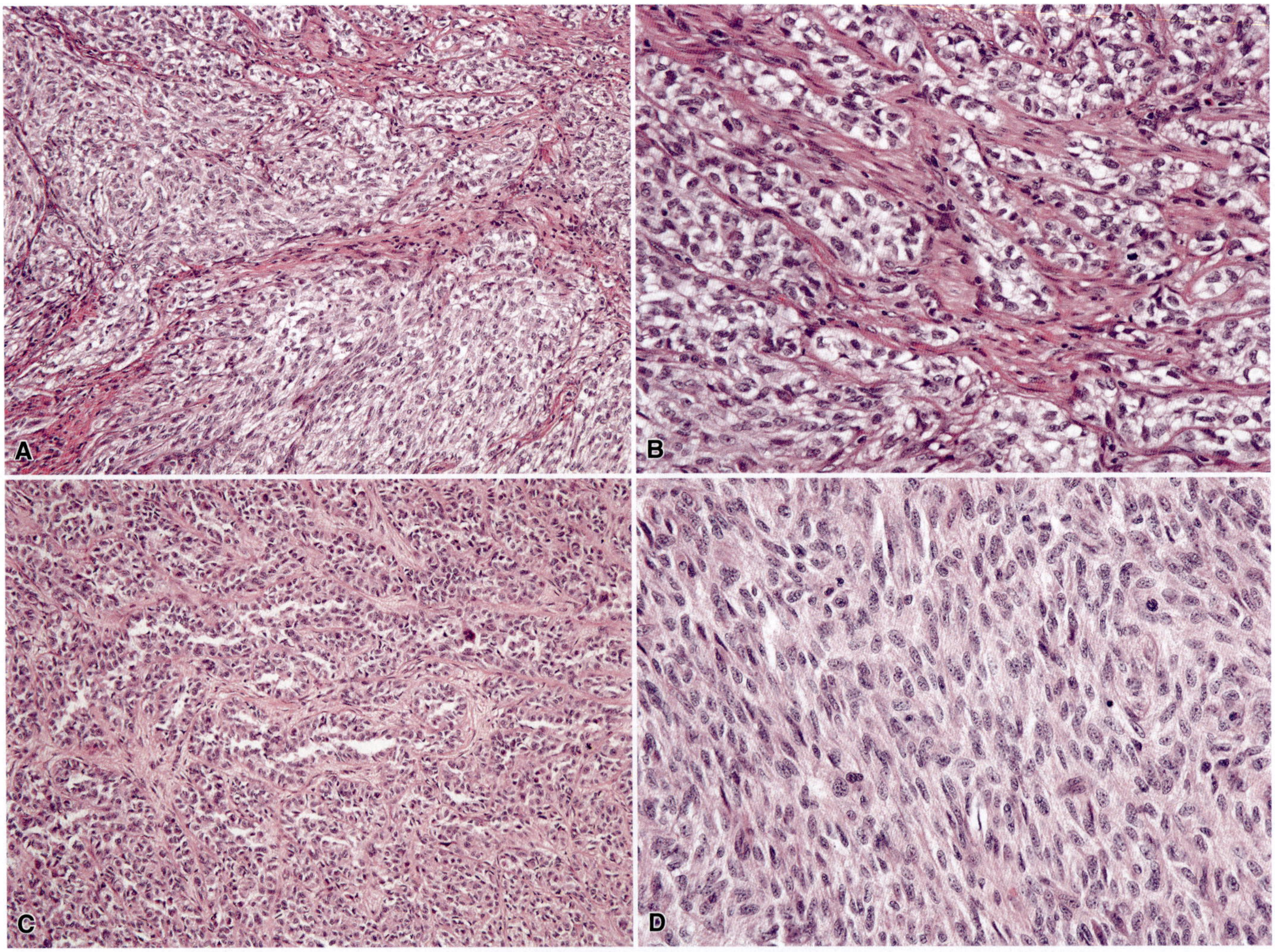

Figure 16.28 Histologic Appearances of Gastrointestinal Clear Cell Sarcoma-Like Tumor. The tumor cells are frequently arranged in sheets, vague fascicles, and nests (A). Focally, the tumor cells have clear cytoplasm (B). Note the nested architecture. Many tumors have a focally pseudopapillary or alveolar growth pattern, somewhat mimicking adenocarcinoma (C). Some tumors contain areas with spindle cell morphology (D).

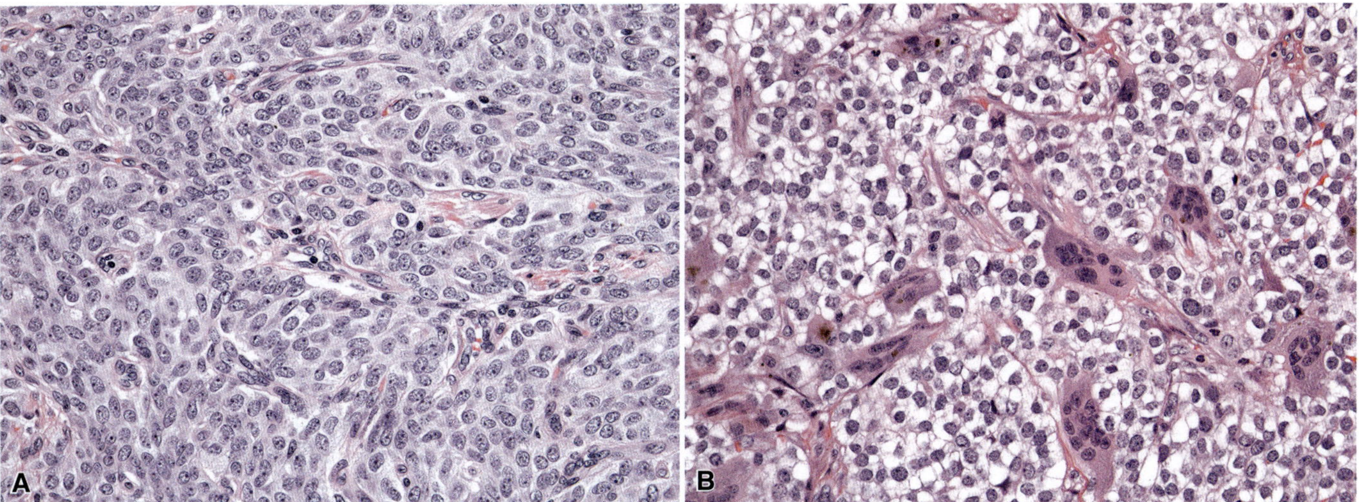

Figure 16.29 **Clear Cell Sarcoma-Like Tumor of the Gastrointestinal Tract.** The tumors usually show uniform cytology (A). Note the ovoid cells with small nucleoli and pale cytoplasm. Some tumors contain prominent osteoclast-like giant cells (B). Note the rounded nuclei and clear cytoplasm.

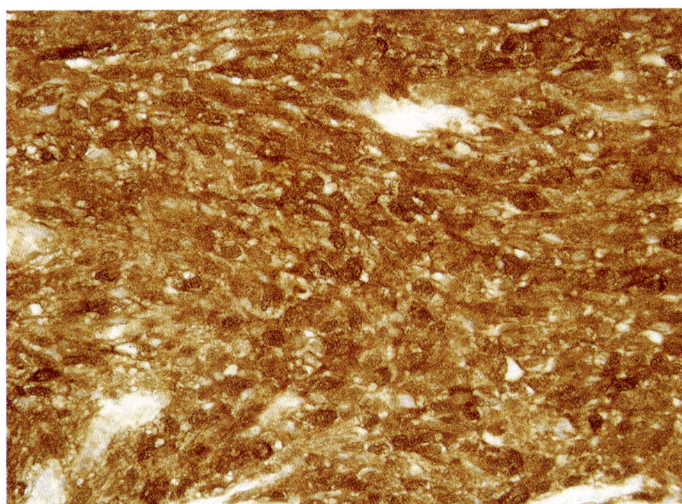

Figure 16.30 **Clear Cell Sarcoma-Like Tumor of the Gastrointestinal Tract.** The tumors are diffusely and strongly positive for S-100.

Electron microscopy reveals features consistent with primitive neuroectodermal cells with secretory vesicles, dense-core granules, and gap junctions.[91] The immunohistochemical and electron microscopic features prompted the suggestion to change the name of this entity from GI CCS-like tumor to malignant GNET.[91]

Molecular Genetics

Some GI CCS-like tumors have the translocation t(12;22)(q13;q12), which is also seen in CCS of soft tissue, resulting in fusion of *EWSR1* and *ATF1*.[88,90,91] Other cases have been shown by reverse transcriptase polymerase chain reaction (RT-PCR) or fluorescence in situ hybridization (FISH) techniques to harbor fusion of *EWSR1* and *CREB1* instead of *EWSR1* and *ATF1*.[87,91] In the distal extremities, about 95% of CCS have *EWSR1-ATF1* fusion[94]; the proportion of GI primary CCS-like tumors with *ATF1* versus *CREB1* gene rearrangements appears to be approximately equal. From a practical standpoint, commercially available *EWSR1* split-apart FISH probes can serve to confirm the diagnosis of GI CCS-like tumors, because all known molecular variants contain rearrangement of the *EWSR1* locus. The genetics of CCS is also discussed in Chapter 18.

Differential Diagnosis

The main differential diagnosis is metastatic melanoma and conventional CCS. GIST and poorly differentiated papillary adenocarcinoma may also be considered. GI CCS-like tumors can have extensive histologic and immunohistochemical overlap with melanoma. The relatively uniform cytology and lack of macronucleoli favor GI CCS-like tumor over melanoma, and only GI CCS-like tumor has rearrangement of the *EWSR1* gene region. Furthermore, lack of a primary diagnosis of cutaneous melanoma favors GI CCS-like tumor. In one series of seven tumors that were originally diagnosed as malignant melanoma of the GI tract, four cases without a history of primary cutaneous malignant melanoma turned out to be CCS-like tumors by molecular analysis.[92] In another retrospective study of 20 GI tumors diagnosed as malignant melanoma, two cases (10%) were found to harbor *EWSR1-ATF1*.[95] The presence of melanin or immunohistochemical evidence of melanocytic differentiation (HMB-45, melan A) allows distinction between conventional CCS and GI CCS-like tumor.[91] Papillary adenocarcinoma is negative for S-100 and positive for epithelial markers. GIST is much more common than GI CCS-like tumor; thus, it is prudent to exclude this entity. Most GISTs are positive for KIT and DOG1 and negative for S-100. However, occasionally, GISTs are positive for S-100, especially in the duodenum; it is therefore mandatory to perform KIT or DOG1 immunohistochemistry to exclude GIST.

Prognosis and Treatment

CCS-like tumor of the GI tract is an aggressive malignant neoplasm with a grim prognosis.[87,88,90,91] Many patients present with regional lymph node, liver, and mesenteric metastases, sometimes with disseminated peritoneal disease. Most patients die within 2 years of diagnosis. Because these tumors are so rare, treatment should be conducted by a multidisciplinary group with considerable experience in the treatment of sarcomas.

Inflammatory Myofibroblastic Tumor

IMT, previously known as *inflammatory pseudotumor*, is a rare neoplasm of intermediate biologic potential that can involve a wide range of anatomic locations but has a predilection for the GI tract.[96] This tumor type is discussed in more detail in Chapters 4 and 10. This section will focus briefly on IMT presenting in the GI tract.

Clinical Features

The largest series of IMT of the GI tract summarized the findings of 38 cases. Patients ranged from 9 months to 84 years of age, with a median of 43 years of age.[97] The highest incidence of IMT was in the fifth decade, with no gender predilection. The lesions arose throughout the GI tract, involving the esophagus (5%), stomach (25%), small intestine (30%), large intestine (37%), and appendix (2%). Abdominal pain was the most common presenting symptom. Some patients reported fever and night sweats. Laboratory results were available in only 10 patients. However, abnormal results were reported in about 50% of the cases and included elevated leukocyte count (eosinophilia and neutrophilia), hypergammaglobulinemia, elevated erythrocyte sedimentation rate, and anemia. There was associated lymphadenopathy in 32% of the patients. A distinctive epithelioid variant of IMT (see subsequent discussion) that mainly affects male patients has a striking predilection for the mesentery and omentum; this variant is known as *epithelioid inflammatory myofibroblastic sarcoma*.[98]

Pathologic Features

GI IMT has a wide size range, with a mean of 8 cm. The majority of tumors are firm and white, tan, or yellow. In the largest series, about 33% of cases were polypoid, one of which was pedunculated.[97] Most of the lesions involve the muscularis propria and extend into the submucosa and mucosa. Some tumors are associated with mucosal ulceration. A subset of IMT cases displays a multinodular gross appearance with involvement of both the mesentery and bowel wall.[96,98]

Histologically, GI IMT has features that are identical to IMT of other sites. The tumors are composed of loose fascicles of plump spindle cells with vesicular tapering nuclei, small nucleoli, and palely eosinophilic cytoplasm, admixed with chronic inflammatory cells. The tumors are set in a collagenous or loose edematous to myxoid stroma (Fig. 16.31). Scattered ganglion-like cells (polygonal cells with eccentric nuclei, prominent nucleoli, and eosinophilic or amphophilic cytoplasm) are commonly seen. Chronic inflammatory cells consist predominantly of lymphocytes and plasma cells (see Fig. 16.31), and there are lymphoid follicles in some cases, often with germinal centers. Eosinophils, neutrophils, and foamy histiocytes are seen in some cases. IMTs are variably cellular, and three basic patterns originally described by Coffin and colleagues can be seen, often in combination in a single tumor: myxoid/vascular (fasciitis-like) pattern, compact spindle cell pattern, and hypocellular fibrous pattern.[96,99] Mitotic activity is generally low. The distinctive, aggressive intraabdominal variant of IMT known as epithelioid inflammatory myofibroblastic sarcoma is composed of sheets of rounded to epithelioid cells with vesicular nuclei, large nucleoli, and eosinophilic to amphophilic cytoplasm, often with a myxoid stroma rich in neutrophils (Fig. 16.32).[98]

Immunohistochemistry

The spindle cells are usually positive for SMA and muscle-specific actin, varying from diffuse to focal. Generally, more cells are positive for SMA than muscle-specific actin. Desmin is positive in 50%–60% of cases, usually only focally.[96] Keratin expression is seen in about 33% of cases. KIT, DOG1, CD34, CD21, and CD35 are negative. ALK is positive in about 50% of cases overall (Fig. 16.33), most often in children and adults younger than 35 years of age.[96,100] Most ALK-positive cases show cytoplasmic staining; epithelioid inflammatory myofibroblastic sarcoma usually shows a nuclear membrane pattern of ALK reactivity, whereas a small subset of such tumors show cytoplasmic staining with perinuclear accentuation, which correspond to specific translocation partners (see later discussion).[98,101,102] Around 5%–10% of IMTs are positive for ROS1, which correlates with *ROS1* gene rearrangements; ROS1-positive tumors are negative for ALK.[103]

Molecular Genetics

About 50% of IMTs contain translocations involving the *ALK* gene, with diverse fusion partners (see Chapters 10 and 18 for more details).[96] Epithelioid inflammatory myofibroblastic sarcomas with a nuclear membrane pattern of ALK staining harbor an *RANBP2-ALK* fusion, whereas those with cytoplasmic staining and perinuclear accentuation harbor an *RRBP1-ALK* fusion.[98,102] Of the IMTs that lack *ALK* gene rearrangements, 5%–10% harbor *ROS1* gene fusions; rare cases harbor *PDGFRB*, *RET*, or *ETV6* rearrangements (including *ETV6-NTRK3* fusion).[104–107]

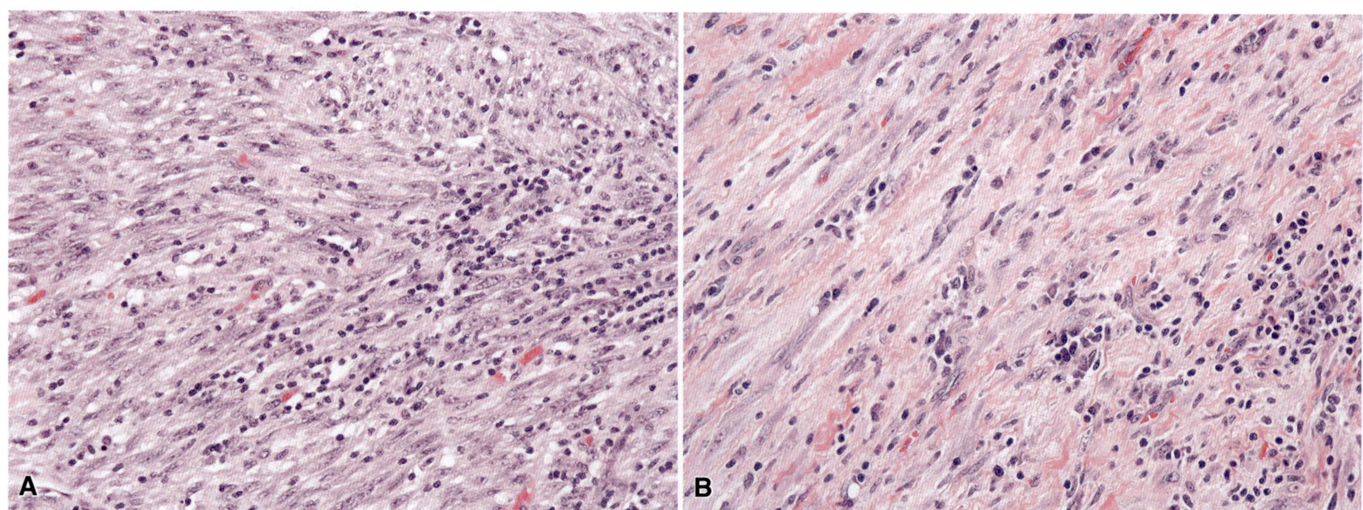

Figure 16.31 Inflammatory Myofibroblastic Tumor. This gastric tumor is composed of fascicles of spindle cells with vesicular nuclei and palely eosinophilic cytoplasm (A). Note the prominent admixed lymphocytes. This colonic inflammatory myofibroblastic tumor contains a collagenous stroma and scattered plasma cells (B).

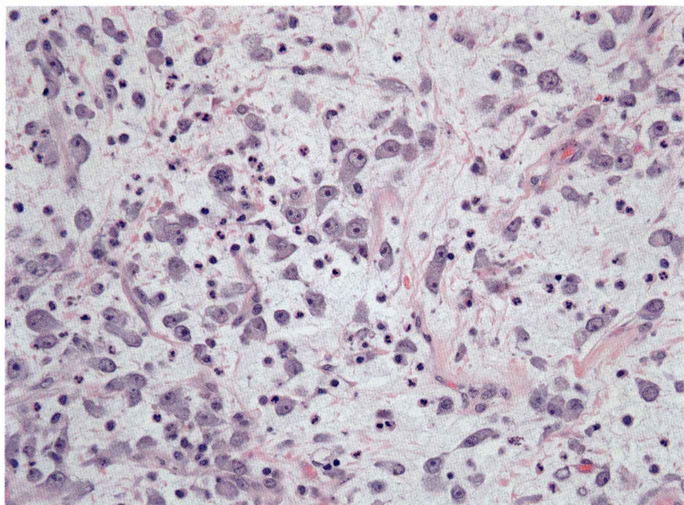

Figure 16.32 Epithelioid Inflammatory Myofibroblastic Sarcoma. This tumor is composed of epithelioid cells with prominent nucleoli and amphophilic cytoplasm. Note the myxoid stroma and prominent neutrophils.

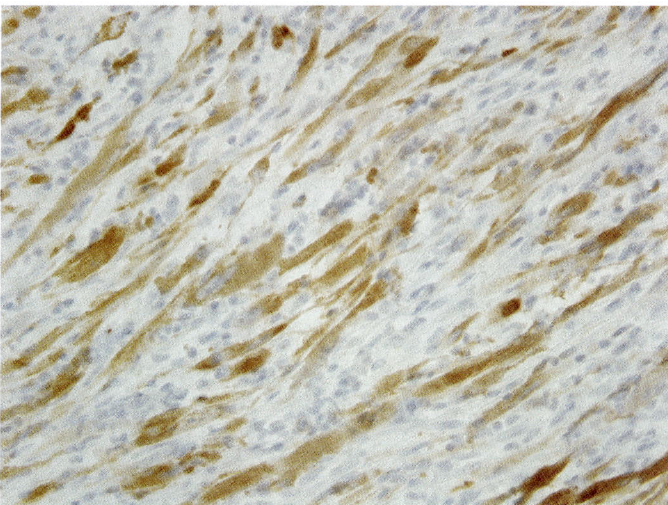

Figure 16.33 Inflammatory Myofibroblastic Tumor. Immunohistochemistry for ALK is positive in 50% of inflammatory myofibroblastic tumors overall, mostly in children and young adults.

Differential Diagnosis

The differential diagnosis is broad, but especially includes inflammatory fibroid polyp, GIST, smooth muscle tumors, follicular dendritic cell sarcoma, and dedifferentiated liposarcoma. Inflammatory fibroid polyps have some of the same clinical and histologic features as IMT. These polyps are most common in the stomach and small intestine and lack the cellular, fascicular appearance of IMT, instead being composed of short spindled to stellate cells in a haphazard pattern within an edematous stroma rich in eosinophils. GISTs are mostly uniformly cellular with fibrillary, syncytial cytoplasm, usually with minimal stroma, generally lack a brisk inflammatory infiltrate, and are positive for KIT and DOG1. Leiomyomas contain blunt-ended nuclei with brightly eosinophilic cytoplasm and are uniformly strongly positive for SMA and desmin and lack an inflammatory component. Leiomyosarcomas display more nuclear atypia and pleomorphism and lack a prominent inflammatory infiltrate. Follicular dendritic cell sarcoma often has a storiform to whorled architecture and is positive for CD21 and CD35. Dedifferentiated liposarcoma not uncommonly involves the wall of the GI tract. The dedifferentiated component characteristically shows considerable morphologic heterogeneity; myofibroblastic differentiation in this component is common (with expression of SMA and desmin), and some cases show a striking resemblance to IMT.[96,100] However, the degree of nuclear atypia is generally greater, and thorough sampling often reveals other histologic patterns (including pleomorphic areas) as well as a well-differentiated liposarcomatous component to allow for proper diagnosis.

Prognosis and Treatment

IMT is a mesenchymal neoplasm of intermediate biologic potential.[96,99,100] Intraabdominal primary tumors have the highest rate of local recurrence (about 25%), although distant metastasis to the liver or other sites is rare (<5%). Histologic features do not reliably predict behavior,[96,100] with the exception of epithelioid inflammatory myofibroblastic sarcoma; this tumor type has an aggressive clinical course with rapid, repeated local recurrences, a significant risk of metastasis, and patient death.[98] Disseminated, aggressive IMTs with *ALK* or *ROS1* gene rearrangements may be treated with receptor tyrosine kinase inhibitor therapies.[104,108]

Desmoid Fibromatosis

Desmoid fibromatosis is a myofibroblastic neoplasm that may arise in the abdominal wall, at extraabdominal sites, or within the abdominal cavity. Intraabdominal desmoid tumors most often affect the mesentery of the small bowel. Desmoid fibromatosis is also discussed in detail in Chapters 3 and 4, and only intraabdominal tumors will be covered briefly in this section.

Clinical Features

Patients with intraabdominal desmoid fibromatosis may present with vague abdominal pain or more rarely with small bowel obstruction. The tumors occur over a broad age range, and there is an equal gender distribution. When desmoid tumors arise in children and young adults, the possibility of familial adenomatous polyposis (Gardner syndrome) should be considered.[109]

Pathologic Features

Mesenteric desmoid fibromatosis is usually large at presentation; most tumors are between 4 and 16 cm in greatest dimension. The tumors have a white, fibrous cut surface with grossly relatively well-circumscribed borders (Fig. 16.34).

Histologically, desmoid fibromatosis is composed of long, sweeping fascicles of elongated spindle cells with ovoid to tapering nuclei, vesicular chromatin, small nucleoli, and palely eosinophilic cytoplasm with ill-defined cell borders, within a variably prominent collagenous stroma (Fig. 16.35). Medium-sized blood vessels are observed between the tumor fascicles. Mesenteric desmoid fibromatosis often shows prominent myxoid stroma and areas with less uniformly fascicular architecture, mimicking nodular fasciitis (Fig. 16.36). The edges of the tumor have infiltrative margins into the bowel wall and mesenteric adipose tissue that may extend to the root of the mesentery (Fig. 16.37).

Immunohistochemistry

Desmoid fibromatosis shows immunoreactivity for SMA (Fig. 16.38A) and occasionally for desmin but is consistently negative for KIT, DOG1, and caldesmon.[28,29,110,111] False positive KIT staining may be seen with excessive antigen retrieval or inadequate antibody dilution.[112,113] Aberrant

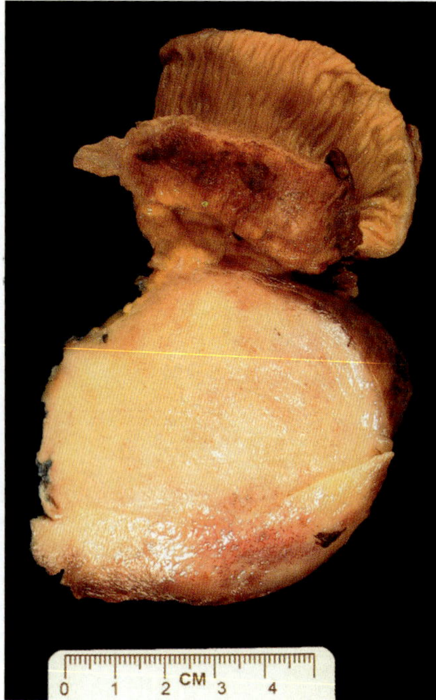

Figure 16.34 **Gross Appearance of Desmoid Fibromatosis.** This large mesenteric tumor shows a fibrous cut surface.

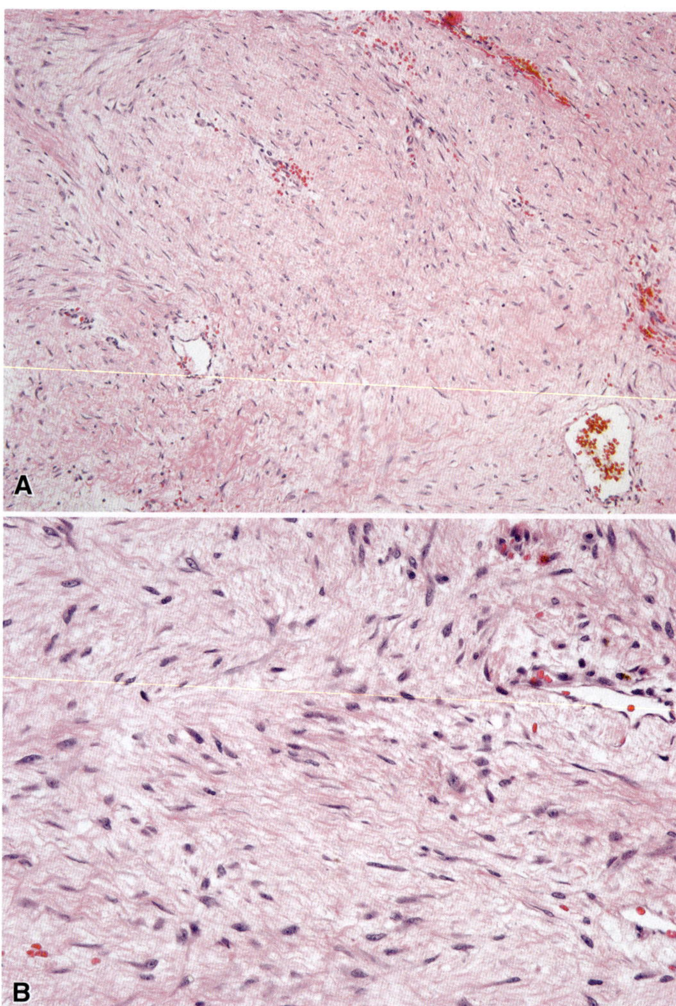

Figure 16.35 **Histologic Appearances of Desmoid Fibromatosis.** The tumor is composed of elongated spindle cells arranged in fascicles with a prominent collagenous stroma (A). The tumor cells are bland with tapering nuclei, small nucleoli, and indistinct cytoplasm (B).

nuclear staining for β-catenin is observed in about 80% of cases (see Fig. 16.38B).[114–116]

Molecular Genetics

Sporadic desmoid fibromatosis usually harbors mutations in *CTNNB1* (β-catenin),[117,118] whereas familial adenomatous polyposis–associated desmoid tumors are caused by germline *APC* gene mutations.[119]

Differential Diagnosis

Mesenteric desmoid fibromatosis should mainly be distinguished from GIST and IMT. Desmoid tumors contain longer fascicles and more collagenous stroma than GISTs, which instead show a hypercellular, syncytial appearance with limited intervening stroma. Only desmoid fibromatosis shows nuclear staining for β-catenin; the GIST markers KIT and DOG1 are negative. IMT has a more loosely fascicular architecture with plumper myofibroblasts than desmoid fibromatosis and contains prominent chronic inflammatory cells, especially plasma cells. Both IMTs and desmoid tumors are positive for SMA, whereas nuclear β-catenin staining is limited to desmoid fibromatosis. Fifty percent of IMTs show immunoreactivity for ALK.

Prognosis and Treatment

Intraabdominal desmoid fibromatosis has a high rate of local recurrence but does not metastasize. The relationship between surgical margin status and recurrence rate is inconsistent. Many different systemic therapies have been administered to patients with desmoid tumors, with variable efficacies (see Chapter 3).[120] Some tumors have an indolent clinical course with slowly progressive growth, whereas other tumors remain stable for years without clinical symptoms. Management must therefore be tailored to the individual patient. Recently, an observational (rather than surgical) strategy has been favored for asymptomatic patients.[121]

PRACTICE POINTS: Intraabdominal Desmoid Fibromatosis

- Most common in mesentery of small bowel
- Often infiltrates bowel wall
- Long fascicles of spindle cells with prominent stromal collagen
- Prominent myxoid stroma common in mesenteric tumors
- SMA positive, nuclear staining for β-catenin, KIT negative

SMA, Smooth muscle actin.

Inflammatory Fibroid Polyp

Inflammatory fibroid polyp is a distinctive benign GI neoplasm originally described by Vanek in 1949 as *gastric submucosal granuloma with eosinophilic infiltration*.[122] Whether inflammatory fibroid polyp is neoplastic or reactive in nature has been a matter of debate for decades.[123] This question has recently been resolved by the identification of activating mutations in *PDGFRA* in this tumor type.[124,125]

Clinical Features

Inflammatory fibroid polyps usually occur in adults over a wide age range, with a peak in the sixth decade and a slight female predominance.[97,123,126–128] The stomach is most often affected, especially the antrum,

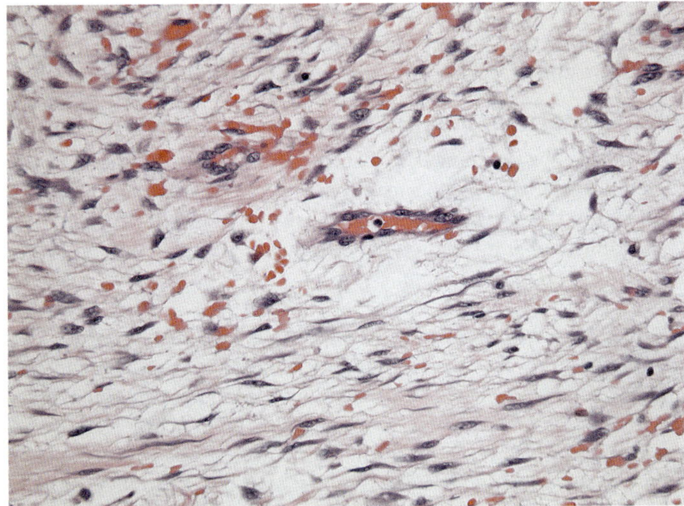

Figure 16.36 Mesenteric Desmoid Fibromatosis. Desmoid tumors at this site often contain prominent myxoid stroma, mimicking nodular fasciitis.

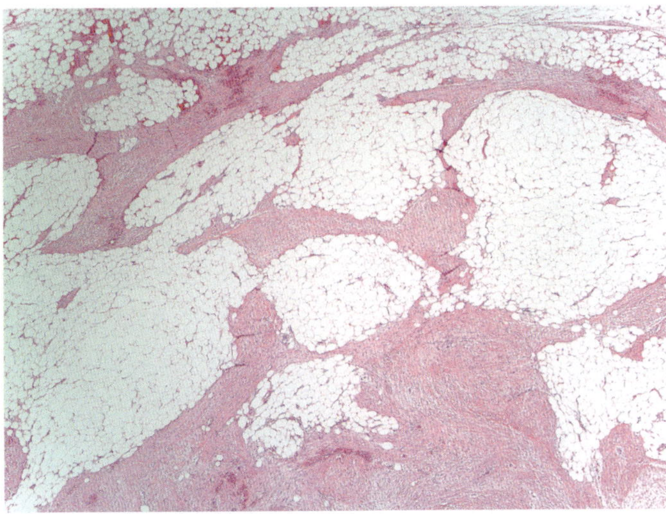

Figure 16.37 Mesenteric Desmoid Fibromatosis. One of the hallmarks of desmoid fibromatosis is an infiltrative growth pattern. This tumor extensively infiltrates mesenteric adipose tissue at the periphery.

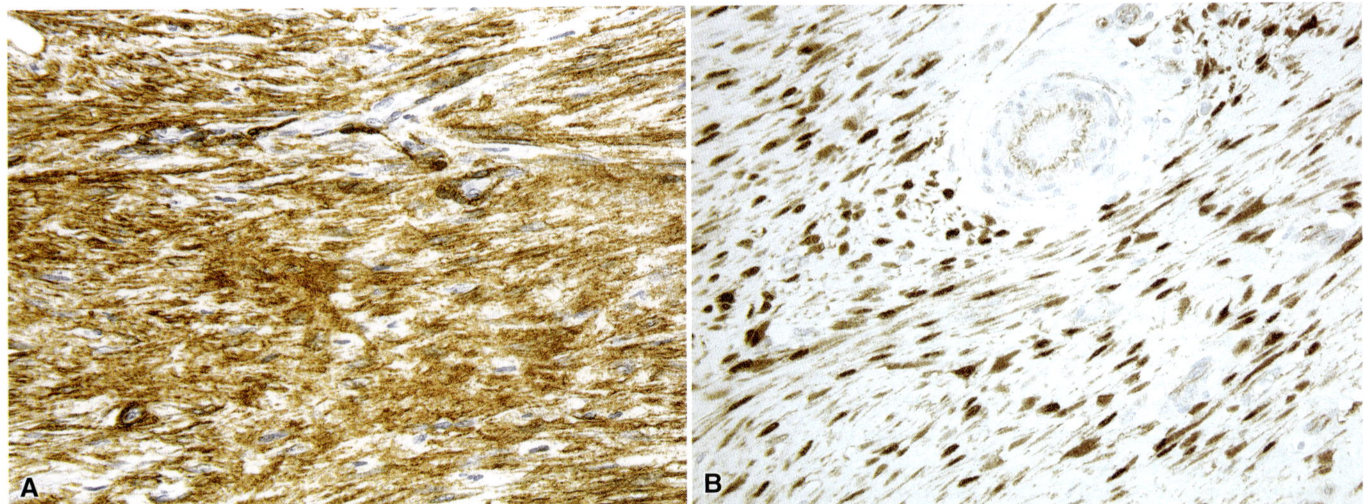

Figure 16.38 Immunophenotypic Features of Desmoid Fibromatosis. The tumor is positive for smooth muscle actin, with extensive staining (A). Aberrant nuclear staining for β-catenin (B).

followed closely by the ileum. Inflammatory fibroid polyps rarely arise in the colon, rectum, or other sites in the GI tract. Patients may present with abdominal pain, anemia, GI bleeding, or obstruction, the latter most often in the case of small intestine tumors, which may present emergently with intussusception. Small gastric or duodenal tumors are sometimes discovered incidentally at the time of endoscopy (Fig. 16.39). The tumors most often appear as pedunculated intraluminal polypoid lesions but may also occur as large mural masses. Overlying mucosal ulceration is common. A familial occurrence of inflammatory fibroid polyps has been reported (Devon polyposis syndrome).[129–131]

Pathologic Features

Inflammatory fibroid polyps show a large range in size, from several millimeters to more than 10 cm in greatest dimension. Gastric tumors are usually between 1 and 3 cm, whereas small intestinal tumors are often larger, between 3 and 8 cm.[123,127,128] The tumors are usually centered in the submucosa and show a tan or white cut surface, often with a glistening or fleshy appearance, and ill-defined margins.

Histologically, inflammatory fibroid polyps are hypocellular lesions composed of bland ovoid, short spindled, stellate, or more epithelioid cells with fine chromatin, inconspicuous nucleoli, and small amounts of eosinophilic cytoplasm haphazardly arranged in a loose, predominantly edematous to myxoid stroma containing a conspicuous inflammatory infiltrate, chiefly of eosinophils, but also histiocytes and lymphocytes (Fig. 16.40). Capillaries and small blood vessels are often prominent, a subset of which show perivascular, lamellar (onion-skin) fibrosis. Occasionally, tumors contain more collagenous stroma (see Fig. 16.40). The tumor often infiltrates and ulcerates the mucosa and may be difficult to distinguish from adjacent granulation tissue, particularly in small biopsies. Larger tumors may infiltrate through the muscularis propria into subserosa.

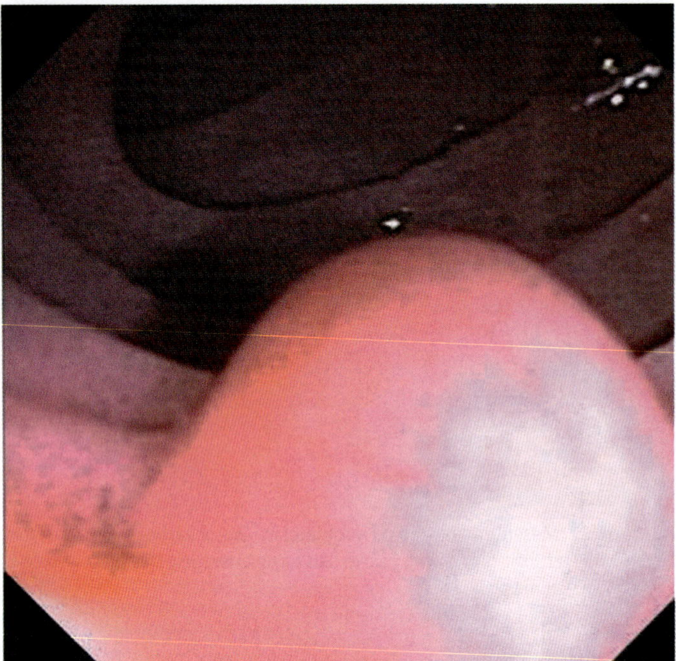

Figure 16.39 Endoscopic Appearance of an Inflammatory Fibroid Polyp. This submucosal tumor of the duodenum is covered by intact mucosa.

Immunohistochemistry

By immunohistochemistry, most inflammatory fibroid polyps are positive for CD34, whereas about 10%–20% of cases show focal reactivity for SMA.[126] Desmin, KIT, DOG1, and S-100 are consistently negative.[29]

Molecular Genetics

Recently, researchers identified activating mutations in *PDGFRA* in the majority of inflammatory fibroid polyps: 70% of inflammatory fibroid polyps of the small intestine[125] and 55% of gastric inflammatory fibroid polyps.[124] Interestingly, nearly all *PDGFRA* mutations in small intestine tumors occurred in exon 12, whereas gastric tumors usually harbor mutations in exon 18, most often the D842V substitution (similar to gastric GISTs). Patients with the very rare familial inflammatory fibroid polyps harbor germline *PDGFRA* mutations.[131]

Differential Diagnosis

The differential diagnosis of inflammatory fibroid polyp primarily includes IMT,[97] GIST, and conventional inflammatory polyps. IMTs are more cellular than inflammatory fibroid polyps, and are composed of plump, elongated spindle cells arranged in fascicles. In terms of the inflammatory infiltrate, plasma cells and lymphocytes usually predominate in IMT, whereas eosinophils are relatively uncommon. IMTs are usually positive for SMA and may also express desmin, whereas CD34 is consistently negative; 50% of tumors show reactivity for ALK, correlating with the presence of *ALK* gene rearrangements. GISTs are generally uniformly cellular and lack the loose, edematous stroma and prominent eosinophils and small blood vessels of inflammatory fibroid polyps. KIT and DOG1 expression are specific for GIST in this differential diagnosis. Small inflammatory fibroid polyps may be mistaken for inflammatory polyps, but inflammatory polyps often contain irregular and dilated crypts containing neutrophils, and the stroma lacks the uniform hypocellularity and stellate to epithelioid cytology of inflammatory fibroid polyps.

Prognosis and Treatment

Inflammatory fibroid polyps are benign. They do not recur.

Plexiform Fibromyxoma

Plexiform fibromyxoma is a recently described, rare, distinctive benign mesenchymal tumor with a marked predilection for the gastric antrum.[132] This tumor type has been previously reported as "myxoma" and "plexiform angiomyxoid myofibroblastic tumor."[133,134]

Clinical Features

About 35 cases of plexiform fibromyxoma have been reported.[132] The tumor occurs over a broad age range, with a peak in young to middle-aged adults and an equal gender distribution. Affected patients often present with anemia or hematemesis. Some large tumors cause gastric outlet obstruction. Nearly all plexiform fibromyxomas arise in the wall of the gastric antrum, and the tumors may extend into the duodenal bulb.[132] The preoperative clinical diagnosis is often GIST.

Pathologic Features

Plexiform fibromyxomas range from 2 to 15 cm in greatest dimension with a mean of 4–5 cm. The tumors are grossly multinodular, with a tan, glistening, often mucoid cut surface.

Histologically, plexiform fibromyxoma has a distinctive multinodular, plexiform architecture through the muscularis propria (Fig. 16.41). The nodules are sharply demarcated from the surrounding tissue and often extend into the subserosa, submucosa, and mucosa. Mucosal ulceration is common. The tumor nodules may extend into the lumina of lymphatic and blood vessels, including large veins. This feature is of no clinical consequence (see the section "Prognosis and Treatment"). Abundant myxoid matrix is usually present (see Fig. 16.41), although a subset of nodules may contain more collagenous stroma. There is a prominent vascular network of small capillaries. The lesional spindle cells contain uniform small nuclei with inconspicuous nucleoli and indistinct eosinophilic cytoplasm (see Fig. 16.41). Mitotic activity is typically scarce.

Immunohistochemistry

By immunohistochemistry, plexiform fibromyxomas are usually positive for SMA, and desmin expression is variable. The tumors are consistently negative for KIT, DOG1, S-100 protein, and CD34.

Molecular Genetics

A subset of plexiform fibromyxomas harbor *MALAT1-GLI1* gene fusions.[135]

Differential Diagnosis

The differential diagnosis for plexiform fibromyxoma includes GIST, inflammatory fibroid polyp, and plexiform neurofibroma. GISTs rarely contain prominent myxoid stroma. Myxoid GISTs usually show epithelioid cytomorphology and lack the plexiform architecture and prominent vascular pattern of plexiform fibromyxoma. Immunohistochemistry for KIT and DOG1 can distinguish among these tumor types. Similar to plexiform fibromyxoma, inflammatory fibroid polyp also shows a predilection for the gastric antrum. However, inflammatory fibroid polyp exhibits a sheet-like (not plexiform) architecture, with tumor cells that are often stellate or more epithelioid, and it contains prominent inflammatory cells, especially eosinophils. Plexiform neurofibroma is essentially diagnostic of NF1 and is composed of expanded, hyperplastic nerve trunks that often contain somewhat myxoid stroma but are in general much more cellular than the nodules in plexiform fibromyxoma. The lesional cells contain elongated, tapering nuclei. An S-100 stain can be used to confirm the diagnosis.

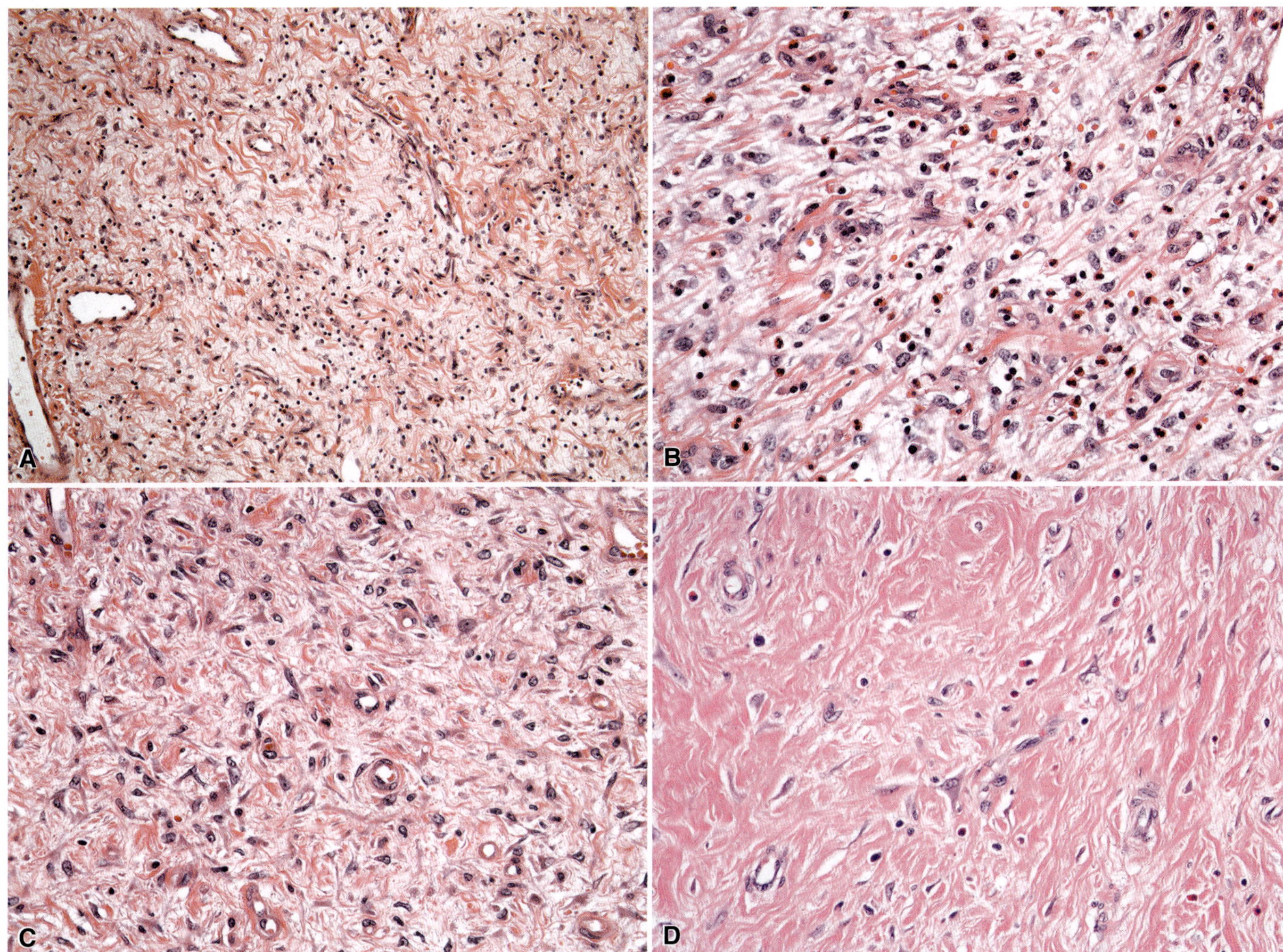

Figure 16.40 **Histologic Appearances of Inflammatory Fibroid Polyp.** Bland short spindle cells haphazardly arranged in an edematous stroma (A). Prominent stromal eosinophils are a typical feature (B). Some tumors contain collagenous stroma (C). Note the stellate cytomorphology. A hypocellular example with prominent stromal hyalinization (D). Note the occasional eosinophils.

Prognosis and Treatment

Plexiform fibromyxoma is a benign tumor. The presence of intravascular growth appears to be of no clinical significance. No recurrences have been reported to date.

Perivascular Epithelioid Cell Tumor

Perivascular epithelioid cell tumors (PEComas) are a family of related mesenchymal neoplasms that include angiomyolipoma, lymphangiomyomatosis, clear cell ("sugar") tumor of the lung, and a group of morphologically and immunophenotypically similar lesions that occur at a wide range of anatomic sites.[136–138] These tumors share a distinctive cell type, the so-called perivascular epithelioid cell. The retroperitoneum, abdomen (mesentery, omentum), and pelvis are relatively commonly involved.[137,138] The most common visceral sites are the uterus and GI tract. This section will focus on PEComas that occur in the GI tract. PEComas are also discussed in detail in Chapter 6.

Clinical Features

GI PEComas occur over a wide age range, with a peak in young to middle-aged adults, and a predilection for female patients.[139] GI PEComas may be discovered incidentally at the time of screening colonoscopy as a small polyp. Alternatively, patients with a large mural mass may present with anemia, hematochezia, abdominal pain, or obstruction. The colon and rectum are the most commonly involved sites in the GI tract (55%–60% of cases), followed by the jejunum and ileum (35%); the stomach and duodenum are particularly rare primary sites.[139] Unlike angiomyolipoma and lymphangiomyomatosis, GI PEComas are rarely associated with the tuberous sclerosis complex (TSC).[139]

Pathologic Features

GI PEComas range from small polyps based in the mucosa and submucosa measuring 0.5–3 cm, to large masses situated in the wall of the bowel, measuring 5–20 cm (median size, 6 cm).[139] Most tumors are

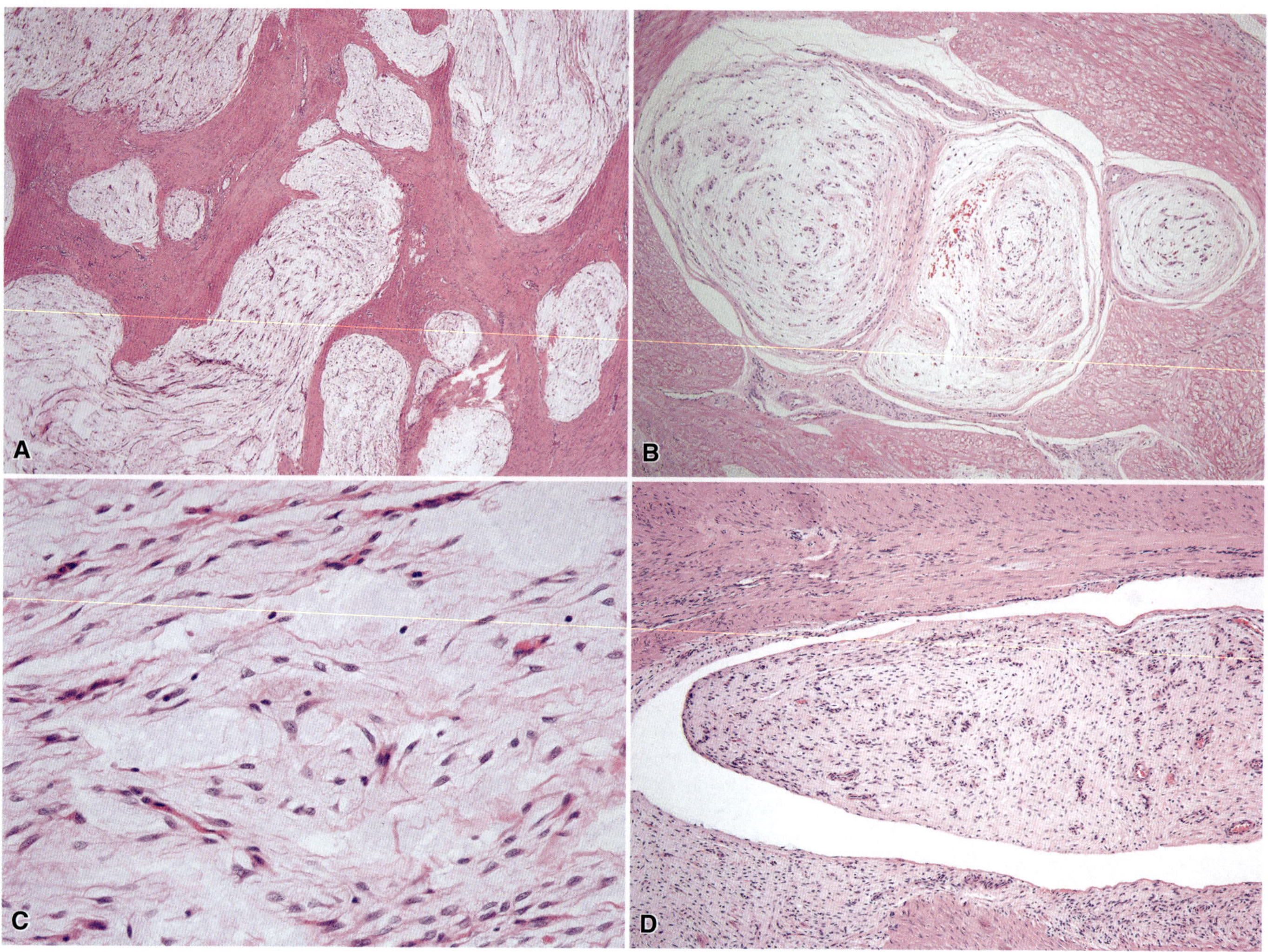

Figure 16.41 **Histologic Appearances of Plexiform Fibromyxoma.** Low-power image showing the plexiform architecture through the gastric wall (A). The individual tumor nodules are sharply demarcated and contain prominent myxoid stroma (B). Note the small, branching blood vessels. The tumor is composed of bland spindle cells with eosinophilic cytoplasm (C). Tumor nodules often extend into the lumina of large dilated veins (D). This finding is of no clinical significance.

grossly well circumscribed, with a tan or yellow, soft and fleshy cut surface. Mucosal ulceration is common, and areas of necrosis and hemorrhage may be seen in large tumors.

Histologically, PEComas are composed of nests and sheets of epithelioid cells with abundant granular eosinophilic to clear cytoplasm, well-defined cell borders, and round to ovoid central nuclei with variably prominent nucleoli (Figs. 16.42 and 16.43). Some PEComas contain a spindle cell component. The nests are surrounded by a delicate capillary vascular network. Cytologically, some PEComas contain uniform, bland nuclei with small nucleoli and rare mitotic figures, whereas others are histologically malignant and show marked nuclear atypia with coarse chromatin, large nucleoli, and a high mitotic rate (Fig. 16.44). Occasionally, multinucleated cells may be observed in otherwise bland tumors. Some PEComas exhibit diffuse and striking pleomorphism. Infiltrative margins are common.

Immunohistochemistry

PEComas show a mixed melanocytic and smooth muscle phenotype. Most GI PEComas are positive for HMB-45, melan A, or both, with a variable extent of expression, ranging from occasional cells to diffuse staining. The tumors are often positive for microphthalmia transcription factor (MiTF), as well as SMA and desmin, and a subset of tumors also expresses caldesmon.[136,138,139] Focal cytoplasmic staining for S-100 protein is seen in 10% of cases. About 10% of PEComas are positive for TFE3.[140] The tumors are consistently negative for KIT, DOG1, keratins, and EMA.[139]

Molecular Genetics

PEComas are usually characterized by loss-of-function mutations in *TSC2* (rarely *TSC1*), leading to activation of the mammalian target of rapamycin (mTOR) pathway; malignant *TSC2*-mutant PEComas often have *TP53* mutations as well.[136,141–143] This can be exploited therapeutically in malignant PEComas through mTOR inhibitors such as sirolimus (see the section "Prognosis and Treatment").[144] Occasionally, PEComas lacking *TSC2* mutations harbor translocations involving *TFE3*.[140,143]

Differential Diagnosis

The differential diagnosis for GI PEComa includes metastatic carcinoma (particularly clear cell renal cell carcinoma), metastatic melanoma,

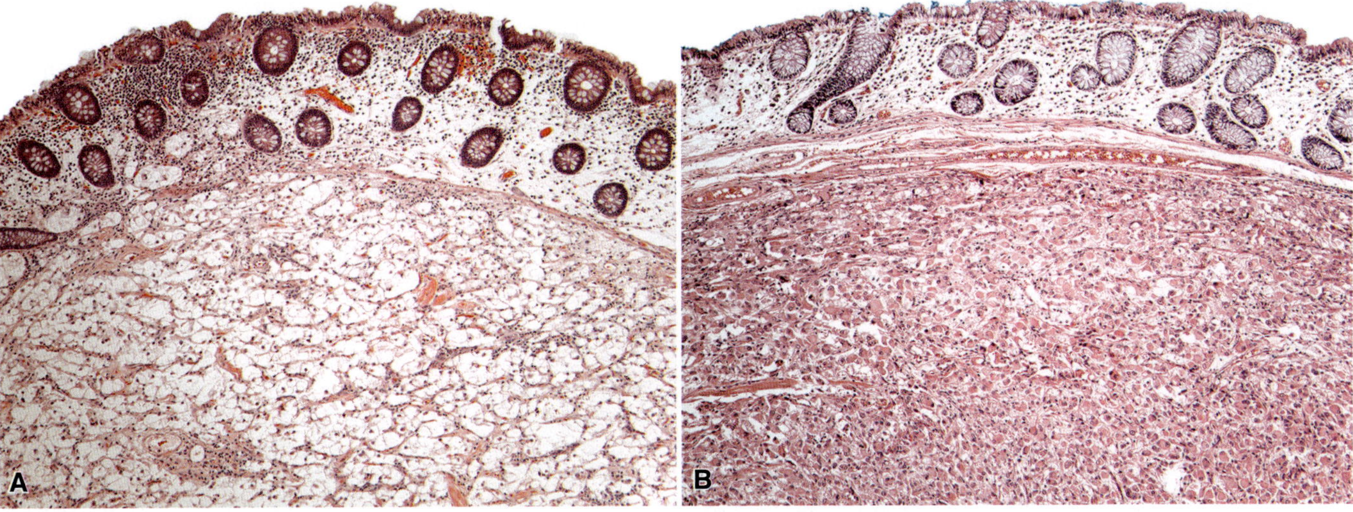

Figure 16.42 **Histologic Appearances of Perivascular Epithelioid Cell Tumors of the Gastrointestinal Tract.** A polypoid perivascular epithelioid cell tumor (PEComa) of the colon (A). Note the abundant clear cytoplasm. This polypoid tumor is composed of epithelioid cells with eosinophilic cytoplasm (B).

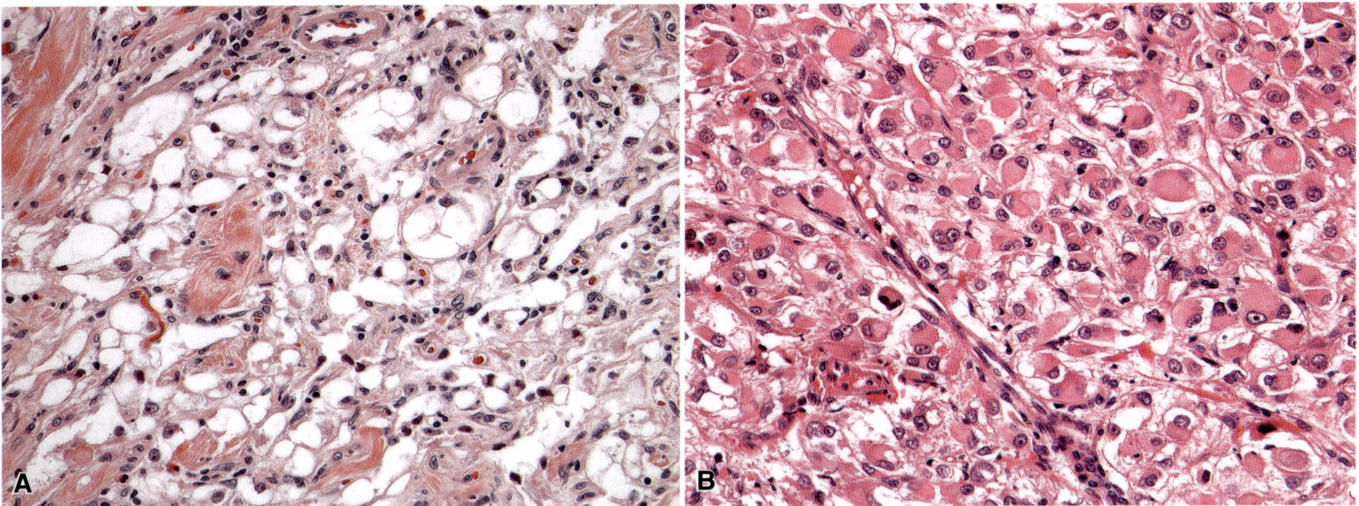

Figure 16.43 **Cytologic Appearances of Perivascular Epithelioid Cell Tumors.** A gastrointestinal perivascular epithelioid cell tumor (PEComa) composed of epithelioid cells with clear cytoplasm and uniform small nuclei (A). A PEComa with granular eosinophilic cytoplasm (B). Note the small nucleoli.

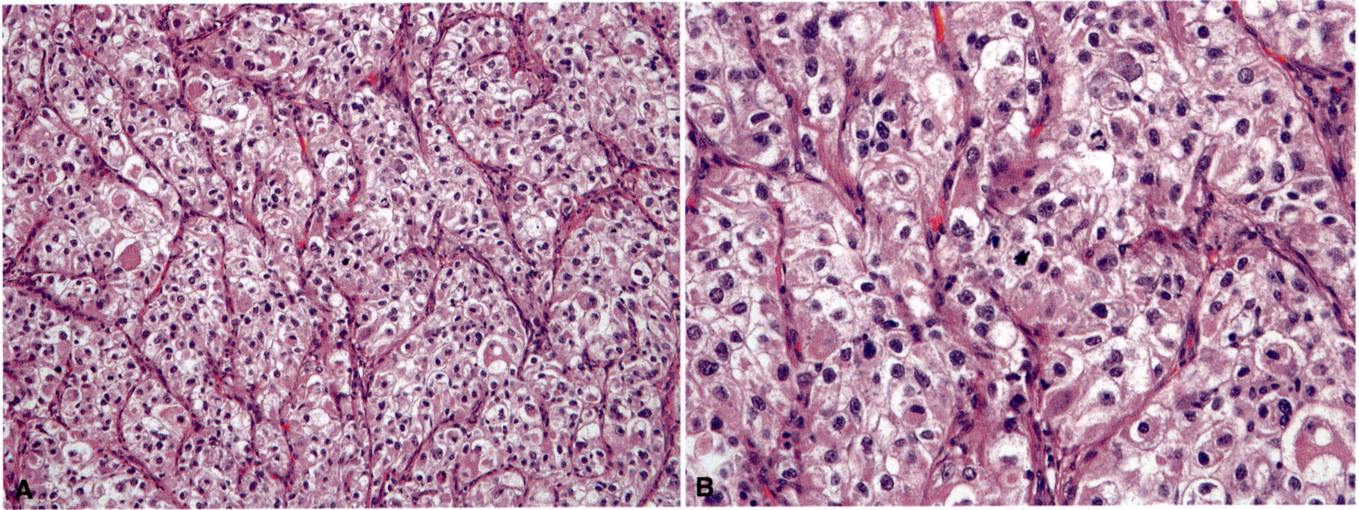

Figure 16.44 **Malignant Perivascular Epithelioid Cell Tumor.** A malignant perivascular epithelioid cell tumor (PEComa) of the colon showing a nested and trabecular architecture (A). The tumor is composed of epithelioid cells with abundant finely granular eosinophilic cytoplasm. Note the nuclear atypia and mitotic activity (B).

metastatic alveolar soft part sarcoma, CCS, paraganglioma, and epithelioid GIST. Metastatic renal cell carcinoma can be distinguished by immunoreactivity for EMA, keratins, and PAX8, whereas metastatic melanoma usually shows strong expression of S-100 protein and lacks muscle markers. Alveolar soft part sarcoma shows significant morphologic overlap with some PEComas, albeit usually with more brightly eosinophilic cytoplasm and more uniformly nested architecture. Alveolar soft part sarcoma is negative for melanocytic markers and positive for TFE3, although the latter marker is also positive in a small subset of PEComas that contain *TFE3* rearrangements. CCS of soft tissue type is usually strongly positive for S-100 protein, in addition to melanocytic markers, and it is negative for SMA and desmin. In addition, the nests and fascicles of tumor cells lack the capillary vasculature of PEComa. The distinctive CCS-like tumor of the GI tract usually shows a more sheet-like growth pattern with alveolar and pseudopapillary areas, and the tumor cells are rounded to epithelioid with small amounts of cytoplasm, in contrast to the abundant cytoplasm in PEComas. Melanocytic markers are negative in this tumor type. Both conventional CCS and the GI CCS-like tumor contain *EWSR1* gene rearrangements (with *ATF1* or *CREB1* fusion partners), the identification of which can be used to confirm the diagnosis. Paragangliomas are positive for chromogranin and synaptophysin and negative for melanocytic and smooth muscle markers. Epithelioid GISTs generally show a more sheet-like architecture, and when a nested growth pattern is observed, the nests lack the vascular pattern of PEComa. The tumor cells in epithelioid GIST contain less abundant cytoplasm than PEComa. KIT and DOG1 expression supports a diagnosis of GIST.

Prognosis and Treatment

GI PEComas range from benign tumors to highly aggressive sarcomas. Criteria for malignancy have not been firmly established at this anatomic site, although the presence of marked nuclear atypia, diffuse pleomorphism, and mitotic activity correlates with aggressive behavior.[137–139] PEComas with mild nuclear atypia and rare mitotic figures are generally benign. Tumor size is not a reliable marker of malignancy, although the majority of malignant PEComas are large (>7 cm). Malignant GI PEComas may present with regional lymph node metastases. Malignant PEComas often have an aggressive clinical course and result in patient death within several years. The most common site of distant metastasis is the liver, followed by peritoneum, lung, and bone. As mentioned earlier, mTOR inhibitors such as sirolimus show some benefit for patients with metastatic PEComa.[144]

Glomus Tumor

Glomus tumors are distinctive, usually benign mesenchymal neoplasms composed of perivascular contractile smooth muscle-like cells. Although glomus tumors most often arise in the skin and subcutaneous tissues of the distal extremities, they may also occur in the GI tract, nearly always in the stomach.[145–147] Glomus tumors are also discussed in Chapter 6. Awareness of the existence of gastric glomus tumors can help avoid misclassification as other tumor types with significant malignant potential.

Clinical Features

GI glomus tumors are very rare, vastly outnumbered by GISTs (100 : 1).[146] These tumors affect adults over a wide age range, with a peak in the sixth decade and a female predominance.[145,146] Nearly all GI glomus tumors occur in the stomach (mostly antrum); the small intestine and colon are very rarely involved. Affected patients often present with upper GI bleeding, melena, abdominal pain, and anemia. Tumors may also be discovered incidentally at the time of endoscopy or abdominal surgery.

Pathologic Features

Gastric glomus tumors range from 1 to 7 cm in size, with a mean of 2–3 cm.[146] Many tumors have a grossly multinodular appearance and a firm or rubbery consistency.

Histologically, gastric glomus tumors consist of cellular nodules separated by bands of smooth muscle of the muscularis propria (Fig. 16.45). Extension to the mucosa with ulceration is common, and serosal involvement may also be seen. The cellular nodules often contain prominent slit-like and dilated hemangiopericytoma-like thin-walled blood vessels, around which the glomus cells are arranged (see Fig. 16.45). The tumor cells are uniform with round nuclei, fine chromatin, inconspicuous nucleoli, and clear to palely eosinophilic cytoplasm with sharply defined cell borders (see Fig. 16.45). Some tumors contain foci with brightly eosinophilic (oncocytic) cytoplasm. Vascular invasion within dilated veins is relatively common, particularly at the periphery of the tumor.[146] Mitotic activity is typically absent or very scant. Occasionally, tumors contain areas with fascicular spindle cell morphology, and some tumors show degenerative nuclear atypia.

Immunohistochemistry

By immunohistochemistry, glomus tumors show strong, diffuse reactivity for SMA (see Fig. 16.45D), and they are often positive for caldesmon.[146] Laminin and type IV collagen show a pericellular staining pattern, but these markers are not widely used for diagnostic purposes. CD34 may be focally positive in occasional cases, and weak, focal staining for synaptophysin may be seen, which can lead to diagnostic confusion (see the section "Differential Diagnosis"). The tumors are consistently negative for desmin, S-100 protein, KIT, DOG1, keratins, and chromogranin.[146]

Molecular Genetics

Glomus tumors often harbor *NOTCH2* gene fusions, most often *MIR143-NOTCH2*; rearrangements of *NOTCH1* and *NOTCH3* are less common.[148]

Differential Diagnosis

The main differential diagnostic considerations for gastric glomus tumor are epithelioid GIST, well-differentiated neuroendocrine (carcinoid) tumor, and rarely lymphoma. Epithelioid GISTs of the stomach may show a multinodular growth pattern and sharply defined cell borders (the latter particularly in tumors with prominent clear cytoplasm), but they typically lack the dilated vessels and subendothelial perivascular growth of glomus tumors. Epithelioid GISTs are usually positive for KIT and/or DOG1, and SMA is at most focally positive. In contrast to glomus tumors, which are centered in the muscularis propria, gastric carcinoid tumors arise in the mucosa and often extend to the submucosa. Carcinoid tumors typically show a prominent trabecular and insular architecture, with less well-defined cell borders and more granular or coarse chromatin than in glomus tumors. Although synaptophysin may show focal, weak staining in glomus tumors, keratins and chromogranin are only positive in carcinoid tumors. Rarely, gastric glomus tumors may be mistaken for lymphoma, especially extranodal marginal zone B-cell lymphoma (mucosa-associated lymphoid tissue [MALT] lymphoma), due to the commonly monocytoid appearance with clear cytoplasm in gastric MALT lymphoma. However, glomus tumors are negative for CD45 (leukocyte common antigen [LCA]) and CD20, which are strongly positive in MALT lymphoma.

Prognosis and Treatment

Gastric glomus tumors are usually clinically benign. Occasionally, histologically typical cases result in metastases.[146,149] Malignant glomus

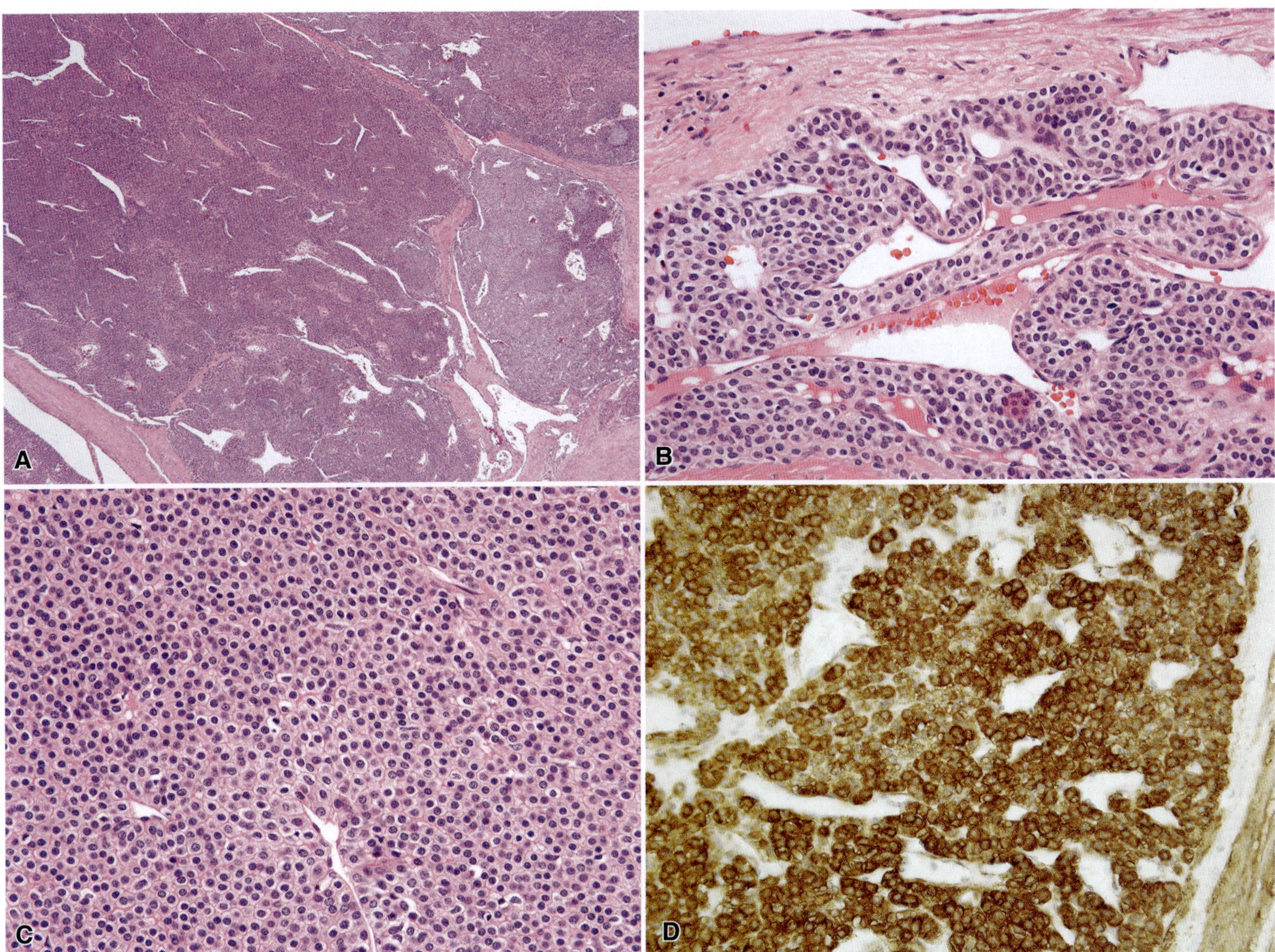

Figure 16.45 Histologic Appearances of Gastric Glomus Tumor. The tumor shows a nodular architecture (A). Note the prominent slit-like and dilated blood vessels. The glomus cells are arranged around dilated blood vessels (B). The tumor is composed of sheets of rounded cells with small nuclei and sharply defined cell borders (C). The tumor cells are strongly positive for smooth muscle actin (D).

tumors are sufficiently rare that firm criteria for malignancy have not been established. The criteria for malignancy derived for glomus tumors of somatic soft tissue (i.e., deep location and size larger than 2 cm or atypical mitotic figures)[149] do not appear to be appropriate for gastric glomus tumors, because many clinically benign tumors at this location are larger than 2 cm. Vascular invasion alone is not an indicator of malignancy for gastric glomus tumors.[146] The rare gastric glomus tumors with spindle cell areas and at least moderate nuclear atypia should be considered malignant. Malignant gastric glomus tumors typically metastasize to the liver.[146]

Polypoid Ganglioneuroma and Ganglioneuromatosis

Ganglioneuromas are benign neuroectodermal lesions that often arise in the retroperitoneum or posterior mediastinum.[150] However, ganglioneuromas may also involve the GI tract. GI ganglioneuromas occur in three settings: (1) solitary polypoid ganglioneuroma, (2) ganglioneuromatous polyposis, and (3) ganglioneuromatosis.[150,151] The latter two disorders are significantly associated with familial syndromes. Ganglioneuromas are also discussed in Chapter 3.

Clinical Features

Solitary polypoid ganglioneuromas are by far the most common form of GI ganglioneuroma.[151] These incidental colorectal lesions are discovered at the time of colonoscopy and endoscopically resemble hyperplastic, juvenile, or adenomatous polyps. They occur over a wide age range, are most common in middle-aged to older adults, and have no gender predilection.

Ganglioneuromatous polyposis is associated with Cowden syndrome (PTEN hamartoma tumor syndrome).[152–154] Nearly all patients with Cowden syndrome have polyps in both the upper and lower GI tract.[152,154,155] Cowden syndrome is a mixed polyposis syndrome; the polyps include not only polypoid ganglioneuromas but also hyperplastic polyps, adenomas, hamartomatous polyps (resembling juvenile polyps or containing cellular stroma or adipose tissue), and inflammatory polyps.[152,154,155] Multiple polypoid ganglioneuromas, and multiple polyps of varied histologic type, should raise the possibility of Cowden syndrome. Ganglioneuromatous polyposis in this syndrome shows a wide range in extent of involvement, from several small polyps to a carpeting of polyps, including large pedunculated examples (Fig. 16.46). Patients with Cowden syndrome also often exhibit glycogenic acanthosis/papillomatosis of the esophagus.[153,155] The incidence of colorectal cancer, breast cancer, and thyroid cancer is significantly increased in patients with Cowden syndrome.[152,154]

Ganglioneuromatosis is associated with both multiple endocrine neoplasia type IIB (MEN2B)[156–158] and NF1.[150,157,159,160] Patients with MEN2B also develop mucosal neuromas, especially on the tongue and lips.[160] Ganglioneuromatosis is common in patients with MEN2B and may involve the intestines (most often) or esophagus.[150,156] Patients may either present in childhood, mimicking Hirschsprung disease, or later in life with constipation, diarrhea, or abdominal pain.[150,156] Megacolon may result. Ganglioneuromatosis may also be discovered incidentally at the time of appendectomy.[150] Because ganglioneuromatosis may be the first presentation of MEN2B, recognition of this association by pathologists is critical so that prophylactic thyroidectomy can be performed before medullary thyroid carcinoma develops.

Ganglioneuromatosis in patients with NF1 is rare.[150,159,160] Other GI manifestations of NF1 include multiple GISTs of the small intestine,[17,18] neurofibromas (including plexiform neurofibromas),[150] and somatostatin-producing neuroendocrine tumors and gangliocytic paraganglioma of the duodenum.[159]

Pathologic Features

Polypoid ganglioneuromas are typically small, sessile polyps ranging in size from 0.5 to 2 cm.[151] Ganglioneuromatosis may present as a discrete mass, or, more often, as an ill-defined thickening of the bowel wall.[150,151,156,157]

Histologically, polypoid ganglioneuromas are composed of an admixture of spindle-shaped Schwann cells with eosinophilic cytoplasm and tapering nuclei (which predominate) and ganglion cells, which entrap and surround colonic crypts (Fig. 16.47). Ganglion cells may be few in number or numerous. The lesion is usually limited to the mucosa but may extend into the superficial submucosa.

The individual polyps in ganglioneuromatous polyposis resemble sporadic polypoid ganglioneuromas. In addition, arbitrary biopsies of endoscopically normal mucosa in patients with Cowden syndrome may also show minute ganglioneural proliferations in the lamina propria.

Ganglioneuromatosis in patients with MEN2B usually involves both the myenteric plexus, which often shows a striking nodular and band-like expansion of Schwann cells, ganglion cells and their processes, and submucosal plexus, and extends in a more subtle fashion through the muscularis propria.[150,156,157] Mucosal involvement is usually only limited and focal. In contrast, ganglioneuromatosis in patients with NF1 is usually centered in the mucosa and submucosa (Fig. 16.48).[150,159]

Immunohistochemistry

By immunohistochemistry, the dominant spindle-shaped Schwann cells are positive for S-100 protein, whereas the ganglion cells can be highlighted by neuron-specific enolase, synaptophysin, PHOX2B, or NFP. The latter also stains the ganglion cell processes. Practically speaking, immunohistochemistry is not required to confirm the diagnosis.

Molecular Genetics

The molecular genetic basis of sporadic polypoid ganglioneuromas is unknown. Cowden syndrome is caused by germline mutation in *PTEN*, located on chromosome 10q23.[152] Patients with MEN2B have germline mutations in *RET* on 10q11,[158] whereas patients with NF1 have mutations in *NF1* (neurofibromin 1) at 17q11.

Differential Diagnosis

Once the distinctive combination of spindle cells and ganglion cells is recognized, there is no realistic differential diagnosis for a polypoid ganglioneuroma. If the ganglion cells are overlooked, the differential diagnosis might include other polyps containing spindle cells that entrap crypts, namely mucosal perineurioma and mucosal Schwann cell hamartoma. In contrast to polypoid ganglioneuroma, the spindle cells in mucosal perineurioma contain small ovoid nuclei and pale indistinct cytoplasm, show a more lamellar and whorled growth pattern around crypts, and are usually associated with a hyperplastic polyp. In perineurioma, EMA is positive, whereas S-100 is negative. Mucosal Schwann cell hamartoma is composed of a pure population of Schwann cells, without the ganglion cells and processes seen in ganglioneuroma.

As mentioned previously, NF1-associated ganglioneuromatosis is usually centered in the mucosa and submucosa, whereas MEN2B-associated ganglioneuromatosis shows diffuse involvement of the myenteric plexus.

Prognosis and Treatment

Polypoid ganglioneuromas and ganglioneuromatosis are benign lesions. Ganglioneuromatosis may require resection of the involved segment of bowel to alleviate obstruction or constipation.

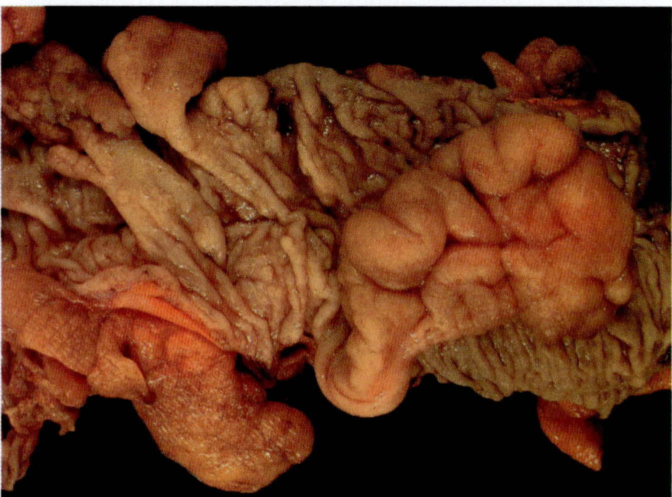

Figure 16.46 **Gross Appearance of the Colon From a Patient With Cowden Syndrome and Ganglioneuromatous Polyposis.** Note the large pedunculated polyps and innumerable small polyps.

PRACTICE POINTS: Polypoid Ganglioneuroma and Ganglioneuromatosis

- Composed of S-100-positive Schwann cells (predominant) and ganglion cells
- Solitary polypoid ganglioneuroma most common (colorectal polyp)
- Ganglioneuromatous polyposis associated with Cowden syndrome (PTEN hamartoma tumor syndrome), along with other types of polyps (hyperplastic, inflammatory, adenomatous) and glycogenic acanthosis/papillomatosis of the esophagus
- Ganglioneuromatosis associated with multiple endocrine neoplasia IIB (ill-defined thickening of bowel wall, based in myenteric plexus/muscularis propria/submucosa) and neurofibromatosis type 1 (often well-circumscribed mass, based in submucosa/mucosa)

Granular Cell Tumor

Granular cell tumor (formerly known as *granular cell myoblastoma*) is a usually benign Schwann cell tumor with a predilection for the oral cavity (especially tongue), skin, and subcutaneous tissues. Occasionally,

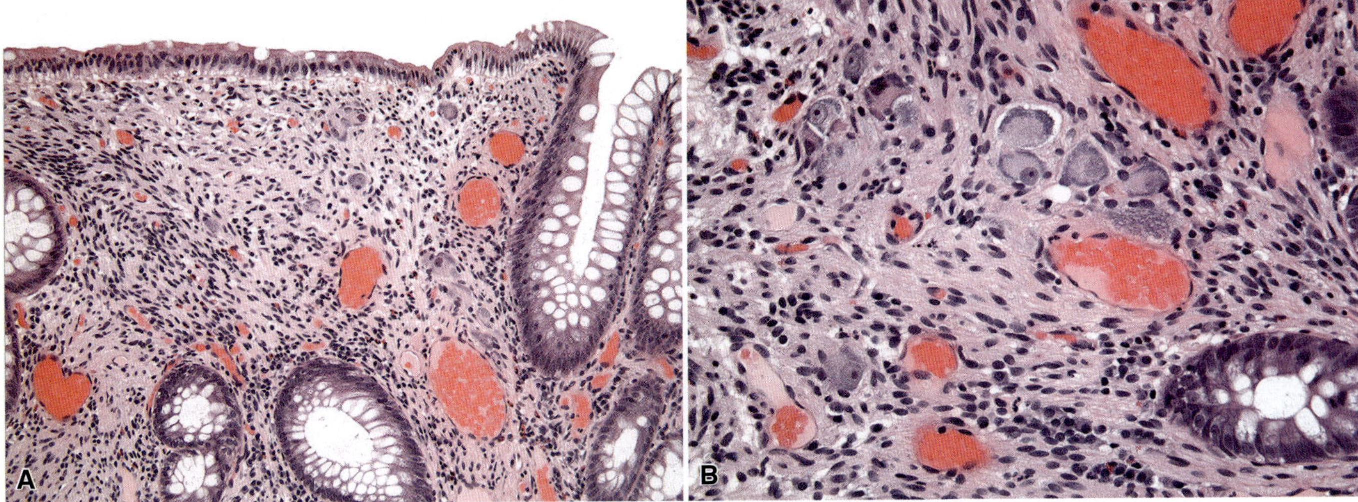

Figure 16.47 Histologic Appearances of a Polypoid Ganglioneuroma. The lesion is composed of an admixture of spindle-shaped Schwann cells with tapering nuclei and eosinophilic cytoplasm and occasional ganglion cells (A). In some cases, ganglion cells are numerous (B).

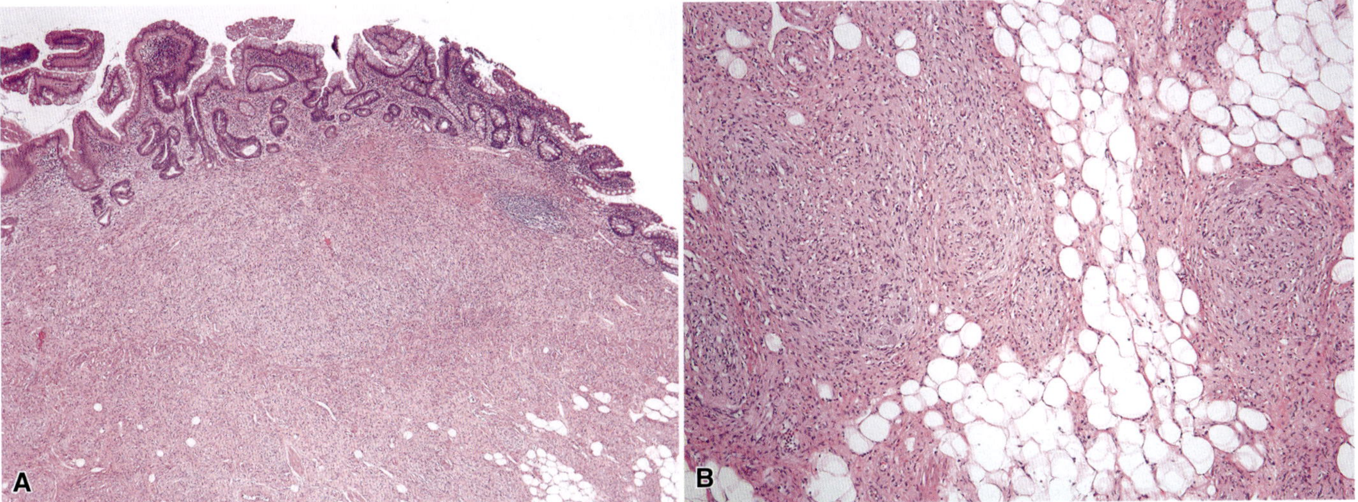

Figure 16.48 Histologic Appearance of Ganglioneuromatosis in a Patient With Neurofibromatosis Type 1. The lesion is centered in the mucosa and submucosa (A). The lesion extends through the submucosa in a nodular fashion (B).

cases occur in the GI tract. Granular cell tumors are also discussed in Chapters 6 and 15.

Clinical Features

Within the GI tract, granular cell tumors are most commonly encountered in the esophagus.[161–165] The colon is much less often involved.[162,166,167] Other organs are very rarely affected. Esophageal granular cell tumors occur over a wide age range, with a peak in middle-aged adults, and a predilection for females and African Americans.[161,162,164] Occasionally, patients present with multiple GI granular cell tumors. Most tumors are discovered incidentally at endoscopy as polyps or small plaque-like lesions, more commonly in the distal esophagus.[161,164] A small subset of patients present with dysphagia. Colonic granular cell tumors have a similar age distribution but no apparent gender or race predilection.[162,166] Although granular cell tumors may be found anywhere in the colon and rectum, the right colon is most often involved.[162,166,167] Colonic granular cell tumors are asymptomatic; incidental lesions are found at screening colonoscopy. The endoscopic appearance may be similar to a hyperplastic polyp or adenoma or, for submucosal lesions, a carcinoid tumor.

Pathologic Features

GI granular cell tumors range from 2 mm to 3 cm in greatest dimension, although most lesions are between 0.3 and 1 cm.[161,162,165,166] They have a yellow or white appearance. Similar to granular cell tumors of other anatomic sites, esophageal granular cell tumors are often associated with overlying acanthosis or pseudoepitheliomatous hyperplasia. The tumors may be well circumscribed or, more often, poorly marginated. Colorectal granular cell tumors more rarely show reactive changes of the overlying epithelium.[166,167]

Histologically, granular cell tumors are composed of plump, polygonal epithelioid cells with abundant granular eosinophilic cytoplasm, ill-defined cell borders, and small, rounded, usually hyperchromatic nuclei with even chromatin and inconspicuous nucleoli, arranged predominantly in sheets and focally in nests (Fig. 16.49). At the infiltrative tumor edges, the lesional cells often encircle small nerves. In the colon, granular cell

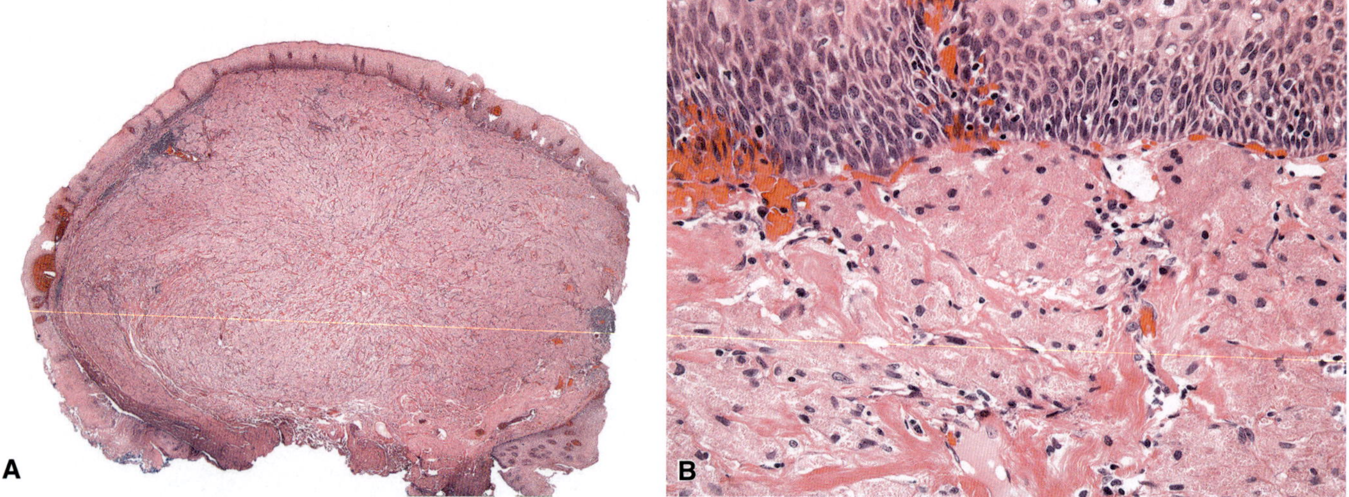

Figure 16.49 **Polypoid Granular Cell Tumor of the Esophagus.** A granular cell tumor with well-circumscribed borders (A). The tumor is composed of large epithelioid cells with abundant granular eosinophilic cytoplasm and small nuclei (B). Note the reactive changes in the overlying squamous epithelium.

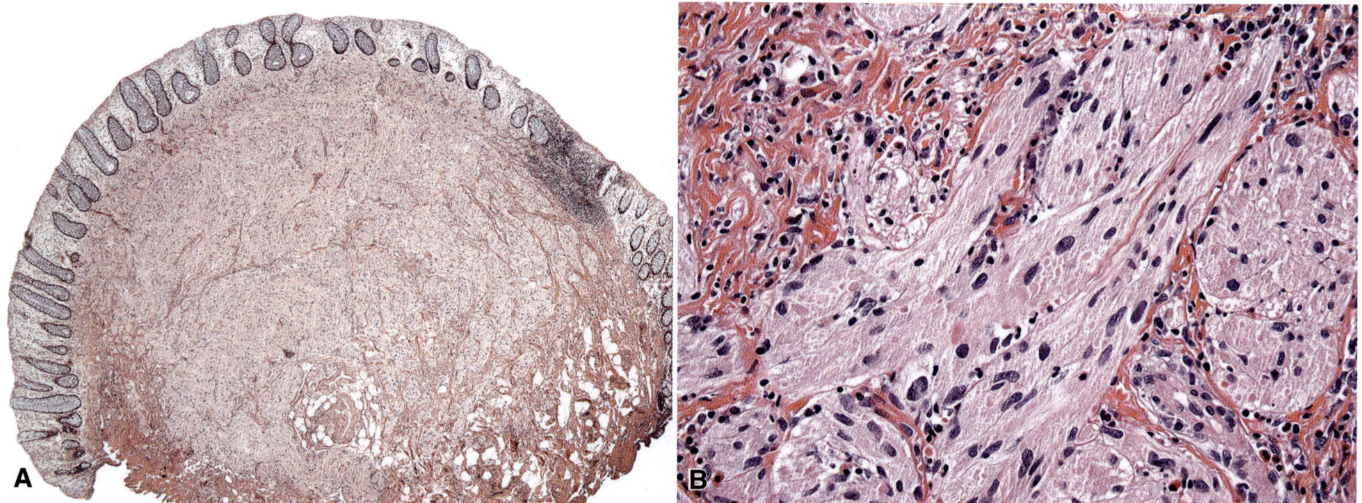

Figure 16.50 **Granular Cell Tumor of the Colon.** The tumor is based in the submucosa and has a sheet-like and vaguely nested architecture with irregular margins (A). Note the nested architecture, spindle cell morphology, and mild nuclear atypia (B).

tumors may show a more nested architecture, more spindled morphology, and mild nuclear atypia with small nucleoli (Fig. 16.50).[167] At this location, some tumors have a peripheral lymphoid infiltrate, dystrophic calcification, and focal degenerative nuclear pleomorphism.[166] Mitoses are very rare, and necrosis is absent.

Immunohistochemistry

By immunohistochemistry, granular cell tumors are strongly and diffusely positive for S-100 protein and SOX10, reflecting their Schwannian nature. They are also often positive for the nonspecific markers CD68, NKI-C3, and neuron-specific enolase, as well as calretinin and inhibin.[165,168,169] Granular cell tumors show nuclear staining for TFE3, although gene rearrangements are absent.[170] They usually show nuclear reactivity for MiTF and may be focally positive occasionally for melan A. HMB-45 is not expressed.[171] The tumors are consistently negative for SMA, desmin, KIT, and GFAP.

Differential Diagnosis

The diagnosis of granular cell tumor is usually straightforward. Due to the presence of overlying pseudoepitheliomatous hyperplasia, superficial biopsies of esophageal squamous mucosa that fail to sample granular cell tumor may rarely be mistaken for squamous cell carcinoma. Colonic granular cell tumors with spindle cell morphology and a peripheral lymphoid infiltrate may be confused with schwannomas, although GI schwannomas are usually larger polyps or mural masses with elongated spindle cells containing eosinophilic cytoplasm that lacks a granular appearance.

Prognosis and Treatment

GI granular cell tumors rarely recur, even after incomplete excision.[161,162,164] Very few malignant granular cell tumors of the esophagus have been reported. As in granular cell tumors of soft tissue, the presence of necrosis and mitotic activity may portend malignant behavior,[172] although there are insufficient cases in the GI tract to establish firm criteria for malignancy. Spindle cell features, mild nuclear atypia, and focal pleomorphism in colonic granular cell tumors are of no clinical significance.[166,167]

Mucosal Perineurioma

Perineuriomas are benign nerve sheath tumors composed of perineurial cells. They include soft tissue, intraneural, and sclerosing variants (see Chapters 3 and 15). Perineuriomas of the GI tract have been relatively recently described.[173] Perineuriomas of soft tissue type may rarely be encountered in the GI tract as mural masses.[173] In contrast, mucosal perineuriomas of the colorectum are commonly encountered on a routine GI biopsy service; in fact, mucosal perineuriomas are the most common spindle cell–containing polyps in the GI tract. These lesions have also been reported as "fibroblastic polyps," which are clinically and histologically indistinguishable from mucosal perineuriomas.[174,175] Recent studies using an expanded panel of immunohistochemical markers have demonstrated that these fibroblastic polyps and mucosal perineuriomas represent the same entity.[176,177]

Clinical Features

Mucosal perineuriomas affect adults over a wide age range, with a peak during middle age. There is a female predominance (female-to-male ratio, 3 : 1).[173,174,177] Mucosal perineuriomas are discovered incidentally at colonoscopy as small sessile lesions resembling hyperplastic polyps or adenomas. Mucosal perineuriomas occur throughout the colon, with a predilection for the rectosigmoid (about 70%).[173,174,177] Similar lesions very rarely arise in the stomach or small intestine. Occasionally, multiple mucosal perineuriomas may be detected.

Pathologic Features

Mucosal perineuriomas are usually between 2 and 8 mm in size, and rarely reach 1 cm. The average size is 3–4 mm.

Histologically, mucosal perineuriomas are composed of uniform, bland spindle cells with ovoid or slender elongated nuclei with fine chromatin, inconspicuous nucleoli, and indistinct palely eosinophilic cytoplasm in a fine, fibrillary collagenous stroma. The lesion entraps and distorts colonic crypts with irregular margins through the lamina propria (Fig. 16.51). The lesional cells often show a focally whorled growth pattern around crypts (see Fig. 16.51) and areas with a lamellar architecture. About 80% of mucosal perineuriomas are associated with a serrated epithelial polyp, usually a hyperplastic polyp (see Fig. 16.51), or less commonly, a sessile serrated polyp/adenoma.[176,178] The relative proportions of the perineurioma and hyperplastic polyp components vary considerably, and some otherwise typical hyperplastic or sessile serrated polyps contain minute perineurial proliferations surrounding the serrated crypts.

Immunohistochemistry

By immunohistochemistry, mucosal perineuriomas are positive for EMA, which can be very weak, requiring examination under high magnification (see Fig. 16.51D). The lesional cells are often positive for the perineurial-associated markers claudin-1 and glucose transporter-1 (GLUT-1).[173,176,177,179] The extent and intensity of staining for each of these markers vary based on antigen retrieval conditions. CD34 is rarely expressed. The lesions are negative for S-100 protein, GFAP, NFP, SMA, desmin, and KIT.

Molecular Genetics

Similar to conventional hyperplastic and sessile serrated polyps, the serrated epithelial component associated with mucosal perineuriomas often contains a typical V600E *BRAF* mutation.[176,178,179] Whether the perineurial component is neoplastic or reactive in nature has not been determined. Mucosal perineuriomas not associated with a serrated polyp lack *BRAF* mutations.[179]

Differential Diagnosis

The differential diagnosis of mucosal perineurioma includes polypoid ganglioneuroma, mucosal Schwann cell hamartoma, neurofibroma, and leiomyoma of the muscularis mucosae (Table 16.3). Similar to mucosal perineuriomas, both ganglioneuroma and mucosal Schwann cell hamartoma entrap crypts with ill-defined margins. However, these lesions contain S-100-positive spindled Schwann cells with larger nuclei and more brightly eosinophilic cytoplasm than mucosal perineurioma; ganglioneuromas also display ganglion cells and occasional NFP-positive axons. Neurofibromas of the GI tract are very rare and are usually associated with NF1. GI neurofibromas are often submucosal tumors that may extend into the overlying mucosa, where the lesional cells entrap crypts in a similar fashion as perineuriomas. In contrast to mucosal perineurioma, neurofibromas are composed of a heterogeneous admixture of cell types, including Schwann cells, fibroblasts, and perineurial-like cells, as well as scattered axons. S-100 protein is positive in the Schwann cell component, which can easily exclude perineurioma. Unlike mucosal perineuriomas, leiomyomas of the muscularis mucosae are well-circumscribed submucosal lesions composed of fascicles of spindle cells with brightly eosinophilic cytoplasm that are positive for SMA, desmin, and caldesmon.

Prognosis and Treatment

Mucosal perineuriomas are benign. They do not recur.

Mucosal Schwann Cell Hamartoma

Mucosal Schwann cell hamartomas are recently described colonic polypoid lesions distinct from neurofibroma and mucosal neuroma.[180] Unlike the latter two lesions, mucosal Schwann cell hamartomas are not associated with an inherited syndrome.

Clinical Features

Mucosal Schwann cell hamartomas affect middle-aged to elderly adults, with a female predominance.[180–182] They are asymptomatic lesions detected at screening colonoscopy as small sessile polyps resembling hyperplastic polyps. The sigmoid colon and rectum are most often involved (60%).[180]

Pathologic Features

Mucosal Schwann cell hamartomas range from 1 to 6 mm in size, with a mean of 3 mm. Histologically, the lesions are composed of uniform, bland spindle cells with elongated, tapering, or wavy nuclei with fine chromatin and indistinct nucleoli. There is abundant, dense eosinophilic cytoplasm and ill-defined cell borders with minimal intervening stroma (Fig. 16.52). The spindle cells entrap crypts and show irregular margins with the adjacent lamina propria. No whorling around crypts is seen.

Immunohistochemistry

By immunohistochemistry, the lesional cells in mucosal Schwann cell hamartomas show strong staining for S-100 protein (Fig. 16.53). The cells are negative for EMA, GFAP, CD34, claudin-1, SMA, and KIT. Most such lesions contain no NFP-positive axons, or at most rare entrapped axons.[180]

Differential Diagnosis

The differential diagnosis for mucosal Schwann cell hamartoma includes polypoid ganglioneuroma, mucosal perineurioma, neurofibroma, mucosal

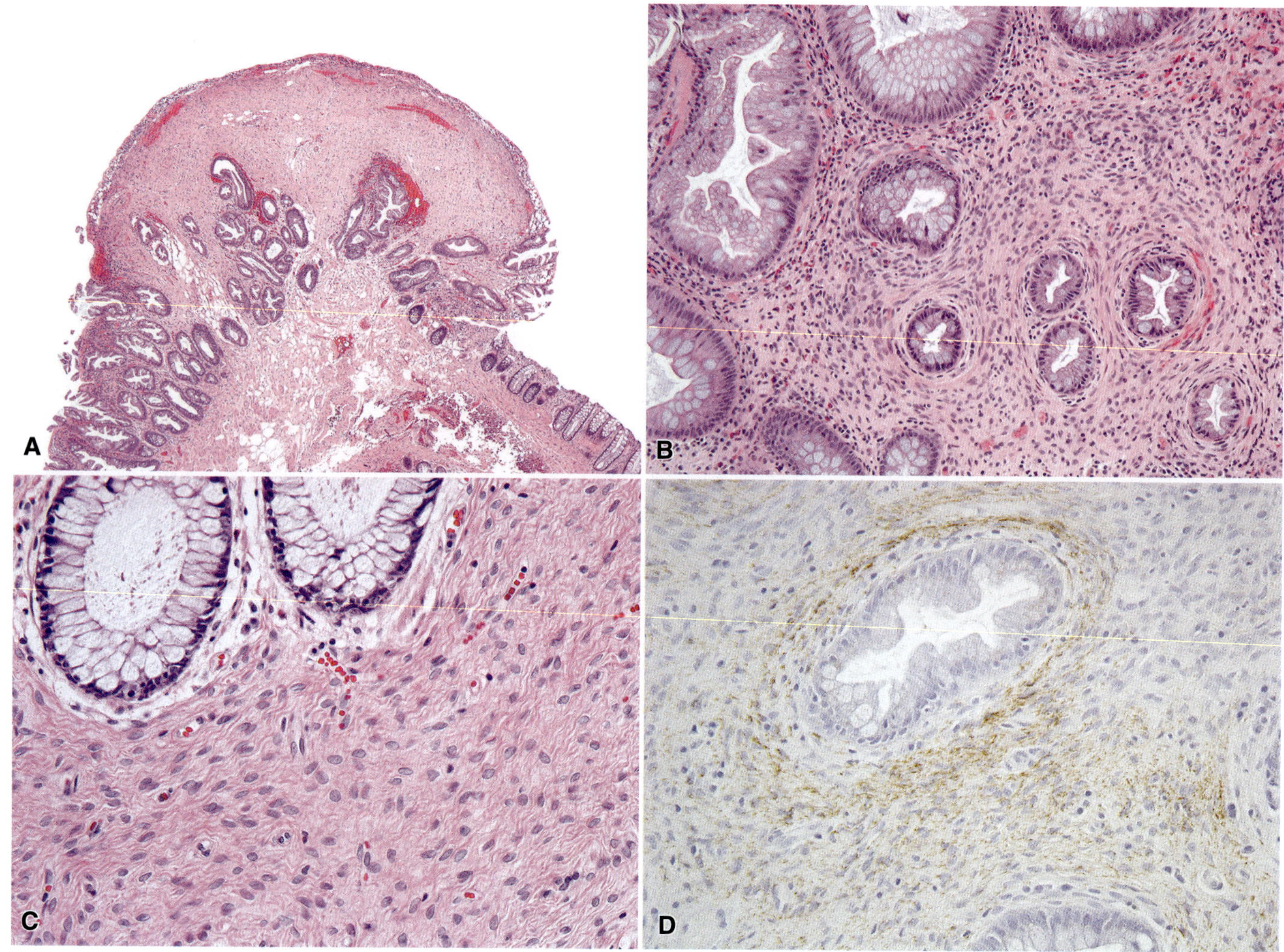

Figure 16.51 Histologic Appearance of Mucosal Perineurioma. The lesion entraps crypts and has irregular margins (A). Note the adjacent hyperplastic polyp. In many cases, the spindle cells focally whorl around crypts (B). This lesion is composed of small cells with ovoid nuclei in a fine fibrillary collagenous stroma (C). Immunohistochemistry for epithelial membrane antigen (EMA) in a mucosal perineurioma (D). The staining intensity can be weak, requiring examination under high magnification.

Table 16.3 Differential Diagnosis of Mesenchymal Polyps

Diagnosis	Anatomic Site	Histologic Features	Immunohistochemistry
Leiomyoma of the muscularis mucosae	Colon/rectum	Well-circumscribed; fascicles of spindle cells with broad (cigar-shaped) or tapering nuclei and brightly eosinophilic cytoplasm	SMA + Desmin + Caldesmon +
Mucosal perineurioma	Colon/rectum	Entrap and distort crypts; focally lamellar and whorled; spindle cells with ovoid or slender, wavy nuclei and pale cytoplasm in a fine fibrillary stroma; 80% associated with hyperplastic or sessile serrated polyps	EMA + (may be weak) Claudin-1 +
Ganglioneuroma	Colon/rectum	Entrap crypts; spindle cells with tapering nuclei and eosinophilic cytoplasm admixed with ganglion cells	S-100 + NFP + (ganglion cells and axons)
Mucosal Schwann cell hamartoma	Colon/rectum	Entrap crypts; spindle cells with tapering nuclei and eosinophilic cytoplasm	S-100 +
Granular cell tumor	Esophagus more often than colon	Well-circumscribed or irregular margins; epithelioid cells with abundant granular eosinophilic cytoplasm; often overlying acanthosis or pseudoepitheliomatous hyperplasia	S-100 +
Inflammatory fibroid polyp	Stomach or ileum	Ill-defined margins; ovoid, short spindled or stellate cells; edematous to myxoid stroma; prominent eosinophils; perivascular fibrosis	CD34 +
Schwannoma	Stomach more often than colon	Well-circumscribed, may be focally infiltrative; spindle cells with tapering nuclei; collagenous stroma; peripheral lymphoplasmacytic infiltrate including germinal centers	S-100 + GFAP +
PEComa	Colon/rectum	Nests and sheets; epithelioid cells with abundant granular eosinophilic or clear cytoplasm; nests surrounded by capillary vascular network	HMB-45 + (often focal) Melan A ± SMA ± Desmin ±

EMA, Epithelial membrane antigen; *GFAP*, glial fibrillary acidic protein; *NFP*, neurofilament protein; *PEComa*, perivascular epithelioid cell tumor; *SMA*, smooth muscle actin.

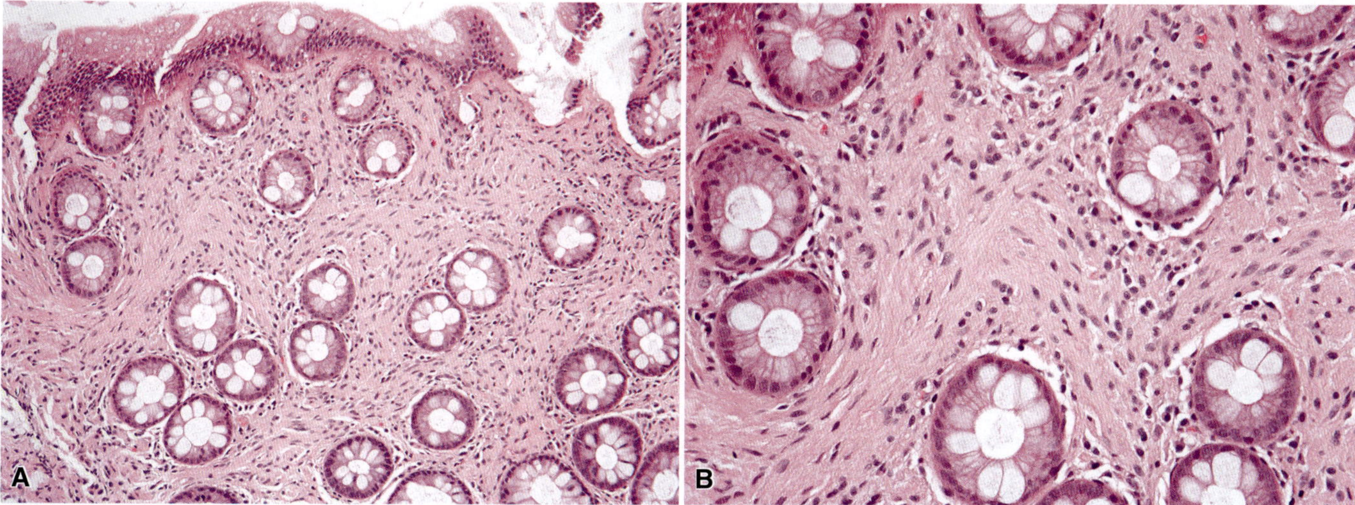

Figure 16.52 Mucosal Schwann Cell Hamartoma. This cellular lesion entraps crypts (A). The lesion is composed of spindle cells with tapering nuclei and eosinophilic cytoplasm (B).

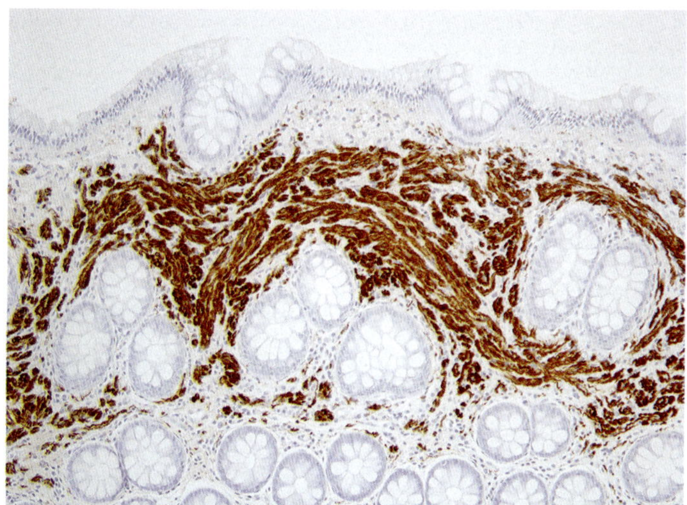

Figure 16.53 Mucosal Schwann Cell Hamartoma. Immunohistochemistry for S-100 is strongly positive.

neuroma, and schwannoma (see Table 16.3). Ganglioneuroma is histologically very similar to Schwann cell hamartoma, except for the presence of ganglion cells in the former lesion. Both perineurioma and Schwann cell hamartoma show irregular margins and entrap colonic crypts. However, the spindle cells in Schwann cell hamartoma are longer and broader than in perineurioma, with more brightly eosinophilic cytoplasm. Only perineuriomas are associated with hyperplastic polyps. Perineuriomas are negative for S-100 but are positive for EMA. Neurofibromas of the GI tract are invariably associated with NF1. In contrast to Schwann cell hamartoma, which is composed of a pure population of S-100-positive Schwann cells, neurofibromas are composed of an admixture of Schwann cells, fibroblasts, perineurial-like cells, and occasional axons. GI neurofibromas are usually submucosal with extension into the mucosa, unlike mucosal Schwann cell hamartomas. Mucosal neuromas are rare lesions that are highly associated with MEN2B. They are found predominantly on the tongue and lips. Mucosal neuromas are composed of hyperplastic nerve fibers arranged in bundles that contain not only S-100-positive Schwann cells but also numerous NFP-positive axons, in contrast to the diffuse, pure Schwann cell proliferation of Schwann cell hamartoma. Schwannomas arising in the GI tract predominate in the stomach and more rarely arise in the colon, show a peripheral lymphoid cuff, and are well circumscribed but unencapsulated. This contrasts with Schwann cell hamartoma, which instead shows irregular margins, crypt entrapment, and a predilection for the rectosigmoid colon.

Prognosis and Treatment

Mucosal Schwann cell hamartomas are entirely benign. They do not recur.

References

1. Corless CL: Gastrointestinal stromal tumors: what do we know now?, *Mod Pathol* 27(Suppl 1):S1–S16, 2014.
2. Doyle LA, Hornick JL: Gastrointestinal stromal tumours: from KIT to succinate dehydrogenase, *Histopathology* 64:53–67, 2014.
3. Miettinen M, Lasota J: Gastrointestinal stromal tumors—definition, clinical, histological, immunohistochemical, and molecular genetic features and differential diagnosis, *Virchows Arch* 438:1–12, 2001.
4. Miettinen M, Sobin LH, Lasota J: Gastrointestinal stromal tumors presenting as omental masses—a clinicopathologic analysis of 95 cases, *Am J Surg Pathol* 33:1267–1275, 2009.
5. Reith JD, Goldblum JR, Lyles RH, et al: Extragastrointestinal (soft tissue) stromal tumors: an analysis of 48 cases with emphasis on histologic predictors of outcome, *Mod Pathol* 13:577–585, 2000.
6. Yamamoto H, Oda Y, Kawaguchi K, et al: c-kit and PDGFRA mutations in extragastrointestinal stromal tumor (gastrointestinal stromal tumor of the soft tissue), *Am J Surg Pathol* 28:479–488, 2004.
7. Agaimy A, Wünsch PH: Gastrointestinal stromal tumours: a regular origin in the muscularis propria, but an extremely diverse gross presentation. A review of 200 cases to critically re-evaluate the concept of so-called extra-gastrointestinal stromal tumours, *Langenbecks Arch Surg* 391:322–329, 2006.
8. Kawanowa K, Sakuma Y, Sakurai S, et al: High incidence of microscopic gastrointestinal stromal tumors in the stomach, *Hum Pathol* 37:1527–1535, 2006.
9. Agaimy A, Wunsch PH, Hofstaedter F, et al: Minute gastric sclerosing stromal tumors (GIST tumorlets) are common in adults and frequently show c-KIT mutations, *Am J Surg Pathol* 31:113–120, 2007.
10. Abraham SC, Krasinskas AM, Hofstetter WL, et al: "Seedling" mesenchymal tumors (gastrointestinal stromal tumors and leiomyomas) are common incidental tumors of the esophagogastric junction, *Am J Surg Pathol* 31:1629–1635, 2007.
11. Prakash S, Sarran L, Socci N, et al: Gastrointestinal stromal tumors in children and young adults: a clinicopathologic, molecular, and genomic study of 15 cases and review of the literature, *J Pediatr Hematol Oncol* 27:179–187, 2005.

12. Pappo AS, Janeway KA: Pediatric gastrointestinal stromal tumors, *Hematol Oncol Clin North Am* 23:15–34, vii, 2009.
13. Miettinen M, Lasota J, Sobin LH: Gastrointestinal stromal tumors of the stomach in children and young adults: a clinicopathologic, immunohistochemical, and molecular genetic study of 44 cases with long-term follow-up and review of the literature, *Am J Surg Pathol* 29:1373–1381, 2005.
14. Zhang L, Smyrk TC, Young WF, Jr, et al: Gastric stromal tumors in Carney triad are different clinically, pathologically, and behaviorally from sporadic gastric gastrointestinal stromal tumors: findings in 104 cases, *Am J Surg Pathol* 34:53–64, 2010.
15. Carney JA, Stratakis CA: Familial paraganglioma and gastric stromal sarcoma: a new syndrome distinct from the Carney triad, *Am J Med Genet* 108:132–139, 2002.
16. Stratakis CA, Carney JA: The triad of paragangliomas, gastric stromal tumours and pulmonary chondromas (Carney triad), and the dyad of paragangliomas and gastric stromal sarcomas (Carney-Stratakis syndrome): molecular genetics and clinical implications, *J Intern Med* 266:43–52, 2009.
17. Miettinen M, Fetsch JF, Sobin LH, et al: Gastrointestinal stromal tumors in patients with neurofibromatosis 1: a clinicopathologic and molecular genetic study of 45 cases, *Am J Surg Pathol* 30:90–96, 2006.
18. Andersson J, Sihto H, Meis-Kindblom JM, et al: NF1-associated gastrointestinal stromal tumors have unique clinical, phenotypic, and genotypic characteristics, *Am J Surg Pathol* 29:1170–1176, 2005.
19. Miettinen M, Sobin LH, Lasota J: Gastrointestinal stromal tumors of the stomach: a clinicopathologic, immunohistochemical, and molecular genetic study of 1765 cases with long-term follow-up, *Am J Surg Pathol* 29:52–68, 2005.
20. Miettinen M, Kopczynski J, Makhlouf HR, et al: Gastrointestinal stromal tumors, intramural leiomyomas, and leiomyosarcomas in the duodenum: a clinicopathologic, immunohistochemical, and molecular genetic study of 167 cases, *Am J Surg Pathol* 27:625–641, 2003.
21. Miettinen M, Makhlouf H, Sobin LH, et al: Gastrointestinal stromal tumors of the jejunum and ileum: a clinicopathologic, immunohistochemical, and molecular genetic study of 906 cases before imatinib with long-term follow-up, *Am J Surg Pathol* 30:477–489, 2006.
22. Miettinen M, Wang Z-F, Sarlomo-Rikala M, et al: Succinate dehydrogenase-deficient GISTs: a clinicopathologic, immunohistochemical, and molecular genetic study of 66 gastric GISTs with predilection to young age, *Am J Surg Pathol* 35:1712–1721, 2011.
23. Rege TA, Wagner AJ, Corless CL, et al: "Pediatric-type" gastrointestinal stromal tumors in adults: distinctive histology predicts genotype and clinical behavior, *Am J Surg Pathol* 35:495–504, 2011.
24. Gill AJ, Chou A, Vilain R, et al: Immunohistochemistry for SDHB divides gastrointestinal stromal tumors (GISTs) into 2 distinct types, *Am J Surg Pathol* 34:636–644, 2010.
25. Antonescu CR, Romeo S, Zhang L, et al: Dedifferentiation in gastrointestinal stromal tumor to an anaplastic KIT-negative phenotype: a diagnostic pitfall: morphologic and molecular characterization of 8 cases occurring either de novo or after imatinib therapy, *Am J Surg Pathol* 37:385–392, 2013.
26. Medeiros F, Corless CL, Duensing A, et al: KIT-negative gastrointestinal stromal tumors: proof of concept and therapeutic implications, *Am J Surg Pathol* 28:889–894, 2004.
27. Miettinen M, Lasota J: Gastrointestinal stromal tumors: review on morphology, molecular pathology, prognosis, and differential diagnosis, *Arch Pathol Lab Med* 130:1466–1478, 2006.
28. Espinosa I, Lee CH, Kim MK, et al: A novel monoclonal antibody against DOG1 is a sensitive and specific marker for gastrointestinal stromal tumors, *Am J Surg Pathol* 32:210–218, 2008.
29. Miettinen M, Wang ZF, Lasota J: DOG1 antibody in the differential diagnosis of gastrointestinal stromal tumors: a study of 1840 cases, *Am J Surg Pathol* 33:1401–1408, 2009.
30. Kang GH, Srivastava A, Kim YE, et al: DOG1 and PKC-theta are useful in the diagnosis of KIT-negative gastrointestinal stromal tumors, *Mod Pathol* 24:866–875, 2011.
31. Gaal J, Stratakis CA, Carney JA, et al: SDHB immunohistochemistry: a useful tool in the diagnosis of Carney-Stratakis and Carney triad gastrointestinal stromal tumors, *Mod Pathol* 24:147–151, 2011.
32. Wagner AJ, Remillard SP, Zhang YX, et al: Loss of expression of SDHA predicts SDHA mutations in gastrointestinal stromal tumors, *Mod Pathol* 26:289–294, 2013.
33. Miettinen M, Killian JK, Wang ZF, et al: Immunohistochemical loss of succinate dehydrogenase subunit A (SDHA) in gastrointestinal stromal tumors (GISTs) signals SDHA germline mutation, *Am J Surg Pathol* 37:234–240, 2013.
34. Hirota S, Isozaki K, Moriyama Y, et al: Gain-of-function mutations of c-kit in human gastrointestinal stromal tumors, *Science* 279:577–580, 1998.
35. Rubin BP, Heinrich MC: Genotyping and immunohistochemistry of gastrointestinal stromal tumors: an update, *Semin Diagn Pathol* 32:392–399, 2015.
36. Patil DT, Rubin BP: Genetics of gastrointestinal stromal tumors: a heterogeneous family of tumors? *Surg Pathol Clin* 8:515–524, 2015.
37. Heinrich MC, Corless CL, Duensing A, et al: PDGFRA activating mutations in gastrointestinal stromal tumors, *Science* 299:708–710, 2003.
38. Tozbikian G, Shen R, Suster S: Signet ring cell gastric schwannoma: report of a new distinctive morphological variant, *Ann Diagn Pathol* 12:146–152, 2008.
39. Corless CL, McGreevey L, Haley A, et al: KIT mutations are common in incidental gastrointestinal stromal tumors one centimeter or less in size, *Am J Pathol* 160:1567–1572, 2002.
40. Hostein I, Faur N, Primois C, et al: BRAF mutation status in gastrointestinal stromal tumors, *Am J Clin Pathol* 133:141–148, 2010.
41. Agaimy A, Terracciano LM, Dirnhofer S, et al: V600E BRAF mutations are alternative early molecular events in a subset of KIT/PDGFRA wild-type gastrointestinal stromal tumours, *J Clin Pathol* 62:613–616, 2009.
42. Agaram NP, Wong GC, Guo T, et al: Novel V600E BRAF mutations in imatinib-naive and imatinib-resistant gastrointestinal stromal tumors, *Genes Chromosomes Cancer* 47:853–859, 2008.
43. Brenca M, Rossi S, Polano M, et al: Transcriptome sequencing identifies ETV6-NTRK3 as a gene fusion involved in GIST, *J Pathol* 238:543–549, 2016.
44. Shi E, Chmielecki J, Tang CM, et al: FGFR1 and NTRK3 actionable alterations in "Wild-Type" gastrointestinal stromal tumors, *J Transl Med* 14:339, 2016.
45. Nannini M, Astolfi A, Urbini M, et al: Integrated genomic study of quadruple-WT GIST (KIT/PDGFRA/SDH/RAS pathway wild-type GIST), *BMC Cancer* 14:685, 2014.
46. Nishida T, Hirota S, Taniguchi M, et al: Familial gastrointestinal stromal tumours with germline mutation of the KIT gene, *Nat Genet* 19:323–324, 1998.
47. Pasini B, McWhinney SR, Bei T, et al: Clinical and molecular genetics of patients with the Carney-Stratakis syndrome and germline mutations of the genes coding for the succinate dehydrogenase subunits SDHB, SDHC, and SDHD, *Eur J Hum Genet* 16:79–88, 2008.
48. Janeway KA, Kim SY, Lodish M, et al: Defects in succinate dehydrogenase in gastrointestinal stromal tumors lacking KIT and PDGFRA mutations, *Proc Natl Acad Sci USA* 108:314–318, 2011.
49. Pantaleo MA, Astolfi A, Indio V, et al: SDHA loss-of-function mutations in KIT-PDGFRA wild-type gastrointestinal stromal tumors identified by massively parallel sequencing, *J Natl Cancer Inst* 103:983–987, 2011.
50. Boikos SA, Pappo AS, Killian JK, et al: Molecular subtypes of KIT/PDGFRA wild-type gastrointestinal stromal tumors: A report from the National Institutes of Health gastrointestinal stromal tumor clinic, *JAMA Oncol* 2:922–928, 2016.
51. Haller F, Moskalev EA, Faucz FR, et al: Aberrant DNA hypermethylation of SDHC: a novel mechanism of tumor development in Carney triad, *Endocr Relat Cancer* 21:567–577, 2014.
52. Killian JK, Miettinen M, Walker RL, et al: Recurrent epimutation of SDHC in gastrointestinal stromal tumors, *Sci Transl Med* 6:268ra177, 2014.
53. von Mehren M, Randall RL, Benjamin RS, et al: Gastrointestinal stromal tumors, version 2.2014, *J Natl Compr Canc Netw* 12:853–862, 2014.
54. Wozniak A, Sciot R, Guillou L, et al: Array CGH analysis in primary gastrointestinal stromal tumors: cytogenetic profile correlates with anatomic site and tumor aggressiveness, irrespective of mutational status, *Genes Chromosomes Cancer* 46:261–276, 2007.
55. Schneider-Stock R, Boltze C, Lasota J, et al: High prognostic value of p16INK4 alterations in gastrointestinal stromal tumors, *J Clin Oncol* 21:1688–1697, 2003.
56. Perrone F, Tamborini E, Dagrada GP, et al: 9p21 locus analysis in high-risk gastrointestinal stromal tumors characterized for c-kit and platelet-derived growth factor receptor alpha gene alterations, *Cancer* 104:159–169, 2005.
57. Deshpande A, Nelson D, Corless CL, et al: Leiomyoma of the gastrointestinal tract with interstitial cells of Cajal: a mimic of gastrointestinal stromal tumor, *Am J Surg Pathol* 38:72–77, 2014.
58. Miettinen M, Lasota J: Gastrointestinal stromal tumors: pathology and prognosis at different sites, *Semin Diagn Pathol* 23:70–83, 2006.
59. Mason EF, Hornick JL: Conventional risk stratification fails to predict progression of succinate dehydrogenase-deficient gastrointestinal stromal tumors: a clinicopathologic study of 76 cases, *Am J Surg Pathol* 40:1616–1621, 2016.
60. Heinrich MC, Corless CL, Demetri GD, et al: Kinase mutations and imatinib response in patients with metastatic gastrointestinal stromal tumor, *J Clin Oncol* 21:4342–4349, 2003.
61. Heinrich MC, Owzar K, Corless CL, et al: Correlation of kinase genotype and clinical outcome in the North American Intergroup Phase III Trial of imatinib mesylate for treatment of advanced gastrointestinal stromal tumor: CALGB 150105 Study by Cancer and Leukemia Group B and Southwest Oncology Group, *J Clin Oncol* 26:5360–5367, 2008.
62. Debiec-Rychter M, Sciot R, Le Cesne A, et al: KIT mutations and dose selection for imatinib in patients with advanced gastrointestinal stromal tumours, *Eur J Cancer* 42:1093–1103, 2006.
63. Falchook GS, Trent JC, Heinrich MC, et al: BRAF mutant gastrointestinal stromal tumor: first report of regression with BRAF inhibitor dabrafenib (GSK2118436) and whole exomic sequencing for analysis of acquired resistance, *Oncotarget* 4:310–315, 2013.
64. Agaram NP, Besmer P, Wong GC, et al: Pathologic and molecular heterogeneity in imatinib-stable or imatinib-responsive gastrointestinal stromal tumors, *Clin Cancer Res* 13:170–181, 2007.
65. Pauwels P, Debiec-Rychter M, Stul M, et al: Changing phenotype of gastrointestinal stromal tumours under imatinib mesylate treatment: a potential diagnostic pitfall, *Histopathology* 47:41–47, 2005.
66. Liegl B, Kepten I, Le C, et al: Heterogeneity of kinase inhibitor resistance mechanisms in GIST, *J Pathol* 216:64–74, 2008.
67. Liegl B, Hornick JL, Antonescu CR, et al: Rhabdomyosarcomatous differentiation in gastrointestinal stromal tumors after tyrosine kinase inhibitor therapy: a novel form of tumor progression, *Am J Surg Pathol* 33:218–226, 2009.
68. Agaimy A, Wunsch PH: True smooth muscle neoplasms of the gastrointestinal tract: morphological spectrum and classification in a series of 85 cases from a single institute, *Langenbecks Arch Surg* 392:75–81, 2007.
69. Miettinen M, Sarlomo-Rikala M, Sobin LH: Mesenchymal tumors of muscularis mucosae of colon and rectum are benign leiomyomas that should be separated from gastrointestinal stromal tumors—a clinicopathologic and immunohistochemical study of eighty-eight cases, *Mod Pathol* 14:950–956, 2001.

70. Miettinen M, Sarlomo-Rikala M, Sobin LH, et al: Esophageal stromal tumors: a clinicopathologic, immunohistochemical, and molecular genetic study of 17 cases and comparison with esophageal leiomyomas and leiomyosarcomas, *Am J Surg Pathol* 24:211–222, 2000.
71. Heidet L, Boye E, Cai Y, et al: Somatic deletion of the 5′ ends of both the COL4A5 and COL4A6 genes in a sporadic leiomyoma of the esophagus, *Am J Pathol* 152:673–678, 1998.
72. Federici S, Ceccarelli PL, Bernardi F, et al: Esophageal leiomyomatosis in children: report of a case and review of the literature, *Eur J Pediatr Surg* 8:358–363, 1998.
73. Lee LS, Nance M, Kaiser LR, et al: Familial massive leiomyoma with esophageal leiomyomatosis: an unusual presentation in a father and his 2 daughters, *J Pediatr Surg* 40:e29–e32, 2005.
74. Miettinen M, Furlong M, Sarlomo-Rikala M, et al: Gastrointestinal stromal tumors, intramural leiomyomas, and leiomyosarcomas in the rectum and anus: a clinicopathologic, immunohistochemical, and molecular genetic study of 144 cases, *Am J Surg Pathol* 25:1121–1133, 2001.
75. Miettinen M, Sobin LH, Lasota J: True smooth muscle tumors of the small intestine: a clinicopathologic, immunohistochemical, and molecular genetic study of 25 cases, *Am J Surg Pathol* 33:430–436, 2009.
76. Katz SC, DeMatteo RP: Gastrointestinal stromal tumors and leiomyosarcomas, *J Surg Oncol* 97:350–359, 2008.
77. Daimaru Y, Kido H, Hashimoto H, et al: Benign schwannoma of the gastrointestinal tract: a clinicopathologic and immunohistochemical study, *Hum Pathol* 19:257–264, 1988.
78. Hou YY, Tan YS, Xu JF, et al: Schwannoma of the gastrointestinal tract: a clinicopathological, immunohistochemical and ultrastructural study of 33 cases, *Histopathology* 48:536–545, 2006.
79. Kwon MS, Lee SS, Ahn GH: Schwannomas of the gastrointestinal tract: clinicopathological features of 12 cases including a case of esophageal tumor compared with those of gastrointestinal stromal tumors and leiomyomas of the gastrointestinal tract, *Pathol Res Pract* 198:605–613, 2002.
80. Miettinen M, Shekitka KM, Sobin LH: Schwannomas in the colon and rectum: a clinicopathologic and immunohistochemical study of 20 cases, *Am J Surg Pathol* 25:846–855, 2001.
81. Prevot S, Bienvenu L, Vaillant JC, et al: Benign schwannoma of the digestive tract: a clinicopathologic and immunohistochemical study of five cases, including a case of esophageal tumor, *Am J Surg Pathol* 23:431–436, 1999.
82. Liegl B, Bennett MW, Fletcher CD: Microcystic/reticular schwannoma: a distinct variant with predilection for visceral locations, *Am J Surg Pathol* 32:1080–1087, 2008.
83. Lasota J, Wasag B, Dansonka-Mieszkowska A, et al: Evaluation of NF2 and NF1 tumor suppressor genes in distinctive gastrointestinal nerve sheath tumors traditionally diagnosed as benign schwannomas: s study of 20 cases, *Lab Invest* 83:1361–1371, 2003.
84. Donner LR, Trompler RA, Dobin S: Clear cell sarcoma of the ileum: the crucial role of cytogenetics for the diagnosis, *Am J Surg Pathol* 22:121–124, 1998.
85. Pauwels P, Debiec-Rychter M, Sciot R, et al: Clear cell sarcoma of the stomach, *Histopathology* 41:526–530, 2002.
86. Taminelli L, Zaman K, Gengler C, et al: Primary clear cell sarcoma of the ileum: an uncommon and misleading site, *Virchows Arch* 447:772–777, 2005.
87. Antonescu CR, Nafa K, Segal NH, et al: EWS-CREB1: a recurrent variant fusion in clear cell sarcoma—association with gastrointestinal location and absence of melanocytic differentiation, *Clin Cancer Res* 12:5356–5362, 2006.
88. Zambrano E, Reyes-Mugica M, Franchi A, et al: An osteoclast-rich tumor of the gastrointestinal tract with features resembling clear cell sarcoma of soft parts: reports of 6 cases of a GIST simulator, *Int J Surg Pathol* 11:75–81, 2003.
89. Rosai J: Editorial: clear cell sarcoma and osteoclast-rich clear cell sarcoma-like tumor of the gastrointestinal tract: one tumor type or two? Melanoma or sarcoma?, *Int J Surg Pathol* 13:309–311, 2005.
90. Kosemehmetoglu K, Folpe AL: Clear cell sarcoma of tendons and aponeuroses, and osteoclast-rich tumour of the gastrointestinal tract with features resembling clear cell sarcoma of soft parts: a review and update, *J Clin Pathol* 63:416–423, 2010.
91. Stockman DL, Miettinen M, Suster S, et al: Malignant gastrointestinal neuroectodermal tumor (GNET): clinicopathologic, immunohistochemical, ultrastructural and molecular analysis of 16 cases with a reappraisal of clear cell sarcoma-like tumors of the gastrointestinal tract, *Am J Surg Pathol* 36:857–868, 2012.
92. Lyle PL, Amato CM, Fitzpatrick JE, et al: Gastrointestinal melanoma or clear cell sarcoma? Molecular evaluation of 7 cases previously diagnosed as malignant melanoma, *Am J Surg Pathol* 32:858–866, 2008.
93. Boland JM, Folpe AL: Oncocytic variant of malignant gastrointestinal neuroectodermal tumor: a potential diagnostic pitfall, *Hum Pathol* 57:13–16, 2016.
94. Hisaoka M, Ishida T, Kuo TT, et al: Clear cell sarcoma of soft tissue: a clinicopathologic, immunohistochemical, and molecular analysis of 33 cases, *Am J Surg Pathol* 32:452–460, 2008.
95. Covinsky M, Gong S, Rajaram V, et al: EWS-ATF1 fusion transcripts in gastrointestinal tumors previously diagnosed as malignant melanoma, *Hum Pathol* 36:74–81, 2005.
96. Gleason BC, Hornick JL: Inflammatory myofibroblastic tumours: where are we now?, *J Clin Pathol* 61:428–437, 2008.
97. Makhlouf HR, Sobin LH: Inflammatory myofibroblastic tumors (inflammatory pseudotumors) of the gastrointestinal tract: how closely are they related to inflammatory fibroid polyps?, *Hum Pathol* 33:307–315, 2002.
98. Mariño-Enríquez A, Wang WL, Roy A, et al: Epithelioid inflammatory myofibroblastic sarcoma: an aggressive intra-abdominal variant of inflammatory myofibroblastic tumor with nuclear membrane or perinuclear ALK, *Am J Surg Pathol* 35:135–144, 2011.
99. Coffin CM, Watterson J, Priest JR, et al: Extrapulmonary inflammatory myofibroblastic tumor (inflammatory pseudotumor). A clinicopathologic and immunohistochemical study of 84 cases, *Am J Surg Pathol* 19:859–872, 1995.
100. Coffin CM, Hornick JL, Fletcher CD: Inflammatory myofibroblastic tumor: comparison of clinicopathologic, histologic, and immunohistochemical features including ALK expression in atypical and aggressive cases, *Am J Surg Pathol* 31:509–520, 2007.
101. Ma Z, Hill DA, Collins MH, et al: Fusion of ALK to the Ran-binding protein 2 (RANBP2) gene in inflammatory myofibroblastic tumor, *Genes Chromosomes Cancer* 37:98–105, 2003.
102. Lee JC, Li CF, Huang HY, et al: ALK oncoproteins in atypical inflammatory myofibroblastic tumours: novel RRBP1-ALK fusions in epithelioid inflammatory myofibroblastic sarcoma, *J Pathol* 241:316–323, 2017.
103. Hornick JL, Sholl LM, Dal Cin P, et al: Expression of ROS1 predicts ROS1 gene rearrangement in inflammatory myofibroblastic tumors, *Mod Pathol* 28:732–739, 2015.
104. Lovly CM, Gupta A, Lipson D, et al: Inflammatory myofibroblastic tumors harbor multiple potentially actionable kinase fusions, *Cancer Discov* 4:889–895, 2014.
105. Alassiri AH, Ali RH, Shen Y, et al: ETV6-NTRK3 is expressed in a subset of ALK-negative inflammatory myofibroblastic tumors, *Am J Surg Pathol* 40:1051–1061, 2016.
106. Yamamoto H, Yoshida A, Taguchi K, et al: ALK, ROS1 and NTRK3 gene rearrangements in inflammatory myofibroblastic tumours, *Histopathology* 69:72–83, 2016.
107. Antonescu CR, Suurmeijer AJ, Zhang L, et al: Molecular characterization of inflammatory myofibroblastic tumors with frequent ALK and ROS1 gene fusions and rare novel RET rearrangement, *Am J Surg Pathol* 39:957–967, 2015.
108. Butrynski JE, D'Adamo DR, Hornick JL, et al: Crizotinib in ALK-rearranged inflammatory myofibroblastic tumor, *N Engl J Med* 363:1727–1733, 2010.
109. Gurbuz AK, Giardiello FM, Petersen GM, et al: Desmoid tumours in familial adenomatous polyposis, *Gut* 35:377–381, 1994.
110. Miettinen MM, Sarlomo-Rikala M, Kovatich AJ, et al: Calponin and h-caldesmon in soft tissue tumors: consistent h-caldesmon immunoreactivity in gastrointestinal stromal tumors indicates traits of smooth muscle differentiation, *Mod Pathol* 12:756–762, 1999.
111. Hornick JL, Fletcher CD: Immunohistochemical staining for KIT (CD117) in soft tissue sarcomas is very limited in distribution, *Am J Clin Pathol* 117:188–193, 2002.
112. Hornick JL, Fletcher CD: Validating immunohistochemical staining for KIT (CD117), *Am J Clin Pathol* 119:325–327, 2003.
113. Lucas DR, al-Abbadi M, Tabaczka P, et al: c-Kit expression in desmoid fibromatosis. Comparative immunohistochemical evaluation of two commercial antibodies, *Am J Clin Pathol* 119:339–345, 2003.
114. Bhattacharya B, Dilworth HP, Iacobuzio-Donahue C, et al: Nuclear beta-catenin expression distinguishes deep fibromatosis from other benign and malignant fibroblastic and myofibroblastic lesions, *Am J Surg Pathol* 29:653–659, 2005.
115. Carlson JW, Fletcher CD: Immunohistochemistry for beta-catenin in the differential diagnosis of spindle cell lesions: analysis of a series and review of the literature, *Histopathology* 51:509–514, 2007.
116. Montgomery E, Folpe AL: The diagnostic value of beta-catenin immunohistochemistry, *Adv Anat Pathol* 12:350–356, 2005.
117. Tejpar S, Nollet F, Li C, et al: Predominance of beta-catenin mutations and beta-catenin dysregulation in sporadic aggressive fibromatosis (desmoid tumor), *Oncogene* 18:6615–6620, 1999.
118. Lazar AJ, Tuvin D, Hajibashi S, et al: Specific mutations in the beta-catenin gene (CTNNB1) correlate with local recurrence in sporadic desmoid tumors, *Am J Pathol* 173:1518–1527, 2008.
119. Lazar AJ, Hajibashi S, Lev D: Desmoid tumor: from surgical extirpation to molecular dissection, *Curr Opin Oncol* 21:352–359, 2009.
120. Lev D, Kotilingam D, Wei C, et al: Optimizing treatment of desmoid tumors, *J Clin Oncol* 25:1785–1791, 2007.
121. Fiore M, MacNeill A, Gronchi A, et al: Desmoid-type fibromatosis: evolving treatment standards, *Surg Oncol Clin N Am* 25:803–826, 2016.
122. Vanek J: Gastric submucosal granuloma with eosinophilic infiltration, *Am J Pathol* 25:397–411, 1949.
123. Johnstone JM, Morson BC: Inflammatory fibroid polyp of the gastrointestinal tract, *Histopathology* 2:349–361, 1978.
124. Lasota J, Wang ZF, Sobin LH, et al: Gain-of-function PDGFRA mutations, earlier reported in gastrointestinal stromal tumors, are common in small intestinal inflammatory fibroid polyps. A study of 60 cases, *Mod Pathol* 22:1049–1056, 2009.
125. Schildhaus HU, Cavlar T, Binot E, et al: Inflammatory fibroid polyps harbour mutations in the platelet-derived growth factor receptor alpha (PDGFRA) gene, *J Pathol* 216:176–182, 2008.
126. Hasegawa T, Yang P, Kagawa N, et al: CD34 expression by inflammatory fibroid polyps of the stomach, *Mod Pathol* 10:451–456, 1997.
127. Kolodziejczyk P, Yao T, Tsuneyoshi M: Inflammatory fibroid polyp of the stomach. A special reference to an immunohistochemical profile of 42 cases, *Am J Surg Pathol* 17:1159–1168, 1993.
128. Ozolek JA, Sasatomi E, Swalsky PA, et al: Inflammatory fibroid polyps of the gastrointestinal tract: clinical, pathologic, and molecular characteristics, *Appl Immunohistochem Mol Morphol* 12:59–66, 2004.
129. Allibone RO, Nanson JK, Anthony PP: Multiple and recurrent inflammatory fibroid polyps in a Devon family ('Devon polyposis syndrome'): an update, *Gut* 33:1004–1005, 1992.

130. Anthony PP, Morris DS, Vowles KD: Multiple and recurrent inflammatory fibroid polyps in three generations of a Devon family: a new syndrome, *Gut* 25:854–862, 1984.
131. Ricci R, Martini M, Cenci T, et al: PDGFRA-mutant syndrome, *Mod Pathol* 28:954–964, 2015.
132. Miettinen M, Makhlouf HR, Sobin LH, et al: Plexiform fibromyxoma: a distinctive benign gastric antral neoplasm not to be confused with a myxoid GIST, *Am J Surg Pathol* 33:1624–1632, 2009.
133. Takahashi Y, Shimizu S, Ishida T, et al: Plexiform angiomyxoid myofibroblastic tumor of the stomach, *Am J Surg Pathol* 31:724–728, 2007.
134. Yoshida A, Klimstra DS, Antonescu CR: Plexiform angiomyxoid tumor of the stomach, *Am J Surg Pathol* 32:1910–1912, 2008.
135. Spans L, Fletcher CD, Antonescu CR, et al: Recurrent MALAT1-GLI1 oncogenic fusion and GLI1 up-regulation define a subset of plexiform fibromyxoma, *J Pathol* 239:335–343, 2016.
136. Folpe AL, Kwiatkowski DJ: Perivascular epithelioid cell neoplasms: pathology and pathogenesis, *Hum Pathol* 41:1–15, 2010.
137. Folpe AL, Mentzel T, Lehr HA, et al: Perivascular epithelioid cell neoplasms of soft tissue and gynecologic origin: a clinicopathologic study of 26 cases and review of the literature, *Am J Surg Pathol* 29:1558–1575, 2005.
138. Hornick JL, Fletcher CD: PEComa: what do we know so far?, *Histopathology* 48:75–82, 2006.
139. Doyle LA, Hornick JL, Fletcher CD: PEComa of the gastrointestinal tract: clinicopathologic study of 35 cases with evaluation of prognostic parameters, *Am J Surg Pathol* 37:1769–1782, 2013.
140. Argani P, Aulmann S, Illei PB, et al: A distinctive subset of PEComas harbors TFE3 gene fusions, *Am J Surg Pathol* 34:1395–1406, 2010.
141. Kenerson H, Folpe AL, Takayama TK, et al: Activation of the mTOR pathway in sporadic angiomyolipomas and other perivascular epithelioid cell neoplasms, *Hum Pathol* 38:1361–1371, 2007.
142. Pan CC, Chung MY, Ng KF, et al: Constant allelic alteration on chromosome 16p (TSC2 gene) in perivascular epithelioid cell tumour (PEComa): genetic evidence for the relationship of PEComa with angiomyolipoma, *J Pathol* 214:387–393, 2008.
143. Agaram NP, Sung YS, Zhang L, et al: Dichotomy of genetic abnormalities in PEComas with therapeutic implications, *Am J Surg Pathol* 39:813–825, 2015.
144. Wagner AJ, Malinowska-Kolodziej I, Morgan JA, et al: Clinical activity of mTOR inhibition with sirolimus in malignant perivascular epithelioid cell tumors: targeting the pathogenic activation of mTORC1 in tumors, *J Clin Oncol* 28:835–840, 2010.
145. Appelman HD, Helwig EB: Glomus tumors of the stomach, *Cancer* 23:203–213, 1969.
146. Miettinen M, Paal E, Lasota J, et al: Gastrointestinal glomus tumors: a clinicopathologic, immunohistochemical, and molecular genetic study of 32 cases, *Am J Surg Pathol* 26:301–311, 2002.
147. Kang G, Park HJ, Kim JY, et al: Glomus tumor of the stomach: a clinicopathologic analysis of 10 cases and review of the literature, *Gut Liver* 6:52–57, 2012.
148. Mosquera JM, Sboner A, Zhang L, et al: Novel MIR143-NOTCH fusions in benign and malignant glomus tumors, *Genes Chromosomes Cancer* 52:1075–1087, 2013.
149. Folpe AL, Fanburg-Smith JC, Miettinen M, et al: Atypical and malignant glomus tumors: analysis of 52 cases, with a proposal for the reclassification of glomus tumors, *Am J Surg Pathol* 25:1–12, 2001.
150. Antonescu CR, Scheithauer BW, Woodruff JM: *AFIP Atlas of tumor pathology: Tumors of the peripheral nervous system*, Series 4, fascicle 19. Washington, DC, 2013, ARP Press.
151. Shekitka KM, Sobin LH: Ganglioneuromas of the gastrointestinal tract. Relation to Von Recklinghausen disease and other multiple tumor syndromes, *Am J Surg Pathol* 18:250–257, 1994.
152. Heald B, Mester J, Rybicki L, et al: Frequent gastrointestinal polyps and colorectal adenocarcinomas in a prospective series of PTEN mutation carriers, *Gastroenterology* 139:1927–1933, 2010.
153. McGarrity TJ, Wagner Baker MJ, Ruggiero FM, et al: GI polyposis and glycogenic acanthosis of the esophagus associated with PTEN mutation positive Cowden syndrome in the absence of cutaneous manifestations, *Am J Gastroenterol* 98:1429–1434, 2003.
154. Stanich PP, Owens VL, Sweetser S, et al: Colonic polyposis and neoplasia in Cowden syndrome, *Mayo Clin Proc* 86:489–492, 2011.
155. Coriat R, Mozer M, Caux E, et al: Endoscopic findings in Cowden syndrome, *Endoscopy* 43:723–726, 2011.
156. Carney JA, Go VL, Sizemore GW, et al: Alimentary-tract ganglioneuromatosis. A major component of the syndrome of multiple endocrine neoplasia, type 2b, *N Engl J Med* 295:1287–1291, 1976.
157. d'Amore ES, Manivel JC, Pettinato G, et al: Intestinal ganglioneuromatosis: mucosal and transmural types. A clinicopathologic and immunohistochemical study of six cases, *Hum Pathol* 22:276–286, 1991.
158. Moline J, Eng C: Multiple endocrine neoplasia type 2: an overview, *Genet Med* 13:755–764, 2011.
159. Fuller CE, Williams GT: Gastrointestinal manifestations of type 1 neurofibromatosis (von Recklinghausen's disease), *Histopathology* 19:1–11, 1991.
160. Thway K, Fisher C: Diffuse ganglioneuromatosis in small intestine associated with neurofibromatosis type 1, *Ann Diagn Pathol* 13:50–54, 2009.
161. Goldblum JR, Rice TW, Zuccaro G, et al: Granular cell tumors of the esophagus: a clinical and pathologic study of 13 cases, *Ann Thorac Surg* 62:860–865, 1996.
162. Johnston J, Helwig EB: Granular cell tumors of the gastrointestinal tract and perianal region: a study of 74 cases, *Dig Dis Sci* 26:807–816, 1981.
163. Parfitt JR, McLean CA, Joseph MG, et al: Granular cell tumours of the gastrointestinal tract: expression of nestin and clinicopathological evaluation of 11 patients, *Histopathology* 48:424–430, 2006.
164. Voskuil JH, van Dijk MM, Wagenaar SS, et al: Occurrence of esophageal granular cell tumors in The Netherlands between 1988 and 1994, *Dig Dis Sci* 46:1610–1614, 2001.
165. An S, Jang J, Min K, et al: Granular cell tumor of the gastrointestinal tract: histologic and immunohistochemical analysis of 98 cases, *Hum Pathol* 46:813–819, 2015.
166. Singhi AD, Montgomery EA: Colorectal granular cell tumor: a clinicopathologic study of 26 cases, *Am J Surg Pathol* 34:1186–1192, 2010.
167. Na JI, Kim HJ, Jung JJ, et al: Granular cell tumours of the colorectum: histopathological and immunohistochemical evaluation of 30 cases, *Histopathology* 65:764–774, 2014.
168. Fine SW, Li M: Expression of calretinin and the alpha-subunit of inhibin in granular cell tumors, *Am J Clin Pathol* 119:259–264, 2003.
169. Chamberlain BK, McClain CM, Gonzalez RS, et al: Alveolar soft part sarcoma and granular cell tumor: an immunohistochemical comparison study, *Hum Pathol* 45:1039–1044, 2014.
170. Schoolmeester JK, Lastra RR: Granular cell tumors overexpress TFE3 without corollary gene rearrangement, *Hum Pathol* 46:1242–1243, 2015.
171. Gleason BC, Nascimento AF: HMB-45 and Melan-A are useful in the differential diagnosis between granular cell tumor and malignant melanoma, *Am J Dermatopathol* 29:22–27, 2007.
172. Fanburg-Smith JC, Meis-Kindblom JM, Fante R, et al: Malignant granular cell tumor of soft tissue: diagnostic criteria and clinicopathologic correlation, *Am J Surg Pathol* 22:779–794, 1998.
173. Hornick JL, Fletcher CD: Intestinal perineuriomas: clinicopathologic definition of a new anatomic subset in a series of 10 cases, *Am J Surg Pathol* 29:859–865, 2005.
174. Eslami-Varzaneh F, Washington K, Robert ME, et al: Benign fibroblastic polyps of the colon: a histologic, immunohistochemical, and ultrastructural study, *Am J Surg Pathol* 28:374–378, 2004.
175. Groisman GM, Polak-Charcon S, Appelman HD: Fibroblastic polyp of the colon: clinicopathological analysis of 10 cases with emphasis on its common association with serrated crypts, *Histopathology* 48:431–437, 2006.
176. Agaimy A, Stoehr R, Vieth M, et al: Benign serrated colorectal fibroblastic polyps/intramucosal perineuriomas are true mixed epithelial-stromal polyps (hybrid hyperplastic polyp/mucosal perineurioma) with frequent BRAF mutations, *Am J Surg Pathol* 34:1663–1671, 2010.
177. Groisman GM, Polak-Charcon S: Fibroblastic polyp of the colon and colonic perineurioma: 2 names for a single entity?, *Am J Surg Pathol* 32:1088–1094, 2008.
178. Pai RK, Mojtahed A, Rouse RV, et al: Histologic and molecular analyses of colonic perineurial-like proliferations in serrated polyps: perineurial-like stromal proliferations are seen in sessile serrated adenomas, *Am J Surg Pathol* 35:1373–1380, 2011.
179. Groisman GM, Hershkovitz D, Vieth M, et al: Colonic perineuriomas with and without crypt serration: a comparative study, *Am J Surg Pathol* 37:745–751, 2013.
180. Gibson JA, Hornick JL: Mucosal Schwann cell "hamartoma": clinicopathologic study of 26 neural colorectal polyps distinct from neurofibromas and mucosal neuromas, *Am J Surg Pathol* 33:781–787, 2009.
181. Pasquini P, Baiocchini A, Falasca L, et al: Mucosal Schwann cell "hamartoma": a new entity?, *World J Gastroenterol* 15:2287–2289, 2009.
182. Rocco EG, Iannuzzi F, Dell'era A, et al: Schwann cell hamartoma: case report, *BMC Gastroenterol* 11:68, 2011.

17

Lower Genital Soft Tissue Tumors

Marisa R. Nucci, MD

Since the initial description of pseudosarcomatous fibroepithelial stromal polyps of the distal female genital tract in the early 1960s, various relatively site-specific mesenchymal lesions of the lower genital tract have been recognized.[1-4] These lesions are often diagnostically challenging because of their morphologic overlap, which in part stems from their likely shared origin from the specialized subepithelial stroma of the distal female genital tract. Ancillary studies such as immunohistochemistry are often not helpful in their distinction; thus one must firmly rely on morphologic features to distinguish among these tumor types.

General Approach to Soft Tissue Lesions of the Lower Genital Tract

Among the relatively site-specific soft tissue tumors of the distal female genital tract discussed herein, the diagnosis of deep (aggressive) angiomyxoma has the greatest impact on the patient with regard to prognosis and potential morbidity; therefore its recognition is of paramount importance. Consequently, a useful approach to spindle cell tumors at this site is to be familiar with the characteristic clinical and pathologic features of deep (aggressive) angiomyxoma and to be aware of how it differs from the other lesions. In general, issues to be considered are the following:

1. Is the lesion myxoid?
2. Is the lesion deep seated (as seen in deep angiomyxoma) or superficial/subcutaneous?
3. If it is superficial, is it polypoid/exophytic, which would argue strongly against deep angiomyxoma?
4. Is the lesion infiltrative (as seen in deep angiomyxoma) or well circumscribed?
5. Does the lesion have a vascular component?
6. If there is a vascular component, is it composed of predominantly medium- to large-caliber blood vessels (typical of deep angiomyxoma), or are they small?

Deep (Aggressive) Angiomyxoma

Since its initial description by Steeper and Rosai in 1983 as a locally infiltrative tumor of adult women, which tends to recur, resulting in significant morbidity (hence the original terminology of *aggressive angiomyxoma*), it has become evident that these lesions have a favorable, less aggressive course if initially completely excised.[5-11] Current terminology therefore favors the designation "deep angiomyxoma" to reflect its tendency to involve deep soft tissue. Deep angiomyxoma is also discussed in Chapter 5.

Clinical Features

Deep angiomyxoma typically occurs in the pelvis and perineum of reproductive-aged women, with a median age in the fourth decade. However, it may also rarely arise in the inguinoscrotal region of men. In women, it may be clinically mistaken for a labial cyst, most commonly a Bartholin gland cyst. Deep angiomyxoma can vary in size but is often relatively large (>10 cm).

Pathologic Features

Deep angiomyxoma is characteristically a soft, gelatinous tumor with ill-defined margins on gross examination. Histologically, it is uniformly paucicellular, composed of bland spindle cells with delicate cytoplasmic processes set within copious myxoid stroma (Fig. 17.1). Evenly distributed throughout are medium- to large-sized vessels, which are often thick walled and hyalinized. Loose fibrillary collagen and collections of smooth muscle cells (so-called myoid bundles) are typically arranged in either loose clusters or tight whorls adjacent to blood vessels (Fig. 17.2). Deep angiomyxoma has deceptively infiltrative borders, and thus its borders are difficult to define both surgically and pathologically. This problem likely explains its propensity to recur, because incomplete excision is associated with a high rate of recurrence.

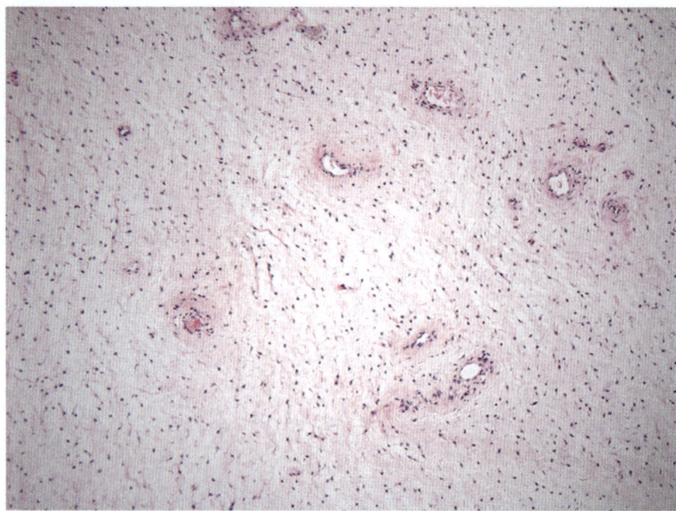

Figure 17.1 Deep Angiomyxoma. Characteristic low-power appearance of bland spindle cells set within a copious myxoid matrix, resulting in a hypocellular appearance. Note the uniformly distributed medium-sized blood vessels.

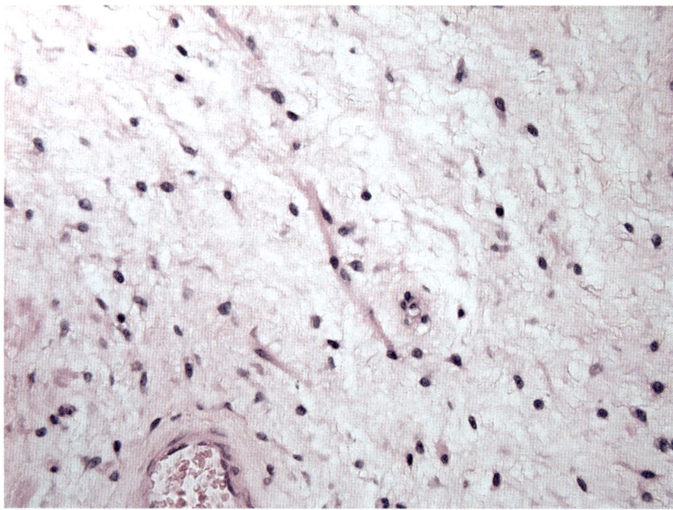

Figure 17.2 Deep Angiomyxoma. Smooth muscle cells (myoid bundles) adjacent to blood vessels are characteristic. Note the bland appearance of the spindle cell component.

Immunohistochemistry

The lesional stromal cells are usually positive for estrogen receptor (ER), progesterone receptor (PR), and desmin, as well as sometimes positive for smooth muscle actin.[12] The myoid bundles are positive for smooth muscle markers. Nuclear expression of HMGA2 is seen in many but not all cases.[13]

Molecular Genetics

Structural rearrangements of the region 12q15 with involvement of *HMGA2* are the most frequent chromosomal aberrations observed in deep (aggressive) angiomyxoma; the break involving 12q15 may occur within or outside of the gene.[14–18] Overall, 12q15 rearrangements occur in approximately 30% of cases.[19] However, detection of HMGA2 expression by immunohistochemistry does not always correlate with gene rearrangement and thus may only be useful in confirming the diagnosis or assessing margin status in a subset of cases.[16]

Differential Diagnosis

Fibroepithelial stromal polyps can sometimes be edematous, usually secondary to torsion, and mimic deep angiomyxoma. However, stromal polyps are superficial lesions that are more commonly polypoid and have a central fibrovascular core rather than the uniformly distributed vascular component of deep angiomyxoma. In addition, stromal polyps characteristically contain multinucleate cells (not a feature of deep angiomyxoma) and lack perivascular cuffing by collagen and myoid bundles (typical features of deep angiomyxoma).

Superficial angiomyxoma (see also Chapters 5 and 15) may be considered in the differential diagnosis of deep angiomyxoma because both are myxoid neoplasms composed of bland spindle cells. However, the former occurs in superficial cutaneous and subcutaneous locations and shows a lobulated growth pattern with well-defined borders, which contrasts with the more deeply situated, ill-defined deep angiomyxoma. In addition, superficial angiomyxoma contains more delicate, thin-walled vessels. Moreover, it is negative for desmin, in contrast to deep angiomyxoma, which is commonly positive for this marker. As a practical point, in some instances, superficial angiomyxoma may be excised without overlying dermis. Its superficial location can usually be determined by the presence of adnexal structures located between the myxoid tumor nodules.

Angiomyofibroblastoma is another relatively site-specific mesenchymal tumor of the distal female genital tract that occurs in reproductive-aged women. It is composed of bland spindle cells and hypocellular areas that may mimic deep angiomyxoma. In contrast to deep angiomyxoma, angiomyofibroblastoma is a nonrecurring, well-circumscribed, typically subcutaneous mass. It classically exhibits areas of alternating cellularity with hypercellular zones merging with less cellular areas, which contrasts with the uniformly hypocellular appearance of deep angiomyxoma. In addition, angiomyofibroblastoma contains more numerous blood vessels, which are typically capillary sized, as opposed to the large thick-walled vessels of deep angiomyxoma. The lesional cells of angiomyofibroblastoma, which are commonly epithelioid in appearance with more abundant eosinophilic cytoplasm, tend to cluster around the vasculature in a characteristic configuration. Because both lesions are often desmin positive, immunohistochemistry is not useful in the differential diagnosis.

Prepubertal vulval fibroma is characterized by a poorly marginated, patternless proliferation of bland spindle cells. In contrast to deep angiomyxoma, this lesion typically occurs in young girls and is more superficially located in submucosal or subcutaneous soft tissue. Although both tumors can have myxoid stroma, deep angiomyxoma is more uniformly myxoid, has a more delicate collagenous matrix, and typically contains myoid bundles. In addition, unlike deep angiomyxoma, the spindle cells of prepubertal vulval fibroma are positive for CD34 and negative for desmin.

Massive vulval edema, most commonly secondary to immobilization or obesity, can mimic deep angiomyxoma because it can form a masslike lesion, lacks circumscription, and has a hypocellular appearance.[20,21] However, massive edema is usually bilateral, has an edematous and not myxoid stroma, often shows perivascular lymphoid inflammation, and typically is negative for ER and HMGA2.

Prognosis and Treatment

Deep angiomyxoma has a propensity for local recurrence, sometimes many years (even decades) after the initial excision. Destructive recurrences may occur, but only if the tumor was initially incompletely excised (hence the previous use of the term *aggressive*). Wide local excision with 1-cm margins is considered optimal treatment. Because these tumors are ER positive, hormonal therapy may play a role in patients with extensive or recurrent disease.[22]

PRACTICE POINTS: Deep (Aggressive) Angiomyxoma

- This infiltrative, hypocellular myxoid tumor of the distal female genital tract has the potential for local, sometimes destructive recurrence
- Typically involves deep soft tissue and is rarely polypoid
- Abundant myxoid stroma, bland spindle cells, and uniformly distributed medium- to large-sized blood vessels with hyalinized walls are characteristic
- Immunohistochemistry is not helpful because most other mesenchymal tumors of the distal female genital tract share the same immunoprofile

Fibroepithelial Stromal Polyp

Fibroepithelial stromal polyps are hormonally responsive lesions that are thought to arise from specialized subepithelial stromal cells of the distal female genital tract.[23–30] Although there is an association with pregnancy, they may occur at any time during the reproductive years and have also been associated with hormonal replacement therapy in perimenopausal and postmenopausal women. Following pregnancy, the polyps typically regress, a finding that suggests they represent a benign reactive proliferation responding to an altered hormonal environment (e.g., pregnancy). Lesions that occur during pregnancy have sometimes been termed *pseudosarcoma botryoides* because of their increased cellularity and atypia. However, consideration of sarcoma botryoides (botryoid embryonal rhabdomyosarcoma) is rarely, if ever, truly a diagnostic concern, given the differences in clinical presentation and lineage.

Clinical Features

Patients typically present with polypoid or pedunculated lesions, which may vary in size, but are generally smaller than 5 cm. They are usually solitary, although multiple polyps may occasionally occur (most commonly during pregnancy).

Pathologic Features

Fibroepithelial stromal polyps are polypoid proliferations of stroma with a variably hyperplastic overlying squamous epithelium and a central fibrovascular core that often contains thick-walled blood vessels (Fig. 17.3). The stroma can be variably cellular but is typically composed of small spindle cells with oval to elongated nuclei and delicate unipolar and bipolar eosinophilic cytoplasmic processes. A characteristic feature is the presence of stellate and multinucleate stromal cells, which are most commonly located near the epithelial-stromal interface or adjacent to the prominent central vasculature (Fig. 17.4). The term *pseudosarcoma botryoides*, which has been used to describe a morphologic subset of stromal polyps that occur during pregnancy, refers to those polyps that exhibit a greater degree of stromal cellularity, nuclear pleomorphism (large, irregularly shaped, hyperchromatic and often multinucleate nuclei), and mitotic activity (Figs. 17.5 and 17.6).

Immunohistochemistry

The stromal cells may be positive for desmin, actin, ER, and PR. Expression of RB1 (retinoblastoma) is intact. This immunoprofile is similar to nonneoplastic vulvovaginal mesenchyme.

Differential Diagnosis

Deep (aggressive) angiomyxoma enters into the differential diagnosis of fibroepithelial stromal polyp because it is also a vascular lesion with a loose spindled stroma. However, deep angiomyxoma characteristically involves deep soft tissue (i.e., not superficial or polypoid), is infiltrative, and has a uniformly distributed vascular component (rather than a vascular core). Myxoid stroma and perivascular cuffing by collagen and

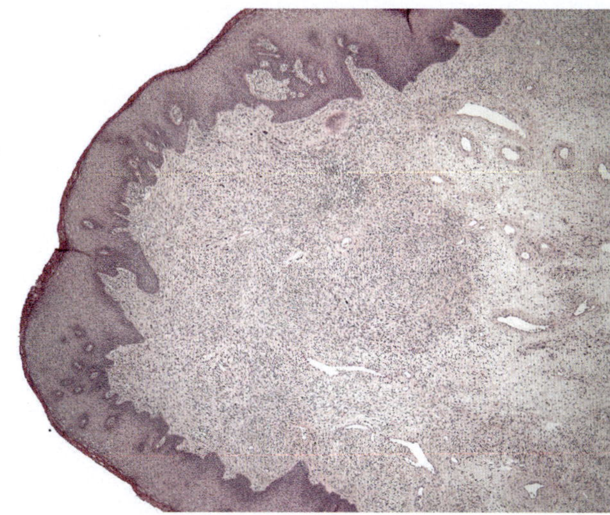

Figure 17.3 Fibroepithelial Stromal Polyp. Polypoid mass with a central fibrovascular core. This polyp is remarkable for hypercellular stroma. Note that there is no clear margin between the spindle cell proliferation and the overlying epithelium.

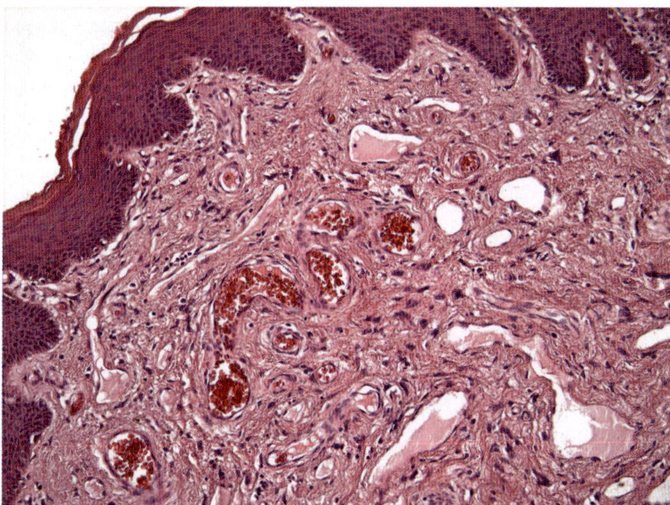

Figure 17.4 Fibroepithelial Stromal Polyp. Stellate and multinucleate cells are a ubiquitous feature and are often adjacent to the overlying epithelium.

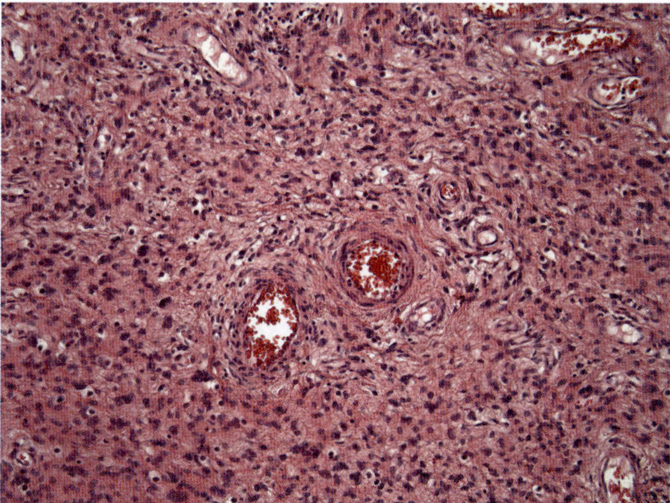

Figure 17.5 Fibroepithelial Stromal Polyp. Pseudosarcomatous change with marked hypercellularity and nuclear enlargement.

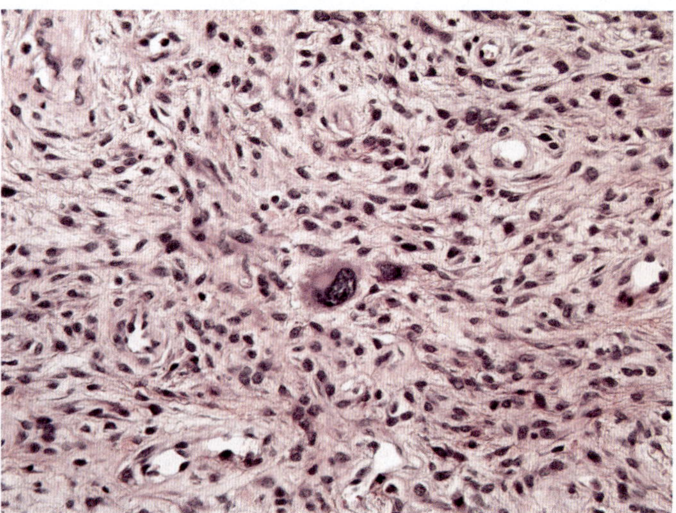

Figure 17.6 **Fibroepithelial Stromal Polyp.** Markedly atypical stromal cells punctuate an otherwise bland-appearing proliferation in this pseudosarcomatous polyp.

myoid bundles are also features of deep angiomyxoma that are not seen in fibroepithelial stromal polyps. Because the stromal cells of both lesions can be positive for desmin and actin, immunohistochemistry is not discriminatory.

Angiomyofibroblastoma and fibroepithelial stromal polyp both typically occur in adult women. However, the former is characteristically a well-circumscribed subcutaneous mass rather than a polypoid mucosal lesion. Histologically, angiomyofibroblastoma has a more prominent vascular component composed of numerous delicate capillary-sized vessels; this differs from the typically centrally located and larger, thicker-walled vessels of stromal polyps. In addition, the stromal cells of angiomyofibroblastoma often have an epithelioid appearance with more abundant eosinophilic cytoplasm that more frequently cluster around the prominent blood vessels. Both lesions can exhibit desmin and, less commonly, actin reactivity; therefore immunohistochemistry is not helpful.

Superficial angiomyxoma and fibroepithelial stromal polyps are superficially located lesions that both occur in adult women. The former has a multinodular growth pattern, an abundant myxoid matrix, and a characteristic neutrophilic infiltrate that does not correlate with erosion or ulceration. In one-third of cases, superficial angiomyxoma is associated with an epithelial component in the form of squamous epithelial-lined cysts (epidermoid cysts), buds of basaloid cells, or strands of squamous cells (likely due to adnexal entrapment, present in either the primary lesion or the recurrence). Furthermore, superficial angiomyxoma lacks the stellate and multinucleate stromal cells characteristic of stromal polyps.

Sarcomas are often considered in the differential diagnosis of stromal polyps with increased cellularity, cytologic atypia, and mitotic activity. Although the pitfall of mistaking pseudosarcomatous polyps during pregnancy may be well known, these worrisome histologic findings are not limited to pregnancy-associated polyps; thus it is important to be aware of features that are helpful in this distinction. Even in the most florid examples of pseudosarcomatous polyps, there is morphologic overlap with their more banal-appearing counterparts, including the (1) lack of an identifiable lesional margin, (2) extension of atypical stromal cells to the stromal-epithelial interface, and (3) frequent presence of multinucleate cells near the stromal-epithelial interface. Although often discussed, pseudosarcomatous polyps are readily distinguished from botryoid embryonal rhabdomyosarcoma (see Chapter 8) because they are rare before puberty and lack a subepithelial hypercellular ("cambium") layer, rhabdomyoblasts, and skeletal muscle marker expression (e.g., myogenin).

Prognosis and Treatment

Fibroepithelial stromal polyps are benign, and local excision is adequate. They may very rarely recur locally, particularly if incompletely excised, or if there is continued hormonal stimulation (e.g., pregnancy).

PRACTICE POINTS: Fibroepithelial Stromal Polyp

- This benign polypoid growth arises from the distinctive subepithelial stroma of the distal female genital tract
- Stellate and multinucleate stromal cells near the epithelial-stromal interface are characteristic
- Some polyps show increased stromal cellularity, nuclear pleomorphism, and mitotic activity ("pseudosarcomatous")
- Pseudosarcomatous stromal changes are commonly, but not always, associated with pregnancy

Angiomyofibroblastoma

Although originally described as occurring exclusively in the vulvovaginal region, angiomyofibroblastoma can also involve the inguinoscrotal region.[31–38]

Clinical Features

Angiomyofibroblastoma is a benign neoplasm that occurs almost exclusively in reproductive-aged women. Tumors are typically small (<5 cm) and well circumscribed and may be mistaken for a cyst on clinical examination. Rarely, they may be pedunculated.[39]

Pathologic Features

Angiomyofibroblastoma is a well-circumscribed, tan to pink, soft tissue mass that usually has a soft or rubbery consistency. Histologically, it is well demarcated from surrounding soft tissue and composed of an admixture of numerous delicate thin-walled capillary-sized vessels and plump, round to spindle-shaped cells. These stromal cells, which are characteristically clustered around the prominent vessels, are set within a variably edematous to collagenous matrix with alternating zones of cellularity (Fig. 17.7). They usually appear somewhat epithelioid (except in postmenopausal patients, where they are more often spindled), with moderate amounts of eosinophilic cytoplasm and nuclei with fine chromatin and inconspicuous nucleoli (Figs. 17.8 and 17.9). Mitoses are uncommon, and intralesional adipose tissue may occasionally be present (Fig. 17.10), and when prominent, the term "lipomatous variant" has been applied.

Immunohistochemistry

The stromal cells are typically positive for desmin, ER and PR and show variable reactivity for actin, although they are usually negative for this marker. CD34 is rarely positive, and expression of RB1 is typically intact.[40] As for the other lower genital soft tissue tumors, immunohistochemistry plays a limited role in diagnosis.

Molecular Genetics

These tumors do not appear to fall within the family of vulvovaginal neoplasms characterized by loss of genetic material at 13q14.[41] The molecular pathogenetic basis for angiomyofibroblastoma has not yet been identified.

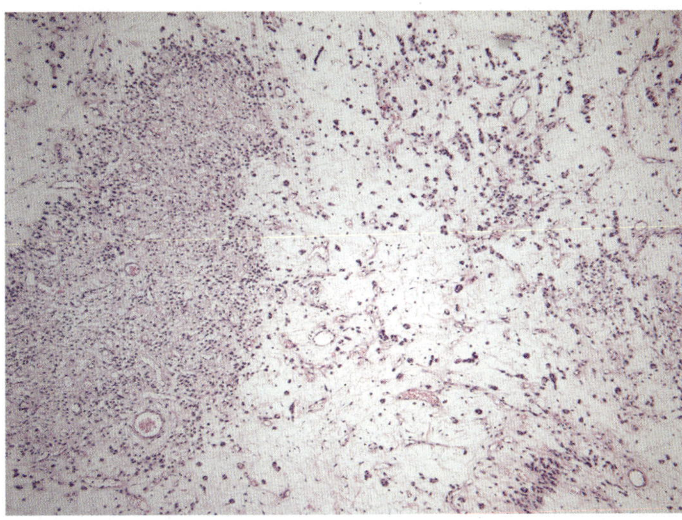

Figure 17.7 Angiomyofibroblastoma. Characteristic low-power appearance with alternating zones of cellularity. Note the numerous capillary-sized vessels.

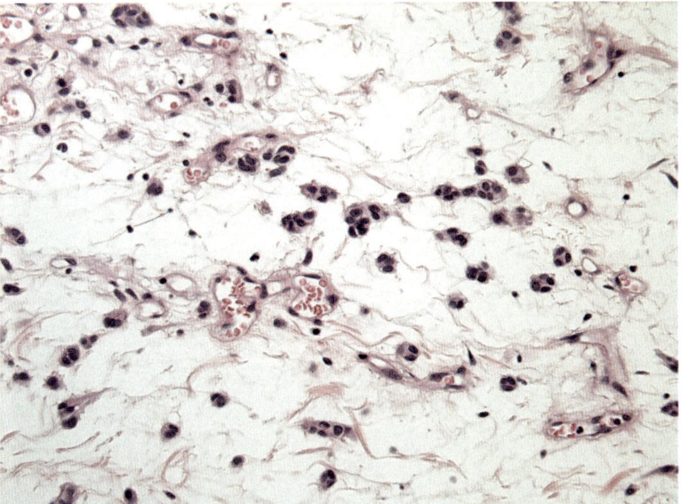

Figure 17.8 Angiomyofibroblastoma. Surrounding the delicate vessels are clusters of epithelioid stromal cells.

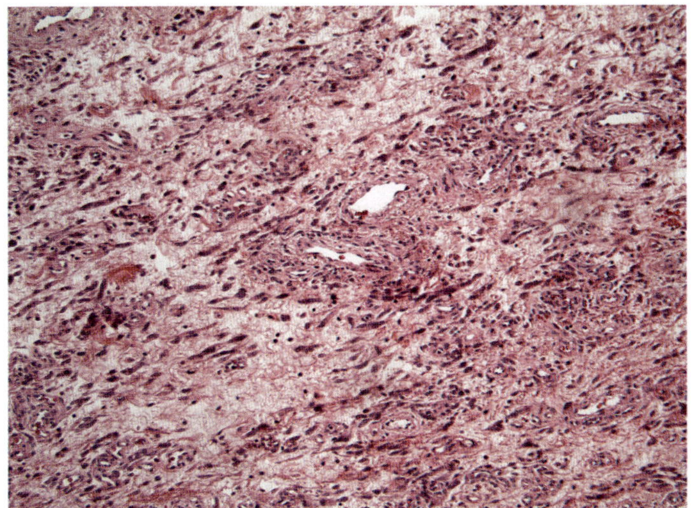

Figure 17.9 Angiomyofibroblastoma. In postmenopausal patients, the tumor cells are more spindled.

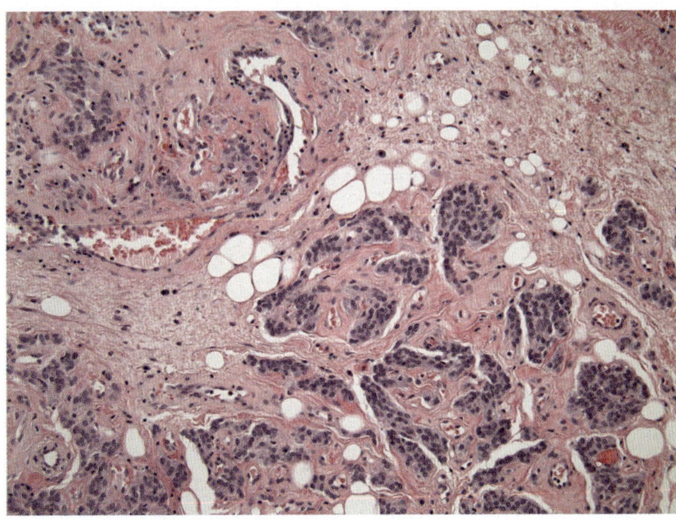

Figure 17.10 Angiomyofibroblastoma. Lipomatous change may occur.

Differential Diagnosis

Deep (aggressive) angiomyxoma should be distinguished from angiomyofibroblastoma because of its recurrent potential, which is closely linked to margin status. In contrast to angiomyofibroblastoma, deep angiomyxoma is uniformly paucicellular and lacks alternating zones of cellularity. In addition, it more often involves deep soft tissue, has an infiltrative margin, and tends to contain larger, thicker-walled vessels. Both tumors have a similar immunophenotype; therefore distinction is based on the morphologic differences alone.

Fibroepithelial stromal polyp is typically polypoid and has an ill-defined interface with the surrounding soft tissue, which is in contrast to the well-defined border of angiomyofibroblastoma. Moreover, stromal polyps have a different vascular pattern, with centrally located larger vessels, and multinucleate cells near the stromal-epithelial interface.

Cellular angiofibroma and angiomyofibroblastoma are both well-circumscribed mesenchymal tumors with a prominent vascular component; however, cellular angiofibroma has numerous small- to medium-sized blood vessels with thickened, often hyalinized walls, in contrast to the delicate capillary-sized vessels of angiomyofibroblastoma. In addition, cellular angiofibroma is uniformly cellular with a spindle cell component that is arranged in short intersecting fascicles. The spindle cells of cellular angiofibroma are typically positive for CD34 and less commonly express desmin. As cellular angiofibroma falls within a family of genetically related tumors showing loss of *RB1*/13q14, there is typically loss of RB1 expression in these tumors.

Prepubertal vulval fibroma is distinguished from angiomyofibroblastoma by its occurrence in young girls, as well as by its ill-defined margins and patternless proliferation of bland spindle cells without increased vascularity. In addition, it is typically positive for CD34 and negative for desmin.

Mammary-type myofibroblastoma is a benign spindle cell lesion that may occur in the genital region. It is morphologically and immunophenotypically identical to myofibroblastoma of the breast. It lacks the prominent vascular component and perivascular distribution of epithelioid cells seen in angiomyofibroblastoma. The spindle cells of both tumors can be positive for desmin; however, mammary-type myofibroblastoma is also positive for CD34. As mammary-type myofibroblastoma falls within the family of genetically related tumors showing loss of *RB1*/13q14, there is typically loss of RB1 expression in these tumors.

Prognosis and Treatment

Angiomyofibroblastoma has no potential for recurrence. Therefore local excision with clear margins is adequate treatment.

PRACTICE POINTS: Angiomyofibroblastoma

- This well-circumscribed, benign, nonrecurring tumor has a prominent capillary component and alternating zones of cellularity
- Clustering of epithelioid cells around the blood vessels is characteristic
- Tumor cells in postmenopausal patients may have a more spindled appearance

Cellular Angiofibroma

Although cellular angiofibroma was initially thought to occur exclusively in women, it is now well known that this condition occurs in the inguinoscrotal region in men with a similar frequency. This tumor may also develop at extragenital sites in both men and women.[42–46]

Clinical Features

Cellular angiofibroma affects both men and women over a wide age range (mean, 53.5 years); however, men tend to be older than women at presentation. Patients most commonly present with a well-circumscribed, painless, subcutaneous mass, often with a long preoperative duration.

Pathologic Features

On gross examination, cellular angiofibroma is typically a well-circumscribed, gray to white mass with a firm, rubbery consistency. Most tumors also have a well-demarcated margin histologically (Fig. 17.11), although occasional examples show limited infiltration of surrounding nonneoplastic soft tissue. It is typically a uniformly cellular neoplasm composed of short, intersecting fascicles of bland spindle cells with ovoid to fusiform nuclei and scant, pale-staining cytoplasm with ill-defined borders (Fig. 17.12). Hyalinized or edematous areas may occasionally contribute to variations in cellularity. Characteristic features also include the presence of numerous small- to medium-sized, thick-walled, and often hyalinized blood vessels and wispy collagen bundles (see Fig. 17.12). A minor component of adipose tissue is often present. Mitoses are typically infrequent, and significant nuclear pleomorphism is usually absent, although multinucleate cells may occur. Rare cases of cellular angiofibroma contain a discrete cytologically atypical or sarcoma-like component, which may mimic atypical lipomatous tumor or pleomorphic liposarcoma.[47] The prognostic significance of this phenomenon is uncertain, although reported examples thus far have pursued a benign clinical course.

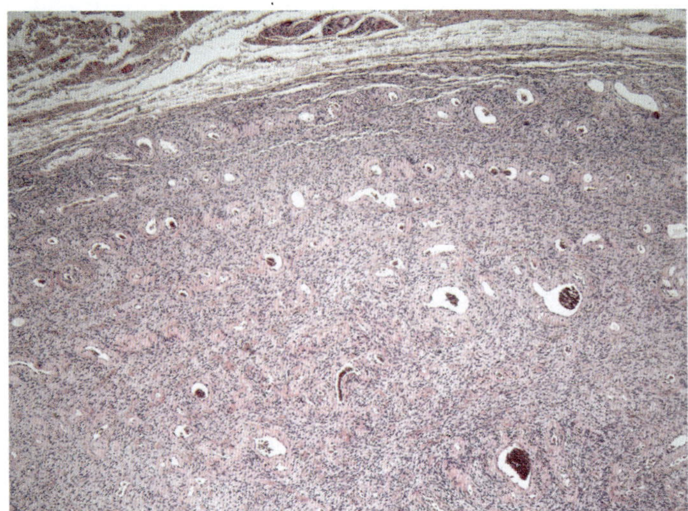

Figure 17.11 Cellular Angiofibroma. These cellular tumors are typically well circumscribed.

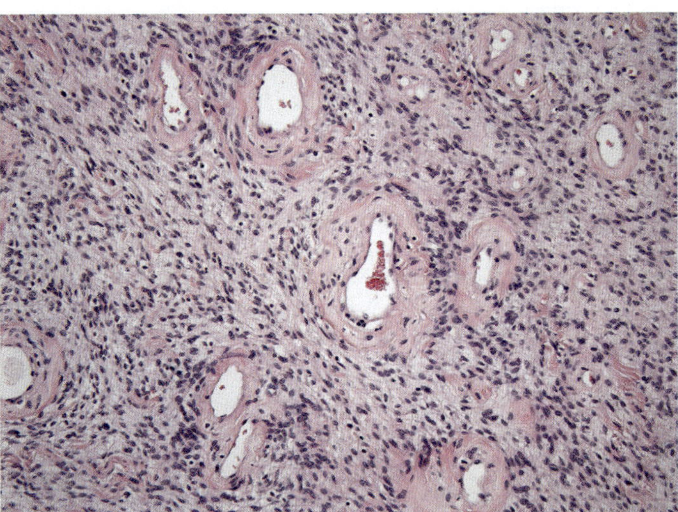

Figure 17.12 Cellular Angiofibroma. Intersecting fascicles of bland spindle cells and numerous medium-sized blood vessels with hyalinized walls are characteristic features.

Immunohistochemistry

Spindle cells are positive for ER and PR and, in approximately half of tumors, CD34. Smooth muscle actin and desmin are less commonly positive, in approximately 20% and 8% of cases, respectively.[44] RB1 expression is deficient (with loss of nuclear staining).[40]

Molecular Genetics

Cellular angiofibroma, which has a similar morphologic appearance as (and immunophenotypic overlap with) spindle cell lipoma (see Chapter 12) and mammary myofibroblastoma, appears to be closely related to the latter tumor types because they all show loss of genetic material at *RB1*/13q14.[48,49]

Differential Diagnosis

Angiomyofibroblastoma and cellular angiofibroma are both relatively site-specific mesenchymal tumors with a prominent vascular component; however, angiomyofibroblastoma has more numerous vessels that are smaller, thin-walled, and more delicate than the medium-sized and often hyalinized vessels of cellular angiofibroma. In addition, angiomyofibroblastoma characteristically exhibits alternating zones of cellularity, a feature that is not common in cellular angiofibroma, which is more often uniformly cellular but occasionally may have zones of decreased cellularity secondary to edema. RB1 expression is typically lost in cellular angiofibroma but intact in angiomyofibroblastoma. Furthermore, desmin expression is uncommon in cellular angiofibroma, and angiomyofibroblastoma is typically negative for CD34.

Mammary-type myofibroblastoma and cellular angiofibroma show similar morphologic features, both being well-circumscribed tumors composed of intersecting fascicles of bland spindle-shaped cells embedded in a collagenous stroma. Although the vessels in mammary-type myofibroblastoma are not as prominent as those seen in cellular angiofibroma, when present, they often contain hyalinized walls. Moreover, both tumors may have an intralesional component of adipose tissue and can be positive for CD34. Desmin is usually positive in mammary-type myofibroblastoma but is uncommon in cellular angiofibroma. These tumors are likely closely related because both have similar genetic findings with loss of 13q14 (and loss of RB1 protein) and probably represent a spectrum of tumors with variable vascularity and cellularity.

Prepubertal vulval fibroma is distinguished from cellular angiofibroma by its more common occurrence in young girls, as well as by its ill-defined margins, hypocellular appearance, and patternless (as opposed to intersecting fascicular) proliferation of bland spindle cells.

Deep (aggressive) angiomyxoma differs from cellular angiofibroma by more often involving deep soft tissue and having an infiltrative margin. In addition, it is characteristically myxoid and paucicellular, in contrast to cellular angiofibroma, which is typically a cellular neoplasm that lacks myxoid stroma. Moreover, RB1 expression is intact.

Prognosis and Treatment

If completely excised, there is no potential for recurrence. Therefore local conservative excision with negative margins is adequate treatment.

PRACTICE POINTS: Cellular Angiofibroma

- Well-circumscribed, benign tumor with a prominent vascular component composed of small- to medium-sized vessels with hyalinized walls, admixed with bland spindle cells arranged in short fascicles
- Most common in vulva and inguinoscrotal region but may occur at extragenital sites
- Majority positive for CD34; subset positive for actin and desmin
- Member of family of tumors characterized by loss of *RB1*/13q14 with associated loss of RB1 expression

Prepubertal Vulval Fibroma

Prepubertal vulval fibroma is mass forming and has the potential to recur, features that favor classification as a neoplasm. However, some have suggested that this process is better classified as a nonneoplastic physiologic response of the vulval mesenchyme to hormonal surges around puberty, resulting in asymmetric enlargement of the labium majus.[50,51]

Clinical Features

Prepubertal vulval fibroma typically occurs in young girls, who usually present with painless, gradual vulval swelling or enlargement, most commonly of the labia majora.

Pathologic Features

Tumors are unilateral, ill-defined submucosal or subcutaneous masses that are typically smaller than 5 cm in greatest dimension. Histologically, they are poorly marginated with no clear interface with the overlying epithelium or surrounding soft tissue. The lesion is hypocellular and composed of a patternless proliferation of bland, uniform spindle cells with ovoid nuclei and palely amphophilic cytoplasm set within a variably myxoid, edematous, or collagenous matrix (Figs. 17.13 and 17.14). The spindle cells permeate into surrounding soft tissue including around adnexal structures, nerves, and into adipose tissue. Small- to medium-sized blood vessels, some with thickened walls, may be present. Mitotic activity is sparse, and nuclear pleomorphism is absent.

Immunohistochemistry

The spindle cells are typically reactive for CD34 but are negative for smooth muscle actin, desmin, and S-100 protein.

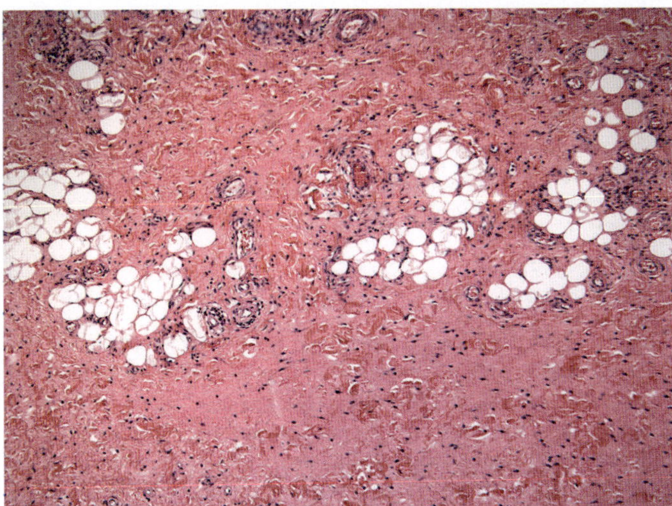

Figure 17.13 **Prepubertal Vulval Fibroma.** A patternless proliferation of bland spindle cells permeate surrounding soft tissue, including adipose tissue as illustrated here.

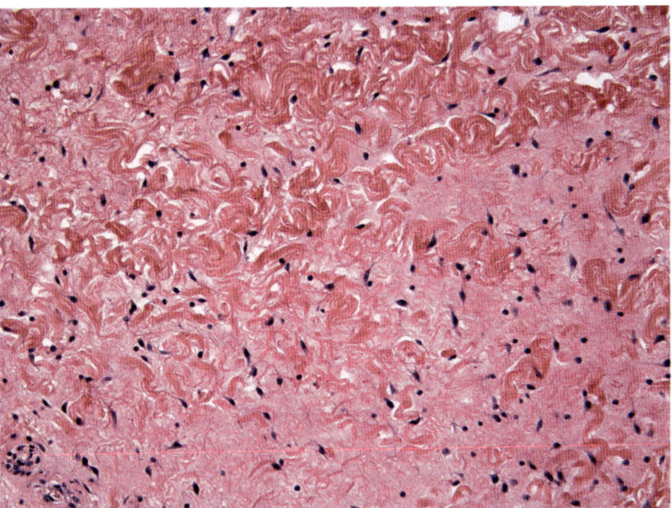

Figure 17.14 **Prepubertal Vulval Fibroma.** The bland spindle cells are set within a variably edematous to collagenous matrix.

Differential Diagnosis

Deep (aggressive) angiomyxoma, also a hypocellular infiltrative process, is distinguished from prepubertal vulval fibroma by occurring in older individuals, being more homogeneously myxoid, and containing uniformly distributed medium- to large-sized vessels with thickened walls. In addition, the presence of myoid bundles and lack of CD34 staining help in its identification.

Cellular angiofibroma is well circumscribed, more uniformly cellular, and more vascular than prepubertal vulval fibroma. In addition, it more commonly occurs in older women and shows loss of RB1 staining.

Angiomyofibroblastoma is distinguished from prepubertal vulval fibroma by its circumscribed margin, alternating zones of cellularity, characteristic clustering of epithelioid cells around the prominent capillary-sized vessels, and lack of staining for CD34.

Prognosis and Treatment

Prepubertal vulval fibromas are benign. However, lesions frequently recur when they are incompletely excised.

PRACTICE POINTS: Prepubertal Vulval Fibroma

- Poorly marginated, hypocellular proliferation of bland spindle cells set within a variably edematous, myxoid, or collagenous matrix
- Controversy over whether this represents a neoplasm or a physiologic response of mesenchyme to hormonal surges during puberty
- Lesional cells are CD34 positive
- Local recurrence if incompletely excised

Mammary-Type Myofibroblastoma

Mammary myofibroblastoma is a benign spindle cell neoplasm initially described to occur in the breast with a predilection for older men. Tumors with a similar morphologic appearance and immunophenotypic characteristics may occur at extramammary sites, particularly the inguinal/groin area, and are termed *mammary-type myofibroblastoma* (see also Chapter 3).[52,53]

Clinical Features

Mammary-type myofibroblastoma more commonly occurs in men, with a median age of 53 years. The neoplasm most often arises in the inguinal/groin area but has also been described (in descending order of frequency) in the chest wall/axilla, trunk, lower and upper extremities, and intraabdominal/retroperitoneal locations. Patients most commonly present with a slowly growing painless mass, or the tumor is discovered incidentally at the time of surgery.

Pathologic Features

Mammary-type myofibroblastomas are usually firm, pink to tan or brown, well-circumscribed tumors that range in size from 2 to 13 cm (median, 6 cm). They often have a whorled, nodular, and occasionally mucoid appearance on cut section. Histologically, they resemble mammary myofibroblastoma, being well-circumscribed, unencapsulated tumors composed of haphazardly arranged, variably sized fascicles of bland spindle to oval cells (Fig. 17.15). The tumor cells are set within a collagenous to myxoid matrix containing interspersed hyalinized collagen bundles, which separate the fascicles (Fig. 17.16). A variable amount of intralesional adipose tissue is typically present, and the relative proportion of adipose tissue and spindle cells varies considerably among tumors (see Figs. 17.16 and 17.17). The mitotic rate is typically low. Less commonly, focal cytologic atypia, epithelioid morphology, or schwannoma-type nuclear palisading may be seen.

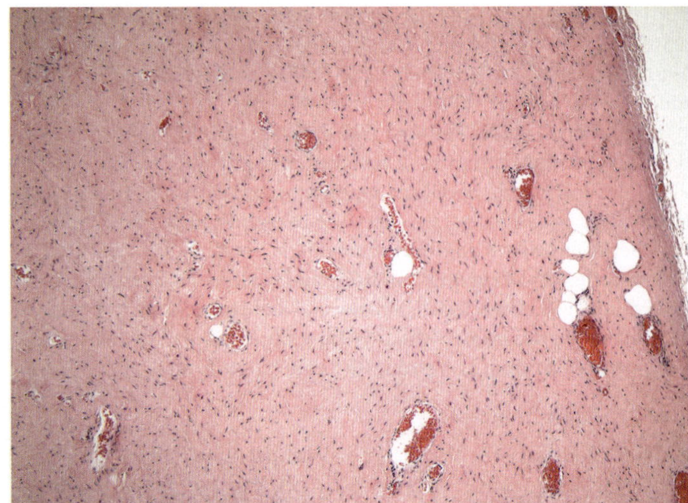

Figure 17.15 Mammary-Type Myofibroblastoma. A well-circumscribed tumor composed of haphazardly arranged fascicles of bland spindle cells.

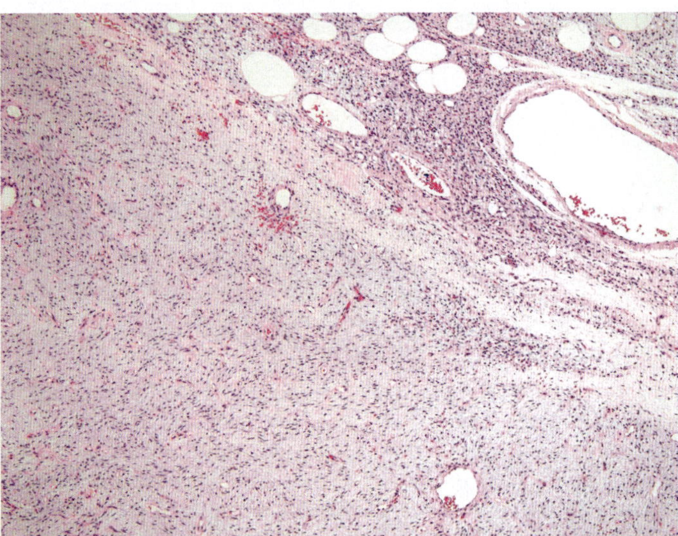

Figure 17.16 Mammary-Type Myofibroblastoma. Collections of adipocytes are present in this example. The amount of adipose tissue varies significantly between tumors.

Immunohistochemistry

The spindle cells are characteristically positive for both desmin and CD34 and occasionally reactive for smooth muscle actin. RB1 expression is lost in the vast majority of cases (>90%).

Molecular Genetics

Mammary-type myofibroblastoma appears to be closely related to spindle cell lipoma (see Chapter 12) and cellular angiofibroma. Evidence has shown that these tumor types, which show overlapping histologic and immunophenotypic features, have similar genetic findings with loss of 13q14, suggesting that they represent points along a single spectrum of genetically related tumors.[49,53]

Differential Diagnosis

Cellular angiofibroma and mammary-type myofibroblastoma are likely closely related tumors that are morphologically, immunophenotypically, and genetically similar. Cellular angiofibroma tends to have a more prominent vascular component and lacks the interspersed hyalinized collagen bundles.

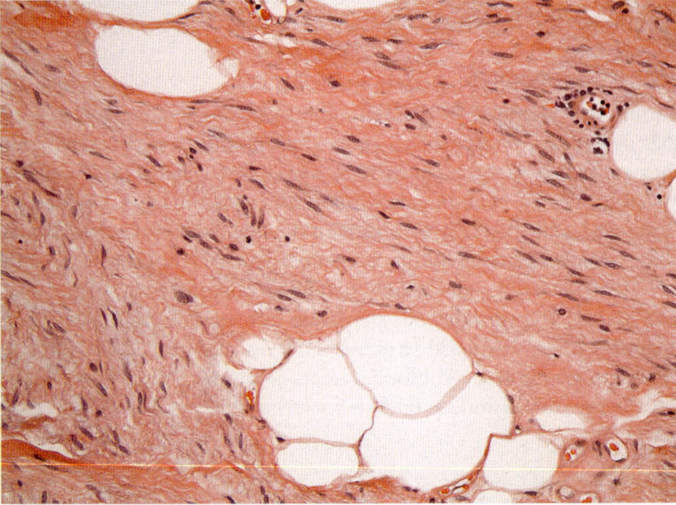

Figure 17.17 Mammary-Type Myofibroblastoma. Bland spindle cells with tapering nuclei in a collagenous stroma.

Angiomyofibroblastoma lacks the intersecting fascicles of bland spindle cells of mammary-type myofibroblastoma and instead is usually composed of rounded or epithelioid cells. Angiomyofibroblastoma has a more prominent vascular component with thin-walled capillaries. In addition, it is typically negative for CD34, and RB1 expression is intact.

Prepubertal vulval fibroma occurs at a younger age, is more infiltrative and less cellular, and lacks the fascicular architecture of mammary-type myofibroblastoma.

Deep (aggressive) angiomyxoma is more uniformly myxoid, paucicellular, and infiltrative than mammary-type myofibroblastoma. Deep angiomyxoma lacks the intersecting fascicles of bland spindle cells separated by hyalinized collagen bundles. In addition, RB1 expression is intact.

Prognosis and Treatment

Mammary-type myofibroblastoma is a benign tumor. Local excision is curative.

PRACTICE POINTS: Mammary-Type Myofibroblastoma

- Morphologically and immunophenotypically similar to its counterpart in the breast
- Benign tumor composed of adipose tissue and variably sized fascicles of bland spindle cells separated by hyalinized collagen bundles
- Relative proportions of adipose tissue and spindle cells vary
- Genetically related to spindle cell lipoma and cellular angiofibroma with shared loss of chromosome 13q14 and loss of RB1 expression

Spindle Cell Epithelioma

Spindle cell epitheliomas were formerly designated as mixed tumors based on their coexpression of keratin and smooth muscle actin, which suggested possible myoepithelial differentiation. However, it is now evident, based on additional immunohistochemical and ultrastructural findings, that these tumors do not in fact show true myoepithelial differentiation, and the term *spindle cell epithelioma* is therefore preferred.[54–56]

Clinical Features

The mean age of presentation with spindle cell epithelioma is the fourth decade. Patients typically present with a painless, submucosal mass that is usually smaller than 5 cm in greatest dimension. This benign tumor most commonly occurs in the distal portion of the vagina near the hymenal ring. This tumor, which also may be discovered during a routine gynecologic examination, is commonly thought clinically to represent a cyst or polyp.

Pathologic Features

Histologically, spindle cell epitheliomas are well-circumscribed, unencapsulated masses that are located adjacent to, but not connected with, the epithelial surface (Fig. 17.18). The tumors are composed of variably cellular proliferations of bland oval to spindle cells with paler hypocellular zones containing fibroblast-like cells separating the more cellular areas into nests and interconnecting islands (Fig. 17.19). Small foci of epithelial differentiation, most commonly nests and interlacing strands of squamous epithelium (which may have a vacuolated or glycogenated appearance), are usually present (Fig. 17.20). Eosinophilic hyaline globules, which likely represent condensation of the stromal matrix, are characteristic (Fig. 17.21).

Immunohistochemistry

The spindle cells are typically positive for keratins and smooth muscle actin and may be positive for desmin, CD34, CD10, and hormone

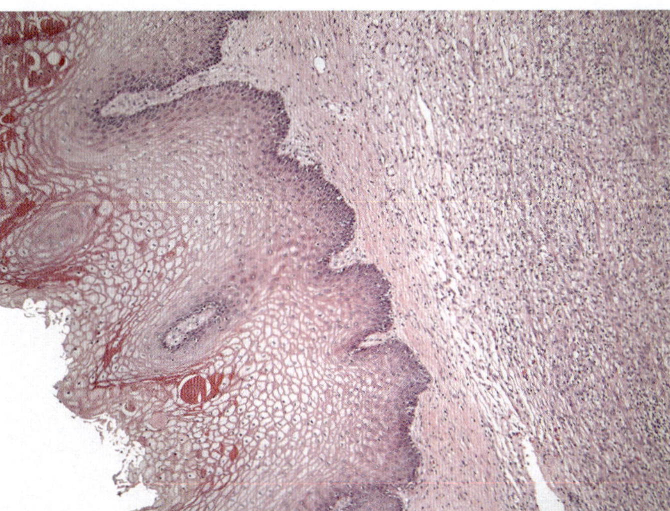

Figure 17.18 Spindle Cell Epithelioma. The tumors are situated close to the overlying epithelium but are not connected to it.

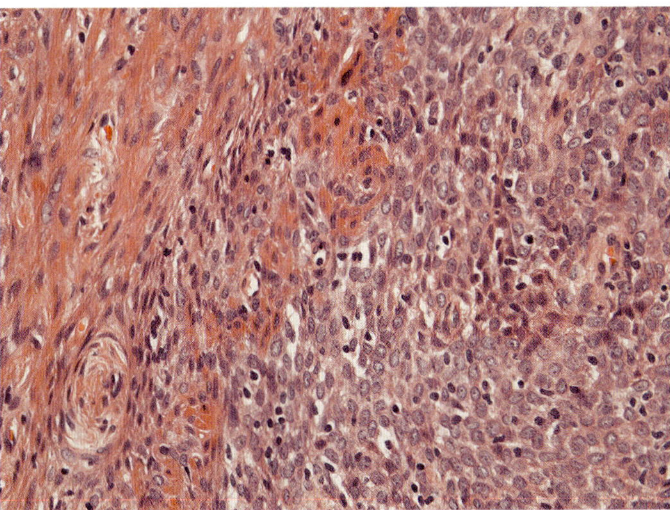

Figure 17.19 Spindle Cell Epithelioma. Alternating hypocellular areas composed of fibroblast-like spindle cells *(left side)* and hypercellular, syncytial areas composed of oval to short spindle cells with bland nuclei.

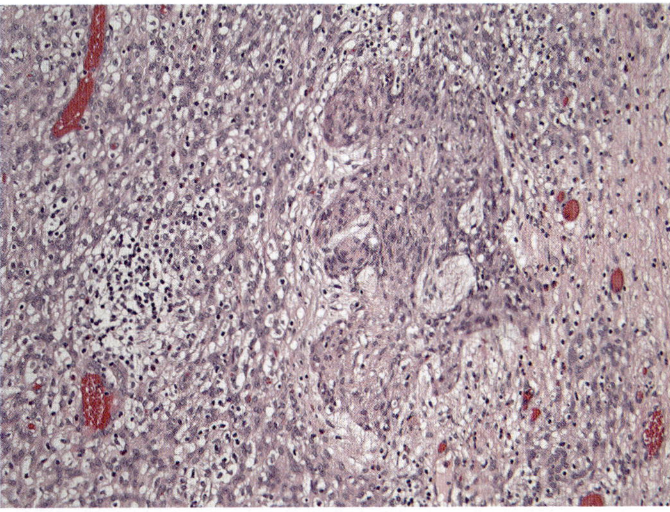

Figure 17.20 Spindle Cell Epithelioma. Small foci of epithelial differentiation are common, most often in the form of squamous nests.

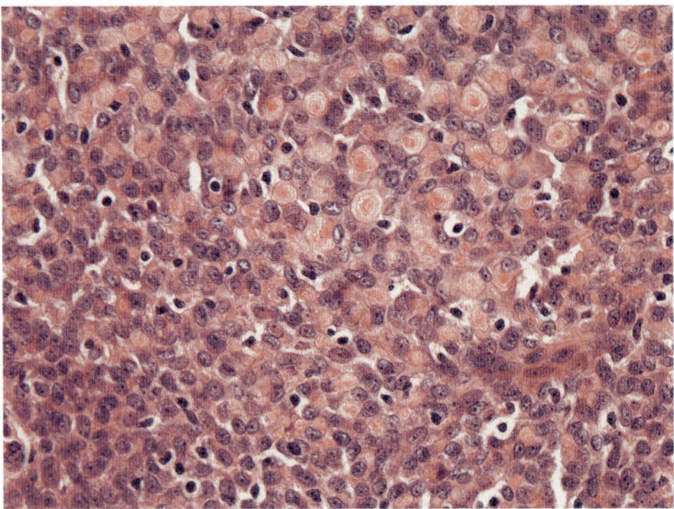

Figure 17.21 Spindle Cell Epithelioma. Eosinophilic hyaline globules are a characteristic finding.

receptors. However, they are negative for S-100 protein and glial fibrillary acidic protein (GFAP).

Differential Diagnosis

Angiomyofibroblastoma is also a well-circumscribed tumor with alternating cellularity. However, it is more vascular than spindle cell epithelioma and also lacks the highly cellular proliferation of spindle cells and foci of epithelial differentiation. In addition, angiomyofibroblastoma is negative for epithelial markers.

Cellular angiofibroma typically exhibits short intersecting fascicles of spindle cells and lacks the biphasic hypocellular and hypercellular areas of spindle cell epithelioma. In addition, cellular angiofibroma contains more prominent blood vessels and lacks the foci of epithelial differentiation. It is also negative for epithelial markers.

Mammary-type myofibroblastoma is composed of spindle cells in haphazardly arranged fascicles, which is not a feature of spindle cell epithelioma. In addition, mammary-type myofibroblastoma has a more collagenous matrix with bundles of hyalinized collagen and lacks expression of epithelial markers. It also shows loss of RB1 staining.

Prognosis and Treatment

Spindle cell epithelioma is a benign tumor, and local excision is curative. One example of a recurrence has been documented 8 years following initial excision.

PRACTICE POINTS: Spindle Cell Epithelioma

- Formerly designated "mixed tumor" but does not show true myoepithelial differentiation
- Most commonly involves distal vagina near hymenal ring
- Well-circumscribed, unencapsulated mass that is near, but not connected to, the epithelial surface
- Biphasic appearance on low-power examination secondary to variably cellular proliferation of spindle cells
- Small foci of epithelial differentiation, most commonly squamous, are typically present
- Spindle cells coexpress keratin and smooth muscle actin

Genital Rhabdomyoma

Genital rhabdomyoma is a benign tumor showing skeletal muscle differentiation. It most commonly occurs in the vagina but may also develop in the vulva and occasionally in the cervix.[57–59]

Clinical Features

Genital rhabdomyoma typically occurs in middle-aged women, with a mean age of 45 years. Patients present with a solitary, polypoid to nodular mass that varies in size (1–11 cm). The overlying mucosa is usually intact. Symptoms are generally related to the mass lesion and include dyspareunia and bleeding.

Pathologic Features

Histologically, genital rhabdomyoma is characterized by a submucosal, somewhat fascicular proliferation of spindle- or strap-shaped cells with plump oval nuclei and abundant, granular eosinophilic cytoplasm containing cross-striations (Fig. 17.22). The tumor cells are surrounded by a variable amount of fibrous stroma. Mitotic activity and nuclear pleomorphism are absent.

Immunohistochemistry

Special stains are rarely indicated, because the morphologic appearances are diagnostic. If necessary, skeletal muscle differentiation can be confirmed with skeletal muscle markers.

Differential Diagnosis

Embryonal rhabdomyosarcoma is the chief differential diagnostic consideration (see Chapter 8). Genital rhabdomyoma is distinguished from embryonal rhabdomyosarcoma by its lack of significant mitotic activity and nuclear atypia, as well as by the lack of a subepithelial cambium layer. In addition, genital rhabdomyoma occurs in an older population.

Prognosis and Treatment

Genital rhabdomyoma is benign. Local excision is curative.

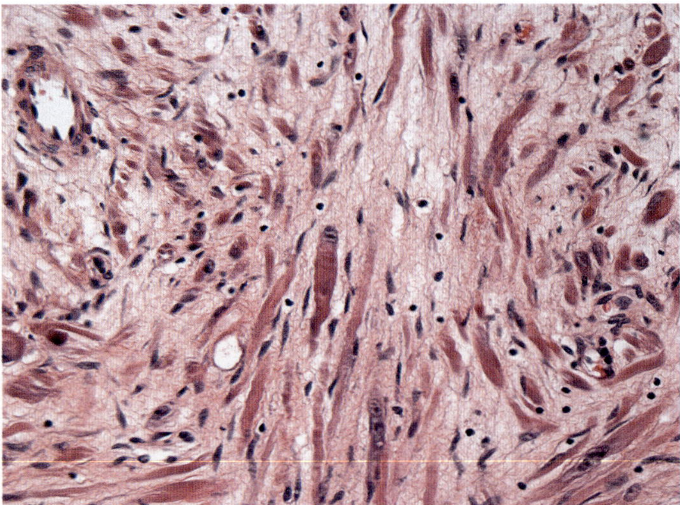

Figure 17.22 Genital Rhabdomyoma. Well-differentiated rhabdomyoblasts without atypia or mitotic activity are haphazardly arranged in a fibrous stroma.

PRACTICE POINTS: Genital Rhabdomyoma

- Benign tumor composed of well-differentiated rhabdomyoblasts
- Somewhat fascicular proliferation of spindle- or strap-shaped cells with easily identifiable cytoplasmic cross-striations
- No nuclear pleomorphism, subepithelial cambium layer, or mitotic activity
- Occurs in an older age group than embryonal rhabdomyosarcoma

Genital Smooth Muscle Tumors

Although genital (vulval and scrotal) smooth muscle tumors were initially considered within the category of superficial smooth muscle tumors, which includes pilar leiomyoma and angioleiomyoma, they are now classified separately based on their distinct clinical behavior, histologic features, and criteria for malignancy. Vulval and scrotal leiomyomas merit separate consideration due to differences in histologic appearances and behavior.[60–64]

Clinical Features

Vulval leiomyomas occur over a wide age range but are most common in the fourth and fifth decades. Patients typically present with a painless, well-circumscribed mass that is usually smaller than 3 cm in greatest dimension. Symptoms are related to a mass. Not uncommonly, the clinical impression is that of a cyst.

Scrotal smooth muscle tumors occur over a wide age range, with a mean in the sixth decade. Patients most commonly present with a painless mass with a mean size of 6.5 cm, which in general is greater than that seen for vulval leiomyoma.

Pathologic Features

Vulval leiomyomas typically exhibit characteristic smooth muscle morphology, being composed of intersecting fascicles of spindle cells with moderate amounts of eosinophilic cytoplasm and elongated to blunt-ended nuclei. Variable deposition of myxohyaline matrix, which imparts a plexiform or lacy appearance, is a morphologic pattern that is more commonly observed in vulval smooth muscle tumors compared with smooth muscle tumors occurring elsewhere in the female genital tract (Fig. 17.23). Due to the relative rarity of smooth muscle tumors of the vulva, in combination with the limited number of published series of cases with long-term follow-up, reliable prediction of which tumors are benign, which have recurrent potential, and which are malignant remains difficult. Although a combination of size, circumscription, nuclear atypia, and mitotic thresholds has been proposed to identify those tumors with recurrent potential, in the author's experience, any mitotic activity, nuclear pleomorphism, or infiltration of surrounding tissue may be associated with local recurrence, sometimes years after the initial excision. These observations suggest that smooth muscle tumors of the distal female genital tract fall along a biologic continuum with regard to their behavior and resist being rigidly classified into benign and malignant categories by currently definable histopathologic criteria. From a practical standpoint, the author advocates use of the term *atypical smooth muscle neoplasm* for those cases that have any of the following three histologic features: (1) any mitotic activity, (2) nuclear pleomorphism, or (3) infiltrative margins. Tumors with three or more of the following criteria should be diagnosed as *leiomyosarcoma*: (1) greater than 5 cm in size, (2) greater than 5 mitoses per 10 high-power fields, (3) infiltrative margins, and (4) moderate to severe cytologic atypia. Although necrosis is not included in this algorithm, its presence should strongly raise the possibility of malignancy.

Scrotal smooth muscle tumors usually have the typical morphologic appearances of smooth muscle neoplasms of other sites, with intersecting fascicles of eosinophilic spindle cells (Fig. 17.24) that may show areas

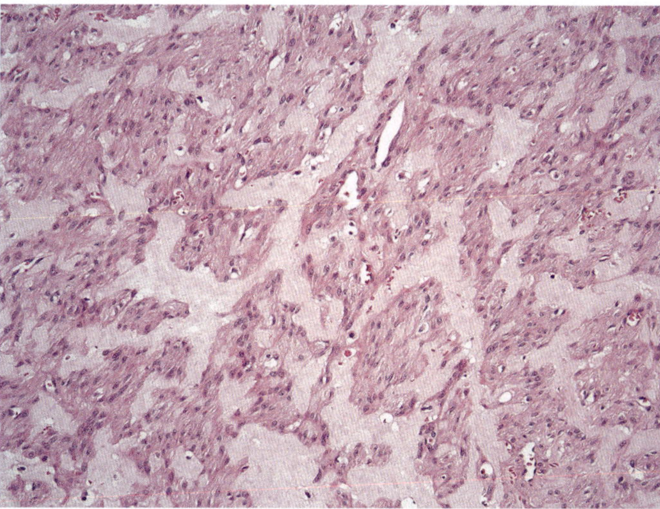

Figure 17.23 Vulval Leiomyoma. Deposition of myxohyaline matrix separates individual muscle fibers and imparts a plexiform appearance.

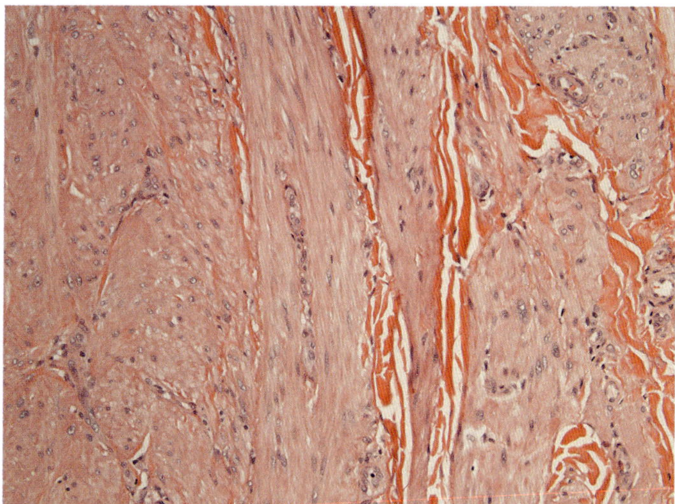

Figure 17.24 Scrotal Leiomyoma. Similar histologic appearances as smooth muscle tumors of other anatomic sites. Note the irregular margins *(right side).*

of hyalinization and degeneration but not the degree of secondary myxohyaline change as seen in vulval leiomyomas. However, unlike vulval tumors, scrotal smooth muscle tumors may show a greater degree of cellularity and often show focally infiltrative margins, which does not correlate with adverse outcome. Bizarre (symplastic) changes of tumor cell nuclei may also be present, which also does not appear to affect clinical outcome. Therefore the criteria for malignancy in scrotal smooth muscle tumors are different than those for vulval smooth muscle tumors, and, at this time, from a practical standpoint, the diagnosis of malignancy should be made when there is any degree of mitotic activity.

Immunohistochemistry

Vulval and scrotal smooth muscle neoplasms are typically positive for smooth muscle markers (smooth muscle actin, desmin, and h-caldesmon), and, in the case of vulval tumors, hormone receptors.

Differential Diagnosis

The main differential diagnostic consideration is the separation between benign smooth muscle tumors and those with recurrent and malignant potential, the criteria for which are outlined in the previous section.

Prognosis and Treatment

For malignant tumors and those associated with recurrent potential, at least a 1-cm margin of excision is recommended whenever possible with close, long-term follow-up.

PRACTICE POINTS: Genital Smooth Muscle Tumors

Vulval and scrotal smooth muscle tumors have differing criteria for malignancy
Scrotal smooth muscle tumors tend to be larger and more commonly have an infiltrative margin compared with vulval smooth muscle tumors
Vulval smooth muscle tumors with three or more of the following criteria should be diagnosed as leiomyosarcoma:
1. >5 cm in size
2. >5 mitoses per 10 high-power fields
3. Infiltrative margins
4. Moderate to severe cytologic atypia

Infiltrative margins, bizarre nuclear pleomorphism ("symplastic" change), and size do not correlate with adverse outcome in scrotal smooth muscle tumors
Scrotal smooth muscle tumors with any degree of mitotic activity should be considered malignant

References

1. Nucci MR, Fletcher CD: Vulvovaginal soft tissue tumours: update and review, *Histopathology* 36:97–108, 2000.
2. McCluggage WG: Recent developments in vulvovaginal pathology, *Histopathology* 54:156–173, 2009.
3. Nielsen GP, Young RH: Mesenchymal tumors and tumor-like lesions of the female genital tract: a selective review with emphasis on recently described entities, *Int J Gynecol Pathol* 20:105–127, 2001.
4. McCluggage WG: A review and update of morphologically bland vulvovaginal mesenchymal lesions, *Int J Gynecol Pathol* 24:26–38, 2005.
5. Steeper TA, Rosai J: Aggressive angiomyxoma of the female pelvis and perineum. Report of nine cases of a distinctive type of gynecologic soft-tissue neoplasm, *Am J Surg Pathol* 7:463–475, 1983.
6. Begin LR, Clement PB, Kirk ME, et al: Aggressive angiomyxoma of pelvic soft parts: a clinicopathologic study of nine cases, *Hum Pathol* 16:621–628, 1985.
7. Fetsch JF, Laskin WB, Lefkowitz M, et al: Aggressive angiomyxoma: a clinicopathologic study of 29 female patients, *Cancer* 78:79–90, 1996.
8. Granter SR, Nucci MR, Fletcher CD: Aggressive angiomyxoma: reappraisal of its relationship to angiomyofibroblastoma in a series of 16 cases, *Histopathology* 30:3–10, 1997.
9. Tsang WY, Chan JK, Lee KC, et al: Aggressive angiomyxoma. A report of four cases occurring in men, *Am J Surg Pathol* 16:1059–1065, 1992.
10. Iezzoni JC, Fechner RE, Wong LS, et al: Aggressive angiomyxoma in males. A report of four cases, *Am J Clin Pathol* 104:391–396, 1995.
11. van Roggen JF, van Unnik JA, Briaire-de Bruijn IH, et al: Aggressive angiomyxoma: a clinicopathological and immunohistochemical study of 11 cases with long-term follow-up, *Virchows Arch* 446:157–163, 2005.
12. McCluggage WG, Patterson A, Maxwell P: Aggressive angiomyxoma of pelvic parts exhibits oestrogen and progesterone receptor positivity, *J Clin Pathol* 53:603–605, 2000.
13. McCluggage WG, Connolly L, McBride HA: HMGA2 is a sensitive but not specific marker of vulvovaginal aggressive angiomyxoma, *Am J Surg Pathol* 34:1037–1042, 2010.
14. Kazmierczak B, Dal Cin P, Wanschura S, et al: Cloning and molecular characterization of part of a new gene fused to HMGIC in mesenchymal tumors, *Am J Pathol* 152:431–435, 1998.
15. Nucci MR, Weremowicz S, Neskey DM, et al: Chromosomal translocation t(8;12) induces aberrant HMGIC expression in aggressive angiomyxoma of the vulva, *Genes Chromosomes Cancer* 32:172–176, 2001.
16. Rabban JT, Dal Cin P, Oliva E: HMGA2 rearrangement in a case of vulvar aggressive angiomyxoma, *Int J Gynecol Pathol* 25:403–407, 2006.
17. Micci F, Panagopoulos I, Bjerkehagen B, et al: Deregulation of HMGA2 in an aggressive angiomyxoma with t(11;12)(q23;q15), *Virchows Arch* 448:838–842, 2006.
18. Rawlinson NJ, West WW, Nelson M, et al: Aggressive angiomyxoma with t(12;21) and HMGA2 rearrangement: report of a case and review of the literature, *Cancer Genet Cytogenet* 181:119–124, 2008.
19. Medeiros F, Erickson-Johnson MR, Keeney GL, et al: Frequency and characterization of HMGA2 and HMGA1 rearrangements in mesenchymal tumors of the lower genital tract, *Genes Chromosomes Cancer* 46:981–990, 2007.
20. McCluggage WG, Nielsen GP, Young RH: Massive vulval edema secondary to obesity and immobilization: a potential mimic of aggressive angiomyxoma, *Int J Gynecol Pathol* 27:447–452, 2008.
21. Fadare O, Brannan SM, Arin-Silasi D, et al: Localized lymphedema of the vulva: a clinicopathologic study of 2 cases and a review of the literature, *Int J Gynecol Pathol* 30:306–313, 2011.
22. Schwartz PE, Hui P, McCarthy S: Hormonal therapy for aggressive angiomyxoma: a case report and proposed management algorithm, *J Low Genit Tract Dis* 18:E55–E61, 2014.
23. Norris HJ, Taylor HB: Polyps of the vagina. A benign lesion resembling sarcoma botryoides, *Cancer* 19:227–232, 1966.
24. Elliott GB, Reynolds HA, Fidler HK: Pseudo-sarcoma botryoides of cervix and vagina in pregnancy, *J Obstet Gynaecol Br Commonw* 74:728–733, 1967.
25. Chirayil SJ, Tobon H: Polyps of the vagina: a clinicopathologic study of 18 cases, *Cancer* 47:2904–2907, 1981.
26. Miettinen M, Wahlstrom T, Vesterinen E, et al: Vaginal polyps with pseudosarcomatous features. A clinicopathologic study of seven cases, *Cancer* 51:1148–1151, 1983.
27. Ostor AG, Fortune DW, Riley CB: Fibroepithelial polyps with atypical stromal cells (pseudosarcoma botryoides) of vulva and vagina. A report of 13 cases, *Int J Gynecol Pathol* 7:351–360, 1988.
28. Mucitelli DR, Charles EZ, Kraus FT: Vulvovaginal polyps. Histologic appearance, ultrastructure, immunocytochemical characteristics, and clinicopathologic correlations, *Int J Gynecol Pathol* 9:20–40, 1990.
29. Nucci MR, Fletcher CD: Fibroepithelial stromal polyps of vulvovaginal tissue: from the banal to the bizarre, *Pathol Case Rev* 3:151–157, 1998.
30. Nucci MR, Young RH, Fletcher CD: Cellular pseudosarcomatous fibroepithelial stromal polyps of the lower female genital tract: an underrecognized lesion often misdiagnosed as sarcoma, *Am J Surg Pathol* 24:231–240, 2000.
31. Fletcher CD, Tsang WY, Fisher C, et al: Angiomyofibroblastoma of the vulva. A benign neoplasm distinct from aggressive angiomyxoma, *Am J Surg Pathol* 16:373–382, 1992.
32. Nielsen GP, Rosenberg AE, Young RH, et al: Angiomyofibroblastoma of the vulva and vagina, *Mod Pathol* 9:284–291, 1996.
33. Ockner DM, Sayadi H, Swanson PE, et al: Genital angiomyofibroblastoma. Comparison with aggressive angiomyxoma and other myxoid neoplasms of skin and soft tissue, *Am J Clin Pathol* 107:36–44, 1997.
34. Fukunaga M, Nomura K, Matsumoto K, et al: Vulval angiomyofibroblastoma. Clinicopathologic analysis of six cases, *Am J Clin Pathol* 107:45–51, 1997.
35. Hisaoka M, Kouho H, Aoki T, et al: Angiomyofibroblastoma of the vulva: a clinicopathologic study of seven cases, *Pathol Int* 45:487–492, 1995.
36. Laskin WB, Fetsch JF, Tavassoli FA: Angiomyofibroblastoma of the female genital tract: analysis of 17 cases including a lipomatous variant, *Hum Pathol* 28:1046–1055, 1997.
37. Cao D, Srodon M, Montgomery EA, et al: Lipomatous variant of angiomyofibroblastoma: report of two cases and review of the literature, *Int J Gynecol Pathol* 24:196–200, 2005.
38. Luis PP, Quinonez E, Nogales FF, et al: Lipomatous variant of angiomyofibroblastoma involving the vulva: report of 3 cases of an extremely rare neoplasm with discussion of the differential diagnosis, *Int J Gynecol Pathol* 34:204–207, 2015.
39. Sims SM, Stinson K, McLean FW, et al: Angiomyofibroblastoma of the vulva: a case report of a pedunculated variant and review of the literature, *J Low Genit Tract Dis* 16:149–154, 2012.
40. Chen BJ, Marino-Enriquez A, Fletcher CD, et al: Loss of retinoblastoma protein expression in spindle cell/pleomorphic lipomas and cytogenetically related tumors: an immunohistochemical study with diagnostic implications, *Am J Surg Pathol* 36:1119–1128, 2012.
41. Magro G, Righi A, Caltabiano R, et al: Vulvovaginal angiomyofibroblastomas: morphologic, immunohistochemical, and fluorescence in situ hybridization analysis for deletion of 13q14, *Hum Pathol* 45:1647–1655, 2014.
42. Nucci MR, Granter SR, Fletcher CD: Cellular angiofibroma: a benign neoplasm distinct from angiomyofibroblastoma and spindle cell lipoma, *Am J Surg Pathol* 21:636–644, 1997.
43. Laskin WB, Fetsch JF, Mostofi FK: Angiomyofibroblastomalike tumor of the male genital tract: analysis of 11 cases with comparison to female angiomyofibroblastoma and spindle cell lipoma, *Am J Surg Pathol* 22:6–16, 1998.
44. Iwasa Y, Fletcher CD: Cellular angiofibroma: clinicopathologic and immunohistochemical analysis of 51 cases, *Am J Surg Pathol* 28:1426–1435, 2004.
45. McCluggage WG, Ganesan R, Hirschowitz L, et al: Cellular angiofibroma and related fibromatous lesions of the vulva: report of a series of cases with a morphological spectrum wider than previously described, *Histopathology* 45:360–368, 2004.
46. Dargent JL, de Saint Aubain N, et al: Cellular angiofibroma of the vulva: a clinicopathological study of two cases with documentation of some unusual features and review of the literature, *J Cutan Pathol* 30:405–411, 2003.
47. Chen E, Fletcher CD: Cellular angiofibroma with atypia or sarcomatous transformation: clinicopathologic analysis of 13 cases, *Am J Surg Pathol* 34:707–714, 2010.
48. Hameed M, Clarke K, Amer HZ, et al: Cellular angiofibroma is genetically similar to spindle cell lipoma: a case report, *Cancer Genet Cytogenet* 177:131–134, 2007.
49. Maggiani F, Debiec-Rychter M, Vanbockrijck M, et al: Cellular angiofibroma: another mesenchymal tumour with 13q14 involvement, suggesting a link with spindle cell lipoma and (extra)-mammary myofibroblastoma, *Histopathology* 51:410–412, 2007.
50. Iwasa Y, Fletcher CD: Distinctive prepubertal vulval fibroma: a hitherto unrecognized mesenchymal tumor of prepubertal girls: analysis of 11 cases, *Am J Surg Pathol* 28:1601–1608, 2004.
51. Vargas SO, Kozakewich HP, Boyd TK, et al: Childhood asymmetric labium majus enlargement: mimicking a neoplasm, *Am J Surg Pathol* 29:1007–1016, 2005.
52. McMenamin ME, Fletcher CD: Mammary-type myofibroblastoma of soft tissue: a tumor closely related to spindle cell lipoma, *Am J Surg Pathol* 25:1022–1029, 2001.
53. Howitt BE, Fletcher CD: Mammary-type myofibroblastoma: clinicopathologic characterization in a series of 143 cases, *Am J Surg Pathol* 40:361–367, 2016.

54. Branton PA, Tavassoli FA: Spindle cell epithelioma, the so-called mixed tumor of the vagina. A clinicopathologic, immunohistochemical, and ultrastructural analysis of 28 cases, *Am J Surg Pathol* 17:509–515, 1993.
55. Wright RG, Buntine DW, Forbes KL: Recurrent benign mixed tumor of the vagina, *Gynecol Oncol* 40:84–86, 1991.
56. Murdoch F, Sharma R, Al Nafussi A: Benign mixed tumor of the vagina: case report with expanded immunohistochemical profile, *Int J Gynecol Cancer* 13:543–547, 2003.
57. Chabrel CM, Beilby JO: Vaginal rhabdomyoma, *Histopathology* 4:645–651, 1980.
58. Hanski W, Hagel-Lewicka E, Daniszewski K: Rhabdomyomas of female genital tract. Report on two cases, *Zentralbl Pathol* 137:439–442, 1991.
59. Iversen UM: Two cases of benign vaginal rhabdomyoma. Case reports, *APMIS* 104:575–578, 1996.
60. Newman PL, Fletcher CD: Smooth muscle tumours of the external genitalia: clinicopathological analysis of a series, *Histopathology* 18:523–529, 1991.
61. Tavassoli FA, Norris HJ: Smooth muscle tumors of the vulva, *Obstet Gynecol* 53:213–217, 1979.
62. Tavassoli FA, Norris HJ: Smooth muscle tumors of the vagina, *Obstet Gynecol* 53:689–693, 1979.
63. Nielsen GP, Rosenberg AE, Koerner FC, et al: Smooth-muscle tumors of the vulva. A clinicopathological study of 25 cases and review of the literature, *Am J Surg Pathol* 20:779–793, 1996.
64. Hornick JL, Fletcher CD: Criteria for malignancy in nonvisceral smooth muscle tumors, *Ann Diagn Pathol* 7:60–66, 2003.

18

Applications of Molecular Testing to Differential Diagnosis

Wei-Lien Wang, MD, and Alexander J. Lazar, MD, PhD

Soft tissue sarcomas are a complex family of rare malignant neoplasms that show mesenchymal differentiation. Benign soft tissue tumors are more common than their malignant counterparts. Both benign and malignant mesenchymal tumors can cause diagnostic confusion. The previous chapters of this book have discussed the characteristics of these tumors as groups based on their morphologic similarities and stressed the features that allow their proper classification primarily based on histologic, immunophenotypic, and clinical features. Classification schemes for sarcomas, on which specific diagnoses are based, have gone through many iterations, with histochemistry, electron microscopy, and immunohistochemistry all making important contributions. Currently, molecular genetic approaches to members of this tumor family play an important role in their classification. More pangenomic approaches—such as comparative genomic hybridization, gene expression arrays, and next-generation sequencing (NGS)—are poised to make important contributions not only to our biologic understanding but also to classification, prognostication, and treatment approaches for these tumors. The basis and role of current clinical molecular testing is presented to demonstrate the practical applications of these methods to the daily practice of a surgical pathologist. Although diagnostic cytogenetic features of benign soft tissue neoplasms are discussed here, this chapter focuses chiefly on malignant tumors, because molecular testing is most commonly used in the differential diagnosis of sarcomas.

Genetic Classification of Sarcomas

Soft tissue sarcomas can be divided broadly into two groups based on their cytogenetic features. One group is made up of sarcomas with simple cytogenetics consisting of relatively normal chromosomal complements and featuring chromosomal translocations (e.g., Ewing sarcoma and synovial sarcoma) or single-gene mutations (e.g., gastrointestinal stromal tumor [GIST] and desmoid fibromatosis), which can be used to support a specific diagnosis. The other group is made up of those with aneuploidy and complex cytogenetic features that lack specificity.[1] The latter sarcomas are listed in Table 18.1. A complex karyotype derived from an undifferentiated pleomorphic sarcoma is depicted in Fig. 18.1. These are commonly associated with *TP53* and/or *RB1* (retinoblastoma) disruption and often show telomere dysfunction. Although they are not specific, the existence of such complex karyotypes can imply malignancy. It is in this tumor family that high-throughput genetic techniques allowing examination of the entire cancer genome may ultimately have great impact. One example of the utility of this approach is the recent discovery that malignant peripheral nerve sheath tumors have loss of histone H3 K27 trimethylation (H3K27me3). Loss of H3K27me3 can be detected by immunohistochemistry, is diagnostically useful, and portends a worse prognosis.[2,3] Other examples in this class of tumors include *IDH* 1/2 and *COL2A1* mutations in chondrosarcomas and *MYC* amplification in radiation-associated angiosarcomas.[4-7]

Within the group of sarcomas with relatively simple cytogenetic changes are some that lack recurrent molecular diagnostic features (e.g., embryonal rhabdomyosarcoma). These are listed in Table 18.2, along with other, mostly benign soft tissue neoplasms for which testing is not generally indicated or utilized. Finally, Table 18.3 includes the group of soft tissue sarcomas (approximately one-third of all soft tissue sarcoma types) associated with genetic changes that are diagnostic when encountered and that provide the molecular basis for commonly used diagnostic tests. With this classification scheme in mind, the chapter presents the types of molecular testing available and then briefly discusses the entities listed in Table 18.3, with a focus on situations where molecular diagnostics are particularly relevant and helpful.

Over the past several decades, there has been a considerable increase in our understanding of the genetic basis of cancer, including sarcomas. Sarcomas have been amenable to a classic cytogenetic approach because, like many hematopoietic malignancies, a considerable subset has

Table 18.1 Sarcomas With Complex Cytogenetic Features

Sarcoma Type	Cytogenetic Alterations	Molecular Alterations
Angiosarcoma	Complex with various recurrent mutations including *MYC* in postradiation cases	The molecular alterations are complex, usually with extensive copy number alterations (deletions > gains), but often involving the *TP53* and/or *RB1* genes and pathways, sometimes combined with telomere dysfunction (± *ATRX* loss-of-function mutations)
Chondrosarcoma	Complex with various recurrent mutations such as *IDH1/2* in conventional chondrosarcomas	
Leiomyosarcoma	Complex with frequent deletion of 1p	
Malignant peripheral nerve sheath tumor	Complex; loss-of-function mutations in *NF1* often with *EED* or *SUZ12*, resulting in loss of histone H3 K27 trimethylation	
Pleomorphic liposarcoma	Complex	
Pleomorphic rhabdomyosarcoma	Complex	
Undifferentiated pleomorphic sarcoma	Complex	

Table 18.2 Soft Tissue Tumors With Simple Cytogenetic Features, Possibly Useful

Tumor Type	Cytogenetic Alterations	Molecular Alterations
Embryonal rhabdomyosarcoma	Trisomies 2q, 8, and 20	LOH at 11p15
Hibernoma	11q13 rearrangements	*MEN1* deletions
Leiomyoma	12q15 rearrangements	*HMGA2* overexpression *MED12* mutation (uterine) *ALK* rearrangement (GI)
Lipoblastoma	8q11–13 rearrangements	*HAS2-PLAG1* fusion *COL1A2-PLAG1* fusion
Spindle cell/sclerosing rhabdomyosarcoma	11p15 mutation	*MYOD1* mutation
Spindle cell/pleomorphic lipoma	13q or 16q deletions	*RB1* locus and unknown
Chondroid lipoma	t(11;16)(q13;p12–13)	*C11orf95-MKL2* fusion
Neurofibroma	Monosomy 17	*NF1* mutation and LOH
Pericytoma	t(7;12)(p21–22;q13–15)	*ACTB-GLI* fusion
Schwannoma	Monosomy 22	*NF2* mutation and LOH
Tenosynovial giant cell tumor	1p13 rearrangements	*CSF1* overexpression

LOH, Loss of heterozygosity.

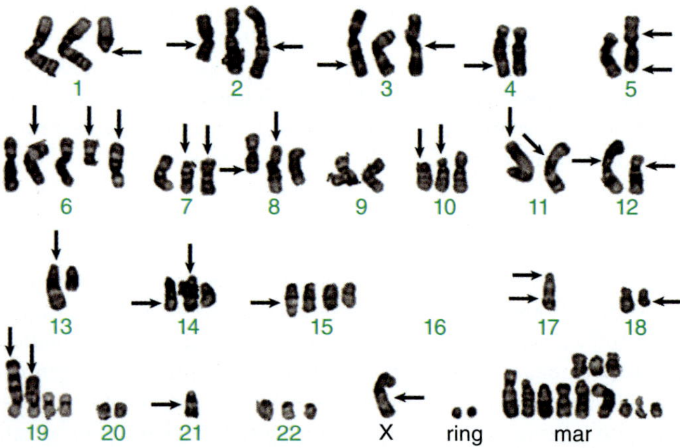

Figure 18.1 **Complex Karyotype.** This karyotype from an undifferentiated pleomorphic sarcoma shows numerous cytogenetic aberrations characteristic of sarcomas with complex cytogenetic features. (Courtesy Dr. Andre Oliveira, Mayo Clinic, Rochester, MN.)

chromosomal translocations that can be detected by standard karyotyping of fresh tumor samples grown in culture. Ewing sarcoma was the first sarcoma and solid tumor noted to harbor such a translocation (Fig. 18.2). For this reason and because the features of this tumor make it an ideal archetype, it is used in the following text to demonstrate the methods and principles of molecular diagnostic testing. Subsequently, an alphabetically ordered discussion of each soft tissue tumor with relevant molecular diagnostic features is briefly presented, including reference to other chapters in this book where the lesions are discussed in more detail.

It is interesting to note that the majority of sarcomas with unique chromosomal translocations tend to occur in younger patients, whereas those with more complex cytogenetic features tend to present in older ones. Furthermore, many soft tissue sarcomas with differentiation patterns that do not clearly recapitulate features of a known mature mesenchymal tissue (e.g., Ewing sarcoma, synovial sarcoma, and alveolar soft part sarcoma) harbor translocations (Box 18.1). The significance of these intriguing associations is unclear. Each of these entities is discussed in detail in the preceding chapters; thus, here the discussion is strictly limited to the relevant molecular diagnostic considerations. The reader is encouraged to refer to the prior chapters and sections covering the individual entities for additional information. The role of these genetic events in the molecular pathogenesis of these neoplasms is a fascinating and rapidly evolving field, but a detailed discussion of each sarcoma presented subsequently is beyond the scope of this chapter.

Approaches to Molecular Diagnostics

The Paradigm of Ewing Sarcoma

Ewing sarcoma was the first sarcoma recognized to have a recurrent cytogenetic abnormality, namely a balanced translocation between chromosomes 11 and 22 (see Fig. 18.2),[8,9] which was initially discovered by chromosomal karyotypic analysis of cultured fresh human tumor. Further analysis refined the genetic intervals to 11q24 and 22q12, which were ultimately shown to contain the *FLI1* and *EWSR1* genes, respectively.[10,11] Because this chromosomal rearrangement involves the transposition of material between two chromosomes without loss of genetic material, it is termed a balanced translocation. The two break points on chromosomes 11 and 22 occur in noncoding DNA introns; thus, when the chromosomes join, the exons from the two genes are in frame and ultimately produce a novel fusion or chimeric gene encoding a protein with an aberrant function (Fig. 18.3). In Ewing sarcoma, this is a novel transcription factor wherein *FLI1* provides the DNA-binding domain and the *EWSR1* portion acts as a transactivator.[12] This transcriptional activation may involve additional protein intermediaries, which is a topic of active research. This translocation is likely an early and necessary pathogenetic event, because the vast majority of well-characterized cases of Ewing sarcoma contain this or an analogous rearrangement.[8] Additional genetic events are probably necessary, with this fusion gene likely relying on a specific cellular compartment to exert its effect (so-called lineage addiction or specificity).

The break points within both *FLI1* and *EWSR1* can involve multiple different introns in each gene; thus, numerous different fusion transcripts

Table 18.3 Soft Tissue Tumors With Simple Cytogenetic Features, Virtually Diagnostic in Appropriate Clinicopathologic Context

Sarcoma Type	Cytogenetic Alterations	Molecular Alterations
Alveolar rhabdomyosarcoma	t(2;13)(q35;q14) t(1;13)(p36;q14), double minutes t(2;2)(q35;p23) t(X;2)(q35;q13)	*PAX3-FOXO1A* fusion *PAX7-FOXO1A* fusion *PAX3-NCOA1* fusion *PAX3-AFX* fusion
Alveolar soft part sarcoma	t(X;17)(p11;q25)	*TFE3-ASPSCR1* fusion[a]
Aneurysmal bone cyst	t(16;17)(q22;p13)	*CDH11-USP6* fusion
Angiomatoid fibrous histiocytoma	t(12;16)(q13;p11) t(12;22)(q13;q12) t(2;22)(q33;q12)	*FUS-ATF1* fusion *EWSR1-ATF1* fusion[a] *EWSR1-CREB1* fusion
Clear cell sarcoma	t(12;22)(q13;q12) t(2;22)(q33;q12)	*EWSR1-ATF1* fusion[a] *EWSR1-CREB1* fusion
Cellular fibroma of tendon sheath	17p13	*USP6* with unknown fusion partners
Desmoid fibromatosis	Trisomies 8 and 20 and loss of 5q21	*CTNNB1* or *APC* mutation[a]
Desmoplastic small round cell tumor	t(11;22)(p13;q12)	*EWSR1-WT1* fusion
Dermatofibrosarcoma protuberans	Ring form of chromosomes 17 and 22 t(17;22)(q21;q13)	*COL1A1-PDGFB* fusion *COL1A1-PDGFB* fusion
Dermatofibroma/fibrous histiocytoma	t(3;11)(p21;q13)	*LAMTOR1-PRKCD* fusion *NUMA1-SFMBT1* fusion
Epithelioid fibrous histiocytoma	2p23	*VCL-ALK* fusion *SQSTM1-ALK* fusion
Endometrial stromal sarcoma	t(7;17)(p15;q21) t(6;7)(p21;7p15) t(6;10)(p21;p11)	*JAZF1-SUZ12* fusion *JAZF1-PHF1* fusion *EPC1-PHF1* fusion
Epithelioid hemangioendothelioma	t(1;3)(p36;q25) t(X;11)(p11;q22)	*WWTR1-CAMTA1* fusion *YAP1-TFE3* fusion
Epithelioid hemangioma of bone with atypical features	t(7;19)(q22;q13)	*ZFP36-FOSB* fusion
Ewing sarcoma	t(11;22)(q24;q12) t(21;22)(q12;q12) t(2;22)(q33;q12) t(7;22)(p22;q12) t(17;22)(q12;q12) inv(22)(q12;q12) t(16;21)(p11;q12) t(19;der)ins.inv(21;22) t(17;22)(q12;q12) t(6;22)(p21;q12) t(1;22)(q36.1;q12) t(2;22)(q31;q12) t(20;22)(q13;q12) t(2;16)(q35;p11) t(15;19)(q14;p13.1)	*EWSR1-FLI1* fusion *EWSR1-ERG* fusion *EWSR1-FEV* fusion *EWSR1-ETV1* fusion *EWSR1-E1AF* fusion *EWSR1-ZSG* fusion *FUS-ERG* fusion[a] *EWSR1-ERG* fusion *EWSR1-ETV4* fusion *EWSR1-POU5F1* fusion *EWSR1-PATZ1* fusion *EWSR1-SP3* fusion *EWSR1-NFATc2* fusion *FUS-FEV* fusion *BRD4-NUT* fusion[a]
Ewing-like tumor	t(4;19)(q35;q13) or t(10;19)(q26;q13) t(X;19)(q13;q13) Inv(X)(p11.4; p11.22) t(X;4)(p1.4;q31.1) t(X;22)(p1.4;q13)	*CIC-DUX4* fusion *CIC-FOXO4* fusion *BCOR-CCNB3* fusion *BCOR-MAML3* fusion *ZC3H7B-BCOR* fusion
Extraskeletal myxoid chondrosarcoma	t(9;22)(q22;q12) t(9;17)(q22;q11) t(9;15)(q22;q21) t(3;9)(q11;q22)	*EWSR1-NR4A3* fusion *TAF2N-NR4A3* fusion *TCF12-NR4A3* fusion *TFG-NR4A3* fusion
Fibrosarcoma, infantile/cellular mesoblastic nephroma	t(12;15)(p13;q26) Trisomies 8, 11, 17, and 20	*ETV6-NTRK3* fusion[a]
Gastrointestinal stromal tumor	Monosomies 14 and 22; deletion on 1p	*KIT* or *PDGFRA* mutation; rarely *BRAF*, *SDHA*, *SDHB*, *SDHC*, or *SDHD* mutations
Inflammatory myofibroblastic tumor	t(1;2)(q22;p23) t(2;19)(p23;p13) t(2;17)(p23;q23) t(2;2)(p23;q13) t(2;2)(p23;q35) t(2;11)(p23;p15) t(2;4)(p23;q21) t(2;12)(p23;p12)	*TPM3-ALK* fusion[a] *TPM4-ALK* fusion *CLTC-ALK* fusion[a] *RANBP2-ALK* fusion *ATIC-ALK* fusion[a] *CARS-ALK* fusion *SEC31L1-ALK* fusion *PPFIBP1-ALK* fusion
Intimal sarcoma	Chromosome 12	Amplification of *MDM2*
Low-grade fibromyxoid sarcoma	t(7;16)(q33;p11) t(11;16)(p11;p11)	*FUS-CREB3L2* fusion *FUS-CREB3L1* fusion
Lipofibromatosis-like neural tumor	1q23	*NTRK1* with various partners including *TFR* and *TPM3*
Mesenchymal chondrosarcoma	t(8;8)(q13;q21)	*HEY1-NCOA2* fusion
Myoepithelial tumors of soft tissue	t(6;22)(p21;q12) t(19;22)(q13;q12) t(1;22)(q23;q12)	*EWSR1-POU5F1* fusion *EWSR1-ZNF444* fusion *EWSR1-PBX1* fusion
Myxoid/round cell liposarcoma	t(12;16)(q13;p11) t(12;22)(q13;q12)	*FUS-DDIT3* fusion *EWSR1-DDIT3* fusion
Myxoinflammatory fibroblastic sarcoma/hemosiderotic fibrolipomatous tumor	t(1;10)(p22;q24) 3p11–12 (ring chromosomes)	*TGFBR3-MGEA5* fusion Amplification of *VGLL3*, *CHMP2B*
Nodular fasciitis	t(17;22)(p13;q13)	*MYH9-USP6* fusion
Ossifying fibromyxoid tumor	6p21	*PHF1* with various partners; one major partner is *EP400*
Primary pulmonary myxoid sarcoma of the lung	t(2;22)(q33;q12)	*EWSR1-CREB1* fusion
Pseudomyogenic hemangioendothelioma	t(7;19)(q22;q13)	*SERPINE1-FOSB* fusion
Sclerosing epithelioid fibrosarcoma	t(11;22)(p11;q12) t(11;16)(p11;p11) t(7;16)(p22;p11)	*EWSR1-CREB3L1* fusion *FUS-CREB3L1* fusion *FUS-CREB3L2* fusion
Solitary fibrous tumor	Inv(12)(q13q13)	*NAB2-STAT6* fusion
Synovial sarcoma		
Biphasic	t(X;18)(p11;q11)	Predominantly *SS18-SSX1* fusion
Monophasic	t(X;18)(p11;q11)	*SS18-SSX1*, *SSX2*, or *SSX4* fusion
Tenosynovial giant cell tumor	t(1;2)(p13;q35)	*COL6A3-CSF1* fusion
Well-differentiated liposarcoma/dedifferentiated liposarcoma	Ring form of chromosome 12	Amplification of *MDM2*, *CDK4*, and others

[a]These alterations are also present in other tumor types (including carcinomas, leukemias, or lymphomas).

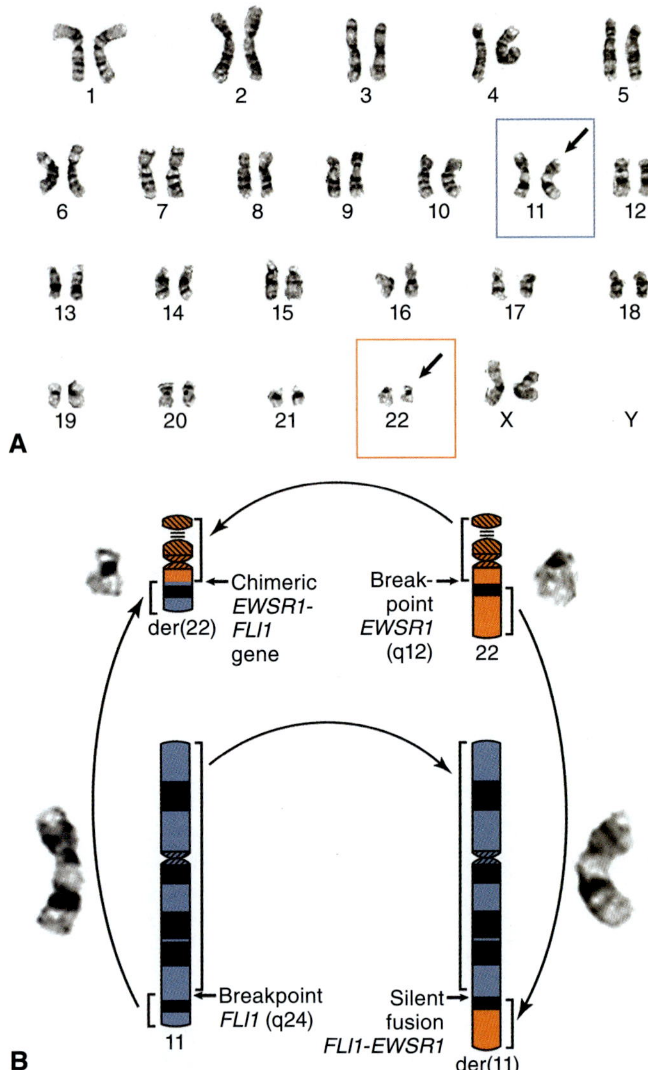

Figure 18.2 **Karyotype and Ideogram of Ewing Sarcoma.** (A) A simple karyotype shows the t(11;22)(q24;q12) in Ewing sarcoma. (B) Portions of chromosomes 11 and 22 involved in the balanced translocation lead to the active fusion gene at derivative chromosome 22 *(upper left)*. (A, Courtesy Dr. Lynne Abruzzo, Ohio State University Wexner Medical Center, Columbus, OH.)

Box 18.1 Soft Tissue Sarcomas and Mesenchymal Neoplasms of Uncertain Histogenesis With Characteristic Translocations

- Alveolar soft part sarcoma
- Angiomatoid fibrous histiocytoma
- Clear cell sarcoma of soft tissue
- Desmoplastic small round cell tumor
- Ewing sarcoma
- Extraskeletal myxoid chondrosarcoma
- Hemosiderotic fibrolipomatous tumor
- Myoepithelioma/myoepithelial carcinoma/mixed tumor
- Ossifying fibromyxoid tumor
- Phosphaturic mesenchymal tumor
- Synovial sarcoma

and corresponding proteins have been described (Fig. 18.4). The *EWSR1* gene occupies approximately 40 kb and is composed of 17 exons that encode a protein with homology to a putative RNA-binding site of RNA polymerase II. The precise function of the native Ewsr1 protein is unclear. Approximately 80% of the break points in *EWSR1* are located

Table 18.4 Estimated Percentages of Fusion Variants in Ewing Sarcoma

Variant	Percentage (%)
EWSR1-FLI1 (all types)	90
EWSR1-ERG	5
EWSR1-FEV	<1
EWSR1-ETV1	<1
EWSR1-ETV4	<1
EWSR1-ZSG	<1
FUS-ERG	<1
EWSR1-POU5F1	<1
EWSR1-PATZ1	<1
EWSR1-SP3	<1
EWSR1-NFATc2	<1
FUS-FEV	<1
BRD4-NUT	<1
None identified	Unknown

in introns 7 or 8 and result in a fusion transcript containing exons 1 to 7. Two particular fusion events are most common, constituting at least 80% of the fusions between these two genes, which are termed type 1 (60%) and type 2 (20%).[13] The remaining *EWSR1-FLI1* fusion types and other fusion variants are relatively rare as single entities (with the exception of *EWSR1-ERG,* about 5%) but as a whole may account for up to 10% of all cases. This may be an overestimate owing to the propensity of researchers to report rare events in the literature (Table 18.4), as many of these variants exist only as single case reports. There also appear to be cases of Ewing sarcoma in which a fusion gene cannot be demonstrated. Some of these tumors are now known, with the help of NGS, to represent histologically similar tumors with alternative translocations, including *CIC-DUX4* and *BCOR-CCNB3*.[14-17] Despite overlapping round cell morphology, these tumors appear to behave differently from Ewing sarcomas (see later discussion) and thus fall broadly under the rubric of unclassified round cell sarcoma in the classification scheme of the World Health Organization (WHO). Additional alternative fusions may be discovered, which might help classify these tumors when traditional morphologic features and immunohistochemical markers are insufficient.

The murine form of *FLI1* contains a Friend murine leukemia retroviral integration site. This gene belongs to the DNA-binding protein superfamily and is rearranged in the erythroleukemias induced by this virus. Human Fli1 shows 70% amino acid sequence homology with Ets1, a gene expressed during cranial neural crest migration and apparently also during vasculogenesis, where it appears to act as a transcription factor.[18,19] The alternative fusion partners that can substitute for *FLI1* are primarily members of the ETS gene family. The DNA-binding domain of Fli1 substitutes for the RNA-binding portion of Ewsr1 in the fusion protein, creating a novel transcription factor. *ERG* (21q22) and four other described members of the ETS gene family can substitute for *FLI1* in a small subset of cases.[20,21] *FUS* (16p11) has been reported to substitute for *EWSR1* in rare cases (see Chapter 8 for additional discussion of Ewing sarcoma). As illustrated in Fig. 18.5, *EWSR1* and *FUS*, a homologous gene, also contribute to multiple fusion genes present in a wide variety of soft tissue sarcomas.

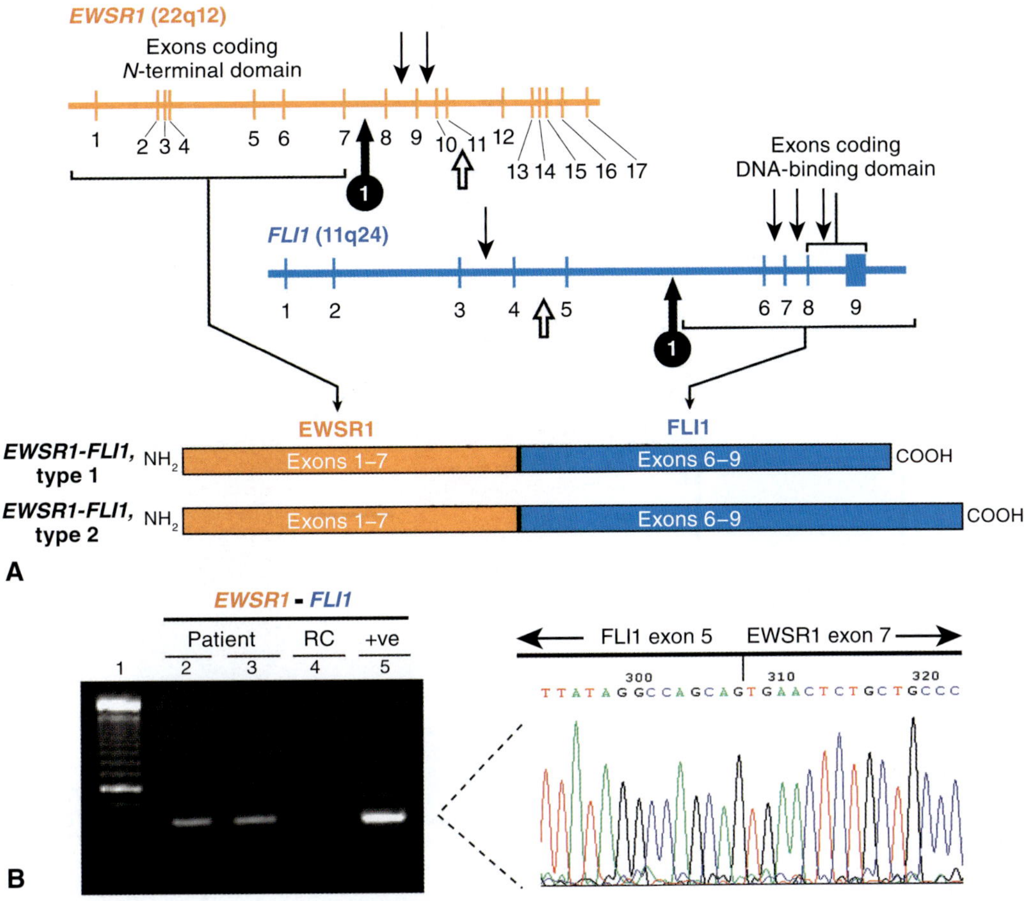

Figure 18.3 **Gene Fusion and Reverse Transcription Polymerase Chain Reaction (RT-PCR) Detection in Ewing Sarcoma.** (A) *EWSR1* and *FLI1* genes are depicted with exons shown as colored cross-hatches, with major intronic break points shown *(large arrows below the gene)* and more minor break points *(arrows above)*. The type 1 fusion transcript depicted below is derived from the break points indicated by the *black arrows* (numbered 1). (B) Gel electrophoresis of the RT-PCR amplicon and confirmation of the type 1 fusion transcript by Sanger sequencing. (B, Courtesy Dr. Dolores López-Terrada, Texas Children's Hospital and Baylor College of Medicine, Houston, TX.)

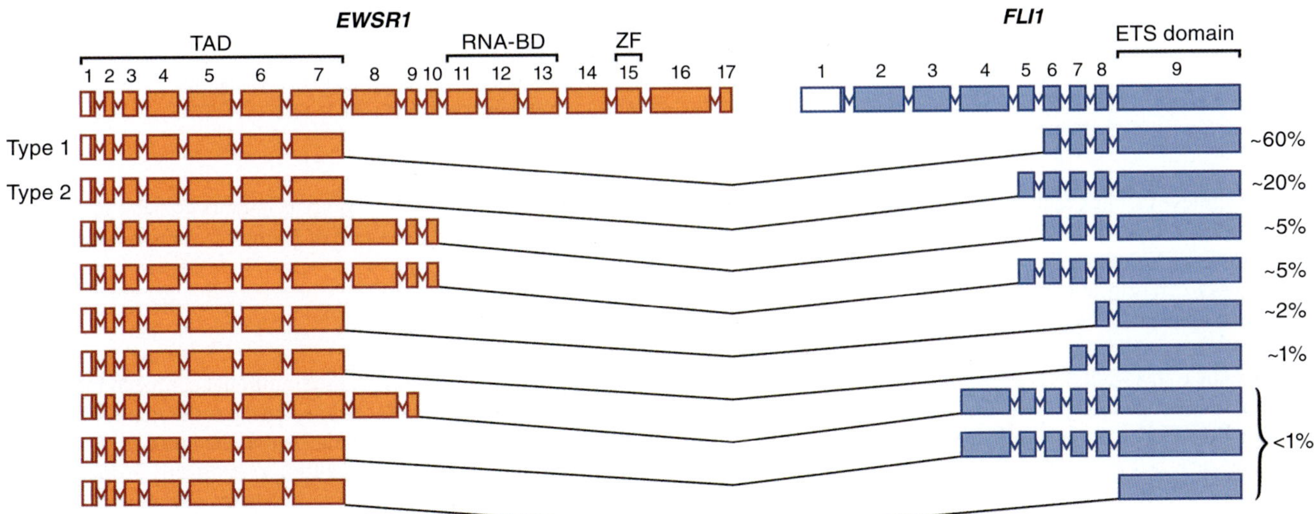

Figure 18.4 **EWSR1-FLI1 Fusion Transcript Types.** *EWSR1* is composed of 17 exons, whereas *FLI1* is composed of 9 exons. With types 1 and 2 dominating, the many fusion types of the *EWSR1-FLI1* fusion variant comprise up to 95% of the fusion events in Ewing sarcoma. *EWSR1-ERG* constitutes up to 5%, and the remaining variants are extremely rare (see Table 18.4). The *EWSR1-FLI1* fusion types retain the transactivation domain of *EWSR1* and the DNA-binding (ETS) domain of *FLI1*. *ETS* domain, highly conserved DNA-binding domain found in the ETS family of transcription factors. *RNA-BD*, RNA-binding domain; *TAD*, transactivation domain; *ZF*, zinc finger domain.

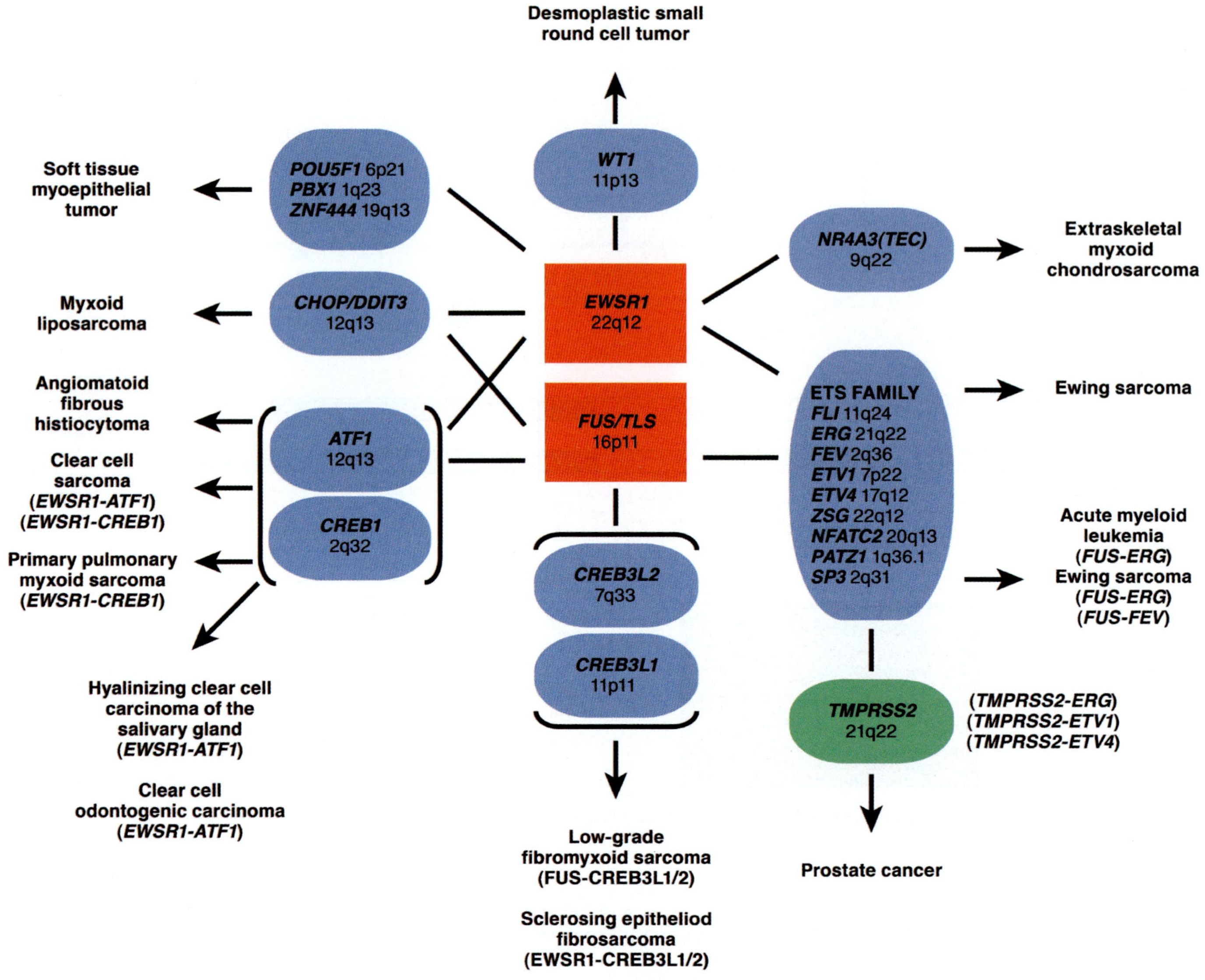

Figure 18.5 **Gene Fusion Variants Involving *EWSR1* and its Homolog *FUS*.** *EWSR1* and *FUS* can substitute for one another in several sarcoma types, but usually one is predominant. For instance, *EWSR1* is dominant in Ewing sarcoma, but *FUS* can be fused with *ERG*. In myxoid liposarcoma, *FUS* is predominantly translocated with *DDIT3*, and *EWSR1* can be a rare substitute. From this diagram, it is clear that there is relative specificity of fusion variant to specific tumor, but the *EWSR1-ATF1* and *EWSR1-CREB1* variants are seen in both clear cell sarcoma and angiomatoid fibrous histiocytoma, whereas *FUS-ERG* is described, albeit rarely, in both Ewing sarcoma and acute myeloid leukemia.

Previously, these fusion events had been considered to be unique to a specific tumor type; however, this assumption is no longer true. One example of this includes a class of tumors that have *EWSR1-CREB1* and *EWSR1-ATF1* translocations. These fusions are found in clear cell sarcoma, gastrointestinal clear cell sarcoma–like tumor, angiomatoid fibrous histiocytoma, and primary pulmonary myxoid sarcoma. Despite sharing the same translocation, these sarcomas have distinct histologic appearances, immunophenotypic findings, and behavior. *EWSR1-ATF1* has also been described in nonmesenchymal tumors and is characteristic of hyalinizing clear cell carcinoma of the salivary gland and clear cell odontogenic carcinoma. Another example of overlap includes Ewing sarcoma and acute myeloid leukemia (*FUS-ERG*). Therefore not all fusion transcripts, nor the genes they involve, are necessarily exclusive to a single entity or to tumors of mesenchymal origin. This highlights the importance of the pathologist to correlate the molecular testing results with the histologic and immunohistochemical findings.

A brief discussion of the various techniques available for the detection of fusion events, using the case of Ewing sarcoma as an example (Box 18.2), follows.

Techniques

Chromosomal Karyotype

Chromosomal karyotyping is the traditional approach for cytogenetic evaluation; historically most chromosomal translocations were discovered in this fashion.[22] In fact, data indicate that the number of translocations discovered in various families of tumors is directly proportional to the number of cases karyotyped.[23,24] In effect, one must look for these alterations to find them. Increasingly, novel methodologies using NGS of RNA or DNA and innovative bioinformatic approaches have yielded exciting, novel discoveries in this area.[25] Nonetheless, karyotype analysis remains an effective diagnostic and discovery approach in many situations. Fresh tumor cells are required for growth in culture and are

Box 18.2 Gene Fusion Terminology

Gene Fusion Variant

Gene fusions occurring in the same neoplasm that involve a single gene such as *EWSR1* with multiple partners such as *FLI1* and *ERG* in Ewing sarcoma. *EWSR1-FLI1* and *EWSR1-ERG* are fusion variants.

Gene Fusion Type

Within a single fusion variant, the different exon combinations between two genes such as *EWSR1* and *FLI1* are known as types. In this example, the type 1 fusion in Ewing sarcoma fuses exon 7 of *EWSR1* to exon 6 of *FLI1*, whereas type 2 combines exons 7 and 5 of these two genes, respectively, when transcribed.

Box 18.3 Clinical Applications of Fluorescence in situ Hybridization

Break-Apart FISH

Can be used to show rearrangement of a particular locus, such as *EWSR1* or *FUS*

Combination or Fusion FISH

Can provide evidence for a particular fusion variant

Amplification FISH

Can provide evidence and rough quantification of the amplification of a locus such as 12q13-15 in well-differentiated liposarcoma

FISH, Fluorescence in situ hybridization.

treated to capture the cells in metaphase, where the chromosomes are condensed and amenable to analysis. Traditionally, the chromosomal spreads are treated with trypsin and stained with Giemsa to produce a G-banding pattern that allows identification of the 22 autosomal pairs and sex chromosomes. These are then formatted into a karyotype, as depicted in Fig. 18.2 for a case of Ewing sarcoma. A complex karyotype is depicted in Fig. 18.1 for comparison. Gross chromosomal abnormalities can be identified in this fashion, although small cryptic deletions, inversions, and translocations can be overlooked. Techniques such as spectral karyotyping and fluorescence in situ hybridization (FISH), discussed further on, can augment this methodology.

The main advantage of karyotyping is that it is open-ended; it evaluates all the chromosomes in a cell and is not targeted to a particular chromosomal event. Disadvantages include the fact that tumor cells, even malignant ones, are surprisingly difficult to grow in culture, and this technique requires highly skilled personnel both for growing cells and for the subsequent interpretation. In addition, as previously mentioned, small chromosomal alterations can be difficult to detect by karyotyping and can be missed.

Fluorescence In Situ Hybridization

FISH can detect chromosomal translocations and also amplifications of a genetic locus. FISH relies on the ability to design DNA probes that specifically hybridize to a unique site on DNA. These probes are labeled with fluorescent dyes, often red and green, so that they can be distinguished from one another. Nuclei are counterstained with 4′,6-diamidino-2-phenylindole (DAPI) which fluoresces blue, so that one can determine which probes are hybridized to the DNA content of an individual cell nucleus. The probes are designed to hybridize to the DNA immediately flanking the adjacent centromeric and telomeric borders of a gene or locus of interest. These regions are in close enough proximity that the overlap of the emission spectra of the green and red probes imparts a single yellow signal. There are normally paired chromosomes, each containing the gene or locus; therefore two yellow signals are observed. In an aneuploid nucleus with chromosomal gains or losses, more or fewer signals can be seen. When the probed locus is rearranged in a balanced translocation, the centromeric probe is retained and the telomeric probe is transferred to the reciprocal chromosome. At this point, the two probes are no longer restricted in close physical proximity, and the red and green probes are separately visualized because they reside on separately segregated chromosomes. This is known as a break-apart FISH probe strategy, which can be used on either interphase nuclei or in cytogenetic metaphase preparations. This technique is illustrated for the example of Ewing sarcoma in Fig. 18.6. It is important to note that although this technique demonstrates that a probed locus is rearranged, it does not provide information regarding the identity of the reciprocal chromosome or fusion gene partner. This can be valuable in the case of Ewing sarcoma, because a number of alternative genes can recombine with *EWSR1*, and FISH detects all of them. However, because it shows an identical pattern of rearrangement for any fusion partner of *EWSR1*, it is not specific for Ewing sarcoma versus the other sarcomas that harbor *EWSR1* gene rearrangements, as illustrated in Fig. 18.5 and Table 18.4. Thus careful correlation with other pathologic features and the clinical setting of any particular case is required to avoid misinterpretation of non–Ewing sarcoma cases, in which *EWSR1* can also be rearranged. This potential pitfall can be avoided using the combination probe strategy, where the two loci are separately probed with red and green hybridization probes, such that a normal cell has two red probes and two green probes, and a cell harboring the rearrangement has one yellow (combined) signal along with single red and green signals (Fig. 18.7). Although this technique has great specificity, a different set of probes is required for each potential binding partner. Virtually all commercially available probes for sarcomas are of the break-apart type.

Another application of FISH is to demonstrate amplification of a gene or chromosomal region. Here, one colored probe is used to hybridize to the centromere, and a second probe is used to hybridize to the potentially amplified region on the same chromosome. The centromeric probe controls for chromosomal copy number. If the ratio of probe to the potentially amplified locus is in excess of the centromeric probe, then amplification is demonstrated. An application of this technique is demonstrating amplification of the 12q13-15 region in well-differentiated or dedifferentiated liposarcoma (see later discussion).

FISH is applicable to standard formalin-fixed paraffin-embedded (FFPE) sections, but it can also be used on touch preparations, karyotype metaphase preparations, and disaggregated nuclei from thick FFPE sections. A modification of the FISH technique allows whole chromosomal painting by numerous individual probes to each chromosome, so that each one is identified by a unique color (spectral karyotyping). A computer system using pseudocoloration enables the interpretation of complex karyotypes, as depicted for desmoplastic small round cell tumor in Fig. 18.8. This technique is basically an unbiased enhancement of the traditional karyotyping method; although not usually necessary, it can be very helpful in complex cases (Box 18.3).

Reverse Transcription Polymerase Chain Reaction

Reverse transcription polymerase chain reaction (RT-PCR) makes use of the precise specificity of PCR primers and the enhanced detection afforded by amplification. Since the completion of the Human Genome Project, the sequences of the intron and exon segments of all human genes are known. Once the two genes involved in a specific translocation have been identified, primers can be designed to amplify the fusion types, which can sometimes be numerous, as for Ewing sarcoma (see Fig. 18.4). Genes are primarily composed of relatively large segments of nontranscribed intronic DNA. It is within these introns that the chromosomal breaks occur, allowing recombination in the nontranscribed DNA, so that when introns are transcribed to RNA, the proper reading

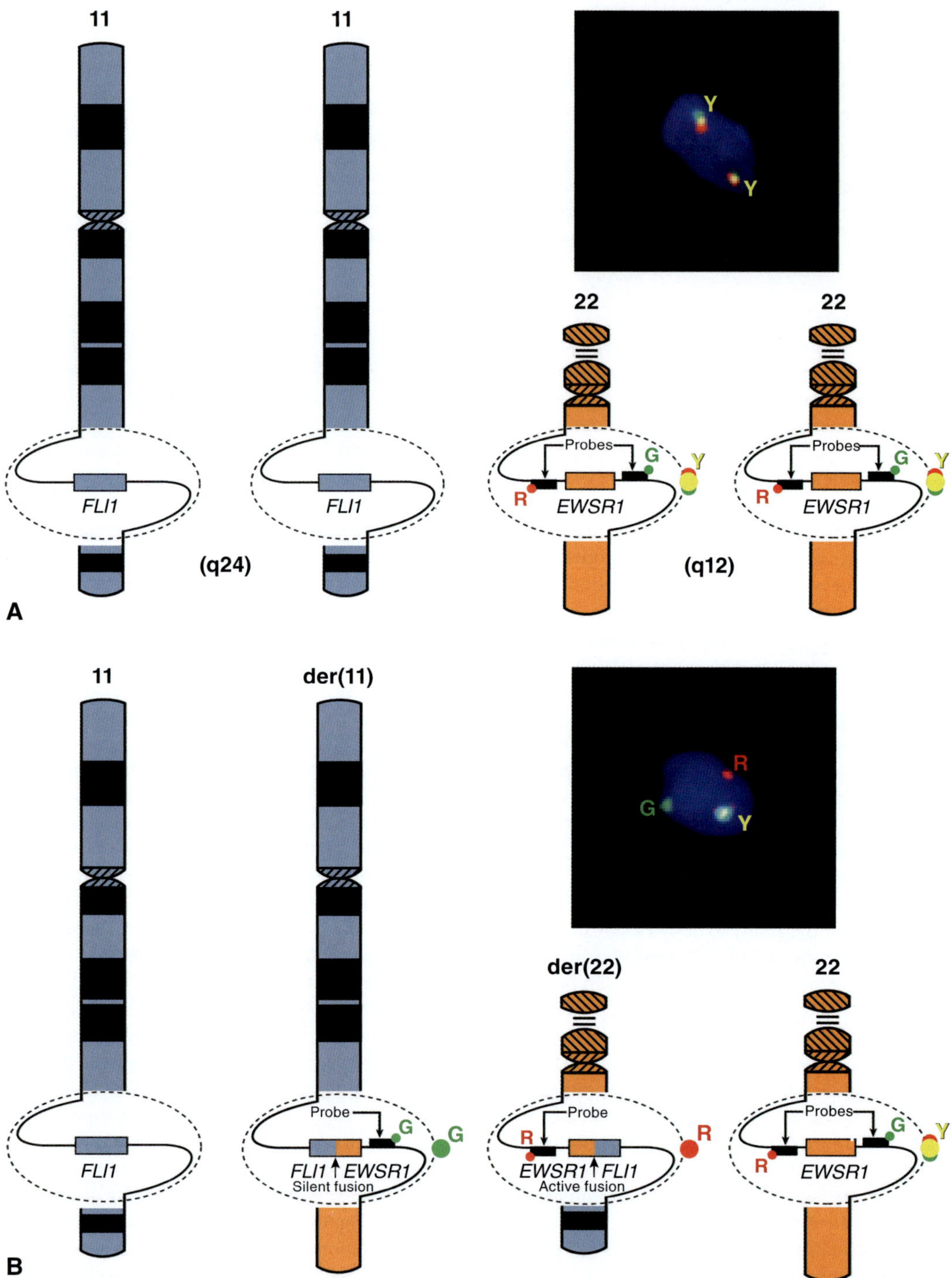

Figure 18.6 **Break-apart Fluorescence In Situ Hybridization (FISH) for the *EWSR1* Locus.** (A) Specific probes that hybridize with the centromeric and telomeric flanking DNA of the *EWSR1* locus are fluorescently labeled red *(R)* and green *(G)*, respectively. The overlapping emission spectra of the two probes when juxtaposed produces a yellow *(Y)* color as depicted within the actual 4′,6-diamidino-2-phenylindole (DAPI)–stained nucleus *(blue)*. Because there are two copies of chromosome 22, two intact yellow signals are seen. (B) When a translocation occurs, the telomeric (G) probe is transferred to the newly formed derivative chromosome 11, and the derivative chromosome 22 retains the centromeric (R) probe. The two probes are no longer juxtaposed on a single chromosome; thus the nucleus reveals a yellow signal for the intact chromosome 22, and the derivative chromosomes show single red and green signals, indicating a positive (break-apart) result for rearrangement. This approach detects a rearrangement of *EWSR1* regardless of the fusion partner.

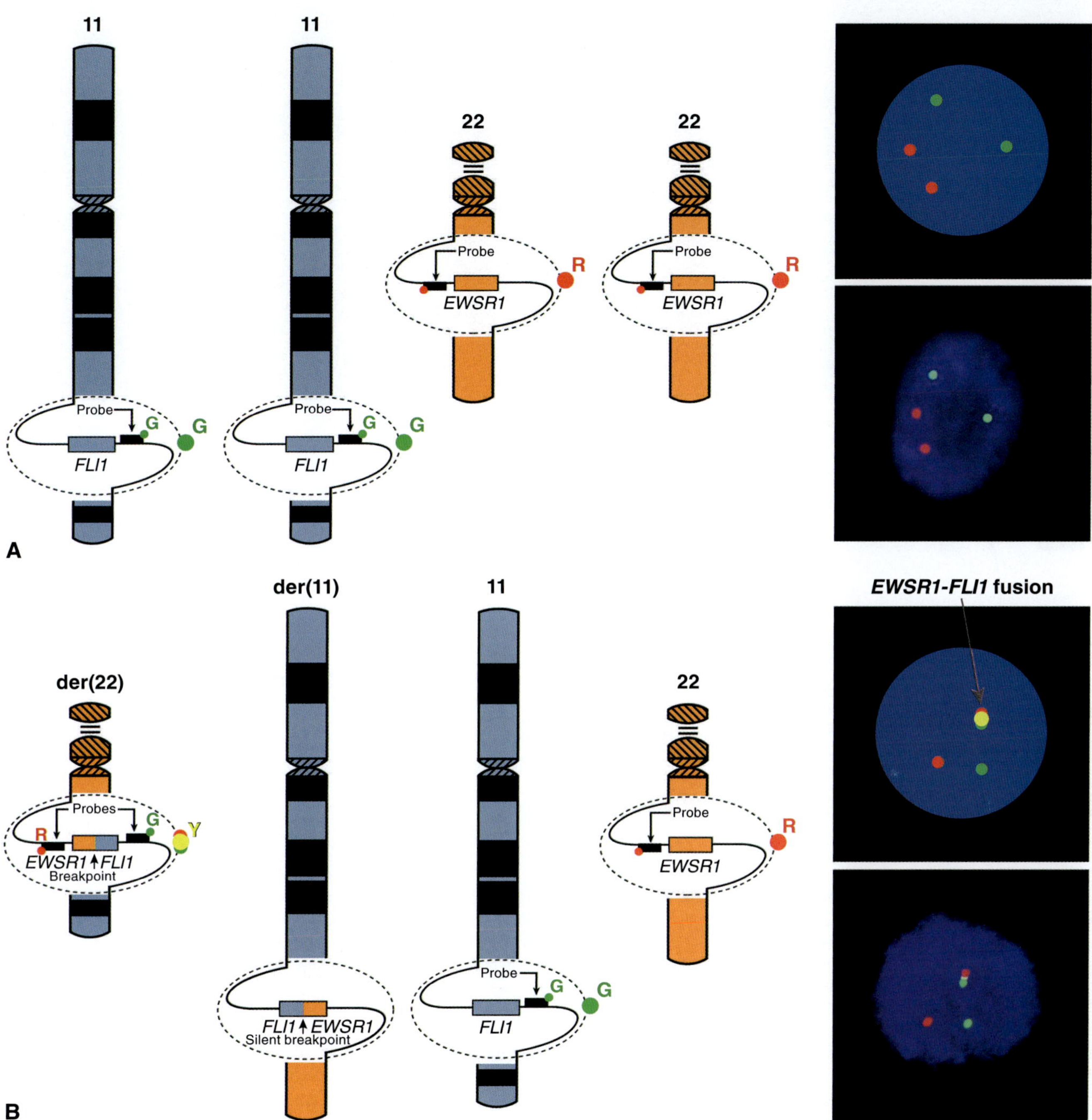

Figure 18.7 **Fusion Fluorescence In Situ Hybridization (FISH) for the *EWSR1* Locus.** (A) The telomeric aspect of *FLI1* on chromosome 11 is labeled with a single green *(G)* fluorescent probe, and the centromeric aspect of the *EWSR1* locus on chromosome 22 is labeled in red *(R)* in this example. In a nonrearranged nucleus, there are thus two green and two red signals indicating two of each of the labeled chromosomes. This is shown in the upper right panel as an idealized figure with an actual 4′,6-diamidino-2-phenylindole (DAPI)-stained nucleus in the panel below. (B) When *EWSR1* is rearranged with *FLI1*, the derivative chromosome 22 now has a juxtaposed centromeric red and telomeric green probes at the active fusion gene site, producing a yellow signal. The two normal chromosomes, 11 and 22, not involved in the rearrangement retain their single green and red signals, respectively. This scheme more directly demonstrates the formation of an actual fusion locus but does not detect fusion of *EWSR1* with loci other than *FLI1*; these other potential fusion partners are not labeled.

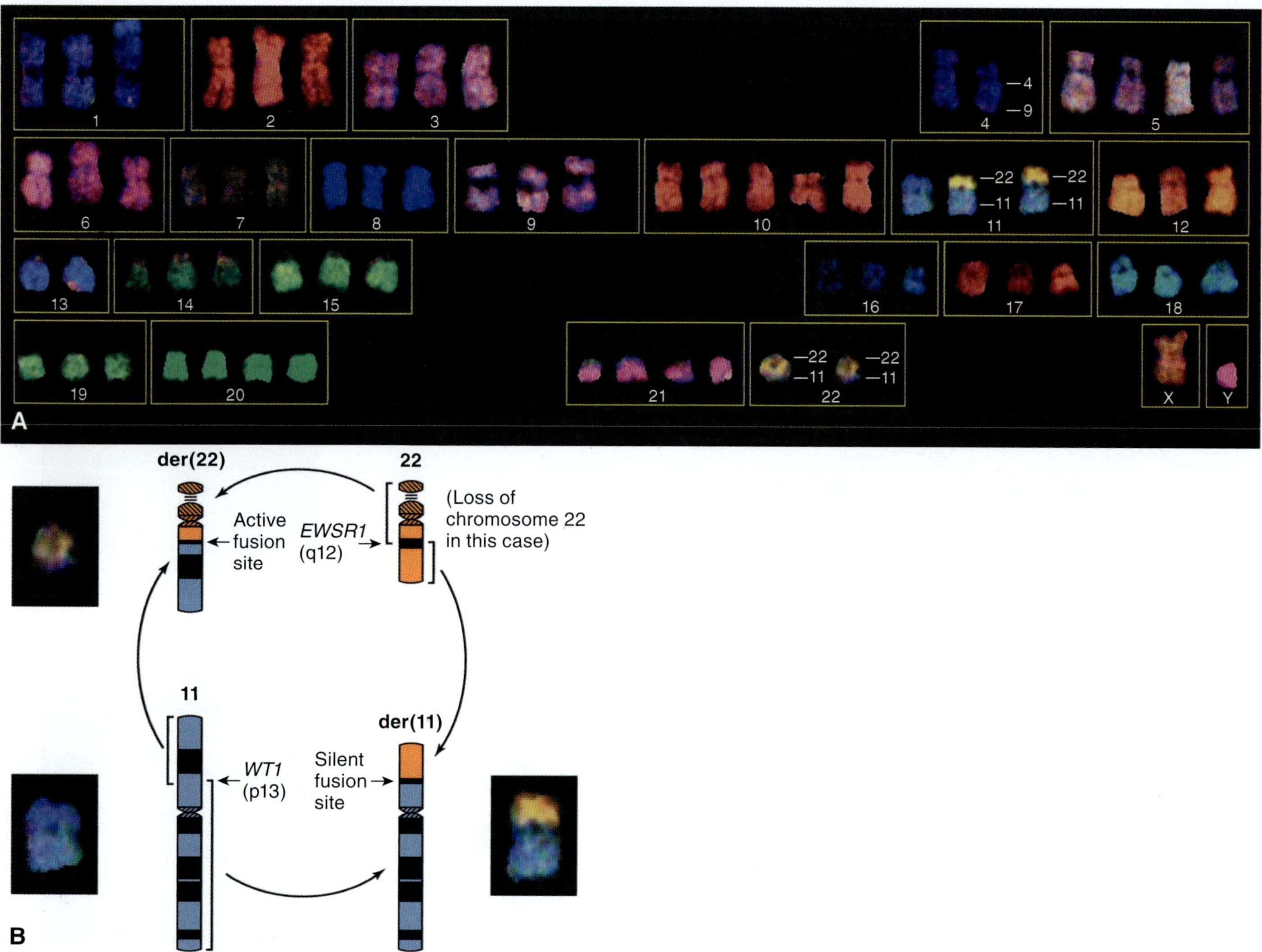

Figure 18.8 **Spectral Karyotyping of Desmoplastic Small Round Cell Tumor.** (A) This complex aneuploid karyotype enhanced by spectral karyotyping reveals a translocation between chromosomes 11 and 22. The fusion chromosomes are duplicated, and the normal chromosome 22 has been lost. (B) An ideogram of t(11;22)(p13;q12) is depicted with isolated chromosomes. Note that the break in this tumor is in the short (p) arm of chromosome 11 rather than the long arm, as noted in Ewing sarcoma (see Fig. 18.2).

frame is maintained, allowing for translation to an active chimeric protein. Because the introns are large, ranging from several to many kilobases, it is not practical to design primers to detect the actual recombination point in the genomic DNA. Recall that only about 1.5% of the ~3 billion base pairs within the human genome is exonic, comprising the ~20,000 genes ultimately transcribed to messenger RNA (mRNA) and then translated to protein. Furthermore, there is a limit to the length of an amplicon that can reliably be produced by PCR. This is further compounded by the fact that genomic DNA is sheared into relatively small fragments because of the cross-linking activity of formalin fixation. For PCR amplification to be consistent in this setting, amplicons cannot be larger than 150 to 200 base pairs, and smaller ones (<100 base pairs) are more reliable. Thus PCR-based strategies take advantage of mRNA instead of DNA because introns are spliced out when mRNA is produced. This juxtaposes the exon from one gene directly to an exon from the other gene when the fusion is present. For PCR to function, one must use a reverse transcriptase (RT) enzyme to convert the extracted RNA to DNA, known as complementary DNA (cDNA); thus the technique is known as RT-PCR. As depicted in Fig. 18.9, one is able to amplify a product only if the primers extend toward each other in an intact fusion transcript. If no fusion gene is present, there is no amplification product. A housekeeping gene such as β-actin is usually also amplified to confirm that the cDNA is of sufficient quality and quantity to allow amplification (see Fig. 18.3B). A variety of techniques can be used to confirm the identity of the amplicon, with direct sequencing being the most specific; but real-time detection, restriction fragment analysis, or other techniques can also be used.

PCR amplification of genomic DNA, followed by Sanger sequencing, can be used to search for mutations in introns such as the deletions, insertions, duplications, and point mutations seen in the *KIT* gene in GIST. These are discussed further later in the chapter. In using Sanger sequencing, it is important to have relatively pure tumor DNA, because there will usually be one nonmutated copy (allele) of a gene in addition to the mutated gene in a tumor cell. The limit of detection of such methods is theoretically about one tumor cell per five total cells (20% tumor; 10% mutated DNA) or better, but for the Sanger method to be reliably effective, tumor should ideally constitute 50% of the sample or greater. Microdissection may be helpful in samples where there is an

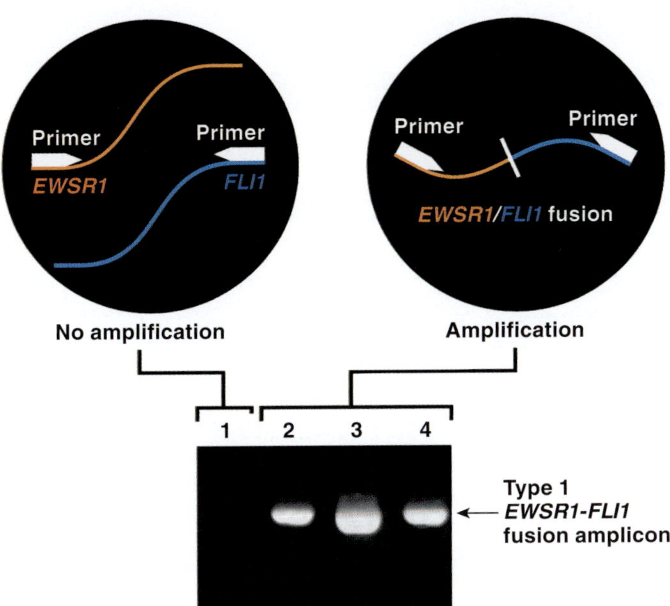

Figure 18.9 Polymerase Chain Reaction (PCR) for Fusion Transcripts. PCR primers specific for *EWSR1* and *FLI1* are used after reverse transcription of mRNA to DNA. When the two primers anneal and extend separate genes, no amplification occurs (lane 1). However, when the fusion gene is present, there is extension between the primer pairs and amplification results (lanes 2 to 4). Multiple primer pairs may be necessary to detect the various fusion types and variants, as seen in Fig. 18.4 and Table 18.4, respectively, for Ewing sarcoma.

abundance of nonneoplastic tissue. Alternative methods such as pyrosequencing or mass spectrometry, which have higher sensitivity, can also be used to evaluate for specific point mutations. The advent of NGS into clinical practice is dramatically reducing the 20% tumor needed as input for reliable results, as noted in the following text.

Use of RT-PCR to detect gene fusions is applicable to fresh and FFPE samples. An advantage of this technique is that the fusion product can be detected even if the tumor DNA is not enriched in the sample (unlike the demonstration of gene mutations in genomic DNA discussed earlier); therefore small samples such as needle biopsies can be used. When there are multiple or numerous different possible fusion types combining various exons between two genes, multiple primer pairs may be required. Similarly, when there are a variety of genes that can recombine in a particular tumor type, at least one primer pair for each of these must be used. As most RT-PCR assays are designed to detect the most common fusions, rare fusions can be missed. Finally, PCR is extremely sensitive, and contamination can be a problem. Thus it is critical to use negative controls and rigorously maintain strict separation of pre-PCR sample preparation and the PCR amplification/postamplification processes to minimize potential contamination.

Next-Generation Sequencing Molecular Assays. Massively parallel DNA sequencing, commonly referred to as NGS, allows a sequencing examination of many genes in parallel.[26,27] Although it is possible to sequence the entire genome or exome of a cancer sample, most clinical panels range from 25 to 500 genes considered important for cancer. In appropriately designed panels, it is also possible to obtain copy number data in addition to sequence. Many of the broad gene panels are developed based on common mutational events in carcinomas and melanoma; thus they are not optimized for sarcoma. Although some sarcomas have characteristic gene sequence mutations, such as *KIT* or *PDGFRA* in GIST or *CTNNB1* (encoding β-catenin) in desmoid-type fibromatosis, many sarcomas lack specific gene sequence mutations that are helpful diagnostically and rather harbor translocations and/or copy number alterations.[27] These single gene mutations can also be readily assessed by more traditional sequencing methods. However, most complex karyotype sarcomas are characterized more by extensive segmental copy number alterations rather than mutations, although *TP53*, *ATRX*, and *RB1* inactivating mutations are often encountered. Because of the broad coverage, NGS can also discover mutations that are rare in sarcomas but occur in potentially targetable genes such as *BRAF* or *PIK3CA*. Characteristic copy number alterations such as the punctuated amplification of the 12q13-15 interval in well-differentiated and dedifferentiated liposarcomas can also be demonstrated on appropriately designed NGS panels. NGS can be readily applied to FFPE specimens. It has additional advantages in that the amounts of DNA needed for sequencing are relatively small and the percent tumor nuclei is lower than that needed for Sanger and other forms of sequencing. Though very powerful, NGS is more complex than traditional sequencing; a germline source of DNA is often needed for comparison to the tumor sample (particularly in large gene panels), and extensive bioinformatic support is needed for definitive interpretation. A full discussion of NGS is beyond the scope of this chapter.

Another exciting application of NGS in sarcoma is RNA sequencing (RNA seq) to demonstrate characteristic gene fusion events in the simple karyotype sarcomas. Like RT-PCR, this method is aided by splicing out the large introns of genes so that only the linked exons remain; thus the junction between two different genes can be more readily detected (Fig. 18.10). A more in-depth description of this technique is beyond the scope of this chapter. Although the entire transcriptome (all coding RNA) can be sequenced, it is usually more practical to examine relevant RNA subsets. Methods have been developed that employ primers based on the known break point of one fusion gene and random primers that will detect any second gene involved in the fusion. Such methods can be very effective for promiscuous genes, which can have many partners and break points and which are challenging to address with RT-PCR due to the many primer sets required. The use of panels that can detect fusions with many genes allows a single test to be used for the detection of many different fusions and can also lead to the discovery of unexpected or novel fusion in clinical cases.[28-30] Gene expression signatures can also be obtained through RNA seq in sarcoma and, combined with copy number data, can convey prognostic information, but clinical implementation remains a future goal.[31,32]

Both RNA seq and DNA NGS testing are transforming the molecular diagnostics landscape, but they require complex bioinformatic processing to support the interpretation of the sequencing results. As many different genes will be sequenced, DNA or RNA (cDNA) libraries incorporating tumor DNA must be constructed. To adequately assess sequence variants and mutations, normal or germline DNA must usually also be sequenced for comparison. Thus the increased sequence information that one gains is earned through more complex, time-consuming, and expensive procedures and extensive bioinformatic interpretation. However, the costs are dropping rapidly, and NGS is quickly becoming the sequencing platform of choice for many applications in molecular testing.[33,34]

PRACTICE POINTS: Using Reverse Transcription Polymerase Chain Reaction to Demonstrate Fusion Transcripts

- Definitively demonstrates a specific fusion variant and type
- Detects only the specific fusion variants and types for which it was designed
- Care must be taken to avoid contamination yielding false positive results
- Technique works well in both fresh and formalin-fixed paraffin-embedded tissue
- RNA from blocks older than 5 years of age or decalcified blocks can be often unreliable due to RNA degradation

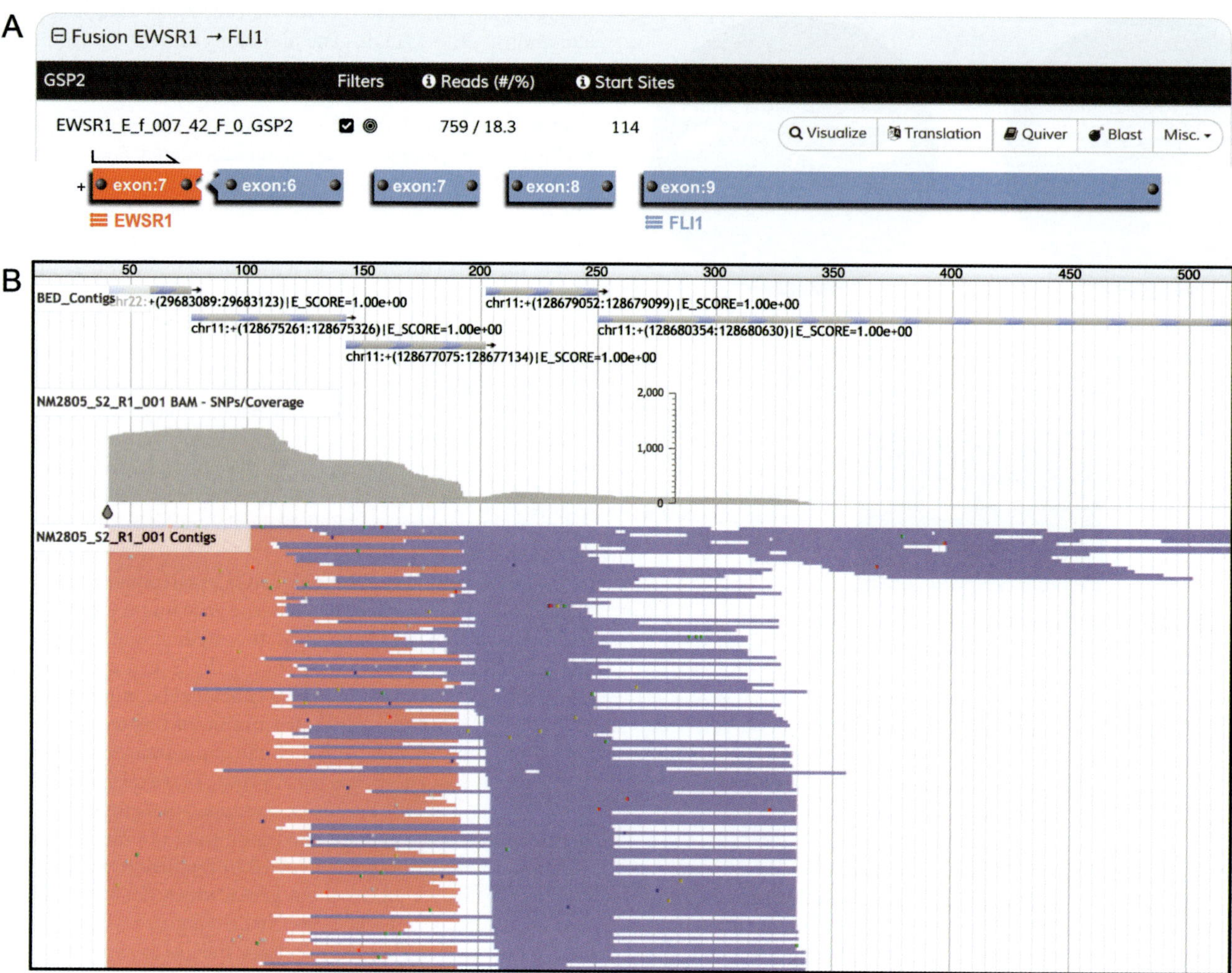

Figure 18.10 **Focused RNA Seq for Fusion Transcript Detection.** (A) Diagram of a detected type 1 EWSR1-FLI1 fusion transcript. (B) Display showing coverage statistics and mapped fusion transcripts. These amplicons were obtained from a cDNA library using primers to EWSR1 break points and random priming for the fusion partner, in this case discovered to be FLI1. (Portions of this figure courtesy Dr. Brian Kudlow, ArcherDX, Boulder, CO.)

From the preceding discussion, it is clear that there are multiple levels at which evidence of a gene fusion event can be identified (Fig. 18.11). Cytogenetics can reveal chromosomal features using a traditional karyotype. FISH allows a more focused look at a specific genetic locus, and spectral karyotyping (essentially whole-genome FISH) provides an unbiased and enhanced view of the entire chromosomal complement. Although translocations can be revealed at the genomic DNA level, these are difficult to detect within large introns and require long-range PCR or NGS that tiles across entire introns. Such approaches are amenable to research applications but are rarely practical for clinical diagnostic work. Transcription to RNA avoids this problem and, using reverse transcription, fusion transcripts can readily be detected. RNA seq is gaining popularity as a sequencing method for fusion detection. Fusion transcripts are ultimately translated into proteins, which, in some cases, can be detected by immunohistochemistry, although the available antibodies are often not completely specific. Finally, many of the soft tissue tumors associated with translocations have unique histologic features. These features are presumably strongly linked to the action of the expressed fusion gene. Thus there are many levels of biologic evidence that directly or indirectly suggest the presence of the fusion gene.

Currently emerging technologies are being applied to sarcomas. These include gene expression arrays, which examine RNA and microRNA production from genes; comparative genomic hybridization, which demonstrates DNA copy numbers of chromosomal regions; DNA methylation studies, which can reveal transcriptionally active and inactive regions of the genome; and proteomic approaches, which examine protein expression and state of activation by a variety of techniques.[35,36] NGS approaches to characterize genomes and transcriptomes have also provided fascinating insights into biology and are increasingly incorporated into the clinical workflow, as discussed earlier. DNA methylation studies are also of increasing interest. These approaches have provided critical insights into the classification and biology of these tumors. These techniques are beginning to be applied to sarcoma for diagnosis and prognosis. Traditional molecular studies are critically important for sarcoma diagnosis and clinical management.[37] Embracing new technologies where appropriate will further assist diagnosis and treatment of this group of diseases.

Molecular Features of Particular Entities

This section contains a discussion of particular soft tissue sarcomas for which molecular features may be evaluated as a diagnostic adjunct.

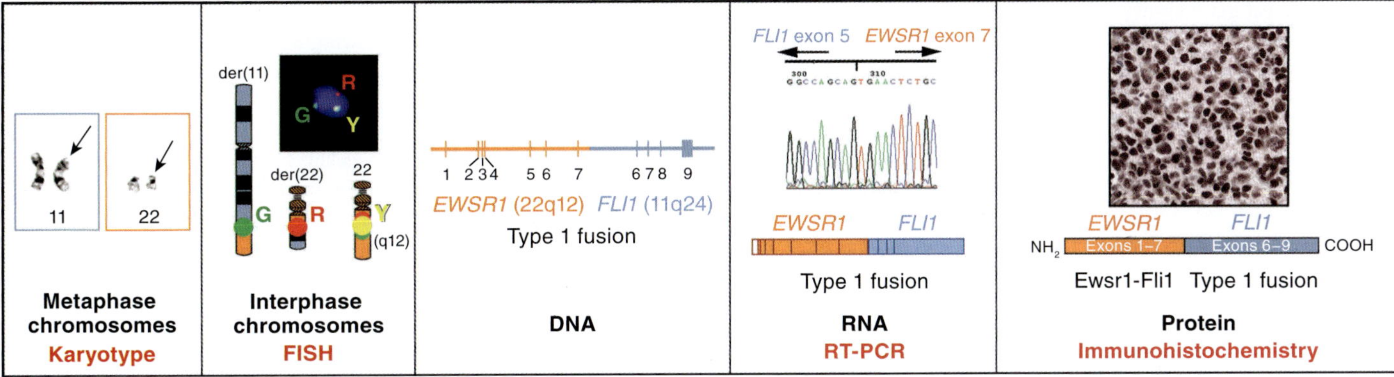

Figure 18.11 Approaches for Fusion Gene Demonstration. Using the example of t(11;22)(q24;q12) in Ewing sarcoma, it is possible to detect this event at the chromosomal level using karyotype analysis of metaphase chromosomes and in interphase (noncondensed) chromosomes using fluorescence in situ hybridization (FISH). Demonstration of fusion genes at the genomic DNA level is difficult because the introns can be large and the break points are not clustered. Long-range polymerase chain reaction (PCR) can be used, but it is not robust for clinical applications. RT (reverse transcription)-PCR can be used to detect the mRNA transcribed from a fusion gene. Finally, some fusion proteins can be detected using immunohistochemistry as seen for Fli1 in Ewing sarcoma, but this also detects the wild-type protein and thus is not specific. Each of these approaches has advantages and challenges in application and interpretation, as detailed in the text.

Although numerous chromosomal alterations and, less commonly, DNA mutations are found in sarcomas, this discussion focuses on those that are diagnostically relevant. This is followed by a discussion of specific differential diagnostic conundrums where molecular diagnostics may be particularly helpful. In keeping with the approach of this book, the focus is on practical applications of molecular characterization; the many recent and exciting research advances for many of these tumors are not discussed unless they are currently germane to diagnostic or prognostic molecular analysis. Future trends in diagnostic testing for certain tumors are presented when relevant. The clinical and morphologic features and diagnostic criteria for these entities are presented in previous chapters; thus the reader is referred there for additional information.

Soft Tissue Sarcomas With Complex Cytogenetic Features

As previously mentioned, sarcomas generally fall into two cytogenetic classes: those with complex karyotypes and those with simple karyotypes, the latter often harboring diagnostically useful translocations or mutations. The neoplasms in the former category have complex karyotypes; some of these complex chromosomal alterations may have prognostic implications, although additional study is needed.[38] Some of these tumors have also now been discovered to have recurrent chromosomal alterations or genetic mutations that can be diagnostically useful, as discussed earlier. A complex karyotype is presented in Fig. 18.1. It is important to recognize that even neoplasms with characteristic genetic alterations may go on to develop complex karyotypes with tumor progression. On the basis of the clinical, morphologic, and immunohistochemical features of the tumor, such investigations can be performed using FISH, spectral karyotyping, or RT-PCR techniques. Soft tissue sarcomas within this group are listed in Table 18.1. Most cytogenetically complex sarcomas have many more copy number alterations than classic activating or inactivating gene mutations. The critical genetic events driving the biology of these sarcomas are largely unknown.[39]

Soft Tissue Sarcomas With Simple Cytogenetic Features

Tumors with simple cytogenetic features often have characteristic molecular findings that can be exploited diagnostically. Although gene fusion producing a novel transcription factor with aberrant activity is the most common pathway, other mechanisms are also involved, as listed in Table 18.5. These are discussed further in the following individual sections.

Table 18.5 Various Types of Molecular Mechanisms for Genetic Drivers in Soft Tissue Sarcomas With Simple Cytogenetic Features

Molecular Feature	Example(s)
Chromosomal Translocation/Gene Fusion	
Novel transcription factor with aberrant function	Ewing sarcoma Synovial sarcoma
Overproduction of a normal growth factor	Dermatofibrosarcoma protuberans
Change in subcellular localization of tyrosine kinase receptor	Inflammatory myofibroblastic tumor
Gene Mutation	
Ligand-independent activation of tyrosine kinase receptor	Gastrointestinal stromal tumor
Decreased degradation of a protein	Desmoid fibromatosis
Increased activation of a signaling molecule	Intramuscular/cellular myxoma

Many sarcomas can be classified according to the cell type or tissue whose lineage they most closely resemble, such as leiomyosarcoma (smooth muscle), angiosarcoma (endothelium), and rhabdomyosarcoma (skeletal muscle). However, there are a group of sarcomas whose lineage is uncertain. Interestingly, chromosomal translocations and resultant fusion genes are especially common in the latter group, as depicted in Box 18.1.

Tumors in the simple cytogenetic group are discussed further in alphabetical order to allow for ease of reference. Table 18.3 lists the tumors in this group, along with their relevant cytogenetic and molecular features. Principles of molecular diagnostics are discussed within these sections as relevant, followed by a discussion of the practical use of molecular testing to resolve examples of particularly problematic differential diagnostic situations.

Alveolar Soft Part Sarcoma

This rare soft tissue sarcoma (see Chapter 6) is associated with an unbalanced translocation der(17)(X;17)(p11;q25).[40,41] Chromosome 17 contains a novel gene known as *ASPSCR1* (formerly *ASPL*), whereas chromosome X contains *TFE3*, which provides the DNA targeting function of the fusion protein. Not much is known about the function of the protein encoded by *ASPSCR1*, but *TFE3* encodes a member of the helix-loop-helix superfamily of DNA-binding proteins, which is normally involved in immunoglobulin gene regulation. *TFE3* is also rearranged with *ASPSCR1* and other genes in rare forms of renal cell carcinoma, which are most common in children.[42] Interestingly, the *TFE3-ASPSCR1* translocations in the renal cell carcinomas tend to be balanced, whereas the translocation is unbalanced in alveolar soft part sarcoma (Fig. 18.12A). *TFE3* has also been found to be rearranged in a small subset of perivascular epithelioid cell tumors (PEComas) (see Chapters 6 and 16).[43] Translocations can be demonstrated by FISH or RT-PCR.[40,44,45] Break-apart FISH probes directed at *TFE3* are generally used. *TFE3* is located on chromosome X; therefore the FISH probe pattern changes depending on whether the patient is male or female and whether the translocation is the most common unbalanced type or a rare instance of a balanced translocation. By RT-PCR, two alternative transcripts are seen that differ by inclusion of one exon from *TFE3*. The break point in *ASPSCR1* is constant. Type 1 does not include exon 3 of *TFE3* and constitutes approximately 75% of reported cases, whereas type 2 includes exon 3 and accounts for 25% of cases (see Fig. 18.12B). Virtually all cases of alveolar soft part sarcoma show evidence of one of these two variant fusion transcripts. Tumors can be tested for reciprocity using PCR primers to the silent fusion site.[46] This is negative in most cases of alveolar soft part sarcoma and positive in the subset of renal cell carcinomas that combine *TFE3* and *ASPSCR1*. Such information could potentially be useful if these two entities needed to be distinguished in a small biopsy, but this would be an uncommon differential diagnosis. Immunohistochemistry demonstrating nuclear TFE3 staining is strongly suggestive of the presence of the fusion transcript,[47] although the available antibodies have been difficult to optimize and can show somewhat inconsistent results.

Angiomatoid Fibrous Histiocytoma

Angiomatoid fibrous histiocytoma (previously referred to as angiomatoid MFH) is a rare tumor of uncertain differentiation and very limited metastatic potential (see Chapters 3 and 10). Several chromosomal translocations have been identified in this neoplasm. The first demonstrated were t(12;16)(q13;p11) and t(12;22)(q13;q12), resulting in *FUS-ATF1* and *EWSR1-ATF1* fusion genes, respectively.[48,49] These findings were very surprising, because the *EWSR1-ATF1* fusion is precisely the same fusion variant seen in clear cell sarcoma, a much more aggressive tumor that will be discussed further in the following paragraphs. This indicates that some fusion genes are not diagnostic of a single entity and must therefore be interpreted in the context of clinical and histologic features. The substitution of *EWSR1* and *FUS* is not surprising because these genes are homologous, and similar substitutions are seen in rare cases of Ewing sarcoma and myxoid liposarcoma (as well as other tumor types), as illustrated in Fig. 18.5. More recently, it has become clear that t(2;22)(q33;q12), resulting in an *EWSR1-CREB1* fusion gene, is the most common genetic event in angiomatoid fibrous histiocytoma.[50,51] Both *ATF1* and *CREB1* belong to the cyclic adenosine monophosphate (cAMP) response element binding a protein family of transcription factors and likely affecting the transcription of similar genes. Interestingly, a *FUS-CREB1* fusion variant has not yet been described. The vast majority of angiomatoid fibrous histiocytomas contain one of these three gene fusions, but additional variants with other homologous genes may eventually be discovered. These rearrangements are readily detected by FISH. RT-PCR is also a viable option, because there is only one type of *EWSR1-CREB1* variant; the other fusion variants result in limited fusion types as well (Fig. 18.13).[50,51] Both *EWSR1-CREB1* and *EWSR1-ATF1* are also shared with other tumor types, most notably clear cell sarcoma. See the following section for more information regarding the fusion types and variants in this family.

Angiosarcoma

Angiosarcoma typically has complex karyotypes. However, recent studies have found recurrent mutations including *PTPRB* and *PLCG1* in a subset of angiosarcomas.[52] Another series revealed recurrent *CIC* gene abnormalities including rearrangements as well as mutations in *PLCG1* and *KDR*. Some of these mutations were associated with site and prognosis.[53] Finally, amplification of *MYC* and sometimes *FLT4* is seen in those tumors that are radiation-associated.[7] This amplification can be detected by FISH or by immunohistochemical studies.[54,55]

Benign Fibrous Histiocytoma (Dermatofibroma)

These common cutaneous tumors (see Chapter 15) have been found to harbor translocations involving the regions encoding for the membrane components of *LAMTOR1* (11q13), podoplanin (*PDPN*; 1p36), *CD63* (12q12-13), and the catalytic domain of the protein kinase C isoforms *PRKCD* (3p21) or *PRKCB* (16p12).[56,57] The fusion proteins are thought to result in aberrant activated kinases in the cell membrane. Another study identified a case of aneurysmal fibrous histiocytoma that harbored the translocation t(3;11)(p21;q13), resulting in two fusions *LAMTOR1-PRKCD* and *NUMA1-SFMBT1*.[58] Although the vast majority of cases are benign and molecular confirmation is not needed for diagnosis, there are rare cases that metastasize (termed by some as benign metastasizing fibrous histiocytoma); these are often deep-seated and large. Tumors with aggressive behavior have increased chromosomal aberrations with frequent gains of 7 and 8q and loss of Xq in metastatic cases, recurrent losses in 9 and 22 in atypical fibrous histiocytoma, and isolated loss of 5q and gains in 20 in cellular benign fibrous histiocytomas.[59] Although previously considered to be a histologic variant of fibrous histiocytoma, the majority of epithelioid fibrous histiocytomas have recently been identified to have *ALK* (2p23) rearrangements. This finding suggests that they may be unrelated to conventional fibrous histiocytomas. Immunohistochemical study for ALK can be useful in these tumors and correlates strongly with *ALK* rearrangement demonstrated by FISH.[60]

Biphenotypic Sinonasal Sarcoma

This rare neoplasm harbors a *PAX3-MAML3* gene fusion in over half of cases.[61] *PAX3-NCOA1* and *PAX3-FOXO1* fusions have also been identified; tumors with such rearrangements sometimes show focal rhabdomyoblastic differentiation.[62] Both *PAX3* break-apart FISH and RNA seq focused on *PAX3* are reasonable diagnostic approaches.

Clear Cell Sarcoma

This neoplasm was previously also known as melanoma of soft parts owing to the presence of melanocytic differentiation and in some cases melanosomes and melanin production (see also Chapter 3). In the clear cell sarcomas that occur in the distal extremities, the predominant chromosomal translocation is t(12;22)(q13;q12), which is detected in almost all such cases.[63] There are four described fusion types, with types 1 and 2 constituting about 95% of reported cases.[64-66] Interestingly, a mixture of both type 1 and type 2 can be detected in many cases by RT-PCR, perhaps indicating alternative splicing of the fusion gene (see Fig. 18.13A).[64] The biologic significance of this finding is unclear, but this phenomenon has not been clearly documented in other fusion genes, including other variants that involve the *EWSR1* gene. More recently, a clear cell sarcoma–like tumor of the gastrointestinal tract has been described, which is often associated with t(2;22)(q33;q12), resulting in an *EWSR1-CREB1* fusion gene (see Fig. 18.13B) (see also Chapter 16).[67] This translocation was initially described in a

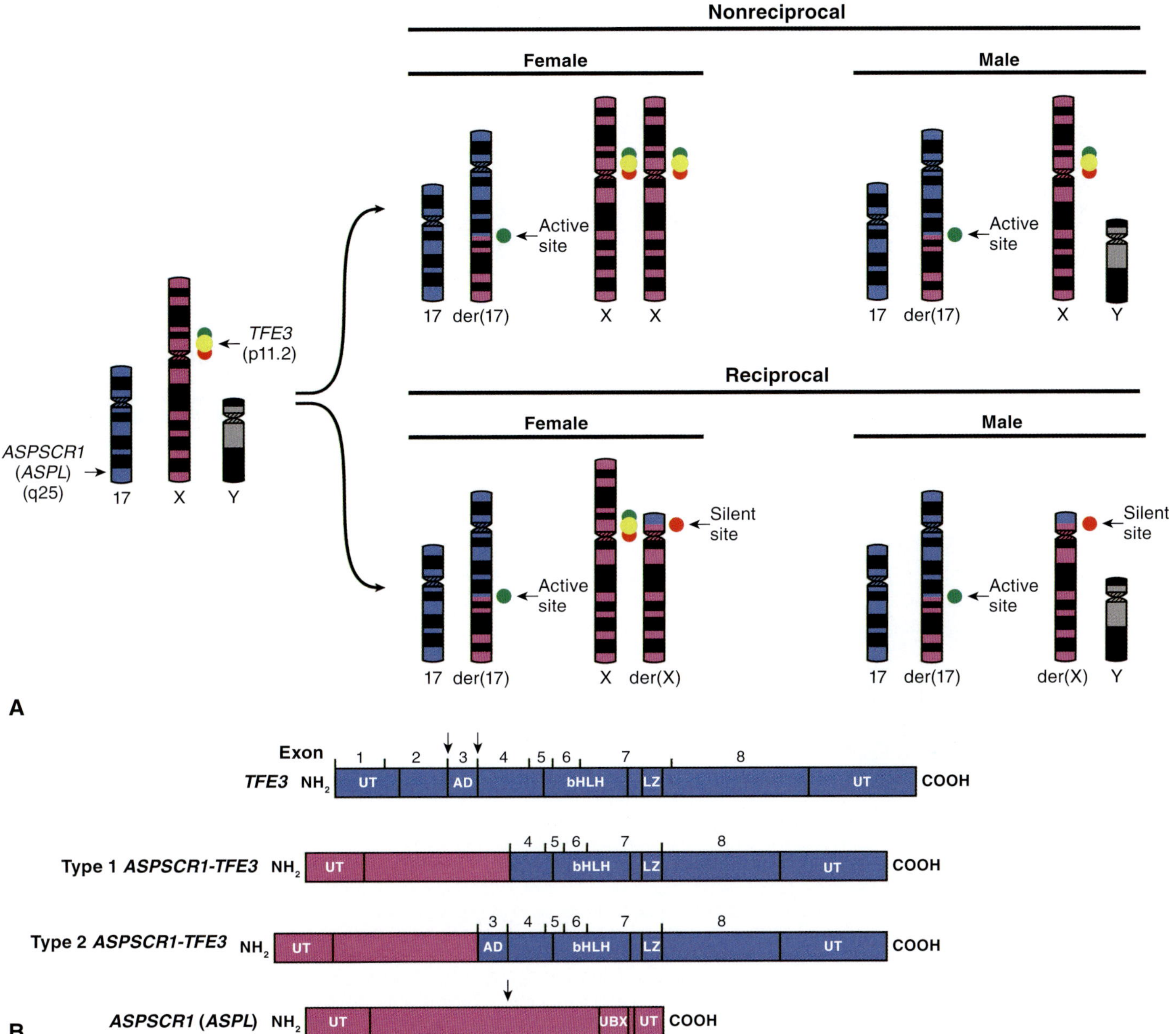

Figure 18.12 **Cytogenetics of Alveolar Soft Part Sarcoma.** (A) A break-apart FISH probe strategy for the *TFE3* locus on chromosome X in alveolar soft part sarcoma (ASPS) is depicted. Because this fusion is most often nonreciprocal in ASPS and *TFE3* is on chromosome X, the pattern is different in males and females. A normal female cell has two fused signals and a male has one based on the expected number of X chromosomes in each gender. A nonreciprocal translocation in a female results in two fused *(yellow)* signals and one split *(green)* probe representing the telomeric probe previously flanking *TFE3* on chromosome X. A nonreciprocal translocation in a male results in only one fused signal and one split *(green)* signal. In the rare reciprocal translocations associated with ASPS, or more often the predominantly pediatric Xp11 translocation renal cell carcinomas, a female with translocation shows one intact fused *(yellow)* locus with split green and red probes on the active derivative 17 and the inactive derivative X chromosomes, respectively. This is the same pattern seen with the use of the *EWSR1* break-apart probe strategy in Ewing sarcoma (see Fig. 18.6). Alternatively, reciprocal rearrangement in a male shows loss of the fused *(yellow)* signal with only single split green and red signals remaining. (B) There is only one break point in *ASPSCR1* and two in *TFE3 (black arrows)*, and thus the design of primers for RT-PCR is relatively straightforward as only two fusion types are produced. Primers at the inactive fusion transcript from the derivative chromosome X can be used to test for a reciprocal translocation by RT-PCR if desired. *AD*, Activation domain; *bHLH*, basic helix-loop-helix domain; *LZ*, leucine zipper; *UBX*, ubiquitin regulatory domain; *UT*, untranslated region.

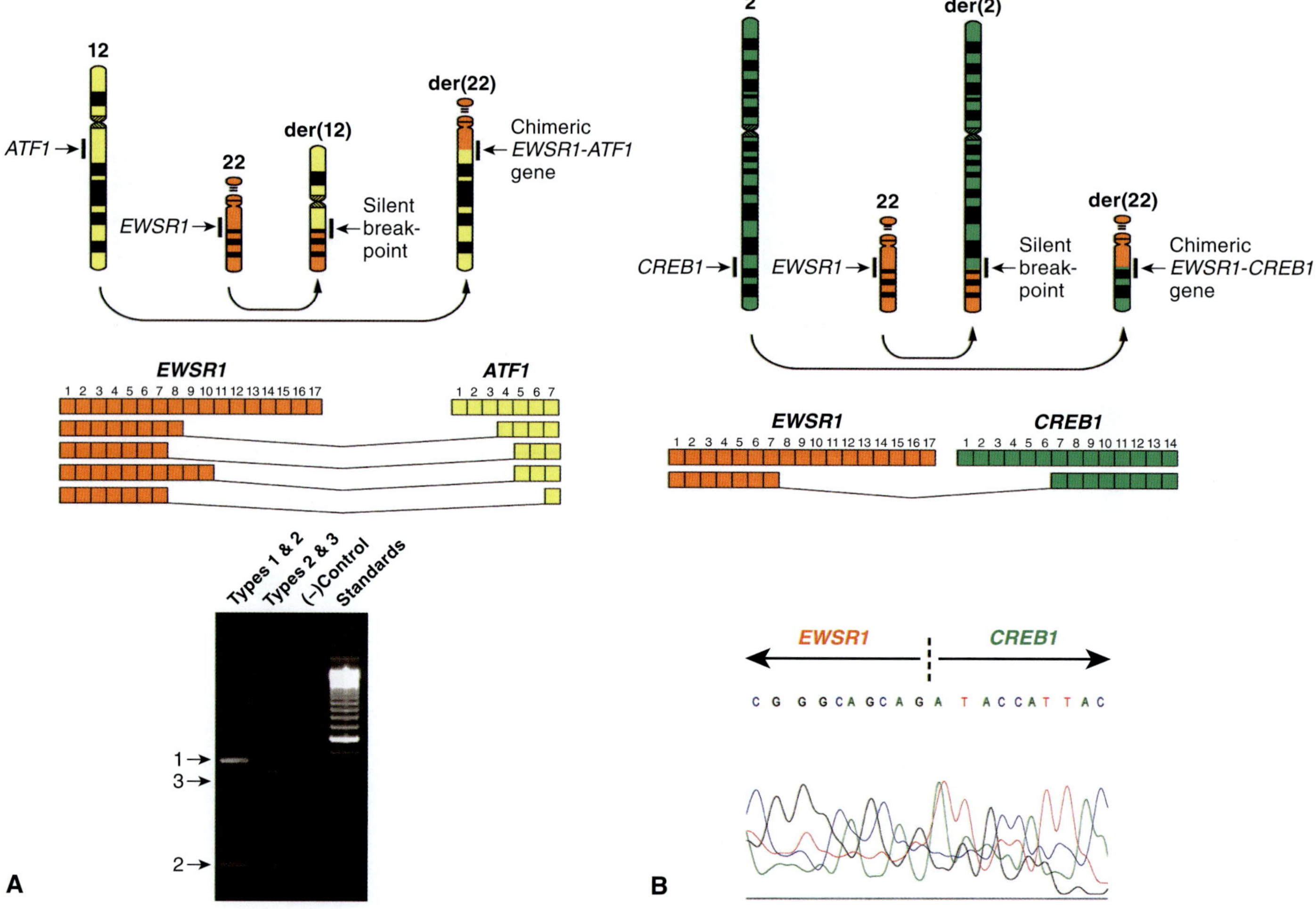

Figure 18.13 **Fusions Variants and Types in Clear Cell Sarcoma.** (A) As with all *EWSR1*-related fusion genes, the active site in clear cell sarcoma is on the derivative chromosome 22. There are four described fusion types, with the first two being predominant. As seen on the polymerase chain reaction (PCR) gel, multiple fusion types can be seen in the same case, with types 1 and 2 and types 2 and 3 present simultaneously. The combination of types 1 and 2 is the most common. This finding is unusual among fusion transcripts and likely due to alternative splicing. (B) The fusion of *CREB1* and *EWSR1* is seen primarily in the rare gastrointestinal clear cell sarcoma-like tumor and exceptionally in extremity clear cell sarcoma. This fusion is the one mostly commonly encountered in angiomatoid fibrous histiocytoma, though *EWSR1-ATF1* and *FUS-ATF1* can also be seen in this tumor (see previous discussion and Fig. 18.5). Only a single fusion type has been described for *EWSR1-CREB1*, making reverse transcription PCR a straightforward option. (Portions of this figure courtesy Dr. Dolores López-Terrada, Texas Children's Hospital and Baylor College of Medicine, Houston, TX.)

gastrointestinal clear cell sarcoma–like tumor and subsequently identified in angiomatoid fibrous histiocytoma (see previous section).[50,51] Only a single type of this fusion gene variant has been described. Interestingly, clear cell sarcoma–like tumors of the gastrointestinal tract, with either *EWSR1-ATF1* or *EWSR1-CREB1*, lack melanocytic differentiation, although they show S-100 protein and SOX10 expression by immunohistochemistry. The majority of such tumors show histologic features distinct from conventional clear cell sarcoma, suggesting that they may represent a unique tumor type (see Chapter 16 for details). The *EWSR1-CREB1* fusion gene has also been reported rarely in distal extremity clear cell sarcoma.[68,69]

It is intriguing that precisely the same fusion genes can be encountered in both the highly malignant clear cell sarcoma and the indolent angiomatoid fibrous histiocytoma. One model of mesenchymal tumor histogenesis suggests that the fusion gene drives the biology of the tumor type with which it is associated, perhaps by occurring in a relatively primitive mesenchymal cell (Fig. 18.14A). This model breaks down in the case of angiomatoid fibrous histiocytoma and clear cell sarcoma (see Fig. 18.14B). Based on the recent work of Capecchi and colleagues on alveolar rhabdomyosarcoma and synovial sarcoma, it seems that the precise cell in which a fusion gene occurs and the differentiation state of that cell are critical factors in tumorigenesis.[70-74] Even within a defined cell lineage, a certain cellular compartment may be permissive to tumorigenesis, whereas a closely related cell may find the fusion gene to have little or no effect or even to be lethal (see Fig. 18.14C). Furthermore, although fusion genes appear to be very early events in tumorigenesis, additional genetic events may also be required. This is an area of active research.

The lack of fusion variant specificity has diagnostic implications as well. Multiple fusion genes involve *EWSR1* or other loci such that detection of rearrangement by break-apart FISH, which does not provide the specific fusion partner, can be a diagnostic pitfall (see Fig. 18.5). In addition, the exact same fusion gene variant and type can be detected in two distinct sarcoma types. The *EWSR1-ATF1* fusion transcript has

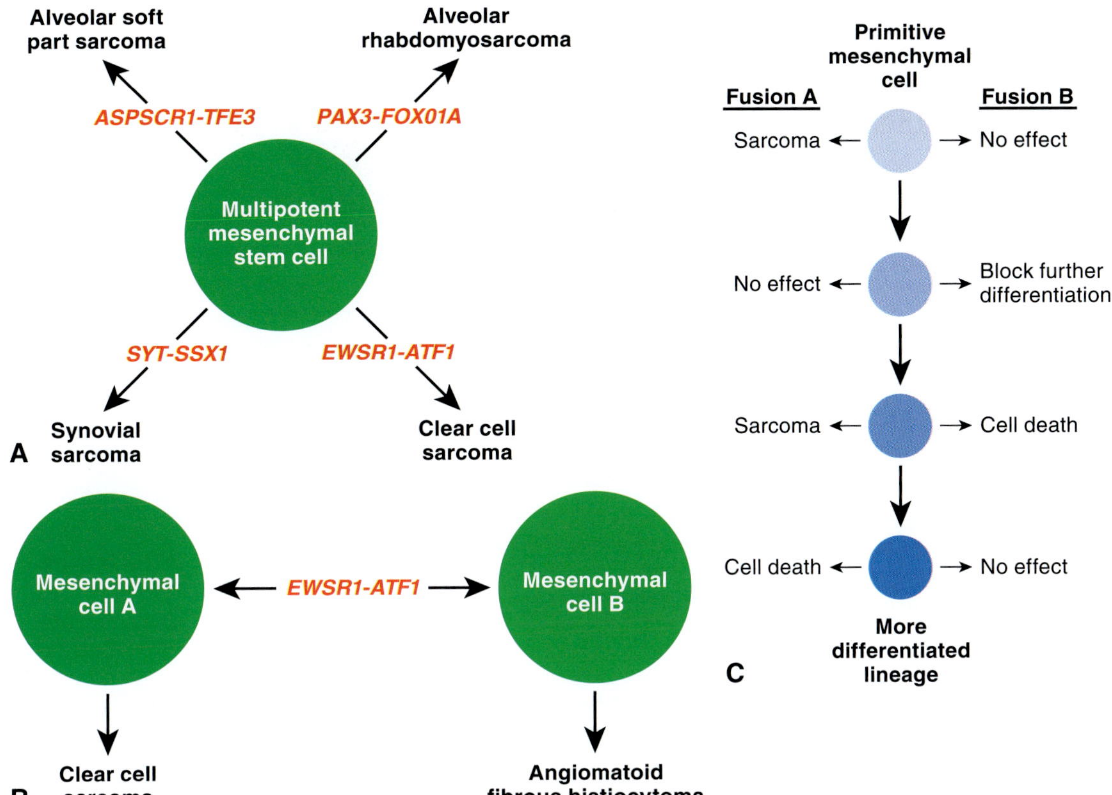

Figure 18.14 **Models of Fusion Gene Function.** (A) The universal applicability of the model of a primitive mesenchymal cell being driven by specific fusion variants to specific sarcomas has been called into question by the finding that clear cell sarcoma and angiomatoid fibrous histiocytoma have the same fusion variants and types. (B) This may indicate that the same fusion events occurring in different cell lineages may produce different tumor types. (C) More recently, the work of Capecchi and colleagues has indicated that only very specific cellular compartments and stages of a lineage are susceptible to fusion gene tumorigenesis and that additional mutations may be required as well.[37-41] In certain cases, the presence of the fusion gene may result in the arrest or death of cellular compartment, rather than tumorigenesis, in their transgenic experimental model.

Box 18.4 Tumors With *EWSR1-CREB1* and/or *EWSR1-ATF1* Fusion Variants

- Clear cell sarcoma
- Angiomatoid fibrous histiocytoma
- Malignant gastrointestinal neuroectodermal tumor (clear cell sarcoma–like tumor of the gastrointestinal tract)
- Hyalinizing clear cell sarcoma of the salivary gland
- Clear cell odontogenic tumor
- Primary pulmonary myxoid tumor of lung
- Novel myxoid mesenchymal tumor with predilection for intracranial location

also been identified in primary pulmonary myxoid sarcoma, hyalinizing clear cell carcinoma of the salivary gland, clear cell odontogenic carcinoma, and recently a novel myxoid mesenchymal tumor with predilection for intracranial locations, further demonstrating the lack of tumor specificity (Box 18.4).[75-78] This can add complexity and nuance to the interpretation of molecular testing in certain instances.

Dermatofibrosarcoma Protuberans

This superficial dermal sarcoma is associated with overexpression of platelet-derived growth factor-β (encoded by *PDGFB*), driven by the strong promoter of *COL1A1*, the gene encoding collagen type 1.[79,80] This fusion gene is formed by a usually unbalanced der(17)(17;22)(q12;q12) and is often expressed as supernumerary ring forms of duplicated segments of chromosomes 17 and 22, resulting in amplification of the fusion gene.[79,80] This fusion gene functions differently than those described previously; the *COL1A1* ultimately provides a promoter function as the amino terminus of the fusion protein is proteolytically processed and the remaining carboxy terminus dimerizes to produce "wild type" PDGF-β (Fig. 18.15). Thus this mechanism serves to overproduce a normal protein rather than producing a novel fusion protein with aberrant function. *COL1A1* comprises 52 exons, and the break points are scattered within any of the intervening introns. The break point in *PDGFB* is invariant, occurring in the intron preceding exon 2, thus allowing for production of the full-length protein after further processing.[80] Because of the many different exons that can be donated by *COL1A1*, RT-PCR primer design is challenging and requires multiple multiplexed amplification reactions.[81] Focused RNA seq is a good potential solution that overcomes the primer design and multiplexing issues. Break-apart FISH probes for the *PDGFB* locus are also used.[81,82] Interpretation can be a bit challenging, because the centromeric probes can be amplified, sometimes prominently, in the ring chromosomes.

Direct demonstration of the *COL1A1-PDGFB* fusion gene is usually not required diagnostically, given the characteristic morphology and diffuse CD34 immunoreactivity in dermatofibrosarcoma protuberans (DFSP) (see Chapter 15). However, the fibrosarcomatous variant and the pediatric giant cell fibroblastoma can be diagnostically challenging. In addition, sometimes the evolution to higher grade in DFSP can adopt unusual morphologic features resembling undifferentiated pleomorphic sarcoma.[83] Copy gains of *COL1A1-PDGFB* can be seen in the

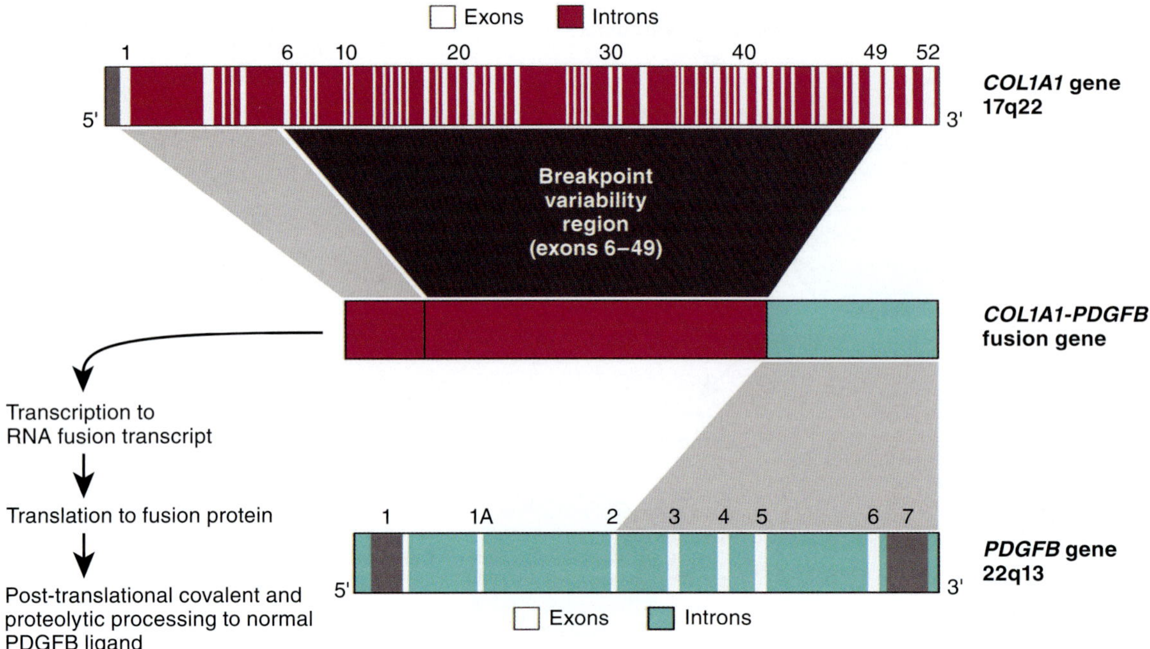

Figure 18.15 Dermatofibrosarcoma Protuberans Fusion Gene. *COL1A1* is composed of 52 exons, and the break points can occur in any intron between exons 6 and 49. The break point in *PDGFB* is invariant (*PDGFB* encodes platelet-derived growth factor-β [PDGFB]). The fusion gene is transcribed under the strong constitutive *COL1A1* promoter, and the fusion protein is ultimately proteolytically processed to a PDGFB dimer that is identical to the wild-type protein. Thus, this fusion gene causes overexpression of a normal protein rather than a protein with novel function. Because of the numerous break points in *COL1A1*, very complex and multiplexed reverse transcription polymerase chain reactions (RT-PCRs) are required, but break-apart fluorescence in situ hybridization (FISH) for the *PDGFB* locus can also be used.

fibrosarcomatous variant, and generally more copies are seen in DFSP than in giant cell fibroblastoma.[82,84] Although DFSP is usually a surgical disease, tumors not amenable to resection can be treated with imatinib mesylate; in this setting, demonstration of the fusion event may be desirable. Imatinib mesylate blocks the kinase function of the PDGF receptor-β and thus inhibits the function of the overproduced ligand, PDGF-β.[85]

Desmoid-Type Fibromatosis

This myofibroblastic tumor has features that resemble various stages of scar tissue (see Chapters 3, 4, and 16). Dysregulation of the Wnt pathway is a characteristic feature of this tumor.[86] Desmoid fibromatosis can been seen in the setting of familial adenomatous polyposis (FAP), which is then termed Gardner syndrome. Germline mutations in the tumor suppressor gene adenomatous polyposis coli (*APC*) are responsible for FAP, and loss of heterozygosity of the remaining wild-type *APC* allele is a key early step in colonic carcinogenesis in both this and the sporadic setting. The same mechanism is seen in desmoid fibromatosis associated with this syndrome and in a small subset (perhaps 5% to 10%) of sporadic desmoid tumors.[87] Interestingly, the type and location of mutation in the inherited mutated *APC* allele is predictive of the likelihood of desmoid tumor development. *CTNNB1*, another gene in the Wnt pathway encoding the protein β-catenin, is mutated in greater than 85% of sporadic desmoid tumors.[88,89] These mutations basically occur at only two codons, 41 and 45, encoding a threonine and serine, respectively. A single mutation is seen at threonine 41 (T41), whereas two mutations may be seen at serine 45 (S45) in the vast majority of cases. This limited repertoire of only three mutations is unusual among tumors with *CTNNB1* mutations, where multiple codons and multiple base pair changes are often detected, although these are most often clustered around four critical codons encoding three important serines and one threonine. The somewhat complex pathway of β-catenin regulation is depicted in Fig. 18.16. Briefly, β-catenin is a multifunctional protein with a role in cell adhesion at the plasma membrane and a cell signaling and transcriptional role in transiting from the cytoplasm to the nucleus.[90] β-catenin is normally constitutively phosphorylated sequentially from amino acids 45, 41, 37, and 33. When fully phosphorylated, β-catenin is targeted for destruction in the proteosome. The protein encoded by *APC* acts as a scaffold for the phosphorylation complex. In the presence of active Wnt signaling, this phosphorylation is disrupted, and β-catenin accumulates in the nucleus, where it acts in a transcription complex with the T-cell factor (TCF) family of transcription factors and other proteins. Disruption of the phosphorylation sequence by mutation prevents the constitutive destruction of the protein and allows for accumulation in the nucleus, which can be detected by immunohistochemistry.[91] Only three specific mutations are observed; detection of these mutations is amenable to pyrosequencing, but other methods are also applicable (Fig. 18.17). Although this test is usually not necessary in resection specimens, it may be useful in needle biopsies and for differentiating local recurrence from scar, which can be difficult in small samples and when immunohistochemistry to demonstrate nuclear accumulation of β-catenin is not definitive. Several large retrospective studies have indicated that the mutation type may be predictive of increased likelihood for recurrence, but this is less clear in other studies.[88,92-96]

Very recently, sporadic desmoid tumors determined to be wild-type for *CTNNB1* by pyrosequencing and/or Sanger sequencing were found to have very low allelic fractions of *CTNNB1* mutation by the more sensitive technique of NGS. Other cases were found to have *APC* mutations or exceptionally yet other mutations predicted to activate the Wnt pathway. These studies suggest that the prevalence of desmoid

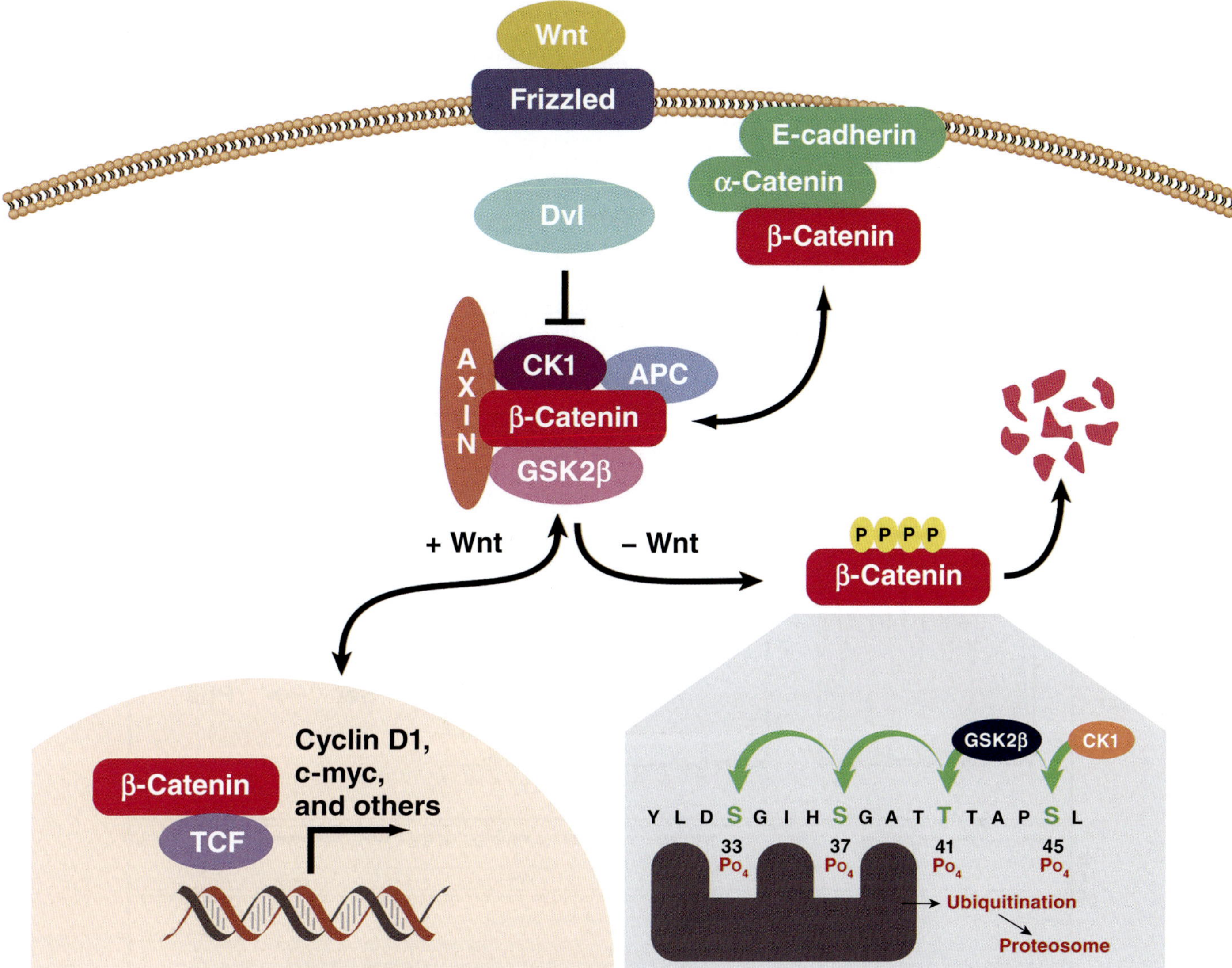

Figure 18.16 **The β-catenin Pathway.** β-catenin is unusual in that it acts both as an adhesion molecule and a signaling molecule. At the cell membrane, it participates in adherens junctions with E-cadherin in epithelial cells. When present in the cytosol, it is normally constitutively phosphorylated by the adenomatous polyposis coli (APC) complex, priming it for ubiquitination and destruction in the proteosome. In the presence of Wnt signaling, the APC complex is inhibited and β-catenin can accumulate in the cytosol and translocate to the nucleus where it acts in concert with other proteins in a transcription complex. β-catenin can also be activated as the result of *APC* mutations and loss of heterozygosity that prevent the function of the APC kinase complex, as seen in familial adenomatous polyposis and many sporadic colon cancers. Normally, β-catenin is sequentially phosphorylated on critical amino acids *(bottom right)* first by CK1 and then GSK3β in the sequential order indicated (45 to 33). Mutations in exon 3 of *CTNNB1*, the gene encoding β-catenin, which prevent phosphorylation at one of these sites, also inhibit phosphorylation of any subsequent sites. Mutations in desmoids tumors are only at positions 41 and 45.

tumors that are wild-type for *CTNNB1* may be exceedingly low. It also raises interesting questions regarding the heterogeneity of mutations (perhaps mosaic in some cases) considered to be driver mutations in these tumors.[97]

Desmoplastic Small Round Cell Tumor

The chromosomal alteration in this tumor type, t(11;22)(p13;q12), is similar to that of Ewing sarcoma except that it involves the *WT1* gene on the short or "p" (for petite arm of chromosome 11) rather than the *FLI1* gene on the long or "q" arm of this same chromosome.[98] A depiction of this translocation along with a karyotype of a complex case resolved with spectral karyotyping is depicted in Fig. 18.8. Although *WT1* is a classic tumor suppressor gene in Wilms tumor, when fused with *EWSR1* it becomes oncogenic. Break-apart *EWSR1* FISH and RT-PCR approaches are available for detection.[99,100] As with most fusions involving *EWSR1*, multiple fusion types are described but no variant partners are known. Virtually all cases of desmoplastic small round cell tumor bear this molecular signature. In small biopsies, care must be taken with the interpretation of *EWSR1* rearrangement demonstrated by break-apart FISH, because this is also seen in Ewing sarcoma (and other tumors; see Fig. 18.5). The clinical setting and immunohistochemical differences can usually resolve this differential diagnosis (see also Chapter 8), but RT-PCR or focused RNA seq to demonstrate the fusion partner can help differentiate between these two round cell sarcomas in equivocal

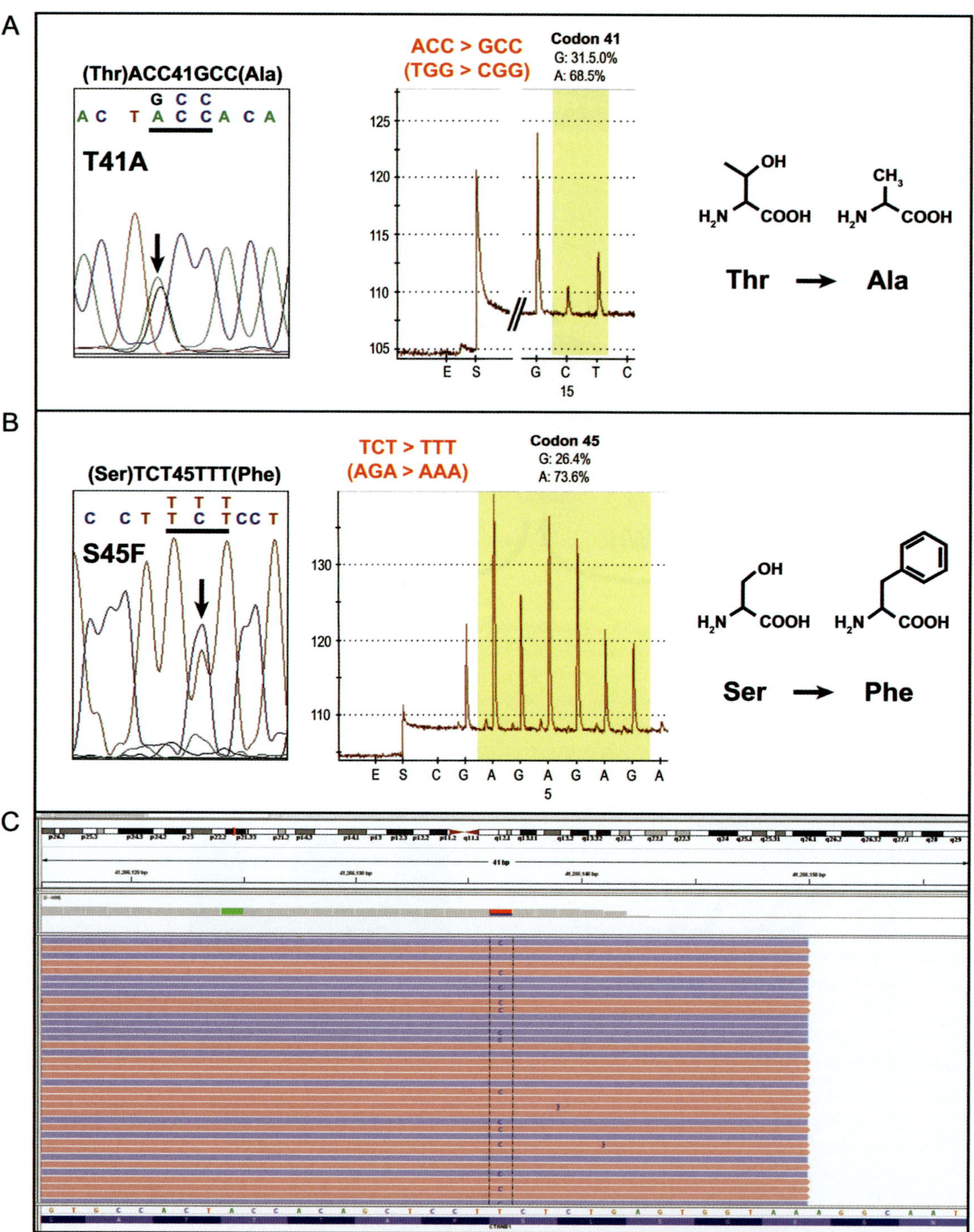

Figure 18.17 ***CTNNB1* Mutations in Desmoid Fibromatosis.** (A and B) The two most common mutations encountered in exon 3 of *CTNNB1*, the gene encoding β-catenin, are shown. Only three mutations are routinely identified in *CTNNB1* in sporadic desmoid tumors and show a combined prevalence of about 85%. These mutations can be demonstrated by both Sanger sequencing *(left)* and pyrosequencing *(middle)* of genomic tumor DNA. Immunohistochemistry to demonstrate nuclear accumulation of β-catenin is often used, but molecular characterization can also be helpful in equivocal cases and in small biopsies or to differentiate between scar and recurrent desmoid. (C) The less common mutation leading to substitution of proline for serine at position 45 (S45P) is demonstrated using next generation sequencing. (Portions of this figure courtesy Dr. Dolores López-Terrada, Texas Children's Hospital and Baylor College of Medicine, Houston, TX & Mark Routbort, MD Anderson Cancer Center, Houston, TX.)

cases. Immunohistochemistry may help demonstrate nuclear WT1 expression, but an antibody that recognizes the C-terminus of the protein must be used (rather than the commonly used monoclonal antibody directed against the N-terminus, which is lost in the fusion protein); such available antibodies show inconsistent results.[101]

Endometrial Stromal Sarcoma

Endometrial stromal tumors are often associated with t(7;17)(p15;q21), resulting in a *JAZF1-SUZ12 (JJAZ1)* fusion.[102-104] This translocation is found in the majority of endometrial stromal nodules and in about 50% of low-grade endometrial stromal sarcomas. *PHF1* on 6p21 can substitute for *SUZ12 (JJAZ1)* on occasion, and few cases of an *EPC1-PHF1* variant have been reported.[105,106] Both break-apart FISH for *JAZF1* and RT-PCR testing are available.[107] Some endometrial stromal sarcomas showing high-grade features have been demonstrated to harbor t(10;17)(q22;p13), resulting in *YWHAE-NUTM2A/B* (*FAM22*) fusion genes.[108,109]

Epithelioid Hemangioendothelioma

The t(1;3)(p36;q25) fuses *WWTR1* and *CAMTA1* in the vast majority of cases of epithelioid hemangioendothelioma (EHE) (see Chapters 6 and 13 for discussion of EHE).[110,111] This fusion appears to be limited to EHE and is not seen in other neoplasms showing vascular differentiation. Both FISH and RT-PCR approaches would be reasonable because the number of fusion types appears to be limited. Interestingly, a subset of EHEs with distinctive morphology (voluminous cytoplasm, focal vasoformative areas) has been described. These tumors have rearrangements involving *YAP1* on 11q22 and *TFE3* on Xp11. Whether these tumors should be retained within the EHE category remains to be determined.[112]

Ewing Sarcoma

The tumor type formerly also designated primitive neuroectodermal tumor (PNET) is now known to be a histologic variant of Ewing sarcoma, with indistinguishable clinical behavior and the same array of fusion gene variants and types (see Chapter 8). The PNET designation is no longer recommended for these tumors; Ewing sarcoma is the preferred diagnostic term. These tumors can occur in both bone and soft tissue and are sometimes referred to as Ewing family tumors. As Ewing sarcoma was discussed earlier as the archetypal translocation-associated sarcoma, the discussion here is abbreviated. Ewing sarcoma is associated with multiple fusion partners, most commonly *EWSR1* (22q12) but rarely also the *EWSR1* homolog *FUS* (16p11). The fusion partner providing the DNA-binding domain is a member of the ETS family of transcription factors, of which *FLI1* on 11q24 is the most common.[8] As mentioned previously, multiple different tumor types use *EWSR1* as a fusion partner, as depicted in Fig. 18.5. *EWSR1* is of uncertain function but comprises 17 exons with the transactivation domain encoded by exons 1 to 7, which is the portion involved in the fusion genes. A domain with homology to the proposed RNA-binding site of RNA polymerase II is encoded by exons 11 to 15, and a DNA-binding zinc finger by exon 15 (see Fig. 18.3). These latter two domains are absent in the active fusion gene. The most common break points in *EWSR1* are in introns 7 and 8, which fall between exons 7 and 8 or 8 and 9, respectively.[13] Exon 8 is spliced out of the transcribed mRNA; thus only exons 1 to 7 are present unless the break point extends beyond intron 8, as shown in Fig. 18.4. Break-apart FISH for *EWSR1* is an efficient way to detect all of the variants that include *EWSR1* and an ETS family member, and *FUS* break-apart FISH can detect most of the other rare variants (see Fig. 18.6).[113] The variants not involving *EWSR1* or *FUS* in Ewing sarcoma are very rare (see Table 18.4); the family of Ewing-like tumors (a subset of undifferentiated round cell sarcomas) that lack involvement of *EWSR1* or *FUS* is addressed further on. However, it must be remembered that multiple other mesenchymal neoplasms are associated with rearrangements of these two genes, and thus recombination or fusion FISH or RT-PCR may be more helpful in certain cases.[114] The vast majority of cases can be detected by RT-PCR that covers the *EWSR1-FLI1* variants (even types 1 and 2 alone detect about 80% of cases). As a practical matter, most RT-PCR assays are designed to detect the most common types of *FLI1* and *ERG* fusion variants because these include more than 95% of cases.[8] The other described fusion variants are extremely rare (see Table 18.4). The variety of fusions makes focused RNA seq a potentially valuable approach. It has been suggested that *EWSR1-FLI1* fusion types 1 and 2 fare better clinically under contemporary treatment protocols than do all the other types, but a recent large European study did not show significant differences between variants and types.[115,116] The clinical value of using RT-PCR to detect minimal residual disease in the peripheral blood and bone marrow has been examined in a retrospective study, which seemed to show that detection of minimal residual disease was associated with an aggressive disease course and shorter clinical remission times.[117] Further confirmation is needed.

Ewing-Like Tumors With Alternative Fusion Transcripts

As mentioned earlier, a subset of round cell sarcomas negative for *EWRS1* rearrangements were discovered to have alternative fusion transcripts including *CIC* on 19q13 and *DUX4* located on both 4q35 and 10q26 or, less commonly, *FOXO4* on Xq13.[16,118-120] *CIC* is part of the high-mobility group (HMG) of transcription factors and is normally expressed in the cerebellum, whereas *DUX4* encodes a double-homeobox transcription factor normally expressed in germ cells in the testis.[16] *FOXO4* encodes a protein that a part of the forkhead family and is homologous to the FKHR protein.[120] The initial report of a round cell sarcoma with *CIC-FOXO4* noted desmoplastic stroma, although this was not seen in a subsequent case.[119,120] As the break point between *DUX4* is variable, FISH for *CIC* is preferable. Although previously lumped together with Ewing sarcoma, studies have suggested that these tumors may behave more aggressively and have gene signatures distinct from Ewing sarcoma, including upregulation of Ets genes (such as *ETV4*) and *WT1*. The detection of expression of these proteins by immunohistochemical studies can be useful.[17,121-123] The distinction between conventional Ewing sarcoma and round cell sarcomas with *CIC* rearrangements is increasingly important (see Chapter 8).

Another subset of Ewing-like sarcomas negative for *EWSR1* and *CIC* rearrangements have been found to have a translocation involving *BCOR* on Xp11.4 and *CCNB3* on Xp11.22. BCOR is a transcriptional repressor associated with BCL6 and is a translocation partner in some acute myeloid leukemias. CCNB3 is expressed in the testis and is involved in sperm development.[14] Interestingly, these tumors most often occur in young adult males, and some show spindle cell morphology, overlapping histologically with synovial sarcoma to some degree. Similar to *CIC-DUX4* round cell sarcomas, some studies suggest that these tumors may behave differently than classic Ewing sarcoma.[15,124,125] The translocation results in the overexpression of CCNB3 and BCOR, both of which can be detected by immunohistochemistry.[126] New discoveries in the category of unclassified round cell sarcomas continue to be reported including *BCOR-MAML3* and *ZC3H7B-BCOR* fusions.[127] RT-PCR and FISH approaches are reasonable for both of these tumor types.

Extraskeletal Myxoid Chondrosarcoma

Extraskeletal myxoid chondrosarcoma is another soft tissue sarcoma that usually utilizes *EWSR1* as a fusion partner (see Chapter 5).[128] As illustrated in Fig. 18.18, *NR4A3* (also known as *TEC* or *CHN*) on 9q22 can combine with *EWSR1* or three alternative *EWSR1* homologs, *TAF2N* (17q11), *TFG* (3q11), and *TCF12* (15p21). Interestingly, *TFG* can also combine with other genes in some cases of papillary thyroid carcinoma

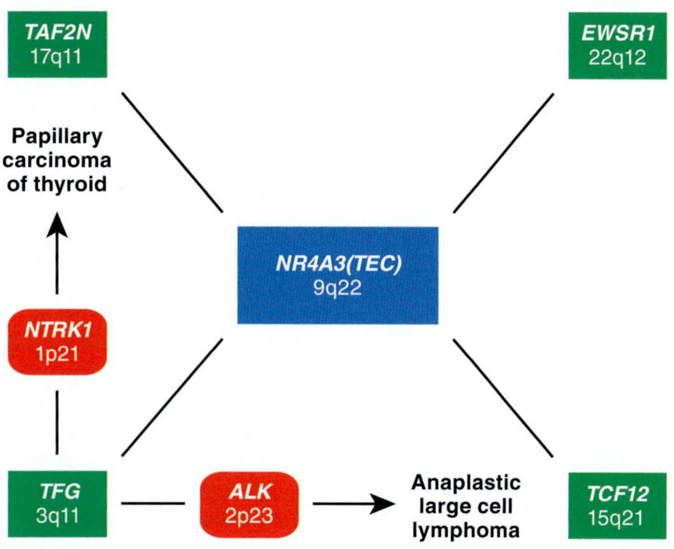

Figure 18.18 Various Fusion Variants Seen in Extraskeletal Myxoid Chondrosarcoma. *NR4A3* can be rearranged with *EWSR1* or three homologs. *EWSR1* is the most commonly encountered fusion partner, and, thus, break-apart *EWSR1* fluorescence in situ hybridization (FISH) is a viable diagnostic approach in most cases. Interestingly, *TFG* is also rearranged in papillary thyroid carcinoma and anaplastic large cell lymphoma.

and anaplastic large-cell lymphoma. Break-apart FISH probes for *NR4A3* have recently been developed, but because *EWSR1* is the fusion partner in 70% of cases, it is the most common break-apart FISH approach used.[129] RT-PCR approaches can also be used to detect the multiple fusion variants and types.[130,131]

Glomus Tumors

Glomus tumors (see Chapters 6 and 16) have recurrent translocations involving the promoter region of miR143 and *NOTCH* (*NOTCH1, 2,* or *3*), with most tumors utilizing *NOTCH2*. Both genes appear to play a role in vascular smooth muscle differentiation. The absence of rearrangement in the vast majority of other perivascular tumors suggests that these tumors are not related, as was previously thought.[132] Familial glomus tumors (glomuvenous malformations) are caused by mutations in *GLMN* (glomulin) on 1p22.1, whereas in patients with neurofibromatosis type 1, digital glomus tumors are secondary to biallelic inactivation of *NF1*.[132-135]

Gastrointestinal Stromal Tumor

GISTs are the most common clinically significant mesenchymal neoplasms of the gastrointestinal tract (see Chapter 16). The relatively simple karyotypes of GISTs lack recurrent structural rearrangements, but losses of particular chromosomal segments are common, although these are not diagnostically relevant at this time. Activating mutations in the gene *KIT*, a receptor tyrosine kinase, are detected in up to 80% of GISTs, with analogous mutations observed in *PDGFRA* in approximately 5% to 10% of cases (Fig. 18.19).[136] The name of this gene is derived from its homology to the feline (*kit*ten) Hardy-Zuckerman 4 sarcoma viral oncogene. Exon 11 encoding the juxtamembrane domain is the most commonly mutated region, seen in 65% of cases. Mutations in this exon include in-frame deletions, point mutations, and in-frame insertions (mostly duplications). Deletions are most commonly encountered and are sometimes seen in combination with point mutations.[137] Duplications are less often seen. Although exon 11 is not large (42 codons or 126 base pairs; codons 550 to 591), there is a rich diversity of deletions, duplications, and point mutations. Fortunately the deletions and insertions must maintain the reading frame, and this aids in interpretation. Interestingly, deletions tend to involve codons 550 to 575 and range from 3 to 42 or more base pairs in length, and duplications tend to involve codons 575 to 591. Point mutations are clustered on codons 557 to 560 and also codon 576, although a variety of codons are involved on occasion. This diversity complicates interpretation of molecular testing of this exon. Homozygous *KIT* mutations in exon 11 appear to portend a poor prognosis.[138]

Exon 9 mutations are detected in about 10% of cases, virtually all of which are duplications of codons 502 and 503. Primary mutations in other exons of *KIT* such as 13 and 17 are rare (1% each) (see Fig. 18.19).[139] In contrast, mutations in *PDGFRA* are most common in the second kinase domain (exon 18).[137]

Although mutational testing is generally not needed for diagnostic purposes, the type of mutation predicts the likelihood of response to imatinib mesylate, a tyrosine kinase inhibitor that inhibits KIT and PDGFRA.[136] GISTs containing mutations in exon 11 are generally highly sensitive to imatinib mesylate, whereas GISTs with exon 9 mutations require higher doses of imatinib to achieve optimal responses.[140] The responsiveness of GISTs harboring the other primary mutations in exons 13 and 17 is less well understood, given their rarity, but appears variable depending on the specific mutation. Tumors with mutations involving *PDGFRA* also have variable imatinib sensitivity depending on mutation type. For example, those tumors with *PDGFRA* D842V tend to be naive in resistance to imatinib.[141] Unfortunately long-term treatment with imatinib mesylate often leads to the emergence of resistance. This has a molecular correlate in the selection of additional point mutations, primarily in exons 13, 14, and 17 (Fig. 18.20).[142,143] The primary mutation is retained; these secondary mutations appear mostly to inhibit the binding of imatinib mesylate to the receptor. The use of mutational testing to guide therapy prospectively has not been universally adopted but is gaining acceptance. With the approval of second- and third-line tyrosine kinase inhibitors (sunitinib malate and regorafenib) and the development of other drugs in the immediate pipeline, it is likely that *KIT* and *PDGFRA* genotyping will increasingly be used to select the most effective therapy for patients with advanced disease.

PCR amplification of genomic DNA with Sanger sequencing is the gold standard for precise determination of *KIT* and *PDGFRA* mutations, given the diversity discussed earlier. Sizing chromatography and high-performance liquid chromatography can also be useful for screening and aid in interpretation (see Fig. 18.19B). These methods can indicate that a certain exon is mutated but are less able to delineate the precise mutation. Therefore precise mutational assessment is becoming more clinically relevant for individual patient management. Techniques such as direct Sanger sequencing or next-generation DNA sequencing approaches increasingly predominate (see Fig. 18.19E).

Mutations in additional genes have been identified in GISTs lacking *KIT* or *PDGFRA* gene mutations (wild-type GISTs). These include activating point mutations (V600E) in the *BRAF* oncogene and also germline mutations in the genes encoding subunits of the succinate dehydrogenase complex (*SDHA*, *SDHB*, *SDHC*, and *SDHD*) with or without other signs of Carney-Stratakis syndrome (i.e., paragangliomas).[144-149] These are also readily detected by immunohistochemistry.[148,150] Other syndromic associations with GIST beyond familial GIST with germline mutations in *KIT* or *PDGFRA* include neurofibromatosis type 1 (germline mutation in *NF1*) and the Carney triad (gastric GIST, extra-adrenal paraganglioma, and pulmonary chondroma), which is not inherited; Carney triad is usually associated with *SDHC* promoter hypermethylation (occasionally with *SDHX* germline mutations).[147,151-155]

Interestingly, an association between GIST and other tumors including desmoid fibromatosis has been identified, suggesting that there may be

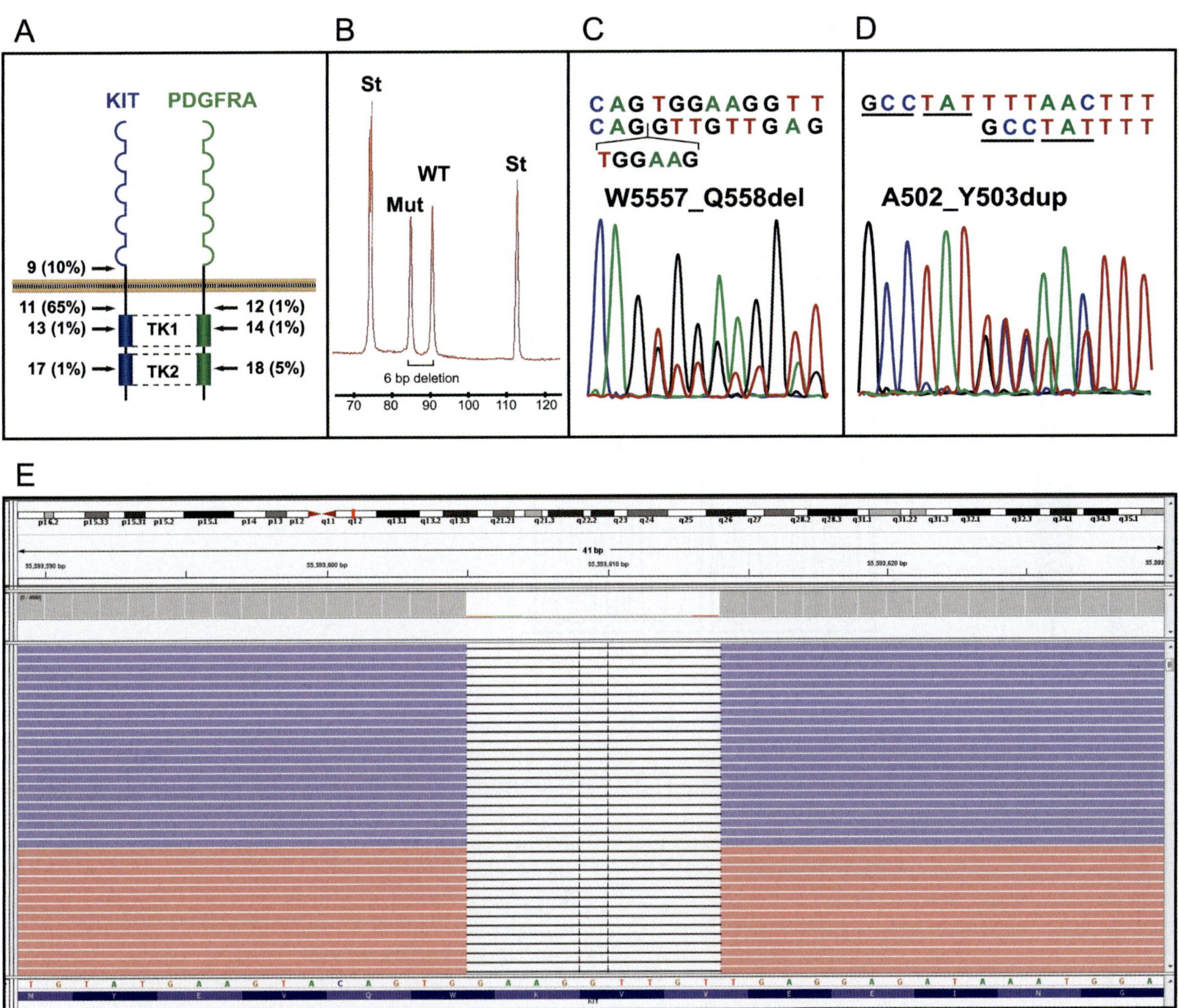

Figure 18.19 **Receptor Tyrosine Kinase Mutations in Gastrointestinal Stromal Tumor (GIST).** (A) The intracellular juxtamembrane domain encoded by exon 11 of KIT is the most common site mutated in GIST. (B) In-frame deletions are the most common mutations encountered. (C) These mutations can also be detected by size fractionation of the polymerase chain reaction (PCR) amplicon with confirmation by Sanger sequencing of the amplified genomic tumor DNA. Point mutations and less commonly insertions (duplications) are seen in exon 11. (D) The extracellular domain encoded by exon 9 is the next most commonly mutated site; virtually all of these mutations are specific duplications (A502_Y503dup). (E) Sequence mapping displays of amplicons showing in-frame deletion of *KIT* exon 11 from next generation sequencing. The tyrosine kinase domains 1 and 2 encoded by exons 13 and 17 of *KIT* are much less common primary mutations (A). Analogous exons are mutated in *PDGFRA*, but extracellular domain mutations are not seen. (Portions of this figure courtesy Mark Routbort, MD Anderson Cancer Center, Houston, TX.)

underlying genetic mechanisms in some patients with GIST that predispose them to the development of other tumors.[156,157]

Infantile Fibrosarcoma

Infantile fibrosarcoma is associated with the recurrent chromosomal aberration t(12;15)(p13;q26) (see Chapter 4).[158] Traditional karyotypic analysis of this event can be difficult because it involves the distal tips of 12p and 15q as well as *ETV6* (also known as *TEL*) and *NTRK3* (also known as *TRCK*).[159] *ETV6* is a transcription factor and *NTRK3* is a receptor tyrosine kinase. The fusion gene is fashioned from the N-terminal oligomerization domain of *ETV6*, which leads to constitutive activation of the associated kinase domain donated by *NTRK3*. Interestingly, a renal neoplasm of infancy, cellular mesoblastic nephroma, harbors the same fusion gene and overlapping histologic features; thus this neoplasm appears to represent a renal form of infantile fibrosarcoma.[160] This fusion gene has also been documented in secretory carcinoma of the breast and mammary analog secretory carcinomas at various sites as well as in rare cases of wild-type GIST, papillary thyroid carcinoma (especially those associated with radiation exposure), inflammatory myofibroblastic tumor, melanocytic Spitz tumors, glioblastoma, colorectal carcinoma, and adult acute myeloid leukemia (Box 18.5).[161-169] Documentation of this fusion is now more relevant given the availability of targeted NTRK inhibitors. That this translocation is detected in small numbers in a variety of tumor types speaks to the strength of using semifocused RNA seq to detected multiple to many fusions in a sample using a single test. *NTRK3* along with *NTRK1* and *NTRK2* can have multiple fusion partners and can be involved in multiple other neoplasms.

Conventional cytogenetics can be useful but challenging, as noted previously. Additional cytogenetic events include trisomies of chromosomes 8, 11, 17, and 20. Chromosome 11 trisomy is particularly

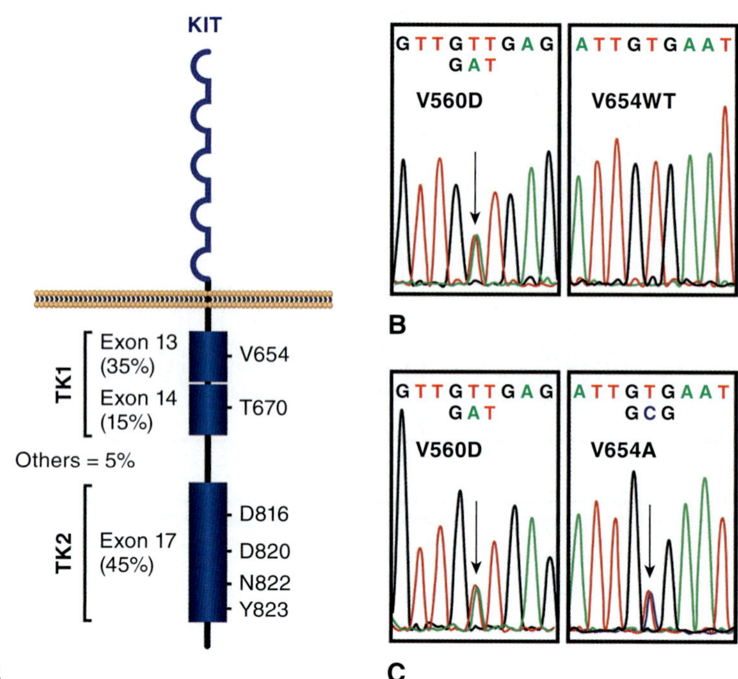

Figure 18.20 **Secondary Resistance Mutations in *KIT*.** Exons 13, 14, and 17 are the most common sites of secondary mutations selected for by treatment of gastrointestinal stromal tumor with the tyrosine kinase inhibitor, imatinib mesylate (A). These are point mutations, and the ones most commonly reported are depicted. The tyrosine kinase domains 1 and 2 encode the ATP-binding and tyrosine kinase catalytic domain of the Kit receptor. The point mutations appear to adversely affect the binding of imatinib to the receptor, reducing its efficacy as an inhibitor, although they may cause ligand-independent receptor activation as well. These point mutations occur in the setting of a primary mutation such as those seen in Fig. 18.19. In the present figure, a tumor with a primary point mutation in exon 11 resulting in a substitution of aspartic acid for valine at amino acid residue 560 (V560D) is present in both the primary tumor (B) and tumor from the same patient who developed resistance to imatinib mesylate treatment (C). The resistance point mutation V654A was not seen in the primary tumor (B) but was selected for by tyrosine kinase inhibitor treatment and detected in the tumor showing treatment resistance (C).

Box 18.5 Neoplasms With *ETV6-NTRK3* Rearrangements

Inflammatory myofibroblastic tumor
"Wild-type" GIST
Adult acute myeloid leukemia
Papillary thyroid carcinoma (especially with radiation exposure)
Colorectal carcinoma
Melanocytic Spitz tumors
Glioblastoma

GIST, Gastrointestinal stromal tumor.

characteristic and may be helpful in the proper setting for the initiation of other methods to demonstrate the fusion gene, such as FISH or RT-PCR.[170]

Inflammatory Myofibroblastic Tumor

The characteristic molecular alterations in this tumor type arise from a variety of balanced structural rearrangements involving the *ALK* gene at 2p23. This tumor type was first described in the lung and subsequently recognized at diverse anatomic sites (see Chapters 4, 10, and 16). *ALK* translocations tend to occur in tumors from pediatric and young adult patients (~50%) and are uncommon in tumors from older adults.[171,172] *ALK* encodes a membrane-bound receptor tyrosine kinase that dimerizes in the presence of ligand to become active. This protein normally has a very limited expression pattern and is seen in certain regions of the brain. Numerous translocation partners exist (see Table 18.3); each donates a domain that causes dimerization and constitutive activation (Fig. 18.21A).[173] These various domains supplied to the fusion variants can cause accumulation of the protein in the cytoplasm, nucleus, or nuclear membrane, as can be demonstrated by immunohistochemistry (see Fig. 18.21B to E). Translocation to the cytoplasm is most common in inflammatory myofibroblastic tumor, resulting from fusion with *TPM3* and other genes. Some of these same translocations are also seen in anaplastic large cell lymphoma. However, the most common *ALK* fusion partner in anaplastic large cell lymphoma, *NPM* (5q35), is not observed in inflammatory myofibroblastic tumor.[174] As previously mentioned, *ALK* rearrangement is also found in epithelioid fibrous histiocytomas (with different fusion partners) and gastrointestinal leiomyomas (see further on). A distinctive epithelioid variant of inflammatory myofibroblastic tumor is usually associated with a *RANBP2-ALK* fusion and less often a *RRBP1-ALK* fusion.[175,176] The former gene fusion leads to a nuclear membrane distribution of the fusion protein detectable by ALK immunohistochemistry (see Fig. 18.21E); the latter leads to a cytoplasmic pattern with perinuclear accentuation.[175] This distinctive variant usually arises in the abdominal cavity and pursues a much more aggressive clinical course than conventional inflammatory myofibroblastic tumor; it is known as epithelioid inflammatory myofibroblastic sarcoma.[175]

Immunohistochemistry for the ALK protein can be helpful, because it is rarely detected in tissues outside the brain.[171] More recently, fusions involving genes other than *ALK* have been documented rarely in inflammatory myofibroblastic tumor, including *ROS1* and *RET* (also seen in lung cancer) as well as *PDGFRB* and *ETV6-NTRK3* (the last seen in infantile fibrosarcoma as well; see Box 18.5).[167,177-179] Break-apart FISH for the *ALK* gene locus is the most commonly used molecular technique. However, given the wide range of fusion partners with this gene and gene substitutions for ALK on rare occasions, focused RNA seq is also a viable option. *ALK* translocations are seen in many other neoplasms as well, with a wide variety of fusion partners (Fig. 18.22).[180-199] For some of these tumors, such as inflammatory myofibroblastic tumor and epithelioid fibrous histiocytoma, ALK overexpression and gene fusions are characteristic; for other neoplasms such as lung adenocarcinoma, only a small subset of tumors have the translocation. Demonstrating these *ALK* translocations can be therapeutically relevant, because effective inhibitors are available clinically.[200,201]

Leiomyoma

Numerous cytogenetic findings have been described in leiomyoma (uterine are the best studied because they are so widespread). The most frequent translocation is t(12;14)(q15;q24) involving *HMGA2* and *RAD51L1*, but this is still relatively uncommon.[202] Interestingly, some rearrangements of the *HMGA2* gene in uterine leiomyomas occur in

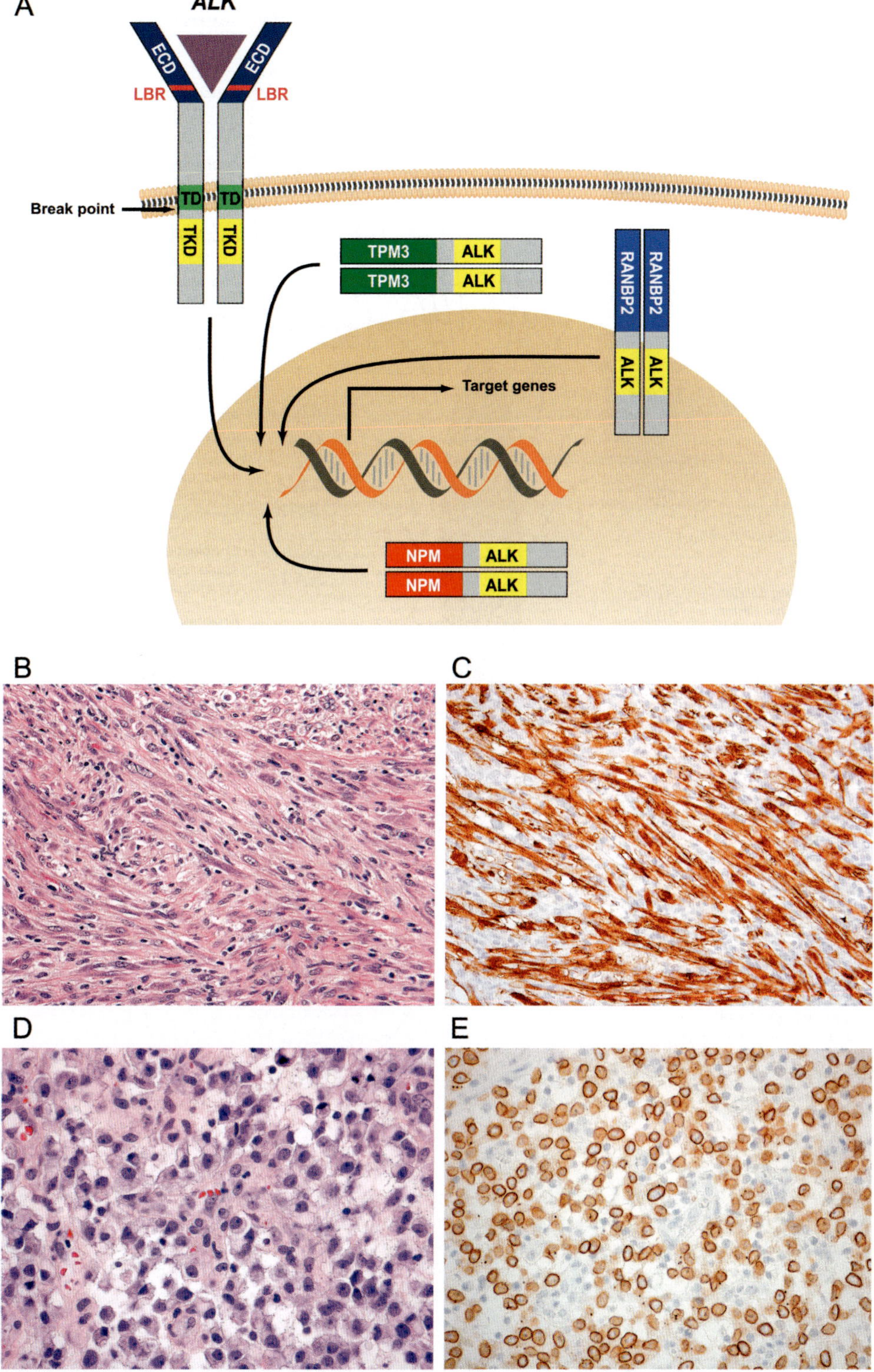

Figure 18.21 **Molecular Alterations Involving *ALK* in Inflammatory Myofibroblastic Tumor.** (A) The protein encoded by *ALK* is a receptor tyrosine kinase that dimerizes in the presence of ligand *(purple triangle)* to release its tyrosine kinase activity and unleash a biochemical cascade resulting in regulation of target genes. The various fusion genes result from the combination of the ALK tyrosine kinase domain with a domain from another protein that promotes dimerization and thus ligand-independent activation. The fusion protein is also targeted to a different cellular compartment such as the cytoplasm for TPM3, the nuclear membrane for RANBP2, or the cytoplasm and nucleus for NPM (the latter seen only in anaplastic large cell lymphoma, not in inflammatory myofibroblastic tumor). (B and C) H&E and immunohistochemistry for ALK showing cytoplasmic staining associated with the *TPM3-ALK* gene fusion, whereas D and E, show H&E and nuclear membrane ALK distribution with the *RANBP2-ALK* translocation. *ECD*, Extracellular domain; *LBR*, ligand binding region; *TD*, transmembrane domain; *TKD*, tyrosine kinase domain.

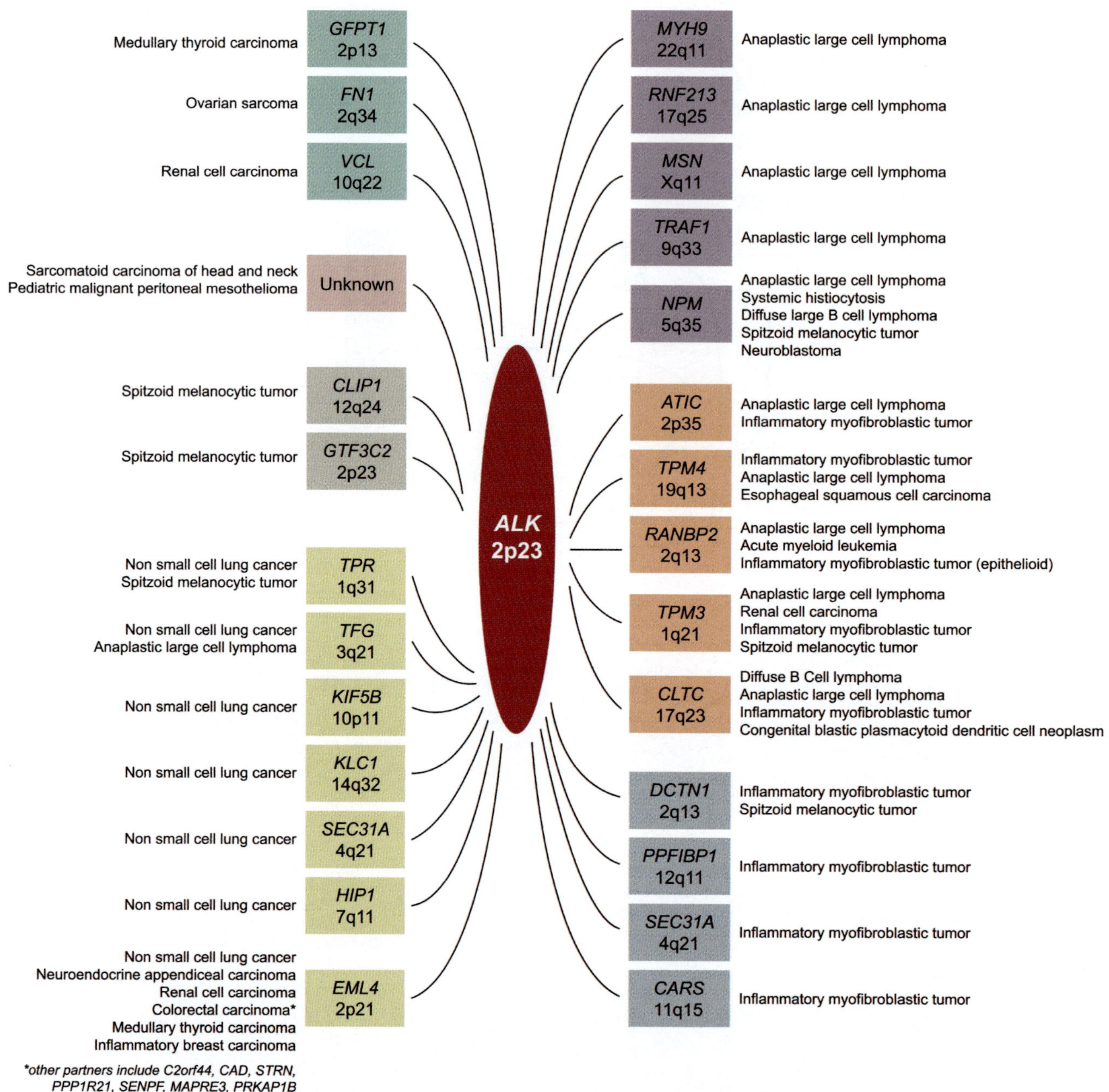

Figure 18.22 Gene Fusion Variants Involving *ALK*. *ALK* is promiscuous with numerous partners involved in translocations in a wide variety of mesenchymal and nonmesenchymal tumor types. In a few neoplasms such as inflammatory myofibroblastic tumor, epithelioid fibrous histiocytoma, and anaplastic large cell lymphoma, such translocations are common and even disease-defining in certain situations. In some other neoplasms, *ALK* translocation and overexpression is seen in only a small subset of cases, such as lung adenocarcinoma. Sometimes *ALK*-translocated tumors have unique clinicopathologic features, whereas in others this is not the case.

DNA 10 to 100 kb upstream (5′) of the gene. Thus no fusion gene is produced, but this does serve to cause overexpression of the encoded protein. Interestingly, specific mutations have been found in leiomyomas of various sites. Uterine leiomyomas have been discovered to harbor mutations in *MED12* (Xq13.1). *MED12* encodes for a protein (mediator complex subunit 12), which is an important component of the transcriptional machinery; mutations in this gene are thought to result in genomic instability. Uterine smooth muscle tumors that harbor *MED12* mutations may have differing morphologic appearances as well.[203] *MED12* mutations are also seen in other tumors, including phyllodes tumors of the breast.[204,205] Recurrent inversion translocations involving *FN1* (2q35), which encodes for fibronectin, and *ALK* (2p23) have been identified in several gastrointestinal leiomyomas.[206]

Hereditary leiomyomatosis and renal cell carcinoma (HLRCC) syndrome are associated with loss-of-function mutations in the *FH* gene encoding fumarate hydratase (1q42); they are inherited in an autosomal dominant fashion.[207,208] Interestingly, this enzyme participates in the Krebs cycle, as does the succinate dehydrogenase (SDH) complex; mutations in SDH subunit genes are detected in a subset of wild-type gastric GISTs. The mechanism by which lack of this mitochondrial

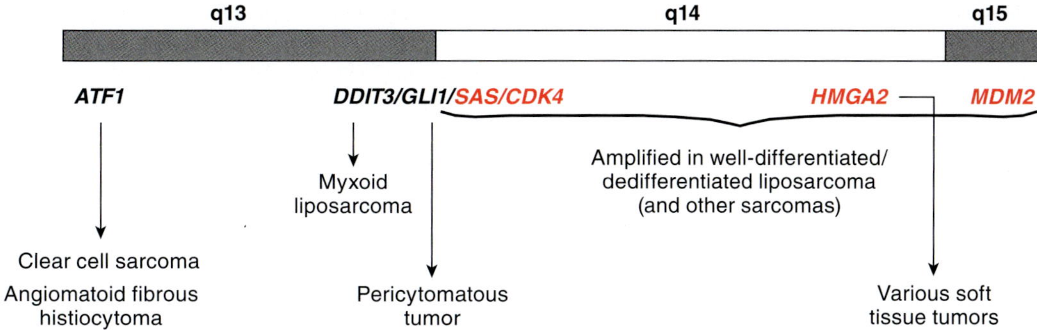

Figure 18.23 Depiction of Chromosome 12q13-15 Interval Involved in Multiple Soft Tissue Tumors. This interval on the long arm of chromosome 12 contains numerous genes involved in sarcomas and other soft tissue tumors. Rearrangements are seen with various genes in this interval, and amplification of this region is seen in well-differentiated and dedifferentiated liposarcomas. The various mesenchymal and other tumors showing *HMGA2* rearrangements are listed in Box 18.6.

metabolic enzyme leads to uterine and dermal leiomyomas and renal cell carcinoma is poorly understood. Germline testing for the HLRCC syndrome is available; this involves the sequencing of germline DNA by NGS or other techniques to demonstrate a variety of inactivating mutations that have been described. Currently, cytogenetics generally plays very little role in the diagnosis of leiomyoma, but a more complex karyotype would favor leiomyosarcoma. However, a distinctive cytogenetic profile has been described for benign metastasizing leiomyoma, indicating the potential usefulness of this approach for studying this group of tumors.[209]

Lipoma Variants (Benign Adipocytic Tumors)

Conventional Lipoma. Multiple lipoma subtypes exist (see Chapter 12). Conventional lipoma is the most common mesenchymal tumor, and more than 75% of cases demonstrate simple yet abnormal karyotypes. The most common alteration is rearrangement with the 12q14-15 chromosomal interval, where *HMGA2* (also known as *HMGIC*), a gene involved in chromatin remodeling, resides.[210,211] This is an interesting chromosomal region that contains multiple genes involved in several sarcoma types, as indicated in Fig. 18.23. In addition to its involvement in conventional lipomas, *HMGA2* is rearranged in many other neoplasms as well (Box 18.6). Many of these neoplasms could be considered overgrowths of normal tissue (fibroadenoma, endometrial stromal polyp, leiomyoma), and the malignant neoplasms show well-defined lines of differentiation (chondrosarcoma, osteosarcoma). In the case of liposarcoma, *HMGA2* can be rearranged on occasion but is more frequently amplified along with other genes in the 12q13-15 interval, as discussed later.

Multiple *HMGA2* fusion genes have been identified in lipomas, and most often the *HMGA2* break point is in the 140-kb intron between exons 3 and 4 of this five-exon gene. This includes the DNA-binding domains (adenine-thymine [AT] hooks) of the encoded protein in the fusion product. The most common chromosomal translocation in lipoma is t(3;12)(q27-28;q14-15), accounting for about 20% of *HMGA2*-rearranged cases.[211] Here the fusion partner is *LPP*, which has an uncertain cellular function but may provide transactivation or protein-binding domains to the fusion gene with *HMGA2*. Multiple other fusion variants are known, and likely others remain to be identified. Other rearrangements not involving *HMGA2* are also known.[212]

Most often, detection of one of the many fusion events described in conventional lipoma is not needed because the diagnosis is straightforward. The most common approach when it is applied is *HMGA2* break-apart FISH. This approach can be complicated by amplification of the 12q13-15 locus seen in other tumors, such as well-differentiated liposarcoma. Focused RNA seq is also applicable here, given the many fusion variants encountered.

Box 18.6 Neoplasms With *HMGA2* Rearrangements

Benign

- Deep ("aggressive") angiomyxoma
- Enchondroma
- Endometrial polyp
- Extraskeletal osteochondroma
- Fibroadenoma of breast
- Lipoma
- Leiomyoma (uterine)
- Myolipoma
- Pleomorphic adenoma
- Polypoid ("mass forming") endometriosis
- Pulmonary chondroid hamartoma

Malignant

- Acute lymphoblastic leukemia (rare)
- Carcinoma ex pleomorphic adenoma
- Chondrosarcoma
- Chronic idiopathic myelofibrosis
- Osteosarcoma
- Polycythemia vera and other myeloproliferative disorders
- Well-differentiated liposarcoma

Other Lipoma Variants. A few cases of chondroid lipoma have been described with a t(11;16)(q13;p13) translocation. This translocation results in the fusion of *C11orf95* (encoding a hypothetical protein) and *MKL2* (myocardin-like 2, which encodes myocardin-related transcription factor B in the megakaryoblastic leukemia gene family).[213] Hibernomas harbor rearrangements of 11q13 with multiple other chromosomal partnering regions. The multiple endocrine neoplasia (*MEN1*) locus on chromosome 11 is often deleted as well.[214] Lipoblastoma shows rearrangements of 8q12 that lead to overexpression of the *PLAG1* gene by placing it under a constitutive promoter at the active fusion site.[215] Spindle cell or pleomorphic lipoma features characteristic losses of 13q12 and 16q13-qter (the distal long arm of 16 from the 13 band), which includes *RB1* (13q14).[216] Interestingly, multiple tumor types showing somewhat overlapping morphologic features with spindle cell/pleomorphic lipoma have also been shown to have loss of *RB1*. These include mammary-type myofibroblastoma, cellular angiofibroma, and superficial acral fibromyxoma (Box 18.7). Immunohistochemistry for Rb1 can be used to demonstrate loss of nuclear expression of this protein; FISH can often demonstrate *RB1* locus deletion.[217]

Box 18.7 Tumors With *RB1* Loss

Spindle cell lipoma
Pleomorphic lipoma
Mammary-type myofibroblastoma
Cellular angiofibroma
Superficial acral fibromyxoma

As with conventional lipoma, identification of these findings is usually not necessary for diagnostic purposes but can be helpful in some cases, as when spindle cell lipoma arises at an unusual site, causing diagnostic confusion with atypical lipomatous tumor. However, given the superficial nature of the vast majority of such cases where uncertainty exists, the clinical approach of complete surgical excision is usually not altered, even without a firm diagnostic category. Most of these various findings are amenable to FISH-based approaches, with RT-PCR also possible but not as widely used.

Liposarcoma

Traditionally, liposarcoma is classified into the diagnostic categories of myxoid and round cell liposarcoma, well-differentiated (and dedifferentiated) liposarcoma, and pleomorphic liposarcoma (see Chapter 12). Pleomorphic liposarcoma is briefly discussed in the initial section of this chapter. Descriptions of the other two types follow.

Myxoid Liposarcoma. Myxoid liposarcoma shares the same genetic alterations as "round cell" liposarcoma; round cell liposarcoma is now regarded as a higher-grade form of myxoid liposarcoma. The most common chromosomal abnormality, t(12;16)(q13;p11), which is present in more than 90% of cases, creates a *FUS-DDIT3* fusion gene.[218-220] *DDIT3* (previously known as *CHOP*) is located in the 12q13-15 region that is prominently involved in soft tissue neoplasms (see Fig. 18.23). It encodes a DNA damage–inducible negative transcriptional regulator that also plays a role in adipocyte differentiation. *FUS* (also called *TLS* [translocated in liposarcoma]) was originally named for its role in this translocation. Multiple *FUS-DDIT3* fusions types are known, but types 1 and 2 constitute the majority (30% and 60% of cases, respectively).[221,222] A less common variant event is t(12;22)(q13;q12), wherein *EWSR1* substitutes for *FUS* (see Fig. 18.5).[223] Progression to more cellular forms of myxoid liposarcoma (previously termed round cell liposarcoma) show the same translocations but can also accumulate activating mutations in *PIK3CA* or loss-of-function mutations in *PTEN*.[224,225] Break-apart FISH for *DDIT3* is a commonly used approach because this rearrangement is demonstrable in virtually all cases. FISH for *FUS* or *EWSR1* is also possible but does not detect all cases, as *DDIT3* does. In the uncommon cases where the differential diagnosis of myxoid liposarcoma versus well-differentiated liposarcoma is entertained, *DDIT3* can be amplified in well-differentiated liposarcoma, potentially causing diagnostic confusion.[226] This can often be resolved by using FISH for *FUS*, because it does not reside within the 12q13-15 amplification region of well-differentiated liposarcoma. RT-PCR approaches are also described and can be helpful in this setting.[227-229]

Well-Differentiated and Dedifferentiated Liposarcoma. Well-differentiated liposarcoma and dedifferentiated liposarcoma are associated with ring and giant marker chromosomes (Fig. 18.24A). The karyotypes can be simple, with only a giant marker or ring chromosome, or they can evolve to show prominent numerical and structural changes similar to what is seen in other pleomorphic sarcomas, particularly in the setting of dedifferentiation.[230] These cases retain the initial giant marker and/or ring chromosomes, which contain amplified sequences from 12q13-15, a region that includes *MDM2*, *SAS*, *HMGA2*, and *CDK4* (see Figs. 18.23 and 18.24B).[218] This region is very interesting as it contains multiple genes involved in a variety of soft tissue and other tumors, both benign and malignant. The protein encoded by *MDM2* binds and inactivates p53, leading to its degradation in the proteosome; thus it is antiapoptotic. *CDK4* promotes cell cycle progression, and *HMGA2* appears to regulate tissue growth and is involved in other tumors by rearrangements or amplification (see Box 18.6).[218] Amplification of this locus can be identified using two colored probes, where one is centromeric and identifies the number of copies of chromosome 12 and the other marks a region within 12q13-15, often including the *MDM2* locus.[231,232] When the number of 12q13-15 region signals is greater than the centromeric 12 signals, amplification is demonstrated (see Fig. 18.24C), which is often seen as ring chromosomes with large numbers of amplified intervals. Low-level amplification (twofold or threefold) can be difficult to detect, but often amplification of *MDM2* and the 12q13-15 locus is very prominent (see Fig. 18.24C, inset).

FISH is the most commonly used method to demonstrate amplification.[231,232] Immunohistochemistry for the MDM2 and CDK4 proteins can sometimes be helpful in the differential diagnosis of (1) lipoma versus atypical lipomatous tumor/well-differentiated liposarcoma and (2) dedifferentiated liposarcoma versus other pleomorphic sarcomas, though it is not considered to be as sensitive or specific as FISH.[233-235] A FISH-based amplification test can be extremely useful in small biopsies because cytologic atypia may be minimal in the adipocytic (lipoma-like) type of well-differentiated liposarcoma. Temperance is needed in the interpretation of amplification in spindle cell sarcomas lacking an identifiable adipocytic component in a biopsy sample because *MDM2* and the 12q13-15 region can rarely be amplified in other sarcomas as well, including parosteal (and low-grade central) osteosarcomas, high-grade osteosarcomas of the jaw, and intimal sarcomas (although the copy number increases in these other tumors tend to be considerably lower).[231,236-240] Correlation with radiologic features can be very helpful in this scenario.

Lipofibromatosis-Like Neural Tumors

Recently a group of rare and unusual superficial tumors with a predilection for children and histologic features reminiscent of lipofibromatosis but with S100 protein and CD34 reactivity have been described. These tumors harbor recurrent translocations involving *NTRK1* (1q23), sometimes with *TPR* and *TPM3*. In contrast, true lipofibromatosis lacks *NTRK1* rearrangements.[241]

Low-Grade Fibromyxoid Sarcoma

Low-grade fibromyxoid sarcoma is associated most commonly with t(7;16)(q33;p11), leading to the *FUS-CREB3L2* fusion gene (see Chapters 3, 4, and 5).[242,243] This fusion is also seen in hyalinizing spindle cell tumor with giant rosettes, a histologic variant of low-grade fibromyxoid sarcoma, as well as in hybrid tumors with components of both low-grade fibromyxoid sarcoma and sclerosing epithelioid fibrosarcoma.[244-246] The prevalence of this translocation in "pure" sclerosing epithelioid fibrosarcoma (lacking a recognizable low-grade fibromyxoid sarcoma component) appears to be very low, and is discussed further on.[247-249] *CREB3L1* on 11p11 has been reported to substitute for *CREB3L2* (7q33) on rare occasions. Other members of this gene family, despite having high rates of identity, have not been described as fusion partners. *FUS*, a homolog of *EWSR1*, substitutes for the latter gene in several fusion events in multiple different tumor types (see Fig. 18.5). The *FUS* gene comprises 15 exons; the fusion gene includes the first 6 or 7 exons of *FUS* and exons 5 through 12 of *CREB3L2* (the last 8 of its 12 total exons), but other rare fusion types have also been reported.[250] The domains donated by *FUS* include its N-terminus, similar to *EWSR1* fusions, whereas the basic leucine zipper (b-ZIP) domain and C-terminus come from *CREB3L2* and thus provide the DNA targeting function of

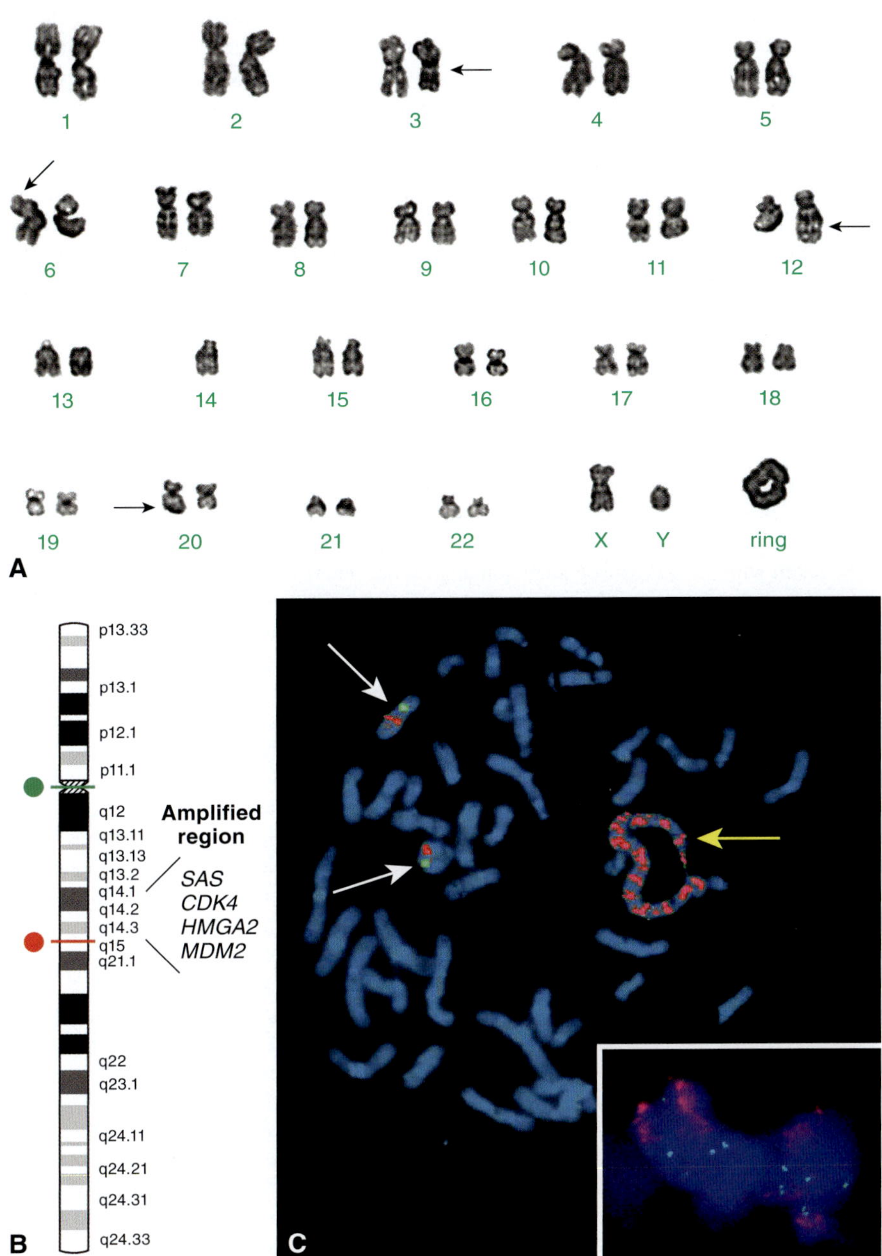

Figure 18.24 Cytogenetics of Well-differentiated Liposarcoma. (A) A relatively simple G-banded karyotype is depicted in the panel showing a ring chromosome. (B) Fluorescence in situ hybridization (FISH) probes in green to the centromere of chromosome 12 and in red to the amplified 12q13-15 region are diagrammed. (C) FISH analysis of the chromosomal spread from (A) reveals that the ring chromosome marked by a *yellow arrow* is composed of multiple copies of the 12q13-15 region. The *white arrows* point to the two copies of chromosome 12. The *inset* depicts another case of dedifferentiated liposarcoma where interphase FISH of tumor nuclei shows multiple copies of chromosome 12 (green probe to the centromere) and extensive amplification of the 12q13-15 region. (Portions of this figure courtesy Dr. Andre Oliveira, Mayo Clinic, Rochester, MN and Dr. Dolores López-Terrada, Texas Children's Hospital and Baylor College of Medicine, Houston, TX.)

the fusion protein. Interestingly, both *CREB3L2* and *CREB3L1* show some homology with the genes *ATF1* and *CREB1* seen in other gene fusion–containing sarcomas (see Fig. 18.5).

FUS is seen in both fusion variants; therefore break-apart FISH is commonly used to detect this rearrangement. As described previously, *FUS* rearrangement is not specific, as it is seen in multiple other soft tissue neoplasms as well. However, within the relevant differential diagnosis of low-grade myxofibrosarcoma, intramuscular/cellular myxoma, soft tissue perineurioma, and some other low-grade spindle cell neoplasms, which do not harbor rearrangements of *FUS*, FISH is extremely helpful to confirm the diagnosis.[251] RT-PCR–based approaches have also been used with success.[252]

Mesenchymal Chondrosarcoma

Mesenchymal chondrosarcoma (see Chapter 14) harbors a *HEY1-NCOA2* gene fusion, identified through an innovative informatics analysis of gene expression data sets.[253] This gene fusion would be expected to correlate with t(8;8)(q13;q21). Such an intrachromosomal translocation would be difficult to detect by traditional cytogenetics. *HEY1* is a downstream effector of Notch signaling, which acts as a transcriptional repressor, whereas *NCOA2* is a coactivator of nuclear hormone receptors. *NCOA2* is also rearranged in a small subset of alveolar rhabdomyosarcomas.[254] Given the nature of this translocation with a relatively close juxtaposition of the two genes on the long arm of chromosome 8, RT-PCR methods would be preferred over FISH approaches.

Myoepithelial Tumors of Soft Tissue

About 50% of myoepithelial tumors of soft tissue, skin, bone, and visceral locations (both myoepitheliomas and myoepithelial carcinomas) are associated with rearrangements of the *EWSR1* gene (22q12) (see Chapters 5 and 6).[255,256] The most common fusion partners are *POU5F1* (6p21) and *PBX1* (1q23), whereas rearrangements involving *ZNF444* (19q13) are rare.[255,256] However, these fusion partners account for only a small fraction of *EWSR1*-rearranged tumors; other fusion partners in these neoplasms remain to be identified. This family of tumors therefore appears to be similar to Ewing sarcoma, in which *EWSR1* can have a variety of fusion partners. *EWSR1* rearrangements are also found in cutaneous myoepithelial tumors (including nearly all cutaneous syncytial myoepitheliomas) and have been reported in several mixed tumors (myoepitheliomas with ductal differentiation; see Chapter 9); the fusion partners in cutaneous syncytial myoepitheliomas have not yet been identified.[257,258] Interestingly, mixed tumors of salivary glands (pleomorphic adenomas) lack *EWSR1* rearrangements, instead frequently harboring *PLAG1* rearrangement or *HMGA2* rearrangement and amplification.[259,260] *PLAG1* rearrangements have also been detected in mixed tumors of skin and soft tissue[261]; *EWSR1* and *PLAG1* rearrangements are mutually exclusive in myoepithelial tumors of these sites.

Break-apart *EWSR1* FISH is likely to be useful for supporting the diagnosis of myoepithelial tumors of soft tissue because this technique is readily available. However, given the numerous tumor types that can show *EWSR1* rearrangements (see Fig. 18.5), care must be taken with this approach. In particular, extraskeletal myxoid chondrosarcoma can be a morphologic mimic, although immunohistochemical studies can aid in this distinction. RT-PCR or focused RNA seq approaches are also possible and might be more definitive in certain cases to differentiate myoepithelial tumors from other tumor types that can also be associated with *EWSR1* rearrangement.

Myxoinflammatory Fibroblastic Sarcoma and Hemosiderotic Fibrolipomatous Tumor

Both myxoinflammatory fibroblastic sarcoma (see Chapters 5 and 7) and hemosiderotic fibrolipomatous tumor (see Chapter 12) have been reported to harbor t(1;10)(p22;q24), resulting in the fusion of *TGFBR3* and *MGEA5*.[262,263] The former is a transforming growth factor-β receptor, whereas the latter is involved in protein glycosylation. Amplification of 3p11-12 is also commonly noted, sometimes in ring chromosomes. These genetic findings, as well as the occurrence of occasional tumors containing both histologic patterns, lead some to speculate that they share a common pathogenetic mechanism.[263,264] However, a recent study has suggested that although these rearrangements are more common in tumors showing hybrid features of both tumor types, rearrangements in "pure" myxoinflammatory fibroblastic sarcomas are rare. Therefore the relationship between these two tumors is not entirely clear.[265] Both FISH and RT-PCR approaches could potentially be used for these tumor types.

Myxomas

Intramuscular myxoma and cellular myxoma are often associated with activating point mutations in *GNAS,* which encodes the $G_{s\alpha}$ subunit of the stimulatory heterotrimeric G-protein complex (see Chapter 5). This protein stimulates adenylyl cyclase to upregulate production of the cAMP second messenger. Mazabraud syndrome is a rare disorder in which patients develop fibrous dysplasia and multiple intramuscular myxomas. Germline mosaic mutations in *GNAS* are the basis for this syndrome. Sporadic myxomas and fibrous dysplasia also often harbor *GNAS* mutations.[266] One series described activating *GNAS* mutations in parosteal osteosarcomas, though other series have failed to demonstrate this.[267-269]

The Carney complex is the combination of primary pigmented nodular adrenocortical disease producing primary hypercortisolism; cutaneous pigmented lesions, including ephelides, lentigines, and cellular blue nevi (sometimes epithelioid); and a variety of endocrine and nonendocrine tumors, including psammomatous melanotic schwannoma and large cell calcifying Sertoli cell tumor, which are rarely encountered outside of this context. Cardiac atrial myxomas, as well as superficial angiomyxomas of the skin and breast, are also seen in this complex.[270] This syndrome is associated with mutations in *PRKAR1A*, a regulatory subunit of protein kinase A, which is a direct target for cAMP activation.[271,272] Rarely, the *MYH8* gene can be associated with the Carney complex.[273]

GNAS mutations are relatively simple to detect by PCR-based methods from tumor genomic DNA because only one major codon and two minor codons are involved.[266] Mutations in *PRKAR1A* can also be detected by such methods. The clinical utility of such testing is not well established outside of confirming the clinical diagnosis of the extremely rare cases of Mazabraud syndrome and Carney complex. The diagnosis of sporadic intramuscular and cellular myxomas is usually relatively straightforward.

Neurofibroma

Neurofibromas are associated with loss of the *NF1* gene (17q11.2), which encodes a protein called neurofibromin that inhibits the action of the proto-oncogene Ras. In the setting of neurofibromatosis type 1 (von Recklinghausen disease), one nonfunctional copy of the gene is inherited, and subsequent somatic loss of heterozygosity allows tumor development.[274] Interestingly, in about half of neurofibromatosis cases, mutations arise as new germline defects without inheritance.[275] There is not generally a role for testing for *NF1* loss, but this can sometimes be done by FISH. Germline DNA sequencing is available to confirm a diagnosis of neurofibromatosis type 1.[276] This gene is composed of 52 exons encoding neurofibromin, a large protein of more than 2800 amino acids. Point mutations account for about 90% of mutations, with intragenic deletions accounting for the other 10%. These mutations do not cluster in this gene; therefore genetic testing is a complex process requiring a large number of multiplexed PCR reactions coupled with extensive sequencing. However, emerging DNA sequencing technologies may simplify this arduous process.

Nodular Fasciitis

Oliveira and colleagues identified a translocation in nodular fasciitis (see Chapters 3 and 4).[277] The t(17;22)(p13;q13) results in a *MYH9-USP6* gene fusion. Interestingly, *USP6* is also involved in rearrangements with a number of other genes, including *CDH11, ZNF9, COL1A1, TRAP150,* and *OMD* (but not *MYH9*), in aneurysmal bone cysts (see Chapter 14).[278-280] All of the translocations in this family result in promoter swaps that drive overexpression of *USP6*.[280] *USP6* encodes a deubiquitinating enzyme involved in cell transformation and other physiologic processes, such as vesicular trafficking, protein turnover, and regulation of inflammatory pathways. *MYH9* encodes a class II nonmuscle myosin involved in cell motility and cell conformation through regulation of actin assembly. Greater than 90% of cases of nodular fasciitis show rearrangement of *USP6*; in about two-thirds of cases, this is fused with *MYH9*. Thus additional gene partners remain to be discovered. *MYH9* germline mutations have been reported in inherited platelet disorders, and fusion with *ALK* has been identified in rare anaplastic large-cell lymphomas.[281-283] The finding of a recurrent translocation in nodular fasciitis is intriguing biologically because this lesion is usually self-limited and resolves over the course of weeks in the absence of surgical intervention. *USP6* is also involved in a subset of cellular fibromas of tendon sheath. These tumors are not known to be partnered with *MYH9* and likely have alternative fusion partners. This finding raises the possibility that cellular fibroma of tendon sheath may be related to nodular fasciitis, although this is not certain.[284] Aneurysmal bone cyst pairs *USP6* with a variety of partners including *COL1A1* (also paired with *PDGFB* in DFSP), *OMD*, *ZNF9*, and *TRAP150*.[284]

The locations of *USP6* and *MYH9* in light-staining terminal bands make visualization by traditional cytogenetic preparations challenging; FISH and RT-PCR approaches are possible avenues of demonstration.

Ossifying Fibromyxoid Tumor

Ossifying fibromyxoid tumor is a mesenchymal tumor of uncertain lineage usually characterized by a peripheral shell of bone and lobules of S100 protein-positive spindled to ovoid cells within a myxoid stroma. These tumors harbor recurrent translocations involving *PHF1* on 6p21 and various fusion partners, most commonly *EP400* on 12q24. As previously discussed, *PHF1* is also involved in endometrial stromal sarcomas. Other gene fusion variants include *EPC1-PHF1*, *MEAF6-PHF1*, and *ZC3H7B-BCOR*, with the latter two variants reported in malignant S100 protein-negative variants.[285-287] Because of the variability in partners, FISH for *PHF1* rearrangement or focused RNA seq would be required.

Pericytoma With t(7;12)

Pericytoma with t(7;12) has a translocation resulting in an *ACTB-GLI* fusion transcript.[288,289] *GLI* lies in the 12q13-15 region commonly involved in soft tissue tumors (see Fig. 18.23).

Pseudomyogenic Hemangioendothelioma

Pseudomyogenic hemangioendothelioma, also known as epithelioid sarcoma–like hemangioendothelioma (see Chapters 3 and 15), harbors a recurrent rearrangement involving *SERPINE1* on 7q22 and *FOSB* on 19q13.[290] SERPINE1 is part of the serine protease inhibitor family expressed in many cells including endothelial cells, whereas FOSB is a member of the FOS family of transcription factors. Interestingly, *FOSB* rearrangements are also observed in a subset of epithelioid hemangiomas, some of which have atypical histologic features. These tumors often have *ZFP36* as a fusion partner instead of *SERPINE1*.[291]

Rhabdomyosarcoma

Rhabdomyosarcoma is classified into alveolar, embryonal, and pleomorphic subtypes. Both botryoid and spindle cell rhabdomyosarcoma have traditionally been considered variants of embryonal rhabdomyosarcoma. However, recent evidence suggests that many spindle cell and sclerosing rhabdomyosarcomas in both children and adults have unique molecular alterations, including L122R mutations in *MYOD1*, which are associated with more aggressive behavior.[292-294] *VGLL2*- and *NCOA2*-related fusions can be seen in infantile cases.[295] Classic embryonal rhabdomyosarcoma can show trisomies of 2, 8, and 20 as well as loss of heterozygosity at 11p15, but these findings are not specific and may also be seen in other sarcomas.[296] Pleomorphic rhabdomyosarcoma falls into the complex karyotype group discussed at the beginning of this chapter. Only alveolar rhabdomyosarcoma has reproducible cytogenetic features helpful in diagnosis (see also Chapter 8) and is the focus of this section.

Alveolar rhabdomyosarcoma is associated with two major chromosomal alterations, t(2;13)(q35;q14) and t(1;13)(p26;q14), as depicted in Fig. 18.25.[297] Both involve rearrangements of the *FOXO1A* gene (previously termed *FKHR*) on 13q14. *PAX3* (2q35) is the partner in about 75% of cases, whereas *PAX7* (1p26) is present in about 25% of the *FOXO1A* rearranged cases. *PAX3* and *PAX7* are homologs important in dorsal neural tube and somite development; *PAX3* is also critical for migration of myoblasts to the limbs. *PAX3*-inactivating mutations are the underlying cause of type I Waardenburg syndrome, where there is loss of skin and hair pigmentation associated with hearing deficits.[298] The fusion genes use the DNA-binding domains of *PAX3* or *PAX7* fused to the activation domain of *FOXO1A*, a transcription factor that appears to regulate cell cycle progression and apoptosis (see Fig. 18.25B). *FOXO1A* acts as a tumor suppressor gene in other tumors, including some carcinomas, but acts as an oncogene when participating in the fusion gene in alveolar rhabdomyosarcoma. More recently, additional very rare variants, including t(2;2)(q35;p23) and t(X;2)(q35;q13), have been described, resulting in the *PAX3-NCOA1* and *PAX3-AFX* fusion genes, respectively.[254,299]

Part of the relevance of these fusion genes is that alveolar rhabdomyosarcoma behaves more aggressively than embryonal rhabdomyosarcoma.[300]

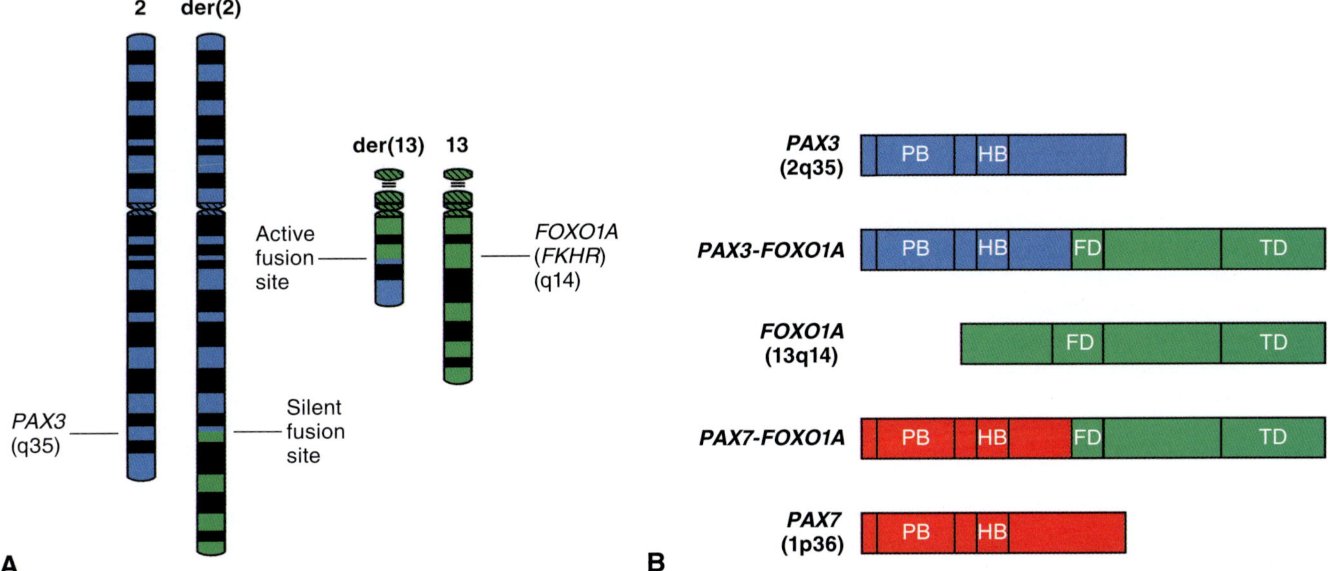

Figure 18.25 Translocations Seen in Alveolar Rhabdomyosarcoma. (A) The most common translocation seen in this tumor is t(2;13)(q35;q14) fusing *PAX3* and *FOXO1A*. The homolog *PAX7* can also be seen. (B) Because of the limited fusion variants and the possibility of prognostic differences between *PAX3* and *PAX7* translocations, reverse transcription polymerase chain reaction (RT-PCR) is often used, although *FOXO1A* break-apart fluorescence in situ hybridization (FISH) is also an excellent option. The fusion genes juxtapose the DNA-binding domains of *PAX3* or *PAX7* to the transactivation domain of *FOXO1A*. *FD*, Forkhead domain; *HB*, homeobox domain; *PB*, paired box domain; *TD*, transactivation domain.

In particular, cases of alveolar rhabdomyosarcoma with a fusion transcript generally behave more aggressively than those without. This is somewhat complicated by retrospective data from pediatric cases suggesting that alveolar rhabdomyosarcoma with *PAX3-FOXO1A* behaves more aggressively, while *PAX7-FOXO1A* behaves more like embryonal rhabdomyosarcoma in metastatic cases.[300] Cases of alveolar rhabdomyosarcoma, including the solid variant, lacking a detectable fusion event behave in a fashion intermediate between *PAX3-FOXO1A* cases and embryonal rhabdomyosarcoma, suggesting that this class of tumors is likely heterogeneous.[301,302] Nonetheless, these findings are retrospective and require validation.

A common approach to diagnosis is the demonstration of *FOXO1A* rearrangement by break-apart FISH.[303] Because there may be prognostic information carried by *PAX3* or *PAX7* involvement, break-apart and combination strategies have been described for these two genes as well.[304,305] The number of *PAX3-FOXO1A* and *PAX7-FOXO1A* fusion types is limited; therefore RT-PCR approaches are readily utilized.[306]

Sclerosing Epithelioid Fibrosarcoma

This is a rare fibroblastic sarcoma that is discussed in Chapter 6. Some sclerosing epithelioid fibrosarcomas have hybrid features of low-grade fibromyxoid sarcoma (LGFMS), whereas others lack any LGFMS areas ("pure" sclerosing epithelioid fibrosarcoma). Molecular studies have demonstrated that rearrangements involving *FUS* in pure sclerosing epithelioid fibrosarcoma are rare, in contrast to LGFMS and hybrid tumors.[247,249] The majority of pure sclerosing epithelioid fibrosarcomas instead have rearrangements involving *EWSR1* and *CREB3L1*.[307,308] Interestingly, isolated cases of small cell osteosarcoma harboring the *EWSR1-CREB3L1* fusion have been reported, although this finding has not been seen in all series.[309,310]

Schwannoma

Schwannomas usually show loss of *NF2* (22q12), which encodes a protein known as merlin. Neurofibromatosis type 2 (bilateral vestibular schwannomas) is associated with inherited (germline) defects in *NF2*, and loss of heterozygosity leads to tumor development. Loss of both *NF2* copies is also seen in sporadic schwannomas. As in neurofibromatosis type 1 and the *NF1* gene, there are indications that the location and type of mutation may have a bearing on tumor development.[311,312] Genetic testing for *NF2* mutations by PCR and sequencing of genomic DNA by NGS and other methods have been described.[313] FISH probes for demonstrating loss of *NF2* are also available.

Another syndrome associated with multiple schwannomas (but not vestibular tumors) is schwannomatosis. Although germline defects in *NF2* are not seen in patients with familial schwannomatosis, germline mutations have been identified in the nearby gene *SMARCB1* (also known as *INI1* and *SNF5*, located at 22q11.23) in a subset of affected patients; some of these mutations are mosaic.[314-316] In addition, *NF2* shows biallelic inactivation in schwannomas with *SMARCB1* mutations, suggesting a "four-hit" model of tumor development in such patients.[315] Some patients with familial schwannomatosis harbor germline mutations in *LZTR1* instead of *SMARCB1*.[317]

Synovial Sarcoma

Synovial sarcoma (see Chapter 3) is associated with t(X;18)(p11;q11), depicted in a complex karyotype resolved by spectral karyotyping in Fig. 18.26.[98,318] *SS18 (SYT)* is located at 18q11 and multiple members of the SSX family of genes reside on chromosome Xp11. *SSX1* is observed in about 65% of fusion events and *SSX2* in about 35% of such events. *SSX4* is rarely detected. Biphasic synovial sarcoma (see Chapter 9) is associated nearly exclusively with *SS18-SSX1*, although given the relative rarity of this variant, most cases of synovial sarcoma with *SS18-SSX1* are monophasic. *SS18-SSX2* cases are virtually always monophasic.[319] The functions of *SS18* and the SSX family are not entirely clear, but the former appears to be a transcriptional coactivator with no direct DNA-binding domain and the latter group appears to encode DNA transcription repressors.[320] The fusion protein appears to perform a bridging function between activating transcription factor 2 (ATF2) and transducin-like enhancer of split 1 (TLE1). Functionally the SS18-SSX protein abrogates the function of ATF2, resulting in repression of genes normally activated by ATF2. Thus dysregulation of ATF2 activity may, in part, drive pathogenesis of this tumor with the attendant pathways representing therapeutic targets.[321] Additional studies have demonstrated that the SS18-SSX fusion protein disrupts the SWI/SNF (BAF) chromatin remodeling complex, reversing polycomb-mediated repression and thereby inducing expression of particular target genes including *SOX2*.[322-325]

SS18 (SYT) break-apart FISH is a commonly used diagnostic approach; however, because there are only single break points in the *SS18* and *SSX* genes, RT-PCR approaches are straightforward as well.[44,326,327] Some studies have suggested that the *SS18-SSX1* fusion is associated with a worse prognosis than *SS18-SSX2*, but further studies that accounted for tumor grade in a multivariate analysis did not confirm fusion type as an independent prognostic factor.[328-332] Genetic confirmation for synovial sarcoma is commonly employed but is not necessary for typical cases.[333,334] Immunohistochemistry for the SYT (SS18) protein has recently been described as a potential diagnostic adjunct,[335] but the available antibodies show inconsistent results with staining of other tumor types as well. As noted earlier, TLE1 is a protein shown to be upregulated in synovial sarcoma using gene expression arrays[336]; TLE1 is a sensitive and moderately specific marker for synovial sarcoma and thus can be helpful in differential diagnosis.[337,338]

Solitary Fibrous Tumor

Previously these tumors were known for relatively simple karyotypes. However, using NGS techniques, an inversion translocation inv(12)(q13q13) involving *NAB2* and *STAT6* was recently described on chromosome 12.[339,340] This explains why the translocation was not detectable (cryptic translocation) by conventional cytogenetics. *NAB2* encodes a protein that helps regulate transcription factors and is normally a transcriptional repressor, whereas *STAT6* is transcription factor. The fusion protein converts NAB2 into a transcriptional activator of various genes involving growth and differentiation.[339] Multiple break points are known and, interestingly, some break-point variants are associated with tumor location (for example, *NAB2* ex4-*STAT6* ex2 is more likely associated with thoracic tumors) and possibly prognosis.[341-344] The rearrangement results in the overexpression of STAT6, which can be detected by immunohistochemical studies.[345-347]

Tenosynovial Giant Cell Tumor

Although many tenosynovial giant cell tumors arise in association with joints or bursae, some arise in extra-articular soft tissues (see Chapter 11). Translocations involving 1p11 containing the colony stimulating factor gene, *CSF1*, are often the only discernible cytogenetic alterations.[348] The most common fusion partner is *COL6A3*, and the strong constitutive promoter of this collagen gene drives the transcription of *CSF1*, probably in a fashion similar to what is seen with *COL1A1* and *PDGFB* in DFSP. Rearrangements at 5q22-31, 8q21-22, 1q21 and 11q11-12 have also been described with *CSF1*, presumably also providing constitutive promoters. Interestingly, only a small subset of cells within the lesion harbors *CSF1* rearrangements, the remainder (predominantly histiocytes) instead express the CSF1 receptor, and are recruited by the presence of CSF1 secreted by the neoplastic cells in a paracrine fashion. This process has been termed "tumor landscaping."[348] Although the histologic diagnosis

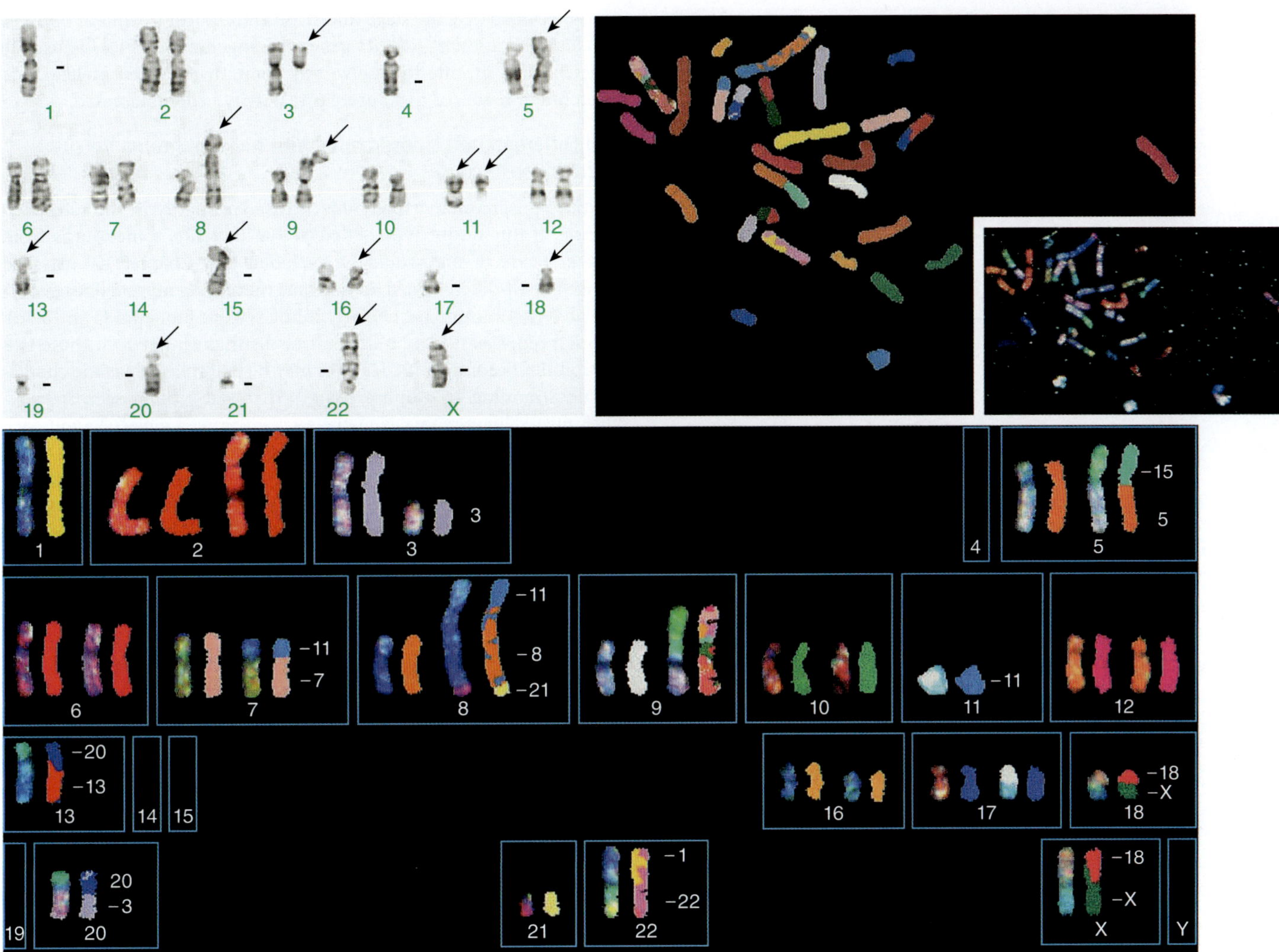

Figure 18.26 **Enhanced Karyotype of Synovial Sarcoma.** This relatively complex G-banded karyotype *(upper left)* was resolved by spectral karyotyping, which in the pseudocolored karyotype clearly revealed a translocation between X and 18 *(lower right)*. This translocation was confirmed to result in an *SS18-SSX1* fusion transcript using reverse transcription polymerase chain reaction.

is generally straightforward, break-apart FISH for *CSF1* in difficult cases is a reasonable approach given the variety of fusion partners, some involving unknown genes.[349] RT-PCR and focused RNA seq for *COL6A3-CSF1* has also been described.[350]

Practical Applications of Molecular Diagnostic Testing

In the preceding sections, the various molecular features helpful in the diagnosis of soft tissue sarcomas have been described. In certain situations, molecular testing may provide specific prognostic or therapeutic response information, such as the type of *KIT* mutation in GIST.[21,333,351] In this final section, a few specific differential diagnostic situations where molecular testing may be particularly useful are discussed.

Desmoplastic Small Round Cell Tumor Versus Ewing Sarcoma

In a small biopsy, it can be difficult to distinguish between desmoplastic small round cell tumor and Ewing sarcoma (see Chapter 8). Although the characteristic clinical setting of a young male with an intra-abdominal tumor expressing keratin, epithelial membrane antigen (EMA), and desmin is characteristic of desmoplastic small round cell tumor, these immunohistochemical findings can be focal, and Ewing sarcoma can also express keratins (Fig. 18.27). Furthermore, the expression of CD99 by Ewing sarcoma can occasionally be unimpressive (Fig. 18.28). It is important to remember that *EWSR1* break-apart FISH does not resolve this differential diagnosis, because both tumors contain *EWSR1* gene rearrangements. Although immunohistochemistry for nuclear Fli1 (for Ewing sarcoma) or nuclear WT1 (for desmoplastic small round cell tumor, using the polyclonal antibody directed against the carboxy terminus of WT1—the N-terminus is absent in the fusion protein) has been described,[101] neither antibody is entirely specific, and the available antibodies directed against the C-terminus of WT1 are difficult to optimize. Thus it is recommended to perform RT-PCR to detect the specific fusion transcripts to distinguish between these two tumor types.

Clear Cell Sarcoma Versus Metastatic Melanoma

Clear cell sarcoma can be very difficult to distinguish from metastatic melanoma. Sometimes primary cutaneous melanoma lacks a recognizable overlying in situ component, and metastatic melanoma of unknown primary is more common than clear cell sarcoma (Fig. 18.29) (see Chapter 3). Although there can be some subtle differences in their immunohistochemical profiles, they essentially overlap. The diagnosis of metastatic melanoma from an unknown primary or primary clear cell

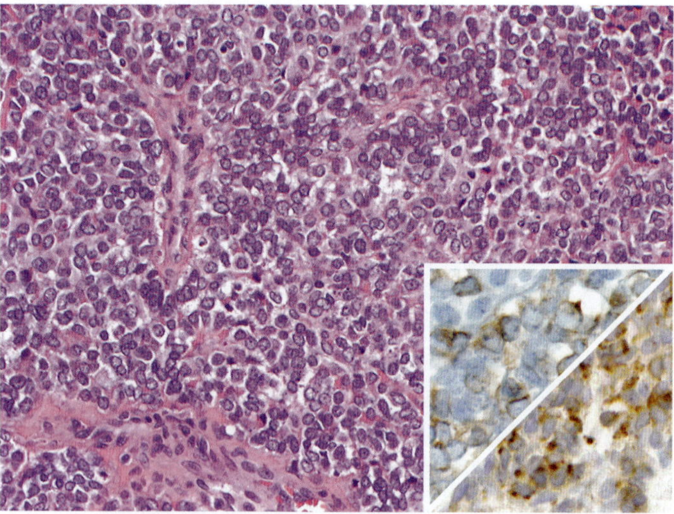

Figure 18.27 Ewing Sarcoma. This case of Ewing sarcoma shows expression of both keratins and epithelial membrane antigen (EMA) (*upper and lower insets*, respectively). Membranous expression of CD99 can occasionally be limited; such results can raise the histologic differential diagnosis of both desmoplastic small round cell tumor and small cell synovial sarcoma.

sarcoma can change the stage of disease and inform treatment options. The demonstration of *EWSR1* gene rearrangement by FISH is usually sufficient and specific to resolve this conundrum when melanocytic differentiation and/or S100 protein reactivity is demonstrated.

Well-Differentiated Liposarcoma With Myxoid Stroma Versus Myxoid Liposarcoma

Myxoid liposarcoma virtually never arises primarily in the retroperitoneum; if this tumor type is detected at that site, a metastasis from another primary site should be excluded (see Chapter 12). Myxoid change in well-differentiated liposarcoma mimicking myxoid liposarcoma is relatively common, particularly in the retroperitoneum (Fig. 18.30). In small biopsies it can be difficult to distinguish between these two possibilities. Radiographic features may be helpful, such as the characteristic stranding in adipose tissue ("dirty fat") often seen in well-differentiated liposarcoma. Nonetheless, sometimes a molecular approach is required. Myxoid liposarcoma shows rearrangement of the *DDIT3* locus on 12q13, whereas well-differentiated liposarcoma shows amplification of the 12q13-15 region containing the *MDM2* and often *CDK4* loci. Both can be detected by FISH. Interestingly, *DDIT3* is contained in the 12q13-15 amplification interval; thus one or both of the two probes flanking this gene can show increased copy numbers (see Fig. 18.23).[226] This can be difficult to quantitate because there is no centromeric

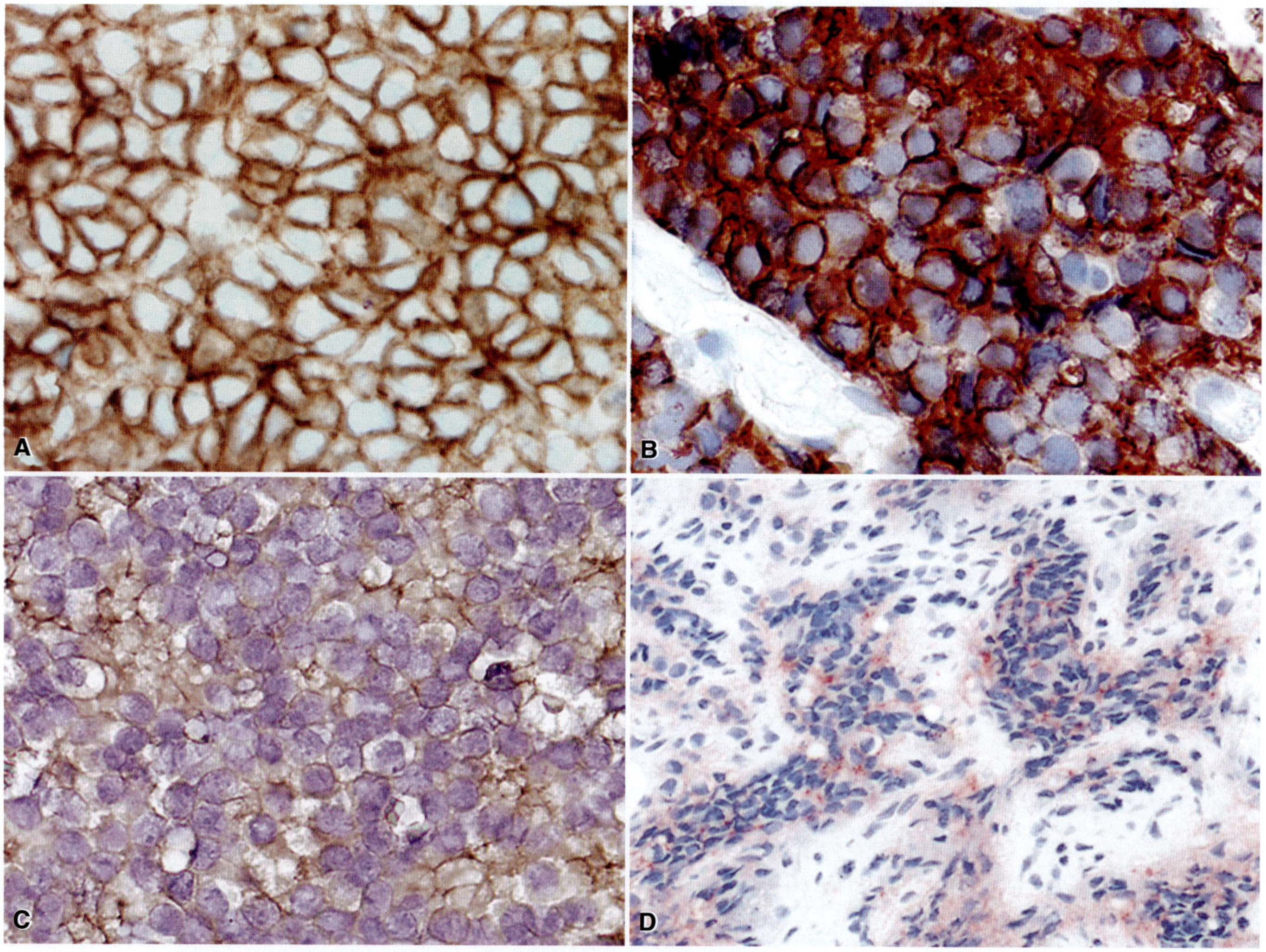

Figure 18.28 CD99 Expression in Four Cases of Molecularly Confirmed Ewing Sarcoma. Although the strong membranous expression of CD99 (A and B) is most often depicted in textbooks, other less dramatic expression patterns (C and D) can also be encountered in daily practice.

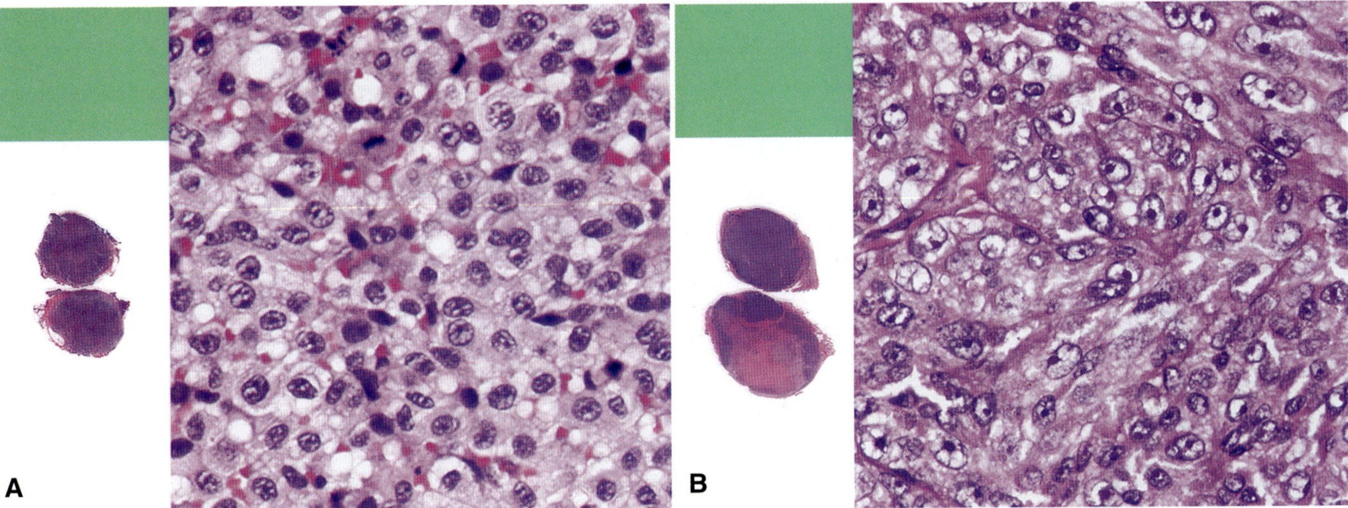

Figure 18.29 Clear Cell Sarcoma and Melanoma. The histologic features of these two entities overlap: a metastatic melanoma of unknown primary (A) and a clear cell sarcoma (B). Both arose at similar anatomic sites and were of similar sizes, as seen in the images.

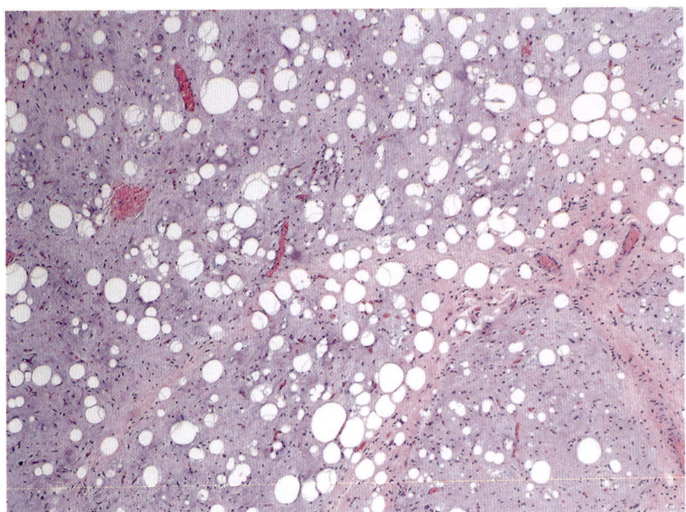

Figure 18.30 Myxoid Features in Well-differentiated Liposarcoma. Extensive myxoid change mimicking myxoid liposarcoma is seen in this cytogenetically confirmed case of retroperitoneal well-differentiated liposarcoma. Focal areas of the tumor show features more characteristic of well-differentiated liposarcoma, adipocytic type.

probe to control for chromosomal copy number, but as the level of amplification of this interval is often high, the increased signals are highly suggestive in this setting. Specific amplification of portions of the 12q13-15 interval such as *MDM2* demonstrated with a control probe to the chromosome 12 centromere (see Fig. 18.24B and C) can also be useful to further investigate such cases. Cases with histologic features of both myxoid and well-differentiated liposarcoma were sometimes termed mixed liposarcomas in the past, but with contemporary molecular methods such cases can now be readily resolved into one of these two diagnostic categories. The diagnostic terminology of mixed liposarcoma is no longer recommended.

Solid Alveolar Rhabdomyosarcoma Versus Embryonal Rhabdomyosarcoma

Although there are usually morphologic differences between the neoplastic cells comprising alveolar and embryonal rhabdomyosarcoma, this distinction is aided by the classic pseudoalveolar architecture in the alveolar subtype as well as diffuse and strong expression of myogenin relative to staining in the embryonal subtype (see Chapter 8). Alveolar architecture may not be apparent in a small biopsy; this pattern can be focal, and completely solid forms are common (Fig. 18.31). This distinction is important because alveolar rhabdomyosarcoma has a worse prognosis, especially in patients with tumors harboring the *PAX3-FOXO1A* translocation, supported by *FOXO1A* break-apart FISH, or direct demonstration of the fusion product by RT-PCR (see Fig. 18.25). Although demonstration of the translocation is important, if a tumor shows classic features of alveolar rhabdomyosarcoma but lacks a *FOXO1A* fusion, it tends to behave more aggressively than embryonal rhabdomyosarcoma but less so than the fusion-positive cases taken in aggregate.[300-302] Some fusion-negative rhabdomyosarcomas with alveolar features may represent cases with the rare alternative fusions not detected by many assays.[352,353]

Extraskeletal Myxoid Chondrosarcoma Versus Soft Tissue Myoepithelioma/Myoepithelial Carcinoma

Extraskeletal myxoid chondrosarcoma is usually composed of lobules of uniform spindled or epithelioid cells with eosinophilic cytoplasm arranged in a reticular pattern, but it can occasionally show more sheet-like growth (Fig. 18.32) (see Chapter 5). This tumor lacks a characteristic immunohistochemical profile but is focally positive for S100 protein in about 20% of cases. Soft tissue myoepithelioma and myoepithelial carcinoma can display a similar range of morphologic features, but they usually show reactivity for S100 protein, keratins, and EMA, as well as glial fibrillary acidic protein (GFAP) in 50% of cases (see Chapters 5 and 6). As described in the previous sections, both myoepithelial tumors of soft tissue and extraskeletal myxoid chondrosarcoma can have *EWSR1* rearrangements, but the fusion partners are different. FISH using probes directed against *NR4A3* (*CHN*) on 9q22 (rather than the traditional *EWSR1*) would be preferable to confirm the diagnosis of extraskeletal myxoid chondrosarcoma in this particular differential diagnosis; FISH also has the advantage of higher sensitivity, because *NR4A3* is the common rearrangement in all extraskeletal myxoid chondrosarcomas (see Fig. 18.18). RT-PCR and focused RNA seq approaches to demonstrate the precise fusion partners are also options.

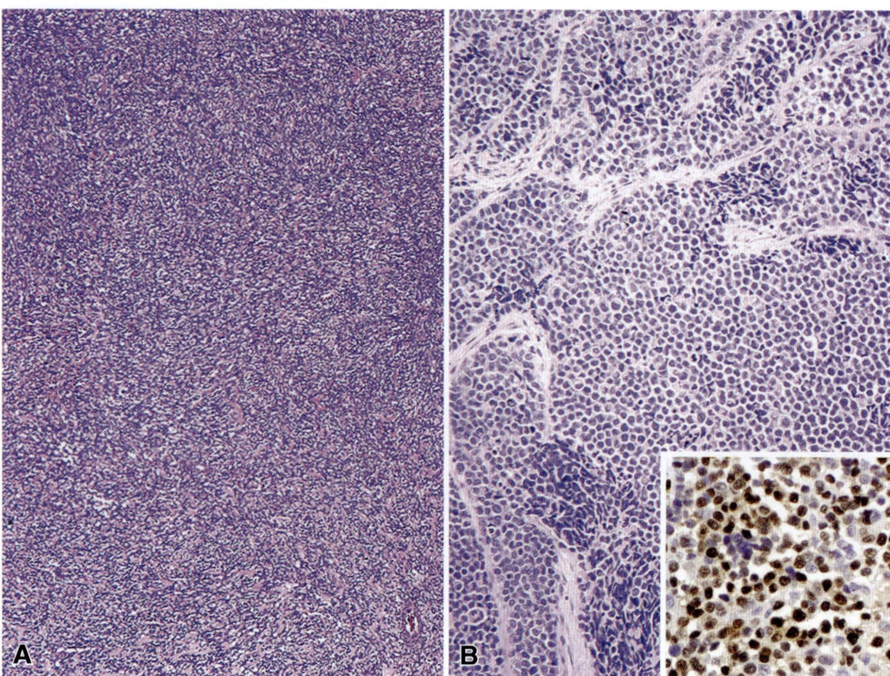

Figure 18.31 Solid Forms of Alveolar Rhabdomyosarcoma. Sheetlike proliferations characterize these two molecularly confirmed cases of alveolar rhabdomyosarcoma (A and B). The *inset* in part B shows immunohistochemistry for myogenin with strong nuclear staining.

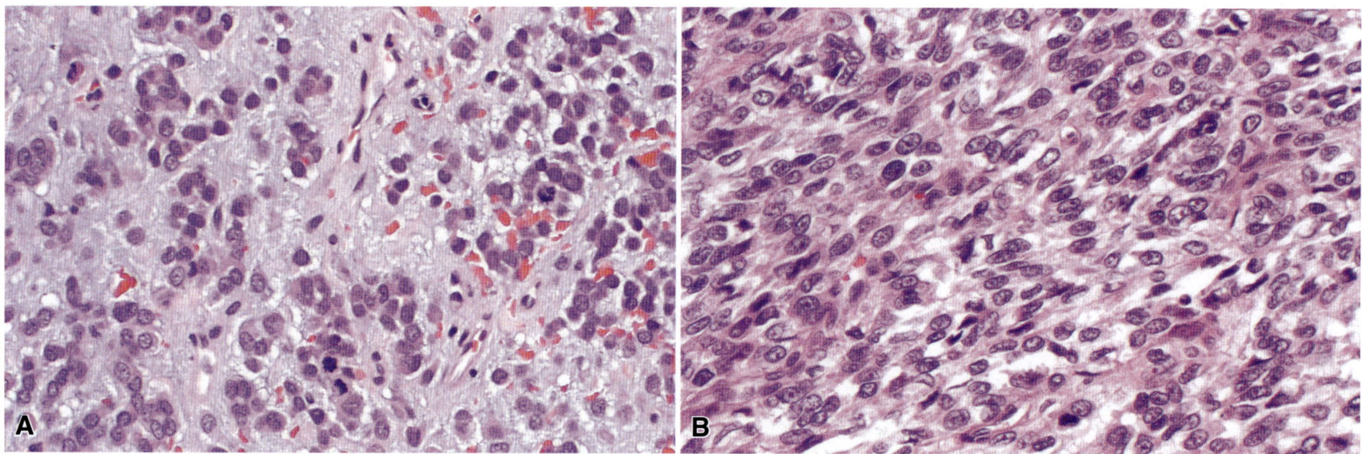

Figure 18.32 Extraskeletal Myxoid Chondrosarcoma. The epithelioid (A) and diffuse spindle cell (B) patterns are less common histologic variants of this tumor and show morphologic overlap with soft tissue myoepithelioma.

Small Cell (Poorly Differentiated) Synovial Sarcoma Versus Ewing Sarcoma

Synovial sarcoma has a small cell variant that can closely mimic Ewing sarcoma (Fig. 18.33) (see Chapter 8). In addition to histologic similarities, these tumor types show immunophenotypic overlap; synovial sarcoma often expresses CD99, and a significant portion of Ewing sarcomas can focally express EMA or keratins (see Fig. 18.27). These similarities can cause diagnostic confusion, particularly in small biopsies. Demonstration of *SS18-SSX* rearrangement confirms the diagnosis of synovial sarcoma, whereas *EWSR1* rearrangement indicates Ewing sarcoma. As noted, if relevant, RT-PCR can be used to distinguish Ewing sarcoma from desmoplastic small round cell tumor or other tumors associated with other *EWSR1* fusion variants.

Gastrointestinal Stromal Tumor With Unusual Features

GIST can lack immunoreactivity for both KIT (CD117) and CD34 ("KIT-negative GIST"; see Chapter 16). These tumors are most often found in the stomach, are predominantly epithelioid in morphology, and are often associated with *PDGFRA* rather than *KIT* mutations. Immunohistochemistry for PDGFRA is not entirely specific, as many laboratories find expression in a variety of soft tissue tumors (Fig. 18.34A), although diffuse, strong expression is more often seen in *PDGFRA*-mutant GISTs. Sequencing of the *PDGFRA* gene in this setting can be extremely helpful to confirm the diagnosis. SDH-deficient GISTs are usually confirmed by immunohistochemistry for SDHB.

GISTs can show significant morphologic changes following tyrosine kinase inhibitor treatment (see Chapter 16). One of these is the emergence of heterologous rhabdomyosarcomatous differentiation (see Fig. 18.34B).[354] If the primary tumor has not been examined, such findings on a biopsy might cause diagnostic confusion, and the more common sarcoma types that can show heterologous rhabdomyoblastic differentiation (i.e., dedifferentiated liposarcoma and malignant peripheral nerve sheath tumor) might be considered. Demonstration of a primary *KIT* mutation in this setting can be helpful (see Fig. 18.19). Tyrosine kinase inhibitor resistance–associated secondary *KIT* mutations have not yet been detected in this form of clonal evolution.[142]

Significance of Detecting an *EWSR1* Gene Rearrangement by Fluorescence In Situ Hybridization

As discussed throughout this chapter, *EWSR1* gene rearrangement can be seen in many different tumor types (see Fig. 18.5). It is important to keep in mind that the demonstration of *EWSR1* rearrangement by FISH is not specific for a particular tumor type; one must interpret this finding in the context of clinical, histologic, and immunophenotypic features. For instance, *EWSR1* rearrangement in a tumor expressing S100 protein by immunohistochemistry could be Ewing sarcoma rather than clear cell sarcoma (Fig. 18.35). Focal desmin and EMA expression in a small round cell tumor showing *EWSR1* rearrangement could be angiomatoid fibrous histiocytoma rather than desmoplastic small round cell tumor. These distinctions can usually be made with careful attention to histologic findings and awareness of the clinical setting in most cases, but small biopsies can be particularly challenging. If diagnostic uncertainty remains, these dilemmas can often be resolved by resorting to RT-PCR or focused RNA seq to demonstrate the expected specific fusion partner.

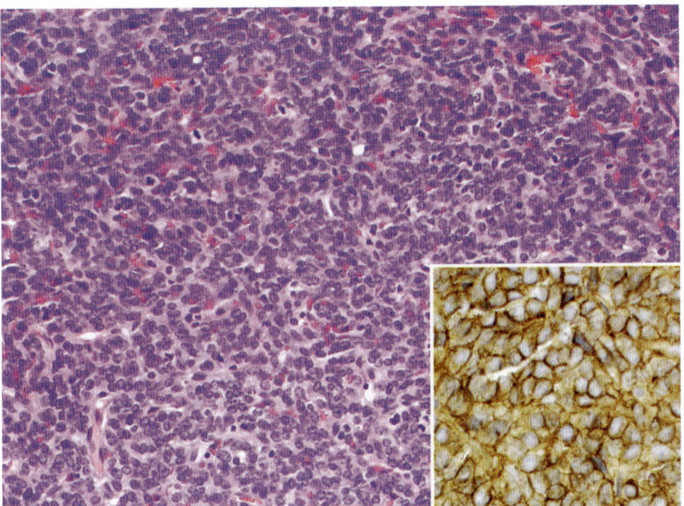

Figure 18.33 Small Cell Variant of Synovial Sarcoma. This molecularly confirmed synovial sarcoma shows strong membranous staining for CD99 *(inset)* along with patchy epithelial membrane antigen (EMA) expression (not shown). Such cases show significant morphologic overlap with Ewing sarcoma and other small round cell tumors and can be very challenging in small biopsies.

PRACTICE POINTS: Interpreting *EWSR1* Break-Apart Fluorescence in situ Hybridization

- Technique recognizes all rearrangements of the *EWSR1* locus
- Provides no insight into the *EWSR1* fusion partner
- Can cause confusion when the differential diagnosis includes two entities with *EWSR1* rearrangements
- RT-PCR to confirm or establish the *EWSR1* fusion partner can be helpful

RT-PCR, Reverse transcription polymerase chain reaction.

Focused RNA seq is emerging as a helpful technique to look for many fusions at once and also to define the fusion partners for promiscuous genes.

Conclusions

When deciding to use a molecular test to support a diagnosis, various considerations should come into play. It is sometimes difficult to render a specific diagnosis based on the very small biopsies that pathologists are often asked to evaluate by current clinical practice styles. Molecular testing in this setting may prevent a diagnostic error or avoid repeat biopsy if a specific diagnosis cannot be rendered otherwise. Poor histologic preservation can complicate interpretation, and in the setting of unusual histologic features or immunohistochemical results, molecular confirmation can provide helpful reassurance. Furthermore, an unusual clinical setting, such as desmoplastic small round cell tumor arising

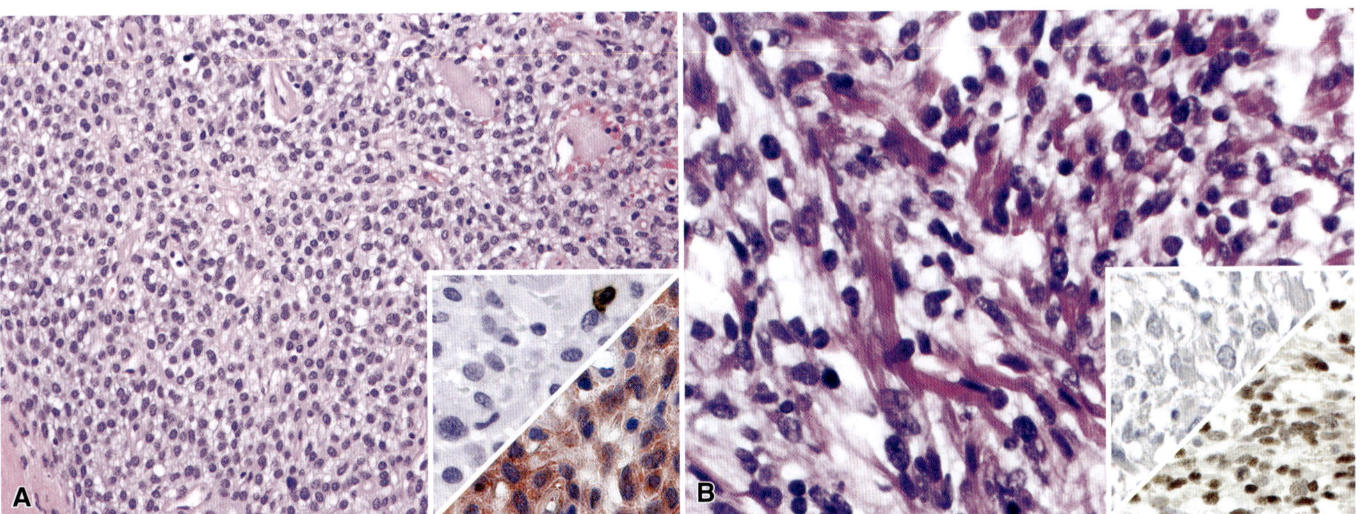

Figure 18.34 Gastrointestinal Stromal Tumor (GIST) Variants. (A) Epithelioid GISTs encountered in the stomach can completely lack KIT expression by immunohistochemistry (*upper inset,* mast cell as internal positive control). Platelet-derived growth factor receptor-α (PDGFRA) staining *(lower inset)* can be seen, but it is not specific. Demonstration of a *PDGFRA* mutation can be helpful in this setting. (B) Long-term treatment with imatinib mesylate can produce unusual morphologic features in GIST, such as rhabdomyosarcomatous differentiation depicted here. The *inset* shows lack of KIT immunoreactivity and nuclear staining for myoD1 (*upper and lower insets,* respectively). Demonstration of a characteristic *KIT* or *PDGFRA* mutation can be diagnostically helpful if the prior GIST was not reviewed.

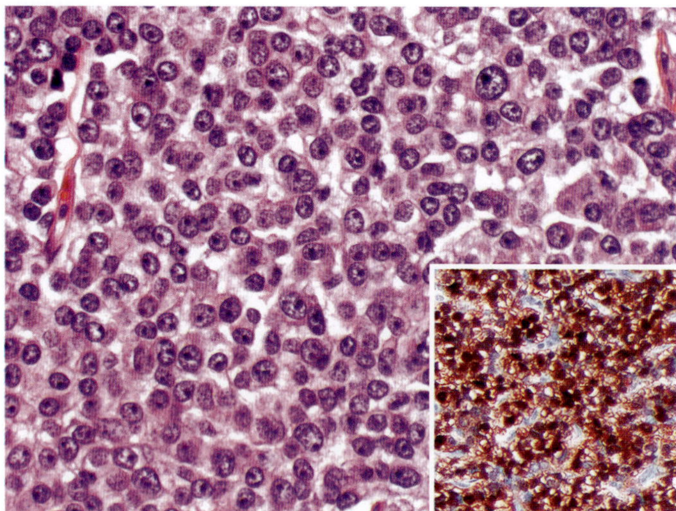

Figure 18.35 Ewing Sarcoma. This case shows more nuclear atypia than is usually encountered in Ewing sarcoma, including prominent nucleoli. Immunoreactivity for S-100 protein *(inset)* could cause confusion with clear cell sarcoma, and *EWSR1* break-apart fluorescence in situ hybridization (FISH) would not distinguish clear cell sarcoma from Ewing sarcoma. Reverse transcription polymerase chain reaction (RT-PCR) approaches can be helpful in such situations.

in an older woman or at an unusual site, can sometimes demand confirmatory molecular testing. Extensive treatment effect without availability of a pretreatment biopsy can also be challenging. In certain settings, the type of treatment may differ significantly based on the diagnosis (e.g., small cell synovial sarcoma vs. Ewing sarcoma). Clinical trials sometimes require molecular testing to ensure homogenous patient populations. Testing can also provide important prognostic information regarding expected natural history or response to treatment, such as *KIT* mutations in GIST. If a particular tumor type is rarely encountered by the diagnosing pathologist such that she or he has little experience with the entity, molecular testing can be very reassuring. In addition, if histology and immunophenotypic results are not sufficient and definitive classification is not possible, it is reasonable to pursue molecular testing. Finally, certain entities such as Ewing sarcoma can be difficult to diagnose with certainty; therefore demonstration of *EWSR1* rearrangement or direct demonstration of an *EWSR1-FLI1* or variant fusion product is becoming the standard of care for diagnosis.[113] In this example, karyotypic analysis, FISH, and RT-PCR methods are all useful methods, but one must use caution in the interpretation of cases because a growing number of tumors involve the same gene or even the same translocation. It is clearly better to delay a diagnosis for additional testing than to issue a potentially significant diagnostic misinterpretation.

PRACTICE POINTS: When to Consider Molecular Diagnostics

- Small biopsy
- Poor histologic preservation
- Unusual morphologic features
- Discordant immunohistochemical results
- Uncharacteristic clinical features:
  - Patient age or gender
  - Rare site of involvement
- Extensive treatment effect
- Necessary for definitive treatment
- Provides prognostic information:
  - Tumor natural history
  - Response to treatment
- Rarely encountered entity for diagnosing pathologist

PRACTICE POINTS: Choosing a Molecular Diagnostic Approach

- Chromosomal karyotyping
  - Expensive and requires expertise to perform and interpret
  - Provides unbiased examination of all chromosomes
  - Can lead to new discoveries but can also miss cryptic events
  - May require FISH or RT-PCR for confirmation of a specific translocation
  - Fresh material is required
- Break-apart FISH
  - Directed technique that detects all rearrangements of a particular locus
  - Does not provide insight into the specific fusion variant or type
  - Cannot distinguish between two tumors that harbor rearrangements of the same locus
  - Fusion or combination FISH can help but is rarely used for sarcomas
  - Can be applied to various preparations of fresh and fixed material
- RT-PCR
  - Directed technique that demonstrates a specific fusion type and variant
  - Can demonstrate a specific fusion transcript for diagnosis or prognosis
  - Can be adapted to track minimal residual disease
  - Sequencing or other techniques are important to confirm the identity of a putative fusion amplicon
  - Various fresh and formalin-fixed tissues can be used
- Real-time PCR
  - The presence of a fusion can be detected rapidly
  - Technique not as widely used as others
- NGS (RNA-seq)
  - Can look for many translocations at once
  - Virtually all fusions partners for the same gene can be detected
  - Technique is very sensitive
  - Sample preparation is more complex
  - Bioinformatic interpretation is involved
  - Various fresh and formalin-fixed tissues can be used
- NGS (DNA-seq)
  - Many genes assessed for mutations, insertions, and deletions and copy number alterations
  - Must make sure that the gene panel is appropriate for sarcoma
  - Translocations are more challenging to detect with this technique
  - Very small amounts of DNA are needed
  - Various fresh and formalin-fixed tissues can be used

FISH, Fluorescence in situ hybridization; *NGS*, next-generation sequencing; *RT-PCR*, reverse transcription polymerase chain reaction.

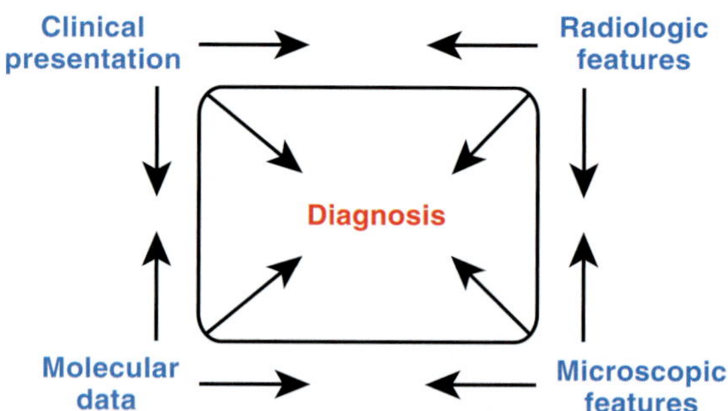

Figure 18.36 Interdependence of Factors Critical for a Specific Diagnosis. No single line of evidence should be taken out of context. Sound diagnosis rests on the careful consideration of all available lines of evidence.

Paramount is the fact that molecular testing cannot be used in isolation; selection of any particular molecular test should be informed by a specific differential diagnosis and relevant pretest probabilities. The final diagnosis should be a coordinated interpretation of a sensible morphologic impression combined with clinical and radiologic data and confirmatory immunohistochemical and molecular findings, as illustrated in Fig. 18.36. Application and interpretation of molecular testing data outside of this framework can lead to diagnostic confusion and significant errors.

References

1. Lahat G, Lazar A, Lev D: Sarcoma epidemiology and etiology: potential environmental and genetic factors, *Surg Clin North Am* 88:451–481, v, 2008.
2. Cleven AH, Sannaa GA, Briaire-de Bruijn I, et al: Loss of H3K27 tri-methylation is a diagnostic marker for malignant peripheral nerve sheath tumors and an indicator for an inferior survival, *Mod Pathol* 29:582–590, 2016.
3. Schaefer IM, Fletcher CD, Hornick JL: Loss of H3K27 trimethylation distinguishes malignant peripheral nerve sheath tumors from histologic mimics, *Mod Pathol* 29:4–13, 2016.
4. Amary MF, Bacsi K, Maggiani F, et al: IDH1 and IDH2 mutations are frequent events in central chondrosarcoma and central and periosteal chondromas but not in other mesenchymal tumours, *J Pathol* 224:334–343, 2011.
5. Tarpey PS, Behjati S, Cooke SL, et al: Frequent mutation of the major cartilage collagen gene COL2A1 in chondrosarcoma, *Nat Genet* 45:923–926, 2013.
6. Manner J, Radlwimmer B, Hohenberger P, et al: MYC high level gene amplification is a distinctive feature of angiosarcomas after irradiation or chronic lymphedema, *Am J Pathol* 176:34–39, 2010.
7. Guo T, Zhang L, Chang NE, et al: Consistent MYC and FLT4 gene amplification in radiation-induced angiosarcoma but not in other radiation-associated atypical vascular lesions, *Genes Chromosomes Cancer* 50:25–33, 2011.
8. Sandberg AA, Bridge JA: Updates on cytogenetics and molecular genetics of bone and soft tissue tumors: Ewing sarcoma and peripheral primitive neuroectodermal tumors, *Cancer Genet Cytogenet* 123:1–26, 2000.
9. Aurias A, Rimbaut C, Buffe D, et al: Translocation involving chromosome 22 in Ewing's sarcoma. A cytogenetic study of four fresh tumors, *Cancer Genet Cytogenet* 12:21–25, 1984.
10. Zucman J, Delattre O, Desmaze C, et al: Cloning and characterization of the Ewing's sarcoma and peripheral neuroepithelioma t(11;22) translocation breakpoints, *Genes Chromosomes Cancer* 5:271–277, 1992.
11. Delattre O, Zucman J, Plougastel B, et al: Gene fusion with an ETS DNA-binding domain caused by chromosome translocation in human tumours, *Nature* 359:162–165, 1992.
12. May WA, Gishizky ML, Lessnick SL, et al: Ewing sarcoma 11;22 translocation produces a chimeric transcription factor that requires the DNA-binding domain encoded by FLI1 for transformation, *Proc Natl Acad Sci USA* 90:5752–5756, 1993.
13. Khoury JD: Ewing sarcoma family of tumors, *Adv Anat Pathol* 12:212–220, 2005.
14. Pierron G, Tirode F, Lucchesi C, et al: A new subtype of bone sarcoma defined by BCOR-CCNB3 gene fusion, *Nat Genet* 44:461–466, 2012.
15. Puls F, Niblett A, Marland G, et al: BCOR-CCNB3 (Ewing-like) sarcoma: a clinicopathologic analysis of 10 cases, in comparison with conventional Ewing sarcoma, *Am J Surg Pathol* 38:1307–1318, 2014.
16. Italiano A, Sung YS, Zhang L, et al: High prevalence of CIC fusion with double-homeobox (DUX4) transcription factors in EWSR1-negative undifferentiated small blue round cell sarcomas, *Genes Chromosomes Cancer* 51:207–218, 2012.
17. Specht K, Sung YS, Zhang L, et al: Distinct transcriptional signature and immunoprofile of CIC-DUX4 fusion-positive round cell tumors compared to EWSR1-rearranged Ewing sarcomas: further evidence toward distinct pathologic entities, *Genes Chromosomes Cancer* 53:622–633, 2014.
18. Ben-David Y, Bernstein A: Friend virus-induced erythroleukemia and the multistage nature of cancer, *Cell* 66:831–834, 1991.
19. Ben-David Y, Giddens EB, Letwin K, et al: Erythroleukemia induction by Friend murine leukemia virus: insertional activation of a new member of the ets gene family, Fli-1, closely linked to c-ets-1, *Genes Dev* 5:908–918, 1991.
20. Sorensen PH, Lessnick SL, Lopez-Terrada D, et al: A second Ewing's sarcoma translocation, t(21;22), fuses the EWS gene to another ETS-family transcription factor, ERG, *Nat Genet* 6:146–151, 1994.
21. Lazar A, Abruzzo LV, Pollock RE, et al: Molecular diagnosis of sarcomas: chromosomal translocations in sarcomas, *Arch Pathol Lab Med* 130:1199–1207, 2006.
22. Bridge JA, Sandberg AA: Cytogenetic and molecular genetic techniques as adjunctive approaches in the diagnosis of bone and soft tissue tumors, *Skeletal Radiol* 29:249–258, 2000.
23. Mitelman F, Johansson B, Mertens F: The impact of translocations and gene fusions on cancer causation, *Nat Rev Cancer* 7:233–245, 2007.
24. Mitelman F, Johansson B, Mertens F: Fusion genes and rearranged genes as a linear function of chromosome aberrations in cancer, *Nat Genet* 36:331–334, 2004.
25. Antonescu CR: Molecular profiling in the diagnosis and treatment of high grade sarcomas, *Ultrastruct Pathol* 32:37–42, 2008.
26. Serrati S, De Summa S, Pilato B, et al: Next-generation sequencing: advances and applications in cancer diagnosis, *Onco Targets Ther* 9:7355–7365, 2016.
27. Sabour L, Sabour M, Ghorbian S: Clinical applications of next-generation sequencing in cancer diagnosis, *Pathol Oncol Res* 23:225–234, 2017.
28. Zheng Z, Liebers M, Zhelyazkova B, et al: Anchored multiplex PCR for targeted next-generation sequencing, *Nat Med* 20:1479–1484, 2014.
29. Guseva NV, Tanas MR, Stence AA, et al: The NAB2-STAT6 gene fusion in solitary fibrous tumor can be reliably detected by anchored multiplexed PCR for targeted next-generation sequencing, *Cancer Genet* 209:303–312, 2016.
30. Li X, Anand M, Haimes JD, et al: The application of next-generation sequencing-based molecular diagnostics in endometrial stromal sarcoma, *Histopathology* 69:551–559, 2016.
31. Chibon F, Lagarde P, Salas S, et al: Validated prediction of clinical outcome in sarcomas and multiple types of cancer on the basis of a gene expression signature related to genome complexity, *Nat Med* 16:781–787, 2010.
32. Lesluyes T, Perot G, Largeau MR, et al: RNA sequencing validation of the complexity INdex in SARComas prognostic signature, *Eur J Cancer* 57:104–111, 2016.
33. Deans ZC, Costa JL, Cree I, et al: Integration of next-generation sequencing in clinical diagnostic molecular pathology laboratories for analysis of solid tumours; an expert opinion on behalf of IQN Path ASBL, *Virchows Arch* 470:5–20, 2017.
34. Luthra R, Chen H, Roy-Chowdhuri S, et al: Next-generation sequencing in clinical molecular diagnostics of cancer: advantages and challenges, *Cancers (Basel)* 7:2023–2036, 2015.
35. Nielsen TO: Microarray analysis of sarcomas, *Adv Anat Pathol* 13:166–173, 2006.
36. Segal NH, Pavlidis P, Antonescu CR, et al: Classification and subtype prediction of adult soft tissue sarcoma by functional genomics, *Am J Pathol* 163:691–700, 2003.
37. Italiano A, Di Mauro I, Rapp J, et al: Clinical effect of molecular methods in sarcoma diagnosis (GENSARC): a prospective, multicentre, observational study, *Lancet Oncol* 17:532–538, 2016.
38. Mertens F, Stromberg U, Mandahl N, et al: Prognostically important chromosomal aberrations in soft tissue sarcomas: a report of the Chromosomes and Morphology (CHAMP) Study Group, *Cancer Res* 62:3980–3984, 2002.
39. Gibault L, Perot G, Chibon F, et al: New insights in sarcoma oncogenesis: a comprehensive analysis of a large series of 160 soft tissue sarcomas with complex genomics, *J Pathol* 223:64–71, 2011.
40. Ladanyi M, Lui MY, Antonescu CR, et al: The der(17)t(X;17)(p11;q25) of human alveolar soft part sarcoma fuses the TFE3 transcription factor gene to ASPL, a novel gene at 17q25, *Oncogene* 20:48–57, 2001.
41. Sandberg A, Bridge J: Updates on the cytogenetics and molecular genetics of bone and soft tissue tumors: alveolar soft part sarcoma, *Cancer Genet Cytogenet* 136:1–9, 2002.
42. Argani P, Antonescu CR, Illei PB, et al: Primary renal neoplasms with the ASPL-TFE3 gene fusion of alveolar soft part sarcoma: a distinctive tumor entity previously included among renal cell carcinomas of children and adolescents, *Am J Pathol* 159:179–192, 2001.
43. Argani P, Aulmann S, Illei PB, et al: A distinctive subset of PEComas harbors TFE3 gene fusions, *Am J Surg Pathol* 34:1395–1406, 2010.
44. Jin L, Majerus J, Oliveira A, et al: Detection of fusion gene transcripts in fresh-frozen and formalin-fixed paraffin-embedded tissue sections of soft-tissue sarcomas after laser capture microdissection and rt-PCR, *Diagn Mol Pathol* 12:224–230, 2003.
45. Aulmann S, Longerich T, Schirmacher P, et al: Detection of the ASPSCR1-TFE3 gene fusion in paraffin-embedded alveolar soft part sarcomas, *Histopathology* 50:881–886, 2007.
46. Lazar AJ, Das P, Tuvin D, et al: Angiogenesis-promoting gene patterns in alveolar soft part sarcoma, *Clin Cancer Res* 13:7314–7321, 2007.
47. Argani P, Lal P, Hutchinson B, et al: Aberrant nuclear immunoreactivity for TFE3 in neoplasms with TFE3 gene fusions: a sensitive and specific immunohistochemical assay, *Am J Surg Pathol* 27:750–761, 2003.
48. Waters BL, Panagopoulos I, Allen EF: Genetic characterization of angiomatoid fibrous histiocytoma identifies fusion of the FUS and ATF-1 genes induced by a chromosomal translocation involving bands 12q13 and 16p11, *Cancer Genet Cytogenet* 121:109–116, 2000.
49. Hallor KH, Mertens F, Jin Y, et al: Fusion of the EWSR1 and ATF1 genes without expression of the MITF-M transcript in angiomatoid fibrous histiocytoma, *Genes Chromosomes Cancer* 44:97–102, 2005.
50. Rossi S, Szuhai K, Ijszenga M, et al: EWSR1-CREB1 and EWSR1-ATF1 fusion genes in angiomatoid fibrous histiocytoma, *Clin Cancer Res* 13:7322–7328, 2007.
51. Antonescu CR, Dal Cin P, Nafa K, et al: EWSR1-CREB1 is the predominant gene fusion in angiomatoid fibrous histiocytoma, *Genes Chromosomes Cancer* 46:1051–1060, 2007.
52. Behjati S, Tarpey PS, Sheldon H, et al: Recurrent PTPRB and PLCG1 mutations in angiosarcoma, *Nat Genet* 46:376–379, 2014.
53. Huang SC, Zhang L, Sung YS, et al: Recurrent CIC gene abnormalities in angiosarcomas: a molecular study of 120 cases with concurrent investigation of PLCG1, KDR, MYC, and FLT4 gene alterations, *Am J Surg Pathol* 40:645–655, 2016.
54. Fernandez AP, Sun Y, Tubbs RR, et al: FISH for MYC amplification and anti-MYC immunohistochemistry: useful diagnostic tools in the assessment of secondary angiosarcoma and atypical vascular proliferations, *J Cutan Pathol* 39:234–242, 2012.
55. Mentzel T, Schildhaus HU, Palmedo G, et al: Postradiation cutaneous angiosarcoma after treatment of breast carcinoma is characterized by MYC amplification in contrast to atypical vascular lesions after radiotherapy and control cases: clinicopathological, immunohistochemical and molecular analysis of 66 cases, *Mod Pathol* 25:75–85, 2012.
56. Plaszczyca A, Nilsson J, Magnusson L, et al: Fusions involving protein kinase C and membrane-associated proteins in benign fibrous histiocytoma, *Int J Biochem Cell Biol* 53:475–481, 2014.
57. Walther C, Hofvander J, Nilsson J, et al: Gene fusion detection in formalin-fixed paraffin-embedded benign fibrous histiocytomas using fluorescence in situ hybridization and RNA sequencing, *Lab Invest* 95:1071–1076, 2015.
58. Panagopoulos I, Gorunova L, Bjerkehagen B, et al: LAMTOR1-PRKCD and NUMA1-SFMBT1 fusion genes identified by RNA sequencing in aneurysmal benign fibrous histiocytoma with t(3;11)(p21;q13), *Cancer Genet* 208:545–551, 2015.
59. Charli-Joseph Y, Saggini A, Doyle LA, et al: DNA copy number changes in tumors within the spectrum of cellular, atypical, and metastasizing fibrous histiocytoma, *J Am Acad Dermatol* 71:256–263, 2014.

60. Doyle LA, Marino-Enriquez A, Fletcher CD, et al: ALK rearrangement and overexpression in epithelioid fibrous histiocytoma, *Mod Pathol* 28:904–912, 2015.
61. Fritchie KJ, Jin L, Wang X, et al: Fusion gene profile of biphenotypic sinonasal sarcoma: an analysis of 44 cases, *Histopathology* 69:930–936, 2016.
62. Huang SC, Ghossein RA, Bishop JA, et al: Novel PAX3-NCOA1 fusions in biphenotypic sinonasal sarcoma with focal rhabdomyoblastic differentiation, *Am J Surg Pathol* 40:51–59, 2016.
63. Sandberg AA, Bridge JA: Updates on the cytogenetics and molecular genetics of bone and soft tissue tumors: clear cell sarcoma (malignant melanoma of soft parts), *Cancer Genet Cytogenet* 130:1–7, 2001.
64. Coindre JM, Hostein I, Terrier P, et al: Diagnosis of clear cell sarcoma by real-time reverse transcriptase-polymerase chain reaction analysis of paraffin embedded tissues: clinicopathologic and molecular analysis of 44 patients from the French sarcoma group, *Cancer* 107:1055–1064, 2006.
65. Panagopoulos I, Mertens F, Debiec-Rychter M, et al: Molecular genetic characterization of the EWS/ATF1 fusion gene in clear cell sarcoma of tendons and aponeuroses, *Int J Cancer* 99:560–567, 2002.
66. Antonescu CR, Tschernyavsky SJ, Woodruff JM, et al: Molecular diagnosis of clear cell sarcoma: detection of EWS-ATF1 and MITF-M transcripts and histopathological and ultrastructural analysis of 12 cases, *J Mol Diagn* 4:44–52, 2002.
67. Antonescu CR, Nafa K, Segal NH, et al: EWS-CREB1: a recurrent variant fusion in clear cell sarcoma–association with gastrointestinal location and absence of melanocytic differentiation, *Clin Cancer Res* 12:5356–5362, 2006.
68. Hisaoka M, Ishida T, Kuo TT, et al: Clear cell sarcoma of soft tissue: a clinicopathologic, immunohistochemical, and molecular analysis of 33 cases, *Am J Surg Pathol* 32:452–460, 2008.
69. Wang WL, Mayordomo E, Zhang W, et al: Detection and characterization of EWSR1/ATF1 and EWSR1/CREB1 chimeric transcripts in clear cell sarcoma (melanoma of soft parts), *Mod Pathol* 22:1201–1209, 2009.
70. Haldar M, Hancock JD, Coffin CM, et al: A conditional mouse model of synovial sarcoma: insights into a myogenic origin, *Cancer Cell* 11:375–388, 2007.
71. Haldar M, Randall RL, Capecchi MR: Synovial sarcoma: from genetics to genetic-based animal modeling, *Clin Orthop Relat Res* 466:2156–2167, 2008.
72. Keller C, Capecchi MR: New genetic tactics to model alveolar rhabdomyosarcoma in the mouse, *Cancer Res* 65:7530–7532, 2005.
73. Keller C, Hansen MS, Coffin CM, et al: Pax3:Fkhr interferes with embryonic Pax3 and Pax7 function: implications for alveolar rhabdomyosarcoma cell of origin, *Genes Dev* 18:2608–2613, 2004.
74. Keller C, Arenkiel BR, Coffin CM, et al: Alveolar rhabdomyosarcomas in conditional Pax3:Fkhr mice: cooperativity of Ink4a/ARF and Trp53 loss of function, *Genes Dev* 18:2614–2626, 2004.
75. Antonescu CR, Katabi N, Zhang L, et al: EWSR1-ATF1 fusion is a novel and consistent finding in hyalinizing clear-cell carcinoma of salivary gland, *Genes Chromosomes Cancer* 50:559–570, 2011.
76. Bilodeau EA, Weinreb I, Antonescu CR, et al: Clear cell odontogenic carcinomas show EWSR1 rearrangements: a novel finding and a biological link to salivary clear cell carcinomas, *Am J Surg Pathol* 37:1001–1005, 2013.
77. Thway K, Nicholson AG, Lawson K, et al: Primary pulmonary myxoid sarcoma with EWSR1-CREB1 fusion: a new tumor entity, *Am J Surg Pathol* 35:1722–1732, 2011.
78. Kao YC, Sung YS, Zhang L, et al: EWSR1 fusions with CREB family transcription factors define a novel myxoid mesenchymal tumor with predilection for intracranial location, *Am J Surg Pathol* 41:482–490, 2017.
79. Pedeutour F, Coindre JM, Sozzi G, et al: Supernumerary ring chromosomes containing chromosome 17 sequences. A specific feature of dermatofibrosarcoma protuberans?, *Cancer Genet Cytogenet* 76:1–9, 1994.
80. Simon MP, Navarro M, Roux D, et al: Structural and functional analysis of a chimeric protein COL1A1-PDGFB generated by the translocation t(17;22)(q22;q13.1) in Dermatofibrosarcoma protuberans (DP), *Oncogene* 20:2965–2975, 2001.
81. Patel KU, Szabo SS, Hernandez VS, et al: Dermatofibrosarcoma protuberans COL1A1-PDGFB fusion is identified in virtually all dermatofibrosarcoma protuberans cases when investigated by newly developed multiplex reverse transcription polymerase chain reaction and fluorescence in situ hybridization assays, *Hum Pathol* 39:184–193, 2008.
82. Abbott JJ, Erickson-Johnson M, Wang X, et al: Gains of COL1A1-PDGFB genomic copies occur in fibrosarcomatous transformation of dermatofibrosarcoma protuberans, *Mod Pathol* 19:1512–1518, 2006.
83. Swaby MG, Evans HL, Fletcher CD, et al: Dermatofibrosarcoma protuberans with unusual sarcomatous transformation: a series of 4 cases with molecular confirmation, *Am J Dermatopathol* 33:354–360, 2011.
84. Macarenco RS, Zamolyi R, Franco MF, et al: Genomic gains of COL1A1-PDFGB occur in the histologic evolution of giant cell fibroblastoma into dermatofibrosarcoma protuberans, *Genes Chromosomes Cancer* 47:260–265, 2008.
85. McArthur GA: Molecular targeting of dermatofibrosarcoma protuberans: a new approach to a surgical disease, *J Natl Compr Canc Netw* 5:557–562, 2007.
86. Kotiligam D, Lazar AJ, Pollock RE, et al: Desmoid tumor: a disease opportune for molecular insights, *Histol Histopathol* 23:117–126, 2008.
87. Lips DJ, Barker N, Clevers H, et al: The role of APC and beta-catenin in the aetiology of aggressive fibromatosis (desmoid tumors), *Eur J Surg Oncol* 35:3–10, 2009.
88. Lazar AJ, Tuvin D, Hajibashi S, et al: Specific mutations in the beta-catenin gene (CTNNB1) correlate with local recurrence in sporadic desmoid tumors, *Am J Pathol* 173:1518–1527, 2008.
89. Amary MF, Pauwels P, Meulemans E, et al: Detection of beta-catenin mutations in paraffin-embedded sporadic desmoid-type fibromatosis by mutation-specific restriction enzyme digestion (MSRED): an ancillary diagnostic tool, *Am J Surg Pathol* 31:1299–1309, 2007.
90. Polakis P: The many ways of Wnt in cancer, *Curr Opin Genet Dev* 17:45–51, 2007.
91. Montgomery E, Folpe AL: The diagnostic value of beta-catenin immunohistochemistry, *Adv Anat Pathol* 12:350–356, 2005.
92. Domont J, Salas S, Lacroix L, et al: High frequency of beta-catenin heterozygous mutations in extra-abdominal fibromatosis: a potential molecular tool for disease management, *Br J Cancer* 102:1032–1036, 2010.
93. Colombo C, Miceli R, Lazar AJ, et al: CTNNB1 45F mutation is a molecular prognosticator of increased postoperative primary desmoid tumor recurrence: an independent, multicenter validation study, *Cancer* 119:3696–3702, 2013.
94. Kasper B, Gruenwald V, Reichardt P, et al: Correlation of CTNNB1 mutation status with progression arrest rate in RECIST progressive desmoid-type fibromatosis treated with imatinib: translational research results from a phase 2 study of the German Interdisciplinary Sarcoma Group (GISG-01), *Ann Surg Oncol* 23:1924–1927, 2016.
95. van Broekhoven DL, Verhoef C, Grunhagen DJ, et al: Prognostic value of CTNNB1 gene mutation in primary sporadic aggressive fibromatosis, *Ann Surg Oncol* 22:1464–1470, 2015.
96. Mullen JT, DeLaney TF, Rosenberg AE, et al: beta-Catenin mutation status and outcomes in sporadic desmoid tumors, *Oncologist* 18:1043–1049, 2013.
97. Crago AM, Chmielecki J, Rosenberg M, et al: Near universal detection of alterations in CTNNB1 and Wnt pathway regulators in desmoid-type fibromatosis by whole-exome sequencing and genomic analysis, *Genes Chromosomes Cancer* 54:606–615, 2015.
98. Sandberg AA, Bridge JA: Updates on the cytogenetics and molecular genetics of bone and soft tissue tumors. Synovial sarcoma, *Cancer Genet Cytogenet* 133:1–23, 2002.
99. Antonescu CR, Gerald WL, Magid MS, et al: Molecular variants of the EWS-WT1 gene fusion in desmoplastic small round cell tumor, *Diagn Mol Pathol* 7:24–28, 1998.
100. Yamaguchi U, Hasegawa T, Morimoto Y, et al: A practical approach to the clinical diagnosis of Ewing's sarcoma/primitive neuroectodermal tumour and other small round cell tumours sharing EWS rearrangement using new fluorescence in situ hybridisation probes for EWSR1 on formalin fixed, paraffin wax embedded tissue, *J Clin Pathol* 58:1051–1056, 2005.
101. Hill DA, Pfeifer JD, Marley EF, et al: WT1 staining reliably differentiates desmoplastic small round cell tumor from Ewing sarcoma/primitive neuroectodermal tumor. An immunohistochemical and molecular diagnostic study, *Am J Clin Pathol* 114:345–353, 2000.
102. Koontz JI, Soreng AL, Nucci M, et al: Frequent fusion of the JAZF1 and JJAZ1 genes in endometrial stromal tumors, *Proc Natl Acad Sci USA* 98:6348–6353, 2001.
103. Sandberg AA: The cytogenetics and molecular biology of endometrial stromal sarcoma, *Cytogenet Genome Res* 118:182–189, 2007.
104. Chiang S, Oliva E: Cytogenetic and molecular aberrations in endometrial stromal tumors, *Hum Pathol* 42:609–617, 2011.
105. Micci F, Panagopoulos I, Bjerkehagen B, et al: Consistent rearrangement of chromosomal band 6p21 with generation of fusion genes JAZF1/PHF1 and EPC1/PHF1 in endometrial stromal sarcoma, *Cancer Res* 66:107–112, 2006.
106. Chiang S, Ali R, Melnyk N, et al: Frequency of known gene rearrangements in endometrial stromal tumors, *Am J Surg Pathol* 35:1364–1372, 2011.
107. Nucci MR, Harburger D, Koontz J, et al: Molecular analysis of the JAZF1-JJAZ1 gene fusion by RT-PCR and fluorescence in situ hybridization in endometrial stromal neoplasms, *Am J Surg Pathol* 31:65–70, 2007.
108. Lee CH, Ou WB, Marino-Enriquez A, et al: 14-3-3 fusion oncogenes in high-grade endometrial stromal sarcoma, *Proc Natl Acad Sci USA* 109:929–934, 2012.
109. Lee CH, Marino-Enriquez A, Ou W, et al: The clinicopathologic features of YWHAE-FAM22 endometrial stromal sarcomas: a histologically high-grade and clinically aggressive tumor, *Am J Surg Pathol* 36:641–653, 2012.
110. Tanas MR, Sboner A, Oliveira AM, et al: Identification of a disease-defining gene fusion in epithelioid hemangioendothelioma, *Sci Transl Med* 3:98ra82, 2011.
111. Errani C, Zhang L, Sung YS, et al: A novel WWTR1-CAMTA1 gene fusion is a consistent abnormality in epithelioid hemangioendothelioma of different anatomic sites, *Genes Chromosomes Cancer* 50:644–653, 2011.
112. Antonescu CR, Le Loarer F, Mosquera JM, et al: Novel YAP1-TFE3 fusion defines a distinct subset of epithelioid hemangioendothelioma, *Genes Chromosomes Cancer* 52:775–784, 2013.
113. Folpe AL, Goldblum JR, Rubin BP, et al: Morphologic and immunophenotypic diversity in Ewing family tumors: a study of 66 genetically confirmed cases, *Am J Surg Pathol* 29:1025–1033, 2005.
114. Bridge RS, Rajaram V, Dehner LP, et al: Molecular diagnosis of Ewing sarcoma/primitive neuroectodermal tumor in routinely processed tissue: a comparison of two FISH strategies and RT-PCR in malignant round cell tumors, *Mod Pathol* 19:1–8, 2006.
115. de Alava E, Lozano MD, Patino A, et al: Ewing family tumors: potential prognostic value of reverse-transcriptase polymerase chain reaction detection of minimal residual disease in peripheral blood samples, *Diagn Mol Pathol* 7:152–157, 1998.
116. Le Deley MC, Delattre O, Schaefer KL, et al: Impact of EWS-ETS fusion type on disease progression in Ewing's sarcoma/peripheral primitive neuroectodermal tumor: prospective results from the cooperative Euro-E.W.I.N.G. 99 trial, *J Clin Oncol* 28:1982–1988, 2010.

117. Avigad S, Cohen IJ, Zilberstein J, et al: The predictive potential of molecular detection in the nonmetastatic Ewing family of tumors, *Cancer* 100:1053–1058, 2004.
118. Graham C, Chilton-MacNeill S, Zielenska M, et al: The CIC-DUX4 fusion transcript is present in a subgroup of pediatric primitive round cell sarcomas, *Hum Pathol* 43:180–189, 2012.
119. Sugita S, Arai Y, Tonooka A, et al: A novel CIC-FOXO4 gene fusion in undifferentiated small round cell sarcoma: a genetically distinct variant of Ewing-like sarcoma, *Am J Surg Pathol* 38:1571–1576, 2014.
120. Solomon DA, Brohl AS, Khan J, et al: Clinicopathologic features of a second patient with Ewing-like sarcoma harboring CIC-FOXO4 gene fusion, *Am J Surg Pathol* 38:1724–1725, 2014.
121. Choi EY, Thomas DG, McHugh JB, et al: Undifferentiated small round cell sarcoma with t(4;19)(q35;q13.1) CIC-DUX4 fusion: a novel highly aggressive soft tissue tumor with distinctive histopathology, *Am J Surg Pathol* 37:1379–1386, 2013.
122. Le Guellec S, Velasco V, Perot G, et al: ETV4 is a useful marker for the diagnosis of CIC-rearranged undifferentiated round-cell sarcomas: a study of 127 cases including mimicking lesions, *Mod Pathol* 29:1523–1531, 2016.
123. Hung YP, Fletcher CD, Hornick JL: Evaluation of ETV4 and WT1 expression in CIC-rearranged sarcomas and histologic mimics, *Mod Pathol* 29:1324–1334, 2016.
124. Peters TL, Kumar V, Polikepahad S, et al: BCOR-CCNB3 fusions are frequent in undifferentiated sarcomas of male children, *Mod Pathol* 28:575–586, 2015.
125. Cohen-Gogo S, Cellier C, Coindre JM, et al: Ewing-like sarcomas with BCOR-CCNB3 fusion transcript: a clinical, radiological and pathological retrospective study from the Societe Francaise des Cancers de L'Enfant, *Pediatr Blood Cancer* 61:2191–2198, 2014.
126. Kao YC, Sung YS, Zhang L, et al: BCOR overexpression is a highly sensitive marker in round cell sarcomas with BCOR genetic abnormalities, *Am J Surg Pathol* 40:1670–1678, 2016.
127. Specht K, Zhang L, Sung YS, et al: Novel BCOR-MAML3 and ZC3H7B-BCOR gene fusions in undifferentiated small blue round cell sarcomas, *Am J Surg Pathol* 40:433–442, 2016.
128. Sandberg AA: Genetics of chondrosarcoma and related tumors, *Curr Opin Oncol* 16:342–354, 2004.
129. Wang WL, Mayordomo E, Czerniak BA, et al: Fluorescence in situ hybridization is a useful ancillary diagnostic tool for extraskeletal myxoid chondrosarcoma, *Mod Pathol* 21:1303–1310, 2008.
130. Sjogren H, Meis-Kindblom JM, Orndal C, et al: Studies on the molecular pathogenesis of extraskeletal myxoid chondrosarcoma-cytogenetic, molecular genetic, and cDNA microarray analyses, *Am J Pathol* 162:781–792, 2003.
131. Antonescu CR, Argani P, Erlandson RA, et al: Skeletal and extraskeletal myxoid chondrosarcoma: a comparative clinicopathologic, ultrastructural, and molecular study, *Cancer* 83:1504–1521, 1998.
132. Mosquera JM, Sboner A, Zhang L, et al: Novel MIR143-NOTCH fusions in benign and malignant glomus tumors, *Genes Chromosomes Cancer* 52:1075–1087, 2013.
133. Brems H, Park C, Maertens O, et al: Glomus tumors in neurofibromatosis type 1: genetic, functional, and clinical evidence of a novel association, *Cancer Res* 69:7393–7401, 2009.
134. Brouillard P, Olsen BR, Vikkula M: High-resolution physical and transcript map of the locus for venous malformations with glomus cells (VMGLOM) on chromosome 1p21-p22, *Genomics* 67:96–101, 2000.
135. Boon LM, Brouillard P, Irrthum A, et al: A gene for inherited cutaneous venous anomalies ("glomangiomas") localizes to chromosome 1p21-22, *Am J Hum Genet* 65:125–133, 1999.
136. Rubin BP, Heinrich MC, Corless CL: Gastrointestinal stromal tumour, *Lancet* 369:1731–1741, 2007.
137. Lasota J, Miettinen M: Clinical significance of oncogenic KIT and PDGFRA mutations in gastrointestinal stromal tumours, *Histopathology* 53:245–266, 2008.
138. Lasota J, vel Dobosz AJ, Wasag B, et al: Presence of homozygous KIT exon 11 mutations is strongly associated with malignant clinical behavior in gastrointestinal stromal tumors, *Lab Invest* 87:1029–1041, 2007.
139. Lasota J, Corless CL, Heinrich MC, et al: Clinicopathologic profile of gastrointestinal stromal tumors (GISTs) with primary KIT exon 13 or exon 17 mutations: a multicenter study on 54 cases, *Mod Pathol* 21:476–484, 2008.
140. Debiec-Rychter M, Sciot R, Le Cesne A, et al: KIT mutations and dose selection for imatinib in patients with advanced gastrointestinal stromal tumours, *Eur J Cancer* 42:1093–1103, 2006.
141. Corless CL, Schroeder A, Griffith D, et al: PDGFRA mutations in gastrointestinal stromal tumors: frequency, spectrum and in vitro sensitivity to imatinib, *J Clin Oncol* 23:5357–5364, 2005.
142. Liegl B, Kepten I, Le C, et al: Heterogeneity of kinase inhibitor resistance mechanisms in GIST, *J Pathol* 216:64–74, 2008.
143. Heinrich MC, Corless CL, Blanke CD, et al: Molecular correlates of imatinib resistance in gastrointestinal stromal tumors, *J Clin Oncol* 24:4764–4774, 2006.
144. Agaram NP, Wong GC, Guo T, et al: Novel V600E BRAF mutations in imatinib-naive and imatinib-resistant gastrointestinal stromal tumors, *Genes Chromosomes Cancer* 47:853–859, 2008.
145. Pasini B, McWhinney SR, Bei T, et al: Clinical and molecular genetics of patients with the Carney-Stratakis syndrome and germline mutations of the genes coding for the succinate dehydrogenase subunits SDHB, SDHC, and SDHD, *Eur J Hum Genet* 16:79–88, 2008.
146. Gill AJ, Chou A, Vilain R, et al: Immunohistochemistry for SDHB divides gastrointestinal stromal tumors (GISTs) into 2 distinct types, *Am J Surg Pathol* 34:636–644, 2010.
147. Gaal J, Stratakis CA, Carney JA, et al: SDHB immunohistochemistry: a useful tool in the diagnosis of Carney-Stratakis and Carney triad gastrointestinal stromal tumors, *Mod Pathol* 24:147–151, 2011.
148. Janeway KA, Kim SY, Lodish M, et al: Defects in succinate dehydrogenase in gastrointestinal stromal tumors lacking KIT and PDGFRA mutations, *Proc Natl Acad Sci USA* 108:314–318, 2011.
149. Pantaleo MA, Astolfi A, Indio V, et al: SDHA loss-of-function mutations in KIT-PDGFRA wild-type gastrointestinal stromal tumors identified by massively parallel sequencing, *J Natl Cancer Inst* 103:983–987, 2011.
150. Wagner AJ, Remillard SP, Zhang YX, et al: Loss of expression of SDHA predicts SDHA mutations in gastrointestinal stromal tumors, *Mod Pathol* 26:289–294, 2013.
151. Miettinen M, Fetsch JF, Sobin LH, et al: Gastrointestinal stromal tumors in patients with neurofibromatosis 1: a clinicopathologic and molecular genetic study of 45 cases, *Am J Surg Pathol* 30:90–96, 2006.
152. Zhang L, Smyrk TC, Young WF, Jr, et al: Gastric stromal tumors in Carney triad are different clinically, pathologically, and behaviorally from sporadic gastric gastrointestinal stromal tumors: findings in 104 cases, *Am J Surg Pathol* 34:53–64, 2010.
153. Kleinbaum EP, Lazar AJ, Tamborini E, et al: Clinical, histopathologic, molecular and therapeutic findings in a large kindred with gastrointestinal stromal tumor, *Int J Cancer* 122:711–718, 2008.
154. Killian JK, Miettinen M, Walker RL, et al: Recurrent epimutation of SDHC in gastrointestinal stromal tumors, *Sci Transl Med* 6:268ra177, 2014.
155. Boikos SA, Xekouki P, Fumagalli E, et al: Carney triad can be (rarely) associated with germline succinate dehydrogenase defects, *Eur J Hum Genet* 24:569–573, 2016.
156. Murphy JD, Ma GL, Baumgartner JM, et al: Increased risk of additional cancers among patients with gastrointestinal stromal tumors: A population-based study, *Cancer* 121:2960–2967, 2015.
157. Dumont AG, Rink L, Godwin AK, et al: A nonrandom association of gastrointestinal stromal tumor (GIST) and desmoid tumor (deep fibromatosis): case series of 28 patients, *Ann Oncol* 23:1335–1340, 2012.
158. Knezevich SR, McFadden DE, Tao W, et al: A novel ETV6-NTRK3 gene fusion in congenital fibrosarcoma, *Nat Genet* 18:184–187, 1998.
159. Sandberg AA, Bridge JA: Updates on the cytogenetics and molecular genetics of bone and soft tissue tumors: congenital (infantile) fibrosarcoma and mesoblastic nephroma, *Cancer Genet Cytogenet* 132:1–13, 2002.
160. Rubin BP, Chen CJ, Morgan TW, et al: Congenital mesoblastic nephroma t(12;15) is associated with ETV6-NTRK3 gene fusion: cytogenetic and molecular relationship to congenital (infantile) fibrosarcoma, *Am J Pathol* 153:1451–1458, 1998.
161. Alessandri AJ, Knezevich SR, Mathers JA, et al: Absence of t(12;15) associated ETV6-NTRK3 fusion transcripts in pediatric acute leukemias, *Med Pediatr Oncol* 37:415–416, 2001.
162. Tognon C, Knezevich SR, Huntsman D, et al: Expression of the ETV6-NTRK3 gene fusion as a primary event in human secretory breast carcinoma, *Cancer Cell* 2:367–376, 2002.
163. Shi E, Chmielecki J, Tang CM, et al: FGFR1 and NTRK3 actionable alterations in "Wild-Type" gastrointestinal stromal tumors, *J Transl Med* 14:339, 2016.
164. Cordioli MI, Moraes L, Bastos AU, et al: Fusion oncogenes are the main genetic events found in sporadic papillary thyroid carcinomas from children, *Thyroid* 27:182–188, 2017.
165. Bishop JA, Taube JM, Su A, et al: Secretory carcinoma of the skin harboring ETV6 gene fusions: a cutaneous analogue to secretory carcinomas of the breast and salivary glands, *Am J Surg Pathol* 41:62–66, 2017.
166. Yeh I, Tee MK, Botton T, et al: NTRK3 kinase fusions in Spitz tumours, *J Pathol* 240:282–290, 2016.
167. Alassiri AH, Ali RH, Shen Y, et al: ETV6-NTRK3 is expressed in a subset of ALK-negative inflammatory myofibroblastic tumors, *Am J Surg Pathol* 40:1051–1061, 2016.
168. Leeman-Neill RJ, Kelly LM, Liu P, et al: ETV6-NTRK3 is a common chromosomal rearrangement in radiation-associated thyroid cancer, *Cancer* 120:799–807, 2014.
169. Amatu A, Sartore-Bianchi A, Siena S: NTRK gene fusions as novel targets of cancer therapy across multiple tumour types, *ESMO Open* 1:e000023, 2016.
170. Bourgeois JM, Knezevich SR, Mathers JA, et al: Molecular detection of the ETV6-NTRK3 gene fusion differentiates congenital fibrosarcoma from other childhood spindle cell tumors, *Am J Surg Pathol* 24:937–946, 2000.
171. Coffin CM, Hornick JL, Fletcher CD: Inflammatory myofibroblastic tumor: comparison of clinicopathologic, histologic, and immunohistochemical features including ALK expression in atypical and aggressive cases, *Am J Surg Pathol* 31:509–520, 2007.
172. Gleason BC, Hornick JL: Inflammatory myofibroblastic tumours: where are we now?, *J Clin Pathol* 61:428–437, 2008.
173. Lawrence B, Perez-Atayde A, Hibbard MK, et al: TPM3-ALK and TPM4-ALK oncogenes in inflammatory myofibroblastic tumors, *Am J Pathol* 157:377–384, 2000.
174. Chiarle R, Voena C, Ambrogio C, et al: The anaplastic lymphoma kinase in the pathogenesis of cancer, *Nat Rev Cancer* 8:11–23, 2008.
175. Marino-Enriquez A, Wang WL, Roy A, et al: Epithelioid inflammatory myofibroblastic sarcoma: An aggressive intra-abdominal variant of inflammatory myofibroblastic tumor with nuclear membrane or perinuclear ALK, *Am J Surg Pathol* 35:135–144, 2011.
176. Lee JC, Li CF, Huang HY, et al: ALK oncoproteins in atypical inflammatory myofibroblastic tumours: novel RRBP1-ALK fusions in epithelioid inflammatory myofibroblastic sarcoma, *J Pathol* 241:316–323, 2017.

177. Lovly CM, Gupta A, Lipson D, et al: Inflammatory myofibroblastic tumors harbor multiple potentially actionable kinase fusions, *Cancer Discov* 4:889–895, 2014.
178. Antonescu CR, Suurmeijer AJ, Zhang L, et al: Molecular characterization of inflammatory myofibroblastic tumors with frequent ALK and ROS1 gene fusions and rare novel RET rearrangement, *Am J Surg Pathol* 39:957–967, 2015.
179. Yamamoto H, Yoshida A, Taguchi K, et al: ALK, ROS1 and NTRK3 gene rearrangements in inflammatory myofibroblastic tumours, *Histopathology* 69:72–83, 2016.
180. Sukov WR, Cheville JC, Carlson AW, et al: Utility of ALK-1 protein expression and ALK rearrangements in distinguishing inflammatory myofibroblastic tumor from malignant spindle cell lesions of the urinary bladder, *Mod Pathol* 20:592–603, 2007.
181. Marino-Enriquez A, Dal Cin P: ALK as a paradigm of oncogenic promiscuity: different mechanisms of activation and different fusion partners drive tumors of different lineages, *Cancer Genet* 206:357–373, 2013.
182. Hayashi H, Nakagawa K: Current evidence in support of the second-generation anaplastic lymphoma kinase (ALK) tyrosine kinase inhibitor alectinib for the treatment of non-small cell lung cancer positive for ALK translocation, *J Thorac Dis* 8:E1311–E1316, 2016.
183. Kim RN, Choi YL, Lee MS, et al: SEC31A-ALK fusion gene in lung adenocarcinoma, *Cancer Res Treat* 48:398–402, 2016.
184. Hong M, Kim RN, Song JY, et al: HIP1-ALK, a novel fusion protein identified in lung adenocarcinoma, *J Thorac Oncol* 9:419–422, 2014.
185. Jeanneau M, Gregoire V, Desplechain C, et al: ALK rearrangements-associated renal cell carcinoma (RCC) with unique pathological features in an adult, *Pathol Res Pract* 212:1064–1066, 2016.
186. Wiesner T, He J, Yelensky R, et al: Kinase fusions are frequent in Spitz tumours and spitzoid melanomas, *Nat Commun* 5:3116, 2014.
187. Ji JH, Oh YL, Hong M, et al: Identification of driving ALK fusion genes and genomic landscape of medullary thyroid cancer, *PLoS Genet* 11:e1005467, 2015.
188. Loharamtaweethong K, Puripat N, Aoonjai N, et al: Anaplastic lymphoma kinase (ALK) translocation in paediatric malignant peritoneal mesothelioma: a case report of novel ALK-related tumour spectrum, *Histopathology* 68:603–607, 2016.
189. Feldman AL, Vasmatzis G, Asmann YW, et al: Novel TRAF1-ALK fusion identified by deep RNA sequencing of anaplastic large cell lymphoma, *Genes Chromosomes Cancer* 52:1097–1102, 2013.
190. Takeoka K, Okumura A, Honjo G, et al: Variant translocation partners of the anaplastic lymphoma kinase (ALK) gene in two cases of anaplastic large cell lymphoma, identified by inverse cDNA polymerase chain reaction, *J Clin Exp Hematop* 54:225–235, 2014.
191. Hoshino A, Nomura K, Hamashima T, et al: Aggressive transformation of anaplastic large cell lymphoma with increased number of ALK-translocated chromosomes, *Int J Hematol* 101:198–202, 2015.
192. Lee SE, Kang SY, Takeuchi K, et al: Identification of RANBP2-ALK fusion in ALK positive diffuse large B-cell lymphoma, *Hematol Oncol* 32:221–224, 2014.
193. Kim SM, Kim MJ, Jung HA, et al: Presence of anaplastic lymphoma kinase translocation in sarcomatoid carcinoma of head and neck and treatment effect of crizotinib: A case series, *Head Neck* 37:E66–E69, 2015.
194. Fransson S, Hansson M, Ruuth K, et al: Intragenic anaplastic lymphoma kinase (ALK) rearrangements: translocations as a novel mechanism of ALK activation in neuroblastoma tumors, *Genes Chromosomes Cancer* 54:99–109, 2015.
195. Tokuda K, Eguchi-Ishimae M, Yagi C, et al: CLTC-ALK fusion as a primary event in congenital blastic plasmacytoid dendritic cell neoplasm, *Genes Chromosomes Cancer* 53:78–89, 2014.
196. Yakirevich E, Resnick MB, Mangray S, et al: Oncogenic ALK fusion in rare and aggressive subtype of colorectal adenocarcinoma as a potential therapeutic target, *Clin Cancer Res* 22:3831–3840, 2016.
197. Busam KJ, Kutzner H, Cerroni L, et al: Clinical and pathologic findings of Spitz nevi and atypical Spitz tumors with ALK fusions, *Am J Surg Pathol* 38:925–933, 2014.
198. Yeh I, de la Fouchardiere A, Pissaloux D, et al: Clinical, histopathologic, and genomic features of Spitz tumors with ALK fusions, *Am J Surg Pathol* 39:581–591, 2015.
199. Werner MT, Zhao C, Zhang Q, et al: Nucleophosmin-anaplastic lymphoma kinase: the ultimate oncogene and therapeutic target, *Blood* 129:823–831, 2017.
200. Butrynski JE, D'Adamo DR, Hornick JL, et al: Crizotinib in ALK-rearranged inflammatory myofibroblastic tumor, *N Engl J Med* 363:1727–1733, 2010.
201. Ou SH, Bartlett CH, Mino-Kenudson M, et al: Crizotinib for the treatment of ALK-rearranged non-small cell lung cancer: a success story to usher in the second decade of molecular targeted therapy in oncology, *Oncologist* 17:1351–1375, 2012.
202. Quade BJ, Weremowicz S, Neskey DM, et al: Fusion transcripts involving HMGA2 are not a common molecular mechanism in uterine leiomyomata with rearrangements in 12q15, *Cancer Res* 63:1351–1358, 2003.
203. Ubago JM, Zhang Q, Kim JJ, et al: Two subtypes of atypical leiomyoma: clinical, histologic, and molecular analysis, *Am J Surg Pathol* 40:923–933, 2016.
204. Lien HC, Huang CS, Yang YW, et al: MED12 exon 2 mutation as a highly sensitive and specific marker in distinguishing phyllodes tumours from other spindle neoplasms of the breast, *APMIS* 124:356–364, 2016.
205. Ng CC, Tan J, Ong CK, et al: MED12 is frequently mutated in breast phyllodes tumours: a study of 112 cases, *J Clin Pathol* 68:685–691, 2015.
206. Panagopoulos I, Gorunova L, Lund-Iversen M, et al: Recurrent fusion of the genes FN1 and ALK in gastrointestinal leiomyomas, *Mod Pathol* 29:1415–1423, 2016.
207. Alam NA, Rowan AJ, Wortham NC, et al: Genetic and functional analyses of FH mutations in multiple cutaneous and uterine leiomyomatosis, hereditary leiomyomatosis and renal cancer, and fumarate hydratase deficiency, *Hum Mol Genet* 12:1241–1252, 2003.
208. Tomlinson IP, Alam NA, Rowan AJ, et al: Germline mutations in FH predispose to dominantly inherited uterine fibroids, skin leiomyomata and papillary renal cell cancer, *Nat Genet* 30:406–410, 2002.
209. Nucci MR, Drapkin R, Dal Cin P, et al: Distinctive cytogenetic profile in benign metastasizing leiomyoma: pathogenetic implications, *Am J Surg Pathol* 31:737–743, 2007.
210. Bartuma H, Hallor KH, Panagopoulos I, et al: Assessment of the clinical and molecular impact of different cytogenetic subgroups in a series of 272 lipomas with abnormal karyotype, *Genes Chromosomes Cancer* 46:594–606, 2007.
211. Sandberg AA: Updates on the cytogenetics and molecular genetics of bone and soft tissue tumors: lipoma, *Cancer Genet Cytogenet* 150:93–115, 2004.
212. Willen H, Akerman M, Dal Cin P, et al: Comparison of chromosomal patterns with clinical features in 165 lipomas: a report of the CHAMP study group, *Cancer Genet Cytogenet* 102:46–49, 1998.
213. Huang D, Sumegi J, Dal Cin P, et al: C11orf95-MKL2 is the resulting fusion oncogene of t(11;16)(q13;p13) in chondroid lipoma, *Genes Chromosomes Cancer* 49:810–818, 2010.
214. Gisselsson D, Hoglund M, Mertens F, et al: Hibernomas are characterized by homozygous deletions in the multiple endocrine neoplasia type I region. Metaphase fluorescence in situ hybridization reveals complex rearrangements not detected by conventional cytogenetics, *Am J Pathol* 155:61–66, 1999.
215. Gisselsson D, Hibbard MK, Dal Cin P, et al: PLAG1 alterations in lipoblastoma: involvement in varied mesenchymal cell types and evidence for alternative oncogenic mechanisms, *Am J Pathol* 159:955–962, 2001.
216. Dal Cin P, Sciot R, Polito P, et al: Lesions of 13q may occur independently of deletion of 16q in spindle cell/pleomorphic lipomas, *Histopathology* 31:222–225, 1997.
217. Chen BJ, Marino-Enriquez A, Fletcher CD, et al: Loss of retinoblastoma protein expression in spindle cell/pleomorphic lipomas and cytogenetically related tumors: an immunohistochemical study with diagnostic implications, *Am J Surg Pathol* 36:1119–1128, 2012.
218. Sandberg AA: Updates on the cytogenetics and molecular genetics of bone and soft tissue tumors: liposarcoma, *Cancer Genet Cytogenet* 155:1–24, 2004.
219. Crozat A, Aman P, Mandahl N, et al: Fusion of CHOP to a novel RNA-binding protein in human myxoid liposarcoma, *Nature* 363:640–644, 1993.
220. Rabbitts TH, Forster A, Larson R, et al: Fusion of the dominant negative transcription regulator CHOP with a novel gene FUS by translocation t(12;16) in malignant liposarcoma, *Nat Genet* 4:175–180, 1993.
221. Antonescu CR, Tschernyavsky SJ, Decuseara R, et al: Prognostic impact of P53 status, TLS-CHOP fusion transcript structure, and histological grade in myxoid liposarcoma: a molecular and clinicopathologic study of 82 cases, *Clin Cancer Res* 7:3977–3987, 2001.
222. Panagopoulos I, Hoglund M, Mertens F, et al: Fusion of the EWS and CHOP genes in myxoid liposarcoma, *Oncogene* 12:489–494, 1996.
223. Panagopoulos I, Mertens F, Isaksson M, et al: A novel FUS/CHOP chimera in myxoid liposarcoma, *Biochem Biophys Res Commun* 279:838–845, 2000.
224. Barretina J, Taylor BS, Banerji S, et al: Subtype-specific genomic alterations define new targets for soft-tissue sarcoma therapy, *Nat Genet* 42:715–721, 2010.
225. Demicco EG, Torres KE, Ghadimi MP, et al: Involvement of the PI3K/Akt pathway in myxoid/round cell liposarcoma, *Mod Pathol* 25:212–221, 2012.
226. Willmore-Payne C, Holden J, Turner KC, et al: Translocations and amplifications of chromosome 12 in liposarcoma demonstrated by the LSI CHOP breakapart rearrangement probe, *Arch Pathol Lab Med* 132:952–957, 2008.
227. Antonescu CR, Elahi A, Healey JH, et al: Monoclonality of multifocal myxoid liposarcoma: confirmation by analysis of TLS-CHOP or EWS-CHOP rearrangements, *Clin Cancer Res* 6:2788–2793, 2000.
228. Antonescu CR, Elahi A, Humphrey M, et al: Specificity of TLS-CHOP rearrangement for classic myxoid/round cell liposarcoma: absence in predominantly myxoid well-differentiated liposarcomas, *J Mol Diagn* 2:132–138, 2000.
229. Powers MP, Wang WL, Hernandez VS, et al: Detection of myxoid liposarcoma-associated FUS-DDIT3 rearrangement variants including a newly identified breakpoint using an optimized RT-PCR assay, *Mod Pathol* 23:1307–1315, 2010.
230. Pedeutour F, Forus A, Coindre JM, et al: Structure of the supernumerary ring and giant rod chromosomes in adipose tissue tumors, *Genes Chromosomes Cancer* 24:30–41, 1999.
231. Weaver J, Downs-Kelly E, Goldblum JR, et al: Fluorescence in situ hybridization for MDM2 gene amplification as a diagnostic tool in lipomatous neoplasms, *Mod Pathol* 21:943–949, 2008.
232. Weaver J, Goldblum JR, Turner S, et al: Detection of MDM2 gene amplification or protein expression distinguishes sclerosing mesenteritis and retroperitoneal fibrosis from inflammatory well-differentiated liposarcoma, *Mod Pathol* 22:66–70, 2009.
233. Binh MB, Sastre-Garau X, Guillou L, et al: MDM2 and CDK4 immunostainings are useful adjuncts in diagnosing well-differentiated and dedifferentiated liposarcoma subtypes: a comparative analysis of 559 soft tissue neoplasms with genetic data, *Am J Surg Pathol* 29:1340–1347, 2005.
234. Clay MR, Martinez AP, Weiss SW, et al: MDM2 and CDK4 immunohistochemistry: should it be used in problematic differentiated lipomatous tumors?: A new perspective, *Am J Surg Pathol* 40:1647–1652, 2016.

235. Clay MR, Martinez AP, Weiss SW, et al: MDM2 amplification in problematic lipomatous tumors: analysis of FISH testing criteria, *Am J Surg Pathol* 39:1433–1439, 2015.
236. Mejia-Guerrero S, Quejada M, Gokgoz N, et al: Characterization of the 12q15 MDM2 and 12q13-14 CDK4 amplicons and clinical correlations in osteosarcoma, *Genes Chromosomes Cancer* 49:518–525, 2010.
237. Dujardin F, Binh MB, Bouvier C, et al: MDM2 and CDK4 immunohistochemistry is a valuable tool in the differential diagnosis of low-grade osteosarcomas and other primary fibro-osseous lesions of the bone, *Mod Pathol* 24:624–637, 2011.
238. Guerin M, Thariat J, Ouali M, et al: A new subtype of high-grade mandibular osteosarcoma with RASAL1/MDM2 amplification, *Hum Pathol* 50:70–78, 2016.
239. Yoshida A, Ushiku T, Motoi T, et al: Immunohistochemical analysis of MDM2 and CDK4 distinguishes low-grade osteosarcoma from benign mimics, *Mod Pathol* 23:1279–1288, 2010.
240. Bode-Lesniewska B, Zhao J, Speel EJ, et al: Gains of 12q13-14 and overexpression of mdm2 are frequent findings in intimal sarcomas of the pulmonary artery, *Virchows Arch* 438:57–65, 2001.
241. Agaram NP, Zhang L, Sung YS, et al: Recurrent NTRK1 gene fusions define a novel subset of locally aggressive lipofibromatosis-like neural tumors, *Am J Surg Pathol* 40:1407–1416, 2016.
242. Vernon SE, Bejarano PA: Low-grade fibromyxoid sarcoma: a brief review, *Arch Pathol Lab Med* 130:1358–1360, 2006.
243. Storlazzi CT, Mertens F, Nascimento A, et al: Fusion of the FUS and BBF2H7 genes in low grade fibromyxoid sarcoma, *Hum Mol Genet* 12:2349–2358, 2003.
244. Folpe AL, Lane KL, Paull G, et al: Low-grade fibromyxoid sarcoma and hyalinizing spindle cell tumor with giant rosettes: a clinicopathologic study of 73 cases supporting their identity and assessing the impact of high-grade areas, *Am J Surg Pathol* 24:1353–1360, 2000.
245. Reid R, de Silva MV, Paterson L, et al: Low-grade fibromyxoid sarcoma and hyalinizing spindle cell tumor with giant rosettes share a common t(7;16)(q34;p11) translocation, *Am J Surg Pathol* 27:1229–1236, 2003.
246. Doyle LA, Moller E, Dal Cin P, et al: MUC4 is a highly sensitive and specific marker for low-grade fibromyxoid sarcoma, *Am J Surg Pathol* 35:733–741, 2011.
247. Wang WL, Evans HL, Meis JM, et al: FUS rearrangements are rare in 'pure' sclerosing epithelioid fibrosarcoma, *Mod Pathol* 25:846–853, 2012.
248. Guillou L, Benhattar J, Gengler C, et al: Translocation-positive low-grade fibromyxoid sarcoma: clinicopathologic and molecular analysis of a series expanding the morphologic spectrum and suggesting potential relationship to sclerosing epithelioid fibrosarcoma: a study from the French Sarcoma Group, *Am J Surg Pathol* 31:1387–1402, 2007.
249. Doyle LA, Wang WL, Dal Cin P, et al: MUC4 is a sensitive and extremely useful marker for sclerosing epithelioid fibrosarcoma: association with FUS gene rearrangement, *Am J Surg Pathol* 36:1444–1451, 2012.
250. Panagopoulos I, Moller E, Dahlen A, et al: Characterization of the native CREB3L2 transcription factor and the FUS/CREB3L2 chimera, *Genes Chromosomes Cancer* 46:181–191, 2007.
251. Downs-Kelly E, Goldblum JR, Patel RM, et al: The utility of fluorescence in situ hybridization (FISH) in the diagnosis of myxoid soft tissue neoplasms, *Am J Surg Pathol* 32:8–13, 2008.
252. Panagopoulos I, Storlazzi CT, Fletcher CD, et al: The chimeric FUS/CREB3l2 gene is specific for low-grade fibromyxoid sarcoma, *Genes Chromosomes Cancer* 40:218–228, 2004.
253. Wang L, Motoi T, Khanin R, et al: Identification of a novel, recurrent HEY1-NCOA2 fusion in mesenchymal chondrosarcoma based on a genome-wide screen of exon-level expression data, *Genes Chromosomes Cancer* 51:127–139, 2012.
254. Sumegi J, Streblow R, Frayer RW, et al: Recurrent t(2;2) and t(2;8) translocations in rhabdomyosarcoma without the canonical PAX-FOXO1 fuse PAX3 to members of the nuclear receptor transcriptional coactivator family, *Genes Chromosomes Cancer* 49:224–236, 2010.
255. Antonescu CR, Zhang L, Chang NE, et al: EWSR1-POU5F1 fusion in soft tissue myoepithelial tumors. A molecular analysis of sixty-six cases, including soft tissue, bone, and visceral lesions, showing common involvement of the EWSR1 gene, *Genes Chromosomes Cancer* 49:1114–1124, 2010.
256. Gleason BC, Fletcher CD: Myoepithelial carcinoma of soft tissue in children: an aggressive neoplasm analyzed in a series of 29 cases, *Am J Surg Pathol* 31:1813–1824, 2007.
257. Flucke U, Palmedo G, Blankenhorn N, et al: EWSR1 gene rearrangement occurs in a subset of cutaneous myoepithelial tumors: a study of 18 cases, *Mod Pathol* 24:1444–1450, 2011.
258. Jo VY, Antonescu CR, Zhang L, et al: Cutaneous syncytial myoepithelioma: clinicopathologic characterization in a series of 38 cases, *Am J Surg Pathol* 37:710–718, 2013.
259. Kas K, Voz ML, Roijer E, et al: Promoter swapping between the genes for a novel zinc finger protein and beta-catenin in pleiomorphic adenomas with t(3;8)(p21;q12) translocations, *Nat Genet* 15:170–174, 1997.
260. Persson F, Andren Y, Winnes M, et al: High-resolution genomic profiling of adenomas and carcinomas of the salivary glands reveals amplification, rearrangement, and fusion of HMGA2, *Genes Chromosomes Cancer* 48:69–82, 2009.
261. Bahrami A, Dalton JD, Krane JF, et al: A subset of cutaneous and soft tissue mixed tumors are genetically linked to their salivary gland counterpart, *Genes Chromosomes Cancer* 51:140–148, 2012.
262. Hallor KH, Sciot R, Staaf J, et al: Two genetic pathways, t(1;10) and amplification of 3p11-12, in myxoinflammatory fibroblastic sarcoma, haemosiderotic fibrolipomatous tumour, and morphologically similar lesions, *J Pathol* 217:716–727, 2009.
263. Antonescu CR, Zhang L, Nielsen GP, et al: Consistent t(1;10) with rearrangements of TGFBR3 and MGEA5 in both myxoinflammatory fibroblastic sarcoma and hemosiderotic fibrolipomatous tumor, *Genes Chromosomes Cancer* 50:757–764, 2011.
264. Elco CP, Marino-Enriquez A, Abraham JA, et al: Hybrid myxoinflammatory fibroblastic sarcoma/hemosiderotic fibrolipomatous tumor: report of a case providing further evidence for a pathogenetic link, *Am J Surg Pathol* 34:1723–1727, 2010.
265. Zreik RT, Carter JM, Sukov WR, et al: TGFBR3 and MGEA5 rearrangements are much more common in "hybrid" hemosiderotic fibrolipomatous tumor-myxoinflammatory fibroblastic sarcomas than in classical myxoinflammatory fibroblastic sarcomas: a morphological and fluorescence in situ hybridization study, *Hum Pathol* 53:14–24, 2016.
266. Idowu BD, Al-Adnani M, O'Donnell P, et al: A sensitive mutation-specific screening technique for GNAS1 mutations in cases of fibrous dysplasia: the first report of a codon 227 mutation in bone, *Histopathology* 50:691–704, 2007.
267. Carter JM, Inwards CY, Jin L, et al: Activating GNAS mutations in parosteal osteosarcoma, *Am J Surg Pathol* 38:402–409, 2014.
268. Salinas-Souza C, De Andrea C, Bihl M, et al: GNAS mutations are not detected in parosteal and low-grade central osteosarcomas, *Mod Pathol* 28:1336–1342, 2015.
269. Tabareau-Delalande F, Collin C, Larousserie F, et al: Comments on Carter et al's "activating GNAS mutations in parosteal osteosarcoma", *Am J Surg Pathol* 39:1010–1013, 2015.
270. Stratakis CA, Kirschner LS, Carney JA: Clinical and molecular features of the Carney complex: diagnostic criteria and recommendations for patient evaluation, *J Clin Endocrinol Metab* 86:4041–4046, 2001.
271. Boikos SA, Stratakis CA: Carney complex: the first 20 years, *Curr Opin Oncol* 19:24–29, 2007.
272. Kirschner LS, Carney JA, Pack SD, et al: Mutations of the gene encoding the protein kinase A type I-alpha regulatory subunit in patients with the Carney complex, *Nat Genet* 26:89–92, 2000.
273. Veugelers M, Bressan M, McDermott DA, et al: Mutation of perinatal myosin heavy chain associated with a Carney complex variant, *N Engl J Med* 351:460–469, 2004.
274. Maertens O, Brems H, Vandesompele J, et al: Comprehensive NF1 screening on cultured Schwann cells from neurofibromas, *Hum Mutat* 27:1030–1040, 2006.
275. McClatchey AI: Neurofibromatosis, *Annu Rev Pathol* 2:191–216, 2007.
276. Upadhyaya M, Spurlock G, Monem B, et al: Germline and somatic NF1 gene mutations in plexiform neurofibromas, *Hum Mutat* 29:E103–E111, 2008.
277. Erickson-Johnson MR, Chou MM, Evers BR, et al: Nodular fasciitis: a novel model of transient neoplasia induced by MYH9-USP6 gene fusion, *Lab Invest* 91:1427–1433, 2011.
278. Oliveira AM, Hsi BL, Weremowicz S, et al: USP6 (Tre2) fusion oncogenes in aneurysmal bone cyst, *Cancer Res* 64:1920–1923, 2004.
279. Oliveira AM, Perez-Atayde AR, Inwards CY, et al: USP6 and CDH11 oncogenes identify the neoplastic cell in primary aneurysmal bone cysts and are absent in so-called secondary aneurysmal bone cysts, *Am J Pathol* 165:1773–1780, 2004.
280. Oliveira AM, Perez-Atayde AR, Dal Cin P, et al: Aneurysmal bone cyst variant translocations upregulate USP6 transcription by promoter swapping with the ZNF9, COL1A1, TRAP150, and OMD genes, *Oncogene* 24:3419–3426, 2005.
281. Lamant L, Gascoyne RD, Duplantier MM, et al: Non-muscle myosin heavy chain (MYH9): a new partner fused to ALK in anaplastic large cell lymphoma, *Genes Chromosomes Cancer* 37:427–432, 2003.
282. Seri M, Pecci A, Di Bari F, et al: MYH9-related disease: May-Hegglin anomaly, Sebastian syndrome, Fechtner syndrome, and Epstein syndrome are not distinct entities but represent a variable expression of a single illness, *Medicine (Baltimore)* 82:203–215, 2003.
283. Kelley MJ, Jawien W, Ortel TL, et al: Mutation of MYH9, encoding non-muscle myosin heavy chain A, in May-Hegglin anomaly, *Nat Genet* 26:106–108, 2000.
284. Carter JM, Wang X, Dong J, et al: USP6 genetic rearrangements in cellular fibroma of tendon sheath, *Mod Pathol* 29:865–869, 2016.
285. Endo M, Kohashi K, Yamamoto H, et al: Ossifying fibromyxoid tumor presenting EP400-PHF1 fusion gene, *Hum Pathol* 44:2603–2608, 2013.
286. Pazienza V, la Torre A, Baorda F, et al: Identification and functional characterization of three NoLS (nucleolar localisation signals) mutations of the CDC73 gene, *PLoS ONE* 8:e82292, 2013.
287. Gebre-Medhin S, Nord KH, Moller E, et al: Recurrent rearrangement of the PHF1 gene in ossifying fibromyxoid tumors, *Am J Pathol* 181:1069–1077, 2012.
288. Dahlen A, Fletcher CD, Mertens F, et al: Activation of the GLI oncogene through fusion with the beta-actin gene (ACTB) in a group of distinctive pericytic neoplasms: pericytoma with t(7;12), *Am J Pathol* 164:1645–1653, 2004.
289. Dahlen A, Mertens F, Mandahl N, et al: Molecular genetic characterization of the genomic ACTB-GLI fusion in pericytoma with t(7;12), *Biochem Biophys Res Commun* 325:1318–1323, 2004.
290. Walther C, Tayebwa J, Lilljebjorn H, et al: A novel SERPINE1-FOSB fusion gene results in transcriptional up-regulation of FOSB in pseudomyogenic haemangioendothelioma, *J Pathol* 232:534–540, 2014.
291. Antonescu CR, Chen HW, Zhang L, et al: ZFP36-FOSB fusion defines a subset of epithelioid hemangioma with atypical features, *Genes Chromosomes Cancer* 53:951–959, 2014.
292. Kohsaka S, Shukla N, Ameur N, et al: A recurrent neomorphic mutation in MYOD1 defines a clinically aggressive subset of embryonal rhabdomyosarcoma associated with PI3K-AKT pathway mutations, *Nat Genet* 46:595–600, 2014.
293. Agaram NP, Chen CL, Zhang L, et al: Recurrent MYOD1 mutations in pediatric and adult sclerosing and spindle cell rhabdomyosarcomas: evidence for a common pathogenesis, *Genes Chromosomes Cancer* 53:779–787, 2014.

294. Rekhi B, Upadhyay P, Ramteke MP, et al: MYOD1 (L122R) mutations are associated with spindle cell and sclerosing rhabdomyosarcomas with aggressive clinical outcomes, *Mod Pathol* 29:1532–1540, 2016.
295. Alaggio R, Zhang L, Sung YS, et al: A molecular study of pediatric spindle and sclerosing rhabdomyosarcoma: identification of novel and recurrent VGLL2-related fusions in infantile cases, *Am J Surg Pathol* 40:224–235, 2016.
296. Bridge JA, Liu J, Qualman SJ, et al: Genomic gains and losses are similar in genetic and histologic subsets of rhabdomyosarcoma, whereas amplification predominates in embryonal with anaplasia and alveolar subtypes, *Genes Chromosomes Cancer* 33:310–321, 2002.
297. Mercado GE, Barr FG: Fusions involving PAX and FOX genes in the molecular pathogenesis of alveolar rhabdomyosarcoma: recent advances, *Curr Mol Med* 7:47–61, 2007.
298. Buckingham M, Relaix F: The role of Pax genes in the development of tissues and organs: Pax3 and Pax7 regulate muscle progenitor cell functions, *Annu Rev Cell Dev Biol* 23:645–673, 2007.
299. Barr FG, Qualman SJ, Macris MH, et al: Genetic heterogeneity in the alveolar rhabdomyosarcoma subset without typical gene fusions, *Cancer Res* 62:4704–4710, 2002.
300. Sorensen PH, Lynch JC, Qualman SJ, et al: PAX3-FKHR and PAX7-FKHR gene fusions are prognostic indicators in alveolar rhabdomyosarcoma: a report from the children's oncology group, *J Clin Oncol* 20:2672–2679, 2002.
301. Parham DM, Qualman SJ, Teot L, et al: Correlation between histology and PAX/FKHR fusion status in alveolar rhabdomyosarcoma: a report from the Children's Oncology Group, *Am J Surg Pathol* 31:895–901, 2007.
302. Barr FG, Smith LM, Lynch JC, et al: Examination of gene fusion status in archival samples of alveolar rhabdomyosarcoma entered on the Intergroup Rhabdomyosarcoma Study-III trial: a report from the Children's Oncology Group, *J Mol Diagn* 8:202–208, 2006.
303. Mehra S, de la Roza G, Tull J, et al: Detection of FOXO1 (FKHR) gene break-apart by fluorescence in situ hybridization in formalin-fixed, paraffin-embedded alveolar rhabdomyosarcomas and its clinicopathologic correlation, *Diagn Mol Pathol* 17:14–20, 2008.
304. Nishio J, Althof PA, Bailey JM, et al: Use of a novel FISH assay on paraffin-embedded tissues as an adjunct to diagnosis of alveolar rhabdomyosarcoma, *Lab Invest* 86:547–556, 2006.
305. Biegel JA, Nycum LM, Valentine V, et al: Detection of the t(2;13)(q35;q14) and PAX3-FKHR fusion in alveolar rhabdomyosarcoma by fluorescence in situ hybridization, *Genes Chromosomes Cancer* 12:186–192, 1995.
306. Fritsch MK, Bridge JA, Schuster AE, et al: Performance characteristics of a reverse transcriptase-polymerase chain reaction assay for the detection of tumor-specific fusion transcripts from archival tissue, *Pediatr Dev Pathol* 6:43–53, 2003.
307. Arbajian E, Puls F, Magnusson L, et al: Recurrent EWSR1-CREB3L1 gene fusions in sclerosing epithelioid fibrosarcoma, *Am J Surg Pathol* 38:801–808, 2014.
308. Prieto-Granada C, Zhang L, Chen HW, et al: A genetic dichotomy between pure sclerosing epithelioid fibrosarcoma (SEF) and hybrid SEF/low-grade fibromyxoid sarcoma: a pathologic and molecular study of 18 cases, *Genes Chromosomes Cancer* 54:28–38, 2015.
309. Debelenko LV, McGregor LM, Shivakumar BR, et al: A novel EWSR1-CREB3L1 fusion transcript in a case of small cell osteosarcoma, *Genes Chromosomes Cancer* 50:1054–1062, 2011.
310. Righi A, Gambarotti M, Longo S, et al: Small cell osteosarcoma: clinicopathologic, immunohistochemical, and molecular analysis of 36 cases, *Am J Surg Pathol* 39:691–699, 2015.
311. Baser ME, Kuramoto L, Woods R, et al: The location of constitutional neurofibromatosis 2 (NF2) splice site mutations is associated with the severity of NF2, *J Med Genet* 42:540–546, 2005.
312. Baser ME, Kuramoto L, Joe H, et al: Genotype-phenotype correlations for nervous system tumors in neurofibromatosis 2: a population-based study, *Am J Hum Genet* 75:231–239, 2004.
313. Baser ME, Contributors to the International NFMD: The distribution of constitutional and somatic mutations in the neurofibromatosis 2 gene, *Hum Mutat* 27:297–306, 2006.
314. Hulsebos TJ, Plomp AS, Wolterman RA, et al: Germline mutation of INI1/SMARCB1 in familial schwannomatosis, *Am J Hum Genet* 80:805–810, 2007.
315. Hadfield KD, Newman WG, Bowers NL, et al: Molecular characterisation of SMARCB1 and NF2 in familial and sporadic schwannomatosis, *J Med Genet* 45:332–339, 2008.
316. Rousseau G, Noguchi T, Bourdon V, et al: SMARCB1/INI1 germline mutations contribute to 10% of sporadic schwannomatosis, *BMC Neurol* 11:9, 2011.
317. Piotrowski A, Xie J, Liu YF, et al: Germline loss-of-function mutations in LZTR1 predispose to an inherited disorder of multiple schwannomas, *Nat Genet* 46:182–187, 2014.
318. Clark J, Rocques PJ, Crew AJ, et al: Identification of novel genes, SYT and SSX, involved in the t(X;18)(p11.2;q11.2) translocation found in human synovial sarcoma, *Nat Genet* 7:502–508, 1994.
319. Antonescu CR, Kawai A, Leung DH, et al: Strong association of SYT-SSX fusion type and morphologic epithelial differentiation in synovial sarcoma, *Diagn Mol Pathol* 9:1–8, 2000.
320. Lim FL, Soulez M, Koczan D, et al: A KRAB-related domain and a novel transcription repression domain in proteins encoded by SSX genes that are disrupted in human sarcomas, *Oncogene* 17:2013–2018, 1998.
321. Su L, Sampaio AV, Jones KB, et al: Deconstruction of the SS18-SSX fusion oncoprotein complex: insights into disease etiology and therapeutics, *Cancer Cell* 21:333–347, 2012.
322. Kadoch C, Crabtree GR: Reversible disruption of mSWI/SNF (BAF) complexes by the SS18-SSX oncogenic fusion in synovial sarcoma, *Cell* 153:71–85, 2013.
323. Kadoch C, Crabtree GR: Mammalian SWI/SNF chromatin remodeling complexes and cancer: Mechanistic insights gained from human genomics, *Sci Adv* 1:e1500447, 2015.
324. Kadoch C, Copeland RA, Keilhack H: PRC2 and SWI/SNF chromatin remodeling complexes in health and disease, *Biochemistry* 55:1600–1614, 2016.
325. Kadoch C, Hargreaves DC, Hodges C, et al: Proteomic and bioinformatic analysis of mammalian SWI/SNF complexes identifies extensive roles in human malignancy, *Nat Genet* 45:592–601, 2013.
326. Amary MF, Berisha F, Bernardi Fdel C, et al: Detection of SS18-SSX fusion transcripts in formalin-fixed paraffin-embedded neoplasms: analysis of conventional RT-PCR, qRT-PCR and dual color FISH as diagnostic tools for synovial sarcoma, *Mod Pathol* 20:482–496, 2007.
327. Shipley J, Crew J, Birdsall S, et al: Interphase fluorescence in situ hybridization and reverse transcription polymerase chain reaction as a diagnostic aid for synovial sarcoma, *Am J Pathol* 148:559–567, 1996.
328. Guillou L, Benhattar J, Bonichon F, et al: Histologic grade, but not SYT-SSX fusion type, is an important prognostic factor in patients with synovial sarcoma: a multicenter, retrospective analysis, *J Clin Oncol* 22:4040–4050, 2004.
329. Kawai A, Woodruff J, Healey JH, et al: SYT-SSX gene fusion as a determinant of morphology and prognosis in synovial sarcoma, *N Engl J Med* 338:153–160, 1998.
330. Ladanyi M: Correlates of SYT-SSX fusion type in synovial sarcoma: getting more complex but also more interesting?, *J Clin Oncol* 23:3638–3639, author reply 3639-3640, 2005.
331. Ladanyi M, Antonescu CR, Leung DH, et al: Impact of SYT-SSX fusion type on the clinical behavior of synovial sarcoma: a multi-institutional retrospective study of 243 patients, *Cancer Res* 62:135–140, 2002.
332. ten Heuvel SE, Hoekstra HJ, Bastiaannet E, et al: The classic prognostic factors tumor stage, tumor size, and tumor grade are the strongest predictors of outcome in synovial sarcoma: no role for SSX fusion type or ezrin expression, *Appl Immunohistochem Mol Morphol* 17:189–195, 2009.
333. Oliveira AM, Fletcher CD: Molecular prognostication for soft tissue sarcomas: are we ready yet?, *J Clin Oncol* 22:4031–4034, 2004.
334. Coindre JM, Pelmus M, Hostein I, et al: Should molecular testing be required for diagnosing synovial sarcoma? A prospective study of 204 cases, *Cancer* 98:2700–2707, 2003.
335. He R, Patel RM, Alkan S, et al: Immunostaining for SYT protein discriminates synovial sarcoma from other soft tissue tumors: analysis of 146 cases, *Mod Pathol* 20:522–528, 2007.
336. Terry J, Saito T, Subramanian S, et al: TLE1 as a diagnostic immunohistochemical marker for synovial sarcoma emerging from gene expression profiling studies, *Am J Surg Pathol* 31:240–246, 2007.
337. Jagdis A, Rubin BP, Tubbs RR, et al: Prospective evaluation of TLE1 as a diagnostic immunohistochemical marker in synovial sarcoma, *Am J Surg Pathol* 33:1743–1751, 2009.
338. Foo WC, Cruise MW, Wick MR, et al: Immunohistochemical staining for TLE1 distinguishes synovial sarcoma from histologic mimics, *Am J Clin Pathol* 135:839–844, 2011.
339. Robinson DR, Wu YM, Kalyana-Sundaram S, et al: Identification of recurrent NAB2-STAT6 gene fusions in solitary fibrous tumor by integrative sequencing, *Nat Genet* 45:180–185, 2013.
340. Chmielecki J, Crago AM, Rosenberg M, et al: Whole-exome sequencing identifies a recurrent NAB2-STAT6 fusion in solitary fibrous tumors, *Nat Genet* 45:131–132, 2013.
341. Chuang IC, Liao KC, Huang HY, et al: NAB2-STAT6 gene fusion and STAT6 immunoexpression in extrathoracic solitary fibrous tumors: the association between fusion variants and locations, *Pathol Int* 66:288–296, 2016.
342. Huang SC, Li CF, Kao YC, et al: The clinicopathological significance of NAB2-STAT6 gene fusions in 52 cases of intrathoracic solitary fibrous tumors, *Cancer Med* 5:159–168, 2016.
343. Tai HC, Chuang IC, Chen TC, et al: NAB2-STAT6 fusion types account for clinicopathological variations in solitary fibrous tumors, *Mod Pathol* 28:1324–1335, 2015.
344. Akaike K, Kurisaki-Arakawa A, Hara K, et al: Distinct clinicopathological features of NAB2-STAT6 fusion gene variants in solitary fibrous tumor with emphasis on the acquisition of highly malignant potential, *Hum Pathol* 46:347–356, 2015.
345. Demicco EG, Harms PW, Patel RM, et al: Extensive survey of STAT6 expression in a large series of mesenchymal tumors, *Am J Clin Pathol* 143:672–682, 2015.
346. Doyle LA, Vivero M, Fletcher CD, et al: Nuclear expression of STAT6 distinguishes solitary fibrous tumor from histologic mimics, *Mod Pathol* 27:390–395, 2014.
347. Cheah AL, Billings SD, Goldblum JR, et al: STAT6 rabbit monoclonal antibody is a robust diagnostic tool for the distinction of solitary fibrous tumour from its mimics, *Pathology* 46:389–395, 2014.
348. West RB, Rubin BP, Miller MA, et al: A landscape effect in tenosynovial giant-cell tumor from activation of CSF1 expression by a translocation in a minority of tumor cells, *Proc Natl Acad Sci USA* 103:690–695, 2006.
349. Cupp JS, Miller MA, Montgomery KD, et al: Translocation and expression of CSF1 in pigmented villonodular synovitis, tenosynovial giant cell tumor, rheumatoid arthritis and other reactive synovitides, *Am J Surg Pathol* 31:970–976, 2007.
350. Moller E, Mandahl N, Mertens F, et al: Molecular identification of COL6A3-CSF1 fusion transcripts in tenosynovial giant cell tumors, *Genes Chromosomes Cancer* 47:21–25, 2008.
351. Lazar AJ, Trent JC, Lev D: Sarcoma molecular testing: diagnosis and prognosis, *Curr Oncol Rep* 9:309–315, 2007.
352. Shern JF, Chen L, Chmielecki J, et al: Comprehensive genomic analysis of rhabdomyosarcoma reveals a landscape of alterations affecting a common genetic axis in fusion-positive and fusion-negative tumors, *Cancer Discov* 4:216–231, 2014.
353. Parham DM, Barr FG: Classification of rhabdomyosarcoma and its molecular basis, *Adv Anat Pathol* 20:387–397, 2013.
354. Liegl B, Hornick JL, Antonescu CR, et al: Rhabdomyosarcomatous differentiation in gastrointestinal stromal tumors after tyrosine kinase inhibitor therapy: a novel form of tumor progression, *Am J Surg Pathol* 33:218–226, 2009.

Index

Note: Page numbers followed by "*f*" refer to illustrations; page numbers followed by "*t*" refer to tables; page numbers followed by "*b*" refer to boxes.

B

C

D

M

O

P

R

T

U

V

W

X